PCF6

KU-415-346

PALLIATIVE CARE FORMULARY

Published by palliativedrugs.com Ltd.

Palliativedrugs.com Ltd
Hayward House Study Centre
Nottingham University Hospitals NHS Trust, City Campus
Nottingham NG5 1PB
United Kingdom

www.palliativedrugs.com

© palliativedrugs.com Ltd 2017

The moral rights of the editors have been asserted.

PCF5+ PDF 2016
PCF5+ PDF 2015
PCF5 2014, reprinted 2015
PCF4+ PDF 2013
PCF4+ PDF 2012
PCF4 2011, reprinted 2012 (twice), 2013
PCF3 2007, reprinted 2008, 2009
PCF2 2002, reprinted 2003
PCF1 1998

All rights reserved. No part of this publication may be reproduced, stored in a retrieval system or transmitted, in any form or by any means, electronic, mechanical, photocopying, recording or otherwise without the prior permission in writing of palliativedrugs.com Ltd or as expressly permitted by law, or under terms agreed with the appropriate reprographics rights organization. Enquiries concerning reproduction outside the scope of the above should be sent to hq@palliativedrugs.com or by ordinary mail to the above address.

British Library Cataloguing in Publication Data

A catalogue record for this book is available from the British Library.

ISBN 978-0-9928467-4-9

Typeset by Anytime Publishing Services, Leicestershire, UK

Printed by Halstan Printing Group, Amersham, UK

DISCLAIMER

Every effort has been made to ensure the accuracy of this text, and that the best information available has been used. However, palliativedrugs.com Ltd neither represents nor guarantees that the practices described herein will, if followed, ensure safe and effective patient care. The recommendations contained in this book reflect the editors' judgement regarding the state of general knowledge and practice in the field as of the date of publication. Information in a book of this type can never be all-inclusive, and therefore will not cover every eventuality.

Thus, those who use this book must make their own determinations regarding specific safe and appropriate patient-care practices, taking into account the personnel, equipment, and practices available at the hospital or other facility at which they are located. Neither palliativedrugs.com Ltd nor the editors can be held responsible for any liability incurred as a consequence of the use or application of any of the contents of this book. Mention of specific product brands does not imply endorsement.

Particularly when prescribing a drug for the first time, a doctor (or other independent prescriber) should study the contents of the manufacturer's Summary of Product Characteristics (SPC), paying particular attention to indications, contra-indications, cautions, drug interactions, and undesirable effects.

EDITORIAL STAFF

Editors-in-Chief

Robert Twycross DM, FRCP
Emeritus Clinical Reader in Palliative Medicine, Oxford University

Andrew Wilcock DM, FRCP
Macmillan Clinical Reader in Palliative Medicine and Medical Oncology, Nottingham University
Consultant Physician, Hayward House, Nottingham University Hospitals NHS Trust

Paul Howard BMedSci, MRCP
Consultant in Palliative Medicine, Earl Mountbatten House, Isle of Wight NHS Trust

Senior Editor

Sarah Charlesworth BPharm, DipClinPharm, MRPharmS
Specialist Pharmacist, Palliative Care Information and Website Management, Hayward House, Nottingham University Hospitals NHS Trust

Editor

Claire Stark Toller MA, MA, MRCP
Consultant in Palliative Medicine, Countess Mountbatten House, University Hospital Southampton NHS Foundation Trust

Associate Editor

Julie Mortimer BPharm, MRPharmS
Malcolm Mortimer Media, Nottingham (former Senior Editor)

Production Editor

Sarah Keeling
Publishing Office Manager, Palliativedrugs.com Ltd. Hayward House, Nottingham University Hospitals NHS Trust

Editorial Board

Jason Boland PhD, FRCP, FHEA
Senior Clinical Lecturer and Honorary Consultant in Palliative Medicine, Hull York Medical School, University Of Hull, UK

Andrew Broadbent BMedSc, MHM, FRACP, FAChPM
Honorary Adjunct Associate Professor, Bond University and Gold Coast Health, Robina Hospital, Australia

Virginia Bray MRCP
Specialist Registrar in Palliative Medicine, Hayward House, Nottingham University Hospitals NHS Trust, Nottingham, UK

Alpna Chauhan MRCP
Consultant in Palliative Medicine, John Eastwood Hospice, Sutton-in-Ashfield, UK

Brian Creedon MMedSci, MRCPI
Consultant in Palliative Medicine, Waterford Regional Hospital, Waterford, Ireland

Vincent Crosby FRCP
Consultant in Palliative Medicine, Hayward House, Nottingham University Hospitals NHS Trust, Nottingham, UK

Andrew Davies MSc, MD, FRCP
Consultant in Palliative Medicine, Royal Surrey County Hospital, St. Luke's Cancer Centre, Guildford, UK

Joanne Droney PhD, MRCPI
Consultant in Palliative Medicine, Royal Marsden Hospital, London, UK

Jo Elverson MA(Ed) MRCP
Consultant in Palliative Medicine, Helen and Douglas House Hospices for Children & Young Adults, Oxford, UK

Ruth England FRCP
Consultant in Palliative Medicine, Derby Hospitals NHS Trust, Derby, UK

Caroline Facey MRCP
Specialist Registrar in Palliative Medicine, Hayward House, Nottingham University Hospitals NHS Trust, Nottingham, UK

Louise Free MSc, MRCP
Consultant in Palliative Medicine, St Wilfrids Hospice and East Sussex NHS Trust, Eastbourne, UK

Catherine Gwilt MA BSc MRCP
Consultant in Palliative Medicine, St Joseph's Hospice, London, UK

Janet Hardy BSc, MD, FRACP
Professor of Palliative Medicine, University of Queensland and Mater Health Services, Brisbane, Australia

Vaughan Keeley PhD, FRCP
Consultant in Palliative Medicine, Derby Hospitals NHS Trust, Derby, UK

Samuel King FRCP
Consultant in Palliative Medicine, St Elizabeth Hospice and Ipswich Hospital Trust, Ipswich, UK

Malgorzata Krajnik MD, PhD
Professor of Palliative Medicine, Nicolaus Copernicus University and University Hospital No 1, Bydgoszcz, Poland

Susie Lapwood MA, DFSRH, DipPallMed, MRCGP
Senior Speciality Doctor, Helen and Douglas House Hospices for Children & Young Adults, Oxford, UK

Mark Lee MD, MRCP
Consultant in Palliative Medicine, St Benedict's Hospice and Specialist Palliative Care Centre, Sunderland, UK

Michael Lucey BMedSc, FRCPI
Consultant in Palliative Medicine, Milford Hospice, Limerick and HSE mid West, Ireland

Staffan Lundstrom MD, PhD
Associate Professor, Karolinska Institutet and Stockholms Sjukhem, Stockholm, Sweden

Louise Lynch FRCA, FFPMRCA
Consultant in Chronic Pain Management, Leeds Teaching Hospitals NHS Trust, UK

Laura Miller MSc, PgDip Dietetics
Team Lead Dietitian, Nottingham University Hospitals NHS Trust, Nottingham, UK

Simon Noble DipPallMed, MD, FRCP
Clinical Professor in Palliative Medicine, Cardiff University, UK

Stephen Oxberry BSc (Hons), PhD, FRCP
Consultant in Palliative Medicine, Kirkwood Hospice and Calderdale and Huddersfield Foundation NHS Trust, Huddersfield, UK

Victor Pace DipPallMed, FRCP, FRCS
Consultant in Palliative Medicine, St Christopher's Hospice, London, UK

Maggie Presswood MRCP
Specialist Registrar in Palliative Medicine, Wales Deanery

Rachel Quibell MRCGP, FRCP
Consultant in Palliative Medicine, Newcastle upon Tyne Hospitals NHS Foundation Trust, Newcastle, UK

Joy Ross PhD, FRCP
Consultant in Palliative Medicine, St Christopher's Hospice, London, UK

Anna Spathis MSc, FRCP, MRCGP, FHEA
Consultant in Palliative Medicine, Cambridge University Hospitals NHS Foundation Trust, Cambridge, UK

Mark Taubert MSc, MRCGP, FRCP
Consultant in Palliative Medicine, Velindre NHS Trust, Cardiff, UK

Jillian Wall MRCP
Specialist Registrar in Palliative Medicine, Hayward House, Nottingham University Hospitals NHS Trust, Nottingham, UK

CONTENTS

PREFACE TO SIXTH EDITION

The target audience for *PCF* comprises doctors, nurses and pharmacists involved in the care of patients receiving palliative/hospice care. *PCF* is a core textbook for registrars in Palliative Medicine in the UK. It is used in some areas to fulfil the NHS National Cancer Standards requirement for specialist palliative care services within a Cancer Centre and Network to have a core palliative care drug formulary and is referred to in many official healthcare documents, e.g. NICE CKS guidelines.

PCF6 has 35 chapters and appendices, an increase of three. In Part 1, some drug monographs have been merged and new ones added. Part 2 has been divided into Parts 2 and 3. The new chapters are all in Part 2: *Prescribing in children*, *Renal impairment* and *Hepatic impairment*. Part 3 covers *Routes of Administration*.

Although written primarily with cancer patients in mind, *PCF* contains specific material relating to a number of other life-limiting diseases, e.g. COPD, congestive heart failure, renal failure, hepatic failure, and Parkinson's disease. However, in relation to the use of strong opioids for analgesia, the focus in *PCF* is on cancer pain. Because the use of strong opioids for chronic *non-cancer* pain is generally associated with lower benefits and higher risks, specialist advice should be followed and/or sought from chronic pain teams.

PCF also includes a number of *Quick Clinical Guides* (listed inside the back cover and in the Topic index). To enhance user-friendliness, each *Guide* is generally limited to no more than two pages, and references are not included. We welcome the donation of clinical guidance from other sources for posting on our website (e-mail copies to hq@palliativedrugs.com).

The production of a book of this nature depends on the help and advice of numerous colleagues, both past and present. We acknowledge with gratitude the support of clinical colleagues, and members of the palliativedrugs.com community who have provided feedback, particularly via surveys, by contributing to the *Syringe Driver Survey Database*, or by postings on the Bulletin Board.

We acknowledge with thanks the advice provided by various correspondents, including: Peter Armstrong, Sabrina Bajwah, Kirsty Bannister, Claudia Bausewein, James Beattie, Jenny Beavis, Sara Booth, Anthony Dickenson, Magnus Ekström, Ronald Elin, Philippa Hawley, Miriam Johnson, Bruce Kennedy, Aleksandra Kotlinska-Lemieszek, Gurminder Mann, Mary Mihalyo, Fliss Murtagh, Russell Portenoy, Constanze Remi, Jan Rémi, Graeme Rocker, Anne Waddington, Sarah Williams, Olivia Worthington, and by Medical Information Departments in the pharmaceutical industry.

We are grateful to Sarah Keeling for type-setting and co-ordinating production and to Karen Isaac for secretarial support.

Robert Twycross
Andrew Wilcock
Paul Howard
Editors-in-chief
September 2017

HOW PCF IS CONSTRUCTED

There is continual review and updating of the contents of *PCF* over a three year cycle. These updates are published regularly on-line, with the whole book published in print every three years.

The *Palliative Care Formulary* (*PCF*) is a unique independent professional publication which provides essential information for prescribers and health professionals involved in palliative and hospice care. *PCF* contains authoritative independent guidance on best practice, and helps to ensure that drugs are used appropriately, safely, and optimally.

Recommended International Non-proprietary Names (rINN) are used for drugs. The chapter order in Part 1 broadly follows that of the print edition of the *British National Formulary* (*BNF*).

Editorial team

The *PCF* editorial team is co-ordinated by three medically qualified Editors-in-chief who are (or have been) accredited specialists in Palliative Medicine and a specialist palliative care pharmacist. For each print edition, every section of *PCF* is reviewed and updated with the help of an Editorial Board. Suggestions for new monographs are discussed by the *PCF* editorial team, and experts identified to assist in the preparation of new documents.

The Editorial Board

The Editorial Board mainly comprises palliative care physicians appointed on the basis of their clinical knowledge and expertise. Editorial Board members have committed to reviewing one or more drug monographs or chapters, and work in liaison with the editorial team. Responsibilities include scrutinizing literature databases such as PubMed, and accessing and studying relevant new publications.

Correspondents

Correspondents are drawn from a range of medical specialties. They include doctors, pharmacists, nurses, and others who provide advice on the text by:

- checking amendments for scientific accuracy, and to enhance clarity
- providing additional expert opinion in areas of controversy or when reliable evidence is lacking
- advising on areas when the *PCF* diverges from a manufacturer's Summary of Product Characteristics (SPC)
- providing additional validation and clinical evidence about unauthorized (off-label) use.

Sources of PCF information

PCF uses various sources for its information, including:

Summary of product characteristics (SPC)

The SPCs are the principal source of product information. Manufacturers are contacted directly when further information is required.

Literature

Research papers and reviews relating to the drugs featured in *PCF* are carefully processed. When a difference between the advice in the *PCF* and a paper is noted, the new information is evaluated for reliability and relevance to UK clinical practice. If necessary, new text is drafted and thoroughly reviewed by the editorial team with support, as needed, from the Editorial Board and/or Correspondents.

PCF also has access to many on-line information resources (see p.xvii). For example, www.azcert.org is used to flag drugs which have the potential to prolong QT interval to a clinically relevant degree, and www.psychotropical.com is used to help adjudicate whether a report about serotonin toxicity is reliable.

Systematic reviews

PCF monitors various databases of systematic reviews, including the *Cochrane Library* and several other web-based resources. Reviews published in *Clinical Evidence* are used to validate *PCF* advice.

Consensus guidelines

The advice in *PCF* is checked against consensus guidelines produced by expert bodies including the National Institute for Health and Care Excellence (NICE), the Scottish Medicines Consortium (SMC), and the Scottish Intercollegiate Guidelines Network (SIGN).

PCF also takes note of other expert bodies which produce clinical guidelines relevant to palliative care, e.g. Association for Palliative Medicine, British Lymphology Society.

Statutory information

PCF routinely processes relevant information from various Government bodies, including Statutory Instruments and regulations affecting the Prescription only Medicines Order, Controlled Drugs and from the Medicines and Healthcare products Regulatory Agency (MHRA). Safety warnings issued by the Commission on Human Medicines (CHM) and guidelines on drug use issued by the UK health departments are routinely processed.

Relevant professional statements issued by the Royal Pharmaceutical Society (RPS), Nursing and Midwifery Council (NMC) and General Medical Council (GMC) are included in *PCF* as are guidelines from the medical Royal Colleges.

Pricing information

Drug prices are obtained from the online edition of the *BNF* at the time of monograph update. When available, the NHS indicative price is used. For non-proprietary (generic) products, the lowest NHS indicative price is used; if unavailable, the price listed in the Drug Tariff is used. Note. Prices for broken bulk, dispensing/sourcing fees and delivery charges are *not* included.

For special order or imported products, prices are obtained from part VIIIB of the Drug Tariff (if listed) or are requested directly from the manufacturer or importing company.

For information on how prices are used, see p.xvii.

GETTING THE MOST OUT OF PCF

Information in a book of this type can never be all-inclusive, and thus will not cover every eventuality. Readers should satisfy themselves as to the appropriateness of the information before applying it in practice.

Particularly when prescribing a drug for the first time, a doctor (or other independent prescriber) should study the contents of the manufacturer's Summary of Product Characteristics (SPC), paying particular attention to indications, contra-indications, cautions, drug interactions, and undesirable effects (also see p.xvi).

PCF often refers to the use of medicinal products beyond the scope of their marketing authorization, e.g. in relation to indication, dose, route of administration. Such use has implications for the prescriber (see p.xix).

A cautious approach is always necessary when prescribing for children, the frail, and the elderly, for those with renal impairment, hepatic impairment, or respiratory insufficiency (see relevant Chapters in Part 2). Further, if caring for a woman who is pregnant or breast-feeding, or for someone with porphyria, it is crucial to check a drug's suitability in both the *BNF* and its SPC.

The literature on the pharmacology of pain and symptom management in end-stage disease is growing continually, and it is impossible for anyone to be familiar with all of it. This is where a book like *PCF* comes into its own as a major accessible resource for prescribing clinicians involved in palliative care.

PCF is not an easy read, indeed it was never intended that it would be read from cover to cover. It is essentially a reference book – to study the monograph of an individual drug, or class of drugs, with specific questions in mind.

Part 1 comprises 145 drug monographs, some covering a class of drugs (e.g. antimuscarinics, bronchodilators, strong opioids) and others restricted to an individual drug (e.g. morphine, fentanyl, ketamine). Drugs marked with an asterisk (*) should generally be used only by, or after consultation with, a specialist palliative care service. A selection of Quick Clinical Guides cover key topics (see inside back cover for index). These are purposefully brief to facilitate everyday use. Before use, it is important to study the associated text in order to fully understand their rationale.

Parts 2 and 3, and the appendices, deal with themes which transcend the drug monographs, e.g. general advice about prescribing in palliative care, anticipatory prescribing in the community, administering drugs to patients with swallowing difficulties or enteral feeding tubes, the use of nebulized drugs, and continuous subcutaneous infusions.

Indications

In *PCF*, generally only those indications relevant to palliative care are listed. The use of medicinal products for indications beyond their Marketing authorization (MA), i.e. off-label, has implications for the prescriber (see p.xx) and *PCF* attempts to highlight such use, applying the following convention:

- the symbol † highlights off-label use when no UK medicinal product containing that drug has a MA for that indication
- the statement 'Authorized indications vary between products; consult SPC for details' is used when variation exists between drugs within a particular class, e.g. bisphosphonates.

However, it is impractical for *PCF* to highlight all cases of off-label use because a MA applies to a specific medicinal product (not the drug *per se*) and is based on what the manufacturer applied for. Thus, there can be variations in the individual SPCs of different medicinal products containing the same drug, i.e. variations in the indications can occur between different:

- manufacturers
- routes of administration
- formulations
- pack sizes.

Pharmacology

The information in the Pharmacology sections is derived from many sources (see How PCF is constructed, p.xii).

Reliable knowledge, levels of evidence and strength of recommendations

Research is the pursuit of reliable knowledge. The gold standard for drug treatment is the randomized controlled trial (RCT) or, better, a systematic review of homogeneous RCTs.

Over the last 20–30 years, numerous systems have been published for categorizing levels of evidence and the strength of the derived recommendations. Box A reproduces the system used by the British Medical Journal. This checklist is based on material published by three main sources, namely the US Agency for Health Care Policy and Research, the NHS Management Executive, and the North of England Guidelines Group.[1–3]

Box A A scheme for categorizing evidence and grading recommendations[4]

Category	*Level of evidence*	*Grade*	*Strength of recommendations*
Ia	Evidence obtained from a meta-analysis of RCTs	A	Directly based on Category I evidence without extrapolation
Ib	Evidence from at least one RCT		
IIa	Evidence obtained from at least one well-designed controlled study without randomization	B	Directly based on Category II evidence or by extrapolation from Category I evidence
IIb	Evidence obtained from at least one other well-designed quasi-experimental study		
III	Evidence obtained from well-designed non-experimental descriptive studies, such as comparative studies, correlation studies and case studies	C	Directly based on Category III evidence or by extrapolation from Category I or II evidence
IV	Evidence obtained from expert committee reports or opinions and/or clinical experiences of respected authorities	D	Directly based on category IV evidence or by extrapolation from Category I, II, or III evidence This grading indicates that directly applicable clinical studies of good quality are absent or not readily available

However, it is important to recognize that an RCT is *not* the only source of reliable knowledge. Broadly speaking, sources of knowledge can be conveniently grouped under three headings:

- *instrumental*, includes RCT data and data from other high-quality studies
- *interactive*, refers to anecdotal data (shared clinical experience), including retrospective and prospective surveys
- *critical*, data unique to the individual in question (e.g. personal choice) and societal/cultural factors (e.g. financial and logistic considerations).[5]

Relying on one type of knowledge alone is *not* good practice. All three sources must be exploited in the process of therapeutic decision-making. This is reflected in the Pharmacology sections.

Pharmaceutical company information

Although the manufacturer's SPC is an important source of information about a drug, it is important to remember that many published studies are sponsored by the drug company in question. This can lead to a conflict of interest between the desire for objective data and the need to make one's own drug as attractive as possible.[6] It is thus best to treat information from company representatives as inevitably biased. The information provided by *PCF* is commercially independent, and should serve as a counterbalance to manufacturer bias.

Remember: it is often safer to stick with an 'old favourite', and not seek to be among the first to prescribe a newly released product – which may simply be a 'me-too' drug rather than true innovation.[6]

Pharmacokinetics

Generally, pharmacokinetic data are taken from *Martindale: the complete drug reference*[7] or from a manufacturer's SPC. Other sources are referenced in the text.

Contra-indications and cautions

Contra-indications and cautions listed in SPCs sometimes vary between different manufacturers of products containing the same drug. Thus, a contra-indication in one SPC may be styled a caution in another, and *vice versa*. *PCF* attempts to collate and standardize contra-indications and cautions between products for individual monographs and across a class of drugs for class monographs.

In *PCF*, we do *not* include universal contra-indications (e.g. history of hypersensitivity to the drug), and have generally *not* included a contra-indication from the SPC if the use of the drug in the stated circumstance is accepted prescribing practice in palliative care, e.g. use of oral morphine as an analgesic in a patient with obstructive airways disease.

As always, a cautious approach is necessary when prescribing for children, the frail, the elderly, and patients with organ impairment or respiratory insufficiency (see relevant chapters in Part 2). If caring for a woman who is pregnant or breast-feeding, or for someone with porphyria, it is crucial to check a drug's suitability in both the *BNF* and SPC, or with a specialist medical information pharmacist.

The effect of sedative drugs on driving ability is covered in Chapter 22, p.743.

Drug interactions

Generally, information on drug interactions is taken from *Stockley's Drug Interactions*[8] or from a manufacturer's SPC. Other sources are referenced in the text.

It is assumed that clinicians are aware of the risk of common sense pharmacodynamic interactions, e.g. that the concurrent prescription of two or more drugs with sedative properties is likely to result in more sedation than if each drug was prescribed alone. Likewise, two drugs with antimuscarinic properties prescribed concurrently will have an additive antimuscarinic effect.

On the other hand, pharmacokinetic interactions (leading to either increased or reduced effect) are generally covered in individual drug monographs and in Chapter 19, p.717.

Undesirable effects of drugs

As recommended by the European Commission, the term 'undesirable effect' is used rather than 'side effect' or 'adverse drug reaction'. Wherever possible, undesirable effects are categorized as:

- very common (>10%)
- common (<10%, >1%)
- uncommon (<1%, >0.1%)
- rare (<0.1%, >0.01%)
- very rare (<0.01%).

PCF generally includes information on the very common and common undesirable effects. Selected other undesirable effects are also included, e.g. uncommon or rare ones which may have serious consequences. The manufacturer's SPC should be consulted for a full list of undesirable effects.

Dose and use

PCF often highlights doses, routes or use in patient populations not covered by the MA of the authorized medicinal products available (off-label use). As with indications (see above), it is impractical for *PCF* to highlight all cases of off-label use, and health professionals must be familiar with the specific SPC of the product they are using and implications for off-label use.

Further, unauthorized medicinal products may feature in this section, e.g. the use of special order or imported products, or the mixing of medicinal products together for administration via CSCI (see p.xix).

Generic and brand prescribing

Generally, *PCF* encourages generic prescribing on the basis of pharmaco-economics.[9] In most instances, branded and generic versions of the same drug will not differ significantly in terms of bio-availability and efficacy. However, there are some important exceptions (see below).[10] Further, in some circumstances, continuity of the same brand is important for patient safety, by reducing the risk of confusion and thereby a dispensing or administration error.[9,11,12] Thus, *PCF* recommends brand prescribing when:

- bio-availability differs significantly between brands, particularly for drugs with a narrow therapeutic index, e.g. some anti-epileptics, m/r formulations of diltiazem, nifedipine, theophylline
- the product range is complex and there is a high risk of error which could be fatal, e.g. m/r opioid analgesics, TD opioid patches[11,12]
- formulation differs significantly between brands, resulting in them not being interchangeable, e.g. some inhaled corticosteroids, TM fentanyl products
- products contain multiple ingredients, and brand name prescribing aids identification, e.g. antacids, compound alginates, macrogols, pancreatin supplements, topical skin products
- administration devices have different instructions for use and patient familiarity with one product is important, e.g. dry powder inhalers or self-injection devices.

Supply

Generally, the list of products indicates the range of formulations and strengths available but is *not* an exhaustive list. Whenever possible, generic products are included; selected brands feature when either a generic product is unavailable, or brand prescribing is important (see above).

Generally, costs reflect a 28 day supply, based on the most convenient strength and cheapest pack size. For short course treatments, p.r.n. or parenteral formulations, costs may be listed either as per course, per dose or per ampoule/vial as appropriate.

Costs are for indicative purposes only, to give a general comparison between available therapeutic options. Generally, costs:

- less than £5 have been rounded to the nearest 25p
- between £5–£10 have been rounded to the nearest 50p
- more than £10 have been rounded to the nearest full pound.

In some cases, e.g. TM fentanyl, to aid closer comparison, exact prices for individual dose units are used.

PCF recognizes that pharmaco-economics is a complicated area, constantly changing in response to various factors, including market demands, hospital and local contracts, and marketing tactics. Costs can also be vastly different in the community compared with hospital, particularly regarding special order products not covered by the part VIIIB of the Drug Tariff. Thus, local circumstances need to be taken into account when cost is a particular consideration.

References

Literature references

In choosing references, articles in hospice and palliative care journals have frequently been selected preferentially. Such journals are likely to be more readily available to our readers, and often contain detailed discussion.

It is not feasible to reference every statement in *PCF*. However, readers are invited to enter into constructive dialogue with the Editors via the Bulletin Board on *www.palliativedrugs.com*. This is currently accessed by >30,000 health professionals in >160 countries.

Online sources of information

Website references are not routinely given for articles available in traditionally published journals. However, various full-text core journals are available free to UK NHS staff with an Athens password through the NHS Evidence Services website at https://www.evidence.nhs.uk.

References to SPCs and PILs are generally *not* included. However, most can be freely accessed from www.medicines.org.uk or obtained directly from the manufacturer.

Online sources of information are referenced when this is the usual route of publication and access is freely available, e.g. UK Department of Health guidelines, MHRA Drug Safety Updates, NICE guidance, SIGN guidance. The website address quoted is for the homepage or the page from which the guidance can be found and downloaded.

Information from the *BNF* and *BNFc* is freely available from the NICE website (https://bnf.nice.org.uk).

Whenever possible, subscription websites have been avoided. However, to ensure that the most current information is included when revising *PCF*, the following standard reference texts are consulted from subscribed access to Medicines Complete (www.medicinescomplete.com):

- American Hospital Formulary Service (AHFS)
- Handbook of drug administration via enteral feeding tubes
- Handbook on injectable drugs
- Martindale: the complete drug reference
- Stockley's drug interactions.

These are available in all UK Medicines Information Services.

1 Eccles M *et al.* (1996) North of England evidence based guidelines development project: methods of guideline development. *British Medical Journal*. **312**: 760–762.

2 DoH (1996) *Clinical Guidelines: Using Clinical Guidelines to Improve Patient Care Within the NHS*. Department of Health: NHS Executive, Leeds.

3 Agency for Health Care Policy and Research (1992) Acute pain management, operative or medical procedures and trauma 92–0032. In: *Clinical Practice Guideline Quick Ref Guide for Clinicians*. AHCPR Publications, Rockville, Maryland, USA, pp. 1–22.

4 BMJ Publishing Group (2009) Resources for authors. Checklists and forms: clinical management guidelines. http://www.bmj.com/about-bmj/resources-authors.

5 Aoun SM and Kristjanson LJ (2005) Challenging the framework for evidence in palliative care research. *Palliative Medicine*. **19**: 461–465.

6 Angell M (2004) *The Truth About the Drug Companies: how they deceive us and what to do about it*. Random House, New York.

7 Sweetman S.C. *Martindale: The Complete Drug Reference*. London: Pharmaceutical Press www.medicinescomplete.com.

8 Baxter K and Preston CL. *Stockley's Drug Interactions*. London: Pharmaceutical Press www.medicinescomplete.com (accessed January 2017).

9 UK Medicines Information (2013) Which medicines should be considered for brand-name prescribing in primary care? *Medicines Q&A* **247.3**. www.evidence.nhs.uk.

10 National Prescribing Centre (2000) Modified-release preparations. *MeReC Bulletin*. **11**: 13–16.

11 Smith J (2004) Building a Safer NHS for Patients - Improving Medication Safety. pp.105–111. Department of Health, London. Available from: www.dh.gov.uk (archived)

12 Care Quality Commission and NHS England (2013) Safer use of controlled drugs - preventing harms from fentanyl and buprenorphine transdermal patches. *Use of controlled drugs supporting information*. www.cqc.org.uk.

Updated September 2017

THE USE OF MEDICINAL PRODUCTS BEYOND (OFF-LABEL) AND WITHOUT (UNAUTHORIZED) MARKETING AUTHORIZATION

The use of medicinal products off-label is widespread. Surveys suggest that up to one quarter of all prescriptions in palliative care come into this category.[1,2] *PCF* attempts to highlight such use, applying the following convention:

- the symbol † highlights off-label use when no UK medicinal product containing that drug has a Marketing authorization (MA) for that indication
- the statement 'Authorized indications vary between products; consult SPC for details' is used when such variation exists between drugs within a particular class, e.g. bisphosphonates.

However, it is impractical for *PCF* to highlight all cases of off-label use, e.g. where the indication varies between different brands or formulations of the same drug, or where the medicinal product is being used in a dose, route or patient population not covered by the MA.

It is important for prescribers to understand that the MA regulates the specific medicinal product (not the drug *per se*) and the *marketing activities* of pharmaceutical companies, and not the prescriber's clinical practice. Even so, off-label use does have implications for health professionals, and these are discussed in this section.

Definitions

Marketing authorization (licence)

A Marketing authorization (MA), previously called a product licence, is granted by a regulatory body to a pharmaceutical company for a specific medicinal product. It specifies the terms of use, including the indications, doses, routes and patient populations for which it can be marketed. *PCF* uses the term authorized in preference to licensed.

Off-label use

Although there is no official definition, generally, 'off-label' describes the use of a medicinal product *beyond the specifications of its MA*, e.g. for an indication, or in a dose, route or patient population not covered by the MA.

Unauthorized (unlicensed) medicinal product

PCF uses the term unauthorized in preference to unlicensed. There is no simple definition of an unauthorized medicinal product. Essentially it is a product which does not have a MA for medicinal use in humans. Unauthorized medicinal products include:

- authorized medicinal products that have been manipulated, thus rendering them unauthorized, e.g. two or more medicinal products mixed together for administration in a syringe for CSCI (see Box A below and p.817)
- 'specials', e.g. special-order manufactured formulations made in the UK by a manufacturer with a 'specials' manufacturing licence (MS) and medicinal products which require importation; for full details see p.751
- medicinal products made in a local pharmacy (extemporaneously prepared) at the request of a prescriber for an individual patient, e.g. dilution of a cream
- new medicinal products undergoing clinical trials or awaiting a MA, e.g. if a patient wishes to continue an investigational product after a clinical trial.

The authorization (licensing) process

Before a medicinal product can be marketed in the UK, it requires a MA (previously product licence). There are four application procedures in the European Union:

- *centralized*, application evaluated by the European Medicines Agency (EMEA); the European Commission grants a single MA valid for the whole European Union
- *decentralized*, simultaneous application made by several member states, with one taking the lead; if successful, a national MA then being granted in each state
- *mutual recognition*, application for authorization in a member state when a MA exists in another member state; the new member state relies on the original member state's evaluation as a basis for its decision
- *national*, application for a MA in only one member state; in the UK the application is evaluated by the Medicines and Healthcare products Regulatory Agency (MHRA) on behalf of the Licensing Authority, a body consisting of UK health ministers.[3]

Certain products, e.g. for HIV/AIDS, cancer, neurodegenerative diseases, must be authorized through the centralized procedure. The UK Parallel Import Licensing Scheme also allows a product authorized in other European Union states to be imported and marketed in the UK, if it has labels and a Patient Information Leaflet (PIL) in English.

In the UK, the MHRA evaluation comprises an evaluation of the efficacy, safety and quality of the product from a medical, pharmaceutical and scientific viewpoint to ensure that it satisfies predefined criteria. Advice is sought from the Commission on Human Medicines (CHM), an independent advisory body, which in turn is assisted by specialist expert advisory groups.

At a European level, the Committee for Medicinal Products for Human Use (CHMP) fulfils a similar role to the CHM. New products will have relatively limited safety information and the pharmaceutical company is generally required to outline a risk management plan.

Restrictions are imposed if evidence of safety and efficacy is unavailable in specific patient groups, e.g. children. A MA is granted for up to 5 years and then renewed following re-evaluation of the risks and benefits.[3]

Thus, the process ensures that in relation to the product's authorized uses, there has been due consideration of its efficacy, safety and quality, that the benefits outweigh the potential risks, and that there is appropriate accompanying product information and labelling.[4] The MA defines the conditions and patient groups for which a pharmaceutical company can market and supply the product, with more information about the authorized uses provided by the manufacturer in the Summary of Product Characteristics (SPC).

However, the MA regulates the marketing activities of the pharmaceutical industry, not the activities of the prescriber, and clinical experience may reveal other indications (i.e. off-label use). For these to be added to the existing MA, additional evidence would need to be gathered and submitted. The considerable expense of this, perhaps coupled with a small market for a new indication, dose or route, often means that a revised application is not made.

Prescribing for off-label use or unauthorized medicinal products

In the UK, the following may legally prescribe for off-label use or unauthorized medicinal products:[5]

- doctors, dentists, specifically safeguarded in the UK Medicines Act 1968
- nurses or pharmacists who are registered as *independent prescribers* if this is accepted clinical practice and within their clinical competence; optometrist, physiotherapist and podiatrist *independent prescribers* may only prescribe for off-label use (for conditions within their clinical competence)
- chiropodists, nurses, optometrists, pharmacists, podiatrists, physiotherapists, midwives and radiographers who are registered as *supplementary prescribers*, provided it is done within the framework of an agreed Clinical Management Plan for a specific patient in partnership with a doctor or dentist.

These prescriptions can be dispensed by pharmacists[6] and administered by nurses or midwives.[7]

The responsibility for the consequences of prescribing under such circumstances lies with the prescriber, who must be competent, operate within the professional codes and ethics of their statutory bodies and the prescribing practices of their employers.[4,6,8–10] The prescriber must be fully informed about the actions and uses of the medicinal product, be assured of the quality of the particular product, and in the light of published evidence, balance both the potential good and the potential harm which might ensue.[10]

In addition to clinical trials, such prescriptions may be justified:

- when prescribing generic formulations for which indications are not described
- with established medicinal products for proven but unauthorized indications
- for conditions for which there are no other treatments (even in the absence of strong evidence)
- when using medicinal products in individuals not covered by the MA, e.g. children
- when mixing medicinal products before administration, e.g. two or more injections in a syringe for administration by CSCI (see Box A).[11,12]

For information relating to the prescription and supply of a 'special', see p.751.

Box A Legislation surrounding the mixing of medicinal products[11]

Any *independent prescriber*, including non-medical prescribers, can mix medicinal products (including those which contain CDs) and direct others to mix, as can *supplementary prescribers* when the preparation is part of the Clinical Management Plan for an individual patient.

Existing good practice recommendations should be followed in relation to mixing all medicinal products.

Preparations resulting from mixing, other than when one product is a vehicle for the administration of the other, cannot be supplied or administered under Patient Group Direction arrangements.

It is possible to draw a hierarchy of degrees of reasonableness relating to off-label and unauthorized use (Figure 1).[13] The more dangerous the medicinal product and the more flimsy the evidence the more difficult it is to justify its prescription.

The GMC recommends that when prescribing either off-label or an unauthorized medicinal product, doctors should:

- be satisfied that such use would better serve the patient's needs than an authorized alternative (if one exists)
- be satisfied that there is sufficient evidence/experience of using the medicinal product to show its safety and efficacy, seeking the necessary information from appropriate sources
- record in the patient's clinical notes the medicinal product prescribed and, when not following common practice, the reasons for the choice
- take responsibility for prescribing the medicinal product and for overseeing the patient's care, including monitoring the clinical effects, or arrange for another suitable doctor to do so.[8]

Non-medical prescribers should ensure that they are familiar with their own profession's prescribing standards, e.g. NMC. Although the advice is broadly similar to that of the GMC, there are some differences.[9,14]

Providing patient information

Prescribers (or those authorizing treatment on their behalf) should provide sufficient information to patients about the expected benefits and potential risks (undesirable effects, drug interactions, etc.) to enable them to make an informed decision (Box B). The PIL supplied by the manufacturer will not contain information about off-label use and may confuse patients.

In palliative care, off-label use is so widespread that concerns have been expressed that a detailed explanation on every occasion is impractical, would be burdensome for the patient and increase anxiety, and could result in the refusal of beneficial treatment.[15] A UK survey of over 220 palliative medicine doctors showed that, when using a drug for a routine off-label indication, <5% *always* mention this to their patients, and 20% *never* do. However, in situations where there is little evidence and limited clinical experience to support a drug's off-label use, these figures change to 75% and 5% respectively.[16]

This is a grey area and each clinician must decide how explicit to be; an appropriate level of counselling and a sensitive approach is essential. Some NHS Trusts and other institutions have policies in place and have produced information cards or leaflets for patients and caregivers (Box C). A joint position statement has also been produced by the British Pain Society and the Association for Palliative Medicine (Box D),[17] together with a patient information booklet.[18]

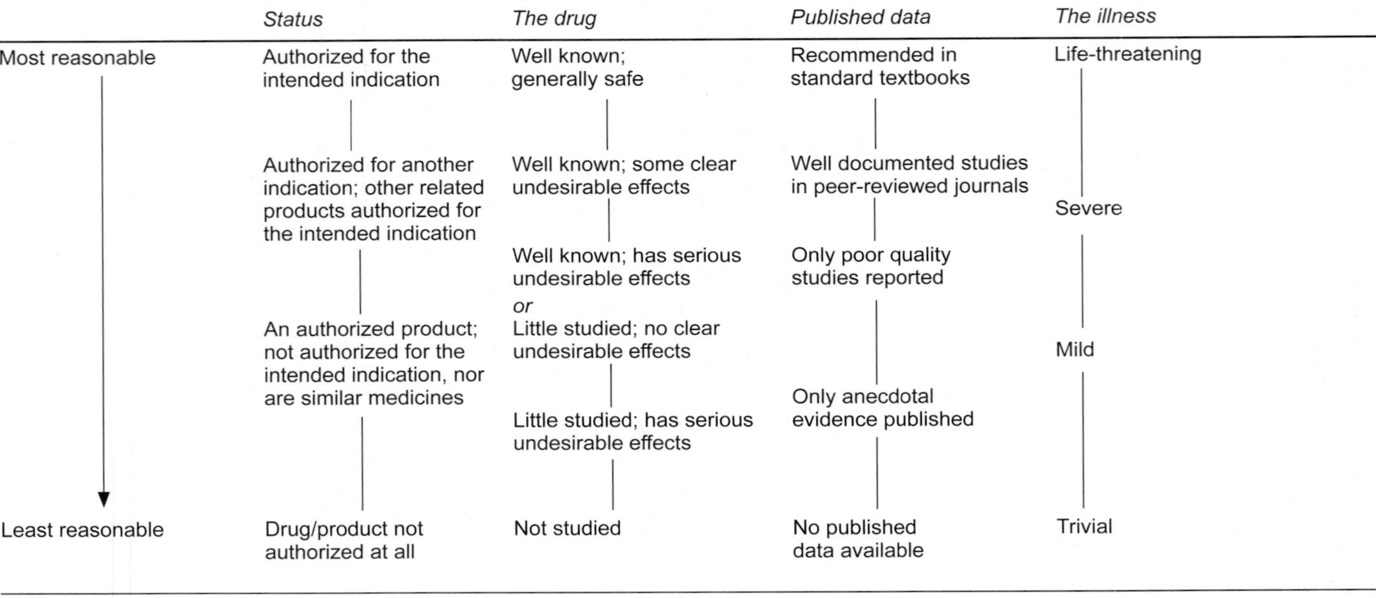

Figure I Factors influencing the reasonableness of prescribing decisions.

Box B Providing information for patients about off-label use and medicinal products without a Marketing authorization[8]

Patients (or their proxy) should be given sufficient information about any proposed treatment to allow them to make an informed decision. Questions must be answered fully and honestly.

Some medicinal products are routinely used beyond their Marketing authorization, e.g. when treating children and in palliative care.

In emergencies, or when there is no realistic alternative treatment and such information is likely to cause distress, it may not be practical or necessary to draw attention to the Marketing authorization.

In other situations, when the prescription of an unauthorized medicinal product is supported by authoritative clinical guidance, it may be sufficient to describe in general terms why it is not authorized for the proposed use.

When prescribing a medicinal product which is unauthorized or off-label in a non-routine way, or when suitable authorized alternatives exist, the reason for this should be explained to the patient.

Box C Example of a patient information leaflet about off-label use

Use of medicines beyond their licence (off-label)

This leaflet contains important information about your medicines, so please read it carefully.

Generally, medicines prescribed by your doctor or bought over-the-counter from a pharmacist are licensed for use by the Medicines and Healthcare products Regulatory Agency (MHRA).

The licence (or marketing authorization) specifies the conditions and patient groups for which the medicine should be used, and how it should be given.

Patient Information Leaflets (PILs) supplied with medicines reflect the licensed uses. When a medicine is used beyond its licence, the information in the PIL may not be relevant to your circumstances.

In palliative care, medicines are commonly used for conditions or in ways that are not specified on the licence.

Your doctor will use medicines beyond the licence only when there is research and experience to back up such use.

Medicines used very successfully beyond the licence include some antidepressants and anti-epileptics (anti-seizure drugs) when given to relieve some types of pain. Also, instead of injecting into a vein or muscle, medicines are often given subcutaneously (under the skin) because this is more comfortable and convenient.

If you would like more information, please ask your doctor or pharmacist.

Alternatively, contact:

Dr/Nurse...

Hospital...

....

....

Tel...

Box D Recommendations of the British Pain Society and Association for Palliative Medicine of Great Britain and Ireland[17]

Use of medicines beyond (off-label) and without (unlicensed) Marketing Authorization (MA) in palliative care and pain medicine

1. This statement should be seen as reflecting the views of a responsible body of opinion within the clinical specialties of palliative medicine and pain medicine.
2. The use of medicines beyond and without a MA in palliative care and pain medicine practice is both necessary and common and should be seen as a legitimate aspect of clinical practice.
3. Organizations providing palliative care and pain medicine services should support therapeutic practices that are underpinned by evidence and advocated by a responsible body of professional opinion.
4. Health professionals involved in prescribing medicines beyond or without MA should select those medicines that offer the best balance of benefit against harm for any given patient.
5. Choice of treatment requires partnership between patients and health professionals, and informed consent should be obtained, whenever possible, before prescribing any medicine.
6. Patients should be offered accurate, clear and specific information that meets their needs about the use of medicines beyond or without a MA in accordance with professional regulatory body guidance. The information needs of carers and other health professionals involved in the care of the patient should also be considered and met as appropriate. The use of information cards or leaflets may help with this. It is often unnecessary to take additional steps when recommending medicines beyond or without MA.
7. Health professionals should inform, change and monitor their practice with regard to medicines beyond or without MA in the light of evidence from audit and published research.
8. The Department of Health should work with health professionals and the pharmaceutical industry to enable and encourage the extension of product licences where there is evidence of benefit in circumstances of defined clinical need.

1 Atkinson C and Kirkham S (1999) Unlicensed uses for medication in a palliative care unit. *Palliative Medicine.* **13**: 145–152.
2 Todd J and Davies A (1999) Use of unlicensed medication in palliative medicine. *Palliative Medicine.* **13**: 466.
3 Anonymous (2009) The licensing of medicines in the UK. *Drug and Therapeutics Bulletin.* **47**: 45–48.
4 Anonymous (2009) Off-label or unlicensed medicines: prescribers' responsibilities. *MHRA Drug Safety Update.* **2 (9)**: 6–7.
5 Royal Pharmaceutical Society (2015) The professional guide for pharmacists. *Medicines, Ethics and Practice Edition 39.* www.rpharms.com
6 Royal Pharmaceutical Society (2015) Professional guidance for the procurement and supply of specials. www.rpharms.com
7 Nursing and Midwifery Council (2008) Standards for medicines management. www.nmc-uk.org
8 General Medical Council (2013) Good practice in prescribing medicines. Available from: www.gmc-uk.org
9 Nursing and Midwifery Council (2006) Standards of proficiency for nurse and midwife prescribers. Available from: www.nmc-uk.org
10 Royal Pharmaceutical Society (2016) Prescribing specials. Guidance for the prescribers of specials. www.rpharms.com
11 Department of Health (2010) Mixing of medicines prior to administration in clinical practice: medical and non-medical prescribing. HMSO, London. Available from: www.dh.gov.uk
12 Home Office (2012) Nurse and pharmacist independent prescribing, 'mixing of medicines', possession authorities under patient group directions and personal exemption provisions for Schedule 4 Part II drugs. Circular 009/2012. https://www.gov.uk
13 MHRA (2014) The supply of unlicensed medicinal products ("specials"). *MHRA Guidance Note 14.* Available from: https://www.gov.uk
14 Royal Pharmaceutical Society of Great Britain (2010) Professional Standards and Guidance for Pharmacist Prescribers. Available from: www.rpharms.com
15 Pavis H and Wilcock A (2001) Prescribing of drugs for use outside their licence in palliative care: survey of specialists in the United Kingdom. *British Medical Journal.* **323**: 484–485.
16 Culshaw J *et al.* (2013) Off-label prescribing in palliative care: a survey of independent prescribers. *Palliative Medicine.* **27**: 314–319.
17 British Pain Society (2012) Use of medicines outside of their UK Marketing Authorization in pain management and palliative care. Available from: www.britishpainsociety.org
18 British Pain Society (2012) Use of medicines outside of their UK Marketing Authorisation in pain management and palliative medicine - information for patients. Available from: www.britishpainsociety.org

Updated March 2017

DRUG NAMES

All drugs marketed in Europe are now known by their recommended International Non-proprietary (generic) Name (rINN). In the past, most publications in the UK used the now outdated British Approved Name (BAN). To aid understanding of the older literature, significant differences between BANs and rINNs are listed in Table 1.

Minor differences, e.g. 'f' instead of 'ph', 'e' instead of 'oe', 't' instead of 'th', have *not* been included.

In the USA, United States Adopted Names (USANs) take precedence over rINNs. USANs are also included in Table 1 where these differ significantly from rINNs.

In the UK, the BANs **adrenaline** and **noradrenaline** are still used in conjunction with the corresponding rINNs, i.e. **adrenaline (epinephrine)** and **noradrenaline (norepinephrine).**

Care should be taken with proprietary drug names in different countries. Some proprietary names are similar in spelling or pronunciation but contain different drugs. Further, some products with identical proprietary names contain different drugs, e.g. Urex® in the USA contains **methenamine** but, in Australia, **furosemide**.[1]

Table 1 Drug names relevant to palliative care for which the rINN, BAN and/or USAN differ

rINN	*BAN*	*USAN*
Alimemazine	Trimeprazine	Trimeprazine
Amobarbital	Amylobarbitone	
Bendroflumethiazide	Bendrofluazide	Bendroflumethiazide
Benzylpenicillin		Penicillin G
Calcitonin (salmon)	Salcatonin	Calcitonin
Carmellose		Carboxymethylcellulose
Chlorphenamine	Chlorpheniramine	Chlorpheniramine
Clomethiazole	Chlormethiazole	
Dexamfetamine	Dexamphetamine	Dextroamphetamine
Dextropropoxyphene		Propoxyphene
Dicycloverine	Dicyclomine	Dicyclomine
Diethylstilbestrol	Stilboestrol	Diethylstilbestrol
Dosulepin	Dothiepin	Dothiepin
Epinephrine	Adrenaline	Epinephrine
Glibenclamide		Glyburide
Glycerol	Glycerine	Glycerin
Glyceryl trinitrate		Nitroglycerin
Hyoscine		Scopolamine
Isoprenaline		Isoproterenol
	Ispaghula	Psyllium
Levomepromazine	Methotrimeprazine	
Levothyroxine	Thyroxine	
Liquid paraffin		Mineral oil
Macrogols	Macrogols	Polyethylene glycols

continued

Table 1 Continued

rINN	*BAN*	*USAN*
Methenamine hippurate	Hexamine hippurate	
Paracetamol		Acetaminophen
Pethidine		Meperidine
Phenobarbital	Phenobarbitone	
Phenoxymethylpenicillin		Penicillin V
Phytomenadione		Phytonadione
Retinol	Vitamin A	Vitamin A
Rifampicin		Rifampin
Salbutamol		Albuterol
Simeticone[a]	Simethicone	Simethicone
Sodium cromoglicate	Sodium cromoglycate	Cromolyn sodium
Tetracaine	Amethocaine	
Torasemide	Torasemide	Torsemide
Trihexyphenidyl	Benzhexol	Trihexyphenidyl

a. silica-activated dimeticone; known in some countries as activated dimethylpolysiloxane.

1 FDA (2006) Consumers filling U.S. prescriptions abroad may get the wrong active ingredient because of confusing drug names. *Public Health Advisory*. www.fda.gov/Drugs/DrugSafety/PostmarketDrugSafetyInformationforPatientsandProviders/DrugSafetyInformationforHeathcareProfessionals/PublicHealthAdvisories/ucm173134.htm.

Updated September 2017

ABBREVIATIONS

Drug administration

In 2005, the Joint Commission on Accreditation of Healthcare Organizations (JCAHO) in the USA published National Patient Safety Goals. These include a series of recommendations about ways in which confusion (and thus errors) can be reduced by avoiding the use of certain abbreviations on prescriptions. The full set of recommendations is available at http://www.jointcommission.org/standards_information/npsgs.aspx.

Although some traditional abbreviations remain acceptable (Table 1), others are not. Thus, it is recommended that, as in *PCF*, the following are written in full:

- at bedtime
- once daily
- each morning
- every other day.

Table 1 Abbreviations in *PCF* for drug administration times

Times	*UK*	*Latin*
Twice per day	b.d.	*bis die*
Three times per day	t.d.s.	*ter die sumendus*
Four times per day	q.d.s.	*quarta die sumendus*
Every 4 hours etc.	q4h	*quaque quarta hora*
Rescue medication (as needed/required)	p.r.n.	*pro re nata*
Give immediately	stat	*stat*

Because of widespread usage, the term 'immediate-release' is now used (without abbreviation) in *PCF*, rather than 'normal-release'. For 'slow-release', 'extended-release' etc., 'm/r' (modified-release) is used generically.

Although the following conventions have *not* been adopted in *PCF*, readers should be aware of the following recommendations for handwritten and printed prescriptions, and other printed medical matter, e.g. packaging, patient records:

- include a space between the drug dose and the unit of measure, e.g. 25 mg, not 25mg
- write 'per' instead of an oblique (mistaken for a figure 1), e.g. 200 mg per day, not 200mg/day
- use 'subcut' or 'subcutaneous' instead of SC (mistaken for SL)
- write 'less than' or 'greater than' instead of < and > (mistaken for a letter L or figure 7; or written the wrong way round and thus signifying the opposite of the intended meaning).

a.c.	ante cibum (before food)
amp	ampoule containing a single dose (cf. vial)
CD	controlled drug; preparation subject to prescription requirements under the Misuse of Drugs Act (UK); for regulations see BNF
CIVI	continuous intravenous infusion
CSCI	continuous subcutaneous infusion
e/c	enteric-coated (gastroresistant)
ED	epidural
IM	intramuscular
IT	intrathecal
IV	intravenous

IVI	intravenous infusion
m/r	modified-release; alternatives, controlled-release, extended-release, prolonged-release, slow-release, sustained-release
NHS	not prescribable on NHS prescriptions
OTC	over the counter (i.e. can be obtained without a prescription)
p.c.	post cibum (after food)
PO	per os, by mouth
POM	prescription-only medicine
PR	per rectum
PV	per vaginam
SC	subcutaneous
SL	sublingual
TD	transdermal
TM	transmucosal
vial	sterile container with a rubber bung containing either a single or multiple doses (cf. amp)
WFI	water for injections

General

*	specialist use only
†	unauthorized (unlicensed) use
ACBS	Advisory Committee on Borderline Substances
AHFS	American Hospital Formulary Service
BNF	British National Formulary
BP	British Pharmacopoeia
CHM	Commission on Human Medicines
CSM	Committee on Safety of Medicines (now part of CHM)
DH	Department of Health (UK)
EMEA	European Medicines Agency
EORTC	European Organisation for Research and Treatment of Cancer
ESRF	End-Stage Renal Failure
FDA	Food and Drug Administration (USA)
IASP	International Association for the Study of Pain
MHRA	Medicines and Healthcare products Regulatory Agency
NICE	National Institute for Health and Care Excellence
NPF	Nurse Prescribers' Formulary
NPSA	National Patient Safety Association
NYHA	New York Heart Association
PCS/PCU	palliative care service/unit
PI	package insert (USA), equivalent to SPC
PIL	Patient Information Leaflet (UK)
rINN	recommended International Non-proprietary Name
RPS	Royal Pharmaceutical Society
SIGN	Scottish Intercollegiate Guidelines Network
SPC	Summary of Product Characteristics (UK)
UK	United Kingdom
UKMI	UK Medicines Information
USA	United States of America
USP	United States Pharmacopoeia
VAS	visual analogue scale, 0–100mm
WHO	World Health Organization

Receptor types

α_1, α_2	alpha adrenergic type 1, 2
β_2	beta adrenergic type 2
δ	delta-opioid
κ	kappa-opioid

μ	mu-opioid
$5HT_{1A}$, $5HT_{2A}$	5-hydroxytryptamine (serotonin) type 1A, 2A etc.
A_1, A_2, A_{2A}	adenosine type 1, 2, 2A
CB_1, CB_2	cannabinoid type 1, 2
D_2	dopamine type 2
$GABA_A$, $GABA_B$	gamma-aminobutyric acid type A, B
H_1, H_2	histamine type 1, 2
M_1, M_2	muscarinic acetylcholine type 1, 2 etc.
MT_1, MT_2	melatonin type 1, 2
SST_1, SST_2	somatostatin type 1,2 etc.

Ion channels

Ca_v	calcium
K_v	potassium
Na_v	sodium

Medical

5HT	5-hydroxytryptamine (serotonin)
ACE	angiotensin-converting enzyme
ADH	antidiuretic hormone (vasopressin)
ATP	adenosine triphosphate
AMPA	α-amino-3-hydroxy-5-methylisoxazole-4-propionic acid
AUC	area under the plasma concentration–time curve
CHF	congestive heart failure
C_{max}	maximum plasma drug concentration
CNS	central nervous system
COPD	chronic obstructive pulmonary disease
COX	cyclo-oxygenase; alternative, prostaglandin synthase
CKD	chronic kidney disease
CRP	C-reactive protein
CSF	cerebrospinal fluid
CT	computed tomography
DIC	disseminated intravascular coagulation
DVT	deep vein thrombosis
ECG (EKG)	electrocardiogram
EFT	enteral feeding tube
ERCP	endoscopic retrograde cholangiopancreatography
FBC	full blood count
FEV_1	forced expiratory volume in 1 second
FRC	functional residual capacity
FSH	follicle-stimulating hormone
FVC	forced vital capacity of lungs
GABA	gamma-aminobutyric acid
GI	gastro-intestinal
Hb	haemoglobin
HIV	human immunodeficiency virus
Ig	immunoglobulin
INR	international normalized ratio
LABA	long-acting β_2-adrenergic receptor agonist
LFTs	liver function tests
LH	luteinizing hormone
LMWH	low molecular weight heparin
MAOI	mono-amine oxidase inhibitor
MARI	mono-amine re-uptake inhibitor
MRI	magnetic resonance imaging
MSU	mid-stream specimen of urine
NaSSA	noradrenergic and specific serotoninergic antidepressant

NDRI	noradrenaline (norepinephrine) and dopamine re-uptake inhibitor
NG	nasogastric
NJ	nasojejunal
NMDA	N-methyl D-aspartate
NNH	number needed to harm, i.e. the number of patients needed to be treated in order to harm one patient sufficiently to cause withdrawal from a drug trial
NNT	number needed to treat, i.e. the number of patients needed to be treated in order to achieve 50% improvement in one patient compared with placebo
NO	nitric oxide
NRI	noradrenaline (norepinephrine) re-uptake inhibitor
NSAID	non-steroidal anti-inflammatory drug
$PaCO_2$	arterial partial pressure of carbon dioxide
PaO_2	arterial partial pressure of oxygen
PCA	patient-controlled analgesia
PE	pulmonary embolus/embolism
PEF	peak expiratory flow
PEG	percutaneous endoscopic gastrostomy
PG	prostaglandin
PPI	proton pump inhibitor
RCT	randomized controlled trial
RIMA	reversible inhibitor of mono-amine oxidase type A
RTI	respiratory tract infection
SaO_2	oxygen saturation
SNRI	serotonin and noradrenaline (norepinephrine) re-uptake inhibitor
SRE	skeletal-related events
SSRI	selective serotonin re-uptake inhibitor
TCA	tricyclic antidepressant
TIBC	total iron-binding capacity; alternative, plasma transferrin concentration
Tl_{CO}	transfer factor of the lung for carbon monoxide
T_{max}	time to reach C_{max}
UTI	urinary tract infection
VEGF	vascular endothelial growth factor
VIP	vaso-active intestinal polypeptide
WBC	white blood cell
w/v	weight of solute (g) per 100mL

Units

cm	centimetre(s)
cps	cycles per sec
dL	decilitre(s)
g	gram(s)
Gy	Gray(s)
h	hour(s)
Hg	mercury
kcal	kilocalories
kg	kilogram(s)
L	litre(s)
mg	milligram(s)
microL	microlitre(s)
micromol	micromole(s)
mL	millilitre(s)
mm	millimetre(s)
mmol	millimole(s)
min	minute(s)
mosmol	milli-osmole(s)
msec	millisecond
nm	nanometre(s)
nmol	nanomole(s)
sec	second(s)

Updated September 2017

1: GASTRO-INTESTINAL SYSTEM

ANTACIDS

Indications: Occasional dyspepsia and/or acid reflux; H_2-receptor antagonists (see p.27) and PPIs (see p.30) are used when continuous gastric acid reduction is indicated.[1]

Pharmacology

Antacids generally contain one or more of the following which neutralize gastric acid:

- magnesium salts
- aluminium hydroxide
- sodium bicarbonate
- calcium carbonate.

These are sometimes combined with other ingredients which work in other ways to relieve the symptoms of dyspepsia, e.g.:

- hydrotalcite (aluminium magnesium carbonate hydroxide hydrate)
- peppermint oil
- alginate (see p.3)
- simeticone (silica-activated **dimeticone**, see p.4).

***Magnesium salts** are laxative and can cause diarrhoea; **aluminium salts** constipate.* Most proprietary antacids contain a mixture of **magnesium salts** and **aluminium salts** so as to have a neutral impact on intestinal transit. With doses of 100–200mL/24h or more, the effect of **magnesium salts** tends to override the constipating effect of **aluminium.**[2]

Aluminium hydroxide binds dietary phosphate. It is of benefit in patients with hyperphosphataemia in renal failure. Long-term complications of phosphate depletion and osteomalacia are not an issue in advanced cancer.

In post-radiation oesophagitis and candidosis which is causing painful swallowing, an **aluminium hydroxide-magnesium hydroxide** suspension containing **oxetacaine**, a local anaesthetic, can be helpful. It is only available as a special order product in the UK. Give 5–10mL (without fluid) 15min before meals & at bedtime, and p.r.n. before drinks. This should be regarded as short-term symptomatic treatment while time and specific treatment of the underlying condition permits healing of the damaged mucosa.

Hydrotalcite, an aluminium-magnesium complex, binds bile salts and is of specific benefit in patients with bile salt reflux, e.g. after certain forms of gastroduodenal surgery. It is available only in combination with **simeticone** in the UK (see p.4).

Peppermint oil is included in some proprietary products. It can help to mask the chalky taste of the antacid and also help belching, by decreasing the tone of the lower oesophageal sphincter.

Cautions

Risk of hypermagnesaemia with magnesium-containing antacids in renal impairment; **calcium carbonate** is preferable.

The relatively high sodium content (e.g. 4–6mmol/10mL) of some antacids and alginate products may be detrimental to patients on salt-restricted diets, e.g. those with hypertension, heart failure or renal impairment; low sodium alternatives (e.g. <1mmol/10mL) are preferable (see Supply).

Sodium bicarbonate: risk of sodium loading and metabolic alkalosis; do not use as a single product antacid. **Calcium carbonate:** rebound acid secretion, about 2h after a dose; also hypercalcaemia, particularly when taken with **sodium bicarbonate**.

Drug interactions

Antacids can impact on the absorption of other PO drugs by:

- temporarily increasing the pH of the stomach contents
- delaying gastric emptying
- forming insoluble complexes in the GI tract
- damaging enteric coating.

Selected interactions where additional caution may be necessary are listed in Table 1. Generally, these can be avoided by separating administration of the antacid and the affected drug by ≥2h. This is particularly important for e/c formulations because direct contact with antacids can result in damage to the enteric coating with consequential exposure of the drug to gastric acid, and of the stomach mucosa to the drug.

Antacids should not be administered by enteral feeding tube as they can cause the feed to coagulate and block the tube (see Chapter 28, Table 2, p.793).

Table 1 Interactions between antacids and other PO drugs[a3]

Drug affected	*Comment*
Bisphosphonates	Avoid antacid for ≥2h before and 30min–2h after the bisphosphonate; see individual SPC
Cefpodoxime	
Dexamethasone[b]	
Fexofenadine	
Gabapentin	Bio-availability reduced ≤20%; of uncertain clinical relevance
Itraconazole	Capsules only
Nitrofurantoin[c]	
Polystyrene sulfonate resin	Creates bicarbonate ions which can lead to metabolic alkalosis; avoid by giving the resin PR
Quinolones	Avoid antacid for ≥4h before and 2h after the quinolone; see individual SPC
Rifampicin	
Tetracyclines	

a. *not* an exhaustive list; limited to drugs most likely to be encountered in palliative care and *excludes* anticancer, HIV and immunosuppressive drugs (seek specialist advice)

b. magnesium trisilicate can reduce dexamethasone absorption by ≤75%

c. magnesium trisilicate can reduce nitrofurantoin absorption by ≤50%.

Large doses of antacids may lead to alkalinzation of the urine and thereby affect the action of other drugs, e.g.:

- **methenamine** action is inhibited at urinary pH >5.5
- the excretion of round-the-clock anti-inflammatory doses of **aspirin** is increased. Occasional doses of **aspirin** are not affected.[3]

Dose and use

Generally, antacids should be taken PO p.r.n. after meals and at bedtime. The dose of liquid formulations is generally 10mL.

Supply

Note. Low Na^+ is defined as <1mmol/tablet or 10mL dose.

Aluminium hydroxide
Alucap® (Meda)
Capsules 475mg, 28 days @ 1 t.d.s. & at bedtime = £13; *low* Na^+.

Magnesium trisilicate mixture BP (generic)
Oral suspension (**magnesium trisilicate** 250mg, **magnesium carbonate** 250mg and **sodium hydrogen carbonate** 250mg/5mL) 28 days @ 10mL t.d.s. & at bedtime = £7; *peppermint flavour, 6mmol* Na^+*/10mL*.

Co-magaldrox
Maalox® (Sanofi-Aventis)
Oral suspension (sugar-free) **co-magaldrox** 195/220 (**magnesium hydroxide** 195mg, **aluminium hydroxide** 220mg/5mL), 28 days @ 10mL t.d.s. & at bedtime = £7.50; *low* Na^+.

Mucogel® (Chemidex)
Oral suspension (sugar-free) **co-magaldrox** 195/220 (**magnesium hydroxide** 195mg, **aluminium hydroxide** 220mg/5mL), 28 days @ 10mL t.d.s. & at bedtime = £7; *low* Na^+.

With **oxetacaine**
Oral suspension **oxetacaine** 10mg, **aluminium hydroxide** 200mg, **magnesium hydroxide** 100mg/5mL, 28 days @ 10mL t.d.s. a.c. & at bedtime = £138; *low* Na^+ (Unauthorized product, available as a special order from Rosemont; see Chapter 24, p.751). *Available as Mucaine® suspension (Wyeth) in some countries.*

Also see Compound alginate products, p.3 and **simeticone**, p.4.

1 NICE (2004) Dyspepsia. Management of dyspepsia in adults in primary care. *Clinical Guideline*. CG17. www.nice.org.uk
2 Morrissey J and Barreras R (1974) Antacid therapy. *New England Journal of Medicine*. **290**: 550–554.
3 Baxter K and Preston CL. *Stockley's Drug Interactions*. London: Pharmaceutical Press www.medicinescomplete.com (accessed April 2015).

Updated May 2015

COMPOUND ALGINATE PRODUCTS

Included for general information. Alginate products are generally *not recommended* as antacids for palliative care patients.

Class: Alginate.

Indications: Acid reflux ('heartburn').

Pharmacology

Antacid products containing alginic acid or sodium alginate prevent oesophageal reflux pain by forming an inert low-density raft on the top of the acidic stomach contents. Both acid and air bubbles are necessary to produce the raft. Compound alginate products may thus be less effective if used with drugs which reduce acid (e.g. an H_2-receptor antagonist or a PPI) or products which reduce air bubbles (i.e. an antifoaming agent/antiflatulent).

Gaviscon® products, Peptac® and Acidex® oral suspensions are sodium alginate products and weak antacids; most of the antacid content adheres to the alginate raft. This neutralizes acid which seeps into the oesophagus around the raft but does nothing to correct the underlying causes, e.g. lax lower oesophageal sphincter, hyperacidity, delayed gastric emptying, obesity. Indeed, alginate-containing products are no better than **simeticone**-containing antacids in the treatment of acid reflux.[1] Compound alginate products have been largely superseded by acid suppression with PPIs (p.30) and H_2-receptor antagonists (p.27).

Onset of action <5min.

Duration of action 1–2h.

Cautions

The relatively high sodium content (e.g. 4–6mmol/10mL) of compound alginate products may be detrimental to patients on salt-restricted diets, e.g. those with hypertension, heart failure or renal impairment.

Drug interactions

Co-administration of antacids with e/c formulations, certain other drugs or via enteral feeding tubes should be avoided, also see Antacids p.2.

Dose and use

Several products are available but none is recommended.

Supply

Gaviscon® products, Peptac® and Acidex® oral suspensions (all sugar-free) contain **sodium alginate** 250mg, **sodium bicarbonate** 133.5mg and **calcium carbonate** 80mg/5mL (for full details see BNF).

Other compound alginate products are also available (see BNF); some have high sugar content. Several compound alginate products are available OTC.

1 Pokorny C *et al.* (1985) Comparison of an antacid/dimethicone mixture and an alginate/antacid mixture in the treatment of oesophagitis. *Gut.* **26**:A574.

Updated May 2015

SIMETICONE

Class: Antifoaming agent (antiflatulent).

Indications: Acid dyspepsia (including acid reflux), gassy dyspepsia, †hiccup (if associated with gastric distension).

Pharmacology

Simeticone (silica-activated dimeticone or dimethylpolysiloxane) is a mixture of liquid dimeticones with silicon dioxide. It is an antifoaming agent, present in some proprietary combination antacids, and more recently available alone. It alters the surface tension of bubbles, causing them to coalesce. This facilitates belching, easing flatulence, distension and postprandial gastric discomfort. Simeticone-containing antacids are as effective as alginate-containing products in the treatment of acid reflux.[1] Simeticone is inert and is not absorbed.

Onset of action <5min.

Duration of action 1–2h.

Cautions

Although Maalox Plus® contains both **aluminium** and **magnesium**, at higher doses (e.g. >100–200mL/day) the laxative effect of **magnesium** tends to override the constipating effect of **aluminium**.[2] Risk of hypermagnesaemia with magnesium-containing antacids in renal impairment.

Drug interactions

Co-administration of antacids with e/c formulations, certain other drugs or via enteral feeding tubes should be avoided, also see Antacids p.2.

Dose and use

Simeticone capsules and chewable tablets are now available:

- start with 100–125mg PO q.d.s or p.r.n after meals and at bedtime
- maximum daily dose 800mg/24h.

When the above are not available, or an antacid effect is also required, prescribe an antacid formulation containing simeticone. Altacite Plus® is preferred because it contains a higher dose of simeticone than Maalox Plus®:

- give 10mL PO p.r.n. or 10 mL after meals and at bedtime.

Supply

Wind-eze® (Teva)
Capsules 125mg, 28 days @ 125mg q.d.s. = £15.
Tablets chewable 125mg, 28 days @ 125mg q.d.s. = £10.

WindSetlers® (Thornton & Ross)
Capsules 100mg, 28 days @ 100mg q.d.s. = £14.

With antacids
Altacite Plus® (Peckforton)
Oral suspension (sugar-free) simeticone 125mg, **hydrotalcite** 500mg/5mL, 28 days @ 10mL q.d.s. = £12; *low Na⁺*.

Maalox Plus® (Sanofi Aventis)
Oral suspension (sugar-free) simeticone 25mg, dried **aluminium hydroxide** 220mg, **magnesium hydroxide** 195mg/5mL, 28days @ 10mL q.d.s = £13; *low Na⁺*.

Note. all simeticone and simeticone-antacid products are available OTC.

1 Pokorny C *et al.* (1985) Comparison of an antacid/dimethicone mixture and an alginate/antacid mixture in the treatment of oesophagitis. *Gut.* **26**:A574.
2 Morrissey J and Barreras R (1974) Antacid therapy. *New England Journal of Medicine.* **290**: 550–554.

Updated (minor change) June 2017

ANTIMUSCARINICS

Indications: Smooth muscle spasm (e.g. bladder, intestine), motion sickness (**hyoscine *hydrobromide***), drying secretions (including surgical premedication, †sialorrhoea, †drooling, †death rattle/noisy rattling breathing, and †inoperable bowel obstruction), †paraneoplastic pyrexia and sweating.

Contra-indications: Narrow-angle glaucoma (unless moribund), tachycardia (heart rate >100 beats/min); see Cautions and **hyoscine *butylbromide*** (p.16), bowel obstruction (unless part of medical management), paralytic ileus, megacolon, prostatic enlargement with urinary retention, myasthenia gravis (unless moribund).

Note. Contra-indications vary between different antimuscarinic drugs (see individual SPCs). When possible, *PCF* collates and standardizes contra-indications across a class of drugs and the above are applicable for antimuscarinics given parenterally, SL, TD and PO. The exception is PO **hyoscine *butylbromide*** (p.16) where low bio-availability reduces the likelihood of systemic antimuscarinic effects.

Pharmacology

Chemically, antimuscarinics are classified as tertiary amines or quaternary ammonium compounds (Box A).

Box A Chemical classification of antimuscarinics

Tertiary amines	**Quaternary ammonium compounds**
Naturally-occurring (belladonna alkaloids)	*Synthetic/semisynthetic*
Atropine	Glycopyrronium
Hyoscine *hydrobromide*	Hyoscine *butylbromide*
Hyoscyamine (l-atropine; not UK)[a]	Ipratropium bromide
	Propantheline
Synthetic/semisynthetic	Tiotropium bromide
Dicycloverine	
Orphenadrine	
Oxybutynin	
Tolterodine	

a. because the d-isomer is virtually inactive, hyoscyamine is twice as potent as racemic atropine.

Numerous other drugs have antimuscarinic effects (Box B). In addition, some drugs generally not considered antimuscarinic have been shown to have detectable antimuscarinic activity by means of a radioreceptor assay, including **codeine**, **digoxin**, **dipyridamole**, **isosorbide**, **loperamide**, **nifedipine**, **prednisolone**, **ranitidine**, **theophylline**, **warfarin**.[1] Thus, potentially, multiple drugs can contribute to the total 'antimuscarinic burden', and thereby exacerbate toxicity, particularly in the frail elderly.[2]

Box B Drugs with antimuscarinic effects used in palliative care

Analgesics	Antipsychotics (typical)
pethidine (*not* recommended)	phenothiazines, e.g.
nefopam (mostly postoperative)	chlorpromazine
Antidepressants	levomepromazine
TCAs, e.g. amitriptyline, imipramine	prochlorperazine
paroxetine (SSRI)	Antisecretory drugs
Antihistamines, e.g.	belladonna alkaloids
chlorphenamine	atropine
cyclizine	hyoscine
dimenhydrinate (not UK)	hyoscyamine (l-atropine, not UK)[a]
promethazine	glycopyrronium
Antiparkinsonians, e.g.	Antispasmodics, e.g.
orphenadrine	dicycloverine
procyclidine	mebeverine
Antipsychotics (atypical)	oxybutynin
clozapine	propantheline
olanzapine	tolterodine

a. hyoscyamine is twice as potent as racemic atropine.

At least five different types of muscarinic receptors have been identified (M_1–M_5).[3] They are widely distributed, but their expression and functional relevance varies between tissues. Most antimuscarinic drugs act as non-selective antagonists, e.g. **atropine**, **glycopyrronium**, **hyoscine *hydrobromide***, **hyoscine *butylbromide***. Newer drugs have aimed to be more selective in their actions, e.g. **oxybutynin** and **tolterodine** are *relatively* selective for M_3 receptors, which predominate in the bladder (see p.567). Nonetheless, undesirable effects are unavoidable because M_3 receptors are also important in other tissues of the body, e.g. salivary gland and bowel, resulting in dry mouth and constipation.

Within the heart, M_2 receptors are mostly responsible for conveying parasympathetic effects on pacemaker activity, atrioventricular conduction and force of contraction. Other subtypes are also present (M_1, M_3, M_5) but their functional significance is uncertain. Further, cardiac disease can alter receptor expression, e.g. the density of M_2 decreases and M_3 increases in chronic atrial fibrillation.[3] Within the coronary arteries in mice, M_3 receptors are the most important in mediating acetylcholine-induced vasodilation; it is not known if this is true in humans, although the genes for M_2 and M_3 receptors are expressed.[3] Thus, although the cardiac toxicity of **hyoscine *butylbromide*** has been the recent focus of attention (see p.17), *all* antimuscarinics have this potential. This is particularly so in patients with cardiac disease associated with a detrimental autonomic nervous system imbalance (increased sympathetic and decreased parasympathetic (vagal) activity).[4] Indeed, *increasing* vagal activity appears beneficial in cardiac disease, and there is growing interest in the use of electrical stimulation or drugs to augment vagal function, e.g. in heart failure.[4,5]

Antimuscarinic effects can be divided into central and peripheral (Box C); undesirable central and peripheral effects have been summarized as:

'Dry as a bone, blind as a bat, red as a beet, hot as a hare, mad as a hatter.'

Box C Antimuscarinic effects

CNS effects

Drowsiness
Cognitive impairment
Delirium
Restlessness
Agitation

Peripheral effects

Visual

Mydriasis
Loss of accommodation
} blurred vision (and thus may impair driving ability)

Cardiovascular

Tachycardia, palpitations
Extrasystoles
Arrhythmias
} also related to noradrenaline (norepinephrine) potentiation and a quinidine-like action

Gastro-intestinal

Dry mouth (inhibition of salivation)
Heartburn (relaxation of lower oesophageal sphincter)
Constipation (decreased intestinal motility)

Urinary tract

Hesitancy of micturition
Retention of urine

Skin

Reduced sweating
Flushing

At *toxic* doses, all the tertiary amines, including **hyoscine *hydrobromide***, cause CNS stimulation resulting in mild central vagal excitation, respiratory stimulation, agitation and delirium. However, at typical *therapeutic* doses, **hyoscine *hydrobromide*** (but *not* **atropine**) causes CNS depression.

Synthetic tertiary amines generally cause less central stimulation than the naturally-occurring alkaloids. Quaternary ammonium compounds do not cross the blood-brain barrier in any significant amount, and accordingly have only peripheral effects (Box C).[6] They are also less well absorbed from the GI tract.

The muscarinic receptors in salivary glands are very responsive to antimuscarinics and inhibition of salivation occurs at lower doses than required for other antimuscarinic effects.[7] In some patients, a reduction in excess saliva results in improved speech.[8]

In the UK, parenteral antimuscarinics are widely used to reduce death rattle (noisy rattling breathing) in those close to death (see QCG: Death rattle (noisy rattling breathing), p.12). Although the use of antimuscarinics for this purpose has been questioned,[9,10] such use is often, although not always, beneficial.[11–13] For example, a prospective clinical survey concluded that antimuscarinics reduce death rattle in 1/2–2/3 of patients.[14]

In relation to death rattle, belladonna alkaloids are generally equally effective,[11,12] and **glycopyrronium** may sometimes be effective when the alkaloids have not been.[15] Although one study reported that **hyoscine *hydrobromide*** acts faster than **glycopyrronium**, there is no detectable difference between the two drugs after 1h.[16] In practice, undesirable effects, availability, fashion, familiarity, and cost are probably the main influences in choice of drug.

Antimuscarinic drugs differ in their pharmacokinetic characteristics (Table 1).

Table 1 Pharmacokinetic details of selected antimuscarinic drugs[7]

	Bio-availability	*Plasma halflife*	*Duration of action (antisecretory)*
Atropine	50% PO	2–2.5h[a]	no data
Glycopyrronium	<5% PO	1–1.5h[a]	7h
Hyoscine *butylbromide*	<1% PO[17]	1–5h[17]	<2h[b,18]
Hyoscine *hydrobromide*	60–80% SL	1–4h[a]	1–9h

a. after IM injection into deltoid muscle
b. in volunteers; possibly longer in moribund patients.

Cautions

After the sudden death of a patient with cardiac disease given an IV bolus of **hyoscine *butylbromide*** at colonoscopy, the MHRA issued a warning highlighting its cardiac toxicity (see p.17).[19]

Cardiac disease, e.g. myocardial infarction, ischaemia, arrhythmia, heart failure, hypertension; other conditions predisposing to tachycardia, e.g. thyrotoxicosis, β agonists. Bladder outflow obstruction (prostatism). Likely to exacerbate acid reflux. Narrow-angle glaucoma may be precipitated in those at risk, particularly the elderly. Use in hot weather or pyrexia may lead to heatstroke.

Use in renal impairment

In end-stage renal failure, do *not* use **hyoscine *hydrobromide*** for death rattle because of an increased risk of delirium. Use **hyoscine *butylbromide*** (dose unchanged) or **glycopyrronium** instead (lower doses may be sufficient).

Antimuscarinics differ in their potential to cause toxicity when renal function is impaired, see Chapter 17 for general information on the choice of antimuscarinic and use in ESRF.

Drug interactions

Concurrent treatment with ≥2 antimuscarinic drugs (including antihistamines, phenothiazines and TCAs; see Box B) will increase the likelihood of undesirable effects, and (when centrally acting) of central toxicity, i.e. restlessness, agitation, delirium (see Box C). Children, the elderly, and patients with renal or hepatic impairment are more susceptible to the central effects of non-quaternary antimuscarinics.

Because antimuscarinics competitively block the final common (cholinergic) pathway through which prokinetics act,[20] concurrent prescription with **metoclopramide** and **domperidone** should be avoided as far as possible.

The increased GI transit time produced by antimuscarinics may allow increased drug absorption from some formulations, e.g. **digoxin** and **nitrofurantoin** tablets and **potassium** m/r tablets, but reduced absorption from others, e.g. **paracetamol** tablets. Dissolution and absorption of SL tablets (e.g. **glyceryl trinitrate**) may be reduced because of decreased saliva production.

Both antimuscarinics and opioids cause constipation (by different mechanisms) and, if used together, will result in an increased need for laxatives, and may even result in paralytic ileus. On the other hand, **morphine** and **hyoscine *butylbromide*** or **glycopyrronium** are sometimes purposely combined in terminally ill patients with inoperable bowel obstruction in order to prevent colic and to reduce vomiting.

Undesirable effects

What is a desired effect becomes an undesirable effect in different circumstances (see Box C). Thus, dry mouth is an almost universal *undesirable* effect of antimuscarinics except when a reduction of oropharyngeal secretions is intended, as in death rattle.

Dose and use

In palliative care patients, there is an association between the number of antimuscarinic drugs used and worsening fatigue and quality of life.[2] Thus, when possible, drugs with antimuscarinic effects should be avoided or discontinued.

By injection, there is no good evidence to recommend one antimuscarinic in preference to another.[12] However, because **atropine** and **hyoscyamine** (not UK) tend to stimulate the CNS rather than sedate, concurrent prescription of **midazolam** or **haloperidol** is more likely to be necessary. In the UK, **glycopyrronium**, **hyoscine *butylbromide*** and **hyoscine *hydrobromide*** are used in preference to **atropine**. Generally, *PCF* favours **hyoscine *butylbromide*** based on its lack of central effects and lower cost.

When given IM, **atropine**, **hyoscine *hydrobromide*** and **glycopyrronium** are all absorbed faster from the deltoid muscle than from the gluteal muscles.[7]

Antispasmodic

Antimuscarinics are used to relieve smooth muscle spasm in the bladder (see **oxybutynin**, p.567) and rectum.

Antispasmodic and antisecretory

Antimuscarinics are used to reduce intestinal colic and intestinal secretions, particularly gastric, associated with inoperable organic bowel obstruction in terminally ill patients (Table 2). Also see QCG: Inoperable bowel obstruction, p.242.

Table 2 Antispasmodic and antisecretory drugs: typical SC doses

Drug	*Stat and p.r.n. doses*	*CSCI dose/24h*
Glycopyrronium	200microgram	600–1,200microgram
Hyoscine *butylbromide*	20mg	20–300mg
Hyoscine *hydrobromide*[a]	400microgram	1,200–2,000microgram

a. atropine doses are generally the same as hyoscine *hydrobromide*.

Antisecretory

Death rattle (noisy rattling breathing)

Treatment regimens are all unauthorized and based mainly on local clinical experience. In the UK antimuscarinic drugs for death rattle are generally given SC/CSCI.[21] See QCG: Death rattle (noisy rattling breathing), p.12.

In some countries the SL route is preferred, particularly in home care because it circumvents the need for injections, e.g. **glycopyrronium**, see p.13).

Drooling (and sialorrhoea)
Seen particularly in patients with ALS/MND, advanced Parkinson's disease and with various disorders of the head and neck. A survey of UK neurologists[22] with a special interest in MND/ALS showed that their preferred first-line drugs for sialorrhoea are:

- **hyoscine *hydrobromide***, e.g. 1mg/3 days TD[23]
- **amitriptyline**, e.g. 10–25mg PO at bedtime
- **atropine**, e.g. 1% ophthalmic solution, 4 drops on the tongue or SL q4h p.r.n.

In relation to the latter, drop size varies with applicator and technique. *Thus, the dose varies from 200–500microgram per drop (800microgram–2mg/dose).* It is important to titrate the dose upwards until there is an adequate effect; in an RCT, 500microgram q.d.s. was no better than placebo.[24]

Glycopyrronium is the most popular second-line drug, typically PO or SL.[22] It is recommended for first-line use in patients with cognitive impairment.[25] It has also been used for drooling in other conditions (see Glycopyrronium, p.13).

In patients in whom antimuscarinics are contra-indicated, ineffective or not tolerated, the parotid ± submandibular glands can be injected with **botulinum toxin**.[22] Injections are generally effective within 2 weeks, and benefit lasts 3–4 months.[26–30] In patients with a relatively long prognosis (years rather than months), radiotherapy and surgery are further options.[22]

Paraneoplastic pyrexia and sweating
Antimuscarinic drugs are used in the treatment of paraneoplastic pyrexia (Box D).

Box D Symptomatic drug treatment of paraneoplastic pyrexia and sweating

Prescribe an antipyretic:

- paracetamol 500–1,000mg PO q.d.s. or p.r.n. (generally less toxic than an NSAID)
- NSAID, e.g. ibuprofen 200–400mg PO t.d.s. or p.r.n. (or the locally preferred alternative).

If the sweating does not respond to an NSAID, prescribe an antimuscarinic drug, e.g.:

- amitriptyline 25–50mg PO at bedtime
- propantheline 15–30mg PO b.d.–t.d.s. on an empty stomach
- hyoscine *hydrobromide* 1mg/3 days TD[31]
- glycopyrronium 200microgram–2mg PO t.d.s.[32]

If an antimuscarinic fails, other PO options include:

- gabapentin, see p.272
- H_2-receptor antagonist, e.g. ranitidine 150mg b.d.[33]
- olanzapine 5mg b.d.[34]
- propranolol 10–20mg b.d.–t.d.s.
- thalidomide 100mg at bedtime.[35,36]

Thalidomide is generally seen as the last resort even though the response rate appears to be high.[36] This is mostly because it can cause an irreversible painful peripheral neuropathy and other undesirable effects (see p.558).

Overdose
In the past, **physostigmine** (not UK), a cholinesterase inhibitor, was sometimes administered to correct antimuscarinic toxicity/poisoning. This is no longer recommended because **physostigmine** itself can cause serious toxic effects, including cardiac arrhythmias and seizures.[37–39]

A benzodiazepine can be given to control marked agitation and seizures. Phenothiazines should *not* be given because they will exacerbate the antimuscarinic effects, and could precipitate an acute dystonia (see Drug-induced movement disorders, p.739).

Anti-arrhythmics are *not* advisable if an arrhythmia develops; but hypoxia and acidosis should be corrected.

1 Tune I *et al.* (1992) Anticholinergic effects of drugs commonly prescribed for the elderly; potential means of assessing risk of delirium. *American Journal of Psychiatry*. **149**: 1393–1394.
2 Hochman MJ *et al.* (2016) Anticholinergic drug burden in noncancer versus cancer patients near the end of life. *Journal of Pain and Symptom Management*. **52**: 737–743.e733.
3 Abrams P *et al.* (2006) Muscarinic receptors: their distribution and function in body systems, and the implications for treating overactive bladder. *British Journal of Pharmacology*. **148**: 565–578.
4 He X *et al.* (2015) Novel strategies and underlying protective mechanisms of modulation of vagal activity in cardiovascular diseases. *British Journal of Pharmacology*. **172**: 5489–5500.
5 He B *et al.* (2016) Autonomic modulation by electrical stimulation of the parasympathetic nervous system: an emerging intervention for cardiovascular diseases. *Cardiovascular Therapeutics*. **34**: 167–171.
6 Sweetman SC (ed) (2005) Martindale: The Complete Drug Reference. (34e). Pharmaceutical Press, London, p. 475.
7 Ali-Melkkila T *et al.* (1993) Pharmacokinetics and related pharmacodynamics of anticholinergic drugs. *Acta Anaesthesiologica Scandinavica*. **37**: 633–642.
8 Rashid H *et al.* (1997) Management of secretions in esophageal cancer patients with glycopyrrolate. *Annals of Oncology*. **8**: 198–199.
9 Wee B and Hillier R (2012) Interventions for noisy breathing in patients near to death. *Cochrane Database of Systematic Reviews*. **1**: CD005177. www.thecochranelibrary.com
10 Lokker ME *et al.* (2014) Prevalence, impact, and treatment of death rattle: a systematic review. *Journal of Pain and Symptom Management*. **47**: 105–122.
11 Likar R *et al.* (2008) Efficacy of glycopyrronium bromide and scopolamine hydrobromide in patients with death rattle: a randomized controlled study. *Wiener Klinische Wochenschrift*. **120**: 679–683.
12 Wildiers H *et al.* (2009) Atropine, hyoscine butylbromide, or scopolamine are equally effective for the treatment of death rattle in terminal care. *Journal of Pain and Symptom Management*. **38**: 124–133.
13 Hugel H *et al.* (2006) Respiratory tract secretions in the dying patient: a comparison between glycopyrronium and hyoscine hydrobromide. *Journal of Palliative Medicine*. **9**: 279–284.
14 Hughes A *et al.* (2000) Audit of three antimuscarinic drugs for managing retained secretions. *Palliative Medicine*. **14**: 221–222.
15 Mirakhur R and Dundee J (1980) A comparison of the effects of atropine and glycopyrollate on various end organs. *Journal of the Royal Society of Medicine*. **73**: 727–730.
16 Back I *et al.* (2001) A study comparing hyoscine hydrobromide and glycopyrrolate in the treatment of death rattle. *Palliative Medicine*. **15**: 329–336.
17 Boehringer Ingelheim GmbH *Data on file*.
18 Herxheimer A and Haefeli L (1966) Human pharmacology of hyoscine butylbromide. *Lancet*. **ii**: 418–421.
19 MHRA (2017) Hyoscine butylbromide (Buscopan) injection: risk of serious adverse effects in patients with underlying cardiac disease. *Drug Safety Update*. www.gov.uk/drug-safety-update
20 Schuurkes JAJ *et al.* (1986) Stimulation of gastroduodenal motor activity: dopaminergic and cholinergic modulation. *Drug Development Research*. **8**: 233–241.
21 Bennett M *et al.* (2002) Using anti-muscarinic drugs in the management of death rattle: evidence based guidelines for palliative care. *Palliative Medicine*. **16**: 369–374.
22 Hobson EV *et al.* (2013) Management of sialorrhoea in motor neuron disease: a survey of current UK practice. *Amyotrophic Lateral Sclerosis Frontotemporal Degeneration*. **14**: 521–527.
23 Talmi YP *et al.* (1990) Reduction of salivary flow with transdermal scopolamine: a four-year experience. *Otolaryngology Head and Neck Surgery*. **103**: 615–618.
24 De Simone GG *et al.* (2006) Atropine drops for drooling: a randomized controlled trial. *Palliative Medicine*. **20**: 665–671.
25 NICE (2016) Motor neurone disease: assessment and management. *NICE Guideline* NG42. www.nice.org.uk
26 Ondo WG *et al.* (2004) A double-blind placebo-controlled trial of botulinum toxin B for sialorrhea in Parkinson's disease. *Neurology*. **62**: 37–40.
27 Jongerius P *et al.* (2004) Effect of botulinum toxin in the treatment of drooling: a controlled clinical trial. *Pediatrics*. **114**: 620–627.
28 Mancini F *et al.* (2003) Double-blind, placebo-controlled study to evaluate the efficacy and safety of botulinum toxin type A in the treatment of drooling in parkinsonism. *Movement Disorders*. **18**: 685–688.
29 Lipp A *et al.* (2003) A randomized trial of botulinum toxin A for treatment of drooling. *Neurology*. **61**: 1279–1281.
30 Ellies M *et al.* (2004) Reduction of salivary flow with botulinum toxin: extended report on 33 patients with drooling, salivary fistulas, and sialadenitis. *Laryngoscope*. **114**: 1856–1860.
31 Mercadante S (1998) Hyoscine in opioid-induced sweating. *Journal of Pain and Symptom Management*. **15**: 214–215.
32 Klaber M and Catterall M (2000) Treating hyperhidrosis. *British Medical Journal*. **321**: 703.
33 Pittelkow M *et al.* (2015) Pruritus and sweating in palliative medicine. In: NI Cherny *et al* (eds). *Oxford Textbook of Palliative Medicine (5e)*. Oxford University Press, Oxford 724–739.
34 Zylicz Z and Krajnik M (2003) Flushing and sweating in an advanced breast cancer patient relieved by olanzapine. *Journal of Pain and Symptom Management*. **25**: 494–495.
35 Deaner P (2000) The use of thalidomide in the management of severe sweating in patients with advanced malignancy: trial report. *Palliative Medicine*. **14**: 429–431.
36 Calder K and Bruera E (2000) Thalidomide for night sweats in patients with advanced cancer. *Palliative Medicine*. **14**: 77–78.
37 Aquilonius SM and Hedstrand U (1978) The use of physostigmine as an antidote in tricyclic anti-depressant intoxication. *Acta Anaesthesiologica Scandinavica*. **22**: 40–45.
38 Caine ED (1979) Anticholinergic toxicity. *New England Journal of Medicine*. **300**: 1278.
39 Newton RW (1975) Physostigmine salicylate in the treatment of tricyclic antidepressant overdosage. *Journal of the American Medical Association*. **231**: 941–943.

Updated July 2017

Quick Clinical Guide: Death rattle (noisy rattling breathing)

Death rattle occurs in about 50% of dying patients. It is caused by fluid collecting in the upper airway, arising from one or more sources:

- saliva (most common)
- bronchial mucosa (e.g. inflammation/infection)
- pulmonary oedema
- gastric reflux.

Rattling breathing can also occur in patients with a tracheostomy.

Non-drug treatment

- if the patient is unconscious, ease the family's distress by explaining that the rattle is not distressing to the patient
- position the patient semiprone to encourage postural drainage; but upright or semirecumbent if the cause is pulmonary oedema or gastric reflux
- suction of the upper airway but, because it can be distressing, generally restrict use to unconscious patients.

Drug treatment

If the rattle is associated with distressing breathlessness in a semiconscious patient, supplement the recommendations below with an opioid (e.g. morphine) and an anxiolytic sedative (e.g. midazolam).

Saliva

Because they do not affect existing secretions, an antimuscarinic drug should be given SC as soon as the rattle begins (Table). Hyoscine *butylbromide* is widely used because it is the cheapest and is free of CNS effects.

CSCI treatment is generally started at the same time as the first or second SC dose; increase the dose if ≥ 2 p.r.n. doses/day are needed.

Antimuscarinic drugs for death rattle

Drug	*Stat and p.r.n. SC dose*	*CSCI dose/24h*
Hyoscine *butylbromide*	20mg	20–120mg
Hyoscine *hydrobromide*	400microgram	1,200–1,600microgram
Glycopyrronium	200microgram	600–1,200microgram

In end-stage renal failure, do *not* use hyoscine *hydrobromide* because of an increased risk of delirium. Use hyoscine *butylbromide* (dose unchanged) or glycopyrronium instead (lower doses may be sufficient).

Respiratory tract infection

Generally, it is *not* appropriate to prescribe an antibacterial in an imminently dying patient. Rarely, one may be indicated if death rattle is caused by profuse purulent sputum in a semiconscious patient.

Pulmonary oedema

Consider furosemide 20–40mg SC/IM/IV q2h p.r.n. Beware precipitating urinary retention.

Gastric reflux

Consider metoclopramide 20mg SC/IV q3h p.r.n. ± ranitidine 50mg SC/IV b.d.–q.d.s.

Antimuscarinics block the prokinetic effect of metoclopramide; avoid concurrent use if possible.

Updated June 2017

GLYCOPYRRONIUM

Class: Antimuscarinic.

Indications: Drying secretions (including surgical premedication, control of upper airway secretions, COPD (Seebri Breezhaler®), †sialorrhoea, †drooling, †death rattle (noisy rattling breathing), †smooth muscle spasm (e.g. intestine, bladder), †inoperable intestinal obstruction), †paraneoplastic pyrexia and sweating, †hyperhidrosis.[1,2]

Contra-indications: See Antimuscarinics (p.000). For tachycardia (heart rate >100 beats/min), also see Pharmacology and **hyoscine *butylbromide*** (p.17).

Pharmacology

Glycopyrronium is a synthetic ionized quaternary ammonium antimuscarinic which penetrates biological membranes slowly and erratically.[3] In consequence it rarely causes sedation or delirium.[4,5] Absorption PO is poor and IV it is about 35 times more potent than PO.[6] Even so, glycopyrronium 200–400microgram PO t.d.s. produces plasma concentrations associated with an antisialogogic effect lasting up to 8h.[7–9]

By injection, glycopyrronium is 2–5 times more potent than **hyoscine *hydrobromide*** as an antisecretory drug,[6] and may be effective in some patients who fail to respond to **hyoscine**. However, the efficacy of parenteral **hyoscine *hydrobromide***, **hyoscine *butylbromide*** and glycopyrronium as antisialogogues is generally similar, with death rattle reduced in 1/2–2/3 of patients.[10] Further, provided that time is taken to explain the cause of the rattle to the relatives and there is ongoing support, relatives' distress is relieved in >90% of cases.[11]

Parenterally, the optimal single dose of glycopyrronium is 200microgram;[12,13] this appears less likely to increase heart rate and cause tachycardia compared with parenteral doses of other antimuscarinic drugs, e.g. **atropine**, **hyoscine *butylbromide*** (see p.16).[14,15] Nonetheless, comparative patient safety data are lacking and, even in young healthy volunteers, changes in cardiac conduction are seen after 200microgram IV.[14] Thus, particularly in those with cardiovascular disease, it would seem appropriate to consider applying similar contra-indications and cautions as for other antimuscarinics (p.5).

Although at standard doses glycopyrronium does not change ocular pressures or pupil size, it can precipitate narrow-angle glaucoma. It is excreted by the kidneys and lower doses may be sufficient in patients with severe renal impairment, see Chapter 17, p.695) [3,16]

Glycopyrronium can also be used in other situations where an antimuscarinic effect is needed, e.g. paraneoplastic pyrexia and sweating (see Antimuscarinics, Box D, p.10), hyperhidrosis, sialorrhoea and drooling.

Glycopyrronium PO or SL has been used to reduce drooling in adults with various conditions, e.g. MND/ALS, Parkinson's disease, cancers of the head and neck or oesophagus.[17–19] An oral solution is now authorized for drooling in children and adolescents ≥3 years with chronic neurological disorders. It has also been given by nebulizer.[19] It is also used as a bronchodilator (inhaled or nebulized) in asthma and COPD.[20,21]

Bio-availability <5% PO.

Onset of action 1min IV; 30–40min SC, PO.

Time to peak plasma concentration immediate IV; no data SC, PO.

Plasma halflife 1–1.5h.

Duration of action 7h.

Cautions

See Antimuscarinics (p.5); renal impairment (also see Chapter 17, p.695).

Drug interactions

Concurrent treatment with ≥2 antimuscarinic drugs (including antihistamines, phenothiazines and TCAs; see Antimuscarinics, Box B, p.6) will increase the likelihood of undesirable effects (see Antimuscarinics, Box C, p.7).

See Antimuscarinics (p.5).

Undesirable effects

Peripheral antimuscarinic effects (see Antimuscarinics, Box C, p.7). The US Product Information lists the following effects, which are not included in the UK SPC:
Very common (>10%): inflammation at the injection site.
Common (<10%, >1%): dysphagia, photosensitivity.

Dose and use

Glycopyrronium is an alternative to **hyoscine *hydrobromide***, **hyoscine *butylbromide*** and **atropine**.[18,22,23] For indications where a parenteral antimuscarinic is required, *PCF* generally prefers **hyoscine *butylbromide***; it is unlikely to cause CNS effects and is cheaper than glycopyrronium.
For CSCI, dilute with WFI, 0.9% saline or 5% glucose.

CSCI compatibility with other drugs: There are 2-drug compatibility data for glycopyrronium in WFI with **alfentanil**, **clonazepam**, **diamorphine**, **haloperidol**, **hydromorphone**, **levomepromazine**, **metoclopramide**, **midazolam**, **morphine sulfate** and **oxycodone**.
Glycopyrronium is *incompatible* with **dexamethasone** and **ketorolac**. For more details and 3-drug compatibility data, see Appendix 3 (p.863).
Compatibility charts for mixing drugs in 0.9% saline can be found in the extended appendix section of the on-line *PCF* on *www.palliativedrugs.com*.

Antispasmodic and inoperable intestinal obstruction

- start with 200microgram SC stat
- continue with 600–1,200microgram/24h CSCI *and/or* 200micorgram SC q2h p.r.n.

Death rattle (noisy rattling breathing)[24]

See QCG: Death rattle (noisy rattling breathing), p.12:
- start with 200microgram SC stat
- continue with 600–1,200microgram/24h CSCI *and/or* 200micorgram SC q1h p.r.n.
- alternatively the SL route can be used; 100microgram SL q6h p.r.n.

Drooling

Administer PO as an oral solution/suspension. Tablets are expensive and only available in higher doses. Various products are available (see Supply), but the only authorized product for drooling is Sialanar® for use in children. When considering an unauthorized product, cost, suitability and availability, particularly in a non-hospital setting, need to be considered (see Chapter 24, p.751).
- start with 200microgram PO stat and q8h
- if necessary, increase dose progressively every 2–3 days to 1mg q8h[25]
- occasionally doses of ≤2mg q8h are needed.

A subsequent reduction in dose may be possible, particularly when initial dose escalation has been rapid. Oral solutions/suspensions can be given by enteral feeding tube (also see p.785).[9,18]

Paraneoplastic pyrexia and sweating

- start with 200microgram PO t.d.s.
- if necessary, increase progressively to 2mg PO t.d.s. (also see Antimuscarinics, Box D, p.10)

Localized hyperhidrosis

- apply topically as a 0.5–4% cream or aqueous solution once daily–b.d. avoiding the nose, mouth and particularly the eyes; do not wash treated skin for 3–4h[2,26]
- if severe, or if alternative treatments fail, 1–2mg PO b.d.–t.d.s., titrated to response (see above and Supply for products available).[1]

Supply

Glycopyrronium *bromide* (generic)
Oral solution 1mg/5mL, 28 days @ 1mg t.d.s = £255. *Authorized as add on therapy in treatment of peptic ulcer.*
Tablets 1mg, 2mg, 28 days @ 1mg t.d.s. = £602. *Authorized as add on therapy in treatment of peptic ulcer.*
Injection 200microgram/mL, 1mL or 3mL amp = £1.50.

Sialanar® (Proveca)
Oral solution 320miorgram/mL glycopyrronium base (equivalent to 400micorgram/mL (2mg/5mL) glycopyrronium bromide), 28 days @ 1mg t.d.s = £270. *Authorized for drooling in children and adolescents ≥3 years.*

Unauthorized oral products
Glycopyrronium *bromide*
Oral solution or oral suspension 200microgram/5mL, 500microgram/5mL, 2.5mg/5mL and 5mg/5mL, 28 days @ 1mg t.d.s. = £68; (available as a special order, see Chapter 24, p.751) price based on 5mg/5mL oral solution specials tariff in community; prices vary significantly between formulations and quantities ordered.

For locally prepared formulations, see Box A.

Unauthorized topical products
Glycopyrronium *bromide*
Cream 2% (20mg/mL) in Cetomacrogol cream (Formula A) 30g = £390; (available as a special order, see Chapter 24, p.751).
For a locally prepared cream, see Box B.

Box A Examples of locally prepared glycopyrronium formulations for PO use

From glycopyrronium powder[27]

Glycopyrronium oral solution 100microgram/mL
Dissolve 100mg of glycopyrronium powder (obtainable from AMCo) in 100mL of sterile or distilled water to produce a 1mg/mL concentrate. This is stable for about 28 days if stored in a refrigerator.

Dilute the required volume of the concentrate 1 part with 9 parts sterile or distilled water (i.e. for every 1mL of concentrate, add 9mL of water) to give a *glycopyrronium oral solution 100microgram/mL.*

To avoid microbial contamination, store in a refrigerator and discard any unused diluted solution after 1 week.

Cost: 28 days @ 1mg (10mL) t.d.s. = £11 worth of glycopyrronium powder (but need to buy 3g = £327).

Glycopyrronium oral suspension 500microgram/mL[28]
Add 5mL of glycerol to 50mg of glycopyrronium powder and mix to form a smooth paste. Add 50mL of Ora-Plus® in portions and mix well. Add sufficient Ora-Sweet® or Ora-Sweet SF® to make a total volume of 100mL.

This suspension is stable for 90 days at room temperature or in a refrigerator.

Cost: 28 days @ 1mg (2mL) t.d.s. = £9 worth of glycopyrronium powder (but need to buy 3g = £327).

From glycopyrronium injection

Glycopyrronium oral suspension 100microgram/mL[29]
Combine 25mL of Ora-Plus® and 25mL of Ora-Sweet®; add to 50mL of preservative-free glycopyrronium injection 200microgram/mL to make up to 100mL, and mix well.

Stable for 35 days at room temperature or in a refrigerator (refrigeration minimizes risk of microbial contamination).

In a taste test, this formulation masked the bitter taste of glycopyrronium better than water or syrup-based vehicles, and was preferred by most patients.

Cost: 28 days @ 1mg (10mL) t.d.s. = £210 worth of glycopyrronium injection.

Box B Example of locally prepared glycopyrronium cream 10mg/mL (1%)[30]

Mix 1g of glycopyrronium powder with propylene glycol to make a paste. Incorporate into a water-washable cream base until smooth, making a total of 100g. Refrigerate after preparation. Stable for 60 days.

Cost: 100g = £109 worth of glycopyrronium *powder* (but need to buy 3g = £327).

1 Solish N *et al.* (2007) A comprehensive approach to the recognition, diagnosis, and severity-based treatment of focal hyperhidrosis: recommendations of the Canadian Hyperhidrosis Advisory Committee. *Dermatologic Surgery*. **33**: 908–923.
2 Kim WO *et al.* (2008) Topical glycopyrrolate for patients with facial hyperhidrosis. *British Journal of Dermatology*. **158**: 1094–1097.
3 Mirakhur R and Dundee J (1983) Glycopyrrolate pharmacology and clinical use. *Anaesthesia*. **38**: 1195–1204.
4 Gram D *et al.* (1991) Central anticholinergic syndrome following glycopyrrolate. *Anesthesiology*. **74**: 191–193.
5 Wigard D (1991) Glycopyrrolate and the central anticholinergic syndrome (letter). *Anesthesiology*. **75**: 1125.
6 Mirakhur R and Dundee J (1980) A comparison of the effects of atropine and glycopyrollate on various end organs. *Journal of the Royal Society of Medicine*. **73**: 727–730.
7 Ali-Melkkila T *et al.* (1989) Glycopyrrolate; pharmacokinetics and some pharmacodynamics findings. *Acta Anaesthesiologica Scandinavica*. **33**: 513–517.
8 Blasco P (1996) Glycopyrrolate treatment of chronic drooling. *Archives of Paediatric and Adolescent Medicine*. **150**: 932–935.
9 Olsen A and Sjogren P (1999) Oral glycopyrrolate alleviates drooling in a patient with tongue cancer. *Journal of Pain and Symptom Management*. **18**: 300–302.
10 Hughes A *et al.* (2000) Audit of three antimuscarinic drugs for managing retained secretions. *Palliative Medicine*. **14**: 221–222.
11 Hughes A *et al.* (1997) Management of 'death rattle'. *Palliative Medicine*. **11**: 80–81.
12 Mirakhur R *et al.* (1978) Evaluation of the anticholinergic actions of glycopyrronium bromide. *British Journal of Clinical Pharmacology*. **5**: 77–84.
13 Back I *et al.* (2001) A study comparing hyoscine hydrobromide and glycopyrrolate in the treatment of death rattle. *Palliative Medicine*. **15**: 329–336.
14 Mirakhur RK (1979) Intravenous administration of glycopyrronium: effects on cardiac rate and rhythm. *Anaesthesia*. **34**: 458–462.
15 Mirakhur R *et al.* (1978) Atropine and glycopyrronium premedication. A comparison of the effects on cardiac rate and rhythm during induction of anaesthesia. *Anaesthesia*. **33**: 906–912.
16 Ali-Melkkila T *et al.* (1993) Pharmacokinetics and related pharmacodynamics of anticholinergic drugs. *Acta Anaesthesiologica Scandinavica*. **37**: 633–642.
17 Hobson EV *et al.* (2013) Management of sialorrhoea in motor neuron disease: a survey of current UK practice. *Amyotrophic Lateral Sclerosis Frontotemporal Degeneration*. **14**: 521–527.
18 Rashid H *et al.* (1997) Management of secretions in esophageal cancer patients with glycopyrrolate. *Annals of Oncology*. **8**: 198–199.
19 UK Medicines Information (2015) Hypersalivation-can glycopyrronium be used to treat it? *Medicines Q&A* 52.7. www.evidence.nhs.uk
20 Hansel TT *et al.* (2005) Glycopyrrolate causes prolonged bronchoprotection and bronchodilatation in patients with asthma. *Chest*. **128**: 1974–1979.
21 Buhl R and Banerji D (2012) Profile of glycopyrronium for once-daily treatment of moderate-to-severe COPD. *International Journal of Chronic Obstructive Pulmonary Disease*. **7**: 729–741.
22 Lucas V and Amass C (1998) Use of enteral glycopyrrolate in the management of drooling. *Palliative Medicine*. **12**: 207.
23 Davis M and Furste A (1999) Glycopyrrolate: a useful drug in the palliation of mechanical bowel obstruction. *Journal of Pain and Symptom Management*. **18**: 153–154.
24 Bennett M *et al.* (2002) Using anti-muscarinic drugs in the management of death rattle: evidence based guidelines for palliative care. *Palliative Medicine*. **16**: 369–374.
25 Arbouw ME *et al.* (2010) Glycopyrrolate for sialorrhea in Parkinson disease: a randomized, double-blind, crossover trial. *Neurology*. **74**: 1203–1207.
26 Kavanagh GM *et al.* (2006) Topical glycopyrrolate should not be overlooked in treatment of focal hyperhidrosis. *British Journal of Dermatology*. **155**: 477–500.
27 Amass C (2007) *Personal communication*. Pharmacist, East and North Hertfordshire NHS Trust.
28 Anonymous (2004) Glycopyrrolate 0.5mg/mL oral liquid. *International Journal of Pharmaceutical Compounding*. **8**: 218.
29 Landry C *et al.* (2005) Stability and subjective taste acceptability of four glycopyrrolate solutions for oral administration. *International Journal of Pharmaceutical Compounding*. **9**: 396–398.
30 Glasnapp A and BJ S (2001) Topical therapy for localized hyperhidrosis. *International Journal of Pharmaceutical Compounding*. **5**: 28–29.

Updated July 2017

HYOSCINE BUTYLBROMIDE

Class: Antimuscarinic.

Indications: Smooth muscle spasm (e.g. bladder, GI tract), †drying secretions (e.g. †death rattle (noisy rattling breathing), †inoperable bowel obstruction).

Contra-indications: ***Parenteral:*** See Antimuscarinics (p.5). For tachycardia (heart rate >100 beats/min), also see Cautions.

Pharmacology

Hyoscine *butylbromide* is an antimuscarinic (see p.16) and has both smooth muscle relaxant (antispasmodic) and antisecretory properties. It is a quaternary compound and, unlike **hyoscine *hydrobromide*** (p.19), it does not cross the blood-brain barrier. Consequently, it does not have a central anti-emetic effect or cause drowsiness.

Oral bio-availability, based on urinary excretion, is <1%.[1] Thus, any antispasmodic effect reported after PO administration probably relates to a local contact effect on the GI mucosa.[2] In an RCT, hyoscine *butylbromide* 10mg t.d.s. PO and **paracetamol** 500mg t.d.s. both significantly reduced the severity of intestinal colic by >50%.[3] However, the difference between the benefit from these two drugs (both given in suboptimal doses) and placebo was only 0.5cm on a 10cm scale of pain intensity. This is of dubious clinical importance.[4] Thus, the therapeutic value of PO hyoscine *butylbromide* for intestinal colic remains debatable.[5]

The main uses for hyoscine *butylbromide* in palliative care are as an antispasmodic and antisecretory drug in inoperable bowel obstruction, and as an antisecretory drug for death rattle (noisy rattling breathing). In bowel obstruction, in comparison with hyoscine *butylbromide* (60–80mg/24h CSCI), **octreotide** (300–800microgram/24h CSCI; p.544) provides more effective and rapid improvements in nausea and vomiting and reduction in NG tube output.[6,7] However, in those patients responding to either drug, after about 3–6 days, overall symptom relief is similar, and NG tube removal is possible with both.[6,7] Further, the presence of colic would favour the use of hyoscine *butylbromide* over **octreotide**. For a suggested management approach, see QCG: Inoperable bowel obstruction (p.242).

In healthy volunteers, 20mg SC has a maximum antisecretory duration of action of 2h.[8] On the other hand, the same dose by CSCI is often effective for 1 day in death rattle. Hyoscine *butylbromide* and **hyoscine *hydrobromide*** act faster than **glycopyrronium** (p.13) for this indication,[9,10] but the overall efficacy is generally the same[11] with death rattle reduced in 1/2–2/3 of patients. However, provided that time is taken to explain the cause of the rattle to the relatives and there is ongoing support, relatives' distress is relieved in >90% of cases.[12]

Bio-availability <1% PO.[1]

Onset of action <10min SC/IM/IV; 1–2h PO.[13]

Time to peak plasma concentration 15min–2h PO.[1]

Plasma halflife 5–10h.

Duration of action <2h in volunteers[8] but possibly longer in moribund patients.

Cautions

The MHRA has issued a warning highlighting the risk of serious undesirable effects with hyoscine *butylbromide* injection in patients with underlying cardiac disease.[14] This followed the death of a patient in 2016 from cardiac arrest after IV hyoscine *butylbromide* during colonoscopy, and the Coroner's recommendation to the MHRA to clarify the cautions in the SPC emphasizing that 'additional caution should be exercised when administering IV hyoscine *butylbromide* to patients with ischaemic heart disease.'

In its own review, the MHRA identified reports of 8 deaths over 16 years associated with the use of IV/IM hyoscine *butylbromide*, and published the following advice:

- hyoscine *butylbromide* injection can cause serious undesirable effects including tachycardia, hypotension and anaphylaxis
- these undesirable effects can result in a fatal outcome in patients with underlying cardiac disease, e.g. heart failure, coronary heart disease, cardiac arrhythmia, hypertension
- hyoscine *butylbromide* injection should be used with caution in patients with cardiac disease
- monitor these patients, and ensure that resuscitation equipment, and personnel who are trained how to use this equipment, are readily available
- hyoscine *butylbromide* injection is contra-indicated in patients with tachycardia.

SPCs have been changed to reflect this advice.

However, full data are not available, and it is difficult to interpret the specific relevance of the reports to use in a palliative care setting, where the SC/CSCI route of administration is more likely than IV/IM.

Nonetheless, in healthy volunteers, an increase in heart rate of ~15 bpm is evident 5min after hyoscine *butylbromide* 20mg SC which lasts about 1h. On the other hand, no effect on heart rate was observed with doses <0.4mg/min CIVI.[8] This equates to <575mg/24h, well above typical doses given CSCI in palliative care.

PCF advises clinicians to remind themselves of the longstanding cautions relating to the use of any antimuscarinic, particularly in patients with cardiovascular disease, and to continue to balance the potential for benefit and harm for each patient individually.

See Antimuscarinics (p.8). PO **hyoscine *butylbromide*** has a low bio-availability reducing the likelihood of systemic antimuscarinic effects.

Drug interactions

Concurrent treatment with ≥2 antimuscarinic drugs (including antihistamines, phenothiazines and TCAs; see Antimuscarinics, Box B, p.6) will increase the likelihood of undesirable effects (see Antimuscarinics, Box C, p.7).

See Antimuscarinics (p.8).

Undesirable effects

Common (<10%,>1%): peripheral antimuscarinic effects (see Antimuscarinics, Box C, p. 7).
Unknown: hypotension (IV), anaphylactic shock (see Cautions).

Dose and use

Hyoscine *butylbromide* is generally used SC/CSCI in palliative care because of poor PO bio-availability ± unsuitability of the PO route. For CSCI dilute with WFI, 0.9% saline or 5% glucose.

CSCI compatibility with other drugs: There are 2-drug compatibility data for hyoscine butylbromide in WFI with **alfentanil**, **clonazepam**, **dexamethasone**, **diamorphine**, **haloperidol**, **hydromorphone**, **levomepromazine**, **midazolam**, **morphine sulfate**, **octreotide** and **oxycodone**.

Incompatibility may occur with **cyclizine**. For more details and 3-drug compatibility data, see Appendix 3 (p.863).

Compatibility charts for mixing drugs in 0.9% saline can be found in the extended appendix of the on-line *PCF* on *www.palliativedrugs.com*.

Inoperable intestinal obstruction with colic

- start with 20mg SC stat and 60mg/24h CSCI and 20mg SC q1h p.r.n.
- if necessary, increase to 120mg/24h
- maximum reported dose 300mg/24h.

Note. The maximum benefit from hyoscine *butylbromide* may be seen only after about 3 days.[6,7] Some centres add **octreotide** 500microgram/24h CSCI if hyoscine *butylbromide* 120mg/24h fails to relieve symptoms adequately, see QCG: Inoperable bowel obstruction (p.242).[15,16]

For patients with obstructive symptoms without colic, **metoclopramide** (see p.244) should be tried before an antimuscarinic drug because the obstruction is often more functional than organic. See QCG: Inoperable bowel obstruction (p.242).

Death rattle (noisy rattling breathing)

See QCG: Death rattle (noisy rattling breathing), p.12:

- start with 20mg SC stat
- continue with 20–60mg/24h CSCI, and/or 20mg SC q1h p.r.n.
- some centres use higher doses, namely 60–120mg/24h CSCI.[10]

Bladder spasm

Use only when more specific bladder antispasmodics (see p.567) are inappropriate, e.g. PO route unavailable.

- start with 20mg SC stat
- continue with 60–120mg/24h CSCI, and/or 20mg SC q1h p.r.n.

Supply

Buscopan® (Boehringer Ingelheim)

Tablets 10mg, 28 days @ 20mg q.d.s. = £12. *Also available OTC as Buscopan® IBS Relief and Buscopan® Cramps.*

Injection 20mg/mL, 1mL amp = £0.25.

1 Boehringer Ingelheim GmbH *Data on file.*
2 Tytgat GN (2007) Hyoscine butylbromide: a review of its use in the treatment of abdominal cramping and pain. *Drugs.* **67**: 1343–1357.
3 Mueller-Lissner S *et al.* (2006) Placebo- and paracetamol-controlled study on the efficacy and tolerability of hyoscine butylbromide in the treatment of patients with recurrent crampy abdominal pain. *Alimentary Pharmacology & Therapeutics.* **23**: 1741–1748.
4 Farrar JT *et al.* (2000) Defining the clinically important difference in pain outcome measures. *Pain.* **88**: 287–294.
5 Thompson DG and Wingate DL (1981) Oral hyoscine butylbromide does not alter the pattern of small intestinal motor activity. *British Journal of Pharmacology.* **72**: 685–687.
6 Mystakidou K *et al.* (2002) Comparison of octreotide administration vs conservative treatment in the management of inoperable bowel obstruction in patients with far advanced cancer: a randomized, double-blind, controlled clinical trial. *Anticancer Research.* **22**: 1187–1192.
7 Peng X *et al.* (2015) Randomized clinical trial comparing octreotide and scopolamine butylbromide in symptom control of patients with inoperable bowel obstruction due to advanced ovarian cancer. *World Journal of Surgical Oncology.* **13**: 50.
8 Herxheimer A and Haefeli L (1966) Human pharmacology of hyoscine butylbromide. *Lancet.* **ii**: 418–421.
9 Back I *et al.* (2001) A study comparing hyoscine hydrobromide and glycopyrrolate in the treatment of death rattle. *Palliative Medicine.* **15**: 329–336.
10 Bennett M *et al.* (2002) Using anti-muscarinic drugs in the management of death rattle: evidence based guidelines for palliative care. *Palliative Medicine.* **16**: 369–374.
11 Hughes A *et al.* (2000) Audit of three antimuscarinic drugs for managing retained secretions. *Palliative Medicine.* **14**: 221–222.
12 Hughes A *et al.* (1997) Management of 'death rattle'. *Palliative Medicine.* **11**: 80–81.
13 Sanches Martinez J *et al.* (1988) Clinical assessment of the tolerability and the effect of IK-19 in tablet form on pain of spastic origin. *Investigacion Medica International.* **15**: 63–65.
14 MHRA (2017) Hyoscine butylbromide (Buscopan) injection: risk of serious adverse effects in patients with underlying cardiac disease. *Drug Safety Update.* www.gov.uk/drug-safety-update
15 Ripamonti CI *et al.* (2008) Management of malignant bowel obstruction. *European Journal of Cancer.* **44**: 1105–1115.
16 Ripamonti C and Mercadante S (2004) How to use octreotide for malignant bowel obstruction. *Journal of Supportive Oncology.* **2**: 357–364.

Updated July 2017

HYOSCINE HYDROBROMIDE

Class: Antimuscarinic.

Indications: Prevention of motion sickness, drying secretions (including surgical premedication, †sialorrhoea, †drooling, †death rattle (noisy rattling breathing) and †inoperable intestinal obstruction), †paraneoplastic pyrexia and sweating, †smooth muscle spasm (e.g. intestine, bladder).

Contra-indications: See Antimuscarinics (p.5). For tachycardia (heart rate >100 beats/min), also see **hyoscine *butylbromide*** (p.17).

Pharmacology

Hyoscine *hydrobromide* is a naturally occurring belladonna alkaloid with smooth muscle relaxant (antispasmodic) and antisecretory properties. Unlike **hyoscine *butylbromide***, hyoscine *hydrobromide* crosses the blood-brain barrier, and repeated administration SC q4h will result in accumulation and may lead to sedation and delirium. On the other hand, a small number of patients are stimulated rather than sedated (also see p.5). For this reason, *PCF* generally prefers **hyoscine *butylbromide***; it is also cheaper.

Despite hyoscine *hydrobromide* having a plasma halflife of several hours, the duration of the antisecretory effect in volunteers after a single dose is only about 2h.[1] On the other hand, particularly after repeated injections in moribund patients, a duration of effect of up to 9h has been observed.[2] Hyoscine *hydrobromide* relieves death rattle in 1/2–2/3 of patients.[3] However, provided that time is taken to explain the cause of the rattle to the relatives and there is ongoing support, relatives' distress is relieved in >90% of cases.[2]

Hyoscine *hydrobromide* can also be used in other situations where an antimuscarinic effect is needed, e.g. sialorrhoea, drooling, paraneoplastic pyrexia and sweating (see p.10) and smooth muscle spasm (e.g. intestine, bladder).

Hyoscine *hydrobromide* has anti-emetic properties (see p.235). However, generally, it is only used as prophylactic treatment for motion sickness PO or by TD patch.[4] The TD patch:

- comprises a reservoir containing hyoscine 1.5mg
- the average amount of hyoscine absorbed *over 3 days* is 1mg
- because of an initial priming dose released from the patch, steady-state is reached after about 6h, and maintained for 3 days[5]
- after a single application of two patches, the average elimination half-life is 9.5h[6]
- after patch removal, because hyoscine continues to be absorbed from the skin, the plasma concentration only decreases to about one third over the next 24h
- absorption is best when the patch is applied on hairless skin behind the ear.[4]

The patch has also been used to control opioid-induced nausea and also oesophageal spasm.[7-9] Other off-label uses include the management of drooling and sialorrhoea in children and adults with various conditions, including disorders of the head and neck.[10-12]

Bio-availability 60–80% SL.[13]
Onset of action 3–5min IM, 10–15min SL.
Time to peak effect 20–60min SL/SC; 24h TD.
Plasma halflife 1–4h IM.[13]
Duration of action IM 15min (spasmolytic), 1–9h (antisecretory).[13]

Cautions

See Antimuscarinics (p.5); renal impairment (see Dose and use and also Chapter 17, p.695).

Drug interactions

Concurrent treatment with ≥2 antimuscarinic drugs (including antihistamines, phenothiazines and TCAs; see Antimuscarinics, Box B, p.6) will increase the likelihood of undesirable effects, and (when centrally acting) of central toxicity, i.e. restlessness, agitation, delirium (see Antimuscarinics, Box C, p.7). Children, the elderly, and patients with renal or hepatic impairment are more susceptible to the central effects of antimuscarinics.

See Antimuscarinics (p.5).

Undesirable effects

Antimuscarinic effects (see Box C, p.7), including central antimuscarinic syndrome, i.e. agitated delirium, drowsiness, ataxia.

TD patch: despite the relatively small dose, delirium has been reported;[14] local irritation ± rash occasionally occurs.

Dose and use

Death rattle (noisy rattling breathing)

See QCG: Death rattle (noisy rattling breathing), p.12:

- start with 400microgram SC stat
- continue with 1,200microgram/24h CSCI, and/or 400microgram SC q1h p.r.n.
- if necessary, increase to 1,600microgram/24h CSCI
- avoid in patients with end-stage renal failure because of an increased risk of delirium.

For CSCI dilute with WFI, 0.9% saline or 5% glucose.

CSCI compatibility with other drugs: There are 2-drug compatibility data for hyoscine *hydrobromide* in WFI with **clonazepam**, **cyclizine**, **dexamethasone**, **diamorphine**, **haloperidol**, **hydromorphone**, **levomepromazine**, **midazolam**, **morphine sulfate** and **oxycodone**.

For more details and 3-drug compatibility data, see Appendix 3 (p.863).

Compatibility charts for mixing drugs in 0.9% saline can be found in the extended appendix of the on-line *PCF* on *www.palliativedrugs.com*.

Note. *PCF* favours **hyoscine *butylbromide*** (see p.16); it is cheaper and is free of CNS effects. Other options include **glycopyrronium** (see p.13) and **atropine** (see p.5).

Drooling and sialorrhoea

- hyoscine *hydrobromide* TD 1mg/3 days; if necessary, use 2 patches concurrently.

Note. An alternative drug PO with antimuscarinic effects may be preferable in some patients because of convenience or concurrent symptom management, e.g. **amitriptyline** (see p.210).

TD patches contain metal and must be removed before MRI to avoid burns (see p.831). Wash hands after handling the TD patch (and the application site after removing it) to avoid transferring hyoscine *hydrobromide* into the eyes (may cause mydriasis and exacerbate narrow-angle glaucoma).

Supply

Kwells® Bayer Consumer Care
Tablets chewable 150microgram, 300microgram, 12 tablets = £2; *also available OTC.*

Scopoderm® (GlaxoSmithKline Consumer Health)
TD (post-auricular) patch 1.5mg (releasing 1mg over 3 days), 1 patch = £2.50.

Hyoscine *hydrobromide* (generic)
Injection 400microgram/mL, 1mL amp = £4.75; 600microgram/mL, 1mL amp = £5.50.

1 Herxheimer A and Haefeli L (1966) Human pharmacology of hyoscine butylbromide. *Lancet.* **ii**: 418–421.
2 Hughes A *et al.* (1997) Management of 'death rattle'. *Palliative Medicine.* **11**: 80–81.
3 Hughes A *et al.* (2000) Audit of three antimuscarinic drugs for managing retained secretions. *Palliative Medicine.* **14**: 221–222.
4 Clissold S and Heel R (1985) Transdermal hyoscine (scopolamine). A preliminary review of its pharmacodynamic properties and therapeutic efficacy. *Drugs.* **29**: 189–207.
5 Novartis (2014). *Personal communication.* Medical affairs.
6 Novartis (2013) Scopoderm TTS. *SPC.* www.medicines.org.uk
7 Ferris FD *et al.* (1991) Transdermal scopolamine use in the control of narcotic-induced nausea. *Journal of Pain and Symptom Management.* **6**: 289–393.
8 Harris SN *et al.* (1991) Nausea prophylaxis using transdermal scopolamine in the setting of patient-controlled analgesia. *Obstetrics and Gynecology.* **78**: 673–677.
9 Murray-Brown F and Davies IL (2016) Oesophageal spasm, vomiting and hyoscine hydrobromide patch. *BMJ Supportive and Palliative Care.* **6**: 125–127.
10 Gordon C *et al.* (1985) Effect of transdermal scopolamine on salivation. *Journal of Clinical Pharmacology.* **25**: 407–412.
11 Becelli R *et al.* (2014) Use of scopolamine patches in patients treated with parotidectomy. *Journal of Craniofacial Surgery.* **25**: e88–89.
12 UK Medicines Information (2015) Hypersalivation - can hyoscine hydrobromide be used to treat it? *Q&A* 51.6. www.evidence.nhs.uk
13 Ali-Melkkila T *et al.* (1993) Pharmacokinetics and related pharmacodynamics of anticholinergic drugs. *Acta Anaesthesiologica Scandinavica.* **37**: 633–642.
14 Wilkinson J (1987) Side-effects of transdermal scopolamine. *Journal of Emergency Medicine.* **5**: 389–392.

Updated July 2017

PROPANTHELINE

Class: Antimuscarinic.

Indications: Smooth muscle spasm (e.g. bladder, intestine), urinary frequency and incontinence, hyperhidrosis, †gustatory sweating in diabetic neuropathy, †paraneoplastic sweating, †drooling and sialorrhoea.

Contra-indications: See Antimuscarinics (p.5). In addition, hiatus hernia associated with reflux oesophagitis, severe ulcerative colitis.

Pharmacology

Propantheline is a quaternary antimuscarinic (see p.5); it does not cross the blood-brain barrier and thus does *not* cause central effects. It doubles gastric half-emptying time[1] and slows GI transit

generally. It has variable effects on drug absorption (see Drug interactions). Propantheline is extensively metabolized in the small intestine before absorption. *If taken with food, the effect of propantheline by mouth is almost abolished.*[2]
Bio-availability <50% PO (much reduced if taken after food).
Onset of action 30–60min.
Time to peak plasma concentration 2h.
Plasma halflife 2–3h.
Duration of action 4–6h.

Cautions

See Antimuscarinics (p.5).

Drug interactions

Concurrent treatment with ≥2 antimuscarinic drugs (including antihistamines, phenothiazines and TCAs; see Antimuscarinics, Box B, p.6) will increase the likelihood of undesirable effects (see Antimuscarinics, Box C, p.7).

See Antimuscarinics (p.5).

Undesirable effects

Peripheral antimuscarinic effects (see Antimuscarinics, Box C, p.7).

Dose and use

Intestinal colic

- start with 15mg t.d.s. *1h before meals* & 30mg at bedtime
- maximum dose 30mg q.d.s.

Urinary frequency

- same as for colic, but largely replaced by **oxybutynin** (see p.567), **amitriptyline** (see p.210) or **imipramine**.

Sweating

One of several alternatives to reduce paraneoplastic sweating (for other options, see Antimuscarinics, Box D, p.10):
- give 15–30mg b.d.–t.d.s. *on an empty stomach.*

Has also been used for hyperhydrosis associated with spinal cord injury.[5]

Drooling and sialorrhoea

Has been used in MND/ALS:
- give 15mg t.d.s.[6] *on an empty stomach.*

However, other options are generally preferred, see p.10.

Supply

Pro-Banthine® (Kyowa Kirin)
Tablets 15mg, 28 days @ 15mg t.d.s. & 30mg at bedtime = £26.

1 Hurwitz A *et al.* (1977) Prolongation of gastric emptying by oral propantheline. *Clin Pharmacol Ther.* **22**: 206–210.
2 Ekenved G *et al.* (1977) Influence of food on the effect of propantheline and L-hyoscyamine on salivation. *Scand J Gastroenterol.* **12**: 963–966.
3 Schuurkes JAJ *et al.* (1986) Stimulation of gastroduodenal motor activity: dopaminergic and cholinergic modulation. *Drug Development Research.* **8**: 233–241.
4 Baxter K and Preston CL. *Stockley's Drug Interactions.* London: Pharmaceutical Press www.medicinescomplete.com (accessed March 2014).
5 Canaday BR and Stanford RH (1995) Propantheline bromide in the management of hyperhidrosis associated with spinal cord injury. *Ann Pharmacother.* **29**: 489-492.
6 Norris FH *et al.* (1985) Motor neurone disease: towards better care. *British Medical Journal.* **291**: 259-262.

Updated July 2017

ORPHENADRINE

Class: Antimuscarinic antiparkinsonian.

Indications: Parkinson's disease, drug-induced parkinsonism, †sialorrhoea (drooling), †extrapyramidal dystonic reactions.

Contra-indications: See Antimuscarinics (p.5) and Tardive dyskinesia (p.739).

Pharmacology

Orphenadrine and other antimuscarinic antiparkinsonian drugs are used primarily in Parkinson's disease.[1] They are less effective than **levodopa** in established Parkinson's disease. However, patients with mild symptoms, particularly tremor, may be treated initially with an antimuscarinic drug (alone or with **selegiline**), and **levodopa** added or substituted if symptoms progress. Antimuscarinics exert their antiparkinsonian effect by correcting the relative central cholinergic excess which occurs in parkinsonism as a result of dopamine deficiency. In most patients, their effects are only moderate, reducing tremor and rigidity to some extent but without significant action on bradykinesia. They exert a synergistic effect when used with **levodopa** and are also useful in reducing sialorrhoea.

Antimuscarinics reduce the symptoms of drug-induced parkinsonism (mainly antipsychotics) but there is no justification for giving them prophylactically. *Tardive dyskinesia is not improved by the antimuscarinic drugs, and they may make it worse.* No major differences exist between antimuscarinic antiparkinsonian drugs, but orphenadrine sometimes has a mood-elevating effect. Some people tolerate one antimuscarinic better than another. **Procyclidine** may be given parenterally, and is effective emergency treatment for severe acute drug-induced dystonic reactions (see Chapter 21, p.739).

Orphenadrine is almost completely metabolized in the liver, producing numerous metabolites which are excreted in the urine.
Bio-availability readily absorbed PO.
Onset of action 30–60min.
Time to peak plasma concentration 2–4h PO.
Plasma halflife 15h single dose but ≤40h with multiple doses.
Duration of action 12–24h.

Cautions

See Antimuscarinics (p.5). Avoid abrupt discontinuation.

Drug interactions

Concurrent treatment with ≥2 antimuscarinic drugs (including antihistamines, phenothiazines and TCAs; see Antimuscarinics, Box B, p.6) will increase the likelihood of undesirable effects, and (when centrally acting) of central toxicity, i.e. restlessness, agitation, delirium (see Antimuscarinics, Box C, p.7). Children, the elderly, and patients with renal or hepatic impairment are more susceptible to the central effects of antimuscarinics.

See Antimuscarinics (p.5).

Undesirable effects

Antimuscarinic effects (see p.5). Nervousness, euphoria, insomnia, confusion, hallucinations occasionally.

Dose and use

Parkinsonism

For treatment of previously unrecognized or untreated symptoms in patients with a prognosis of <6 months:

- start with 50mg PO b.d.–t.d.s.
- if necessary, increase by 50mg every 2–3 days
- normal dose range 150–300mg daily in divided doses
- maximum recommended daily dose 400mg.

Propranolol, a non-selective β-adrenergic receptor antagonist (β-blocker), is the treatment of choice for akathisia. Antimuscarinic antiparkinsonian drugs are *contra-indicated* in tardive dyskinesia because they may exacerbate the condition (see Chapter 21, p.739).

Supply

Orphenadrine (generic)
Tablets 50mg, 28 days @ 50mg t.d.s. = £67.
Oral solution (sugar-free) 50mg/5mL, 28 days @ 50mg t.d.s. = £100.

1 Katzenschlager R *et al.* (2003) Anticholinergics for symptomatic management of Parkinson's disease. *Cochrane Database of Systematic Reviews*. CD003735. www.thecochranelibrary.com

Updated July 2017

PROKINETICS

Pharmacology

Prokinetics accelerate GI transit and include:

- D_2 antagonists, e.g. **domperidone** (p.247), **metoclopramide** (p.244)
- $5HT_4$ agonists, e.g. **metoclopramide, prucalopride**
- motilin agonists, e.g. **erythromycin**.

Clinical trials are underway of cholinesterase inhibitors and drugs acting at other receptors, e.g. ghrelin agonists.[1]

Drugs which enhance intestinal transit indirectly are not considered prokinetics (e.g. bulk-forming agents, other laxatives, and drugs such as **misoprostol** which cause diarrhoea by increasing GI secretions). Some drugs increase contractile motor activity but not in a co-ordinated fashion, and so do not reduce transit time, e.g. **bethanechol**. Such drugs are promotility but not prokinetic.[2]

D_2 antagonists and $5HT_4$ agonists act by triggering a cholinergic system in the wall of the GI tract (Table 1, Figure 1).[3] This action is impeded by opioids. Further, antimuscarinic drugs competitively block cholinergic receptors on the intestinal muscle fibres (and elsewhere).[4] Thus, all drugs with antimuscarinic properties reduce the impact of prokinetic drugs. The extent of this depends on several factors, including the respective doses of the interacting drugs and times of administration. Thus, the concurrent administration of prokinetics and antimuscarinic drugs is generally best avoided. On the other hand, even if the peripheral prokinetic effect is completely blocked, **domperidone** and **metoclopramide** will still exert an anti-emetic effect at the dopamine receptors in the area postrema (see p.235).

Table 1 Comparison of gastric prokinetic drugs[5]

Drug	*Erythromycin*	*Domperidone*	*Metoclopramide*
Mechanism of action			
Motilin agonist	+	–	–
D_2 antagonist	–	+	+
$5HT_4$ agonist	–	–	+
Response to treatment[a, b]			
Gastric emptying (mean % acceleration)	45	30	20
Symptom relief (mean % improvement)	50	50	40

a. all percentages rounded to nearest 5%
b. although acceleration in gastric emptying is a useful indicator of the efficacy of a prokinetic drug, it correlates poorly with symptom relief in gastroparesis.[6]

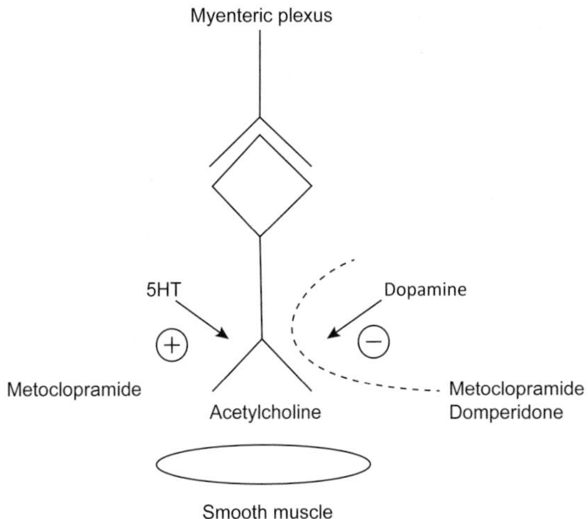

Figure 1 Schematic representation of drug effects on antroduodenal co-ordination via a postganglionic effect on the cholinergic nerves from the myenteric plexus.
(+) stimulatory effect of 5HT triggered by metoclopramide;
(−) inhibitory effect of dopamine;
– – – blockade of dopamine inhibition by metoclopramide and domperidone.

Erythromycin is reported to improve symptoms in about half of patients. A review suggested that, overall, its prokinetic effect was greater than that of **metoclopramide** (Table 1). However, the studies, mainly in diabetic gastroparesis, were small and open to bias.[7] Further, **erythromycin** can cause intestinal colic and diarrhoea. There are concerns about the possible development of bacterial resistance or tolerance to its prokinetic effects, although there are reports of **erythromycin** 250mg b.d. given for more than a year without apparent loss of efficacy.[8,9] Thus, **erythromycin** is generally used second-line when **metoclopramide** and **domperidone** have been ineffective.

Compared with **erythromycin**, **azithromycin** has a longer halflife and the potential for fewer drug interactions and undesirable effects. However, there are few trials to support its use.[10] Non-antibacterial motilin agonists are also undergoing trials, e.g. **atilmotin** and **mitemcinal**.

Use of prokinetics in palliative care

Prokinetics are used in various situations in palliative care (Box A). D_2 antagonists block the dopaminergic 'brake' on gastric emptying induced by stress, anxiety, and nausea from any cause. In contrast, $5HT_4$ agonists have a direct excitatory effect. However, when used for dysmotility dyspepsia, dual-action **metoclopramide** is no more potent than **domperidone** in standard doses.[11,12]

Box A Indications for prokinetics in palliative care

Gastro-oesophageal reflux
Delayed gastric emptying
Hiccup
Gastroparesis
  dysmotility dyspepsia
  paraneoplastic autonomic neuropathy
  spinal cord compression
  diabetic autonomic neuropathy
Functional GI obstruction
  drug-induced, e.g. opioids
  cancer of head of pancreas
  linitis plastica (locally diffuse mural infiltration by cancer)

Table 2 Drug treatment of hiccup (PO unless stated otherwise)

Class of drug	*Drug*	*Acute relief*	*Maintenance regimen*
Reduce gastric distension ± gastro-oesophageal reflux			
Antiflatulent (carminative)	Peppermint water[a,b]	10mL	Probably best used p.r.n. only
Antiflatulent (defoaming agent)	Simeticone	See p.4	See p.4
Prokinetic	Metoclopramide[b,c]	10mg	10mg t.d.s.[15]
PPI	Lansoprazole	30mg	30mg each morning
Central suppression of the hiccup reflex			
First-line options			
GABA agonist	Baclofen	5mg	5–20mg t.d.s., occasionally more[16,17]
Anti-epileptic	Gabapentin	'Burst gabapentin', i.e. 400mg t.d.s. for 3 days, then 400mg once daily for 3 days, then stop; repeat if necessary[d,18]	400mg t.d.s.[19,20]
Second-line options			
Dopamine antagonist	Metoclopramide	As above	As above
Third-line options			
L-type calcium-channel blocker	Nifedipine	10mg PO/SL	10–20mg t.d.s., occasionally more[21,22]
Anti-epileptic	Valproate	200–500mg	15mg/kg/24h in divided doses[23]
Dopamine antagonist	Haloperidol	1.5–3mg b.d.–t.d.s. (≤5mg t.d.s if severe)	500microgram–1mg t.d.s. (≤3mg t.d.s. if severe)
Benzodiazepine	Midazolam	2mg IV, followed by 1–2mg increments every 3–5min	10–60mg/24h by CSCI if patient in last days of life[24]

a. facilitates belching by relaxing the lower oesophageal sphincter; an old-fashioned remedy, can result in gastro-oesophageal reflux
b. peppermint water and metoclopramide should not be used concurrently because of their opposing actions on the gastro-oesophageal sphincter
c. tightens the lower oesophageal sphincter and hastens gastric emptying
d. a smaller dose advisable in elderly frail patients and those with renal impairment, e.g. start with 100mg t.d.s.

Doses are given in individual monographs for **metoclopramide** (p.244) and **domperidone** (p.247). For **erythromycin**:

- start with 50–100mg PO q.d.s (use suspension)
- if necessary, increase every few days by 25–50mg to a maximum dose of 250mg q.d.s.[3]

Metoclopramide is also used to relieve hiccup associated with delayed gastric emptying and/or oesophageal reflux (Table 2).[13]

For patients with refractory symptoms, seek advice from a gastroenterologist. In some settings, patients may benefit from **clonidine** (p.77), intrapyloric **botulinum toxin** or gastric electrical stimulation.[14] Ultimately, some patients may require a venting gastrostomy and/or a feeding jejunostomy.[1]

1 Stevens JE *et al.* (2013) Pathophysiology and pharmacotherapy of gastroparesis: current and future perspectives. *Expert Opinion on Pharmacotherpy.* **14**: 1171–1186.
2 Rayner CK and Horowitz M (2005) New management approaches for gastroparesis. *Nature Clinical Practice Gastroenterology and Hepatology.* **2**: 454–462.
3 Patrick A and Epstein O (2008) Review article: gastroparesis. *Alimentary Pharmacology and Therapeutics.* **27**: 724–740.
4 Schuurkes JAJ *et al.* (1986) Stimulation of gastroduodenal motor activity: dopaminergic and cholinergic modulation. *Drug Development Research.* **8**: 233–241.
5 Sturm A *et al.* (1999) Prokinetics in patients with gastroparesis: a systematic analysis. *Digestion.* **60**: 422–427.
6 Janssen P *et al.* (2013) The relation between symptom improvement and gastric emptying in the treatment of diabetic and idiopathic gastroparesis. *American Journal Gastroenterology.* **108**: 1382–1391.
7 Maganti K *et al.* (2003) Oral erythromycin and symptomatic relief of gastroparesis: a systematic review. *American Journal of Gastroenterology.* **98**: 259–263.
8 Dhir R and Richter JE (2004) Erythromycin in the short- and long-term control of dyspepsia symptoms in patients with gastroparesis. *Journal of Clinical Gastroenterology.* **38**: 237–242.
9 Hunter A *et al.* (2005) The use of long-term, low-dose erythromycin in treating persistent gastric stasis. *Journal of Pain and Symptom Management.* **29**: 430–433.
10 Potter TG and Snider KR (2013) Azithromycin for the treatment of gastroparesis. *Annals of Pharmacotherapy.* **47**: 411–415.
11 Loose FD (1979) Domperidone in chronic dyspepsia: a pilot open study and a multicentre general practice crossover comparison with metoclopramide and placebo. *Pharmatheripeutica.* **2**: 140–146.
12 Moriga M (1981) A multicentre double blind study of domperidone and metoclopramide in the symptomatic control of dyspepsia. In: G Towse (ed) *International congress and symposium series: Progress with Domperidone, a gastrokinetic and anti-emetic agent* (No. 36). Royal Society of Medicine, London, pp. 77–79.
13 Twycross R and Wilcock A (eds) (2016) *Introducing Palliative Care* (5e). palliativedrugs.com Ltd, Nottingham, pp. 166–170.
14 Haans JJ and Masclee AA (2007) Review article: The diagnosis and management of gastroparesis. *Alimentary Pharmacology and Therapeutics.* **26 (Suppl 2)**: 37–46.
15 Wang T and Wang D (2014) Metoclopramide for patients with intractable hiccups: a multicentre, randomised, controlled pilot study. *Internal Medicine Journal.* **44**: 1205–1209.
16 Ramirez FC and Graham DY (1992) Treatment of intractable hiccup with baclofen: results of a double-blind randomized, controlled, crossover study. *American Journal of Gastroenterology.* **87**: 1789–1791.
17 Guelaud C *et al.* (1995) Baclofen therapy for chronic hiccup. *European Respiratory Journal.* **8**: 235–237.
18 Moretti R *et al.* (2004) Gabapentin as a drug therapy of intractable hiccup because of vascular lesion: a three-year follow up. *Neurologist.* **10**: 102–106.
19 Schuchmann JA and Browne BA (2007) Persistent hiccups during rehabilitation hospitalization: three case reports and review of the literature. *American Journal of Physical Medicine and Rehabilitation.* **86**: 1013–1018.
20 Tegeler ML and Baumrucker SJ (2008) Gabapentin for intractable hiccups in palliative care. *American Journal of Hospice and Palliative Care.* **25**: 52–54.
21 Lipps DC *et al.* (1990) Nifedipine for intractable hiccups. *Neurology.* **40**: 531–532.
22 Brigham B and Bolin T (1992) High dose nifedipine and fludrocortisone for intractable hiccups. *Medical Journal of Australia.* **157**: 70.
23 Jacobson P *et al.* (1981) Treatment of intractable hiccups with valproic acid. *Neurology.* **31**: 1458–1460.
24 Wilcock A and Twycross R (1996) Case report: midazolam for intractable hiccup. *Journal of Pain and Symptom Management.* **12**: 59–61.

Updated August 2017

H_2-RECEPTOR ANTAGONISTS

Class: Gastroprotective drugs.

Indications: Chronic episodic dyspepsia, acid reflux, prevention and treatment of peptic ulceration (including NSAID-related ulceration), reduction of malabsorption and fluid loss in short bowel syndrome (**cimetidine**), prevention of degradation of pancreatin supplements (**cimetidine**), †reduction of gastric secretions in bowel obstruction, †paraneoplastic sweating.

Pharmacology

H_2-receptor antagonists (H_2 antagonists) include **cimetidine**, **famotidine**, **nizatidine** and **ranitidine**. All are equally effective at gastric acid suppression.[1] However, because of their greater acid suppression and/or tolerability, PPIs (p.30) are generally preferred over H_2 antagonists and **misoprostol**, which is now rarely used.[2]

Other effects include increasing lower oesophageal sphincter pressure and reducing the volume of gastric secretions.[3,4] H_2 antagonists are more effective than PPIs in reducing the volume of gastric secretions which has led some to recommend the use of **ranitidine** in patients with bowel obstruction.[4,5] Further, injection formulations of **ranitidine** (unlike PPIs) can be mixed with other drugs, making administration by CSCI more convenient (see Dose and use).

Anecdotally, H_2 antagonists are of benefit in paraneoplastic sweating.[6,7] The mechanism is unknown. An early therapeutic trial of **ranitidine** is reasonable on the basis that it is likely to be better tolerated than the other drugs used this setting (see Box D, Antimuscarinics, p.10).

Cimetidine, alone among H_2 antagonists, can cause serious CYP450-related drug interactions (see Table 1 and Chapter 19, Table 8, p.725). **Ranitidine** is a good choice in terms of cost and lack of drug interactions.

Bio-availability **ranitidine** 50% PO.
Onset of action <1h.
Time to peak plasma concentration, **ranitidine** 2–3h PO, 15min IM.
Plasma halflife **ranitidine** 2–3h.
Duration of action **ranitidine** 8–12h.

Cautions

Hepatic impairment, renal impairment (dose reduction required, see SPCs).

Gastric acid suppression is associated with an increased risk of *Clostridium difficile* infection (p.496); H_2 antagonists have a lower risk than PPIs (p.30).[8]

Drug interactions

H_2 antagonists increase gastric pH and this reduces the absorption of some drugs and formulations. Clinically important examples include **itraconazole** (capsules only), **posaconazole**, antivirals and protein kinase inhibitors (seek specialist advice); see respective SPCs for full details. Rarely, absorption is increased, e.g. **saquinivir**.[9]

Cimetidine is the only H_2 antagonist that affects the CYP450 enzyme system. It is classified as a weak inhibitor of multiple CYP enzymes involved in drug metabolism (CYP1A2, CYP2D6, CYP2C19, CYP3A4/5). Thus, caution is required with concurrent use of drugs which are metabolised by these enzymes (see Chapter 19, Table 8, p.725). Table 1 lists interactions where close monitoring ± dose adjustment are required.

Table 1 Clinically important CYP450-related interactions with cimetidine[a,9,10]

Drug group	*Drug effect ↑ by cimetidine*[b]
Anticoagulants	Warfarin and other coumarins
Anti-epileptics	Carbamazepine (transient), phenytoin
Benzodiazepines	Alprazolam, diazepam, chlordiazepoxide, flurazepam, midazolam[c], nitrazepam, triazolam (not UK)
Calcium antagonists	Potentially all, including diltiazem and nifedipine
Local anaesthetics	Flecainide, lidocaine (IV), procainamide
Opioids	Alfentanil, fentanyl, methadone
SSRIs	All
TCAs	Potentially all
Xanthines	Aminophylline, theophylline
Miscellaneous	Erythromycin, mirtazapine, moclobemide, quinine, quinidine (not UK), zaleplon, zolmitriptan

a. *not* an exhaustive list; limited to drugs most likely to be encountered in palliative care and *excludes* anticancer, antiviral, HIV and immunosuppressive drugs (seek specialist advice)
b. either specifically reported or likely based on pharmacokinetic studies
c. midazolam reports inconsistent.

Undesirable effects

Cimetidine occasionally causes gynaecomastia.

Possible increased risk of pneumonia (gastric acid suppression leads to bacterial overgrowth in the upper-GI and respiratory tracts); association stronger for PPIs (p.30).[11]

Dose and use

NICE guidance: in the treatment of uninvestigated dyspepsia or proven gastro-oesophageal reflux disease, H_2 antagonists are a second-line option after PPIs (p.30). In all other acid-related disorders, where efficacy may be similar, PPIs remain generally preferable to H_2 antagonists.[2]

Dose recommendations are limited to **ranitidine** because of its low cost and lack of drug interactions. **Ranitidine** is more effective if taken at bedtime rather than with the evening meal.[12]

In renal impairment (creatinine clearance <50mL/min) the dose of **ranitidine** should be reduced to 150mg at bedtime but increased to 150mg b.d. if an ulcer fails to respond at the lower dose.

Uninvestigated dyspepsia or reflux-like symptoms

- **ranitidine** 150mg PO b.d. or 300mg at bedtime for 6 weeks.

Proven gastro-oesophageal reflux disease

- **ranitidine** 150mg PO b.d. or 300mg at bedtime for 8–12 weeks.

Proven severe oesophagitis

- **ranitidine** 150mg PO q.d.s. or 300mg b.d. for up to 12 weeks.

Peptic ulcer (including NSAID-related)

- stop the NSAID; if continuation is necessary, use long-term gastric protection after ulcer healing (see below)
- test for *H pylori*:
  - ▷ if negative, use **ranitidine** 150mg PO b.d. or 300mg at bedtime for 4–8 weeks (8 weeks if continuing an NSAID)
  - ▷ if positive, and the ulcer is NSAID-related, use **ranitidine** 150mg PO b.d. or 300mg at bedtime for 8 weeks, followed by eradication therapy (see BNF) *or*
  - ▷ if positive, and the ulcer is *not* NSAID-related, use eradication therapy first and then review (see BNF)
- if symptoms recur, use the lowest effective dose either as long-term maintenance or, when symptoms infrequent, p.r.n.

Gastric protection in patients taking an NSAID at high risk of peptic ulcer disease

- **ranitidine** 300mg PO b.d. *and*
- consider use of a COX-2 selective NSAID (continue gastric protection;[2] also see p.325).

Bowel obstruction

See parenteral administration.

Paraneoplastic sweating

- **ranitidine** 150mg PO b.d.; benefit is generally seen within 2–3 days.[7]

Parenteral administration

If the PO route is unavailable, **ranitidine** 50mg can be administered IM/IV t.d.s–q.d.s. Although unauthorized, some centres use the SC route:

- **ranitidine** 50mg SC b.d.–q.d.s. *or*
- **ranitidine** 150–200mg/24h CSCI, using WFI or 0.9% saline as diluent.

CSCI compatibility with other drugs: limited clinical experience suggests that **ranitidine** is compatible with **diamorphine**, **fentanyl**, **haloperidol**, **hydromorphone**, **hyoscine butylbromide**, **methadone**, **metoclopramide**, **morphine sulfate**, **octreotide** and **oxycodone**.

There are mixed reports of *incompatibility* with **levomepromazine** and **midazolam**. Successful combinations at lower concentrations are reported; to minimize the risk of precipitation, **ranitidine** should always be the last drug added to an already diluted combination of drugs.

For more information, see the www.palliativedrugs.com SDSD; we encourage members to submit more combinations containing **ranitidine**.

Supply

Ranitidine (generic)
Tablets 150mg, 300mg, 28 days @ 150mg b.d. or 300mg at bedtime = £1.75.
Tablets effervescent 150mg, 300mg, 28 days @ 150mg b.d. or 300mg at bedtime = £29; *may contain* Na^+.
Oral solution 75mg/5mL, 28 days @ 150mg b.d. or 300mg at bedtime = £15; *may contain alcohol. Sugar-free versions available.*
Injection 25mg/mL, 2mL amp = £0.50.

Zantac® (GSK)
Tablets 150mg, 300mg, 28 days @ 150mg b.d. or 300mg at bedtime = £1.25.
Oral solution (sugar-free) 75mg/5mL, 28 days @ 150mg b.d. or 300mg at bedtime = £39; *contains 8% alcohol.*
Injection 25mg/mL, 2mL amp = £0.50.

Ranitidine tablets are available as an OTC measure for acid dyspepsia and heartburn.

1 Tougas G and Armstrong D (1997) Efficacy of H2 receptor antagonists in the treatment of gastroesophageal reflux disease and its symptoms. *Canadian Journal of Gastroenterology*. **11 Suppl B**: 51B–54B.
2 NICE (2014) Dyspepsia and gastro-oesophageal reflux disease. *Clinical Guideline*. CG184 www.nice.org.uk
3 Iwakiri K *et al.* (2011) The effects of nizatidine on transient lower esophageal sphincter relaxations (TLESRs) and acid reflux in healthy subjects. *Journal of Smooth Muscle Research*. **47**: 157–166.
4 Clark K *et al.* (2009) Reducing gastric secretions–a role for histamine 2 antagonists or proton pump inhibitors in malignant bowel obstruction? *Supportive Care in Cancer*. **17**: 1463–1468.
5 Currow DC *et al.* (2015) Double-blind, placebo-controlled, randomized trial of octreotide in malignant bowel obstruction. *Journal of Pain and Symptom Management*. **49**: 814–821.
6 Pittelkow M *et al.* (2015) Pruritus and sweating in palliative medicine. In: NI Cherny *et al* (eds). *Oxford Textbook of Palliative Medicine (5e)*. Oxford University Press, Oxford 724–739.
7 Howard P (2015) Personal communication.
8 Tleyjeh IM *et al.* (2013) The association between histamine 2 receptor antagonist use and Clostridium difficile infection: a systematic review and meta-analysis. *PLoS One*. **8**: e56498.
9 Baxter K and Preston CL. *Stockley's Drug Interactions*. London: Pharmaceutical Press www.medicinescomplete.com (accessed May 2015).
10 Sorkin E and Ogawa C (1983) Cimetidine potentiation of narcotic action. *Drug Intelligence and Clinical Pharmacy*. **17**: 60–61.
11 Fohl AL and Regal RE (2011) Proton pump inhibitor-associated pneumonia: Not a breath of fresh air after all? *World Journal of Gastrointestinal Pharmacology and Therapeutics*. **2**: 17–26.
12 Johnston DA and Wormsley KG (1988) The effect of food on ranitidine-induced inhibition of nocturnal gastric secretion. *Alimentary Pharmacology and Therapeutics*. **2**: 507–511.

Updated (minor change) August 2016

PROTON PUMP INHIBITORS

Class: Gastroprotective drugs.

Indications: Authorized indications vary between products; consult the manufacturers' SPCs for details; they include acid dyspepsia, acid reflux, peptic ulceration, prevention and treatment of NSAID-related ulceration and eradication of *H. pylori* (with antibacterials), †prevention of degradation of pancreatin supplements (see Pancreatin, p.58).

Pharmacology

Proton pump inhibitors (PPIs) include **esomeprazole** (the *S*-enantiomer of **omeprazole**), **lansoprazole**, **omeprazole**, **pantoprazole** and **rabeprazole**. Following absorption they are selectively taken up by gastric parietal cells and converted into active metabolites which irreversibly inhibit the proton pump (H^+/K^+-ATPase), thereby blocking gastric acid secretion.

PPIs provide symptomatic relief of acid dyspepsia and acid reflux, help prevent and heal peptic ulcers (including those associated with NSAIDs), and reduce the risk of recurrent ulceration and rebleeding.[1–3] Because of their greater acid suppression and/or tolerability, PPIs are generally preferred over H_2 antagonists (p.27) and **misoprostol**, which is now rarely used.[4] However, H_2 antagonists are more effective than PPIs in reducing the volume of gastric secretions, which may be an advantage in some situations, e.g. bowel obstruction (see p.27).

There is relatively little comparative data to guide the choice of one PPI over another on the basis of efficacy and thus factors such as patient preference, risk of drug interaction, cost, and local guidelines will determine choice.[4]

Because PPIs are rapidly degraded by acid, they are formulated as e/c granules or tablets. These dissolve in the duodenum where the drug is rapidly absorbed. The bio-availability of **lansoprazole** is reduced by food and the manufacturer recommends that it should be given ≥30min before food. However, the reduced bio-availability appears not to reduce efficacy.[5–7]

The plasma halflives of PPIs are mostly <2h but, because they irreversibly inhibit the proton pump, the antisecretory activity continues for several days until new proton pumps are synthesized.

Elimination is predominantly by metabolism in the liver to inactive derivatives excreted mostly in the urine. Most PPIs are metabolized via CYP2C19 and to a variable extent CYP3A4; the exception is **rabeprazole** which mostly undergoes non-enzymatic metabolism. CYP2C19 is subject to genetic polymorphism (see Chapter 19, p.719) with higher levels of activity associated with lower plasma concentrations of **omeprazole**, **lansoprazole** and **pantoprazole**, and higher rates of treatment failure, e.g. in *H pylori* eradication.[8,9]

Pharmacokinetic data are shown in Table 1.

Onset of action <2h.

Duration of action >24h.

Table 1 Pharmacokinetic details of PPIs given PO

	Bio-availability (%)	*Time to peak plasma concentration (h)*	*Plasma halflife (h)*
Esomeprazole	68 (20mg dose) 89 (40mg dose)	1–2	1.3
Lansoprazole	80–90	1.5–2	1–2
Omeprazole	60	3–6	0.5–3
Pantoprazole	77	2–2.5	1[a]
Rabeprazole	52	1.6–5	1[b]

a. increases to 3–6h in cirrhosis

b. increases to 2–3h in hepatic impairment.

Cautions

The dose should be reduced in severe hepatic impairment (see Dose and use).

PPIs are an independent risk factor for *Clostridium difficile* infection (see p.496); and the association is stronger than for other acid-reducing agents.[10] Patients are at risk of recurrent *Clostridium difficile* colitis, up to nearly 5 times more likely.[11–16] Although the spores of *Clostridium difficile* are resistant to gastric acid, reduced acidity allows bacteria to survive. Counts of *Clostridium difficile* organisms, which cannot survive at normal stomach pH, increase when the pH is >5, and go on to infect the bowel. Further, the spores can live up to 6h on moist surfaces, long enough to allow transmission between patients.[17] The concomitant use of PPIs and antibacterials further increases the risk of *Clostridium difficile* infection.[18]

Drug interactions

PPIs increase gastric pH and this can affect the absorption of some drugs and formulations; generally, absorption is reduced, e.g. **itraconazole** (capsules only), **posaconazole**, antivirals and protein kinase inhibitors (seek specialist advice). However, rarely it can be increased, e.g. **digoxin** (high dose PPIs in the elderly) and **saquinivir;**[9] see respective SPCs for full details.

Esomeprazole and **omeprazole** are weak–moderate inhibitors of CYP2C19 (see Chapter 19, p.717). Important interactions include:

- inhibition of the metabolism of **citalopram** and **escitalopram**, increasing the risk of QT interval prolongation (see SSRIs, p.212 and Chapter 20, p.731); the maximum daily dose should be reduced (see SPC)[19]
- a reduction in the antithrombotic effect of **clopidogrel** (a pro-drug activated by CYP2C19); avoid concurrent use with any PPI, use an H_2 antagonist instead[20]
- inhibition of the metabolism of **diazepam**
- inhibition of the metabolism of **warfarin**; isolated reports of raised INR with all PPIs.[9]

Undesirable effects

Common (<10%, >1%): headache, abdominal pain, nausea, vomiting, diarrhoea or constipation, flatulence.

Severe hypomagnesaemia: rare and generally with prolonged use, i.e. >1 year. The measurement of serum magnesium before starting a PPI and periodically thereafter has been suggested for patients using a PPI long-term.[21] However, a routine annual measurement in every patient appears unnecessary and should be reserved for older patients, particularly those taking **digoxin** or drugs which can cause hypomagnesaemia, e.g. diuretics (see p.588).[22]

Observational studies suggest a modest increase in the risk of hip and vertebral fracture in the elderly with prolonged use of PPIs. Those at risk of osteoporosis should ensure an adequate intake of vitamin D and calcium, using supplements if necessary.[23]

Possible increased risk of pneumonia (gastric acid suppression leads to bacterial overgrowth in the upper-GI and respiratory tracts); association weaker for H_2 antagonists.[24]

Ocular damage has been reported, mostly with IV **omeprazole**.[25,26] PPIs possibly cause vasoconstriction by blocking H^+/K^+-ATPase. Because the retinal artery is an end-artery, anterior ischaemic optic neuropathy may result. If the PPI is stopped, visual acuity may improve but some patients have become permanently blind, in some instances after only 3 days. Impaired hearing and deafness have also been reported, again mostly with IV **omeprazole**.

Dose and use

Dose recommendations are limited to **lansoprazole** and **omeprazole** (**esomeprazole** and **rabeprazole** are more expensive) and are mostly based on NICE guidance (see Table 2), which can differ from the SPC and BNF.[4]

The SPC for **lansoprazole** states that administration should be ≥30min before food in order to achieve 'optimal acid inhibition'. However, this precaution is unnecessary (see Pharmacology).

Table 2 NICE dose recommendations[4]

	Low-dose	*Standard dose*	*Double-dose*[a]
Lansoprazole	15mg once daily	30mg once daily	30mg b.d.
Omeprazole	10mg once daily	20mg once daily	40mg once daily

a. in severe hepatic impairment, do not exceed the standard dose.

Uninvestigated dyspepsia or reflux-like symptoms

- use standard dose PPI for 4 weeks; consider testing for *H pylori* in patients with dyspepsia
- subsequently, use the lowest effective dose either as long-term maintenance or, when symptoms infrequent, p.r.n.
- if there is an inadequate response to a PPI, switch to an H_2 antagonist.

Proven gastro-oesophageal reflux disease

- use standard dose PPI for 4–8 weeks
- subsequently, use the lowest effective dose either as long-term maintenance or, when symptoms infrequent, p.r.n.
- if there is an inadequate response to a PPI, switch to an H_2 antagonist.

Proven severe oesophagitis

- use **lansoprazole** 30mg PO or **omeprazole** 40mg once daily for 8 weeks
- if inadequate, increase the dose to b.d. or switch to an alternate PPI
- subsequently, use the lowest effective dose as long-term maintenance as necessary.

Peptic ulcer (including NSAID-related)

- stop any NSAIDs; if continuation is necessary, use long-term gastric protection after ulcer healing (see below)
- test for *H pylori*:
  - ▷ if negative, use standard dose PPI (or H_2 antagonist) for 4–8 weeks (8 weeks if continuing an NSAID)
  - ▷ if positive, and the ulcer is NSAID-related, use standard dose PPI (or H_2 antagonist) for 8 weeks, followed by eradication therapy (see BNF) *or*
  - ▷ if positive, and the ulcer is *not* NSAID-related, use eradication therapy first and then review (see BNF)
- if symptoms recur, use the lowest effective dose either as long-term maintenance or, when symptoms infrequent, p.r.n.

Gastric protection in patients taking an NSAID at high risk of peptic ulcer disease

- use standard dose PPI (or double-dose H_2 antagonist) *and*
- consider use of a COX-2 selective NSAID (continue gastric protection;[4] also see p.325).

Non-variceal upper-GI haemorrhage

- when bleeding or stigmata of recent bleeding is confirmed at endoscopy, use high-dose **omeprazole** 80mg PO/IV stat, followed by 8mg/h IVI (or 40mg b.d. PO) for 72h.[27]

For patients with swallowing difficulties, **lansoprazole** and **omeprazole** can be given as orodispersible or dispersible tablets respectively (Note. there is *no* SL absorption from orodispersible tablets). Some capsules containing e/c granules can be opened and the e/c granules swallowed with water or fruit juice, or mixed with apple sauce or yoghurt; check with the specific manufacturer's SPC. *Care must be taken not to crush or chew the e/c granules* (see Chapter 28, p.785).

Specific procedures are available from the manufacturers for administration by enteral feeding tubes (see Chapter 28, p.791). For patients with obstructive dysphagia and acid dyspepsia or with severe gastritis and vomiting, the rectal route has also been used.[28]

Parenteral administration

IV **omeprazole** (and **esomeprazole**) have been used in palliative care to treat painful reflux oesophagitis in patients unable to take PO medication.

Although PPIs are unauthorized for CSCI administration, there are case reports of such use:[29,30]

- **omperazole** 40mg for infusion diluted as per IVI (see supply) given by CSCI over 3–4h as a single daily dose for ≤4 days
- **esomeprazole** 40mg for infusion diluted in 50mL 0.9% normal saline and given by CSCI over 20min–1h as a single daily dose for ≤13 days.

After reconstitution, PPI injections/infusions are alkaline (pH 9–10.5) and should not be mixed with other drugs.

Ranitidine given IV, SC or CSCI is an alternate, see p.28.

Supply

Lansoprazole (generic)
Capsules enclosing e/c granules 15mg, 30mg, 28 days @ 30mg each morning = £1.50.
Tablets orodispersible 15mg, 30mg, 28 days @ 30mg each morning = £5.50.

Zoton® (Pfizer)
Tablets orodispersible (FasTab®) 15mg, 30mg, 28 days @ 30mg each morning = £5.50.

Omeprazole (generic)
Capsules enclosing e/c granules or hard e/c capsule 10mg, 20mg, 40mg, 28 days @ 20mg each morning = £1.25.
Tablets e/c 10mg, 20mg, 40mg, 28 days @ 20mg each morning = £6.50.

Tablets dispersible enclosing e/c pellets 10mg, 20mg, 40mg, 28 days @ 20mg each morning = £12.
Infusion powder for reconstitution in 5mL of infusion fluid 0.9% saline or 5% glucose. Further dilute to 100mL and give IVI over at least 20–30min. 40mg vial = £6.50.

Losec® (AstraZeneca)
Capsules enclosing e/c granules 10mg, 20mg, 40mg, 28 days @ 20mg each morning = £14.
Tablets dispersible (multiple-unit pellet system, MUPS®) ***enclosing e/c pellets*** 10mg, 20mg, 40mg, 28 days @ 20mg each morning = £12.

Omeprazole e/c tablets are available as an OTC measure for heartburn.

For details of ***esomeprazole, pantoprazole*** *and* ***rabeprazole,*** *see BNF; Combination products of* ***omeprazole*** *with* ***ketoprofen*** *and* ***esomeprazole*** *with* ***naproxen*** *are also available.*

1 Frech EJ and Go MF (2009) Treatment and chemoprevention of NSAID-associated gastrointestinal complications. *Therapeutics and Clinical Risk Management.* **5**: 65–73.
2 Leontiadis GI *et al.* (2007) Systematic reviews of the clinical effectiveness and cost-effectiveness of proton pump inhibitors in acute upper gastrointestinal bleeding. *Health Technology Assessment.* **11**: iii-iv, 1–164.
3 Leontiadis GI *et al.* (2005) Systematic review and meta-analysis of proton pump inhibitor therapy in peptic ulcer bleeding. *British Medical Journal.* **330**: 568.
4 NICE (2014) Dyspepsia and gastro-oesophageal reflux disease. *Clinical Guideline.* CG184 www.nice.org.uk
5 Moules I *et al.* (1993) Gastric acid inhibition by the proton pump inhibitor lansoprazole is unaffected by food. *British Journal of Clinical Research.* **4**: 153–161.
6 Delhotal-Landes B *et al.* (1991) The effect of food and antacids on lansoprazole absorption and disposition. *European Journal of Drug Metabolism and Pharmacokinetics.* **3**: 315–320.
7 Andersson T (1990) Bioavailability of omeprazole as enteric coated (EC) granules in conjunction with food on the first and seventh days of treatment. *Drug Investigations.* **2**: 184–188.
8 Shi S and Klotz U (2008) Proton pump inhibitors: an update of their clinical use and pharmacokinetics. *European Journal of Clinical Pharmacology.* **64**: 935–951.
9 Baxter K and Preston CL. *Stockley's Drug Interactions.* London: Pharmaceutical Press www.medicinescomplete.com (accessed June 2016).
10 Tleyjeh IM *et al.* (2013) The association between histamine 2 receptor antagonist use and *Clostridium difficile* infection: a systematic review and meta-analysis. *PLoS One.* **8**: e56498.
11 Kim JW *et al.* (2010) Proton pump inhibitors as a risk factor for recurrence of Clostridium difficile-associated diarrhea. *World Journal of Gastroenterology.* **16**: 3573–3577.
12 Cunningham R and Dial S (2008) Is over-use of proton pump inhibitors fuelling the current epidemic of Clostridium difficile-associated diarrhoea? *Journal of Hospital Infection.* **70**: 1–6.
13 Yearsley KA *et al.* (2006) Proton pump inhibitor therapy is a risk factor for Clostridium difficile-associated diarrhoea. *Alimentary Pharmacology and Therapeutics.* **24**: 613–619.
14 Dial S *et al.* (2005) Use of gastric acid suppressive agents and the risk of community acquired Clostridium difficile-associated diarrhoea. *Journal of the American Medical Association.* **294**: 2984–2995.
15 Cadle RM *et al.* (2007) Association of proton-pump inhibitors with outcomes in Clostridium difficile colitis. *American Journal of Health System Pharmacy.* **64**: 2359–2363.
16 Garey KW *et al.* (2008) Meta-analysis to assess risk factors for recurrent Clostridium difficile infection. *Journal of Hospital Infection.* **70**: 298–304.
17 Jump RL *et al.* (2007) Vegetative Clostridium difficile survives in room air on moist surfaces and in gastric contents with reduced acidity: a potential mechanism to explain the association between proton pump inhibitors and C. difficile-associated diarrhea? *Antimicrobial Agents and Chemotherapy.* **51**: 2883–2887.
18 Kwok CS *et al.* (2012) Risk of Clostridium difficile infection with acid suppressing drugs and antibiotics: meta-analysis. *American Journal of Gastroenterology.* **107**: 1011–1019.
19 MHRA (2011) Citalopram and escitalopram: QT interval prolongation - new maximum daily dose restrictions (including in elderly patients), contraindications, and warnings. *Drug Safety Update.* **5**: www.gov.uk/drug-safety-update
20 MHRA (2010) Clopidogrel and proton pump inhibitors: interaction - updated advice. *Drug Safety Update* **3**: www.gov.uk/drug-safety-update
21 MHRA (2012) Proton pump inhibitors in long term use: reports of hypomagnesaemia. *Drug safety update.* **5**: www.gov.uk/drug-safety-update
22 Begley J *et al.* (2016) Proton pump inhibitor associated hypomagnasaemia - a cause for concern? *British Journal of Clinical Pharmacology.* **81**: 753–758.
23 MHRA (2012) Proton pump inhibitors in long-term use: recent epidemiological evidence of increased risk of bone fracture *Drug Safety Update.* **5**: www.gov.uk/drug-safety-update
24 Fohl AL and Regal RE (2011) Proton pump inhibitor-associated pneumonia: Not a breath of fresh air after all? *World Journal of Gastrointestinal Pharmacology and Therapeutics.* **2**: 17–26.
25 Schonhofer P (1994) Intravenous omeprazole and blindness. *Lancet.* **343**: 665.
26 Schonhofer P *et al.* (1997) Ocular damage associated with proton pump inhibitors. *British Medical Journal.* **314**: 1805.
27 NICE (2012) Acute upper gastrointestinal bleeding management. *Clinical Guideline* **CG141**: www.nice.org.uk
28 Zylicz Z and van Sorge A (1998) Rectal omeprazole in the treatment of reflux pain in esophageal cancer. *Journal of Pain and Symptom Management.* **15**: 144–145.

29 Desmidts T and Constans T (2009) Subcutaneous infusion of esomeprazole in elderly patients in palliative care: A report of two cases. *Journal of the American Geriatrics Society*. **57**: 1724–1725.
30 Agar M *et al.* (2004) The use of subcutaneous omeprazole in the treatment of dyspepsia in palliative care patients. *Journal of Pain and Symptom Management*. **28**: 529–531.

Updated (minor change) July 2016

LOPERAMIDE

Class: Antimotility drug.

Indications: Acute and chronic diarrhoea, †ileostomy (to improve faecal consistency).[1]

Contra-indications: Colitis (ulcerative, infective, or antibiotic-associated); acute dysentery; conditions where inhibition of peristalsis should be avoided because of a risk of ileus, megacolon or toxic megacolon.

Pharmacology

Loperamide is a potent μ-opioid receptor agonist (μ agonist).[2] Although well absorbed from the GI tract, loperamide is almost completely extracted and metabolized by cytochrome P450 in the liver (particularly CYP3A4) where it is conjugated, and the conjugates excreted in the bile. Because of this extensive first-pass metabolism, in normal circumstances, little loperamide reaches the systemic circulation.

The antidiarrhoeal action of loperamide results from direct absorption into the gut wall. Like **morphine** and other μ agonists, loperamide increases intestinal transit time by decreasing propulsive activity and increasing non-propulsive activity via its effect on the myenteric plexus in the longitudinal muscle layer.[3,4] Loperamide also increases anal sphincter tone and improves night-time continence in patients with ileo-anal pouches.[5]

Loperamide also modifies the intestinal transport of water and electrolytes by stimulating absorption,[6] and by an anti-secretory action mediated by calmodulin antagonism, a property not shared by other opioids.[7–9]

Paradoxically, loperamide reduces the sodium-dependent uptake of glucose and other nutrients from the small bowel.[10] The development of tolerance to the GI effects of loperamide has been demonstrated in animal studies.[11] However, loperamide has been successfully used in patients with chronic diarrhoea for several years without evidence of tolerance.[12]

Loperamide is a substrate for P-glycoprotein, the efflux membrane transporter in the blood-brain barrier, and, although highly lipophilic,[4] loperamide is actively excluded from the CNS.[13,14] Consequently, unlike **morphine** which has both central and peripheral constipating effects, loperamide generally acts only peripherally when used within the recommended dose range[2] (but see Drug interactions and Undesirable effects).

Unlike other drugs used for diarrhoea, e.g. **diphenoxylate** (in **co-phenotrope**) and **codeine**, loperamide has no analgesic effect in therapeutic or supratherapeutic doses. The lack of CNS effects is one reason why loperamide is a popular first-line choice for the control of diarrhoea, including that associated with short-bowel syndrome, radiotherapy or chemotherapy.[15,16]

However, **octreotide** (see p.544) is recommended first-line for chemotherapy or radiotherapy-induced diarrhoea when severe (i.e. an increase of ≥7 stools/24h over baseline, hospital admission and IV fluids required for >24h), and second-line for less severe diarrhoea which does not respond to loperamide 16–24mg/24h.[15–17]

As an antidiarrhoeal, loperamide is about 3 times more potent mg for mg than **diphenoxylate** and 50 times more potent than **codeine**.[18] It is longer acting and, if used regularly, generally needs to be given only b.d. However, its maximum therapeutic impact may not manifest for 16–24h; this has implications for initial dosing.[14] The following regimens are approximately equivalent:

- loperamide 2mg b.d.
- **diphenoxylate** 2.5mg q.d.s. (in **co-phenotrope**)
- **codeine phosphate** 60mg q.d.s.

Loperamide is available in a range of formulations. Orodispersible tablets (Imodium® Instants), which melt on the tongue, are bio-equivalent to the capsules and are preferred by some patients.

A combination product with **simeticone** provides more rapid relief of diarrhoea and abdominal discomfort from bloating in acute non-specific diarrhoea than either loperamide or **simeticone** alone.[19,20] One suggested explanation is that the surfactant effect of **simeticone** enhances the contact of loperamide with the gut mucosa. However, both these formulations are relatively expensive (see Supply).

Bio-availability ~0.3%.

Onset of action about 1h; maximum effect 16–24h.[21]

Time to peak plasma concentration 2.5h (oral solution); 5h (capsules).[22]

Plasma halflife 11h[22] but up to 41h with doses of ≥16 mg/24h.[23]

Duration of action up to 3 days.[12]

Cautions

A patient on **clozapine** (an atypical antipsychotic) died of toxic megacolon after taking loperamide during an episode of food poisoning; additive inhibition of intestinal motility was considered the precipitating cause.[24]

Patients with AIDS are at risk of toxic megacolon if loperamide is used in viral or bacterial colitis.

Severe hepatic impairment (see Chapter 18, p.703) can increase plasma concentrations of loperamide and the risk of undesirable effects, including suppression of consciousness.[25] This may also occur in children, particularly <2 years, who receive excessive doses.[26–28] If **naloxone** is considered necessary, repeated doses may be needed because loperamide has a longer duration of action than **naloxone** (see, p.457).

Loperamide should be used with caution in patients who are at risk of *torsade de pointes* or other cardiac arrhythmias, and in patients who are using drugs which can alter the absorption or metabolism of loperamide.

Loperamide has become a drug of abuse, both to prevent withdrawal from other opioids and also to bring about euphoria in high doses.[29] High doses are associated with QT prolongation and potentially fatal cardiac arrhythmias, e.g. Torsade de Pointes (see Chapter 20, p.731).

Many of the reports of loperamide-induced cardiac arrhythmias occurred when taken in higher than recommended doses (median 250mg/24h, range 70–1600mg), either for the treatment of diarrhoea or as a drug of abuse.[30] Cardiac arrhythmias have also been reported rarely in patients taking therapeutic doses when taking a CYP3A4 inhibitor concurrently (see below).[23]

Cardiac arrhythmias may occur if absorption is enhanced or metabolism inhibited (see Drug interactions below). *Loperamide should be considered in any case of unexplained cardiac arrhythmia.* Blood concentrations can be measured.[23]

Drug interactions

Loperamide triples the PO bio-availability of **desmopressin**, possibly by both reducing GI enzymic degradation and slowing GI motility.[31]

Some CYP3A4 and P-glycoprotein inhibitors, e.g. **itraconazole**, increase plasma concentrations of loperamide significantly. Generally, these increases have not been associated with significant CNS effects. However, because of the risk of cardiac arrhythmia with high loperamide plasma concentrations, caution should be taken with potent CYP3A4 or P-glycoprotein inhibitors (see Chapter 19, Table 8, p.725).

Undesirable effects

Common (<10%, >1%): headache, dizziness, nausea, flatulence, constipation.

Uncommon (<1%, >0.1%): drowsiness, dry mouth, dyspepsia, vomiting, abdominal pain or discomfort, rash.

Rare (<0.1%, >0.01%): fatigue, depression of consciousness, unco-ordination, hypertonia, abdominal distension, ileus, faecal impaction, megacolon, urinary retention, angioedema, pruritus, urticaria, bullous skin eruptions.

Dose and use

Confirm that the diarrhoea is not secondary to faecal impaction.

In severe diarrhoea, ensure adequate fluid and electrolyte replacement is given, e.g. by using oral rehydration salts or IV fluids.

Note. For patients on a sodium-restricted diet, Imodium® *oral solution* contains Na^+ 4.85mg/5mL.

Acute diarrhoea

- start with 4mg PO stat
- continue with 2mg after each loose bowel action for up to 5 days
- maximum recommended dose 16mg/24h.

Chemotherapy- or radiotherapy-induced diarrhoea

- if mild–moderate, give 4mg stat and 2mg after each loose bowel action
- if not responding to doses of 24mg/24h, switch to **octreotide** (see p.544)
- if severe, use **octreotide** first-line.

Chronic diarrhoea

If symptomatic treatment is appropriate, the same initial approach is used for 2–3 days, after which a prophylactic b.d. regimen is instituted based on the needs of the patient during the previous 24h, plus 2mg after each loose bowel action. The effective dose varies widely. It is occasionally necessary to increase the dose to 32mg/24h; *this is twice the recommended maximum daily dose.* Such doses should *not* be used in conjunction with a CYP3A4 inhibitor (see Drug interactions above), or in someone at risk of a cardiac arrhythmia.

High-output stoma/ileostomy or intestinal fistula

Above-recommended doses of loperamide, e.g. 10mg q.d.s., may be necessary to reduce stoma or fistula output to manageable volumes. In specialist centres in the UK, 64mg/24h is regarded as the usual maximum dose, while recognizing that it may occasionally be beneficial to increase the dose to 96mg/24h.[1] Such doses should *not* be used in conjunction with a CYP3A4 inhibitor (see Drug interactions above), or in someone at risk of a cardiac arrhythmia. However, **octreotide** (± lower-dose loperamide) is probably a better option (see p.544).

Supply

Loperamide (generic)
Capsules 2mg, 5 days @ 2mg p.r.n., max 16mg/24h = £1.25.
Tablets 2mg, 5 days @ 2mg p.r.n., max 16mg/24h = £3.

Imodium® (Janssen)
Orodispersible tablets 2mg, 5 days @ 2mg p.r.n., max 16mg/24h = £5.
Oral solution (sugar-free) 1mg/5mL, 5 days @ 2mg p.r.n., max 16mg/24h = £11; *contains alcohol; also contains Na^+ 4.85mg/5mL.*

With **simeticone**
Imodium® Plus (McNeil)
Caplets (capsule-shaped tablets) containing loperamide 2mg, **simeticone** 125mg, 5 days @ 1 p.r.n., max 4 caplets/24h = £6.

Loperamide capsules are available to purchase OTC for acute diarrhoea.

1 UK Medicines Information (2013) Can high dose loperamide be used to reduce stoma output? *Medicines Q&A* 185.4. www.evidence.nhs.uk
2 Shannon H and Lutz E (2002) Comparison of the peripheral and central effects of the opioid agonists loperamide and morphine in the formalin test in rats. *Neuropharmacology*. **42**: 253–261.
3 Van Nueten JM *et al.* (1979) Distribution of loperamide in the intestinal wall. *Biochemical Pharmacology*. **28**: 1433–1434.
4 Ooms L *et al.* (1984) Mechanisms of action of loperamide. *Scandinavian Journal of Gastroenterology*. **19 (Suppl 96)**: 145–155.
5 Hallgren T *et al.* (1994) Loperamide improves anal sphincter function and continence after restorative proctocolectomy. *Digestive Diseases and Sciences*. **39**: 2612–2618.
6 Dashwood MR *et al.* (1990) Autoradiographic demonstration of [3H] loperamide binding to opioid receptors in rat and human small intestine. *Progress in Clinical and Biological Research*. **328**: 165–169.
7 Merritt J *et al.* (1982) Loperamide and calmodulin. *Lancet*. **1**: 283.
8 Zavecz J *et al.* (1982) Relationship between anti-diarrheal activity and binding to calmodulin. *European Journal of Pharmacology*. **78**: 375–377.

9 Daly J and Harper J (2000) Loperamide: novel effects on capacitative calcium influx. *Celluar and Molecular Life Sciences*. **57**: 149–157.
10 Klaren P *et al.* (2000) Effect of loperamide on Na+/D-glucose cotransporter activity in mouse small intestine. *Journal of Pharmacy and Pharmacology*. **52**: 679–686.
11 Tan-No K *et al.* (2003) Development of tolerance to the inhibitory effect of loperamide on gastrointestinal transit in mice. *European Journal of Pharmaceutical Sciences*. **20**: 357–363.
12 Heel R *et al.* (1978) Loperamide: A review of its pharmacological properties and therapeutic efficacy in diarrhoea. *Drugs*. **15**: 33–52.
13 Heykants J *et al.* (1974) Loperamide (R 18553), a novel type of antidiarrheal agent. Part 5: The pharmacokinetics of loperamide in rats and man. *Arzneimittel-Forschung*. **24**: 1649–1653.
14 Sadeque A *et al.* (2000) Increased drug delivery to the brain by P-glycoprotein inhibition. *Clinical Pharmacology and Therapeutics*. **68**: 231–237.
15 Maroun JA *et al.* (2007) Prevention and management of chemotherapy-induced diarrhea in patients with colorectal cancer: a consensus statement by the Canadian Working Group on Chemotherapy-Induced Diarrhea. *Current Oncology*. **14**: 13–20.
16 Benson AB *et al.* (2004) Recommended guidelines for the treatment of cancer treatment-induced diarrhea *Journal of Clinical Oncology*. **22**: 2918–2926.
17 Bhattacharya S (2009) Octreotide in chemotherapy induced diarrhoea in colorectal cancer: a review article. *Acta Gastroenterologica Belgica*. **72**: 289–295.
18 Schuermans V *et al.* (1974) Loperamide (R18553), a novel type of antidiarrhoeal agent. Part 6: clinical pharmacology. Placebo-controlled comparison of the constipating activity and safety of loperamide, diphenoxylate and codeine in normal volunteers. *Arzneimittel-Forschung Drug Research*. **24**: 1653–1657.
19 Kaplan MA *et al.* (1999) Loperamide-simethicone vs loperamide alone, simethicone alone, and placebo in the treatment of acute diarrhea with gas-related abdominal discomfort. A randomized controlled trial. *Archives of Family Medicine*. **8**: 243–248.
20 Hanauer SB *et al.* (2007) Randomized, double-blind, placebo-controlled clinical trial of loperamide plus simethicone versus loperamide alone and simethicone alone in the treatment of acute diarrhea with gas-related abdominal discomfort. *Current Medical Research Opinion*. **23**: 1033–1043.
21 Dreverman JWM and van der Poel AJ (1995) Loperamide oxide in acute diarrhoea: a double-blind placebo-controlled trial. *Alimentary Pharmacology and Therapeutics*. **9**: 441–446.
22 Killinger J *et al.* (1979) Human pharmacokinetics and comparative bioavailability of loperamide hydrochloride. *Journal of Clinical Pharmacology*. **19**: 211–218.
23 FDA (2016) Drug safety communication: FDS warns about serious heart problems with high doses of the antidiarrheal medicine loperamide (Imodium), including from abuse and misuse. Available from: https://www.fda.gov/Drugs/DrugSafety/ucm504617.htm
24 Eronen M *et al.* (2003) Lethal gastroenteritis associated with clozapine and loperamide. *American Journal of Psychiatry*. **160**: 2242–2243.
25 Baker DE (2007) Loperamide: a pharmacological review. *Reviews in Gastroenterological Disorders*. **7 (Suppl 3)**: S11–18.
26 Friedli G and Haenggeli CA (1980) Loperamide overdose managed by naloxone. *Lancet*. **ii**: 1413.
27 Minton N and Smith P (1987) Loperamide toxicity in a child after a single dose. *British Medical Journal*. **294**: 1383.
28 Litovitz T *et al.* (1997) Surveillance of loperamide ingestions: an analysis of 216 poison center reports. *Journal of Toxicology and Clinical Toxicology*. **35**: 11–19.
29 Vakkalanka JP *et al.* (2017) Epidemiologic trends in loperamide abuse and misuse. *Annals of Emergency Medicine*. **69**: 73–78.
30 Swank KA *et al.* (2017) Adverse event detection using the FDA post-marketing drug safety surveillance system: Cardiotoxicity associated with loperamide abuse and misuse. *Journal of the American Pharmacists Association*. **57**: S63-S67.
31 Callreus T *et al.* (1999) Changes in gastrointestinal motility influence the absorption of desmopressin. *European Journal of Clinical Pharmacology*. **55**: 305–309.

Updated July 2017

LAXATIVES

There is limited RCT evidence about laxative use in palliative care patients.[1] Consequently, guidelines for the management of constipation in palliative care are based largely on consensus best practice and expert opinion.[1–4]

Constipation is common in advanced cancer,[5] and is generally caused by multiple factors, e.g. poor diet, weakness, the underlying disease, drugs (particularly opioids). It can be defined as the passage of small hard faeces infrequently and with difficulty,[2] and is characterized by:

- *slow GI transit:* prolonged transit time allows more absorption of water from the faeces by the GI tract, manifesting as decreased frequency of bowel movements and small hard faeces[6,7]
- *disordered rectal evacuation:* the need to strain when defaecating.[6]

The aims of drug management of constipation are:

- to restore the amount of water in the faeces by:
  - ▷ reducing bowel transit time
  - ▷ increasing faecal water
  - ▷ increasing the ability of the faeces to retain water
- to improve rectal evacuation by improving faecal consistency and promoting peristalsis.

There are two broad classes of laxatives: those acting predominantly as *faecal softeners* and those acting predominantly as *bowel stimulants* (Table 1).

Table 1 Classification of commonly used laxatives

Class of laxative	*General mode of action*	*Common laxatives*
Faecal softeners		
Surface-wetting agents	Act as a detergent, lowering surface tension, thereby allowing water and fats to penetrate hard, dry faeces	Docusate sodium[a] Poloxamer 188 (in co-danthramer)
Osmotic laxatives	Water is retained in the gut lumen with a subsequent increase in faecal volume	Lactulose syrup Magnesium hydroxide suspension (Phillips' Milk of Magnesia®); sometimes combined with liquid paraffin (a lubricant), e.g. Mil-Par® Magnesium sulfate (Epsom Salts) Macrogols (e.g. Movicol®)
Stimulant laxatives	Act via direct contact with the submucosal and myenteric plexus in the large bowel, resulting in rhythmic muscle contractions and improved intestinal motility. Also increase water secretion into the bowel lumen, thereby adding a degree of softening	Bisacodyl Dantron Senna Sodium picosulfate
Lubricants	Coat the surface of the stool to make it more slippery and easier to pass	Liquid paraffin[b] Arachis oil
Bulk-forming agents (fibre)	Increase faecal bulk through water-binding and increasing bacterial cell mass. This causes intestinal distension and thereby stimulates peristalsis; only a limited role in palliative care	Ispaghula (psyllium) husk (e.g. Fybogel®) Methylcellulose (e.g. Celevac®) Sterculia (e.g. Normacol®)

a. reflects predominant action; at doses >400mg/24h also has a stimulant effect

b. limited role in palliative care due to potentially serious undesirable effects.

Faecal softeners also increase faecal mass, and can thereby stimulate peristalsis. Further, **lactulose** (an osmotic laxative) is converted by colonic fermentation to organic acids which act as contact stimulants in the large bowel (see p.50).[8] Conversely, stimulant laxatives reduce water absorption from the faeces and thus have a softening action (see p.46).

At doses commonly used, **docusate sodium** (≤400mg/24h) acts mainly by lowering surface tension (enabling water and fats to penetrate into the substance of the faeces) but at higher doses it also acts as a stimulant laxative (see p.49).

To date, RCTs of laxatives in palliative care patients have failed to show clinically meaningful differences (Table 2). A Cochrane review has concluded that there is inadequate experimental evidence to guide the optimal treatment of constipation with laxatives.[1]

There is evidence for the benefit of some laxatives, e.g. **bisacodyl**, **sodium picosulphate**, **macrogols**, compared with placebo. However, these laxatives are rarely used as the comparator arm in RCTs of new medications.[9]

Given the limited RCT evidence, the following should be noted:

- an appreciation of the pathophysiology of constipation (particularly opioid-induced),[2,16] and of how different laxatives work, and their cost will guide laxative choice
- generally, all laxatives given in sufficient quantities are capable of normalizing bowel function in constipated patients[17,18]
- compliance with laxative therapy may be limited in individual patients by palatability, undesirable effects (e.g. colic, flatulence), volume required, and polypharmacy. Patient preference and drug tolerability should be taken into account
- the concurrent prescription of several different laxatives should be avoided
- laxative doses should be titrated every 1–2 days according to response up to the maximum recommended or tolerable dose before changing to an alternative

- immobile patients with faecal incontinence are at risk of perineal skin irritation from **dantron**-containing laxatives
- anal seepage with associated irritation can be problematic with **liquid paraffin**. Absorption of **liquid paraffin** can also cause granulomatous reaction formation. Absorption is enhanced by concomitant use of **docusate sodium**
- traditionally a combination of a bowel stimulant with a faecal softener has been recommended in palliative care patients.[2,19] However, the results of the RCT which compared **senna** alone with **senna** and **docusate** in hospice patients (see Table 2)[15] and comparable results from a non-randomized non-blinded sequential cohort study in cancer inpatients[10] suggest that it is reasonable to prescribe a stimulant laxative alone, at least initially[20]
- if an adequate result is not achieved after 3–4 days using a stimulant laxative alone despite dose titration, consider adding a faecal softener
- if colic occurs, a softener should be added
- if faecal leakage occurs, the dose of the faecal softener will need to be reduced.[2,3]

Table 2 RCTs of laxatives in palliative care patients

Interventions	*Sample size*	*Outcome*
Senna and lactulose vs. co-danthramer (dantron and poloxamer)[10]	N=51	Participants on high-dose strong opioids; those receiving senna and lactulose had more bowel evacuations compared with those receiving co-danthramer, but there was no difference in patient preference
Senna and lactulose vs. magnesium hydroxide and liquid paraffin (unpublished data)[11]	N=118	No significant difference in efficacy outcomes between interventions
Senna vs. lactulose[12]	N = 75	No significant difference in efficacy outcomes between interventions
Senna vs. misrakasneham (Ayurvedic herbal remedy)[13]	N=36	No significant difference in efficacy outcomes between interventions
Senna vs. senna and docusate[14]	N=74	No significant difference between the groups, suggesting no benefit in routinely adding docusate. However, a high proportion of patients in each group required rescue rectal interventions (74% and 69%), suggesting neither treatment was very effective. Although the dose of senna could be titrated to response, the dose of docusate was fixed, and thus may not always have been optimal[15]

Rectal interventions

Rectal products available for the management of constipation include suppositories and enemas (see Rectal products, p.55). As far as possible, rectal interventions should be avoided in patients who are neutropenic or thrombocytopenic because of the risk, respectively, of infection or bleeding.

About one third of palliative care patients need rectal measures[21,22] either because of failed oral treatment or electively, e.g. in bedbound frail elderly patients, patients with paralysis (see p.44).

A Cochrane review of the management of constipation and faecal incontinence in patients with central neurological disease included 22 trials and 902 patients with diagnoses such as Parkinson's disease, multiple sclerosis and spinal cord injuries. The review concluded that there was limited evidence supporting bulk-forming laxatives (**ispaghula**) or **macrogols** (and also abdominal massage and transanal irrigation).[23]

Opioid-induced constipation

Opioids are a major contributory factor for constipation in palliative care patients, reducing quality of life, and sometimes resulting in opioid discontinuation.[24–26] Opioids cause constipation by increasing ring contractions, decreasing propulsive intestinal activity, and by enhancing the resorption of fluid and electrolytes.[27,28] Tolerance does not develop to these effects.[29] Although some strong opioids are possibly less constipating than **morphine** (e.g. **buprenorphine**, **fentanyl**, **methadone**), most patients receiving any opioid regularly will need a laxative concurrently.[30] Thus, as a general rule, all patients prescribed **morphine** (or other opioid) should also be prescribed a laxative (see p. 42).

Methylnaltrexone, a peripherally-acting opioid antagonist, represents an additional approach to the management of opioid-induced constipation (see p.42 and p.466). A recent Cochrane review concluded that there is some evidence that, compared with placebo, **methylnaltrexone** is effective in patients taking opioids who have not had a good response with conventional laxatives.[1]

1 Candy B *et al.* (2015) Laxatives for the management of constipation in people receiving palliative care. *Cochrane Database of Systematic Reviews.* **19**: CD003448. www.thecochranelibrary.com

2 Larkin PJ *et al.* (2008) The management of constipation in palliative care: clinical practice recommendations. *Palliative Medicine.* **22**: 796–807.

3 NICE (2013) Palliative cancer care - constipation. Clinical Knowledge Summaries. http://cks.nice.org.uk

4 Librach SL *et al.* (2010) Consensus recommendations for the management of constipation in patients with advanced, progressive illness. *Journal of Pain and Symptom Management.* **40**: 761–773.

5 Droney J *et al.* (2008) Constipation in cancer patients on morphine. *Supportive Care in Cancer.* **16**: 453–459.

6 Soligo M *et al.* (2006) Patterns of constipation in urogynecology: clinical importance and pathophysiologic insights. *American Journal of Obstetrics and Gynecology.* **195**: 50–55.

7 Lewis SJ and Heaton KW (1997) Stool form scale as a useful guide to intestinal transit time. *Scandinavian Journal of Gastroenterology.* **32**: 920–924.

8 Jouet P *et al.* (2008) Effects of therapeutic doses of lactulose vs. polyethylene glycol on isotopic colonic transit. *Alimentary Pharmacology and Therapeutics.* **27**: 988–993.

9 Ford AC (2013) Death knell for placebo-controlled trials in chronic idiopathic constipation? *Gastroenterology.* **145**: 897–898.

10 Sykes N (1991) A clinical comparison of laxatives in a hospice. *Palliative Medicine.* **5**: 307–314.

11 Sykes N (1991) A clinical comparison of lactulose and senna with magnesium hydroxide and liquid paraffin emulsion in a palliative care population. [cited in Candy B et *al.* (2011) Laxatives or methylnaltrexone for the management of constipation in palliative care patients. *Cochrane Database of Systematic Reviews.* CD003448. www.thecochranelibrary.com

12 Agra Y *et al.* (1998) Efficacy of senna versus lactulose in terminal cancer patients treatment with opioids. *Journal of Pain and Symptom Management.* **15**: 1–7.

13 Ramesh P *et al.* (1998) Managing morphine-induced constipation: a controlled comparison of an Ayurvedic formulation and senna. *Journal of Pain and Symptom Management.* **16**: 240–244.

14 Tarumi Y *et al.* (2013) Randomized, double-blind, placebo-controlled trial of oral docusate in the management of constipation in hospice patients. *Journal of Pain and Symptom Management.* **45**: 2–13.

15 Sykes N (2013) Emerging evidence on docusate: commentary on Tarumi et al. *Journal of Pain Symptom Management.* **45**: 1.

16 Fallon M and Hanks G (1999) Morphine, constipation and performace status in advanced cancer patients. *Palliative Medicine.* **13**: 159–160.

17 Sykes NP (1996) A volunteer model for the comparison of laxatives in opioid-related constipation. *Journal of Pain and Symptom Management.* **11**: 363–369.

18 Portenoy RK (1987) Constipation in the cancer patient: causes and management. *Medical Clinics of North America.* **71**: 303–311.

19 Hawley PH and Byeon JJ (2008) A comparison of sennosides-based bowel protocols with and without docusate in hospitalized patients with cancer. *Journal of Palliative Medicine.* **11**: 575–581.

20 Clemens KE and Klaschik E (2008) Management of constipation in palliative care patients. *Current Opinion in Supportive and Palliative Care.* **2**: 22–27.

21 Twycross RG and Lack SA (1986) *Control of Alimentary Symptoms in Far Advanced Cancer.* Churchill Livingstone, Edinburgh, pp. 173–174.

22 Twycross RG and Harcourt JMV (1991) The use of laxatives at a palliative care centre. *Palliative Medicine.* **5**: 27–33.

23 Coggrave M *et al.* (2014) Management of faecal incontinence and constipation in adults with central neurological diseases. *Cochrane Database of Systematic Reviews.* **13**: CD002115. www.thecochranelibrary.com

24 Sykes N (1998) The relationship between opioid use and laxative use in terminally ill cancer patients. *Palliative Medicine.* **12**: 375–382.

25 Bell T *et al.* (2009) Opioid-induced constipation negatively impacts pain management, productivity, and health-related quality of life: findings from the National Health and Wellness Survey. *Journal of Opioid Management.* **5**: 137–144.

26 Candrilli SD *et al.* (2009) Impact of constipation on opioid use patterns, health care resource utilization, and costs in cancer patients on opioid therapy. *Journal of Pain and Palliative Care Pharmacotherapy.* **23**: 231–241.

27 Beubler E (1983) Opiates and intestinal transport: in vivo studies. In: LA Turnberg (ed) *Intestinal secretion.* Smith Kline and French, Hertfordshire, pp. 53–55.

28 Kurz A and Sessler DI (2003) Opioid-induced bowel dysfunction: pathophysiology and potential new therapies. *Drugs.* **63**: 649–671.

29 Ross GR *et al.* (2008) Morphine tolerance in the mouse ileum and colon. *Journal of Pharmacology and Experimental Therapeutics.* **327**: 561–572.

30 Radbruch L *et al.* (2000) Constipation and the use of laxatives: a comparison between transdermal fentanyl and oral morphine. *Palliative Medicine.* **14**: 111–119.

Updated August 2017

Quick Clinical Guide: Opioid-induced constipation

Generally, all patients prescribed an opioid should also be prescribed a stimulant laxative, with the aim of achieving bowel movement without straining every 1–3 days. A standardized protocol aids management.

Sometimes, rather than automatically changing to the local standard laxative, it may be more appropriate to optimize a patient's existing regimen.

These guidelines can also be followed in patients who are not on opioids, although smaller doses may well suffice.

1 Ask about the patient's past and present bowel habit and use of laxatives; record the date of last bowel action.

2 Palpate for faecal masses in the line of the colon; examine the rectum digitally if the bowels have not been open for ≥3 days or if the patient reports rectal discomfort or has diarrhoea suggestive of faecal impaction with overflow.

3 For inpatients, keep a daily record of bowel actions.

4 Encourage fluids generally, and fruit juice and fruit specifically.

5 When an opioid is prescribed, prescribe bisacodyl or senna and titrate the dose according to response:

Bisacodyl

If *not* constipated:
- generally start with 5mg at bedtime
- if no response after 24–48h, increase to 10mg at bedtime.

If already constipated:
- generally start with 10mg at bedtime
- if no response after 24–48h, increase to 20mg at bedtime
- if no response after a further 24–48h, consider adding a second daytime dose
- if necessary, consider increasing to a maximum of 20mg t.d.s.

Senna

If *not* constipated:
- generally start with 15mg at bedtime
- if no response after 24–48h, increase to 15mg at bedtime and each morning.

If already constipated:
- generally start with 15mg at bedtime and each morning
- if no response after 24–48h, increase to 22.5mg at bedtime and each morning
- if no response after a further 24–48h, consider adding a third daytime dose
- if necessary, consider increasing to a maximum of 30mg t.d.s.

An oral solution (7.5mg/5mL) is an alternative to tablets; it is tasteless and generally cheaper.

6 During dose titration and subsequently, if ≥3 days since last bowel action, give suppositories, e.g. bisacodyl 10mg and glycerol 4g, or a micro-enema. If these are ineffective, administer a phosphate enema and possibly repeat the next day.

7 If the maximum dose of the stimulant laxative is ineffective and/or there has been no bowel evacuation within 3–4 days of commencing a stimulant, add a faecal softener laxative and titrate as necessary, e.g.:
- macrogols (e.g. Movicol®) one sachet each morning *or*
- lactulose 15mL once daily–b.d.

8 In a patient receiving opioids, if adequately titrated oral laxatives + rectal interventions fail to produce the desired response, consider SC methylnaltrexone.

Methylnaltrexone

Methylnaltrexone is a peripherally acting opioid antagonist administered as a SC injection. It is relatively expensive and should be considered in patients with opioid-induced constipation only when the optimum use of laxatives is ineffective. In patients with advanced disease, because constipation is generally multifactorial in origin, methylnaltrexone is added to the existing laxative regimen.

- dose recommendations:
  - ▷ for patients weighing 38-61kg, start with 8mg on alternate days
  - ▷ for patients weighing 62–114kg, start with 12mg on alternate days
  - ▷ outside this range, give 150microgram/kg on alternate days
  - ▷ the interval between administrations can be varied, either extended or reduced, but not more than once daily
- in severe renal impairment (creatinine clearance <30mL/min) reduce the dose:
  - ▷ for patients weighing 62–114kg, reduce to 8mg
  - ▷ outside this range, reduce to *75microgram/kg*, rounding up the dose volume to the nearest 0.1mL
- methylnaltrexone is contra-indicated in cases of known or suspected bowel obstruction. It should be used with caution in patients with conditions which may predispose to perforation
- common undesirable effects include abdominal pain/colic, diarrhoea, flatulence, and nausea and vomiting; these generally resolve after a bowel movement; postural hypotension can also occur
- about 1/3–1/2 of patients given methylnaltrexone have a bowel movement within 4h. The bowel movement can occur rapidly, consider having pads and a commode in place, particularly in those with poor mobility.

9 If the stimulant laxative causes bowel colic, divide the total daily dose into smaller more frequent doses or change to a faecal softener (see above), and titrate as necessary.

10 As initial treatment, a faecal softener is preferable in patients with a history of colic with stimulant laxatives.

Updated August 2016

Quick Clinical Guide: Bowel management in paraplegia and tetraplegia

Theoretically, management is determined by the level of the spinal cord lesion:

- above T12–L1 = cauda equina intact → spastic GI tract with preserved sacral reflex; generally responds to digital stimulation of the rectum; the presence of an anal reflex suggests an intact sacral reflex
- below T12–L1 = cauda equina involved → flaccid GI tract; generally requires digital evacuation of the rectum
- a lesion at the level of the conus medullaris (the cone shaped distal end of the spinal cord, surrounded by the sacral nerves) may manifest a mixture of clinical features.

However, in practice, management tends to follow a common pathway.

Aims

1 Primary: to achieve the controlled regular evacuation of normal formed faeces:
   - every day in long-term paraplegia/tetraplegia, e.g. post-traumatic
   - every 1–3 days in advanced cancer.

2 Secondary: to prevent both incontinence (faeces too soft, over-treatment with laxatives) and an anal fissure (faeces too hard, under-treatment with laxatives).

Oral measures

3 In debilitated patients with a poor appetite, a bulking agent is unlikely to be helpful, and may result in a soft impaction.

4 Particularly if taking morphine or another constipating drug, an oral stimulant laxative should be prescribed, e.g. senna 15mg b.d., bisacodyl tablets 5–10mg b.d. The dose should be carefully titrated to a level which results in normal faeces *in the rectum* but without causing an uncontrolled evacuation.

5 In relatively well patients with a good appetite (probably the minority):
   - maintain a high fluid intake
   - encourage a high roughage diet, e.g. wholegrain cereals, wholemeal foods, greens, bran or a bulk-forming laxative, e.g. ispaghula.

6 Beware:
   - the prescription of docusate sodium, a faecal softener, may result in a soft faecal impaction of the rectum, and faecal leakage through a patulous anus
   - oral bisacodyl in someone not on opioids may cause multiple uncontrolled evacuations, at the wrong time and in the wrong place.

Rectal measures

7 Initially, if impacted with faeces, empty the rectum digitally. Then, develop a daily routine:
   - as soon as convenient after waking up in the morning, insert 2 glycerol suppositories, or 1–2 bisacodyl suppositories (10–20mg), or an osmotic micro-enema deep into the rectum, and wait for 1.5–2h
   - because the bisacodyl acts only after absorption and biotransformation, bisacodyl suppositories must be placed against the rectal wall, and not into faeces
   - the patient should be encouraged to have a hot drink after about 1h in the hope that it will stimulate a gastro-colonic reflex
   - if there is a strong sacral reflex, some faeces will be expelled as a result of the above two measures
   - to ensure complete evacuation of the rectum and sigmoid colon, digitally stimulate the rectum:
     - ▷ insert gloved and lubricated finger (either soap or gel)
     - ▷ rotate finger 3–4 times
     - ▷ withdraw and wait 5min
     - ▷ if necessary, repeat 3–4 times
     - ▷ check digitally that rectum is fully empty.

8 Patients who are unable to transfer to the toilet or a commode will need nursing assistance. Sometimes it is easiest for a patient to defaecate onto a pad while in bed in a lateral position.

9 If the above measures do not achieve complete evacuation of the rectum and sigmoid colon, proceed to digital evacuation (more likely with a flaccid bowel). A pattern will emerge for each patient, allowing the rectal measures to be adjusted to the individual patient's needs and response.

Updated August 2017

ISPAGHULA (PSYLLIUM) HUSK

Ispaghula husk is *not recommended* for patients taking constipating drugs, and in those with decreasing dietary intake and activity. However, it can be helpful in regulating the consistency of faeces (making them more formed) in a patient with a colostomy/distal ileostomy.

Class: Bulk-forming laxative.

Indications: Colostomy/ileostomy regulation, anal fissure, haemorrhoids, diverticular disease, irritable bowel syndrome, ulcerative colitis.

Contra-indications: Dysphagia, bowel obstruction, colonic atony, faecal impaction.

Pharmacology

Ispaghula (psyllium) is derived from the husks of an Asian plant, *Plantago ovata*. It has very high water-binding capacity, is partly fermented in the colon, and increases bacterial cell mass, thereby further increasing faecal bulk. Like other bulk-forming laxatives, ispaghula stimulates peristalsis by increasing faecal mass. Its water-binding capacity also helps to make loose faeces more formed in some patients with a colostomy/distal ileostomy.
Onset of action full effect obtained only after several days.
Duration of action best taken regularly to obtain a consistent ongoing effect; may continue to act for 2–3 days after the last dose.

Cautions

Adequate fluid intake should be maintained to avoid bowel obstruction.

Undesirable effects

Flatulence, abdominal distension, faecal impaction, bowel obstruction.

Dose and use

Ispaghula swells in contact with fluid and needs to be drunk quickly before it absorbs water. Stir the granules or powder briskly in 150mL of water and swallow immediately; carbonated water can be used if preferred. Alternatively, the granules can be swallowed dry, or mixed with a vehicle such as jam, but must be followed by 100–200mL of water. Give 1 sachet each morning–t.d.s., preferably after meals; not immediately before going to bed.

Supply

Ispaghula husk (generic)
Oral granules 3.5g/sachet, 28 days @ 1 sachet b.d. = £5; *low* Na^+*; sugar- and gluten-free; plain, lemon or orange flavour.*

Updated (minor change) July 2017

STIMULANT LAXATIVES

Indications: Prevention and treatment of constipation.

Contra-indications: Severe dehydration, acute inflammatory bowel disease, large bowel obstruction.

Pharmacology

Stimulant laxatives act through direct contact with the submucosal (Meissner's) plexus and the deeper myenteric (Auerbach's) plexus, resulting in both a motor and a secretory effect in the large intestine. The motor effect precedes the secretory effect, and is the more important laxative action. There is a decrease in segmenting muscular activity and an increase in propulsive waves.

Senna (sennosides) is a naturally-occurring plant-derived anthranoid and a pro-drug. It passes unabsorbed and unchanged through the small intestine as an inactive glycoside and is hydrolyzed by *bacterial glycosidases* in the large intestine to yield active compounds.[1] Thus, **senna** has no effect on the small intestine but becomes active in the large intestine. Differences in bacterial flora may be partly responsible for differences in individual responses.

Dantron is a synthetic anthranoid. It is not a glycoside, and has a direct action on the large intestine.[2] Whereas systemic absorption of **senna** or its metabolites is small, **dantron** is absorbed to some extent from the small intestine with subsequent significant urinary excretion.

Bisacodyl and **sodium picosulfate** are phenolics and are both pro-drugs. They are hydrolyzed to the same active metabolite bis-(p-hydroxyphenyl)-pyridyl-2-methane (BHPM).[1] **Bisacodyl** is hydrolyzed by *intestinal enzymes* and, when applied directly to the intestinal mucosa in normal subjects, it induces powerful propulsive motor activity within minutes.[3] To ensure a laxative effect in the colon after oral intake, **bisacodyl** is formulated as an e/c tablet. **Sodium picosulfate** is hydrolyzed by *colonic bacteria*, and thus potentially has a more uncertain action because of its dependence on bacterial flora.

Bisacodyl is often given by suppository. The laxative effect is the result of local direct contact with the rectal mucosa after dissolution of the suppository and after activation by hydrolysis. Thus the minimum time for response is generally >20min.[4]

There is convincing evidence supporting the efficacy of **bisacodyl** versus placebo and **sodium picosulphate** versus placebo in patients with chronic constipation.[5–7]

Phenolphthalein (not UK) is a stimulant laxative that is present in some proprietary laxatives, e.g. Fam-Lax. It is generally *not* recommended for use in palliative care as it can cause a drug rash or photosensitivity. Rarely, it causes encephalitis which can be fatal. It is also associated with increased risk of developing cancer. Laxatives containing this are prohibited in many countries.[8]

To date, RCTs of stimulant laxatives in palliative care patients have failed to show clinically meaningful differences (see Laxatives, Table 2, p.40). A small non-blinded dose-ranging study in palliative care patients with opioid-induced constipation, showed that **sodium picosulfate** alone yielded a satisfactory result in 15/20 patients (normal stool consistency, no need for enemas, suppositories or manual evacuation, and no noteworthy undesirable effects).[9]

In the past, a combination of a bowel stimulant with a stool softener was often prescribed in palliative care patients.[10,11] However, the results of the RCT which compared **senna** alone with **senna** and **docusate** in hospice patients (see Laxatives, Table 2, p.40)[12] and comparable results from a non-randomized non-blinded sequential cohort study in cancer inpatients suggest that *generally a stimulant laxative alone will be satisfactory.*[13] In countries where combined products are not available, this will also reduce the patient's tablet load.[14]

If a stimulant laxative is used alone but a satisfactory result is not achieved despite dose titration in a week, consider adding **docusate**. If faecal leakage occurs, the dose of this will need to be reduced.[10,15]

Onset of action

Bisacodyl tablets 6–12h;[4] suppositories 10–45min.[1]

Dantron 6–12h.

Senna 8–12h.

Sodium picosulfate 6–24h (median 12h).[9]

Cautions

Because very high doses in rodents revealed a carcinogenic risk,[16–18] UK marketing authorizations for laxatives containing **dantron** are limited to constipation in terminally ill patients.

Undesirable effects

Intestinal colic, diarrhoea. **Bisacodyl** suppositories may cause local rectal inflammation. **Dantron** discolours urine, typically red but sometimes green or bluish. It may also stain the peri-anal skin. Prolonged contact with skin (e.g. in urinary or faecally incontinent patients) may cause a **dantron** burn (a red erythematous rash with a definite edge); if ignored, this may cause painful excoriation.

Dose and use

The doses recommended here for opioid-induced constipation are often higher than those featured in the BNF and SPCs. For frail patients not receiving opioids or other constipating drugs, the PO starting doses of a stimulant laxative will generally be lower.

Because round-the-clock opioids constipate, b.d. or t.d.s. laxatives may well be necessary, rather than the traditional once daily dose (at bedtime or each morning). Requirements do not correlate closely with the opioid dose; individual titration is necessary.

All palliative care services should have a protocol for the management of opioid-induced constipation (see QCG: Opioid-induced constipation, p.42).[19–22] Likewise, there is need for a protocol for patients with paraplegia and tetraplegia (see QCG: Bowel management in paraplegia and tetraplegia, p.44).

Bisacodyl

If *not* constipated:

- generally start with 5mg PO at bedtime
- if no response after 24–48h, increase to 10mg at bedtime.

If already constipated:

- generally start with 10mg PO at bedtime
- if no response after 24–48h, increase to 20mg at bedtime
- if no response after a further 24–48h, consider adding a second daytime dose
- if necessary, consider increasing to a maximum of 20mg t.d.s.

By suppository: give 10–20mg PR once daily. For an optimal result, it is best to give **bisacodyl** suppositories *30min after breakfast* and thereby co-ordinate the drug response with the gastrocolonic reflex.[23]

Dantron

Because of the undesirable effects and cost (see Supply), other stimulant laxatives are preferred.

Senna

If *not* constipated:

- generally start with 15mg at bedtime
- if no response after 24–48h, increase to 15mg at bedtime and each morning.

If already constipated:

- generally start with 15mg at bedtime and each morning
- if no response after 24–48h, increase to 22.5mg at bedtime and each morning
- if no response after a further 24–48h, consider adding a third daytime dose
- if necessary, consider increasing to a maximum of 30mg t.d.s.

Senna oral solution (7.5mg/5mL) can be used instead of tablets; it is tasteless and odourless.

Sodium picosulfate

- start with 5–10mg (5–10mL of oral solution) at bedtime; 10mg if taking regular opioids
- if necessary, increase daily by 5mg until a satisfactory result is achieved
- median satisfactory dose = 15mg at bedtime
- typical maximum dose = 30mg.[9]

Consider a lower dose b.d. in the frail elderly.

Supply

Bisacodyl (generic)

Tablets e/c 5mg, 28 days @ 10mg at bedtime = £2.

Suppositories 5mg, 10mg, 28 days @ 10mg once daily = £8.

Dantron

Co-danthramer (dantron and **poloxamer 188)** (generic)

Oral suspension **co-danthramer** 25/200 in 5mL (**dantron** 25mg, **poloxamer 188** 200mg/5mL), 28 days @ 10mL at bedtime = £136.

Strong oral suspension **co-danthramer** 75/1000 in 5mL (**dantron** 75mg, **poloxamer 188** 1g/5mL), 28 days @ 5mL at bedtime = £136.

Co-danthrusate (dantron and **docusate sodium)** (generic)

Capsules **co-danthrusate** 50/60 (**dantron** 50mg, **docusate sodium** 60mg), 28 days @ 2 at bedtime = £46.

Oral suspension **co-danthrusate** 50/60 in 5mL (**dantron** 50mg, **docusate sodium** 60mg/5mL), 28 days @ 10mL at bedtime = £126.

Senna (generic)

Tablets total **sennosides**/tablet 7.5mg, 28 days @ 15mg b.d. = £3.75.

Senokot® (Reckitt Benckiser)

Oral solution (sugar-free) total **sennosides** 7.5mg/5mL, 28 days @ 10mL b.d.= £5.50.

Sodium picosulfate (generic)

Oral solution (elixir) 5mg/5mL, 28 days @ 10mL at bedtime = £6.50; *contains alcohol.*

Note. **Sodium picosulfate** oral solution 5mg/5mL is available as Dulcolax® Pico liquid. The proprietary name Dulcolax® (NHS) is also used for **bisacodyl** tablets and suppositories.

1 Jauch R *et al.* (1975) Bis-(p-hydroxyphenyl)-pyridyl-2-methane: the common laxative principle of bisacodyl and sodium picosulfate. *Arzneimittel-Forschung Drug Research.* **25**: 1796–1800.

2 Lennard-Jones J (1994) Clinical aspects of laxatives, enemas and suppositories. In: M Kamm and J Lennard-Jones (eds) *Constipation.* Wrightson Biomedical Publishing, Petersfield, pp. 327–341.

3 De Schryver AM *et al.* (2003) Effects of a meal and bisacodyl on colonic motility in healthy volunteers and patients with slow-transit constipation. *Digestive Diseases Sciences.* **48**: 1206–1212.

4 Flig E *et al.* (2000) Is bisacodyl absorbed at all from suppositories in man? *International Journal of Pharmaceutics.* **196**: 11–20.

5 Kamm MA *et al.* (2011) Oral bisacodyl is effective and well-tolerated in patients with chronic constipation. *Clinical Gastroenterology and Hepatology.* **9**: 577–583.

6 Mueller-Lissner S *et al.* (2010) Multicenter, 4-week, double-blind, randomized, placebo-controlled trial of sodium picosulfate in patients with chronic constipation. *American Journal of Gastroenterology.* **105**: 897–903.

7 Nelson AD *et al.* (2016) Comparison of efficacy of pharmacological treatments for chronic idiopathic constipation: a systematic review and network meta-analysis. *Gut.* **66**: 1611–1622.

8 Cooper GS *et al.* (2000) Risk of ovarian cancer in relation to use of phenolphthalein-containing laxatives. *British Journal of Cancer.* **83**: 404–406.

9 Twycross RG *et al.* (2006) Sodium picosulfate in opioid-induced constipation: results of an open-label, prospective, dose-ranging study. *Palliative Medicine.* **20**: 419–423.

10 Larkin PJ *et al.* (2008) The management of constipation in palliative care: clinical practice recommendations. *Palliative Medicine.* **22**: 796–807.

11 Portenoy RK (1987) Constipation in the cancer patient: causes and management. *Medical Clinics of North America.* **71**: 303–311.

12 Tarumi Y *et al.* (2013) Randomized, double-blind, placebo-controlled trial of oral docusate in the management of constipation in hospice patients. *Journal of Pain and Symptom Management.* **45**: 2–13.

13 Sykes N (2013) Emerging evidence on docusate: commentary on Tarumi et al. *Journal of Pain Symptom Management.* **45**: 1.

14 Hawley PH and Byeon JJ (2008) A comparison of sennosides-based bowel protocols with and without docusate in hospitalized patients with cancer. *Journal of Palliative Medicine.* **11**: 575–581.

15 NICE (2013) Palliative cancer care - constipation. Clinical Knowledge Summaries. http://cks.nice.org.uk

16 Mori H *et al.* (1985) Induction of intestinal tumours in rats by chrysazin. *British Journal of Cancer.* **52**: 781–783.

17 Mori H *et al.* (1986) Carcinogenicity of chrysazin in large intestine and liver of mice. *Japanese Journal of Cancer Research (Gann).* **77**: 871–876.

18 CSM (Committee on Safety of Medicines and Medicines Control Agency) (2000) Danthron restricted to constipation in the terminally ill. *Current Problems in Pharmacovigilance.* **26 (May)**: 4.

19 Levy MH (1996) Pharmacologic treatment of cancer pain. *N Engl J Med.* **335**: 1124–1132.

20 Pappagallo M (2001) Incidence, prevalence, and management of opioid bowel dysfunction. *American Journal of Surgery.* **182 (Suppl 5A)**: 11s–18s.

21 Bouvy ML *et al.* (2002) Laxative prescribing in relation to opioid use and the influence of pharmacy-based intervention. *Journal of Clinical Pharmacy and Therapeutics.* **27**: 107–110.

22 Herndon CM *et al.* (2002) Management of opioid-induced gastrointestinal effects in patients receiving palliative care. *Pharmacotherapy.* **22**: 240–250.

23 Bharucha AE *et al.* (2013) American Gastroenterological Association technical review on constipation. *Gastroenterology.* **144**: 218–238.

Updated August 2017

DOCUSATE SODIUM

Class: Surface-wetting agent (faecal softener).

Indications: Constipation, haemorrhoids, anal fissure, bowel preparation before abdominal radiography, †partial bowel obstruction.

Contra-indications: Fructose or sorbitol intolerance (capsules contain sorbitol).

Pharmacology

Although sometimes classified as a stimulant laxative, docusate sodium is principally an emulsifying and wetting agent. In most patients, it has a relatively weak effect on GI transit at doses commonly used (≤400mg/24h). Other wetting agents include **poloxamer 188** (in **co-danthramer**). Docusate lowers surface tension, thereby allowing water and fats to penetrate hard, dry faeces. It also stimulates fluid secretion by the small and large intestines.[1,2] Docusate does not interfere with protein or fat absorption.[3] Docusate has been evaluated in several groups of elderly patients; frequency of defaecation increased and the need for enemas decreased almost to zero.[4–6] Given these clinical results, it is surprising that, in a study in normal subjects, docusate did not increase faecal weight.[7]

In palliative care, docusate is generally *not* recommended as the sole laxative except in patients with partial bowel obstruction. The routine combination of docusate (or alternative surface-wetting agent) and a stimulant laxative has been criticized because of a lack of published data supporting such a regimen.[8] A non-randomized non-blinded sequential cohort study in cancer inpatients failed to show any benefit when docusate was added to **senna**.[9] A more recent 10-day blinded RCT in hospice patients of docusate and **senna** vs **senna** alone likewise showed no significant difference.[10] However, a high proportion of patients in each group required rescue rectal interventions (around 70%), suggesting neither treatment was fully effective. The dose of **senna** could be titrated to response but the dose of docusate was fixed (200mg b.d.), and this may not have been optimal for some patients.[11] On the other hand, it is a high dose in terms of typical UK practice with stimulant-softener laxative combination regimens (e.g. **co-danthrusate**) for opioid-induced constipation.
Onset of action 1–2 days.

Cautions

Docusate enhances the absorption of **liquid paraffin**;[12] combined preparations of these substances are prohibited in some countries.

Undesirable effects

Diarrhoea, nausea, abdominal cramp, rashes. Docusate oral solution may cause a bitter aftertaste or burning sensation, minimized by drinking plenty of water after taking the solution.

Dose and use

Despite evidence suggesting it is generally unnecessary, many centres still routinely use docusate in combination with a stimulant laxative, e.g. **senna, bisacodyl** (see p.46). Docusate is often used alone for patients with persistent partial bowel obstruction. Dose varies according to individual need:

- generally start with 100mg PO b.d.
- if necessary, increase to 200mg b.d.–t.d.s.; *the latter is higher than the authorized maximum dose of 500mg/day.*

Docusate can also be used as an enema (see Rectal products, p.55).

Supply

Docusate sodium (generic)
Capsules 100mg, 28 days @ 100mg b.d. = £4.
Oral solution (sugar-free) 12.5mg/5mL, 50mg/5mL, 28 days @ 100mg b.d. = £15.

For combination products containing docusate and **dantron** (**co-danthrusate**) or **poloxamer 188** and **dantron** (**co-danthramer**), see Stimulant laxatives, p.46.

1 Donowitz M and Binder H (1975) Effect of dioctyl sodium sulfosuccinate on colonic fluid and electrolyte movement. *Gastroenterology*. **69**: 941–950.
2 Moriarty K *et al.* (1985) Studies on the mechanism of action of dioctyl sodium sulphosuccinate in the human jejunum. *Gut*. **26**: 1008–1013.
3 Wilson J and Dickinson D (1955) Use of dioctyl sodium sulfosuccinate (aerosol O.T.) for severe constipation. *Journal of the American Medical Association*. **158**: 261–263.
4 Cass L and Frederik W (1956) Doxinate in the treatment of constipation. *American Journal of Gastroenterology*. **26**: 691–698.
5 Harris R (1957) Constipation in geriatrics. *American Journal of Digestive Diseases*. **2**: 487–492.
6 Hyland C and Foran J (1968) Dicotyl sodium sulphosuccinate as a laxative in the elderly. *Practitioner*. **200**: 698–699.
7 Chapman R *et al.* (1985) Effect of oral dioctyl sodium sulfosuccinate on intake-output studies of human small and large intestine. *Gastroenterology*. **89**: 489–493.
8 Hurdon V *et al.* (2000) How useful is docusate in patients at risk for constipation? A systematic review of the evidence in the chronically ill. *Journal of Pain and Symptom Management*. **19**: 130–136.
9 Hawley PH and Byeon JJ (2008) A comparison of sennosides-based bowel protocols with and without docusate in hospitalized patients with cancer. *Journal of Palliative Medicine*. **11**: 575–581.
10 Tarumi Y *et al.* (2013) Randomized, double-blind, placebo-controlled trial of oral docusate in the management of constipation in hospice patients. *Journal of Pain and Symptom Management*. **45**: 2–13.
11 Sykes N (2013) Emerging evidence on docusate: commentary on Tarumi et al. *Journal of Pain Symptom Management*. **45**: 1.
12 Godfrey H (1971) Dangers of dioctyl sodium sulfosuccinate in mixtures. *Journal of the American Medical Association*. **215**: 643.

Updated August 2017

LACTULOSE

Class: Osmotic laxative.

Indications: Constipation, hepatic encephalopathy.

Contra-indications: Intestinal obstruction, galactosaemia.

Pharmacology

Lactulose is a synthetic disaccharide, a combination of galactose and fructose, which is not absorbed by the small intestine.[1] It is a 'small bowel flusher', i.e. through an osmotic effect lactulose deposits a large volume of fluid into the large intestine. Lactulose is fermented by colonic bacteria to organic acids which act as contact stimulants in the large bowel.

The low pH discourages the proliferation of ammonia-producing organisms and thus reduces the absorption of ammonium ions and other nitrogenous compounds; hence its use in hepatic encephalopathy.[2]

Lactulose has been shown to be more effective than increasing dietary fibre.[3] It also increases colonic bacterial flora, i.e. is prebiotic (whereas **macrogols** are not).[4] Lactulose does not affect the management of diabetes mellitus; 15mL of Duphalac® (NHS) contains 14 calories. However, because bio-availability is negligible, the number of calories absorbed is negligible. (Note. Other generic products may differ.)

In a small RCT in palliative care patients receiving high-dose strong opioids, those given a combination of lactulose and **senna** had more bowel evacuations compared with those given **co-danthramer**, but there was no difference in patient preference.[5] In healthy volunteers, lactulose alone was effective in opioid-induced constipation, but the volumes required (mean 55mL b.d.) is likely to preclude widespread use.[6]

A Cochrane review of lactulose and **macrogols** for chronic constipation concluded that **macrogols** are better than lactulose in terms of bowel movements per week, faecal consistency, relief of abdominal pain, and the need for additional products.[7] This review included 10 trials, with a total of nearly 900 patients, aged 3 months to 70 years. However, the volume per dose of **macrogols** is 5–10 times greater than lactulose (see p.51), which will be unacceptable to many patients. Lactulose is also cheaper.

Bio-availability negligible.

Onset of action up to 48h.

Cautions

Lactose intolerance.

Undesirable effects

Abdominal bloating, flatulence (generally only in the first few days of treatment), nausea (may be reduced if diluted with water or fruit juice, or taken with meals), intestinal colic.

Dose and use

Lactulose can be used in patients who experience intestinal colic with stimulant laxatives, or who fail to respond to stimulant laxatives alone:

- start with 15mL b.d. and adjust according to need
- in hepatic encephalopathy, start with 30–50mL t.d.s. and adjust the dose to produce 2–3 soft evacuations per day.

Supply

Lactulose (generic)
Oral solution 10g/15mL, 28 days @ 15mL b.d. = £5.
Oral solution (sachets) 10g/15mL sachet, 28 days @ one sachet b.d. = £14.

1 Schumann C (2002) Medical, nutritional and technological properties of lactulose. An update. *European Journal of Nutrition.* **41 (Suppl 1)**: 117–25.
2 Zeng Z *et al.* (2006) Influence of lactulose on the cognitive level and quality of life in patients with minimal hepatic encephalopathy. *Chinese Journal of Clinical Rehabilitation.* **10**: 165–167.
3 Quah HM *et al.* (2006) Prospective randomized crossover trial comparing fibre with lactulose in the treatment of idiopathic chronic constipation. *Techniques in Coloproctology.* **10**: 111–114.
4 Bouhnik Y *et al.* (2004) Prospective, randomized, parallel-group trial to evaluate the effects of lactulose and polyethylene glycol-4000 on colonic flora in chronic idiopathic constipation. *Alimentary Pharmacology and Therapeutics.* **19**: 889–899.
5 Sykes N (1991) A clinical comparison of laxatives in a hospice. *Palliative Medicine.* **5**: 307–314.
6 Sykes NP (1996) A volunteer model for the comparison of laxatives in opioid-related constipation. *Journal of Pain and Symptom Management.* **11**: 363–369.
7 Lee-Robichaud H *et al.* (2010) Lactulose versus polyethylene glycol for chronic constipation. *Cochrane Database of Systematic Reviews.* **7**: CD007570. www.thecochranelibrary.com

Updated August 2017

MACROGOLS (POLYETHYLENE GLYCOLS)

Class: Osmotic laxative.

Indications: Constipation, faecal impaction (macrogol 3350 sachets).

Contra-indications: Acute inflammatory bowel disease, bowel obstruction, paralytic ileus.

Pharmacology

Macrogol 3350 is available in the UK (the number refers to the molecular weight). It acts by virtue of an osmotic action in the intestines. Due to the large molecular structure of the macrogol, water is not transported across the bowel wall out of the lumen and hence the volume of the macrogol solution is retained within the lumen to soften the stool directly and stimulate peristalsis indirectly (by producing an increase in faecal volume).

Macrogols are unchanged in the GI tract, virtually unabsorbed and have no known pharmacological activity. Any absorbed macrogols are excreted via the urine; no reduction is required in renal impairment. Macrogols reduce colonic bacterial flora, whereas **lactulose** causes an increase.[1]

Most studies have used isotonic solutions. Adding more water to make a hypotonic (dilute) solution of macrogols is as effective as an isotonic solution in treating constipation but causes hyponatraemia.[2] There are no data on the effect on appetite of the volume of fluid needed with macrogols.

There are no studies in chronic constipation comparing macrogols with stimulant laxatives. However, when clearing the colon before colonoscopy, macrogols are inferior to stimulant laxatives.[3,4]

In an RCT in opioid-induced constipation, macrogols were found to be no better than **lactulose**.[5] On the other hand, a Cochrane review of macrogols and **lactulose** for chronic constipation in adults and in children concluded that macrogols are better than **lactulose** in terms of bowel movements per week, faecal consistency, relief of abdominal pain (children only), and the need for additional products.[6] However, the volume per dose of macrogols is 5–10 times greater than **lactulose** (see p.50); this will be unacceptable to many patients.

A systematic review in children suggested that macrogols may be better than other treatments but the evidence is poor.[7] However, in faecal impaction in children, macrogols are no better than enemas, and cause more faecal incontinence.[8] Children also find macrogols less palatable than **lactulose**.[9] They are also more expensive.

Onset of action 1–2 days for constipation; 1–3 days for faecal impaction.

Cautions

Stop treatment if symptoms of fluid and electrolyte shift occur (see Undesirable effects).

Macrogol 3350 *concentrated oral liquid* contains ethanol and a large amount of benzyl alcohol. Because the dose required for faecal impaction would exceed the maximum acceptable daily intake of benzyl alcohol, this formulation is not authorized for faecal impaction, and the manufacturer's maximum recommended dose for constipation is 25mL (diluted with 100mL of water) t.d.s.

Drug interactions

There are reports of decreased effect of other drugs when taken at the same time as macrogols, e.g. anti-epileptics. Accordingly, other drugs should not be taken within an hour of taking macrogol.[10]

Undesirable effects

Uncommon (<1%, >0.1%): abdominal bloating, discomfort, borborygmi, hyponatraemia (when used as a hypotonic solution), nausea.

Very rare (<0.01%): severe electrolyte shift (oedema, shortness of breath, heart failure, dehydration).

Frequency unknown: hyper- or hypokalaemia (macrogol 3350 with electrolytes).

Dose and use

Macrogol 3350 is generally formulated with electrolyes and is available as an oral powder sachet, a concentrated oral liquid and an oral solution sachet. The powder and concentrated liquid products need to be dissolved or diluted in water:

- dissolve one sachet of oral powder in half a glass of water (about 125mL) *or*
- dilute 25mL of the concentrated oral liquid with 100mL water (total volume 125mL).

Half-strength macrogol 3350 (with electrolytes) and Paediatric oral powder sachets are available for fine-tuning the dose and should be dissolved in a quarter of a glass of water (about 60mL).

The solution is generally used immediately after reconstitution or dilution. However, reconstituted powder sachets can be kept (covered) for up to 6h in a refrigerator, and the diluted oral liquid can be kept (covered) for 24h at room temperature.

Note. Although the 25mL oral solution sachet (Movicol® Ready to Take) does not require further dilution, it is recommended that patients drink 2–2.5L fluid/24h to maintain good health.

Constipation

- start with one sachet or 125mL of *diluted* oral liquid concentrate PO once daily
- if necessary, increase to b.d. or t.d.s.

Faecal impaction

The concentrated oral liquid is not authorized for faecal impaction (see Cautions).

- start with eight sachets PO on day 1, taken in <6h
- patients with cardiovascular impairment should restrict intake to two sachets/h
- if necessary, repeat on days 2 and 3; most patients do not need the full dose on the second day.

For convenience, all eight oral powder sachets can be made up together in 1L of water and kept in a refrigerator for a maximum of 6h, after which any remaining solution should be discarded.

Note. For Movicol® Ready to take sachets, although the product itself does not require dilution, patients are recommended to take an additional 1L fluid.

I

Supply

Macrogol 3350 with electrolytes: sodium bicarbonate, sodium chloride and potassium chloride *(Containing per sachet or 25mL dose of oral liquid: Na^+ = 8mmol, K^+ = 0.7mmol, Cl^- = 7mmol and bicarbonate = 2mmol).*

Movicol® (Norgine)
Oral powder macrogol 3350 = 13.125g, 28 days @ one sachet once daily = £7; *available in plain (sugar-free), lime-lemon and chocolate flavour. Other brands include CosmoCol®, Laxido®, Macilax®, Molaxole®, Molative®; not all have the full range of flavours available.*
Concentrated oral liquid macrogol 3350 = 13.125g/25mL, 28 days @ 25mL (diluted with 100mL water) once daily = £7; *orange flavour, contains ethanol and benzyl alcohol.*

Movicol® Ready to take (Norgine)
Oral solution (sachet) macrogol 3350 = 13.125g, 25mL sachet, 28 days @ one sachet once daily = £3.50

Movicol-Half® (Norgine)
Oral powder macrogol 3350 = 6.563g, 28 days @ one sachet once daily = £4: *lime-lemon flavour (sugar-free).*
Other brands include CosmoCol-Half®.

Paediatric sachets are also available for children aged ≤12 years (see *BNFc*).

Note. Magrogol 3350 (with other salts and electrolytes) is available as Moviprep® and Klean-prep®; authorized for bowel cleansing before radiological examination, colonoscopy or surgery.

1 Bouhnik Y *et al.* (2004) Prospective, randomized, parallel-group trial to evaluate the effects of lactulose and polyethylene glycol-4000 on colonic flora in chronic idiopathic constipation. *Alimentary Pharmacology and Therapeutics.* **19**: 889–899.
2 Seinela L *et al.* (2009) Comparison of polyethylene glycol with and without electrolytes in the treatment of constipation in elderly institutionalized patients: a randomized, double-blind, parallel-group study. *Drugs and Aging.* **26**: 703–713.
3 Radaelli F *et al.* (2005) High-dose senna compared with conventional PEG-ES lavage as bowel preparation for elective colonoscopy: a prospective, randomized, investigator-blinded trial. *American Journal of Gastroenterology.* **100**: 2674–2680.
4 Valverde A *et al.* (1999) Senna vs polyethylene glycol for mechanical preparation the evening before elective colonic or rectal resection: a multicenter controlled trial. French Association for Surgical Research. *Archives of Surgery.* **134**: 514–519.
5 Freedman MD *et al.* (1997) Tolerance and efficacy of polyethylene glycol 3350/electrolyte solution versus lactulose in relieving opiate induced constipation: a double-blinded placebo-controlled trial. *Journal of Clinical Pharmacology.* **37**: 904–907.
6 Lee-Robichaud H *et al.* (2010) Lactulose versus polyethylene glycol for chronic constipation. *Cochrane Database of Systematic Reviews.* **7**: CD007570. www.thecochranelibrary.com
7 Gordon M *et al.* (2016) Osmotic and stimulant laxatives for the management of childhood constipation. *Cochrane Database of Systematic Reviews.* **8**: CD009118. www.thecochranelibrary.com
8 Bekkali NL *et al.* (2009) Rectal fecal impaction treatment in childhood constipation: enemas versus high doses oral PEG. *Pediatrics.* **124**: e1108–1115.
9 Voskuijl W *et al.* (2004) PEG 3350 (Transipeg) versus lactulose in the treatment of childhood functional constipation: a double blind, randomised, controlled, multicentre trial. *Gut.* **53**: 1590–1594.
10 Galen (2015) Laxido orange, powder for oral solution SPC, www.medicines.org.uk

Updated August 2017

MAGNESIUM SALTS

Class: Osmotic laxative.

Indications: Constipation, particularly in patients who experience intestinal colic with stimulant laxatives, or who fail to respond to the latter.

Contra-indications: Severe renal impairment.

Pharmacology

Magnesium ions are poorly absorbed from the gut. Their action is mainly osmotic but other factors may be important, e.g. the release of cholecystokinin.[1,2] Magnesium ions also decrease absorption or increase secretion in the small bowel.

Magnesium salts are generally not used first line in palliative care patients as they may be unpredictably effective. Magnesium sulfate is more potent than magnesium hydroxide and tends to produce a large volume of liquid faeces. In patients with idiopathic constipation, magnesium salts often lead to a sense of distension and the sudden passage of offensive liquid faeces which is socially inconvenient; it is difficult to adjust the dose to produce a normal soft result. However, when used as an osmotic laxative in conjunction with a stimulant laxative in opioid-induced constipation, this is not generally a problem.

An RCT of magnesium hydroxide and **liquid paraffin** vs. **senna** and **lactulose** failed to differentiate between the two combination treatments.[3]

Cautions

Risk of hypermagnesaemia in patients with renal impairment (see p.589).

Drug interactions

Oral magnesium salts act as antacids and the resulting increase in gastric pH may affect the absorption of several drugs if taken concurrently (see p.1).

Dose and use

For the treatment of hypomagnesaemia, see p.588.
For use of magnesium in antacids, see p.1.

Magnesium hydroxide

For opioid-induced constipation (see QCG: Opioid-induced constipation, p.42), as an alternative to **lactulose** when an osmotic laxative is indicated:

- if the maximum dose of a stimulant laxative (e.g. **dantron, senna**) is ineffective, halve the dose and add magnesium hydroxide 15–30mL b.d., and titrate as necessary; mix with water before administration
- alternatively, switch completely to magnesium hydroxide 15–60mL b.d.

Magnesium hydroxide (or **lactulose**) may be preferable in patients with a history of colic with stimulant laxatives (see p.46).

Magnesium sulfate

A typical dose is 5–10g of crystals/powder (one or two 5mL spoonfuls) once daily *before breakfast*; dissolve in about 250mL of warm water.

Supply

All the preparations below are available OTC.

Magnesium hydroxide

Oral suspension hydrated magnesium oxide 415mg (7.1mmol elemental magnesium)/5mL, 28 days @ 15mL b.d. = £14; available OTC as Phillips' Milk of Magnesia®; *do not store in a cold place*.

Magnesium sulfate

Oral powder (Epsom Salts) 4mmol/g elemental magnesium, 28 days @ 5g once daily = £1; also Original Andrew's Salts® (magnesium sulfate, citric acid, sodium bicarbonate).

1 Donowitz M (1991) Magnesium-induced diarrhea and new insights into the pathobiology of diarrhea. *New England Journal of Medicine*. **324**: 1059–1060.

2 Harvey R and Read A (1975) Mode of action of the saline purgatives. *American Heart Journal*. **89**: 810–813.

3 Sykes N (1991) A clinical comparison of lactulose and senna with magnesium hydroxide and liquid paraffin emulsion in a palliative care population. [cited in Candy B et *al*. (2011) Laxatives or methylnaltrexone for the management of constipation in palliative care patients. *Cochrane Database of Systematic Reviews*. CD003448. www.thecochranelibrary.com

Updated August 2017

RECTAL PRODUCTS FOR CONSTIPATION

Indications: Constipation and faecal impaction if oral laxatives are ineffective or not feasible.

Pharmacology

The evidence base for laxative suppositories and enemas in palliative care is generally limited to clinical experience and retrospective studies. Survey data indicate that about one third of palliative care patients receiving opioids require rectal measures (laxative suppositories, enemas and/or digital evacuation) either regularly and electively, or intermittently and p.r.n., generally in addition to laxatives PO (Table 1)[1] However, the need for enemas and digital evacuation has decreased since the introduction of **macrogols** (see p.51).[2,3]

Table 1 Rectal measures for the relief of constipation or faecal impaction[a]

Rectal laxative	*Dose/volume*	*Predominant mode of action*	*Time to effect[b]*
Suppositories[c]			
Bisacodyl	10mg	Stimulates propulsive activity after hydrolysis by enteric enzymes[4]	10–45min
Glycerol	4g	Hygroscopic; softens and lubricates	15–30min
Enemas[d]			
Osmotic micro-enema	5mL	Faecal softener and osmotic effect (see text below)	15min
Osmotic standard phosphate enema	118–128mL	Osmotic effect	2–5min
Docusate sodium micro-enema	120mg in 10g	Faecal softener (surface-wetting agent), some direct stimulant action	5–20min
Arachis (peanut) oil retention enema	130mL	Faecal softener	Overnight retention enema

a. PR digital examination will indicate the most appropriate intervention

b. as stated in SPC

c. suppositories should be administered only if there are faeces in the rectum; place in contact with the rectal mucosa

d. warm enemas to room temperature before use.

There is evidence supporting the use of **bisacodyl** suppositories in postoperative ileus[5] and in pre-colonoscopy preparations,[6] and of **docusate sodium** enemas in spinal injury patients.[7] In practice, for soft faeces, a **bisacodyl** suppository is given on its own; and, for hard faeces, **glycerol** alone or **glycerol** plus **bisacodyl**.

The laxative effect of **bisacodyl** is the result of local direct contact with the rectal mucosa after dissolution of the suppository and after activation by enteric enzymes (see p.46). The minimum time for response is thus generally >20min, and may be up to 3h.[8] Defaecation a few minutes after the insertion of a **bisacodyl** suppository is the result of anorectal stimulation. **Bisacodyl** suppositories occasionally cause faecal leakage, even after a successful evacuation.

Osmotic *micro-enemas* contain **sodium citrate** and **sodium lauryl sulfoacetate** with several excipients, including **glycerol** and **sorbitol**. **Sodium lauryl sulfoacetate** is a faecal softener (surface-wetting agent) similar to **docusate sodium** (see p.49), whereas **sodium citrate** draws fluid into the bowel by osmosis, an action enhanced by **sorbitol**.

Osmotic *standard enemas* contain phosphates. These should be used with caution in elderly patients because of a risk of serious electrolyte disturbances. Fatalities have been reported.[9]

When treating a hard faecal impaction, a **docusate sodium** micro-enema will help to soften the faecal mass. This should be instilled into the rectum and retained overnight before giving a stimulant suppository (**bisacodyl**) or an osmotic enema (Table 1).

An **arachis (peanut) oil** retention enema is sometimes used in patients with a hard faecal impaction: instil and leave overnight before giving a stimulant laxative suppository or an osmotic enema. *Do not use in patients with peanut allergy.*

Digital evacuation is the ultimate approach to faecal impaction but is a distressing procedure and may need sedation. Distress can be reduced by explaining the procedure, using plenty of lubrication, and encouraging the patient to respond to any urge to defaecate.

Supply

Suppositories
Bisacodyl (generic)
Suppositories 5mg, 10mg, 12 = £3.50.

Glycerol (generic)
Suppositories glycerol 700mg/1g, gelatin 140mg/1g, adult suppositories 4g, 12= £1.25.

Enemas
Docusate sodium (generic)
Norgalax® (Essential Pharma)
Micro-enema 120mg in 10g single-use disposable pack, one enema = £4.50.

Sodium citrate (generic)
Micro-enema 90mg/mL with **sodium lauryl sulfoacetate**, **glycerol** and **sorbitol**, supplied in 5mL single-dose disposable packs with nozzle, 5mL = £0.50.

Phosphate enema BP Formula B (generic)
Enema **sodium phosphate** 10.24g, **sodium acid phosphate** 12.8g, in 128mL, standard tube = £4, long rectal tube = £28.

Cleen Ready-to-use® (Casen Recordati)
Enema **sodium phosphate** 9.4g, **sodium acid phosphate** 21.4g, in 118mL, standard tube = £0.75.

Arachis (peanut) oil (generic)
Retention enema 1mg/mL, single-dose disposable pack, 130mL = £48; *do not use in patients with peanut allergy.*

1 Twycross RG and Harcourt JMV (1991) The use of laxatives at a palliative care centre. *Palliative Medicine*. **5**: 27–33.
2 Goldman M (1993) Hazards of phosphate enemas. *Gastroenterology Today*. **3**: 16–17.
3 Culbert P *et al.* (1998) Highly effective oral therapy (polyethylene glycol/electrolyte solution) for faecal impaction and severe constipation. *Clinical Drug Investigation*. **16**: 355–360.
4 von Roth W and von Beschke K (1988) Pharmakokinetik und laxierende wirkung von bisacodyl nach gabe verschiedener zubereitungsformen. *Arzneimittel Forschung Drug Research*. **38**: 570–574.
5 Wiriyakosol S *et al.* (2007) Randomized controlled trial of bisacodyl suppository versus placebo for postoperative ileus after elective colectomy for colon cancer. *Asian Journal of Surgery*. **30**: 167–172.
6 Rapier R and Houston C (2006) A prospective study to assess the efficacy and patient tolerance of three bowel preparations for colonoscopy. *Gastroenterology Nursing*. **29**: 305–308.
7 Amir I *et al.* (1998) Bowel care for individuals with spinal cord injury: comparison of four approaches. *Journal of Spinal Cord Medicine*. **21**: 21–24.
8 Flig E *et al.* (2000) Is bisacodyl absorbed at all from suppositories in man? *International Journal of Pharmaceutics*. **196**: 11–20.
9 Ori Y *et al.* (2012) Fatalities and severe metabolic disorders associated with the use of sodium phosphate enemas: a single center's experience. *Archives of Internal Medicine*. **172**: 263–265.

Updated August 2017

PRODUCTS FOR HAEMORRHOIDS

Because haemorrhoids can be more troublesome if associated with the evacuation of hard faeces, constipation must be corrected (see Laxatives, p.38).

Peri-anal pruritus, soreness and excoriation are generally best treated by the application of a bland ointment or cream. Suppositories are often not effective because they are inserted into the rectum, bypassing the anal canal where the medication is needed.

For haemorrhoids, products containing mild astringents (e.g. **bismuth subgallate, zinc oxide, hamamelis (witch hazel)**) often provide symptomatic relief. Some products, not featured here, also contain vasoconstrictors and/or antiseptics.

Lidocaine ointment is used mainly to relieve pain associated with an anal fissure, but will also relieve pruritus ani. Alternative local anaesthetics include **pramocaine (pramoxine)** and **cinchocaine (dibucaine)**. Painful spasm of the internal anal sphincter is often eased by topical **glyceryl trinitrate** ointment (off-label use; see p.81).

Local anaesthetic ointments are absorbed through the anal mucosa but, given the amount of ointment likely to be used, there is no realistic risk of systemic toxicity.[1] However, local anaesthetic ointments should be used for only a few days because all 'caines' can cause contact dermatitis.

Corticosteroids may be helpful if local inflammation is exacerbating discomfort. Infection (bacterial, viral, e.g. *Herpes simplex* or fungal, e.g. candidosis) must first be excluded, and treatment generally limited to 7–10 days because prolonged use with excessive amounts can lead to atrophy of the anal skin. However, this is unlikely with low concentration hydrocortisone.

Dose and use

Topical products should be applied:

- t.d.s.–q.d.s. for the first 24h
- then b.d. and after defaecation for 5–7 days, or longer if necessary
- then daily for 3–5 days after symptoms have cleared.

Products containing a local anaesthetic (to ease painful defaecation) are best applied 15–20min before defaecation, and p.r.n.

Supply

The following list is highly selective. Other OTC products are also available.

Astringent
Anusol® (McNeil)
Ointment **zinc oxide**, **bismuth subgallate**, **Peru balsam**, **bismuth oxide** 25g. (Available OTC).

Local anaesthetic
Lidocaine (generic)
Ointment 5%, 15g = £6.25.

Corticosteroid plus astringent
Anusol HC® (McNeil)
Ointment **hydrocortisone acetate** 0.25%, **zinc oxide**, **benzyl benzoate**, **bismuth oxide**, **bismuth subgallate**, **Peru balsam** 30g = £2.50. (Also available OTC as Anusol Plus HC ointment).

Corticosteroid plus local anaesthetic
Scheriproct® (Bayer)
Ointment **prednisolone hexanoate** 0.19%, **cinchocaine hydrochloride** 0.5%, 30g = £3.

Corticosteroid plus local anaesthetic and astringent
Xyloproct® (Astra Zeneca)
Ointment (water miscible) **hydrocortisone acetate** 0.275%, **lidocaine** 5%, **aluminium acetate** 3.5%, **zinc oxide**, 20g (with applicator) = £4.25.

1 Brosh-Nissimov T *et al.* (2004) Central nervous system toxicity following topical skin application of lidocaine. *European Journal of Clinical Pharmacology*. **60**: 683–684.

Updated May 2015

PANCREATIN

Class: Enzyme supplement.

Indications: †Symptomatic steatorrhoea caused by biliary and/or pancreatic obstruction.

Pharmacology

Steatorrhoea (the presence of undigested faecal fat) typically results in pale, bulky, offensive, frothy and greasy faeces which flush away with difficulty, associated with abdominal distension, increased flatus, weight loss, and mineral and vitamin deficiency (A, D, E and K).

Pancreatin is a preparation of porcine lipase, protease and amylase. Pancreatin hydrolyzes fats to glycerol and fatty acids, degrades protein into amino acids, and converts starch into dextrin and sugars. Because it is inactivated by gastric acid, pancreatin is best taken with food (or immediately before or after food).

Reducing gastric acid by concurrently prescribing a PPI leads to greater efficacy.[1] With gastro-resistant (e/c) granules, acid reduction is generally unnecessary provided the granules are swallowed whole without chewing.[2] However, in patients who are not adequately controlled on high-dose gastro-resistant pancreatin (e.g. ≥120,000 units of lipase/24h), concurrent prescription of a PPI generally leads to improvement.[3,4]

On the other hand, mixing e/c granules with alkaline foods or drinks, or crushing or chewing them before swallowing, destroys the gastro-resistant coating. This causes release of the enzymes in the mouth, possible stomatitis, and reduced efficacy.

Pancreatin has been used to clear feed-related blockages in enteral feeding tubes. However, this should only be considered when other options have failed (see Chapter 28, p.791).[5]

Cautions

Fibrotic strictures of the colon have developed in children with cystic fibrosis who have used certain high-strength pancreatin products. This has not been reported in adults or in patients without cystic fibrosis; higher strength Creon® 25,000 and Creon® 40,000 have not been implicated.

Undesirable effects

Very common (>10%): abdominal pain.
Common (<10%, >1%): nausea and vomiting, constipation or diarrhoea.

Dose and use

There are several different pancreatin products, all derived from pigs. Creon® is a good choice in terms of cost and range of strengths available. The dose is adjusted upwards according to faecal size, consistency, and frequency:

- generally start with Creon® 10,000 1–2 capsules with each meal
- if a smaller dose is required, use Creon® Micro; this contains 5,000 units of lipase in 100mg of granules
- if necessary, change to a higher strength capsule.

The granules in the capsules are gastro-resistant (e/c). The capsules may be swallowed whole, or the contents sprinkled onto slightly acidic fluid or soft food, e.g. fruit juice or apple sauce, and *swallowed without chewing:*

- avoid very hot food or drinks because heat inactivates pancreatin
- do not mix the capsule contents with alkaline foods or drinks, e.g. dairy products, because this degrades the gastro-resistant coating
- take immediately after mixing because the gastro-resistant coating starts to dissolve if left to stand.

Extra capsules may be needed if snacks are taken between meals. If the pancreatin continues to be ineffective, prescribe a PPI or H_2-receptor antagonist concurrently, and review.

Supply

Creon® (Abbott Healthcare)

Granules **(*gastro-resistant*)** Creon® Micro, lipase 5,000 units, amylase 3,600 units, protease 200 units in 100mg (measuring scoop provided), 28 days @ 100mg t.d.s. = £13.

Capsules (enclosing gastro-resistant granules) Creon® 10,000, lipase 10,000 units, amylase 8,000 units, protease 600 units, 28 days @ 2 t.d.s. = £22.

Higher strength capsules (enclosing gastro-resistant granules)

Creon® 25,000, lipase 25,000 units, amylase 18,000 units, protease 1,000 units, 28 days @ 2 t.d.s. = £47.

Creon® 40,000, lipase 40,000 units, amylase 25,000 units, protease 1,600 units, 28 days @ 2 t.d.s. = £70.

See BNF for other products available.

1 Vecht J *et al.* (2006) Efficacy of lower than standard doses of pancreatic enzyme supplementation therapy during acid inhibition in patients with pancreatic exocrine insufficiency. *Journal of Clinical Gastroenterology*. **40**: 721–725.

2 Stead RJ *et al.* (1988) Treatment of steatorrhoea in cystic fibrosis: a comparison of enteric-coated microspheres of pancreatin versus non-enteric-coated pancreatin and adjuvant cimetidine. *Alimentary Pharmacology and Therapeutics*. **2**: 471–482.

3 Proesmans M and De Boeck K (2003) Omeprazole, a proton pump inhibitor, improves residual steatorrhoea in cystic fibrosis patients treated with high dose pancreatic enzymes. *European Journal of Pediatrics*. **162**: 760–763.

4 Dominguez-Munoz JE *et al.* (2006) Optimising the therapy of exocrine pancreatic insufficiency by the association of a proton pump inhibitor to enteric coated pancreatic extracts. *Gut*. **55**: 1056–1057.

5 White R and Bradnam V. *Handbook of Drug Administration via Enteral Feeding Tubes*. London: Pharmaceutical Press www.medicinescomplete.com (accessed June 2015).

Updated July 2015

2: CARDIOVASCULAR SYSTEM

2

This chapter features cardiovascular drugs used in palliative *cancer* care. It does *not* include guidance about the drug treatment of end-stage congestive heart failure (CHF). *For guidance about simplifying medication in patients with end-stage CHF who appear to be imminently dying,* *see p.665.*

More detailed guidance about caring for patients with end-stage CHF is available from NICE[1] and various other authorities.[2–4] Additional resources include:

- *Heart failure: from advanced disease to bereavement*[5]
- *Supportive care in heart failure*[6]
- *Heart failure and palliative care: a team approach.*[7]

Unlike cancer, where disease-specific treatment tends to become increasingly burdensome and futile (and possibly counterproductive), the continued disease-specific treatment of CHF continues to be essential for symptom management even when end-stage.

Note. CHF can be a concurrent cause of breathlessness in some cancer patients, which needs to be recognized and treated appropriately.

1 NICE (2010) Chronic heart failure in adults: management. *Clinical Guideline* CG108. www.nice.org.uk
2 Arnold JM *et al.* (2006) Canadian Cardiovascular Society consensus conference recommendations on heart failure 2006: diagnosis and management. *Canadian Journal of Cardiology.* **22**: 23–45.
3 Hunt SA *et al.* (2005) Guideline update for the diagnosis and management of chronic heart failure in the adult. *Circulation.* **112**: e154–235.
4 Ponikowski P *et al.* (2016) 2016 ESC Guidelines for the diagnosis and treatment of acute and chronic heart failure: The Task Force for the diagnosis and treatment of acute and chronic heart failure of the European Society of Cardiology (ESC). Developed with the special contribution of the Heart Failure Association (HFA) of the ESC. *European Journal of Heart Failure.* **18**: 891–975.
5 Johnson M *et al.* (2013). *Heart failure: from advanced disease to bereavement.* Oxford University Press, Oxford.
6 Beattie J and Goodlin S (2008). *Supportive care in heart failure.* Supportive Care Series, Oxford University Press.
7 Johnson MJ and Lehman R (2006). *Heart failure and palliative care: a team approach.* Radcliffe Publishing Ltd, Oxford.

Updated February 2017

FUROSEMIDE

Class: Loop diuretic.

Indications: Oedema, hypertension (unresponsive to usual treatments), †malignant ascites associated with portal hypertension and hyperaldosteronism (with **spironolactone**).

Contra-indications: Hepatic encephalopathy, anuric renal failure.

Pharmacology

Loop diuretics inhibit Na^+ (and hence water) resorption from the ascending limb of the loop of Henlé in the renal tubule. They also increase urinary excretion of K^+, Mg^{2+}, H^+ and Cl^-. Loop diuretics, of which furosemide is the most commonly prescribed, are used to treat fluid overload in CHF and ESRF in order to improve symptoms of breathlessness and oedema.[1–4]

A diuretic-induced reduction in plasma volume can activate several neurohumoral systems, e.g. renin-aldosterone-angiotensin, resulting in impaired renal perfusion and increased Na^+ and water resorption. These changes contribute towards a reduced effect of the diuretic ('diuretic resistance') and also renal impairment. Strategies to overcome 'resistance' to furosemide include:

- a progressive increase in dose and b.d. administration
- switching to a loop diuretic with a higher/more consistent bio-availability
- adding a thiazide diuretic
- switching to parenteral administration.

Other loop diuretics include **bumetanide** and **torasemide**, with respective PO doses of 1mg and 10mg equivalent to 40mg of furosemide.[5–7] Compared with furosemide, they are more expensive, but they have a higher (≥80%) and more consistent PO bio-availability.[5,6] Thus, some patients may have a better diuresis when switched to them from furosemide.

In the UK, furosemide is the only loop diuretic available in a parenteral formulation. When switching from PO to IV because of fluid overload, a 1:1 conversion is generally used.[8] Based on bio-availability, this represents an increase in dose. Thus, although some use the same PO:IV conversion ratio in patients with *controlled oedema* no longer able to take drugs PO at the end of life, a conversion ratio of 2:1 may be sufficient. *Whatever the circumstance and dose used, patients receiving parenteral furosemide require close monitoring.*

Thiazide-type diuretics, e.g. **bendroflumethiazide**, **indapamide**, **metolazone** (not UK, but see Supply), block distal tubule Na^+ resorption and thereby antagonize part of the renal adaptations to a loop diuretic. All thiazides are equally effective when added to a PO/IV loop diuretic, and the combination can avoid the need for parenteral administration of a loop diuretic in both CHF and ESRF.[4,9] Close monitoring of plasma electrolytes and renal function is required, particularly because of the increased risk of hypokalaemia ± hypomagnesaemia. Initially, when diuresis is likely to be at its greatest, daily monitoring may be necessary. An aldosterone antagonist, e.g. **spironolactone**, is sometimes also added to augment the diuresis and conserve K^+.[9]

Compared with bolus IV doses, furosemide by CIVI appears to provide a greater diuresis with a similar or better safety profile.[10] However, the data are inconsistent and insufficiently robust to specifically recommend one approach rather than the other.[3]

Furosemide is effective when given by SC injection (off-label). However, because the concentration of the injection is 10mg/mL, volume considerations may limit feasibility. Diuresis reaches a maximum at 2–3h and lasts for about 4h.[11,12] Furosemide has been successfully given SC/CSCI as a means of avoiding hospital admission, and for when oral medication becomes problematic in the last days of life.[13,14] In a report of 47 episodes of the use of furosemide CSCI in 37 patients with end-stage CHF, the majority benefited (>80%), with mild or severe site reactions seen in one quarter and one episode respectively.[13]

Nebulized furosemide has been used in a patient at home with decompensated CHF as a temporary measure when IV access could not be established. A dose of 80mg resulted in a rapid improvement in pulmonary oedema and breathlessness, diuresis and a weight loss of 1kg. However, despite repeated daily doses, overall there was insufficient diuresis to prevent admission for central line insertion and IV furosemide.[15]

Ascites: when caused by a *transudate* associated with portal hypertension, e.g. from cirrhosis, extensive liver metastases, furosemide alone has little effect, even when used in total daily doses of 100–200mg PO.[16,17] Thus, furosemide in ascites is best limited to concurrent use with **spironolactone**, when the latter alone is insufficient (see p.67).

Octreotide 300microgram SC b.d. (see p.544) can suppress the diuretic-induced activation of the renin-aldosterone-angiotensin system and its addition has improved renal function and Na^+ and water excretion in patients with cirrhosis and ascites receiving furosemide and **spironolactone**.[18,19]

Breathlessness: There is current interest in the use of *nebulized* furosemide for the treatment of breathlessness (Box A). However, a review of 42 trials concluded that there was insufficient evidence to currently support its routine use.[20] Further, in one study,[21] 5/7 patients reported a deterioration in their breathing after furosemide. Thus, ideally, nebulized furosemide should be used only in a clinical trial.

Pharmacokinetic data are summarized in Table 1.

2

Box A Nebulized furosemide and breathlessness

Experimentally-induced cough and breathlessness

Allergen-induced asthma

Nebulized furosemide 20–40mg attenuates cough and breathlessness,[22–24] possibly via an effect on vagal sensory nerve endings.

The reduction in breathlessness may result from increasing sensory traffic to the brain stem from sensitized slowly adapting pulmonary stretch receptors. However, the effect:

- has not been demonstrated consistently
- shows wide interindividual variability
- is of short duration (generally <2h)
- systemic absorption can be sufficient to induce a diuresis.[25–27]

COPD

Compared with placebo in moderate–severe COPD, nebulized furosemide has reduced breathlessness ± increased exercise time during endurance testing,[28,29] but *not* incremental exercise testing.

The mechanism underlying the benefit is unclear, but improvements are seen in airway function (e.g. slow vital capacity at rest) and dynamic ventilatory mechanics (e.g. inspiratory capacity and breathing pattern).[29] Although small but significant bronchodilation was seen in one study,[28] this is unlikely to be a direct effect of nebulized furosemide.

When given alongside initial 'standard' treatment for an exacerbation of COPD, nebulized furosemide results in additional improvement in breathlessness and various respiratory parameters.[30] However, it does not have an established role in this setting.

Cancer

In patients with cancer, nebulized furosemide has been used to relieve severe breathlessness.[31,32] However, RCTs have failed to show benefit.[21,33]

Table 1 Pharmacokinetic details[34–36]

Drug	*Bumetanide*	*Furosemide*	*Torasemide*
Bio-availability PO (%)	80–95%	60–70%[a]	~80%
Onset of action (min)	30–60 PO ≤2 IV (not UK)	30–60 PO 30 SC 2–5 IV	≤60 PO ≤10 IV (not UK)
Tmax (h)	0.5–2 PO	1.5 PO	≤1 PO
Plasma halflife (h)	1–2	0.5–2 (healthy) 1–6 (CHF) 10 (ESRF)	3.5
Duration of action (h)	4–6 PO 2 IV	4–6 PO 4 SC 2 IV	≤8 PO/IV

a. varies widely due to erratic absorption and can be as low as 10%.

Cautions

Severe electrolyte disturbances (correct before treatment and monitor during use); elderly (lower doses); renal impairment (monitor during use); hepatic impairment; diabetes, hypoproteinaemia.

Some patients receive long-term diuretic therapy for hypertension or non-heart failure ankle oedema. This often becomes inappropriate as physical deterioration progresses, and may lead to postural hypotension and prerenal failure. In such circumstances the dose of furosemide should be reduced and possibly discontinued altogether. However, the withdrawal of diuretics requires careful monitoring to prevent the subsequent insidious onset of CHF.[37]

Drug interactions

Serious drug interactions: furosemide-induced electrolyte disturbances, particularly hypokalaemia, can increase the risk of:

- cardiac arrhythmia and death with drugs known to prolong the QT interval, e.g. **citalopram**, **methadone** (see p.731)
- **digoxin** toxicity
- **lithium** toxicity (possibly).[38]

Plasma electrolytes, drug concentrations, and the patient's clinical condition should be monitored closely.

Concurrent use of furosemide with **risperidone** is associated with an increased risk of death in elderly patients with dementia. The reason is unclear, but the manufacturer advises avoiding this combination unless the benefits clearly outweigh the risks.

Furosemide can *decrease* **vancomycin** levels by up to 50%.

Aliskiren, **phenytoin** (up to 50% reduction), **indometacin** and possibly other NSAIDs can reduce the diuretic effect of furosemide; a larger dose of furosemide may be required.

Additive pharmacodynamic interactions with furosemide increase the risk of:

- hypokalaemia with other K^+ depleting drugs, e.g. corticosteroids, β_2 agonists, and **theophylline**
- hyponatraemia with other Na^+ depleting drugs, e.g. **carbamazepine**
- hypotension with other drugs that lower blood pressure, e.g. ACE inhibitors, angiotensin II receptor antagonists, TCAs
- nephrotoxicity with other renally toxic drugs, e.g. NSAIDs, aminoglycosides
- ototoxicity, e.g. aminoglycosides, **vancomycin**.

Colestyramine, **colestipol** and **sucralfate** decrease absorption of furosemide; give furosemide 2–3h before these drugs.

Undesirable effects

Transient pain at the site of SC injection.[36]

Frequency not stated: dyspepsia, thirst, dizziness, dehydration, drowsiness, weakness, muscle cramps.
Rare: tinnitus and deafness (generally after rapid injection; may be permanent).
Biochemical disturbances: hyperglycaemia, hyperuricaemia, hypocalcaemia, hypokalaemia, hypomagnesaemia, hyponatraemia, metabolic alkalosis.

Dose and use

Ascites

Use only as a supplement to **spironolactone** (see p.67):

- start with 40mg PO each morning
- increase in steps of 40mg each morning every 3–5 days
- maximum dose 160mg each morning.

Symptomatic relief of fluid overload in CHF and ESRF

- start with 40mg PO each morning
- if necessary, increase the dose progressively in 40mg increments
- usual maximum daily dose 160mg, generally given as 80mg each morning and noon
- in patients admitted to hospital with decompensated CHF, much higher doses are sometimes used, e.g. ≤600mg/24h.[7]

The Frusol® brand of furosemide oral solution is authorized for administration via NG or PEG tubes, see SPC and also Chapter 28, p.785.

Once the excess fluid has been cleared, attempts can be made to reduce the furosemide to the lowest effective maintenance dose. Excessive diuresis is generally indicated by worsening renal function. Conversely, weight gain is an early indicator of fluid overload. Some patients are taught to adjust their diuretic dose according to changes in body weight.

Addition of a thiazide diuretic

Seek specialist advice: When there is an inadequate response to an optimally titrated dose of furosemide PO/IV, benefit may be obtained from the addition of a thiazide diuretic (see Pharmacology). A typical starting dose for **bendroflumethiazide**, **indapamide** and **metolazone** is 2.5mg PO given each morning or less frequently (see above); other thiazide diuretics can also be used.[9]

Close monitoring of plasma electrolytes, renal function, and clinical response (e.g. blood pressure, body weight, diuresis) is generally required. Particularly for outpatients, or with ongoing use, alternate day or even less frequent dosing is preferable, e.g. 1–2 times weekly.[7]

In ESRF, prolonged benefit has been obtained from short courses, e.g. **metolazone** 2.5–5mg once daily for 2–5 days.[4]

Parenteral administration

This may be necessary when the response to PO diuretics is inadequate in a patient with fluid overload, or when a patient is no longer able to take PO diuretics, e.g. at the end of life.

Patients with fluid overload

When switching from furosemide PO to IV a 1:1 conversion is generally used. Although data are mixed, the largest study to date suggests bolus IV and CIVI administration result in similar changes in patient's symptoms and renal function, and guidelines recommend either.[3,8] However, many centres only switch to CIVI when the maximum dose of bolus IV is insufficient, e.g.:

- start with *bolus IV:* 40–80mg b.d. (morning and noon); dilute with 0.9% saline to a suitable volume, e.g. 20mL, and give at a maximum rate of 4mg/min (2.5mg/min in severe renal impairment)
- if insufficient, switch to *CIVI:* 200–250mg/24h; dilute in a convenient volume of 0.9% saline
- generally, the fluid overload takes 3–5 days to clear; a switch back to the patient's usual PO maintenance dose of furosemide is then attempted.

Some palliative care services have used CSCI furosemide as a way of managing decompensated CHF in the hospice or community setting:[14]

- start with the same dose CSCI as the patient's current PO total daily dose
- weigh the patient daily
- after 48h, if the daily weight loss is not ≥1kg/day, consider obtaining cardiologist/heart failure nurse specialist advice; options include:
  - ▷ increasing the furosemide dose by 50%
  - ▷ adding a thiazide diuretic PO (see above)
  - ▷ adding or increasing the dose of an aldosterone antagonist, e.g. PO **spironolactone**
- because furosemide injection is 10mg/mL, practical daily dose limits for a CME T34 syringe driver are 200mg and 300mg for a 30mL and 50mL syringe respectively
- if CSCI furosemide fails to provide the necessary weight loss, admission to hospital/hospice for IV furosemide may be unavoidable.

Patients unable to take PO furosemide

For patients with CHF in the last days of life, unless anuric or clinically hypovolaemic, a loop diuretic should generally be continued for symptom management. Once unable to take furosemide PO:

- *if fluid overloaded*, switch to IV bolus or CSCI furosemide using a PO to IV conversion of 1:1 (this represents an increase in dose; see Pharmacology)
- if *not* fluid overloaded, although some use a 1:1 conversion, using half the PO dose IV may suffice.

Alternatively, in a patient without fluid overload, some clinicians will monitor the situation *daily* and only commence parenteral furosemide if fluid overload develops. *This approach requires the whole team to have the necessary expertise to monitor for symptoms and signs of pulmonary oedema.*

Incompatibility: Furosemide injection is alkaline and there is a high risk of *incompatibility* when mixed with acidic drugs. Because of this and the lack of compatibility data, *furosemide should not be mixed in the same syringe with any other drugs* (see p.822).[39]

If further dilution is required, 0.9% saline is recommended; do *not* mix or dilute with glucose solutions or other acidic fluids.

Supply

Furosemide (generic)
Tablets 20mg, 40mg, 500mg, 28 days @ 40mg each morning = £0.75.
Oral solution (sugar-free) 20mg/5mL, 40mg/5mL, 50mg/5mL, 28 days @ 40mg each morning = £17; *some formulations may contain alcohol.*
Injection 10mg/mL, 2mL amp = £0.25, 5mL amp = £0.75, 25mL amp = £2.50.

Bumetanide (generic)
Tablets 1mg, 5mg, 28 days @ 1mg each morning = £1.50.
Oral solution (sugar-free) 1mg/5mL, 28 days @ 1mg each morning = £157.

Torasemide (generic)
Tablets 5mg, 10mg, 28 days @ 10mg each morning = £19.
Torem (Meda)
Tablets 2.5mg, 5mg, 10mg, 28 days @ 10mg each morning = £8.

For thiazide diuretics, e.g. **bendroflumethiazide, indapamide** and **metolazone**, see the BNF.

Note. Although there is no authorized **metolazone** product available in the UK it is widely used, obtained as an imported special order product (see Chapter 24, p.751); it costs more than other thiazides, particularly the 2.5mg tablet.

1 NICE (2010) Chronic heart failure: management of chronic heart failure in adults in primary and secondary care *Clinical Guideline.* CG108. www.nice.org.uk
2 McMurray JJ *et al.* (2012) ESC Guidelines for the diagnosis and treatment of acute and chronic heart failure 2012: The Task Force for the Diagnosis and Treatment of Acute and Chronic Heart Failure 2012 of the European Society of Cardiology. Developed in collaboration with the Heart Failure Association (HFA) of the ESC. *European Heart Journal.* **33**: 1787–1847.
3 Yancy CW *et al.* (2013) 2013 ACCF/AHA guideline for the management of heart failure: a report of the American College of Cardiology Foundation/American Heart Association Task Force on practice guidelines. *Circulation.* **128**: e240–327.
4 Cheng HW *et al.* (2014) Combination therapy with low-dose metolazone and furosemide: a "needleless" approach in managing refractory fluid overload in elderly renal failure patients under palliative care. *International Urology and Nephrology.* **46**: 1809–1813.
5 Ward A and Heel RC (1984) Bumetanide. A review of its pharmacodynamic and pharmacokinetic properties and therapeutic use. *Drugs.* **28**: 426–464.
6 Vargo DL *et al.* (1995) Bioavailability, pharmacokinetics, and pharmacodynamics of torsemide and furosemide in patients with congestive heart failure. *Clinical Pharmacology and Therapeutics.* **57**: 601–609.
7 Heart Failure Society of America (2010) Comprehensive heart failure practice guideline. *Journal of Cardiac Failure.* **16**: e1–194.
8 Felker GM *et al.* (2011) Diuretic strategies in patients with acute decompensated heart failure. *New England Journal of Medicine.* **364**: 797–805.
9 Jentzer JC *et al.* (2010) Combination of loop diuretics with thiazide-type diuretics in heart failure. *Journal of the American College of Cardiology.* **56**: 1527–1534.
10 Amer M *et al.* (2012) Continuous infusion versus intermittent bolus furosemide in ADHF: an updated meta-analysis of randomized control trials. *Journal of Hospital Medicine.* **7**: 270–275.
11 Goenaga MA *et al.* (2004) Subcutaneous furosemide. *Annals of Pharmacotherpy.* **38**: 1751.
12 Farless LB *et al.* (2012) Intermittent subcutaneous furosemide: parentral diuretic rescue for hospice patients with congestive heart failure resistant to oral diuretic. *American Journal of Hospice and Palliative Care.* **30**: 791–792.
13 Zacharias H *et al.* (2011) Is there a role for subcutaneous furosemide in the community and hospice management of end-stage heart failure? *Palliative Medicine.* **26**: 658–663.
14 Galindo-Ocana J *et al.* (2013) Subcutaneous furosemide as palliative treatment in patients with advanced and terminal-phase heart failure. *British Medical Journal Supportive and Palliative Care.* **3**: 7–8.
15 Towers KA *et al.* (2010) Nebulised frusemide for the symptomatic treatment of end-stage congestive heart failure. *Medical Journal of Australia.* **193**: 555.
16 Amiel S *et al.* (1984) Intravenous infusion of frusemide as treatment for ascites in malignant disease. *British Medical Journal.* **288**: 1041.
17 Fogel M *et al.* (1981) Diuresis in the ascitic patient: a randomized controlled trial of three regimens. *Journal of Clinical Gastroenterology.* **3**: 73–80.
18 Kalambokis G *et al.* (2006) The effects of treatment with octreotide, diuretics, or both on portal hemodynamics in nonazotemic cirrhotic patients with ascites. *Journal of Clinical Gastroenterology.* **40**: 342–346.
19 Kalambokis G *et al.* (2005) Renal effects of treatment with diuretics, octreotide or both, in non-azotemic cirrhotic patients with ascites. *Nephrology, Dialysis, Transplantation.* **20**: 1623–1629.
20 Newton PJ *et al.* (2008) Nebulized furosemide for the management of dyspnea: does the evidence support its use? *Journal of Pain and Symptom Management.* **36**: 424–441.
21 Stone P *et al.* (2002) Re: nebulized furosemide for dyspnea in terminal cancer patients. *Journal of Pain and Symptom Management.* **24**: 274–275; author reply 275–276.
22 Ventresca P *et al.* (1990) Inhaled furosemide inhibits cough induced by low-chloride solutions but not by capsaicin. *American Review of Respiratory Disease.* **142**: 143–146.
23 Bianco S *et al.* (1989) Protective effect of inhaled furosemide on allergen-induced early and late asthmatic reactions. *New England Journal of Medicine.* **321**: 1069–1073.
24 Nishino T *et al.* (2000) Inhaled furosemide greatly alleviates the sensation of experimentally induced dyspnea. *American Journal of Respiratory and Critical Care Medicine.* **161**: 1963–1967.

25 Laveneziana P *et al.* (2008) Inhaled furosemide does not alleviate respiratory effort during flow-limited exercise in healthy subjects. *Pulmonary Pharmacology and Therapeutics*. **21**: 196–200.
26 Newton PJ *et al.* (2012) The acute haemodynamic effect of nebulised frusemide in stable, advanced heart failure. *Heart Lung Circulation*. **21**: 260–266.
27 Moosavi SH *et al.* (2006) Effect of inhaled furosemide on air hunger induced in healthy humans. *Respiritory Physiology and Neurobiology*. **156**: 1–8.
28 Ong KC *et al.* (2004) Effects of inhaled furosemide on exertional dyspnea in chronic obstructive pulmonary disease. *American Journal of Respiratory and Critical Care Medicine*. **169**: 1028–1033.
29 Jensen D *et al.* (2008) Mechanisms of dyspnoea relief and improved exercise endurance after furosemide inhalation in COPD. *Thorax*. **63**: 606–613.
30 Sheikh Motahar Vahedi H *et al.* (2013) The adjunctive effect of nebulized furosemide in acute treatment of patients with chronic obstructive pulmonary disease exacerbation: A randomized controlled clinical trial. *Respiratory Care*. **58**: 1873–1877.
31 Shimoyama N and Shimoyama M (2002) Nebulized furosemide as a novel treatment for dyspnea in terminal cancer patients. *Journal of Pain and Symptom Management*. **23**: 73–76.
32 Kohara H *et al.* (2003) Effect of nebulized furosemide in terminally ill cancer patients with dyspnea. *Journal of Pain and Symptom Management*. **26**: 962–967.
33 Wilcock A *et al.* (2008) Randomised, placebo-controlled trial of nebulised furosemide for breathlessness in patients with cancer. *Thorax*. **63**: 872–875.
34 Haegeli L *et al.* (2007) Sublingual administration of furosemide: new application of an old drug. *British Journal of Clinical Pharmacology*. **64**: 804–809.
35 Murray MD *et al.* (1997) Variable furosemide absorption and poor predictability of response in elderly patients. *Pharmacotherapy*. **17**: 98–106.
36 Verma AK *et al.* (2004) Diuretic effects of subcutaneous furosemide in human volunteers: a randomized pilot study. *Annals of Pharmacotherapy*. **38**: 544–549.
37 Walma E *et al.* (1997) Withdrawal of long term diuretic medication in elderly patients: a double blind randomised trial. *British Medical Journal*. **315**: 464–468.
38 Baxter K and Preston CL *Stockley's Drug Interactions*. London: Pharmaceutical Press www.medicinescomplete.com (accessed July 2014).
39 Trissel LA (2013) *Handbook on Injectable Drugs*. Maryland, USA: Society of Health-System Pharmacists www.medicinescomplete.com (accessed October 2013).

Updated June 2016

SPIRONOLACTONE

Class: Potassium-sparing diuretic; aldosterone antagonist.

Indications: Ascites and peripheral oedema associated with portal hypertension and hyperaldosteronism (i.e. cirrhosis, hepatocellular cancer, extensive hepatic metastases), CHF, nephrotic syndrome, primary hyperaldosteronism, †hypertension.

Contra-indications: Hyperkalaemia, Addison's disease, anuria, severe renal impairment, concurrent use with potassium supplements or potassium-sparing diuretics.

Pharmacology

Spironolactone and two metabolites (7α-thiomethyl-spironolactone and canrenone) bind to cytoplasmic mineralocorticoid receptors and function as aldosterone antagonists. This results in a potassium-sparing diuretic effect in the distal tubules of the kidney.

A diuretic-induced reduction in plasma volume can activate several neurohumoral systems, e.g. the renin-aldosterone-angiotensin system, sympathetic nervous system, ADH secretion, resulting in impaired renal perfusion and increased Na^+ and water resorption. These changes contribute towards a reduced effect of the diuretic ('diuretic resistance') and also renal impairment.

In patients with cirrhosis receiving spironolactone ± **furosemide**, improved renal function and diuresis is seen with co-administration of **octreotide** 300microgram SC b.d. (see p.544) or **clonidine** 75microgram PO b.d. (see p.77) due to inhibition of the renin-aldosterone-angiotensin (**octreotide** and **clonidine**) and sympathetic nervous (**clonidine**) systems.[1–3] Patients in the **clonidine** study were considered to have an overactive sympathetic nervous system based on a higher than normal serum noradrenaline (norepinephrine) level.[3]

Spironolactone also binds to the androgen receptor and to a lesser extent oestrogen and progesterone receptors. The resultant anti-androgenic effect is used to treat acne and hirsutism in women, particularly when associated with polycystic ovary syndrome. It can also result in undesirable effects such as menstrual disorders and, in men, gynaecomastia, breast pain or impotence. **Eplerenone**, an aldosterone antagonist with greater selectively for the mineralocorticoid receptor, has been used as an alternative in these circumstances;[4,5] it is substituted for spironolactone on a 1:1 basis.[6]

Caution is required when using spironolactone in patients with prostate cancer. Although there are reports of cancer regression in keeping with an androgen blocking effect, disease progression has also been reported.[7] It is suggested that spironolactone acts as an androgen receptor modulator and thus can exert both anti- and pro-androgenic effects.

Aldosterone binds to the mineralocorticoid receptor and activates pro-inflammatory and other cell pathways.[8–11] Thus, by preventing the binding of aldosterone, spironolactone has anti-inflammatory and other effects. Although the full therapeutic potential of this remains to be determined, benefit is seen with spironolactone in various experimental and clinical settings, with reductions in cancer growth, cancer cachexia and insulin resistance, for example.[12–14]

Ascites: Hyperaldosteronism is a concomitant of ascites associated with portal hypertension (a *transudate* with a relatively low albumin concentration, best indicated by a serum–ascites albumin difference of ≥11g/L) as seen in cirrhosis, hepatocellular cancer, extensive hepatic metastases.[15,16] Most evidence comes from cirrhosis, but spironolactone in a median daily dose of 200–300mg is successful in most patients with these conditions (90% in cirrhosis).[15–20]

In patients with cirrhosis, the combined use of spironolactone + **furosemide** provides a more rapid effect than spironolactone alone, but requires closer monitoring and more frequent dose adjustments.[18] Thus, particularly in outpatients, the initial use of spironolactone alone may be preferable.[20] In contrast, treatment with even large PO doses of a loop diuretic alone, e.g. **furosemide** 200mg, generally fails to reduce ascites.[21]

Note. Paracentesis is used for patients failing to respond to or tolerate diuretic therapy. Paracentesis is also preferable for patients with predominantly peritoneal ascites (an *exudate* with relatively high albumin concentration, best indicated by a serum–ascites albumin gradient of ≤11g/L) or chylous ascites as these are unlikely to respond to diuretics,[17,19] and also for patients with a tense distended abdomen in need of rapid relief.

For patients requiring frequent paracentesis and a prognosis of >1 month, an indwelling tunnelled drain can be considered, e.g. Pleurx® catheter. Patients are taught to drain off fluid using special drainage sets with vacuum bottles, initially up to 2L every day for 1–2 weeks, and then as required, generally alternate days.

CHF: Spironolactone improves morbidity and mortality in patients with CHF and a reduced left ventricular ejection fraction. It is added in low dose (e.g. 12.5mg–25mg) to standard treatment.[6,22,23] Its aldosterone antagonist action helps reduce vascular and myocardial fibrosis, sympathetic nervous system activation, baroreceptor dysfunction and K^+ and Mg^{2+} depletion.[24]

Hypertension: aldosterone antagonists are used as a fourth-line add-on therapy in patients with hypertension failing to respond to more usual antihypertensive drugs.[25,26]

Spironolactone is extensively metabolized. The 7α-thiomethyl-spironolactone and canrenone metabolites have long halflives and are excreted in the urine. Consequently, because of their accumulation and increased risk of hyperkalaemia, the use of spironolactone requires caution in mild–moderate renal impairment, and is generally contra-indicated in severe renal impairment.

Bio-availability 60–90%.

Onset of action 2–4h.

Maximum effect 7h (single dose), 2–3 days (multiple doses).

Time to peak plasma concentration 2–3h; active metabolites 3–4.5h PO.

Plasma halflife 1–1.5h; active metabolites 14–17h (multiple doses).

Duration of action >24h (single dose), 2–3 days (multiple doses).

Cautions

Prostate cancer (see Pharmacology).

Elderly; hepatic impairment, may induce reversible hyperchloraemic metabolic acidosis in patients with decompensated hepatic cirrhosis; renal impairment (see Dose and use). Initial drowsiness and dizziness (may impair driving).

Drug interactions

Serious additive pharmacodynamic interactions with other drugs, notably *hyperkalaemia* with potassium supplements (avoid concurrent use), table salt substitutes (contain both potassium and sodium chlorides), potassium-sparing diuretics, ACE inhibitors, angiotensin II receptor antagonists, certain antimicrobials (**trimethoprim**, **nitrofurantoin**), **ciclosporin**, LMWH and **tacrolimus**, particularly if other risk factors also present, e.g. elderly, renal impairment, diabetes.[27–29]

May induce *hyponatraemia*, particularly if used with other diuretics. Natriuretic effect reduced by **aspirin**, **indometacin** and possibly other NSAIDs.

Spironolactone increases the plasma concentration of digoxin by up to 25% and can interfere with digoxin plasma concentration assays; measure free digoxin levels using a chemiluminescent assay.[28]

Undesirable effects

Very common (>10%): CNS disturbances (drowsiness, lethargy, confusion, headache, fever, ataxia, fatigue), GI disturbances (anorexia, dyspepsia, nausea, vomiting, peptic ulceration, colic).
Common (<10%, >1%): gastritis, hyperkalaemia, gynaecomastia, breast pain.[30]

Dose and use

To reduce the risk of gastric irritation, advise patient to take with food. If, despite this, once daily spironolactone causes nausea and vomiting, try giving in divided doses.

For patients with swallowing difficulties, although an unauthorized oral suspension is available, it is expensive. A cheaper (and authorized) alternative is to disperse generic spironolactone tablets in water (also see p.785).

In patients with ascites and moderate renal impairment (e.g. eGFR 30–59mL/min/1.73m^2), halve the recommended dose.

Cirrhotic or malignant ascites associated with portal hypertension

Most experience comes from cirrhotic ascites.[15,16,18,20,21,31] Elimination of ascites may take 10–28 days:

- when close monitoring is possible (e.g. inpatients) spironolactone 100mg PO and **furosemide** 40mg PO each morning are started together. If necessary, both are increased every 3–5 days maintaining the 100mg:40mg ratio, up to a usual maximum of 400mg and 160mg respectively
- when close monitoring is *not* possible (e.g. outpatients) or when minimal fluid overload:
  - ▷ start with spironolactone alone 100–200mg PO each morning
  - ▷ if necessary, increase by 100mg every 3–5 days
  - ▷ typical maintenance dose 200–300mg/24h; maximum dose 400–600mg/24h
  - ▷ if not achieving the desired weight loss with spironolactone 300–400mg/24h, consider adding **furosemide** 40–80mg each morning.

Monitor body weight and renal function:

- adjust doses to achieve a weight loss of 0.5–1kg/24h (<0.5kg/24h when peripheral oedema absent)
- if Na^+ falls to <120mmol/L, temporarily stop diuretics
- if K^+ falls to <3.5mmol/L, temporarily stop or decrease the dose of **furosemide**
- if K^+ rises to >5.5mmol/L, halve the dose of spironolactone; if >6mmol/L, temporarily stop spironolactone
- if creatinine rises to >150micromol/L, temporarily stop diuretics.

Even if paracentesis becomes necessary, diuretics should be continued because they reduce the rate of recurrence. (Note. When >5L are to be removed, stop diuretics 2 days before paracentesis and start again 1–2 days afterwards.)[32]

Severe CHF (NYHA class III or IV disease)

Seek specialist advice. The following is based on several sets of published guidelines:

- do *not* prescribe spironolactone unless serum K^+ <5mmol/L and creatinine <200micromol/L or eGFR >30mL/min/1.73m^2
- start with 12.5–25mg PO once daily; check serum K^+ and creatinine after 4–7 days
- if necessary, *after 1 month*, increase to 25–50mg once daily; check serum K^+ and creatinine after 1 week
- if K^+ rises to >5mmol/L, halve the dose; if >5.5mmol/L, stop spironolactone completely
- occasionally, higher doses are used
- it is particularly important to monitor potassium levels when spironolactone and an ACE inhibitor are prescribed concurrently.[22,24,29,33,34]

Resistant hypertension

Seek specialist advice. Used as a fourth-line add-on therapy for hypertension not responding to the combination of three more usual antihypertensive drugs:

- do not prescribe if serum K^+ is >4.5mmol/L
- start with 25mg PO once daily; check serum Na^+, K^+ and creatinine within 1 month and repeat at intervals thereafter
- typical dose 25–50mg once daily, maximum dose 100mg.[25,35]

Supply

Spironolactone (generic)

Tablets 25mg, 50mg, 100mg, 28 days @ 200mg each morning = £4.25.

Oral suspension (sugar-free) 5mg/5mL, 10mg/5mL, 25mg/5mL, 50mg/5mL, 100mg/5mL; 28 days @ 200mg each morning = £142. (Unauthorized, available as a special order; see p.751) *Note price based on community specials tariff.*

Spironolactone oral suspension can also be prepared locally for individual patients.[36]

Spironolactone is also available in fixed dose combinations with hydroflumethiazide or furosemide. However, these are more expensive and do not allow titration of the individual drugs.

1 Kalambokis G *et al.* (2005) Renal effects of treatment with diuretics, octreotide or both, in non-azotemic cirrhotic patients with ascites. *Nephrology, Dialysis, Transplantation.* **20**: 1623–1629.

2 Kalambokis G *et al.* (2006) The effects of treatment with octreotide, diuretics, or both on portal hemodynamics in nonazotemic cirrhotic patients with ascites. *Journal of Clinical Gastroenterology.* **40**: 342–346.

3 Lenaerts A *et al.* (2006) Effects of clonidine on diuretic response in ascitic patients with cirrhosis and activation of sympathetic nervous system. *Hepatology.* **44**: 844–849.

4 Barnes BJ and Howard PA (2005) Eplerenone: a selective aldosterone receptor antagonist for patients with heart failure. *Annals of Pharmacotherapy.* **39**: 68–76.

5 Dimitriadis G *et al.* (2011) Eplerenone reverses spironolactone-induced painful gynaecomastia in cirrhotics. *Hepatology International.* **5**: 738–739.

6 Ponikowski P *et al.* (2016) ESC guidelines for the diagnosis and treatment of acute and chronic heart failure: The Task Force for the diagnosis and treatment of acute and chronic heart failure of the European Society of Cardiology (ESC) developed with the special contribution of the Heart Failure Association (HFA) of the ESC. *European Heart Journal.* **37**: 2129–2200.

7 Sundar S and Dickinson PD (2012) Spironolactone, a possible selective androgen receptor modulator, should be used with caution in patients with metastatic carcinoma of the prostate. *BMJ Case Reports.* doi:10.1136/bcr.1111.2011.5238.

8 Chantong B *et al.* (2012) Mineralocorticoid and glucocorticoid receptors differentially regulate NF-kappaB activity and pro-inflammatory cytokine production in murine BV-2 microglial cells. *Journal of Neuroinflammation.* **9**: 260.

9 Syngle A *et al.* (2009) Effect of spironolactone on endothelial dysfunction in rheumatoid arthritis. *Scandinavian Journal of Rheumatology.* **38**: 15–22.

10 Syngle A *et al.* (2013) Spironolactone improves endothelial dysfunction in ankylosing spondylitis. *Clinical Rheumatology.* **32**: 1029–1036.

11 Sun YE *et al.* (2012) Intrathecal injection of spironolactone attenuates radicular pain by inhibition of spinal microglia activation in a rat model. *PLoS One.* **7**: e39897.

12 King S *et al.* (2014) Evidence for aldosterone-dependent growth of renal cell carcinoma. *International Journal of Experimental Pathology.* **95**: 244–250.

13 Springer J *et al.* (2014) Prevention of liver cancer cachexia-induced cardiac wasting and heart failure. *European Heart Journal.* **35**: 932–941.

14 Ogino K *et al.* (2014) Spironolactone, not furosemide, improved insulin resistance in patients with chronic heart failure. *International Journal of Cardiology.* **171**: 398–403.

15 Greenway B *et al.* (1982) Control of malignant ascites with spironolactone. *British Journal of Surgery.* **69**: 441–442.

16 Fernandez-Esparrach G *et al.* (1997) Diuretic requirements after therapeutic paracentesis in non-azotemic patients with cirrhosis. A randomized double-blind trial of spironolactone versus placebo. *Journal of Hepatology.* **26**: 614–620.

17 Pockros P *et al.* (1992) Mobilization of malignant ascites with diuretics is dependent on ascitic fluid characteristics. *Gastroenterology.* **103**: 1302–1306.

18 Moore KP *et al.* (2003) The management of ascites in cirrhosis: report on the consensus conference of the International Ascites Club. *Hepatology.* **38**: 258–266.

19 Becker G *et al.* (2006) Malignant ascites: systematic review and guideline for treatment. *European Journal of Cancer.* **42**: 589–597.

20 Runyon BA (2012) Management of adult patients with ascites due to cirrhosis: Update 2012. *American Association for the Study of Liver Diseases.* https://www.aasld.org

21 Fogel M *et al.* (1981) Diuresis in the ascitic patient: a randomized controlled trial of three regimens. *Journal of Clinical Gastroenterology.* **3**: 73–80.

22 NICE (2010) Chronic heart failure in adults: management. *Clinical Guideline.* CG108. www.nice.org.uk

23 Yancy CW *et al.* (2013) 2013 ACCF/AHA guideline for the management of heart failure: a report of the American College of Cardiology Foundation/American Heart Association Task Force on practice guidelines. *Circulation.* **128**: e240–327.

24 Swedberg K *et al.* (2005) Guidelines for the diagnosis and treatment of chronic heart failure: full text (update 2005). European Heart Journal. Available from: 10.1093/eurheartj/ehi205

25 NICE (2011) Hypertension in adults: diagnosis and management. *Clinical Guideline.* CG127. www.nice.org.uk

26 Wang C *et al.* (2016) Efficacy and safety of spironolactone in patients with resistant hypertension: a meta-analysis of randomised controlled trials. *Heart Lung Circulation.* **25**: 1021–1030.
27 Antoniou T *et al.* (2015) Trimethoprim-sulfamethoxazole and risk of sudden death among patients taking spironolactone. *Canadian Medical Association Journal.* **187**: e138–143.
28 Baxter K, Preston CL *Stockley's Drug Interactions*. London: Pharmaceutical Press www.medicinescomplete.com (accessed January 2017).
29 MHRA (2016) Spironolactone and renin-angiotensin system drugs in heart failure: risk of potentially fatal hyperkalaemia. *Drug Safety Update*. www.gov.uk/drug-safety-update
30 Williams EM *et al.* (2006) Use and side-effect profile of spironolactone in a private cardiologist's practice. *Clinical Cardiology*. **29**: 149–153.
31 Sharma S and Walsh D (1995) Management of symptomatic malignant ascites with diuretics: two case reports and a review of the literature. *Journal of Pain and Symptom Management.* **10**: 237–242.
32 Twycross R and Wilcock A (eds) (2016) *Introducing Palliative Care* (5e). Palliativedrugs.com Ltd. Nottingham. UK. 138–142.
33 Arnold JM *et al.* (2006) Canadian Cardiovascular Society consensus conference recommendations on heart failure 2006: diagnosis and management. *Canadian Journal of Cardiology*. **22**: 23–45.
34 Shchekochikhin D *et al.* (2013) Increased spironolactone in advanced heart failure: effect of doses greater than 25 mg/day on plasma potassium concentration. *Cardiorenal Medicine*. **3**: 1–6.
35 Dahal K *et al.* (2015) The effects of aldosterone antagonists in patients with resistant hypertension: a meta-analysis of randomized and nonrandomized studies. *American Journal of Hypertension*. **28**: 1376–1385.
36 Allen LV Jr and Erickson MA 3rd (1996) Stability of ketoconazole, metolazone, metronidazole, procainamide hydrochloride, and spironolactone in extemporaneously compounded oral liquids. *American Journal of Health System Pharmacy*. **53**: 2073–2078.

Updated February 2017

SYSTEMIC LOCAL ANAESTHETICS

Local anaesthetics and their orally administered congeners are sometimes useful as third- or fourth-line drugs in the treatment of neuropathic pain. An analgesic effect has been reported when such drugs have been administered systemically:[1]

- **lidocaine** CSCI, IVI (and also TD)[2,3]
- **flecainide** PO
- **mexiletine** PO (not UK; may be imported as a special order)
- **tocainide** PO (not UK).

The mechanism by which they provide relief is not fully understood, but probably includes blockade of sodium channels. This stabilizes the nerve membrane and thus suppresses injury-induced hyperexcitability in the peripheral and central nervous systems. Antidepressants and anti-epileptics which benefit neuropathic pain also have membrane stabilizing properties, e.g. **amitriptyline**, **carbamazepine**.[4]

Other actions may be relevant and can occur at lower concentrations than necessary for sodium channel blockade. These include anti-inflammatory effects, interaction with other receptors (e.g. NMDA-receptor channel complex) and increased inhibitory neurotransmission (e.g. a **lidocaine** metabolite increases glycine levels).[5,6]

A systematic review of 32 RCTs, mostly of IV **lidocaine** and PO **mexiletine**, for neuropathic pain of various causes concluded that systemic local anaesthetics are better than placebo and as effective as **amantadine**, **carbamazepine**, **gabapentin**, **morphine** (Box A).[1]

Even so, despite the occasional impressive anecdotal account, RCT evidence of benefit is not overwhelming. The overall degree of improvement is small, and some studies suggest that not all components of neuropathic pain are relieved, e.g. constant pain and touch allodynia improve but cold-induced allodynia does not.[7,8] The systematic review found benefit to be inconsistent in some types of pain, e.g. diabetic neuropathy, and absent in others, e.g. cancer-related neuropathic pain.[1,9,10] Further, in a study of elderly patients (mean age 77 years), **lidocaine** 5mg/kg IVI over 2h provides no greater analgesic benefit than 1mg/kg, despite producing higher serum levels which were potentially toxic in some patients.[11]

Thus, generally in cancer-related neuropathic pain, systemic local anaesthetics should be considered for use only when the combination of a strong opioid + NSAID + TCA + anti-epileptic is ineffective or poorly tolerated. Even then, **ketamine** (see p.641) may be preferable because:

- the serum level does not need to be monitored
- it can be given PO
- it is more effective than **lidocaine** in spinal cord injury pain.[12]

Systemic **lidocaine** has been explored in various other pains, e.g. postoperative, critical limb ischaemia, colic (renal, bowel),[13–16] and also persistent hiccup and status epilepticus.[17,18] Although benefit is reported, the evidence is insufficient to support its routine use in these settings.

Box A Systemic local anaesthetics and neuropathic pain[1]

Of overall benefit in:
- trigeminal neuralgia
- post-herpetic neuralgia
- diabetic neuropathy
- lumbosacral radiculopathy
- post-stroke pain
- chronic post-surgery pain
- chronic post-trauma pain
- spinal cord injury pain
- complex regional pain syndrome
- cancer-related neuropathy.

Not of benefit in:
- cancer-related neuropathy (but see main text)
- HIV-related neuropathy.

Lidocaine dose used ranged from 1mg/kg IV over 2–3min to 1–5mg/kg IVI over 30min–2h.

Mexiletine median dose 600mg/24h PO (range 300–1200mg/24h).

Improvement equivalent to a reduction of 10mm on a 100mm VAS, but about 50% of patients achieve an improvement of ≥30%.

*Systemic lidocaine

*The use of systemic **lidocaine** is limited to specialist palliative care or pain services. Ideally, there should be an agreed protocol to ensure appropriate safety considerations are followed, including patient monitoring and staff training to manage toxicity.*[19]

Lidocaine has a narrow therapeutic index, and there are important contra-indications and cautions to be observed (see manufacturer's SPC). Contra-indications include patients at greater risk of cardiac arrhythmias, e.g. any type of cardiac disease, electrolyte abnormalities, and those already taking an anti-arrhythmic drug. Cautions include factors which increase the risk of toxicity, e.g. patients who are elderly, cachectic, or have renal or hepatic impairment.

A normal 12-lead ECG is a mandatory prerequisite. When administering IV **lidocaine** as a day case, particularly in non-cancer pain, some services monitor heart rhythm continuously and blood pressure/SpO_2 frequently, e.g. every 8 minutes, and ensure immediate access to resuscitation equipment. However, because of limited access to heart rhythm monitors, some palliative care centres follow IV **lidocaine** protocols that do not require it.[20]

Non-cancer pain

In non-cancer pain, improvement lasting 4–20 weeks following a single dose of IV **lidocaine** has been reported in patients with, e.g. central pain syndrome, diabetic neuropathy.[21,22] However, benefit is mostly limited to a few hours or days.[21,23] Some services repeat the dose weekly, as long as beneficial.[5] Alternatively, ongoing relief will necessitate CIVI or CSCI **lidocaine** or the use of an oral analogue, e.g. **flecainide, mexiletine** (not UK). However, the response to IV **lidocaine** does not reliably predict subsequent benefit from PO **mexiletine** and undesirable effects can limit its chronic use.[7,22] For example, in a cohort of patients with non-cancer neuropathic pain treated with **mexiletine**, the median time to discontinuation (for any reason) was 6 weeks with only 20% persisting with its use >1 year.[24] Further, recent specialist guidelines were strongly against **mexiletine** on the basis of lack of evidence.[25]

Cancer pain

In cancer-related neuropathic pain, subsequent to the systematic review,[1] there has been one positive RCT of IV **lidocaine**.[26] Compared with placebo, pain relief with **lidocaine** was faster (40 vs. 75min), of greater magnitude (75 vs. 25% reduction) and duration (9 vs. 4 days). Otherwise, reports of benefit are limited to case reports. Regimens include:
- IV 2mg/kg over 20min followed by 2mg/kg over 1h[26]
- IV 1–2mg/kg over 15–20min[27]

- IV 5mg/kg over 1h; progressively increased to a maximum of 10mg/kg[20]
- CIVI 0.5–1mg/kg/h[27,28]
- CSCI 4 or 10% **lidocaine** hydrochloride solution, generally 10–80mg/h; 100–160mg/h reported in patients aged ~ 60 years.[28,29]

Continuous infusions have been given for up to 6 months.[29] There is limited published experience in children.[30,31]

Monitoring use

Analgesia is generally seen with serum levels of 1.5–5microgram/mL and severe neurotoxicity with levels ≥10microgram/mL.[2,32] As a minimum, some suggest monitoring serum levels 1–3 days after starting or a dose increase and when toxicity is suspected.[28] However, there is large interindividual variation and the beneficial/toxic effect relates more to the amount of free **lidocaine** (unbound to protein), rather than the total serum level (bound plus unbound).[33]

With a continuous infusion, accumulation of **lidocaine** and its active metabolites, e.g. monoethylglycinexylidide and glycinexylidide, can occur and lead to toxicity. Particular caution is required in the elderly in whom clearance is already reduced.[33–35] For example, two elderly patients (≥70 years) despite normal renal/liver function and receiving a relatively small dose of **lidocaine** (200–300mg/day), developed severe drowsiness after 10 days.[36]

Generally, developing toxicity should be clinically obvious because as serum levels rise, there is a progressive worsening of neurotoxicity:

- lightheadedness, dizziness
- circumoral numbness
- tinnitus
- visual changes
- dysarthria
- muscle spasm
- seizures
- coma
- respiratory arrest.

However, monitoring serum levels is the most effective way of maintaining a consistent and safe **lidocaine** dose.[32,34]

Cardiovascular toxicity is more likely to lead to serious harm or death. Generally, it appears after neurotoxicity and is suggested by changes in heart rate, blood pressure, ECG (widening of QRS complex, ST segment changes, ventricular ectopics) and cardiac arrhythmia.

Note. Prolonged toxicity has also been reported when 10mL of 2% viscous **lidocaine** (not UK) was used hourly for a painful mouth ulcer (twice the recommended daily dose), and was probably partly caused by accumulation of metabolites.[35]

Lidocaine medicated plasters

These are authorized for post-herpetic neuralgia (Box B). Sufficient high-quality data are lacking to recommend them for first-line use in this setting.[3,25,37] Indeed, NICE considers the data insufficient to make any recommendation on their use.[38] Thus, in post-herpetic neuralgia, the plasters are best reserved for situations where tricyclic antidepressants (e.g. **amitriptyline**) and anti-epileptics (e.g. **gabapentin**) are contra-indicated, ineffective or poorly tolerated.

The analgesic effect of the **lidocaine** plasters is considered to be local via a non-selective block of peripheral sodium channels on sensory afferents in the epidermis.[39] However, neither the density of epidermal nerve fibres nor the results of quantitative sensory testing/nerve conduction studies predict pain relief from the plasters.[40,41] Indeed, some patients with a complete loss of epidermal nerve fibres report benefit. Thus, the exact mechanism of effect is unclear.[40,42]

There is also a strong placebo effect. In chronic back pain, active and placebo plasters provide similar reductions in pain intensity, sensory and affective scores and pain-related brain activity (functional MRI).[43] If the main effect of the **lidocaine** plasters is physical protection in patients with allodynia, they are an unnecessarily expensive form of plaster.

Situations in which **lidocaine** plasters have been used include:

- diabetic polyneuropathy[44]
- post-surgical neuropathic pain[41,45]
- post-traumatic neuropathic pain[41]

- osteo-arthritis[46]
- carpal tunnel syndrome[47]
- erythromelalgia[48]
- myofascial pain[49]
- cancer-related neuropathic pain[50,51]
- back pain[52]
- trigeminal neuralgia.[53]

Most evidence of benefit comes from low-quality open studies, case series or reports. RCTs have shown benefit in peripheral neuropathic pain (mostly post-surgical/post-traumatic),[41] mixed results in traumatic rib fracture,[54,55] and no benefit in post-surgical neuropathic pain, post-herniorrhapy or back pain.[43,45,56] Even when beneficial, the treatment effect size is small–medium (0.3–0.4) and the NNT for 50% pain relief ranges between 4–20.[41,57]

A survey showed that, in palliative care, the main use of the plasters is neuropathic pain associated with invasion of the chest wall by mesothelioma, breast or lung cancer. They were considered acceptable, well tolerated and beneficial to most patients. On the other hand, there were concerns about an unpredictable or variable response, and high cost.[58]

Box B Use of lidocaine 5% medicated plaster

Each plaster contains 700mg lidocaine. *Only about 5% of the plaster dose is absorbed.* Steady-state is achieved after three days. Maximum concentrations (0.07–0.19microgram/mL) are well below systemic analgesic (1.5–5microgram/mL) and serious toxic levels (≥10microgram/mL).

Caution is required in patients with severe renal impairment because accumulation of lidocaine and active metabolites can occur, and CNS toxicity has been reported, e.g. delirium.[59]

A recommended maximum of three plasters are applied to the painful area on a 12h on–off basis. The plasters can be cut if required but must not be applied close to the eyes or mouth, or on inflamed/broken skin or wounds.

Similar considerations apply as for other medical transdermal products, e.g. skin hair should be clipped rather than shaved, fold plasters in half and dispose of safely (>660mg remains in the plasters), remove before MRI scans (see p.831).

The 12h off periods are to help reduce the risk of skin reactions, but these still occur in about 15% of patients. The skin over the head and neck appears most susceptible.[60] The skin can be rested for longer when necessary, but up to 5% of patients have to discontinue.

Generally, high quality data are lacking. Experience with post-herpetic neuralgia suggests that overall <50% of patients will obtain sufficient benefit to warrant continuing with the plasters,[61] that a two-week trial may be required to identify responders[62] and, for those who respond, sustained benefit (≥4 years) has been reported. [63] The magnitude of the benefit appears similar to that obtained with pregabalin but the plasters are better tolerated.[44]

Anaphylaxis is a very rare complication (≤1:10,000).

*Flecainide

The use of ***flecainide*** *is limited to specialist palliative care or pain services.*

Flecainide is a class 1C anti-arrhythmic authorized for use primarily in the prevention and treatment of supraventricular and ventricular arrhythmias. Rarely, it is used to treat nerve injury pain. There are important contra-indications and cautions to be observed (see manufacturer's SPC). **Flecainide** has a narrow therapeutic index, and some patients experience psychoneurological and cardiac toxicity within the recommended therapeutic range (also see **lidocaine** above).[64,65] Flecainide is both metabolized by and inhibits CYP2D6 (see Chapter 19, Table 8, p.725).

Response rate for neuropathic pain in non-controlled studies in cancer and AIDS patients varies between 30–60%.[66–69] Generally, tricyclic antidepressants should be stopped at least 48h before starting **flecainide**. Initial doses are comparable to those used in cardiology:

- start with 50mg PO b.d.
- usual dose 100mg b.d.
- maximum dose 200mg b.d.[66,69]

Supply

Lidocaine hydrochloride (generic)
Medicated plaster 5%, 30 = £72.
Injection solution (preservative-free) 5mg/mL (0.5%), 10mg/mL (1%), 20mg/mL (2%) 2mL, 5mL, 10mL and 20mL = £1.

Versatis® (Grunenthal)
Medicated plaster 5% 30 = £72.

For topical use of **lidocaine** in oral inflammation and ulceration or in wound care see p.619 and p.638 respectively.

Flecainide (generic)
Tablets 50mg, 100mg, 28 days @100mg b.d. = £4.

1 Challapalli V *et al.* (2005) Systemic administration of local anesthetic agents to relieve neuropathic pain. *Cochrane Database of Systematic Reviews*. CD003345. www.thecochranelibrary.com
2 Devulder J *et al.* (1993) Neuropathic pain in a cancer patient responding to subcutaneously administered lignocaine. *Clinical Journal of Pain*. **9**: 220–223.
3 Derry S *et al.* (2014) Topical lidocaine for neuropathic pain in adults. *Cochrane Database of Systematic Reviews*. CD010958. www.thecochranelibrary.com
4 Devor M (2006) Sodium channels and mechanisms of neuropathic pain. *Journal of Pain*. **7**: S3–S12.
5 Przeklasa-Muszynska A *et al.* (2016) Intravenous lidocaine infusions in a multidirectional model of treatment of neuropathic pain patients. *Pharmacological Reports*. **68**: 1069–1075.
6 Werdehausen R *et al.* (2015) The lidocaine metabolite N-ethylglycine has antinociceptive effects in experimental inflammatory and neuropathic pain. *Pain*. **156**: 1647–1659.
7 Attal N *et al.* (2000) Intravenous lidocaine in central pain: a double-blind, placebo-controlled, psychophysical study. *Neurology*. **54**: 564–574.
8 Attal N *et al.* (2004) Systemic lidocaine in pain due to peripheral nerve injury and predictors of response. *Neurology*. **62**: 218–225.
9 Bruera E *et al.* (1992) A randomized double-blind crossover trial of intravenous lidocaine in the treatment of neuropathic cancer pain. *Journal of Pain and Symptom Management*. **7**: 138–140.
10 Ellemann K *et al.* (1989) Trial of intravenous lidocaine on painful neuropathy in cancer patients. *Clinical Journal of Pain*. **5**: 291–294.
11 Baranowski AP *et al.* (1999) A trial of intravenous lidocaine on the pain and allodynia of postherpetic neuralgia. *Journal of Pain and Symptom Management*. **17**: 429–433.
12 Kvarnstrom A *et al.* (2004) The analgesic effect of intravenous ketamine and lidocaine on pain after spinal cord injury. *Acta anaesthesiologica Scandinavica*. **48**: 498–506.
13 Kranke P *et al.* (2015) Continuous intravenous perioperative lidocaine infusion for postoperative pain and recovery. *Cochrane Database of Systematic Reviews*. CD009642. www.thecochranelibrary.com
14 Vahidi E *et al.* (2015) Comparison of intravenous lidocaine versus morphine in alleviating pain in patients with critical limb ischaemia. *Emergency Medical Journal*. **32**: 516–519.
15 Firouzian A *et al.* (2016) Does lidocaine as an adjuvant to morphine improve pain relief in patients presenting to the ED with acute renal colic? A double-blind, randomized controlled trial. *American Journal of Emergency Medicine*. **34**: 443–448.
16 Bafuma PJ *et al.* (2015) Opiate refractory pain from an intestinal obstruction responsive to an intravenous lidocaine infusion. *American Journal of Emergency Medicine*. **33**: 1544.e1543–1544.
17 Kaneishi K and Kawabata M (2013) Continuous subcutaneous infusion of lidocaine for persistent hiccup in advanced cancer. *Palliative Medicine*. **27**: 284–285.
18 Zeiler FA *et al.* (2015) Lidocaine for status epilepticus in adults. *Seizure*. **31**: 41–48.
19 Dickerson DM and Apfelbaum JL (2014) Local anesthetic systemic toxicity. *Aesthetic Surgery Journal*. **34**: 1111–1119.
20 Peixoto RD and Hawley P (2015) Intravenous lidocaine for cancer pain without electrocardiographic monitoring: a retrospective review. *Journal of Palliative Medicine*. **18**: 373–377.
21 Backonja M and Gombar KA (1992) Response of central pain syndromes to intravenous lidocaine. *Journal of Pain and Symptom Management*. **7**: 172–178.
22 Viola V *et al.* (2006) Treatment of intractable painful diabetic neuropathy with intravenous lignocaine. *Journal of Diabetes and Its Complications*. **20**: 34–39.
23 Kosharskyy B *et al.* (2013) Intravenous infusions in chronic pain management. *Pain Physician*. **16**: 231–249.
24 Carroll IR *et al.* (2008) Mexiletine therapy for chronic pain: survival analysis identifies factors predicting clinical success. *Journal of Pain and Symptom Management*. **35**: 321–326.
25 Finnerup NB *et al.* (2015) Pharmacotherapy for neuropathic pain in adults: a systematic review and meta-analysis. *Lancet Neurology*. **14**: 162–173.
26 Sharma S *et al.* (2009) A phase II pilot study to evaluate use of intravenous lidocaine for opioid-refractory pain in cancer patients. *Journal of Pain and Symptom Management*. **37**: 85–93.
27 Thomas J *et al.* (2004) Intravenous lidocaine relieves severe pain: results of an inpatient hospice chart review. *Journal of Palliative Medicine*. **7**: 660–667.
28 Ferrini R (2000) Parenteral lidocaine for severe intractable pain in six hospice patients continued at home. *Journal of Palliative Medicine*. **3**: 193–200.
29 Massey GV *et al.* (2002) Continuous lidocaine infusion for the relief of refractory malignant pain in a terminally ill pediatric cancer patient. *Journal of Pediatric Hematology/Oncology*. **24**: 566–568.
30 Berde C *et al.* (2016) Lidocaine infusions and other options for opioid-resistant pain due to pediatric advanced cancer. *Pediatric Blood and Cancer*. **63**: 1141–1143.

31 Gibbons K *et al.* (2016) Continuous lidocaine infusions to manage opioid-refractory pain in a series of cancer patients in a pediatric hospital. *Pediatric Blood and Cancer.* **63**: 1168–1174.
32 Ferrante FM *et al.* (1996) The analgesic response to intravenous lidocaine in the treatment of neuropathic pain. *Anesthesia and Analgesia.* **82**: 91–97.
33 Rosenberg PH *et al.* (2004) Maximum recommended doses of local anesthetics: a multifactorial concept. *Regional Anesthesia and Pain Medicine.* **29**: 564–575; discussion 524.
34 Brose W and Cousins M (1991) Subcutaneous lidocaine for treatment of neuropathic pain. *Pain.* **45**: 145–148.
35 Yamashita S *et al.* (2002) Lidocaine toxicity during frequent viscous lidocaine use for painful tongue ulcer. *Journal of Pain and Symptom Management.* **24**: 543–545.
36 Tei Y *et al.* (2005) Lidocaine intoxication at very small doses in terminally ill cancer patients. *Journal of Pain and Symptom Management.* **30**: 6–7.
37 Scottish Medicines Consortium (2008) Lidocaine 5% medicated plaster (Versatis(R)). 334/06. Available from: www.scottishmedicines.org.uk
38 NICE (2013) Pharmacological management of neuropathic pain in adults in non-specialist setting. *Clinical Guideline.* CG173. www.nice.org.uk
39 Madsen CS *et al.* (2013) Differential effects of a 5% lidocaine medicated patch in peripheral nerve injury. *Muscle Nerve.* **48**: 265–271.
40 Herrmann DN *et al.* (2006) Skin biopsy and quantitative sensory testing do not predict response to lidocaine patch in painful neuropathies. *Muscle Nerve.* **33**: 42–48.
41 Demant DT *et al.* (2015) Pain relief with lidocaine 5% patch in localized peripheral neuropathic pain in relation to pain phenotype: a randomised, double-blind, and placebo-controlled, phenotype panel study. *Pain.* **156**: 2234–2244.
42 Campbell JN (2012) How does topical lidocaine relieve pain? *Pain.* **153**: 255–256.
43 Hashmi JA *et al.* (2012) Lidocaine patch (5%) is no more potent than placebo in treating chronic back pain when tested in a randomised double blind placebo controlled brain imaging study. *Molecular Pain.* **8**: 29.
44 Baron R *et al.* (2009) 5% lidocaine medicated plaster versus pregabalin in post-herpetic neuralgia and diabetic polyneuropathy: an open-label, non-inferiority two-stage RCT study. *Current Medical Research and Opinion.* **25**: 1663–1676.
45 Cheville AL *et al.* (2009) Use of a lidocaine patch in the management of postsurgical neuropathic pain in patients with cancer: a phase III double-blind crossover study (N01CB). *Supportive Care in Cancer.* **17**: 451–460.
46 Burch F *et al.* (2004) Lidocaine patch 5% improves pain, stiffness, and physical function in osteoarthritis pain patients. A prospective, multicenter, open-label effectiveness trial. *Osteoarthritis and Cartilage.* **12**: 253–255.
47 Nalamachu S *et al.* (2006) A comparison of the lidocaine patch 5% vs naproxen 500 mg twice daily for the relief of pain associated with carpal tunnel syndrome: a 6-week, randomized, parallel-group study. *Medscape General Medicine.* **8**: 33.
48 Davis MD and Sandroni P (2005) Lidocaine patch for pain of erythromelalgia: follow-up of 34 patients. *Archives of Dermatology.* **141**: 1320–1321.
49 Lin YC *et al.* (2012) Therapeutic effects of lidocaine patch on myofascial pain syndrome of the upper trapezius: a randomized, double-blind, placebo-controlled study. *American Journal of Physical Medicine and Rehabilitation.* **91**: 871–882.
50 Fleming JA and O'Connor BD (2009) Use of lidocaine patches for neuropathic pain in a comprehensive cancer centre. *Pain Research and Management.* **14**: 381–388.
51 Garzon-Rodriguez C *et al.* (2013) Lidocaine 5 % patches as an effective short-term co-analgesic in cancer pain. Preliminary results. *Supportive Care in Cancer.* **21**: 3153–3158.
52 Likar R *et al.* (2015) Treatment of localized neuropathic pain of different etiologies with the 5% lidocaine medicated plaster - a case series. *International Journal of General Medicine.* **8**: 9–14.
53 Tamburin S *et al.* (2014) Effect of 5% lidocaine medicated plaster on pain intensity and paroxysms in classical trigeminal neuralgia. *Annals of Pharmacotherpy.* **48**: 1521–1524.
54 Ingalls NK *et al.* (2010) Randomized, double-blind, placebo-controlled trial using lidocaine patch 5% in traumatic rib fractures. *Journal of the American College of Surgeons.* **210**: 205–209.
55 Cheng YJ (2016) Lidocaine skin patch (Lidopat(R) 5%) is effective in the treatment of traumatic rib fractures: a prospective double-blinded and vehicle-controlled study. *Medical Principles and Practice.* **25**: 36–39.
56 Bischoff JM *et al.* (2013) Lidocaine patch (5%) in treatment of persistent inguinal postherniorrhaphy pain: a randomized, double-blind, placebo-controlled, crossover trial. *Anesthesiology.* **119**: 1444–1452.
57 Meier T *et al.* (2003) Efficacy of lidocaine patch 5% in the treatment of focal peripheral neuropathic pain syndromes: a randomized, double-blind, placebo-controlled study. *Pain.* **106**: 151–158.
58 Palliativedrugs.com Ltd Lidocaine 5% medicated plasters - What is your experience? *Latest additions: Survey results (October 2012).* www.palliativedrugs.com
59 Byun EK *et al.* (2016) Delirium associated with lidocaine patch administration: a case presentation. *Physical Medicine and Rehabilitation.* **8**: 597–601.
60 Nalamachu S *et al.* (2013) Influence of anatomic location of lidocaine patch 5% on effectiveness and tolerability for postherpetic neuralgia. *Patient Prefer Adherence.* **7**: 551–557.
61 Binder A *et al.* (2009) Topical 5% lidocaine (lignocaine) medicated plaster treatment for post-herpetic neuralgia: results of a double-blind, placebo-controlled, multinational efficacy and safety trial. *Clinical Drug Investigation.* **29**: 393–408.
62 Katz NP *et al.* (2002) Lidocaine patch 5% reduces pain intensity and interference with quality of life in patients with postherpetic neuralgia: an effectiveness trial. *Pain Medicine.* **3**: 324–332.
63 Sabatowski R *et al.* (2012) Safety and efficacy outcomes of long-term treatment up to 4 years with 5% lidocaine medicated plaster in patients with post-herpetic neuralgia. *Current Medical Research and Opinion.* **28**: 1337–1346.
64 Nestico PF *et al.* (1988) New antiarrhythmic drugs. *Drugs.* **35**: 286–319.
65 Bennett M (1997) Paranoid psychosis due to flecainide toxicity in malignant neuropathic pain. *Pain.* **70**: 93–94.
66 von Gunten CF *et al.* (2007) Flecainide for the treatment of chronic neuropathic pain: a Phase II trial. *Palliative Medicine.* **21**: 667–672.
67 Chong S *et al.* (1997) Pilot study evaluating local anesthetics administered systemically for treatment of pain in patients with advanced cancer. *Journal of Pain and Symptom Management.* **13**: 112–117.
68 Sinnott C *et al.* (1991) Flecainide in cancer nerve pain. *Lancet.* **337**: 1347.
69 Dunlop R *et al.* (1988) Analgesic effects of oral flecainide. *Lancet.* **1**: 420–421.

Updated November 2016

*CLONIDINE

Class: α-Adrenergic receptor agonist (α agonist).

Indications: Hypertension, migraine prophylaxis, menopausal flushing, †pain poorly responsive to epidural or intrathecal **diamorphine/morphine** and **bupivacaine**, †spasticity, †diarrhoea or †gastroparesis related to autonomic dysfunction in diabetes mellitus, †sweating, †ascites, †opioid withdrawal.

Contra-indications: Cardiac conduction defects.

Pharmacology

Clonidine is a mixed α_1 and α_2 agonist (mainly α_2). It acts centrally to inhibit the release of noradrenaline (norepinephrine) which decreases sympathetic tone. This reduces cardiac output and peripheral vascular resistance, lowering blood pressure. However, its use as an antihypertensive has been eclipsed by the development of other drugs. Clonidine has a range of other clinical effects:

Analgesia: Clonidine analgesia is probably mediated by an effect at α_2-receptors resulting in:

- peripheral and/or central suppression of sympathetic transmitter release[1,2]
- peripheral and central inhibition of nociceptive afferents[3,4]
- post-synaptic inhibition of spinal cord neurones[5,6]
- facilitation or inhibition of brain stem pain modulating systems.[7]

Postoperatively, clonidine given IV or IT augments the analgesic effects of opioids.[8,9] Clonidine also enhances the analgesic effects of local anaesthetics administered ED, IT or peripherally (e.g. single nerve or plexus blocks or applied directly to the wound).[10–16] Further, treatment with high-dose ED clonidine alone (a bolus of 10microgram/kg followed by an infusion of 6microgram/kg/h) can provide effective postoperative analgesia.[17] However, clonidine given PO pre-operatively ± TD postoperatively does not reduce pain or opioid requirements.[18]

In neuropathic pain, clonidine provides reproducible pain relief in some patients, particularly when given via the ED or IT routes.[1,19–25] There is limited evidence to suggest clonidine (0.1%) gel applied topically improves painful diabetic neuropathy.[26]

ED clonidine is effective in cancer-related neuropathic pain, generally as an 'add-on' drug to spinal **morphine** plus **bupivacaine** (see Spinal analgesia, p.839).[27,28] A typical dose is 150–300microgram/24h ED, but benefit has been reported in some patients on higher IT doses, up to 1mg/24h.[24] Benefit has also been reported in patients receiving clonidine by CSCI, with increasing benefit in a few patients with doses of up to 1.5mg/24h.[29]

ED clonidine is absorbed into the systemic circulation producing significant plasma concentrations (reflected clinically by drowsiness and cardiovascular effects), reaching a peak after 20min. IT clonidine produces similar effects; sedation occurs within 15–30min and lasts 1–2h.[24,30,31] The analgesic effect of clonidine can be reversed by α antagonists but not by **naloxone**.[1] Clonidine can thus be used in the management of unexpected acute pain in addicts receiving **naltrexone** (see p.460).

An alternative to clonidine in some settings is **dexmedetomidine**, a more selective α_2 agonist. When given with local anaesthetics IT, **dexmedetomidine** provides a more rapid onset and prolonged sensory block than clonidine.[32]

Spasticity: In patients with spinal cord injury, the addition of TD clonidine reduces muscle spasticity which has failed to respond to maximal doses of **baclofen**.[33,34] In healthy volunteers, clonidine induces muscular relaxation and reduces pain caused by distension in the stomach, colon and rectum.[35,36]

Diabetic GI autonomic neuropathy: Clonidine improves symptoms of gastroparesis and chronic diarrhoea.[37,38] The improvement in diarrhoea is due partly to the stimulation of α_2-adrenergic receptors on enterocytes, which promotes intestinal fluid and electrolyte absorption, inhibits anion secretion and decreases bowel transit time. Benefit is also reported in other causes of intractable diarrhoea, e.g. neuroendocrine tumours, short bowel syndrome.[38]

Sweats and hot flushes: There is RCT evidence that clonidine relieves sweating and hot flushes resulting from hormonal manipulation in women with breast cancer, but not in men with prostate cancer.[39,40] More recent trials in patients with breast cancer and hot flushes have found benefit from SSRIs, **venlafaxine** (p.216) and **gabapentin** (see p.272).[41] Comparative trials suggest **venlafaxine** works faster than clonidine, and participants prefer **venlafaxine** over

gabapentin.[41] Despite the lack of data, some suggest that SSRIs, **gabapentin** or clonidine could also be tried in men with hot flushes resulting from medical or surgical castration.[42]

Ascites: In patients with cirrhosis and ascites refractory to **spironolactone** ± **furosemide**, the addition of clonidine 75–100microgram PO b.d. can improve the response to diuretic therapy by inhibiting the renin-aldosterone-angiotensin and sympathetic nervous systems (see p.67).[43,44]

Opioid withdrawal: Increased sympathetic (noradrenergic) activity has been implicated in various symptoms of opioid withdrawal, e.g. shivering, sweating, anxiety, diarrhoea. Clonidine reduces these symptoms and has been used alone to manage opioid withdrawal. However, although as effective as reducing doses of **methadone**, clonidine is associated with more undesirable effects, e.g. hypotension.[45]

Nausea and vomiting: Premedication with clonidine (IV, PO) can reduce postoperative nausea and vomiting. This may relate to a reduced sympathetic outflow or analgesic requirement, or general sedative effect.[8,46] However, the effect is inconsistent and inferior to more standard approaches, e.g. $5HT_3$ antagonists.[47]

Other uses: Clonidine is used in dystonia[48] and also to reduce symptoms in several psychiatric conditions, e.g. attention-deficit/hyperactivity disorder, post-traumatic stress disorder, autism.[49]

About half of a dose of clonidine is excreted unchanged by the kidneys, and most of the remainder is metabolized by the liver to inactive metabolites. Accumulation occurs in renal impairment, extending its halflife up to 40h.

Bio-availability 75–100% PO; 60% TD.[50]

Onset of action 30–60min IV, PO; 2–3 days TD.

Time to peak plasma concentration 1.5–5h PO; 20min ED; 2 days TD.

Plasma halflife 12–16h.

Duration of action 8–24h PO; 24h TD.

Cautions

Severe coronary insufficiency, recent myocardial infarction, stroke, peripheral vascular disease, renal impairment (also see Chapter 17, p.681). May precipitate depression in susceptible patients; occasionally precipitates delirium.[51] Abrupt curtailment of long-term treatment likely to cause agitation, sympathetic overactivity, rebound hypertension (worsened if also taking a β-blocker); withdraw treatment progressively over 2–4 days (ED) or 1 week (PO). Discontinue any β-blocker several days before discontinuing clonidine.

Drug interactions

Effects reduced or abolished by drugs with α antagonist activity, e.g. **mirtazapine**, TCAs, and antipsychotic drugs, although the hypotensive effects of the phenothiazines can be additive. Concerns regarding serious undesirable effects with concurrent use of **methylphenidate** (see SPC) appear unfounded.[52]

Undesirable effects

Very common (>10%): sedation and dry mouth (initially), dizziness, orthostatic hypotension, transient pruritus and erythema (TD route).

Common (<10%, >1%): headache, fatigue, depression (long-term use), disturbed sleep, nausea, vomiting, constipation, erectile dysfunction, salivary gland pain, local reactions with TD route (e.g. rash, hyperpigmentation, excoriation).

Rare (<0.1%, ≥0.01%): decreased lacrimation.

$Alpha_2$ agonists (clonidine and **dexmedetomidine**) promote breast cancer cell growth and spread *in vitro* and in animal models;[53] the clinical relevance of this is unknown.

Dose and use

Clonidine can be given PO, TD (not UK, but see Supply),[23,54] CSCI and spinally.

Spinal analgesia

ED clonidine is generally given with **diamorphine/morphine** and **bupivacaine** (see Chapter 32, p.839). A typical ED regimen would be:

- a test bolus dose of 50–150microgram in 5mL 0.9% saline injection over 5min
- if relief obtained, 150–300microgram/24h by infusion.

Clonidine is also used IT. A typical IT regimen would be:

- a test bolus dose of 50microgram in 5mL 0.9% saline injection over 5min
- if relief obtained, 50–150microgram/24h by infusion.

Spasticity

Generally used as an adjunct to maximum dose of **baclofen**:

- start with 50microgram PO b.d.
- if necessary, increase by 50microgram every 3–7 days
- usual maximum dose 200microgram b.d.

Gastroparesis or diarrhoea related to autonomic dysfunction in diabetes mellitus

- start with 50microgram PO b.d.
- if necessary, increase by 50microgram every 24h
- usual maintenance dose 150microgram b.d.
- usual maximum dose for diabetic gastroparesis 300microgram b.d.
- usual maximum dose for diabetic diarrhoea 600microgram b.d.

For other causes of intractable diarrhoea, use similar doses.

Hormonal/menopausal sweating

- start with 50microgram PO b.d.
- after 2 weeks, if necessary, increase to 75microgram b.d.
- for some patients, the optimum dose is 100microgram b.d.

TD

TD patches (not UK) contain metal and must be removed before MRI to avoid burns (see Chapter 30, p.831).

TD is generally better tolerated than PO, but the relationship between effective doses of PO and TD clonidine is not predictable.

- start with a patch delivering 100microgram/24h applied once every 7 days and review.

Supply

Clonidine (generic)
Tablets 25microgram, 28 days @ 50microgram b.d. = £5.50.

Catapres® (Boehringer Ingelheim)
Tablets (scored) 100microgram, 28 days @ 50microgram b.d. = £2.25.
Injection 150microgram/mL, 1mL amp = £0.50. *Available but not listed in the BNF as no longer recommended for use in hypertensive crisis.*

Catapres® TTS
Transdermal patch 2.5mg (100microgram/24h), 5mg (200microgram/24h) 1 patch (7 days treatment) = £10 (not UK, available to import via IDIS as an unauthorized UK product, see Chapter 24, p.751).

1 Quan D *et al.* (1993) Clonidine in pain management. *Annals of Pharmacotherapy*. **27**: 313–315.
2 Langer SZ *et al.* (1980) Recent developments in noradrenergic neurotransmission and its relevance to the mechanism of action of certain antihypertensive agents. *Hypertension*. **2**: 372–382.
3 Calvillo O and Ghignone M (1986) Presynaptic effect of clonidine on unmyelinated afferent fibers in the spinal cord of the cat. *Neuroscience Letters*. **64**: 335–339.
4 Riedl MS *et al.* (2009) Coexpression of alpha 2A-adrenergic and delta-opioid receptors in substance P-containing terminals in rat dorsal horn. *Journal of Comparative Neurology*. **513**: 385–398.
5 Yaksh T (1985) Pharmacology of spinal adrenergic systems which modulate spinal nociceptive processing. *Pharmacology, Biochemistry and Behaviour*. **22**: 845–858.
6 Michel MC and Insel PA (1989) Are there multiple imidazoline binding sites? *TIPS*. **10**: 342–344.
7 Bie B *et al.* (2003) Roles of alpha1- and alpha2-adrenoceptors in the nucleus raphe magnus in opioid analgesia and opioid abstinence-induced hyperalgesia. *Journal of Neuroscience*. **23**: 7950–7957.
8 Samantaray A *et al.* (2012) The effect on post-operative pain of intravenous clonidine given before induction of anaesthesia. *Indian Journal of Anaesthesia*. **56**: 359–364.
9 Engelman E and Marsala C (2013) Efficacy of adding clonidine to intrathecal morphine in acute postoperative pain: meta-analysis. *British Journal of Anaesthesia*. **110**: 21–27.

10 Elia N *et al.* (2008) Clonidine as an adjuvant to intrathecal local anesthetics for surgery: systematic review of randomized trials. *Regional Anesthesia and Pain Medicine.* **33**: 159–167.
11 Popping DM *et al.* (2009) Clonidine as an adjuvant to local anesthetics for peripheral nerve and plexus blocks: a meta-analysis of randomized trials. *Anesthesiology.* **111**: 406–415.
12 Ya Deau JT *et al.* (2008) Clonidine and analgesic duration after popliteal fossa nerve blockade: Randomized, double-blind, placebo-controlled study. *Anesthesia and Analgesia.* **106**: 1916–1920.
13 Schnabel A *et al.* (2011) Efficacy and safety of clonidine as additive for caudal regional anesthesia: a quantitative systematic review of randomized controlled trials. *Paediatric Anaesthesia.* **21**: 1219–1230.
14 Mohamed SA and Abdel-Ghaffar HS (2013) Effect of the addition of clonidine to locally administered bupivacaine on acute and chronic postmastectomy pain. *Journal of Clinical Anesthesia.* **25**: 20–27.
15 Bharti N *et al.* (2013) Postoperative analgesic effect of intravenous (i.v.) clonidine compared with clonidine administration in wound infiltration for open cholecystectomy. *British Journal of Anaesthesia.* **111**: 656–661.
16 Mohammad W *et al.* (2015) A randomized double-blind study to evaluate efficacy and safety of epidural magnesium sulfate and clonidine as adjuvants to bupivacaine for postthoracotomy pain relief. *Anesthesia Essays and Researches.* **9**: 15–20.
17 Abd-Elsayed AA *et al.* (2015) A double-blind randomized controlled trial comparing epidural clonidine vs bupivacaine for pain control during and after lower abdominal surgery. *Ochsner Journal.* **15**: 133–142.
18 Turan A *et al.* (2016) Clonidine does not reduce pain or opioid consumption after noncardiac surgery. *Anesthesia and Analgesia.* **123**: 749–757.
19 Siddall PJ *et al.* (2000) The efficacy of intrathecal morphine and clonidine in the treatment of pain after spinal cord injury. *Anesthesia and Analgesia.* **91**: 1493–1498.
20 Walters JL *et al.* (2012) Idiopathic peripheral neuropathy responsive to sympathetic nerve blockade and oral clonidine. *Case Reports in Anesthesiology.* Article ID 407539.
21 Glynn C *et al.* (1988) A double-blind comparison between epidural morphine and epidural clonidine in patients with chronic noncancer pain. *Pain.* **34**: 123–128.
22 Max MB *et al.* (1988) Association of pain relief with drug side effects in postherpetic neuralgia: a single-dose study of clonidine, codeine, ibuprofen and placebo. *Clinical Pharmacology and Therapeutics.* **43**: 363–371.
23 Zeigler D *et al.* (1992) Transdermal clonidine versus placebo in painful diabetic neuropathy. *Pain.* **48**: 403–408.
24 Ackerman LL *et al.* (2003) Long-term outcomes during treatment of chronic pain with intrathecal clonidine or clonidine/opioid combinations. *Journal of Pain and Symptom Management.* **26**: 668–677.
25 Rauck RL *et al.* (2015) Intrathecal clonidine and adenosine: effects on pain and sensory processing in patients with chronic regional pain syndrome. *Pain.* **156**: 88–95.
26 Wrzosek A *et al.* (2015) Topical clonidine for neuropathic pain. *Cochrane Database of Systematic Reviews.* **8**: CD010967. www.thecochranelibrary.com
27 Eisenach JC *et al.* (1995) Epidural clonidine analgesia for intractable cancer pain. The Epidural Clonidine Study Group. *Pain.* **61**: 391–399.
28 Chen H *et al.* (2004) Contemporary management of neuropathic pain for the primary care physician. *Mayo Clinic Proceedings.* **79**: 1533–1545.
29 Glynn C (1997) Personal communication.
30 Wells J and Hardy P (1987) Epidural clonidine. *Lancet.* **i**: 108.
31 Malinovsky JM *et al.* (2003) Sedation caused by clonidine in patients with spinal cord injury. *British Journal of Anaesthesia.* **90**: 742–745.
32 Zhang C *et al.* (2016) Comparison of dexmedetomidine and clonidine as adjuvants to local anesthetics for intrathecal anesthesia: a meta-analysis of randomized controlled trials. *Journal of Clinical Pharmacology.* **56**: 827–834.
33 Weingarden S and Belen J (1992) Clonidine transdermal system for treatment of spasticity in spinal cord injury. *Archives of Physical Medicine and Rehabilitation.* **73**: 876–877.
34 Yablon S and Sipski M (1993) Effect of transdermal clonidine on spinal spasticity: a case series. *American Journal of Physical Medicine and Rehabilitation.* **72**: 154–156.
35 Thumshirn M *et al.* (1999) Modulation of gastric sensory and motor functions by nitrergic and alpha2-adrenergic agents in humans. *Gastroenterology.* **116**: 573–585.
36 Viramontes BE *et al.* (2001) Effects of an alpha(2)-adrenergic agonist on gastrointestinal transit, colonic motility, and sensation in humans. *American Journal of Physiology Gastrointestinal and Liver Physiology.* **281**: G1468–1476.
37 Rosa-Silva L *et al.* (1995) Treatment of diabetic gastroparesis with oral clonidine. *Alimentary Pharmacology and Therapeutics.* **9**: 179–183.
38 Fragkos KC *et al.* (2016) What about clonidine for diarrhoea? A systematic review and meta-analysis of its effect in humans. *Therapeutic Advances in Gastroenterology.* **9**: 282–301.
39 Frisk J (2010) Managing hot flushes in men after prostate cancer--a systematic review. *Maturitas.* **65**: 15–22.
40 Rada G (2010) Non-hormonal interventions for hot flashes in women with a history of breast cancer. *Cochrane Database of Systematic Reviews.* **2**: CD004923. www.thecochranelibrary.com
41 Johns C *et al.* (2016) Informing hot flash treatment decisions for breast cancer survivors: a systematic review of randomized trials comparing active interventions. *Breast Cancer Research and Treatment.* **156**: 415–426.
42 Loprinzi CL *et al.* (2011) Nonestrogenic management of hot flashes. *Journal of Clinical Oncology.* **29**: 3842–3846.
43 Yang YY *et al.* (2010) Association of the G-protein and alpha2-adrenergic receptor gene and plasma norepinephrine level with clonidine improvement of the effects of diuretics in patients with cirrhosis with refractory ascites: a randomised clinical trial. *Gut.* **59**: 1545–1553.
44 Singh V *et al.* (2013) Midodrine and clonidine in patients with cirrhosis and refractory or recurrent ascites: a randomized pilot study. *American Journal Gastroenterology.* **108**: 560–567.
45 Gowing L *et al.* (2016) Alpha2-adrenergic agonists for the management of opioid withdrawal. *Cochrane Database of Systematic Reviews.* CD002024. www.thecochranelibrary.com
46 Yadav G *et al.* (2013) A prospective, randomized, double blind and placebo-control study comparing the additive effect of oral midazolam and clonidine for postoperative nausea and vomiting prophylaxis in granisetron premedicated patients undergoing laparoscopic cholecystecomy. *Journal of Anaesthesiology, Clinical Pharmacology.* **29**: 61–65.
47 Shilpa SN *et al.* (2015) Comparison of efficacy of clonidine versus ondansetron for prevention of nausea and vomiting post thyroidectomy: a double blind randomized controlled trial. *Journal of Clinical and Diagnostic Research.* **9**: UC01–UC03.
48 McCluggage HL (2016) Changing from continuous SC to transdermal clonidine to treat dystonia in a teenage boy with end-stage leucodystrophy. *BMJ Supportive and Palliative Care* (Epub ahead of print).
49 Dowben JS *et al.* (2011) Clonidine: diverse use in pharmacologic management. *Perspectives in Psychiatric Care.* **47**: 105–108.
50 Toon S *et al.* (1989) Rate and extent of absorption of clonidine from a transdermal therapeutic system. *Journal of Pharmacy and Pharmacology.* **41**: 17–21.

51 Delaney J *et al.* (2006) Clonidine-induced delirium. *International Journal of Cardiology*. **113**: 276–278.
52 Baxter K, Preston CL *Stockley's Drug Interactions*. London: Pharmaceutical Press www.medicinescomplete.com (accessed January 2017).
53 Xia M *et al.* (2016) Dexmedetomidine regulate the malignancy of breast cancer cells by activating alpha2-adrenoceptor/ERK signaling pathway. *European Review for Medical and Pharmacological Sciences*. **20**: 3500–3506.
54 Davis K *et al.* (1991) Topical application of clonidine relieves hyperalgesia in patients with sympathetically maintained pain. *Pain*. **47**: 309–317.

Updated August 2017

GLYCERYL TRINITRATE

Class: Nitrate.

Indications: Angina, left ventricular failure, anal fissure, †smooth muscle spasm pain (particularly of the oesophagus, rectum and anus or cutaneous leiomyomas),[1] †biliary and †renal colic, †painful diabetic neuropathy,[2,3] †symptomatic relief of breathlessness in acute pulmonary oedema (in conjunction with diuretics)[4] or paroxysmal nocturnal dyspnoea. ***TD patch (selected brands):*** maintenance of venous patency, prevention of phlebitis, treatment of drug extravasation.

Contra-indications: Severe hypotension (systolic <90mmHg), or severe aortic or mitral stenosis, cardiac tamponade, constrictive pericarditis, hypertrophic obstructive cardiomyopathy, marked anaemia, severe hypovolaemia, raised intracranial pressure, narrow-angle glaucoma. Concurrent use of **avanafil, sildenafil, tadalafil** and **vardenafil** (may precipitate hypotension and myocardial infarction).[5]

Pharmacology

Glyceryl trinitrate (GTN) relaxes smooth muscle in blood vessels and the GI tract. This effect is mediated via its metabolism to nitric oxide (NO), which stimulates guanylate cyclase. This leads to an increase in cyclic guanosine monophosphate which reduces the amount of intracellular calcium available for muscle contraction.[6]

Endogenous NO is produced when the NMDA-receptor is stimulated by excitatory amino acids (see **ketamine**, p.641), and NO synthase inhibitors attenuate the development of opioid tolerance.[7] This points to a wider role of NO in pain modulation. GTN has a range of clinical effects:

Smooth muscle relaxant/antispasmodic: NO is involved in the regulation of distal oesophageal peristalsis and relaxation of the lower oesophageal sphincter. Thus, GTN can improve dysphagia and odynophagia associated with oesophagitis and oesophageal spasm.[8–10]

NO is also the major inhibitory neurotransmitter in the internal anal sphincter. In patients with acute anal fissure, GTN ointment 0.2–0.4% applied b.d. to the anal canal relieves painful spasm, improves quality of life and aids healing.[11] However, 30% of patients experience headache which, although transient, can be severe enough to discontinue treatment. **Diltiazem** 2% cream is an alternative; it is as effective as GTN ointment but causes less headache and less anal irritation.[12] Injections of **botulinum toxin** into the internal sphincter have also been used, but their exact role remains to be clarified. About 90% of acute anal fissures resolve with non-surgical approaches. However, for chronic fissures, i.e. those persisting >6 weeks, surgery is the most effective approach.[11]

Analgesic: GTN administered systemically using a TD patch enhances pain relief in cancer patients; when applied directly as a gel or TD patch, it also reduces local pain and inflammation, e.g. from thrombophlebitis, tendinopathies.[13–18] In a RCT for diabetic neuropathic pain affecting the feet, locally applied GTN spray reduced mean pain scores significantly from 7.5 to 4.6 (NNT=4).[2] In a second RCT, the concurrent use of PO **valproate** provided no additional benefit.[3]

Vasodilator: Nitrates cause venous then arterial dilation in a dose-related manner. Nitrates such as GTN and **isosorbide dinitrate** are thus given by IVI in *acute* heart failure to reduce pre- and after-load, which helps to relieve breathlessness. Generally, nitrates are given in conjunction with IV diuretics; they can be used alone when hypertension is the cause of acute heart failure.[4] Nitrates are not suitable for patients with hypotension (systolic <90mmHg), severe obstructive valvular disease, or long-term use (nitrate tolerance generally develops after 24–48h).

Short-acting nitrates such as GTN and **isosorbide dinitrate** are used SL to treat or prevent angina episodes.[19] Because of tolerance, the chronic use of nitrates in cardiovascular disease is best reserved for specific circumstances, such as nocturnal angina or paroxysmal nocturnal dyspnoea. In this setting, p.r.n. GTN spray SL may be helpful or, if a frequent occurrence, a regular bedtime dose of a longer-acting nitrate PO. In those unable to swallow tablets, a bedtime application of TD GTN can be used. All these approaches permit a daily nitrate-free period of ≥10h.

TD GTN appears to improve outcomes in acute stroke, potentially via its vasodilator effects improving peri-lesional perfusion along with lowering and stabilization of systolic blood pressure.[20]

In cancer, the use of TD GTN could potentially improve perfusion of the tumour, thereby increasing anticancer drug delivery or decreasing hypoxia, which is associated with invasion, metastasis, and drug resistance.[21] Studies in various settings are ongoing; however, initial findings of benefit from TD GTN alongside chemotherapy in patients with lung cancer have not been replicated.[22,23] Use of a low dose (i.e. application of one sixth of a 5mg TD patch daily) in patients with prostate cancer and an increasing PSA after surgery or radiotherapy, increased the PSA doubling time from 13 to 32 months.[24]

GTN is rapidly absorbed through the buccal mucosa but orally it is inactivated by extensive first-pass metabolism in the GI mucosa and liver. Many patients on long-acting or TD nitrates develop tolerance, i.e. experience a reduced therapeutic effect. Tolerance is generally prevented if nitrate levels are allowed to fall for ≥10h in every 24h (a 'nitrate holiday'). This may not be possible for patients with persistent pain. If tolerance develops, it will be necessary to increase the dose to restore efficacy.

Bio-availability 40% SL.
Onset of action 1–3min SL; 30–60min ointment or TD patch.
Time to peak plasma concentration 3–6min SL; 2h TD.
Plasma halflife 1–3min SL; 2–4min TD.
Duration of action 30–60min SL; 8h ointment; 24h TD patch.

Cautions

Severe hepatic or renal impairment, hypothyroidism, hypovolaemia, hypoxaemia, hypothermia, recent myocardial infarction. Topically applied GTN can be absorbed in sufficient quantities to cause undesirable systemic effects.

Drug interactions

Serious drug interactions: Concurrent use of **avanafil**, **sildenafil**, **tadalafil** and **vardenafil** may precipitate profound hypotension and myocardial infarction and is contra-indicated.

Exacerbates the hypotensive effect of other drugs. Drugs causing dry mouth may reduce the effect of sublingual nitrates.

Undesirable effects

Very common (>10%): headache (sometimes severe).
Common (<10%, >1%): flushing, dizziness, nausea.
Uncommon (<1%, >0.1%): local stinging, itching or burning sensation after SL spay, TD or rectal administration.
Rare (<0.1%, >0.01%): postural hypotension, tachycardia (paradoxical bradycardia also reported); may be more frequent with IV use.
These effects generally settle with continued use.

Dose and use

TD patches: some contain metal and must be removed before MRI to avoid burns (see Chapter 30, p.831.
Injection: glass, polyethylene or polypropylene apparatus should be used with parenteral GTN as loss of potency will occur if PVC is used.

If necessary, **paracetamol** can be used for headache.

Intermittent dysphagia and/or odynophagia

- start with 400–500microgram SL 5–15min before eating
- if necessary, increase to a maximum single dose of 1mg
- instruct the patient to swallow or spit out tablet once pain relief is obtained (or if headache develops)
- repeat p.r.n.

Persistent smooth muscle spasm

Consider:

- GTN TD patches, starting with 5mg/24h *or*
- orally active nitrates, e.g. **isosorbide mononitrate**, start with 20mg PO b.d. (8am and 3pm).

If a 'nitrate holiday' is not possible, a TD patch may have to remain in place for 24h, or m/r **isosorbide mononitrate** considered instead (see Pharmacology).

Anal fissure pain

- use 0.2–0.4% rectal ointment
- using a covered finger, gently insert a 2.5cm length (or pea-sized quantity) of ointment about 1cm into the anal canal b.d. for 6 weeks.[25]

Painful diabetic neuropathy

- apply GTN spray locally to the painful extremity: 1 spray/sole of foot/day.

Angina on effort

The patient should stop and rest sitting down; tablets/spray are placed/directed under the tongue and should not be swallowed:

- start with one SL tablet (300 or 600microgram) or spray (400microgram)
- the dose is repeated every 5min until the pain goes or the maximum dose reached (1,200microgram/15min)
- if there is no relief, immediate medical attention should be sought.

For prophylactic use, take immediately before the activity known to cause angina.

Acute pulmonary oedema in conjunction with diuretics

Use under the guidance of a cardiologist:

- start with 10–20microgram/min IVI, titrate every 3–5min as needed in 5–10microgram/min increments, up to a maximum of 200microgram/min.

Supply

Because GTN is an explosive substance, spray formulations contain additives (e.g. medium-chain partial glycerides or alcohol) to stabilize the solution and minimize the potential for explosion.

Glyceryl trinitrate (generic)
Tablets SL 300microgram, 500microgram, 100 = £2.25 and £6 respectively; *store in the original glass container; because of degradation, unused tablets should be discarded after 8 weeks.*
Aerosol SL spray 400microgram/metered dose, 200-dose unit = £3.50, *contains alcohol.*
Injection 1mg/mL, 50mL vial = £16.
Injection 5mg/mL, 5mL and 10mL amps = £6.50 and £13 respectively; *must be diluted before use. Contains propylene glycol; maximum recommended use of 3 days.*

Nitrocine (UCB Pharma)
Injection 1mg/mL, 10mL amp = £6.

Nitronal (Merk Serono)
Injection 1mg/mL, 5mL amp and 50mL vial = £2 and £15 respectively.

TD products
Nitro-Dur® (Schering-Plough)
TD patch 200microgram/h (5mg/24h), 400microgram/h (10mg/24h), 600microgram/h (15mg/24h), 28 days @ 1 patch daily = £11, £12 and £13 respectively.

Topical products
Ointment 0.2%, 30g = £23 (Unauthorized, available as a special order; see Chapter 24, p.751). *Note. Price based on specials tariff in community.*

Rectogesic® (ProStrakan)
Rectal ointment 0.4%, 30g = £40. *Discard 8 weeks after opening. Contains propylene glycol and lanolin (irritants).*

This is not a complete list; see BNF for more information.

Diltiazem
Ointment or cream 2%, 30g = £36 or £61 respectively (Unauthorized, available as a special order; see Chapter 24, p.751). *Note. Price based on specials tariff in community.*

Isosorbide mononitrate
Tablets 10mg, 20mg, 40mg, 28 days@ 20mg b.d. = £3.50.
Tablets m/r 25mg, 40mg, 50mg, 60mg, 28 days @ 40mg once daily = £7.
Capsules m/r 25mg, 40mg, 50mg, 60mg, 28 days @ 40mg once daily = £6.50.

1 George S *et al.* (1997) Pain in multiple leiomyomas alleviated by nifedipine. *Pain.* **73**: 101–102.
2 Agrawal RP *et al.* (2007) Glyceryl trinitrate spray in the management of painful diabetic neuropathy: a randomized double blind placebo controlled cross-over study. *Diabetes Research and Clinical Practice.* **77**: 161–167.
3 Agrawal RP *et al.* (2009) Management of diabetic neuropathy by sodium valproate and glyceryl trinitrate spray: a prospective double-blind randomized placebo-controlled study. *Diabetes Research and Clinical Practice.* **83**: 371–378.
4 Ponikowski P *et al.* (2016) 2016 ESC Guidelines for the diagnosis and treatment of acute and chronic heart failure: The Task Force for the diagnosis and treatment of acute and chronic heart failure of the European Society of Cardiology (ESC). Developed with the special contribution of the Heart Failure Association (HFA) of the ESC. *European Journal of Heart Failure.* **18**: 891–975.
5 Baxter K and Preston CL. *Stockley's Drug Interactions.* London: Pharmaceutical Press www.medicinescomplete.com (accessed January 2017).
6 Hashimoto S and Kobayashi A (2003) Clinical pharmacokinetics and pharmacodynamics of glyceryl trinitrate and its metabolites. *Clinical Pharmacokinetics.* **42**: 205–221.
7 Elliott K *et al.* (1994) The NMDA receptor antagonists, LY274614 and MK-801, and the nitric oxide synthase inhibitor, NG-nitro-L-arginine, attenuate analgesic tolerance to the mu-opioid morphine but not to kappa opioids. *Pain.* **56**: 69–75.
8 McDonnell F and Walsh D (1999) Treatment of odynophagia and dysphagia in advanced cancer with sublingual glyceryl trinitrate. *Palliative Medicine.* **13**: 251–252.
9 Tutuian R and Castell DO (2006) Review article: oesophageal spasm - diagnosis and management. *Alimentary Pharmacology and Therapeutics.* **23**: 1393–1402.
10 Maradey-Romero C *et al.* (2014) Treatment of esophageal motility disorders based on the chicago classification. *Current Treatment Options Gastroenterology.* **12**: 441–455.
11 Nelson RL *et al.* (2012) Non surgical therapy for anal fissure. *Cochrane Database of Systematic Reviews.* **2**: CD003431. www.thecochranelibrary.com
12 Sajid MS *et al.* (2013) Systematic review of the use of topical diltiazem compared with glyceryltrinitrate for the nonoperative management of chronic anal fissure. *Colorectal Disease.* **15**: 19–26.
13 Ferreira S *et al.* (1992) Blockade of hyperalgesia and neurogenic oedema by topical application of nitroglycerin. *European Journal of Pharmacology.* **217**: 207–209.
14 Berrazueta J *et al.* (1994) Local transdermal glyceryl trinitrate has an antiinflammatory action on thrombophlebitis induced by sclerosis of leg varicose veins. *Angiology.* **5**: 347–351.
15 Lauretti G *et al.* (1999) Oral ketamine and transdermal nitroglycerin as analgesic adjuvants to oral morphine therapy and amitriptyline for cancer pain management. *Anesthesiology.* **90**: 1528–1533.
16 Lauretti GR *et al.* (2002) Double-blind evaluation of transdermal nitroglycerine as adjuvant to oral morphine for cancer pain management. *Journal of Clinical Anesthesia.* **14**: 83–86.
17 El-Sheikh SM and El-Kest E (2004) Transdermal nitroglycerine enhanced fentanyl patch analgesia in cancer pain management. *Egyptian Journal of Anaesthesia.* **20**: 291–294.
18 Gambito ED *et al.* (2010) Evidence on the effectiveness of topical nitroglycerin in the treatment of tendinopathies: a systematic review and meta-analysis. *Archives of Physical Medicine and Rehabilitation.* **91**: 1291–1305.
19 Montalescot G *et al.* (2013) 2013 ESC guidelines on the management of stable coronary artery disease: the Task Force on the management of stable coronary artery disease of the European Society of Cardiology. *European Heart Journal.* **34**: 2949–3003.
20 Appleton JP *et al.* (2017) Therapeutic potential of transdermal glyceryl trinitrate in the management of acute stroke. *CNS Drugs.* **31**: 1–9.
21 Sukhatme V *et al.* (2015) Repurposing Drugs in Oncology (ReDO)-nitroglycerin as an anti-cancer agent. *Ecancermedicalscience.* **9**: 568.
22 Yasuda H *et al.* (2006) Randomized phase II trial comparing nitroglycerin plus vinorelbine and cisplatin with vinorelbine and cisplatin alone in previously untreated stage IIIB/IV non-small-cell lung cancer. *Journal of Clinical Oncology.* **24**: 688–694.
23 Davidson A *et al.* (2015) A phase III randomized trial of adding topical nitroglycerin to first-line chemotherapy for advanced nonsmall-cell lung cancer: the Australasian lung cancer trials group NITRO trial. *Annals of Oncology.* **26**: 2280–2286.
24 Siemens DR *et al.* (2009) Phase II study of nitric oxide donor for men with increasing prostate-specific antigen level after surgery or radiotherapy for prostate cancer. *Urology.* **74**: 878–883.
25 Gagliardi G *et al.* (2010) Optimal treatment duration of glyceryl trinitrate for chronic anal fissure: results of a prospective randomized multicenter trial. *Techniques in Coloproctology.* **14**: 241–248.

Updated August 2017

NIFEDIPINE

Class: Calcium-channel blocker.

2

Indications: Prophylaxis of stable angina, hypertension, Raynaud's phenomenon (immediate-release only authorized formulation), †severe smooth muscle spasm pain (particularly of the oesophagus, rectum and anus, cutaneous leiomyomas),[1–5] †intractable hiccup.[6]

Contra-indications: Cardiogenic shock, severe aortic stenosis, acute or unstable angina (immediate-release capsules PO or SL may cause hypotension and reflex tachycardia precipitating myocardial or cerebrovascular ischaemia). *Do not use within one month of myocardial infarction.*
Adalat® LA: hepatic impairment; previous or current GI obstruction or stenosis, inflammatory bowel disease.

Pharmacology

Nifedipine inhibits the influx of calcium through L-type channels into cells, thereby modifying cell function, e.g. smooth muscle contraction and neural transmission.[7] It has a range of clinical effects:
Smooth muscle relaxant/antispasmodic: Nifedipine is used to relieve dysphagia and chest pain associated with oesophageal spasm.[8–10] It also relieves painful spasm associated with an anal fissure. Topical application of nifedipine cream is more effective and better tolerated than PO administration.[11] However, topical treatment with either **glyceryl trinitrate** or **diltiazem** are generally preferred in practice (see p.81).

Nifedipine may help hiccup by relieving oesophageal spasm or by interference with nerve pathways involved in hiccup.[6,12] However, other alternatives are generally tried before nifedipine (See Prokinetics, Table 2, p.26).
Analgesic: In animal studies, nifedipine and other calcium-channel blockers augment the analgesic effects of **paracetamol**, **morphine** and anti-epileptics.[13–15] The clinical relevance of this is uncertain; inconsistent benefit has been found from the addition of calcium-channel blockers to postoperative pain regimens.[16–18]
Vasodilator: Nifedipine is used to treat angina, hypertension and Raynaud's phenomenon. It has a relatively greater effect on blood vessels than the myocardium and has no anti-arrhythmic activity. It rarely precipitates heart failure because any negative inotropic effect is offset by a reduction in left ventricular work.

Nifedipine promotes cancer proliferation *in vitro* and in animal models of breast cancer, via activation of a cellular growth pathway.[19] The relevance of these findings to patients is unknown.

Nifedipine undergoes extensive first-pass metabolism in the liver to inactive metabolites which are excreted in the urine. Higher plasma concentrations are seen in slow metabolizers, which are more prevalent in South American, South Asian and black African populations.[20,21] Hepatic impairment increases bio-availability and halflife.
Bio-availability 45–75% PO (immediate-release capsules).
Onset of action 15min (immediate-release capsules); 1.5h (m/r tablets, Adalat® Retard).
Time to peak plasma concentration 30min PO (immediate-release capsules).
Plasma halflife about 2h (immediate-release capsules); 2–2.5h (m/r tablets, Adalat® Retard).
Duration of action 8h (immediate-release capsules); 12 or 24h (m/r tablets, depending on brand).

Cautions

May exacerbate angina; discontinue nifedipine if angina occurs 30–60min after the first dose. Rarely, it may precipitate or worsen heart failure; avoid in patients with significantly impaired cardiac function or heart failure. Hepatic impairment. May impair glucose tolerance and worsen diabetes mellitus.

Drug interactions

Serious drug interactions: augments the hypotensive and negative inotropic effects of other drugs, e.g. α and β antagonists, **chlorpromazine**.[22]

Nifedipine is metabolized by and inhibits CYP3A4 and CYP2D6; it also inhibits CYP1A2 and CYP2C8/9. Caution is required with concurrent use of drugs which inhibit or induce these enzymes, particularly in poor CYP2D6 metabolizers (see Chapter 19, Table 8, p.725).[22] Reports of interactions where dose adjustment or close monitoring are needed are listed in Table 1.

Table 1 CYP450 interactions with nifedipine which can alter drug plasma concentrations

Nifedipine plasma concentration		*Drug plasma concentration*	
increased by	*decreased by*	*increased by nifedipine*	*decreased by nifedipine*
Azole antifungals	Carbamazepine	Digoxin	Quinidine
Cimetidine[a]	Phenobarbital	Quinidine	
Fluoxetine	Phenytoin	Sertindole (not UK)	
Grapefruit juice	Rifampicin[b]	Tacrolimus	
Imatinib	St Johns wort	Theophylline	
Macrolide antibacterials			
Protease inhibitors			
Quinupristin/dalfopristin (not UK)			

a. reduce nifedipine dose by 50%

b. manufacturer considers that rifampicin renders nifedipine ineffective.

Undesirable effects

Common (<10%, >1%): headache, dizziness, vasodilation, peripheral oedema, constipation.
Uncommon (<1%, >0.1%): asthenia, lethargy, malaise, agitation, nervousness, sleep disorder, tremor, vertigo, abnormal vision, chest pain, tachycardia, palpitations, postural hypotension, oedema, dyspnoea, dry mouth, dyspepsia, abdominal pain, nausea, rash, pruritus, sweating, transient increase in liver enzymes.

Dose and use

Patients with angina should not bite into or use an immediate-release capsule SL because of the risk of rapid-onset hypotension and reflex tachycardia, which could lead to myocardial or cerebrovascular ischaemia.

For SL administration, patients should bite into and use the liquid contents of the immediate-release capsules immediately (unauthorized use). *Modified release formulations must not be used SL or chewed.*

- start with 10mg PO/SL stat and 10–20mg t.d.s. or m/r 20mg PO b.d. or 30–60mg PO once daily
- for achalasia, start with 10–20mg SL 30–45min before food; usual maximum dose 60–80mg/24h
- for painful spasm associated with anal fissure, use m/r 20mg PO b.d.; *topical treatments preferred*, see Pharmacology
- for intractable hiccup, ≤160mg/24h PO has been used with concurrent **fludrocortisone** 0.5–1mg PO to overcome associated orthostatic hypotension.[6]

Remains of some m/r tablets (Adalat® LA) may appear in the patient's faeces ('ghost tablets'), but these are inert residues, and do not affect the efficacy of the products.

Supply

Immediate-release products
Nifedipine (generic)
Capsules 5mg, 10mg, 28 days @ 10mg t.d.s. = £10.
Oral Solution 10mg/5mL, 28 days @ 10mg t.d.s. = £730. (Unauthorized, available as a special order; see Chapter 24). *Note. Price based on specials tariff in community.*
Oral solution (drops) 20mg/mL, 30mL = £30. (Unauthorized, available as a special order imported via The Specials Laboratory; see Chapter 24, p.751).

Modified-release products
Because of their different dosing regimens and concern over possible non-bio-equivalence, the BNF recommends that m/r formulations of nifedipine should be prescribed by brand name.[23]

Adalat® Retard (Bayer)
Tablets m/r 10mg, 20mg, 28 days @ 20mg b.d. = £9.

Adalat® LA (Bayer)
Tablets m/r 20mg, 30mg, 60mg, 28 days @ 30mg once daily = £7.

Adipine® MR (Chiesi)
Tablets m/r 10mg, 20mg, 28 days @ 20mg b.d. = £5.

Adipine® XL (Chiesi)
Tablets m/r 30mg, 60mg, 28 days @ 30mg once daily = £5.

This is not a complete list; see BNF for more information.

1 McLoughlin R and McQuillan R (1997) Using nifedipine to treat tenesmus. *Palliative Medicine*. **11**: 419–420.
2 George S *et al.* (1997) Pain in multiple leiomyomas alleviated by nifedipine. *Pain*. **73**: 101–102.
3 Cargill G *et al.* (1982) Nifedipine for relief of esophageal chest pain. *New England Journal of Medicine*. **307**: 187–188.
4 Al-Waili N (1990) Nifedipine for intestinal colic. *Journal of the American Medical Association*. **263**: 3258.
5 Celik A *et al.* (1995) Hereditary proctalgia fugax and constipation: report of a second family. *Gut*. **36**: 581–584.
6 Brigham B and Bolin T (1992) High dose nifedipine and fludrocortisone for intractable hiccups. *Medical Journal of Australia*. **157**: 70.
7 Castell DO (1985) Calcium-channel blocking agents for gastrointestinal disorders. *American Journal of Cardiology*. **55**: 210B–213B.
8 Achem SR and Gerson LB (2013) Distal esophageal spasm: an update. *Current Gastroenterology Reports*. **15**: 325.
9 Cross-Adame E *et al.* (2013) Treatment of esophageal (noncardiac) chest pain: Review. *Clinical Gastroenterology and Heptology*. **12**: 1224–1245.
10 Maradey-Romero C *et al.* (2014) Treatment of esophageal motility disorders based on the chicago classification. *Current Treatment Options Gastroenterology*. **12**: 441–455.
11 Golfam F *et al.* (2014) Comparison of topical nifedipine with oral nifedipine for treatment of anal fissure: a randomized controlled trial. *Iran Red Crescent Medical Journal*. **16**: e13592.
12 Steger M *et al.* (2015) Systemic review: the pathogenesis and pharmacological treatment of hiccups. *Alimentary Pharmacology and Therapeutics*. **42**: 1037–1050.
13 Koleva M and Dimova S (2000) Effects of nifedipine, verapamil, diltiazem and trifluoperazine on the antinociceptive activity of acetaminophen. *Methods and Findings in Experimental and Clinical Pharmacology*. **22**: 741–745.
14 Michaluk J *et al.* (1998) Effects of various Ca2+ channel antagonists on morphine analgesia, tolerance and dependence, and on blood pressure in the rat. *European Journal of Pharmacology*. **352**: 189–197.
15 El-Azab MF and Moustafa YM (2012) Influence of calcium channel blockers on anticonvulsant and antinociceptive activities of valproic acid in pentylenetetrazole-kindled mice. *Pharmacological Reports*. **64**: 305–314.
16 Carta F *et al.* (1990) Effect of nifedipine on morphine-induced analgesia. *Anesthesia and Analgesia*. **70**: 493–498.
17 Zarauza R *et al.* (2000) A comparative study with oral nifedipine, intravenous nimodipine, and magnesium sulfate in postoperative analgesia. *Anesthesia and Analgesia*. **91**: 938–943.
18 Casey G *et al.* (2006) Perioperative nimodipine and postoperative analgesia. *Anesthesia and Analgesia*. **102**: 504–508.
19 Guo DQ *et al.* (2014) Nifedipine promotes the proliferation and migration of breast cancer cells. *PLoS One*. **9**: e113649.
20 Sowunmi A *et al.* (1995) Ethnic differences in nifedipine kinetics: comparisons between Nigerians, Caucasians and South Asians. *British Journal of Clinical Pharmacology*. **40**: 489–493.
21 Castaneda-Hernandez G *et al.* (1996) Interethnic variability in nifedipine disposition: reduced systemic plasma clearance in Mexican subjects. *British Journal of Clinical Pharmacology*. **41**: 433–434.
22 Baxter K and Preston CL. *Stockley's Drug Interactions (online edition)*. Pharmaceutical Press, London: www.medicinescomplete.com (accessed June 2017).
23 British National Formulary. London: BMJ Group and Pharmaceutical Press www.bnf.org (accessed June 2017).

Updated August 2017

ANTICOAGULANTS

Anticoagulants are used predominantly to prevent or treat venous thrombo-embolism (VTE).[1] There is a range of drugs which act at various points in the coagulation cascade (Figure 1). In patients with cancer, **LMWH** (see p.911) and **warfarin** are still generally the most frequently used.

LMWH (derived from porcine heparin) and **fondaparinux** (a synthetic heparin pentasaccharide) both inhibit factor Xa.[3] LMWH is the current gold standard anticoagulant for cancer patients; compared with **warfarin**, it halves the rate of recurrent VTE (8% vs. 14%).[4,5] **Fondaparinux** is a useful alternative in those patients who need to avoid LMWH because of hypersensitivity, history of heparin induced thrombocytopenia, or for religious or cultural reasons.[6–8] The use of **unfractionated heparin** is limited to specific circumstances, e.g. severe renal impairment (eGFR <30mL/min/1.73m^2), increased risk of bleeding.

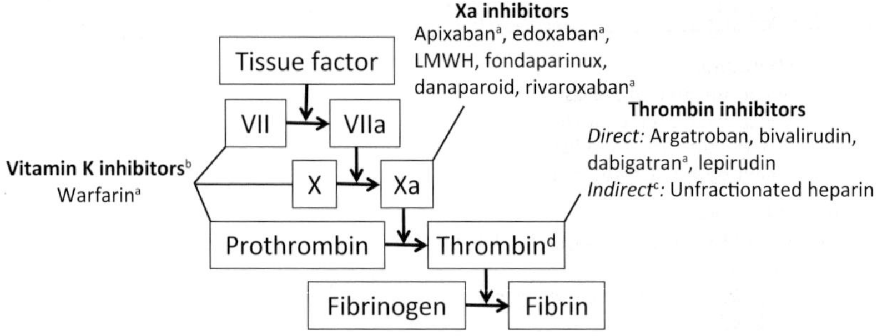

Figure 1 Sites of action of anticoagulants. Unless indicated otherwise, administration is parenteral, e.g. SC, IV, CIVI (see individual SPC). Heparins are antagonized by protamine sulfate, warfarin by vitamin K_1 (phytomenadione).[2] Specific antidotes have recently become available for the direct oral anticoagulants (see text).

a. administered PO
b. vitamin K inhibitors also reduce factor IX synthesis, inhibiting coagulation amplification pathways
c. indirect thrombin inhibitors activate antithrombin III, a regulator of coagulation
d. thrombin also triggers several amplification pathways (factors V, VIII, IX and XI) which promote further factor X activation and thus further thrombin generation.

In patients without cancer, **warfarin** is being increasingly replaced by direct oral anticoagulants (DOAC) such as **apixaban**, **edoxaban** and **rivaroxaban** (direct Xa inhibitors) or **dabigatran etexilate** (direct thrombin inhibitor). Potential advantages of DOAC include standard doses and no need to monitor levels of anticoagulation.

In the treatment of VTE, **apixaban**, **dabigatran etexilate**, **edoxaban** and **rivaroxaban** are non-inferior to **warfarin** with respect to recurrent VTE and bleeding.[9–12] All are authorized for both treatment of VTE and secondary prevention of recurrent VTE, and recommended by NICE.[13] However, in cancer patients, their use requires caution because efficacy and safety data are limited in this group.[5,14] Indeed, some currently recommend against the use of DOAC in cancer patients because of:

- non-inferiority with LMWH has not been demonstrated
- the risk of significant drug–drug interactions, e.g. with CYP3A4 inducers or inhibitors (these include several chemotherapy drugs), which could lead to clinically important changes in plasma concentrations of DOAC, and result in therapeutic failure or bleeding
- major bleeding is more likely in patients with cancer who are anticoagulated,[15] and the lack of standardized methods of monitoring DOAC and availability of antidotes could cause problems.[16]

Further, there is risk of accumulation in renal impairment. Nonetheless, DOAC are likely to be increasingly used in cancer patients unwilling to tolerate daily SC injections of LMWH. Seek advice from a haematologist about such use, and urgently if bleeding occurs during use (Box A).

Box A Management of bleeding in patients on DOAC[17,18]

General principles

For most bleeds, supportive care measures, e.g. local haemostatic control, haemodynamic support and blood transfusions will be sufficient. Reversal strategies are reserved for severe or life-threatening bleeds and include:

- drug removal: activated charcoal, haemodialysis (dabigatran etexilate)
- specific antidotes: sequestering and neutralizing agents, e.g. idarucizumab (dabigatran etexilate), andexanet alfa, ciparantag (apixaban, edoxaban, rivaroxaban)
- non-specific antidotes: prohaemostatic agents, e.g. prothrombin complex concentrates.

continued

Box A Continued

Minor bleeding
- document the time of the last dose of DOAC
- apply local haemostatic measures, if feasible
- if bleeding continues, consider tranexamic acid (see below)
- delay next dose of DOAC or stop.

Major bleeding
- apply local haemostatic measures, if feasible
- give IV fluid replacement
- *obtain advice from haematologist urgently*
- stop DOAC
- document the time of the last dose; if taken <2h ago, consider giving activated charcoal PO
- arrange laboratory tests *as recommended by haematologist*, e.g. FBC, prothrombin time (PT), APTT, eGFR
- give tranexamic acid 15mg/kg IV t.d.s–q.d.s. (or 25mg/kg PO t.d.s.); reduce dose in renal impairment (see p.103)
  - ▷ if feasible, apply topically to bleeding point, e.g. mouthwash, nasal drops
- consider also other possible causes of a coagulopathy, e.g. DIC
- give IV blood product support as indicated by Hb, other coagulopathy, platelets (if count <75 x 10^9/L).

If ongoing life- or limb- threatening bleeding
- obtain further advice from haematologist urgently regarding use of specific or non-specific antidotes (see above).

General considerations in patients with cancer

Compared with non-cancer patients, those with cancer are three times more likely to experience recurrent VTE (21% vs. 7%), *despite optimal treatment with **warfarin**.*[19] The increased risk results from a cancer-related pro-inflammatory state associated with:
- activation of the coagulation cascade by procoagulant proteins expressed by the cancer
- damage to blood vessel walls
- venous stasis
- other general risk factors (Box B).

Box B Main risk factors for VTE in medical patients[7,20–27]

Age ≥40 years, particularly >60 years

Immobility

Dehydration

Obesity

Cancer, particularly metastatic, especially of the pancreas, stomach, bladder, ovary, uterus, kidney or lung; also haematological

Chronic respiratory or cardiac disease

Other serious medical conditions, e.g. sepsis, lower limb weakness (including spinal cord compression), inflammatory bowel disease, collagen disorder

Varicose veins/chronic venous insufficiency

Previous VTE

Cancer chemotherapy, e.g. platinum compounds, 5-FU, mitomycin-C, thalidomide

Growth factors, e.g. granulocyte colony stimulating factor, erythropoietin

Radiation therapy, e.g. to the pelvis

Hormone therapy, e.g. oral contraceptives, hormone replacement, tamoxifen, anastrozole, and possibly progestins

Thrombophilia

In palliative care, LMWH is preferable because haemorrhagic complications with **warfarin** may occur in up to 50% of patients, possibly related to poor performance status, drug interactions and hepatic impairment. Those patients agreeing to the indefinite use of LMWH have found it acceptable.[28–31] Compared with **warfarin**, treatment with LMWH is more straightforward: no need to check INR, and little need for dose adjustments. However, compared with **warfarin**, LMWH is much more expensive (Table 1). The specific antidotes for DOACs are also expensive, e.g. idarucizumab costs >£2,400 per dose.

Table 1 Cost of anticoagulants

Drug	*Route*	*Dose[a]*	*Approximate 28 day cost*
Apixaban	PO tablets	1 tablet b.d.	£53
Dabigatran etexilate	PO capsules	1 capsule b.d.	£48
Edoxaban	PO tablets	1 tablet once daily	£52
LMWH	SC injection	1 injection daily	£84–98
Rivaroxaban	PO tablets	1 tablet once daily	£50
Warfarin	PO tablets	Based on INR, 0.5–1 tablet once daily	£1–2[b]
	PO suspension	Based on INR, 1–5mL once daily	£17–84[b]

a. actual dose can depend on age, weight ± renal impairment; consult specific SPCs

b. does not include cost of checking INR.

Specialist guidelines recommend that thromboprophylaxis should be considered if an acute medical illness is likely to render a cancer patient bedbound for ≥3 days, particularly in the presence of one or more additional risk factors (Box B).[6,26,32] This includes patients admitted to a palliative care unit with a potentially reversible acute medical illness. Duration of treatment is generally about 2 weeks.[24]

If anticoagulation is contra-indicated, mechanical measures, e.g. graduated compression stockings, intermittent pneumatic compression, should be considered.[26] However, the evidence in medical patients is limited, and there have been reports of harm.[33,34]

Patients admitted to a palliative care unit for end-of-life care should not be routinely offered any form of thromboprophylaxis.[26]

1 Farge D *et al.* (2013) International clinical practice guidelines for the treatment and prophylaxis of venous thromboembolism in patients with cancer. *Journal of Thrombosis and Haemostasis.* **11**: 56–70.

2 Noble S and Johnson M (2012) Management of cancer associated thrombosis in people with advanced disease. *BMJ Supportive and Palliative Care.* **2**: 163–167.

3 Hoppensteadt D *et al.* (2003) Heparin, low-molecular-weight heparins, and heparin pentasaccharide: basic and clinical differentiation. *Hematology Oncology Clinics of North America.* **17**: 313–341.

4 Kearon C *et al.* (2016) Antithrombotic therapy for VTE disease: chest guideline and expert panel report. *Chest.* **149**: 315–352.

5 Noble S and Sui J (2016) The treatment of cancer associated thrombosis: does one size fit all? Who should get LMWH/warfarin/DOACs? *Thrombosis Research.* **140 (Suppl 1)**: S154–159.

6 Baglin T *et al.* (2006) Guidelines on the use and monitoring of heparin. *British Journal of Haematology.* **133**: 19–34.

7 Blann AD and Lip GY (2006) Venous thromboembolism. *British Medical Journal.* **332**: 215–219.

8 Cohen AT *et al.* (2006) Efficacy and safety of fondaparinux for the prevention of venous thromboembolism in older acute medical patients: randomised placebo controlled trial. *British Medical Journal.* **332**: 325–329.

9 Schulman S *et al.* (2009) Dabigatran versus warfarin in the treatment of acute venous thromboembolism. *New England Journal of Medicine.* **361**: 2342–2352.

10 Bauersachs R *et al.* (2010) Oral rivaroxaban for symptomatic venous thromboembolism. *New England Journal of Medicine.* **363**: 2499–2510.

11 Agnelli G *et al.* (2013) Oral apixaban for the treatment of acute venous thromboembolism. *New England Journal of Medicine.* **369**: 799–808.

12 Buller HR *et al.* (2013) Edoxaban versus warfarin for the treatment of symptomatic venous thromboembolism. *New England Journal of Medicine.* **369**: 1406–1415.

13 NICE (2016) Anticoagulants, including non-vitamin K antagonist oral anticoagulants (NOACs). *Key therapeutic topic.* KTT16: www.nice.org.uk

14 Gerotziafas GT *et al.* (2014) New orally active anticoagulant agents for the prevention and treatment of venous thromboembolism in cancer patients. *Therapeutics and Clinical Risk Managemnt.* **10**: 423–436.

15 Streiff MB (2006) Long-term therapy of venous thromboembolism in cancer patients. *Journal of the National Comprehensive Cancer Network*. **4**: 903–910.
16 Carrier M *et al.* (2013) Management of challenging cases of patients with cancer-associated thrombosis including recurrent thrombosis and bleeding: guidance from the SSC of the ISTH. *Journal of Thrombosis and Haemostasis*. **12**: 116–117.
17 NICE (2016) Reversal of the anticoagulant effect of dabigatran: idarucizumab. evidence summary ESNM 73.www.nice.org.uk
18 Samuelson BT and Cuker A (2017) Measurement and reversal of the direct oral anticoagulants. *Blood Reviews*. **31**: 77–84.
19 Prandoni P *et al.* (2002) Recurrent venous thromboembolism and bleeding complications during anticoagulant treatment in patients with cancer and venous thrombosis. *Blood*. **100**: 3484–3488.
20 Samama MM *et al.* (1999) A comparison of enoxaparin with placebo for the prevention of venous thromboembolism in acutely ill medical patients. Prophylaxis in Medical Patients with Enoxaparin Study Group. *New England Journal of Medicine*. **341**: 793–800.
21 De Cicco M (2004) The prothrombotic state in cancer: pathogenic mechanisms. *Critical Reviews in Oncology Hematology*. **50**: 187–196.
22 Deitcher SR and Gomes MP (2004) The risk of venous thromboembolic disease associated with adjuvant hormone therapy for breast carcinoma: a systematic review. *Cancer*. **101**: 439–449.
23 Leizorovicz A *et al.* (2004) Randomized, placebo-controlled trial of dalteparin for the prevention of venous thromboembolism in acutely ill medical patients. *Circulation*. **110**: 874–879.
24 Leizorovicz A and Mismetti P (2004) Preventing venous thromboembolism in medical patients. *Circulation*. **110**: 13–19.
25 Chew HK *et al.* (2006) Incidence of venous thromboembolism and its effect on survival among patients with common cancers. *Archives of Internal Medicine*. **166**: 458–464.
26 NICE (2015) Reducing the risk of venous thromboembolism (deep vein thrombosis and pulmonary embolism) in patients admitted to hospital. *Clinical Guideline* 92. www.nice.org.uk
27 Kahn SR *et al.* (2012) Prevention of VTE in nonsurgical patients: Antithrombotic Therapy and Prevention of Thrombosis, 9th ed: American College of Chest Physicians Evidence-Based Clinical Practice Guidelines. *Chest*. **141**: e195S–e226S.
28 Johnson M (1997) Problems of anticoagulation within a palliative care setting: an audit of hospice patients taking warfarin. *Palliative Medicine*. **11**: 306–312.
29 Johnson M and Sherry K (1997) How do palliative physicians manage venous thromboembolism? *Palliative Medicine*. **11**: 462–468.
30 Noble SI and Finlay IG (2005) Is long-term low-molecular-weight heparin acceptable to palliative care patients in the treatment of cancer related venous thromboembolism? A qualitative study. *Palliative Medicine*. **19**: 197–201.
31 Noble SI *et al.* (2006) Acceptability of low molecular weight heparin thromboprophylaxis for inpatients receiving palliative care: qualitative study. *British Medical Journal*. **332**: 577–580.
32 Cunningham MS *et al.* (2006) Prevention and management of venous thromboembolism in people with cancer: a review of the evidence. *Clinical Oncology (Royal College of Radiologists)*. **18**: 145–151.
33 Dennis M *et al.* (2009) Effectiveness of thigh-length graduated compression stockings to reduce the risk of deep vein thrombosis after stroke (CLOTS trial 1): a multicentre, randomised controlled trial. *Lancet*. **373**: 1958–1965.
34 Dennis M *et al.* (2013) Effectiveness of intermittent pneumatic compression in reduction of risk of deep vein thrombosis in patients who have had a stroke (CLOTS 3): a multicentre randomised controlled trial. *Lancet*. **382**: 516–524.

Updated August 2017

LOW MOLECULAR WEIGHT HEPARIN (LMWH)

Class: Parenteral anticoagulant.

Indications: Authorized indications vary between products; consult SPCs for details. Thromboprophylaxis, initial treatment of venous thrombo-embolism (VTE), treatment of cancer-associated thrombosis, †thrombophlebitis migrans, †disseminated intravascular coagulation (DIC).

Contra-indications: IM use (risk of injection site haematoma); active major bleeding; suspected or confirmed heparin-induced thrombocytopenia (HIT) with LMWH; known bleeding diathesis (including bleeding peptic ulcer); severe uncontrolled hypertension; haemorrhagic stroke; diabetic or haemorrhagic retinopathy; bacterial endocarditis; injury or surgery to brain, spinal cord, eyes or ears.
Stated contra-indications and cautions vary; see individual SPCs.

Pharmacology

Three low molecular weight heparins (LMWHs) are available in the UK, **dalteparin**, **enoxaparin**, **tinzaparin**, all derived from porcine heparin. Some patients need to avoid the use of LMWH because of known hypersensitivity, or for religious or cultural reasons; the most appropriate parenteral alternative is **fondaparinux**, a non-porcine synthetic heparin pentasaccharide.

LMWH acts mainly by potentiating the inhibitory effect of antithrombin III on factor Xa. The dose of LMWH is determined by the patient's weight, and routine monitoring of an anticoagulant effect is not necessary. However, in cases where the patient is considered at risk of bleeding, has renal impairment (CrCl <30mL/min) or a history of recurrent thrombosis, anti-factor Xa activity levels can be measured.

LMWH is as effective as unfractionated heparin (UFH) for the treatment of DVT and pulmonary embolism (PE) and is now considered the initial treatment of choice. Advantages include a longer duration of action permitting once daily administration, and possibly a better safety profile (fewer major haemorrhages).[1,2]

In cancer patients, LMWH is more effective than **warfarin** for the treatment of VTE, with a similar or reduced risk of bleeding.[3,4] LMWH is the anticoagulant of choice for long-term use in patients for whom maintaining a stable INR is difficult (risking either therapeutic failure or haemorrhagic complications) or in those who have recurrent VTE despite a therapeutic INR.

Experimental models suggest that LMWH has an anticancer effect via the inhibition of metastatic spread.[5] However, clinical trials in a range of cancers have overall failed to demonstrate an improvement in survival ± time to disease progression.[5] Thus, LMWH is *not* recommended as routine adjunctive treatment.[4]

LMWHs are primarily renally excreted and can accumulate in renal impairment (see Dose and use below). For pharmacokinetic details, see Table 1.

Table 1 LMWH pharmacokinetics[6–10]

	Dalteparin	*Enoxaparin*	*Tinzaparin*
Bio-availability SC[a]	87%	100%	87%
Onset of action	3min IV	5min IV	5min IV
	2–4h SC	3h SC	2–3h SC
Time to peak plasma activity[a]	4h SC	2–6h SC	4–5h SC
Plasma activity halflife[a]	2h IV	2–4.5h IV	1.5h IV
	3–5h SC	4.5–7h SC	3–4h SC
Duration of action	10–24h SC	>24h SC	24h

a. based on anti-factor Xa activity.

Cautions

Contra-indications and cautions vary between manufacturers; see individual SPCs.

Risk factors for bleeding include serious concurrent illness, severe renal and hepatic impairment (see Dose and use below), chronic heavy consumption of alcohol, age, and possibly female gender.

Monitor closely if spinal analgesia is used in a patient receiving LMWH *thromboprophylaxis*; and, because of the risk of a spinal haematoma, spinal analgesia should be avoided in a patient receiving *therapeutic* doses of LMWH.

Drug interactions

Enhanced bleeding tendency with NSAIDs (particularly **ketorolac**) and other drugs with anticoagulant/antiplatelet effect.

Inhibition of aldosterone secretion by heparin/LMWH may cause hyperkalaemia. The risk appears to increase with duration of therapy and is higher in patients with diabetes mellitus, chronic renal failure, acidosis and those taking potassium supplements or potassium-sparing drugs. The CSM recommends measuring plasma potassium in such patients before starting heparin and regularly thereafter, particularly if heparin is to be continued for >1 week, although a specific frequency is not stated.

Undesirable effects

Common (<10%, >1%): headache, dizziness, pain at the injection site, minor bleeding (haematoma at the injection site), major bleeding in surgical patients receiving thromboprophylaxis and patients being treated for VTE, tachycardia, chest pain, oedema, hypotension, hypertension, anaemia, nausea, constipation, reversible increases in liver transaminases, back pain, haematuria.

Uncommon (<1%, >0.1%): major bleeding in patients receiving thromboprophylaxis, immune-mediated heparin-induced thrombocytopenia (see QCG: Heparin-induced thrombocytopenia, p.100),[11] abdominal pain, diarrhoea.

Dose and use

Routine platelet count monitoring

All patients should have a baseline platelet count before starting LMWH (or any other heparin). Postoperative patients receiving UFH (any surgery) or LMWH (cardiopulmonary bypass only) should have their platelet count checked every 2–3 days for 2 weeks, or until heparin is stopped.

Postoperative patients and cardiopulmonary bypass patients receiving any type of heparin who have been exposed to heparin in the last 3 months should have a repeat platelet count after 24h to exclude rapid-onset HIT caused by pre-existing cross-reacting antibodies.

Medical and postoperative (other than cardiopulmonary bypass) patients receiving LMWH do not need routine platelet monitoring.[11]

Renal impairment

In severe renal impairment (creatinine clearance <30mL/min) accumulation of **dalteparin**, **enoxaparin** and **tinzaparin** occurs to a variable degree, increasing overall exposure and prolonging anti-factor Xa activity halflife. Monitoring of anti-factor Xa activity is advised to guide dosing, particularly in those at increased risk of bleeding (see specific SPCs). For example, the dose of **tinzaparin** should be reduced if anti-factor Xa activity exceeds 1.5 units/mL (usual range 0.5–1.5 units/mL). For **enoxaparin**, the manufacturer recommends specific dose reduction for both prophylaxis and treatment (see SPC).

Although doses recommended for prophylaxis against DVT (and thrombus formation in extracorporeal circuits) are well tolerated in patients with ESRF, the doses recommended for treatment of VTE have been associated with severe, sometimes fatal, bleeding. Thus, specialist guidelines suggest using UFH IV instead of LMWH for treatment of VTE in severe renal impairment.[12,13]

Severe hepatic impairment

Reduced synthesis of clotting factors increases the risk of bleeding. Consider dose reduction for **dalteparin**, **enoxaparin** (also possible risk of accumulation) and **tinzaparin**.

SC injections

May cause transient stinging and local bruising.[14] Long-term treatment is not acceptable to some cancer patients (about 15%).[15]

Rotate injection sites daily, e.g. between different abdominal quadrants (see SPCs for the manufacturers' recommendations). Create a skin fold by squeezing the skin between thumb and forefinger, and insert the total length of the needle vertically into the thickest part of the fold; do *not* rub the injection site.

Thromboprophylaxis in patients with cancer

Recommendations vary between guidelines.[16] *PCF* reflects NICE and British Committee for Standards in Haematology guidance.[4,13]

Generally, patients with cancer admitted for surgical or medical reasons should be offered thromboprophylaxis, except where likely benefit is outweighed by the associated bleeding risk.

Undergoing surgery

Patients with cancer undergoing major surgery are at high risk of VTE; they have twice the risk of developing a DVT and three times the risk of a fatal PE.[17] Abdominal and pelvic surgery is particularly high-risk.

Standard mechanical measures are recommended, e.g. graduated compression stockings, intermittent pneumatic compression, until mobility is regained.[13]

For those who have undergone major cancer surgery in the abdomen or pelvis, or hip surgery, an extended period of thromboprophylaxis is more effective than the usual ~1 week (Table 2).[13]

Reduced mobility because of an intercurrent illness

Hospitalized cancer patients are at high risk of VTE. NICE guidelines recommend thromboprophylaxis is considered in patients who have ≥3 days reduced mobility relative to their normal state, when there are ≥1 risk factors, such as cancer (see p.89).[18] Duration of treatment is generally ≤2 weeks (Table 2).[19]

Table 2 Thromboprophylaxis with LMWH in patients with cancer[13]

	Dalteparin	*Enoxaparin*	*Tinzaparin*
Undergoing surgery involving the abdomen, pelvis or hip[a]	5,000 units SC once daily; start evening before surgery; continue for 4 weeks	40mg SC once daily; start 12h before surgery; continue for 4 weeks	4,500 units 12h before surgery, then once daily; continue for 4 weeks
Reduced mobility because of an intercurrent illness[a]	5,000 units SC once daily	40mg SC once daily	4,500 units SC once daily
Cost per dose (pre-filled syringe)	5,000 units/0.2mL = £3	40mg/0.4mL = £3	4,500 units/0.45mL = £3.50

a. for other types of major surgery and in medical patients, LMWH is continued until the patient no longer has significantly reduced mobility (generally 1–2 weeks).

In patients receiving palliative care, thromboprophylaxis is generally acceptable,[20] and should be offered to those with potentially reversible acute pathology.[13] The decision to start should take into account the views of patients, family/informal carers and the multiprofessional team, and be kept under review. NICE guidance suggests reviewing daily, but this seems excessive and will often be impractical.

If anticoagulation is contra-indicated, mechanical measures, e.g. graduated compression stockings, intermittent pneumatic compression, should be considered.[13] However, the evidence in medical patients is limited, and there have been reports of harm.[21,22]

However, thromboprophylaxis is less relevant for patients with a poor performance status in their last weeks–days of life, at a stage when symptom relief alone is more appropriate. Thus, patients admitted to a palliative care unit for end-of-life care should *not* be routinely offered any form of thromboprophylaxis.[13]

Outpatient chemotherapy

Thromboprophylaxis should *not* be offered routinely to patients with cancer receiving chemotherapy as an outpatient. However, it may be considered in those at very high thrombotic risk (Box A).[4]

Thromboprophylaxis should also be considered in patients with multiple myeloma receiving **lenolidamide** or **thalidomide** (see p.558).

Box A Predictive model for chemotherapy-associated VTE[4]

Calculate score:

	Score
Site of cancer:	
Pancreas, stomach	2
Bladder, gynaecological, lung, lymphoma, testicular	1
Haemoglobin <100g/L or use of erythropoietic drug, e.g. epoetin	1
Pre-chemotherapy WBC >11 x 10^9/L	1
Pre-chemotherapy platelets ≥350 x 10^9/L	1
BMI ≥35 Kg/m^2	1

Interpretation:

Score		*Thrombosis rate per 2.5 months (%)*
Low	0	0.3–0.8
Intermediate	1–2	1.8–2
High	>2	6.7–7.1

2

Indwelling venous catheters

The presence of a central (subclavian) or peripheral indwelling venous catheter can lead to catheter-related thrombosis. However, routine thromboprophylaxis with LMWH or **warfarin** does not reduce the risk of thrombosis and is *not* recommended.[4,13] NICE guidelines suggest thromboprophylaxis may be considered in patients at increased risk of VTE.[13,18]

Long-distance air travel

The evidence for an association between prolonged travel and venous VTE is controversial. Overall, the risk appears to be extremely low, but is greater in journeys of >6h and in those travellers with pre-existing risk factors (see Box B, p.89).[23]

Although there is insufficient evidence to support routine thromboprophylaxis for all travellers, it is generally advisable in patients with cancer undertaking a continuous journey >6h:

- prescribe three injections (one each for the outward and return journeys, and one spare)
- provide a covering letter for the use of the injections (along with any other drugs required, see p.749) to ease passage through Security, Immigration and Customs
- provide training in the correct administration of the injection (see the information on self-administration included in the patient information leaflet)
- self-administer **dalteparin** 5,000 units, **enoxaparin** 40mg or **tinzaparin** 4,500 units SC 2–4h before departure
- if there is a stop-over followed by another long flight, another injection is not necessary unless the second flight is more than 24h after the first.

In addition, patients should be advised to:

- wear properly fitted below-knee graduated compression stockings, providing 14–17mmHg of pressure at the ankle (unless contra-indicated, e.g. peripheral arterial disease)
- avoid prolonged immobility; stretch the calf muscles frequently by moving the feet up and down, walk around
- avoid constrictive clothing around the waist and lower limbs.

Treatment

Recommendations vary between guidelines.[16] *PCF* reflects NICE and British Committee for Standards in Haematology guidance.[4,12]

DVT and PE in cancer patients: initial treatment

Confirm the diagnosis radiologically (e.g. ultrasound, CT pulmonary angiography). Treat DVT and PE presenting either symptomatically or as an incidental finding with LMWH for 6 months:

- **dalteparin** maximum daily dose 18,000 units/24h; give 200 units/kg SC once daily for the first month, followed by 150 units/kg SC once daily thereafter *or*
- **enoxaparin** 1.5mg/kg SC once daily *or*
- **tinzaparin** 175 units/kg SC once daily.[12]

Note. In the UK, only **dalteparin** and **tinzaparin** are authorized for extended (6 months) treatment of cancer-associated VTE.

In patients for whom LMWH is contra-indicated or not tolerated, **warfarin** can be considered. Although a DOAC is a potential alternative to **warfarin**, there are less supporting data and concerns exist regarding their use in this population (see p.87).

'Grade 2' compression stockings should *not* be used routinely to reduce post-thrombotic syndrome or recurrent DVT. However, they can be trialled in patients with symptomatic post-thrombotic syndrome.[12]

An inferior vena caval filter should only be used when there is a strong contra-indication to anticoagulation. It should be removed as soon as anticoagulation becomes possible.

DVT and PE cancer patients: ongoing treatment

Indefinite anticoagulation beyond 6 months should be considered for patients who have a DVT or PE and have an ongoing major risk factor for VTE such as cancer (see Box B, p.89).[4,12]

In cancer patients, the evidence that LMWH is more effective than **warfarin** relates to the first 3–6 months of anticoagulation.[4] Although probable that LMWH would continue to remain more effective than **warfarin**, efficacy and safety data are lacking to guide the choice of anticoagulant for indefinite use in this population. Thus, an increasing practice is to discuss this uncertainty with patients, along with the potential benefits and harms of continuing with LMWH vs. switching to **warfarin**.[24] Although a DOAC is a potential alternative to **warfarin**, there are less supporting data and concerns exist regarding their use in this population (see p.87).

When a switch to **warfarin** is considered in a patient with stable or cured cancer, LMWH should be continued until a therapeutic INR has been achieved on two consecutive days.

VTE in a seemingly cured cancer patient may be an indication of occult recurrence. If truly idiopathic, a minimum of 6–12 months of anticoagulation is recommended, and indefinite anticoagulation considered.

Provided no contra-indications develop, indefinite anticoagulation is generally continued in patients with cancer until they reach the stage when symptom relief alone becomes more appropriate, e.g. in the last few weeks or days of life.

Special circumstances

There is no standard approach to the following circumstances; seek specialist advice.[4,24,25]

Recurrent VTE despite anticoagulation

Consider:

- is patient adhering to treatment?
- is the dose of anticoagulant correct? Measure anti-factor Xa activity levels (LMWH), INR (**warfarin**)
- excluding HIT, see QCG: Heparin-induced thrombocytopenia, p.100
- possible mechanical compression from tumour masses
- for those on LMWH:
  - ▷ ensure on full weight-based therapeutic dose
  - ▷ if already on full dose, increase dose by 20–33% and give b.d., e.g. increase **enoxaparin** from 1.5mg/kg SC once daily → 1mg/kg SC b.d.
  - ▷ if necessary, make further increases guided by anti-factor Xa activity levels
- for those on **warfarin** or a DOAC, switch to LMWH.

Note. Insertion of an inferior vena caval filter is *not* recommended for recurrence alone.

Bleeding while anticoagulated

Consider:

- bleeding source, severity, impact and reversibility
- supportive measures, **tranexamic acid** (p.102), blood transfusion
- in a major or life-threatening bleed:
  - ▷ withholding anticoagulation and the use of reversal agents (also see Anticoagulants, p.87)
  - ▷ use of a retrievable inferior vena caval filter (in acute or subacute VTE only); remove when bleeding has stopped and recommencing anticoagulation appropriate.

VTE in thrombocytopenia

- when platelet count >50 x10^9/L, use normal LMWH dose
- when platelet count <50 x10^9/L:
  - ▷ in acute VTE, during the highest risk of recurrence, use normal LMWH dose and give platelet transfusions to maintain platelet count >50 x10^9/L; if persistent thrombocytopenia or other bleeding risk prevents anticoagulation, consider insertion of a temporary inferior vena caval filter
  - ▷ in subacute/chronic VTE, use half normal LMWH dose
  - ▷ omit LMWH if platelet count <25 x10^9/L
- if thrombocytopenia develops during LMWH treatment, exclude HIT, see QCG: Heparin-induced thrombocytopenia, p.100.

Thrombophlebitis migrans

- *do not use **warfarin** because it is ineffective*
- generally responds rapidly to small doses of LMWH:
  - ▷ **dalteparin**: 2,500–5,000 units SC once daily; if necessary, titrate to maximum permitted dose, 200 units/kg once daily *or*
  - ▷ **enoxaparin**: ≤60mg once daily; if necessary, titrate to maximum permitted dose, 1.5mg/kg SC once daily
- continue treatment indefinitely.[26]

Disseminated intravascular coagulation (DIC)

Confirm the diagnosis

This is made on the basis of the presence of a clinical condition known to be associated with DIC, together with various haematological indices:

- thrombocytopenia (platelet count <150 x 10^9/L in 98% of cases)
- elevated plasma D-dimer concentration, a fibrin degradation product (85% of cases)
- prolonged prothrombin time and/or partial thromboplastin time (50–60% of cases)
- decreased plasma fibrinogen concentration (40% of cases).

These can be scored to indicate the likelihood of overt DIC, with scores predictive of mortality (Box B).[27] Overt DIC represents a stressed and decompensated haemostatic system generally resulting in clinical consequences. In non-overt DIC, the haemostatic system is under stress but compensated.

DIC is a dynamic state and serial laboratory tests, e.g. daily, are required to fully evaluate the clinical situation.

Box B Diagnostic scoring system for DIC[27]

Risk assessment

If the patient has an underlying disorder known to be associated with DIC, proceed to measure and score the haematological indices below:

	Score			
	0	*1*	*2*	*3*
Platelets (x 10^9/L)	>100	<100	<50	
D-dimer increase (ng/mL)	none		moderate (250–5,000)	strong (>5,000)
Prolonged PT (sec)	<3	3–6	>6	
Fibrinogen (g/L)	>1	<1		

Calculate total score:

≥5 Compatible with overt DIC, repeat score daily

<5 Suggestive (not affirmative) for non-overt DIC, repeat score in 1–2 days

Management

When possible, correct the underlying cause, e.g. sepsis.

Seek specialist advice:

- on the use of platelet transfusions, fresh frozen plasma, other coagulation factors and **tranexamic acid**, in patients actively bleeding, requiring an invasive procedure, or at risk of bleeding complications
- on the use of anticoagulants, e.g. UFH, LMWH, prophylactically in those not bleeding, or when thrombosis predominates.

Note. Generally, antifibrinolytic drugs, e.g. **tranexamic acid** and **aminocaproic acid** (not UK), should *not* be used in DIC because they increase the risk of end-organ damage from microvascular thromboses.

LMWH is the anticoagulant of choice in the treatment of *chronic* DIC; this commonly presents as recurrent thromboses in both superficial and deep veins which do not respond to **warfarin**.

Overdose

See individual SPCs for details.

With recommended doses of LMWH, there should be no need for an antidote. However, an accidental overdose may result in haemorrhagic complications.

Protamine sulfate partially reverses the effects of LMWH on factor Xa (**dalteparin** 25%, **enoxaparin** 60%, **tinzaparin** 65–80%). Because **protamine** in excess can have an anticoagulant effect[28] and, because the effect of LMWH may outlast that of **protamine** (this will depend on the interval between the last dose of LMWH and administering **protamine**), it should be used only in an emergency and in accordance with the recommendations in the individual LMWH SPCs. However, typically:

- for each 100 units (or 1mg **enoxaparin**) of LMWH, **protamine sulfate** 1mg is given
- a maximum of 50mg by slow IV injection is given *over 10min.*

Decisions regarding the necessity and dose of subsequent **protamine** injections are based on clinical response.

Alternatively, recombinant **activated factor VIIa concentrate** can be used. In three patients who bled after surgery or an invasive procedure, a single IV dose of 20–30microgram/kg successfully reversed anticoagulation from LMWH. It did not precipitate thrombosis, despite the patients all having a risk factor for hypercoagulation, e.g. cancer-related surgery.[29]

Supply

Dalteparin (generic)
Injection (single-dose graduated syringe for SC injection) 10,000 units/mL, 1mL syringe = £6.
Injection (single-dose syringe for SC injection) 2,500 units/0.2mL = £2.
Injection (single-dose syringe for SC injection) 5,000 units/0.2mL = £3, 7,500 units/0.3mL = £4, 10,000 units/0.4mL = £5.50, 12,500 units/0.5mL = £7, 15,000 units/0.6mL = £8.50, 18,000 units/0.72mL = £10.

Fragmin® (Pfizer)
Injection (single-dose ampoule for SC or IV injection) 10,000 units/4mL, 4mL amp = £5.
Injection (single-dose ampoule for SC or IV injection) 10,000 units/mL 1mL amp = £5.
Injection (multiple-dose vial for SC injection), 100,000 units/4mL, 4mL vial = £49.

Enoxaparin
Note. Enoxaparin 1mg = 100 units.
Clexane® (Sanofi)
Injection (single-dose syringe for SC injection) 20mg/0.2mL = £2, 40mg/0.4mL = £3, 60mg/0.6mL = £4, 80mg/0.8mL = £5.50, 100mg/1mL = £7.
Injection (Clexane® Forte; single-dose syringe for SC injection) 120mg/0.8mL = £9, 150mg/1mL = £10.
Injection (Clexane® Multidose; multiple-dose vial for SC or IV injection) 300mg/3mL, 3mL vial = £21.

Tinzaparin (generic)
Injection (single-dose syringe for SC injection), 2,500 units/0.25mL = £2, 3,500 units/0.35mL = £3, 4,500 units/0.45mL = £3.50.

Innohep® (Leo)
Injection (single-dose syringe for SC injection), 8,000 units/0.4mL = £5, 10,000 units/0.5mL = £6, 12,000 units/0.6mL = £7, 14,000 units/0.7mL = £8, 16,000 units/0.8mL = £9.50, 18,000 units/0.9mL = £11.
Injection (multiple-dose vial for SC injection) 20,000 units/2mL, 2mL vial = £11.
Injection (multiple-dose vial for SC injection) 40,000 units/2mL, 2mL vial = £34.

Protamine sulfate (generic)
Injection 50mg/5mL, 5mL amp = £5.

1 Quinlan D *et al.* (2004) Low-molecular weight heparin compared with intravenous unfractionated heparin for treatment of pulmonary embolism. *Annals of Internal Medicine.* **140**: 175–183.
2 Van Dongen CJ *et al.* (2004) Fixed dose subcutaneous low molecular weight heparins versus adjusted dose unfractionated heparin for venous thromboembolism. *Cochrane Database of Systematic Reviews.* **4**: CD001100. www.thecochranelibrary.com
3 Kearon C *et al.* (2016) Antithrombotic therapy for VTE disease: chest guideline and expert panel report. *Chest.* **149**: 315–352.
4 Watson HG *et al.* (2015) Guideline on aspects of cancer-related venous thrombosis. *British Journal of Haematology.* **170**: 640–648.
5 Zhang N *et al.* (2016) Low molecular weight heparin and cancer survival: clinical trials and experimental mechanisms. *Journal of Cancer Research and Clinical Oncology.* **142**: 1807–1816.
6 Fossler MJ *et al.* (2001) Pharmacodynamics of intravenous and subcutaneous tinzaparin and heparin in healthy volunteers. *American Journal of Health System Pharmacy.* **58**: 1614–1621.
7 Fareed J *et al.* (1990) Pharmacologic profile of a low molecular weight heparin (enoxaparin): experimental and clinical validation of the prophylactic antithrombotic effects. *Acta Chirurgica Scandinavica Suppl.* **556 (Suppl)**: 75–90.
8 Dawes J (1990) Comparison of the pharmacokinetics of enoxaparin (Clexane) and unfractionated heparin. *Acta Chirurgica Scandinavica Supplementum.* **556 (Suppl)**: 68–74.

9 Bara L and Samama M (1990) Pharmacokinetics of low molecular weight heparins. *Acta Chirurgica Scandinavica Supplementum*. **556 (Suppl)**: 57–61.

10 Hirsh J *et al.* (2001) Heparin and low-molecular-weight heparin: mechanisms of action, pharmacokinetics, dosing, monitoring, efficacy, and safety. *Chest*. **119 (Suppl)**: 64s–94s.

11 Watson H *et al.* (2012) Guidelines on the diagnosis and management of heparin-induced thrombocytopenia: second edition. *British Journal of Haematology*. **159**: 528–540.

12 NICE (2012) Venous thromboembolic diseases: the management of venous thromboembolic diseases and the role of thrombophilia testing. *Clinical Guideline*. CG144. www.nice.org.uk (updated 2015).

13 NICE (2015) Reducing the risk of venous thromboembolism (deep vein thrombosis and pulmonary embolism) in patients admitted to hospital. *Clinical Guideline* 92. www.nice.org.uk

14 Noble SI and Finlay IG (2005) Is long-term low-molecular-weight heparin acceptable to palliative care patients in the treatment of cancer related venous thromboembolism? A qualitative study. *Palliative Medicine*. **19**: 197–201.

15 Wittkowsky AK (2006) Barriers to the long-term use of low-molecular weight heparins for treatment of cancer-associated thrombosis. *Journal of Thrombosis and Haemostasis*. **4**: 2090–2091.

16 Ay C *et al.* (2017) Cancer-associated venous thromboembolism: Burden, mechanisms, and management. *Thrombosis Haemostasis*. **117**: 219–230.

17 Kakkar AK and Williamson RC (1999) Prevention of venous thromboembolism in cancer patients. *Seminars in Thrombosis and Hemostasis*. **25**: 239–243.

18 Cunningham MS *et al.* (2006) Prevention and management of venous thromboembolism in people with cancer: a review of the evidence. *Clinical Oncology (Royal College of Radiologists)*. **18**: 145–151.

19 Leizorovicz A and Mismetti P (2004) Preventing venous thromboembolism in medical patients. *Circulation*. **110**: 13–19.

20 Noble SI *et al.* (2006) Acceptability of low molecular weight heparin thromboprophylaxis for inpatients receiving palliative care: qualitative study. *British Medical Journal*. **332**: 577–580.

21 Dennis M *et al.* (2013) Effectiveness of intermittent pneumatic compression in reduction of risk of deep vein thrombosis in patients who have had a stroke (CLOTS 3): a multicentre randomised controlled trial. *Lancet*. **382**: 516–524.

22 Dennis M *et al.* (2009) Effectiveness of thigh-length graduated compression stockings to reduce the risk of deep vein thrombosis after stroke (CLOTS trial 1): a multicentre, randomised controlled trial. *Lancet*. **373**: 1958–1965.

23 NICE (2013) DVT prevention for travellers. *Clinical Knowledge Summaries*. http://cks.nice.org.uk

24 Noble S and Sui J (2016) The treatment of cancer associated thrombosis: does one size fit all? Who should get LMWH/warfarin/DOACs? *Thrombosis Research*. **140 (Suppl 1)**: S154–159.

25 Carrier M *et al.* (2013) Management of challenging cases of patients with cancer-associated thrombosis including recurrent thrombosis and bleeding: guidance from the SSC of the ISTH. *Journal of Thrombosis and Haemostasis*. **12**: 116–117.

26 Walsh-McMonagle D and Green D (1997) Low-molecular weight heparin in the management of Trousseau's syndrome. *Cancer*. **80**: 649–655.

27 British Committee for Standards in Haematology (2010) Guidelines for the diagnosis and management of disseminated intravascular coagulation. *British Journal of Haematology*. **145**: 24–33.

28 British National Formulary Section 2.8.3. Protamine sulfate. London: BMJ Group and Pharmaceutical Press www.medicinescomplete.com (accessed August 2017).

29 Firozvi K *et al.* (2006) Reversal of low-molecular-weight heparin-induced bleeding in patients with pre-existing hypercoagulable states with human recombinant activated factor VII concentrate. *American Journal of Hematology*. **81**: 582–589.

Updated August 2017

Quick Clinical Guide: Heparin-Induced Thrombocytopenia (HIT)

Consistent with the Guidelines of the Haemostasis and Thrombosis Task Force of the British Committee for Standards in Haematology

1 Both unfractionated heparin (UFH) and low molecular weight heparin (LMWH) can cause thrombocytopenia (platelet count $<100 \times 10^9$/L).

2 An early mild fall in platelet count is often seen after starting heparin (<4 days), particularly postoperatively. This is asymptomatic, and corrects spontaneously despite continuing heparin.

3 In <1% of patients, *immune* HIT develops 5–10 days after starting heparin. Can occur sooner or later; rarely several days after heparin has been stopped.

4 If a patient has had treatment with heparin within the last 3 months, HIT can manifest <1 day after restarting treatment.

5 HIT is less common with:
- LMWH than UFH
- medical than surgical patients.

6 Heparin-dependent IgG antibody–platelet factor 4 complexes bind to the platelet surface, causing disruption and release of procoagulant material.

7 HIT manifests as *venous* or *arterial* thrombo-embolism, and can be fatal.

8 **Diagnosis**
The probability of HIT is initially judged on clinical grounds, aided by a scoring system (Box).

Box '4Ts' score to predict probability of HIT

4Ts	*Clinical findings*			*Score*
Thrombocytopenia	Platelet count fall[a]		Platelet nadir[b]	
	<30%	*or*	$<10 \times 10^9$/L	0
	30–50%	*or*	$10–19 \times 10^9$/L	1
	>50%	*and*	$\geq 20 \times 10^9$/L	2
Timing of platelet count fall or other sequelae[c]	≤4 days (without recent heparin exposure)			0
	Consistent with immunization but unclear (missing counts), or onset >10 days, or ≤1 day (if heparin exposure 30–100 days ago)			1
	Clear onset within 5–10 days, or ≤1 day (if heparin exposure within last 30 days)			2
Thrombosis or other sequelae	None			0
	Progressive or recurrent thrombosis; erythematous skin lesions; suspected thrombosis			1
	New thrombosis; skin necrosis; post-heparin bolus acute systemic reaction			2
Other cause for thrombocytopenia	Definite			0
	Possible			1
	None			2

a. to determine % fall, compare the highest platelet count with the lowest
b. severe thrombocytopenia (platelet count $<15 \times 10^9$/L) is unusual in HIT
c. day 0 = first day of heparin exposure; the day the platelet count starts to fall is considered the day of onset of thrombocytopenia (it generally takes 1–3 days more until the arbitrary threshold defining thrombocytopenia is passed).

continued

Box B Continued

Calculate total score (maximum 8):

Score	Probability	*Implications*
6–8	high	Stop heparin, commence alternative anticoagulant and perform further tests
4–5	intermediate	Stop heparin, commence alternative anticoagulant and perform further tests
0–3	low	HIT excluded, no need for further tests

9 Treatment

Stop heparin immediately if high or intermediate probability of HIT and obtain advice from a haematologist urgently.

While awaiting laboratory results (e.g. platelet activation assay, antigen assay):

- prescribe a treatment-dose of a non-heparin (e.g. argatroban, danaparoid) or synthetic heparin (e.g. fondaparinux) parenteral anticoagulant, whether or not there is clinical evidence of a DVT
- only when the platelet count has recovered to ≥150 x 10^9/L, prescribe warfarin
- continue the non-heparin anticoagulant until the INR reaches a therapeutic level, typically 5–7 days. Note. Argatroban can falsely increase the INR
- when a thrombotic complication has occurred, continue anticoagulation for 3 months; when no thrombosis, 1 month is sufficient.

Do *not* use warfarin alone (risk of skin necrosis and venous limb gangrene).
Consider platelet transfusion when there is bleeding, but *not* prophylactically.

10 Preventing recurrence

- record the diagnosis in the patient's notes as a serious allergy
- issue antibody card (but most patients are antibody negative after 3 months)
- if possible, avoid surgery for >3 months after HIT
- although cross-reactivity between UFH and LMWH is uncommon, advise the patient not to have injections of any type of heparin in the future
- if subsequent anticoagulation is required, a non-heparin (e.g. argatroban, danaparoid) or synthetic heparin (e.g. fondaparinux) parenteral anticoagulant should be used; in certain situations, a DOAC may be an option, e.g. orthopaedic surgery.

11 For patients with a history of HIT requiring renal dialysis or cardiac surgery, seek specialist advice.

Updated August 2017

HAEMOSTATICS

Indications: Prevention/treatment of bleeding (authorized indications vary between products; consult SPC for details), †subarachnoid haemorrhage, †surface bleeding from, e.g. ulcerating tumours on the skin, in the nose, mouth, pharynx and other hollow organs (lungs, stomach, rectum, bladder, uterus).

Contra-indications: Active thrombo-embolic disease, e.g. recent thrombo-embolism, DIC, history of convulsions; severe renal impairment (**tranexamic acid**, but see below).

Pharmacology

Tranexamic acid and **aminocaproic acid** (not UK) are synthetic antifibrinolytic drugs derived from lysine. They bind to plasminogen and prevent its interaction as plasmin with fibrin, thereby preventing dissolution of haemostatic plugs.[1] **Tranexamic acid** has a longer duration of action and causes fewer undesirable GI effects than **aminocaproic acid**.[2]

Systemic or topical use of antifibrinolytics reduces blood loss in various circumstances, e.g. menorrhagia (PO), major injury (IV) and peri-operatively (IV, topical).[3–5] They are used in cancer patients to control surface bleeding. In patients with leukaemia and thrombocytopenia, antifibrinolytics appear to reduce bleeding and platelet transfusion requirements, but supporting data are too limited to routinely recommend such use.[6,7] Although sometimes used for haemoptysis caused by lung cancer, supporting data are lacking.[8]

The evidence that antifibrinolytics may increase the risk of thrombosis is generally limited to case reports, with many RCTs identifying no such concerns.[3] However, this has not been well evaluated in patients with cancer and other diseases associated with an underlying prothrombotic tendency. On the other hand, it is suggested that **tranexamic acid** could be antithrombotic by inhibiting the wider effects of prothrombin and plasmin which include promoting inflammation, platelet aggregation and coagulation.[9]

Antifibrinolytics are generally contra-indicated in DIC, even when haemorrhagic manifestations (ecchymoses, haematomas) are predominant, because clot formation is the trigger for further intravascular coagulation and platelet consumption, and an increased risk of end-organ damage from microvascular thromboses.[10] Rarely, they have been used in DIC when there is severe bleeding due to a marked hyperfibrinolytic state;[10] *seek specialist advice*.

Tranexamic acid and **aminocaproic acid** are excreted in the urine mainly unchanged. Because of accumulation, dose reduction will be necessary in renal impairment. Although the SPC gives severe renal impairment as a contra-indication to **tranexamic acid**, there are reports of its use in this circumstance in reduced doses (see Table 2 below).[11,12]

Etamsylate (not UK, see Supply) acts by increasing capillary vascular wall resistance and platelet adhesiveness in the presence of a vascular lesion. This is achieved by inhibiting the biosynthesis and actions of those PGs which cause platelet disaggregation, vasodilation and increased capillary permeability, thereby promoting platelet activation and aggregation, and also by increasing communication between platelets, leucocytes and endothelial cells via the cell adhesion molecule P-selectin.[13] Thus, **etamsylate** is of limited value in thrombocytopenia. It does not cause vasoconstriction, nor does it affect normal coagulation; it has no effect on prothrombin time, fibrinolysis, or platelet count.

Studies have mainly explored the use of **etamsylate** for menorrhagia or peri-ventricular haemorrhage in premature infants.[13] In palliative care, it is used for surface bleeding ± **tranexamic acid**. Rarely, parenteral use may be necessary, e.g. in patients with bleeding and complete dysphagia due to oesophageal cancer. **Etamsylate** is excreted in the urine mainly unchanged.

Pharmacokinetic details are listed in Table 1.

Table 1 Pharmacokinetics of antifibrinolytic and haemostatic drugs

	Tranexamic acid	*Aminocaproic acid*	*Etamsylate*
Bio-availability PO	30–50%[a]	'complete'	'complete'
Onset of action (route-dependent)	1–3h	1–3h	30min IV
Time to peak plasma concentration	3h PO	2h	4h PO; 1h IV
Plasma halflife	2h	2h	5–17h PO; 2–2.5h IM/IV
Duration of action	24h	12–18h	no data

a. systemic bio-availability minimal with oral rinse when not swallowed.

Cautions

History of thrombo-embolism, renal impairment. In both microscopic and macroscopic haematuria there is a risk of clot formation causing ureteric obstruction or urinary retention.[14] Nonetheless, **tranexamic** acid has been used successfully in patients with polycystic kidneys and severe haematuria.[15]

Undesirable effects

Tranexamic acid and aminocaproic acid: hypotension, bradycardia, arrhythmia (give slowly IV), possible increased risk of thrombosis; nausea, vomiting, abdominal pain, diarrhoea (generally settle if the dose is reduced); muscle weakness; seizures (generally following high dose IV use, e.g. 100mg/kg).[16]
Tranexamic acid: disturbances in colour vision (discontinue drug).
Etamsylate: fever, headache, rash.

Dose and use

Generally, antifibrinolytics should be used as one part of a multimodal approach to the management of surface bleeding (see Box A below). Where available, **aminocaproic acid** can be used instead of **tranexamic acid**.

Tranexamic acid

Topical use

When using **tranexamic acid** 5% solutions, generally, it is cheaper to dilute the contents of standard 500mg/5mL (10%) ampoules with 5mL water rather than use special order mouthwash (see supply). Ideally, give instillations at body temperature.

The following recommendations are mainly from anecdotal reports. Apart from fungating wounds and anterior epistaxis, topical **tranexamic acid** is generally used only if other options, including PO **tranexamic acid**, have failed:

- *fungating cancer in the skin:* soak the undiluted contents of a 500mg/5mL (10% solution) ampoule into gauze and apply with pressure for 10min; leave *in situ* covered with a dressing[17]
- *nose (anterior epistaxis):* soak the undiluted contents of a 500mg/5mL (10% solution) ampoule into a cotton pledget/gauze and insert into nostril for 10min[18]
- *mouth:* use as mouthwash, 500mg/10mL (5% solution), 10mL q.d.s. and swallow after use[3,19]
- *rectum:* instil as enema, 500mg/10mL (5% solution), 100mL (10 ampoules + 50mL water) once daily or b.d.[20]
- *lungs:* use 500mg/5mL (10% solution):
  - ▷ haemoptysis: nebulize contents of an undiluted 5mL ampoule t.d.s–q.d.s.[21,22]
  - ▷ pleural haemorrhage: instil 10 x 5mL ampoules (50mL) intrapleurally via a thoracic drain once daily, clamping drain for 1h; benefit seen after 1–2 instillations[23]
- *bladder:* see Haematuria below.

Systemic treatment for surface bleeding from any site[24]

- give 1.5g PO stat and 1g t.d.s.
- if bleeding not subsiding after 3 days, increase dose to 1.5–2g t.d.s. (manufacturer's recommended maximum dose is 1.5g t.d.s., but doses of ≤2g q.d.s. have been used)
- discontinue 1 week after cessation of bleeding or reduce to 500mg t.d.s.
- restart if bleeding occurs, and possibly continue indefinitely.

IV use may occasionally be necessary, e.g. in patients with bleeding and complete dysphagia, 15mg/kg IV over 5–10min t.d.s.–q.d.s. The dose should be reduced in renal impairment (Table 2).

Table 2 Tranexamic acid doses in renal impairment

Plasma creatinine (micromol/L)	*Creatinine clearance (mL/min)*	*PO dose*	*IV dose*
120–249	50–80	15mg/kg b.d.	10mg/kg b.d.
250–500	10–50	15mg/kg once daily	10mg/kg once daily
>500	<10	7.5mg/kg once daily or 15mg/kg every 2 days[4,5]	5mg/kg once daily or 10mg/kg every 2 days

Aminocaproic acid (not UK)

In oliguria or end-stage renal disease, give 15–25% of the normal dose.[12]

Acute bleeding syndromes due to elevated fibrinolytic activity[25]

- stat dose of 5g PO (or 4–5g IVI in 250mL of diluent) during the first hour of treatment, then 1.25g/h PO (or 1g/h IVI in 50mL of diluent) for 8h or until bleeding stops; suitable diluents for IVI are 0.9% saline or 5% glucose
- manufacturer's maximum recommended dose = 30g/24h PO/IV.

Chronic bleeding tendency

- give 5–30g PO daily in divided doses at 3–6h intervals
- when bleeding controlled, adjust to the lowest effective dose.

Bleeding from oral cancers[26]

- give 500mg PO q.d.s. until bleeding stops
- then discontinue by tapering dose frequency every 2–3 days.

Box A Other measures for bleeding in addition to tranexamic acid

Review drugs

- discontinue anticoagulants (e.g. LMWH, warfarin), anti-platelet drugs (e.g. aspirin, clopidogrel) and other drugs which impair platelet function (e.g. most NSAIDs, SSRIs)
- prescribe paracetamol or an NSAID which does *not* impair platelet function (see p.315).

Topical

- *bleeding points (nose, mouth, wounds):* apply silver nitrate stick
- *wounds:* adrenaline (epinephrine) (1 in 1,000) 1mg in 1mL (short-term only because of risk of ischaemic necrosis and rebound vasodilation)
- *wounds:* sucralfate paste, 2 x 1g tablets crushed in 5mL water-soluble gel, e.g. KY jelly[27]
- *mouth, rectum:* sucralfate suspension 2g in 10mL b.d.[28]
- *fungating cancer in the skin:* use alginate haemostatic dressings (e.g. Kaltostat®, Sorbsan®)
- *posterior epistaxis:* sympathomimetic vasoconstrictors, e.g. xylometazoline nasal spray;[29] also applied directly onto malignant wounds,[30] but short-term use only (risk of rebound vasodilation after several days application).

Systemic drugs

- *second-line:* switch from first-line tranexamic acid/aminocaproic acid (not UK) to, or combine with, etamsylate (not UK):
  - ▷ give 500mg PO q.d.s. either indefinitely or until 1 week after cessation of bleeding
  - ▷ if it causes nausea, vomiting or diarrhoea, take after food
- *third-line:* desmopressin (see p.528).[31]

Note. Etamsylate and desmopressin augment platelet function, and thus of limited value in thrombocytopenia.

Specialist measures

- radiotherapy, e.g. skin, lung, oesophagus, rectum, bladder, uterus, vagina[32]
- coagulation, e.g. diathermy, cryotherapy, LASER
- embolization.[33,34]

Haematuria

Haematuria in advanced cancer is generally associated with urinary tract cancer, most commonly bladder. It may also be caused by chronic radiation cystitis which can develop several years after pelvic radiotherapy. In many cases haematuria is mild, and no intervention is necessary.

Correct the correctable:

- can the cancer be modified? If the patient is well enough, consider cystoscopy for diathermy and resection
- can other factors be modified?
  - ▷ instead of a non-selective NSAID, prescribe **paracetamol** or an NSAID which does not impair platelet function (see p.315)
  - ▷ consider checking PT, APTT and FBC
  - ▷ culture urine; treat infection if present.

Drug treatment

If the haematuria is marked, **tranexamic acid** (PO, or if this fails, by a 5% intravesical instillation, 100mL once daily–b.d.) may be used, although there is a risk of clot retention until the bleeding has completely stopped, and this may necessitate removal under general anaesthetic. Other options are shown in Table 3.

Daily bladder instillations of **carboprost tromethamine**, a PGE_1 analogue, are occasionally used in **cyclophosphamide**-induced haematuria, second-line to **alum**. No anaesthesia is required, but **carboprost** is expensive and requires close monitoring.[35]

Non-drug treatment

Rarely, it may be necessary to consider:

- cauterization
- arterial embolization
- urinary diversion, e.g. nephrostomy
- hyperbaric oxygen.[36]

Table 3 Bladder irrigations and instillations for haemorrhagic cystitis[37]

Treatment	*Administration*	*Comment*
0.9% Saline (*preferred option*)	Continuous irrigation until urine is clear	No undesirable effects but not effective in severe cases
Alum 1% (*if saline fails*)	Continuous irrigation 250–300mL/h until urine is clear	No anaesthesia required. Solution is acidic and may cause bladder spasms; treat with antispasmodics. Expensive, 1L costs about £24. Recurrence common; aluminium toxicity rare
Formalin 1–3% (*rarely necessary*)	Instillation, retain for 20–30min; repeat if no response	General anaesthesia required. Often successful but risk of ureteric stenosis and obstruction if formalin refluxes into the ureters

Supply

Tranexamic acid (generic)
Tablets 500mg, 28 days @ 1g t.d.s. = £20.
Oral solution or suspension 500mg/5mL (10%), 28 days @ 1g t.d.s. = £232 or £277 respectively, (unauthorized products available as a special order; see Chapter 24, p.751). *Price based on Specials tariff in community.*
Mouthwash 500mg/10mL (5%), 28 days @ 10mL q.d.s. = £270, (unauthorized product available as a special order; see Chapter 24, p.751). *Price based on Specials tariff in community.*
Injection 100mg/mL (10%), 5mL amp = £1.50.

Etamsylate
Tablets 500mg, 28 days @ 500mg q.d.s. = £126 (unauthorized product, obtainable as an import from IDIS; see Chapter 24, p.751).
Injection 125mg/mL, 2mL amp = £1 (unauthorized product, obtainable as an import from IDIS; see Chapter 24, p.751).

Sucralfate
Antepsin® (Chugai)
Tablets 1g, 50 = £7.
Oral suspension 1g/5mL, 250mL = £7.

1 Mannucci PM (1998) Hemostatic drugs. *New England Journal of Medicine*. **339**: 245–253.
2 Okamoto S *et al.* (1964) An active stereoisomer (trans form) of AMCHA and its antifibrinolytic (antiplasminic) action in vitro and in vivo. *Keio Journal of Medicine*. **13**: 177–185.
3 McCormack PL (2012) Tranexamic acid: a review of its use in the treatment of hyperfibrinolysis. *Drugs*. **72**: 585–617.
4 Ker K *et al.* (2012) Effect of tranexamic acid on surgical bleeding: systematic review and cumulative meta-analysis. *British Medical Journal*. **344**: e3054.
5 Roberts I *et al.* (2013) The CRASH-2 trial: a randomised controlled trial and economic evaluation of the effects of tranexamic acid on death, vascular occlusive events and transfusion requirement in bleeding trauma patients. *Health Technol Assess*. **17**: 1–79.
6 Wardrop D *et al.* (2013) Antifibrinolytics (lysine analogues) for the prevention of bleeding in patients with haematological disorders. *Cochrane Database of Systematic Reviews*. **7**: CD009733. www.thecochranelibrary.com
7 Antun AG *et al.* (2013) Epsilon aminocaproic acid prevents bleeding in severely thrombocytopenic patients with hematological malignancies. *Cancer*. **119**: 3784–3787.
8 Prutsky G *et al.* (2012) Antifibrinolytic therapy to reduce haemoptysis from any cause. *Cochrane Database of Systematic Reviews*. **4**: CD008711. www.thecochranelibrary.com
9 Godier A *et al.* (2012) Tranexamic acid: less bleeding and less thrombosis? *Critical Care*. **16**: 135.
10 Wada H *et al.* (2013) Guidance for diagnosis and treatment of DIC from harmonization of the recommendations from three guidelines. *Journal of Thrombosis and Haemostasis*. **11**: 761–767.
11 Andersson L *et al.* (1978) Special considerations with regard to the dosage of tranexamic acid in patients with chronic renal diseases. *Urological Research*. **6**: 83–88.
12 Lacy C *et al.* (eds) (2003) Lexi-Comp's Drug Information Handbook. (11e). Lexi-Comp and the American Pharmaceutical Association, Hudson, Ohio.
13 Garay RP *et al.* (2006) Therapeutic efficacy and mechanism of action of ethamsylate, a long-standing hemostatic agent. *American Journal of Therapeutics*. **13**: 236–247.
14 Schultz M and van der Lelie H (1995) Microscopic haematuria as a relative contraindication for tranexamic acid. *British Journal of Haematology*. **89**: 663–664.
15 Peces R *et al.* (2012) Medical therapy with tranexamic acid in autosomal dominant polycystic kidney disease patients with severe haematuria. *Nefrologia*. **32**: 160–165.
16 Murkin JM *et al.* (2010) High-dose tranexamic Acid is associated with nonischemic clinical seizures in cardiac surgical patients. *Anesthesia and Analgesia*. **110**: 350–353.
17 Palliativedrugs.com (2013). Topical Tranexamic Acid - What do you do? *Survey*. March-April: Available from www.palliativedrugs.com.
18 Zahed R *et al.* (2013) A new and rapid method for epistaxis treatment using injectable form of tranexamic acid topically: a randomized controlled trial. *American Journal of Emergency Medicine*. **31**: 1389–1392.
19 Dunn CJ and Goa KL (1999) Tranexamic acid: a review of its use in surgery and other indications. *Drugs*. **57**: 1005–1032.
20 McElligott E *et al.* (1991) Tranexamic acid and rectal bleeding. *Lancet*. **337**: 431.
21 Solomonov A *et al.* (2009) Pulmonary hemorrhage: A novel mode of therapy. *Respiratory Medicine*. **103**: 1196–1200.
22 Hankerson MJ *et al.* (2015) Nebulized tranexamic acid as a noninvasive therapy for cancer-related hemoptysis. *Journal of Palliative Medicine*. **18**: 1060–1062.
23 deBoer W *et al.* (1991) Tranexamic acid treatment of haemothorax in two patients with malignant mesothelioma. *Chest*. **100**: 847–848.
24 Seto AH and Dunlap DS (1996) Tranexamic acid in oncology. *Annals of Pharmacology*. **30**: 868–870.
25 Roberts SB *et al.* (2010) Palliative use of aminocaproic acid to control upper gastrointestinal bleeding. *Journal of Pain and Symptom Management*. **40**: e1–3.
26 Setla J (2004) Duration of aminocaproic acid therapy in bleeding for malignant wounds. In: *Bulletin Board*. Palliativedrugs.com Ltd. Available from: www.palliativedrugs.com
27 Regnard C and Makin W (1992) Management of bleeding in advanced cancer: a flow diagram. *Palliative Medicine*. **6**: 74–78.
28 Kochhar R *et al.* (1988) Rectal sucralfate in radiation proctitis. *Lancet*. **332**: 400.
29 Krempl GA and Noorily AD (1995) Use of oxymetazoline in the management of epistaxis. *Annals of Otology, Rhinology, and Laryngology*. **104**: 704–706.
30 Recka K *et al.* (2012) Management of bleeding associated with malignant wounds. *Journal Palliative of Medicine*. **15**: 952–954.
31 Hedges SJ *et al.* (2006) Evidence-based treatment recommendations for uremic bleeding. *Nature Clinical Practice Oncology*. **3**: 138–153.
32 Cihoric N *et al.* (2012) Clinically significant bleeding in incurable cancer patients: effectiveness of hemostatic radiotherapy. *Radiation Oncololgy*. **7**: 132.
33 Rankin E *et al.* (1988) Transcatheter embolisation to control severe bleeding in fungating breast cancer. *European Journal of Surgical Oncology*. **14**: 27–32.
34 Broadley K *et al.* (1995) The role of embolization in palliative care. *Palliative Medicine*. **9**: 331–335.
35 Denton AS *et al.* (2002) Non-surgical interventions for late radiation cystitis in patients who have received radical radiotherapy to the pelvis. *Cochrane Database Systematic Reviews*. CD001773. www.thecochranelibrary.com
36 Corman JM *et al.* (2003) Treatment of radiation induced hemorrhagic cystitis with hyperbaric oxygen. *Journal of Urology*. **169**: 2200–2202.
37 Abt D *et al.* (2013) Therapeutic options for intractable hematuria in advanced bladder cancer. *International Journal of Urology*. **20**: 651–660.

Updated August 2016

3: RESPIRATORY SYSTEM

BRONCHODILATORS

Palliative care clinicians caring for patients with end-stage COPD need to be aware of the latest management guidelines. Further, some patients with cancer also suffer from COPD or asthma, and occasionally both. Concurrent COPD can be a major cause of breathlessness, notably in lung cancer, but may be unrecognized, and so go untreated.

The guidelines provided here (Box A–Box C, Table 1) for the use of bronchodilators in patients with asthma and COPD are based on the recommendations of the British Thoracic Society/Scottish Intercollegiate Guidelines Network Guidelines on Asthma[1] and the National Institute for Health and Clinical Excellence COPD Guidelines.[2] These have much in common with international guidelines produced by the Global Initiative for Asthma (GINA) and the Global Initiative for Chronic Obstructive Lung Disease (GOLD), although there are some differences in emphasis.[3,4]

Generally, the guidelines should be followed. However, for patients in the last weeks or days of life, particularly those having difficulties with metered-dose inhalers (MDIs), the regular use of short-acting nebulized bronchodilators may be preferable.

Further, if a patient is receiving long-term PO corticosteroids for another indication (see p.513), it is often possible to discontinue inhaled corticosteroids.

Inhalation delivers the drug directly to the bronchi and enables a smaller dose to work more quickly and with fewer undesirable systemic effects. β_2-Adrenergic receptor agonists (β_2 agonists), e.g. **salbutamol** (p.117) and **salmeterol** (p.119), act directly on bronchial smooth muscle to cause bronchodilation whereas antimuscarinics, e.g. **ipratropium** (p.107) and **tiotropium** (p.115), act by reducing the vagal tone to the airways. Both classes of drug improve breathlessness by airway bronchodilation and/or reducing air-trapping at rest (static hyperinflation) and on exertion (dynamic hyperinflation). A reduction in hyperinflation probably explains why clinical benefit may be seen in patients with COPD with little or no change in the FEV_1.[5]

β_2 Agonists are used in both asthma and COPD; antimuscarinic drugs in COPD and *acute* asthma. Their use is often combined in *acute* asthma and COPD (Table 1, Box B). In asthma and in severe COPD, bronchodilators are generally combined with inhaled corticosteroids (Box A, Box B; also see p.126).

In asthma and COPD, if the optimal use of inhaled therapy provides inadequate relief, a third class of bronchodilators, the methylxanthines, are sometimes used systemically, e.g. PO m/r **theophylline** (p.123). Because of a narrow therapeutic index, their use requires careful monitoring to avoid toxicity.

β-Adrenergic receptor blocking drugs (β-blockers), both cardioselective and non-selective, are contra-indicated in patients with asthma. They should also be avoided in patients with COPD, unless there are compelling reasons for their use, e.g. severe glaucoma. In such circumstances, a cardioselective β-blocker should be used with extreme caution under specialist guidance.

Table 1 Summary of the immediate management of an acute asthma attack in adults[1,a]

	Severity of attack		
	Moderate	*Severe*	*Life-threatening*[b]
Assessment		Any of the following:	
PEF[c]	>50–75%	33–50%	<33%
SpO_2 (pulse oximeter)		≥92%	<92%; check blood gases
General condition	No features of severe asthma	Unable to complete sentence in one breath; respirations ≥25/min, pulse ≥110/min	Silent chest, poor respiratory effort, cyanosis, PaO_2<8kPa, normal or raised $PaCO_2$[d], arrhythmia, hypotension, exhaustion, altered consciousness
Chest radiograph	Necessary if pneumothorax, pneumomediastinum or consolidation suspected, life-threatening asthma, failure to respond to treatment or ventilation required		
Place of care	Hospital for life-threatening; severe or moderate when, e.g. failure to respond to treatment or psychosocial concerns. Intensive care if life-threatening or when severe and failing to respond to treatment and ventilation required		
Treatment			
Oxygen	Not needed	via face/venturi mask or nasal cannulae at flow rate which maintains SpO_2 94–98%	
Bronchodilators[e]	Salbutamol or terbutaline MDI 4 puffs via spacer (give one puff at a time), followed by 2 puffs every 2min, up to a maximum of 10 puffs *or* salbutamol 5mg or terbutaline 10mg via oxygen-driven nebulizer		Use nebulized β_2 agonist as for moderate–severe but give with ipratropium 500microgram via an oxygen-driven nebulizer; use spacer only if nebulizer unavailable
	If inadequate response after 15min, give nebulized β_2 agonist		Repeat above
	If inadequate response after 15min:		
		Use nebulized β_2 agonist + ipratropium (if not already given) or consider continuous nebulization of salbutamol 5–10mg/h (requires specific nebulizer)	
Corticosteroid[f]	Prednisolone 40–50mg PO stat & once daily for 5 days or until recovery		
Other treatments[g]		IV magnesium sulfate 1.2–2g over 20min	
		IV aminophylline 5mg/kg over 20min, followed by 500–700microgram/kg/h[h]	

a. full guidance available on www.brit-thoracic.org.uk

b. obtain senior/intensive care unit help as soon as life-threatening asthma recognized

c. % of best peak expiratory flow (PEF) within last two years or, if unavailable, predicted PEF

d. termed near-fatal asthma when $PaCO_2$ is raised and/or mechanical ventilation is required with raised inflation pressures

e. IV β_2 agonists are reserved for patients in whom inhaled route unreliable (see full guidance)

f. the earlier corticosteroids are given, the better the outcome; where PO not possible, give hydrocortisone 100mg IV stat & q.d.s.

g. when poor response to standard bronchodilator therapies; requires guidance from senior/experienced staff (see full guidance)

h. monitor plasma levels daily (aim for 10–20mg/L or 55–110micromol/L); in patients already taking regular PO theophylline, omit loading dose and measure plasma level on admission.

Box A Summary of the management of chronic asthma in adults[1]

Start treatment at the level most appropriate to the initial severity of asthma. The aim is to achieve control as soon as possible, defined as:
- no daytime symptoms
- no night-time awakening due to asthma
- no need for rescue medication
- no asthma attacks
- no limitations on activity including exercise
- normal lung function, i.e. FEV_1 ± PEF >80% predicted or best
- minimal undesirable effects from drugs.

Before initiating a new drug, check adherence, inhaler technique and eliminate trigger factors.

Intermittent reliever therapy

Inhaled short-acting β_2-adrenergic receptor agonist (β_2 agonist) p.r.n., e.g. salbutamol.

Move to regular preventer therapy if:
- symptomatic/inhaler needed ≥3 times a week
- night-time symptoms ≥1 times a week
- asthma attack requiring PO corticosteroids in the last 2 years.

Regular preventer therapy

Low-dose inhaled corticosteroid, i.e. beclometasone 400microgram/24h or equivalent[a]
+ inhaled short-acting β_2 agonist p.r.n.
If there is insufficient response, consider initial add-on therapy.

Initial add-on therapy

Inhaled long-acting β_2 agonist (LABA), e.g. salmeterol 50microgram b.d. or formoterol 12microgram b.d.[b]
+ low-dose inhaled corticosteroid[a]
+ inhaled short-acting β_2 agonist p.r.n.

If there is:
- *insufficient response*, continue the LABA and increase the inhaled corticosteroid to a medium-dose, i.e. beclometasone 800microgram/24h or equivalent
- *no response*, discontinue the LABA and increase the inhaled corticosteroid to a medium-dose

When there is insufficient response to the increase in inhaled corticosteroid, consider additional add-on therapies.

Additional add-on therapies

Continue medium-dose inhaled corticosteroid.
+ inhaled LABA (when of known benefit)[b]
+ inhaled short-acting β_2 agonist p.r.n.

Consider therapeutic trials of the following:
- PO leukotriene receptor antagonist
- inhaled long-acting muscarinic antagonist, e.g. tiotropium
- PO m/r theophylline
- PO m/r β_2 agonist (use with caution if already on inhaled LABA).

If add-on drug ineffective, discontinue.
If asthma not controlled, consider referral to asthma clinic before proceeding to high-dose therapies.

High-dose therapies

Consider therapeutic trials of the following:
- high-dose inhaled corticosteroid, i.e. beclometasone 1,600microgram/24h or equivalent
- PO leukotriene receptor antagonist
- PO m/r theophylline
- PO m/r β_2 agonist (use with caution if already on inhaled LABA)
- inhaled long-acting muscarinic antagonist, e.g. tiotropium.

If add-on drug ineffective, discontinue or, in the case of inhaled corticosteroid, reduce to original dose.
Refer to asthma clinic.

continued

Box A Continued

Continuous or frequent use of oral corticosteroids
High-dose inhaled corticosteroid, i.e. beclometasone 1,600microgram/24h or equivalent.
+ one or more add-on therapy (see previous levels)
+ regular PO prednisolone at lowest effective dose once daily (monitor blood/urine glucose, blood pressure, cholesterol and bone mineral density, and for cataracts/glaucoma)
+ inhaled short-acting β_2 agonist p.r.n.
Consider corticosteroid-sparing treatments, e.g. anti-IgE monoclonal antibody.
Refer to asthma clinic.

Moving up or down treatment levels
Review treatment regularly, moving up a treatment level if control inadequate or use of ≥3 doses of short-acting β_2 agonist/week. Conversely, if control good, consider going down a level. The most appropriate drug to reduce first may be influenced by individual patient circumstances. Reduce dose of inhaled corticosteroid slowly, e.g. ≤50% every 3 months.

a. doses of inhaled corticosteroids are expressed as low, medium or high (see p.126); high doses are used only after specialist assessment
b. inhaled LABAs should *not* be used without inhaled corticosteroids because of concern over an increase in severe asthma exacerbations and asthma-related deaths; combination inhalers are thus recommended to ensure the LABA is taken with an inhaled corticosteroid and to improve adherence.

Diagnosing asthma and COPD

The diagnosis of asthma or COPD is based mainly on the history and examination, supported by objective tests and, ultimately, the response to treatment.

In asthma, there are recurrent episodes of respiratory symptoms (>1 of wheeze, cough, breathlessness, chest tightness) caused by variable airflow obstruction. Airflow should be compared objectively during both symptomatic and asymptomatic periods using spirometry preferably or peak expiratory flow rate. Patients with airflow obstruction and a high probability of asthma can start a trial of treatment (Box A).

Those with an intermediate probability should be further investigated, initially with reversibility testing using inhaled **salbutamol** 400microgram. In those with obstruction, an improvement in FEV_1 of ≥12% and ≥200mL is considered a positive result. An improvement in FEV_1 >400mL strongly suggests asthma.

If there is incomplete response, prescribe corticosteroids, generally inhaled, e.g. **beclometasone** 200microgram b.d. or equivalent for 6 weeks and reassess degree of response.[1]

Further tests are recommended for patients without obstruction and an intermediate probability of asthma, and when there is only a low probability of asthma.[1]

In suspected COPD, post-bronchodilator spirometry is generally sufficient to indicate the presence of airflow obstruction (FEV_1/FVC <0.7) and its severity. COPD is now classified as:

- stage 1 (mild; FEV_1 ≥80% of predicted)
- stage 2 (moderate; FEV_1 50–79%)
- stage 3 (severe; FEV_1 30–49%)
- stage 4 (very severe; FEV_1 <30%).[2]

In palliative care, when airflow obstruction is suspected, evaluating the impact on symptoms of a 1–2 week trial of a bronchodilator is probably the most pragmatic and relevant approach.

Delivery devices

Pressurized metered-dose inhalers (MDIs) are the most commonly prescribed delivery device and the correct inhaler technique should be carefully explained to the patient and subsequently checked.[1] The patient should be instructed to inhale slowly and then, if possible, hold their breath for 10sec. Even with a good MDI technique, 80% of the dose is deposited in the mouth and oropharynx.

If inhaler technique does not improve with training or in patients with poor respiratory effort, consider using an MDI plus a large-volume (650–850mL) spacer device to deliver single-dose actuations. There should be minimal delay between actuation and inhalation, but normal (tidal) breathing is as effective as taking a single breath.

Box B Summary of palliative drug therapy in COPD[2]

Smoking and β-blockers may cause bronchoconstriction and should be avoided.

The choice of drug(s) is informed by the degree of benefit obtained from a therapeutic trial, patient preference, undesirable effects, potential to reduce exacerbations and cost. Assess benefit in terms of improvement in symptoms, activities of daily living, exercise capacity, and rapidity of symptom relief; discontinue if ineffective.

Breathlessness and/or exercise limitation
Short-acting β_2 agonist, e.g. salbutamol, or short-acting antimuscarinic bronchodilator, e.g. ipratropium, p.r.n.

Exacerbations or persistent breathlessness
Short-acting β_2 agonist p.r.n. +

- *if* FEV_1 *≥50%*, regular LABA *or* long-acting antimuscarinic bronchodilator, e.g. tiotropium
- *if* FEV_1 *<50%*, regular LABA + corticosteroid combination inhaler *or*, if corticosteroid declined or not tolerated, LABA + long-acting antimuscarinic bronchodilator, *or* long-acting antimuscarinic bronchodilator.

Persistent exacerbations or breathlessness (irrespective of FEV_1)
Short-acting β_2 agonist p.r.n. +

- if previously only on LABA, regular LABA + corticosteroid combination inhaler, *or*, if corticosteroid declined or not tolerated, LABA + long-acting antimuscarinic bronchodilator, *or ultimately*
- regular LABA + corticosteroid combination inhaler + long-acting antimuscarinic bronchodilator.

Patients with distressing or disabling breathlessness despite maximal use of inhalers (with spacer if appropriate) should be considered for nebulizer therapy.

Other drugs
Reserved for patients with distressing symptoms despite maximal inhaled therapy:

- oral corticosteroids; when unavoidable in advanced COPD keep dose to a minimum and in patients >65 years provide routine osteoporosis prophylaxis; in those <65 years, monitor for osteoporosis and treat if required
- theophylline; requires caution, particularly in the elderly, monitoring of serum concentration and for risk of drug–drug interaction; can be used earlier in patients unable to use inhaled therapy
- mucolytics; can be considered in patients with chronic productive cough
- for the role of oxygen in COPD, see p.130
- for the role of opioids and benzodiazepines for breathlessness in advanced COPD and the last days of life, see p.382.

Build up of static on plastic and polycarbonate spacers attracts drug particles and reduces drug delivery. To reduce static, spacers should be washed once a month with detergent, rinsed and left to dry without wiping.[1] Spacers should be replaced every 6–12 months.[1]

Dry powder inhalers, e.g. Turbohalers® and breath-actuated MDIs, are other options; but they are no more effective than MDI ± a spacer.[1,6] Patients generally prefer Turbohalers® over an MDI ± a spacer, but they are not suited to patients with poor inspiratory effort. Compared to MDIs, actuation of a dry powder inhaler causes less sensation in the oropharynx and patients should be informed of this to avoid inadvertent overuse. Breath-actuated MDIs are triggered at low inspiratory flow rates, are popular with patients, and are the easiest to use correctly.[7]

Nebulizers are more expensive and less convenient than an MDI but may be preferable in patients with a poor inhaler technique, e.g. children, the frail, and patients with end-stage disease. Because of improved drug delivery, there may be better symptom relief in this group of patients.[8] However, the higher doses administered can increase the risk of undesirable effects and their use should be carefully monitored (also see Nebulized drugs, p.835).

Box C Summary of the initial management of exacerbations of COPD[2]

Diagnosis

A sustained worsening of symptoms of acute onset, beyond the normal day-to-day variation experienced by the patient. Commonly reported symptoms are:

- worsening breathlessness, cough
- increased sputum volume
- change in sputum colour.

Management

Optimize bronchodilator use (see Box B); for patients with distressing or disabling breathlessness despite maximal use of inhalers:

- consider use of a nebulizer
- PO corticosteroid, e.g. prednisolone 30mg once daily for 1–2 weeks (Note. The trend is toward shorter courses of a higher dose, e.g. 40mg once daily for 5 days)
- antibacterials if purulent sputum.

Admission to hospital should be considered if:

- rapid onset of symptoms
- acute confusion or impaired consciousness
- severe breathlessness, cyanosis, SpO_2 <90%, PaO_2 <7kPa, arterial pH <7.35
- already receiving long-term oxygen
- increasing peripheral oedema
- living alone or unable to cope at home
- poor ± deteriorating general condition and level of activity
- significant co-morbidity (particularly cardiac disease, insulin-dependent diabetes mellitus)
- changes on chest radiograph.

For those requiring hospitalization, investigations will include:

- chest radiograph, ECG
- arterial blood gases
- serum theophylline concentration, if already taking theophylline
- if sputum purulent, sputum microscopy and culture
- if pyrexial, blood cultures.

For those requiring hospitalization, management will also include:

- oxygen to keep SaO_2 within an individualized target range, according to local protocols
- consideration of the need for:
  - ▷ IV aminophylline if poor response to other bronchodilators
  - ▷ non-invasive ventilation (NIV)
  - ▷ a respiratory stimulant, e.g. doxapram (if NIV unavailable)
  - ▷ intubation.

However, overall, there is no evidence to suggest that a nebulizer is superior to any inhaler device for the delivery of a β_2 agonist or corticosteroid for the treatment of stable asthma, or to a MDI + spacer in the initial treatment of acute asthma, unless there are life-threatening features. In patients with COPD and a good inhaler technique, nebulized bronchodilator therapy is indicated only in severe acute exacerbations or when there is distressing or disabling breathlessness despite maximal therapy using inhalers.[2]

In patients with lung cancer, concurrent COPD can be a major cause of breathlessness but may be unrecognized and so go untreated.[9] Breathlessness can be improved in most patients with lung cancer and COPD by a combination of a β_2 agonist and an antimuscarinic bronchodilator; this is equally effective when given by a MDI + a spacer or by nebulizer (see Nebulized drugs, p.835).[9]

Supply

Spacer devices are not interchangeable; prescribe a device that is compatible with the pressurized MDI.

Inhaler and spacer devices
AeroChamber Plus® (GSK)
Spacer medium-volume for use with all pressurized MDIs, standard adult device = £5, with mask = £8.

Haleraid® (A&H)
Inhaler device to aid operation of manually actuated pressurized MDIs by patients with impaired strength in hands. For use with *Flixotide*®, *Seretide*®, *Serevent*®, and *Ventolin*® inhalers, available for 120 and 200-dose inhalers. NHS.

Volumatic® (A&H)
Spacer large-volume for use with *Clenil Modulite*®, *Flixotide*®, *Seretide*®, *Serevent*®, and *Ventolin*® pressurized MDIs = £4, with paediatric mask = £7.

This is not a complete list; see BNF for more information including devices for paediatric use.

1 BTS/SIGN (2016) British Guideline on the Management of Asthma. A National Clinical Guideline. Revised edition September 2016. British Thoracic Society and Scottish Intercollegiate Guidelines Network. Available from: www.brit-thoracic.org.uk

2 NICE (2010) Chronic obstructive pulmonary disease in over 16s: diagnosis and management. *Clinical Guideline*. CG101. www.nice.org.uk

3 NHLBI/WHO (2017) Global Initiative for Asthma (GINA). Pocket guide for asthma management and prevention. Available from: www.ginasthma.com

4 NHLBI/WHO (2017) Global Initiative for Chronic Obstructive Lung Disease. Global strategy for the diagnosis, management and prevention of chronic obstructive pulmonary disease. www.goldcopd.com

5 Laveneziana P *et al.* (2012) New physiological insights into dyspnea and exercise intolerance in chronic obstructive pulmonary disease patients. *Expert Reviews in Respiratory Medicine*. **6**: 651–662.

6 Anonymous (2003) Inhaler devices for the management of asthma and COPD. *Effective Health Care Bulletins*. **8**: 1–12.

7 Lenney J *et al.* (2000) Inappropriate inhaler use: assessment of use and patient preference of seven inhalation devices. *Respiratory Medicine*. **94**: 496–500.

8 Tashkin DP *et al.* (2007) Comparing COPD treatment: nebulizer, metered dose inhaler, and concomitant therapy. *American Journal of Medicine*. **120**: 435–441.

9 Congleton J and Muers MF (1995) The incidence of airflow obstruction in bronchial carcinoma, its relation to breathlessness, and response to bronchodilator therapy. *Respiratory Medicine*. **89**: 291–296.

Updated July 2017

IPRATROPIUM BROMIDE

Class: Quaternary ammonium antimuscarinic bronchodilator.

Indications: Reversible airways obstruction, particularly in COPD.

Contra-indications: Hypersensitivity to atropine or its derivatives.

Pharmacology

Ipratropium is a short-acting antimuscarinic which blocks all muscarinic receptor subtypes with equal affinity. In patients with COPD, cholinergic vagal efferent nerves to the airways activate muscarinic receptors, resulting in increased resting bronchial tone and mucus secretion.[1] Antimuscarinics block these effects and cause bronchodilation. Short-acting antimuscarinics increase FEV_1 but have less consistent benefit on breathlessness, need for rescue medication, walking distance and quality of life.[2]

For patients with COPD-related breathlessness and exercise limitation, an inhaled short-acting antimuscarinic bronchodilator *or* a short-acting β_2 agonist are recommended as initial treatment on a p.r.n. basis. However, a short-acting β_2 agonist is generally preferred as it has a more rapid onset of action and, unlike a short-acting antimuscarinic bronchodilator, can also be prescribed concurrently with a long-acting antimuscarinic bronchodilator (e.g. **tiotropium**, p.115), which subsequently may be required (see Bronchodilators, Box B, p.111). For persistent symptoms, compared with the regular use of ipratropium, **tiotropium** is safer and more effective across a range of outcomes.[3]

In acute exacerbations of COPD when there is insufficient relief with an inhaled short-acting β_2 agonist, a short-acting antimuscarinic bronchodilator is often added despite limited evidence to support this (also see Bronchodilators, Box C, p.112).[4]

In asthma, long-acting but not short-acting antimuscarinic bronchodilators have a role in the management of chronic asthma (see Bronchodilators, Box A, p.109). However, nebulized ipratropium bromide is used in severe or life-threatening asthma attacks (see Bronchodilators, Table 1, p.108).[5]

Bio-availability most of the 10–30% of the inhaled dose which reaches the lower airways is absorbed.

Onset of action 3–30min asthma; 15min COPD.

Peak response 1.5–3h asthma; 1–2h COPD.

Plasma halflife 2.3–3.8h.

Duration of action 4–8h.

Cautions

Nebulized solution reaching the eye may precipitate narrow-angle glaucoma in susceptible patients; bladder neck obstruction, prostatic hypertrophy.

Undesirable effects

A small increase in cardiovascular events (e.g. myocardial infarction, heart failure, cardiac arrhythmia, stroke) has been reported in patients with COPD using ipratropium regularly and requires further investigation.[6]

Common (<10%, >1%): headache, dizziness, dry mouth, oropharyngeal irritation, cough, bronchoconstriction, vomiting, GI motility changes.

Uncommon (<1%, >0.1%): visual accommodation changes, tachycardia.

Rare (<0.1%, >0.01%): cardiac arrhythmia, e.g. atrial fibrillation, laryngospasm, nausea, urinary retention.

Nebulized drug droplets may reach the eye and there have been uncommon reports of precipitation of narrow-angle glaucoma and rare reports of eye pain, mydriasis and increased intra-ocular pressure.

Dose and use

In most patients, administration t.d.s. is sufficient.

Pressurized metered-dose inhaler

- give 20–40microgram (1–2 puffs) p.r.n. up to t.d.s.–q.d.s.
- give 20–40microgram (1–2 puffs) before exercise in exercise-induced bronchoconstriction.

Nebulizer solution

- use with a mouthpiece to minimize any nebulized drug entering the eye
- give 250–500microgram p.r.n. up to t.d.s.–q.d.s in COPD; generally given q.d.s. in an exacerbation of COPD
- give 500microgram q6h–q4h in acute exacerbation of asthma (see Bronchodilators, Table 1, p.108).[5]

Also see nebulized drugs, p.835.

Supply

Ipratropium bromide (generic)

Pressurized metered-dose inhaler 20microgram/puff, 28 days @ 40microgram (2 puffs) t.d.s. = £5.50.

Nebulizer solution (single-dose units) 250microgram/mL, 20 x 1mL (250microgram) = £4.50, 20 x 2mL (500microgram) = £2.75; *may be diluted with sterile 0.9% saline.*

With **salbutamol** (generic)

Nebulizer solution (single-dose units) ipratropium bromide 500microgram, salbutamol 2.5mg/2.5mL, 60 x 2.5mL = £24.

1 Gross NJ *et al.* (1989) Cholinergic bronchomotor tone in COPD. Estimates of its amount in comparison with that in normal subjects. *Chest.* **96**: 984–987.
2 NICE (2010) Chronic obstructive pulmonary disease in over 16s: diagnosis and management. *Clinical Guideline*. CG101. www.nice.org.uk
3 Cheyne L *et al.* (2016) Tiotropium versus ipratropium bromide for chronic obstructive pulmonary disease. *Cochrane Database of Systematic Reviews*. **9**: CD009552. www.thecochranelibrary.com
4 McCrory D and Brown CD (2008) Anticholinergic bronchodilators versus beta2-sympathomimetic agents for acute exacerbations of chronic obstructive pulmonary disease. *Cochrane Database of Systematic Reviews*. **4**: CD003900. www.thecochranelibrary.com
5 BTS/SIGN (2016) British guideline on the management of asthma. A National Clinical Guideline. Revised edition September 2016. British Thoracic Society and Scottish Intercollegiate Guidelines Network. Available from: www.brit-thoracic.org.uk
6 NHLBI/WHO (2017) Global initiative for chronic obstructive lung disease. Global strategy for the diagnosis, management and prevention of chronic obstructive pulmonary disease. www.goldcopd.com

Updated July 2017

3

TIOTROPIUM

Class: Quaternary ammonium antimuscarinic bronchodilator.

Indications: Maintenance treatment of airways obstruction in COPD; add-on therapy in chronic asthma (Spiriva® Respimat®).

Contra-indications: Hypersensitivity to **atropine** or its derivatives, including ipratropium, lactose intolerance (dry powder formulation).

Pharmacology

Tiotropium bromide is structurally related to **ipratropium bromide** but is longer acting and thus has the convenience of once daily administration.[1–3] Its main effect is to inhibit muscarinic M_3-receptors in airway smooth muscle and mucous glands, and M_1-receptors in parasympathetic ganglia. Because it is a quaternary compound, relatively little tiotropium is absorbed into the systemic circulation. However, a small amount of tiotropium is excreted renally unchanged and, theoretically, accumulation could occur in patients with moderate–severe renal impairment.

In patients with COPD, tiotropium is safer and more effective than the use of regular ipratropium in improving lung function, relieving breathlessness, reducing exacerbations, exacerbation-related hospitalizations, and improving quality of life.[4,5] Compared with **salmeterol**, tiotropium has similar efficacy, but appears better tolerated.[6]

Tiotropium can be introduced and used alone when symptoms are unrelieved by the use of p.r.n. short-acting bronchodilators, or as an add-on therapy when other regular long-acting bronchodilator approaches are insufficient (see Bronchodilators, Box B, p.111).[7] The combination of tiotropium and a LABA leads to a small improvement in quality of life and spirometry, compared to either drug given alone.[8]

Alternative antimuscarinic bronchodilators authorized for maintenance treatment in COPD are **aclidinium**, **glycopyrronium** (p.13), **umeclidinium**.

In patients with chronic asthma, tiotropium is used when the response to adding a LABA to an inhaled corticosteroid is insufficient (see Bronchodilators, Box A, p.109).[9]

Tiotropium should *not* be used for an acute asthma attack. Compared with a short-acting β_2 agonist, e.g. **salbutamol**, tiotropium-induced bronchodilation is relatively slow onset (≤30 vs. 5min).[10] Further, **ipratropium** should *not* be used as rescue medication in patients on regular tiotropium because the muscarinic receptors will already be occupied.[11]

Bio-availability 20% dry powder inhalation, 33% solution for inhalation (soft mist inhaler).
Onset of action ≤30min.
Peak response 1–3h.
Plasma halflife 5–6 days.
Duration of action >24h.

Cautions

Powder or solution accidentally sprayed into the eye may precipitate narrow-angle glaucoma in susceptible patients; cardiac arrhythmia, bladder neck obstruction, prostatic hypertrophy, moderate–severe renal impairment (creatinine clearance ≤50mL/min).

Undesirable effects

Common (<10%, >1%): dry mouth (generally mild and improves with continued use).
Uncommon (<1%, >0.1%): dizziness, headache, cardiac arrhythmia, e.g. atrial fibrillation, tachycardia, epistaxis, oral candidosis, pharyngitis, cough, dysphagia, dysphonia, constipation, dysuria, urinary retention, pruritus, rash.
Rare (<0.1%, >0.01%): blurred vision, increased intra-ocular pressure, glaucoma, oropharyngeal irritation, bronchoconstriction, gastro-oesophageal reflux, dry skin.

Dose and use

Increased mortality from cardiovascular disease and from all causes has been reported with use of the Spiriva® Respimat® pressurized metered-dose inhaler (MDI).[12] Data are mixed, with no excess deaths seen in a large study comparing the MDI and dry powder inhalers.[13] However, because those with unstable cardiovascular disease (defined as myocardial infarction within 6 months; hospitalized for Class III or IV heart failure, or had unstable or life-threatening arrhythmia requiring new treatment within 12 months) or moderate–severe renal impairment were excluded, tiotropium is best avoided in these groups.

Dry powder inhaler

For maintenance treatment of COPD:
- give 1 capsule once daily via the dedicated inhalation device.

Note. In the UK there are two different brands of dry powder capsules, both delivering 10microgram, but differences in labelling may cause confusion (see Supply).

Pressurized metered-dose inhaler

For maintenance treatment of COPD or add-on therapy in chronic asthma:
- give 5microgram (2 puffs) once daily via the Spiriva® Respimat® inhalation device.

Supply

Spiriva® (Boehringer Ingelheim)
Dry powder inhaler capsules for use with the HandiHaler® device, 28 days @ 1 capsule (delivering 10microgram/inhalation) once daily = £35; *contains lactose. Note. Labelled as 18microgram capsules.*
Pressurized metered-dose inhaler (Spiriva® Respimat®) 2.5microgram/puff, 28 days @ 5microgram once daily = £23.

Braltus® (Teva)
Dry powder inhaler capsules for use with the Zonda® device, 28 days @ 1 capsule (delivering 10microgram/inhalation) once daily = £25; *contains lactose.*

1 Barnes PJ (2000) The pharmacological properties of tiotropium. *Chest.* **117 (Suppl)**: 63s–66s.
2 Hvizdos KM and Goa KL (2002) Tiotropium bromide. *Drugs.* **62**: 1195–1203; discussion 1204–1195.
3 Gross NJ (2004) Tiotropium bromide. *Chest.* **126**: 1946–1953.
4 Cheyne L *et al.* (2016) Tiotropium versus ipratropium bromide for chronic obstructive pulmonary disease. *Cochrane Database of Systematic Reviews.* **9**: CD009552. www.thecochranelibrary.com
5 Barr RG *et al.* (2006) Tiotropium for stable chronic obstructive pulmonary disease: A meta-analysis. *Thorax.* **61**: 854–862.
6 Chong J *et al.* (2012) Tiotropium versus long-acting beta-agonists for stable chronic obstructive pulmonary disease. *Cochrane Database of Systematic Reviews.* **9**: CD009157. www.thecochranelibrary.com
7 NICE (2010) Chronic obstructive pulmonary disease in over 16s: diagnosis and management. *Clinical Guideline.* CG101. www.nice.org.uk
8 Farne HA and Cates CJ (2015) Long-acting beta$_2$-agonist in addition to tiotropium versus either tiotropium or long-acting beta$_2$-agonist alone for chronic obstructive pulmonary disease. *Cochrane Database of Systematic Reviews.* **10**: CD008989. www.thecochranelibrary.com
9 BTS/SIGN (2016) British guideline on the management of asthma. A National Clinical Guideline. Revised edition September 2016. British Thoracic Society and Scottish Intercollegiate Guidelines Network. Available from: www.brit-thoracic.org.uk
10 Calverley PMA (2000) The timing and dose pattern of bronchodilation with tiotropium in stable COPD [abstract P523]. *European Respiratory Journal.* **16 (Suppl 31)**: 56s.
11 Sutherland ER and Cherniack RM (2004) Management of chronic obstructive pulmonary disease. *New England Journal of Medicine.* **350**: 2689–2697.
12 Jenkins CR and Beasley R (2013) Tiotropium Respimat increases the risk of mortality. *Thorax.* **68**: 5–7.
13 Wise RA *et al.* (2013) Tiotropium Respimat inhaler and the risk of death in COPD. *New England Journal of Medicine.* **369**: 1491–1501.

Updated July 2017

SALBUTAMOL

Class: β_2-Adrenergic receptor agonist (β_2 agonist, sympathomimetic).

Indications: Asthma and other conditions associated with reversible airways obstruction.

3

Contra-indications: Lactose intolerance (dry powder formulation).

Pharmacology

Short-acting β_2 agonists (salbutamol, **terbutaline**) have an important role in the management of chronic asthma and COPD and acute exacerbations of both (see Bronchodilators, p.107).[1,2] At low doses, they have predominantly a β_2 agonist bronchodilator effect and no major impact on the heart. However, with increasing dose, tachycardia can occur and rarely prolongation of the QT interval, which may predispose to *torsade de pointes*, a ventricular tachyarrhythmia (see Chapter 20, p.731).

In chronic asthma, short-acting β_2 agonists should be used only p.r.n.[1] They are not recommended for regular use because little benefit has been shown in RCTs. Further, regular use has also been associated with poorer asthma control.[3] Thus, p.r.n. use ≥3 times a week is one indication for the need for prophylactic therapy with an inhaled corticosteroid (see Bronchodilators, Box A, p.109).[1]

In chronic COPD, for breathlessness and exercise limitation, either a short-acting β_2 agonist or a short-acting antimuscarinic bronchodilator can be used p.r.n. If symptoms persist, a regular long-acting bronchodilator is recommended (see Bronchodilators, Box B, p.111).[2] Thus, for p.r.n. symptom relief, a short-acting β_2 agonist is generally preferred; it has a more rapid onset of action and, unlike a short-acting antimuscarinic bronchodilator, can also be prescribed concurrently with a long-acting antimuscarinic bronchodilator (see **Tiotropium**, p.115).

Plasma potassium concentration should be monitored in severe asthma because β_2 agonists, particularly in combination with **theophylline** and inhaled corticosteroids, can cause *hypokalaemia* which further increases the QT interval and risk of arrhythmia.

For details of the use of salbutamol in the treatment of *hyperkalaemia*, see **Potassium**, p.585.

Bio-availability 10–20% of the dose reaches the lower airways.
Onset of action 5min inhaled; 3–5min nebulized.
Peak response 0.5–2h inhaled; 1.2h nebulized.
Plasma halflife 4–6h inhaled and nebulized.
Duration of action 4–6h inhaled and nebulized.

Cautions

Hyperthyroidism, myocardial insufficiency, cardiac arrhythmia, susceptibility to QT prolongation, hypertension, diabetes mellitus (risk of keto-acidosis if given by CIVI).

Drug interactions

Serious drug interaction: increased risk of hypokalaemia with corticosteroids, diuretics, **theophylline**.[4]

Undesirable effects

Common (<10%, >1%): tremor, headaches, tachycardia.
Uncommon (<1%, >0.1%): mouth and throat irritation from dry powder inhalation.

Dose and use

Also see Nebulized drugs, p.835.

Asthma

In moderate–severe asthma attacks, β_2 agonists can be given by MDI + spacer or nebulizer, and repeated until symptoms improve. In life-threatening asthma, they should be nebulized and combined with **ipratropium** (see Bronchodilators, Table 1, p.108).

Pressurized metered-dose inhaler (MDI) and Dry powder inhaler

Chronic asthma:

- give 100–200microgram p.r.n. up to q.d.s.
- give 200microgram before exercise in exercise-induced bronchoconstriction.

Acute asthma (see, Bronchodilators, Table 1, p.108):

- give 400microgram via a spacer, given one puff at a time and inhaled separately, followed by 200microgram every 2min, up to a maximum of 1mg.[1]

Note. MDI deliver 100microgram/puff; Dry powder inhalers deliver 100microgram or 200microgram/inhalation.

Nebulizer solution

Chronic asthma:

- give 2.5–5mg p.r.n. up to q.d.s. in patients for whom inhalers are unsuitable.

Acute asthma (see Bronchodilators, Table 1, p.108):

- give 5mg up to every 15–30min via an oxygen-driven nebulizer
- give 5–10mg/h by continuous nebulization (requires specific nebulizer).[1]

COPD

In acute exacerbations of COPD, bronchodilator use should be optimized (see Bronchodilators, Box B, p.111); both nebulizers and inhalers can be used to administer inhaled therapy during exacerbations (see Bronchodilators, Box B, p.111 and Box C, p.112).

In stable COPD, patients with distressing or disabling breathlessness despite maximal bronchodilator therapy using inhalers should be considered for nebulizer therapy (also see Delivery devices, p.110).[2]

Pressurized metered-dose inhaler and Dry powder inhaler

- give 100–200microgram p.r.n. up to q.d.s.

Note. MDI deliver 100microgram/puff; Dry powder inhalers deliver 100microgram or 200microgram/inhalation.

Nebulizer solution

- give 2.5–5mg p.r.n. up to q.d.s. via an oxygen-driven nebulizer, unless the patient is hypercapnic or acidotic, when compressed air should be used. If oxygen therapy is required by such patients, administer simultaneously by nasal cannulae.

Supply

Salbutamol (generic)

Pressurized metered-dose inhaler 100microgram/puff, 28 days @ 200microgram p.r.n. up to q.d.s. = £1.50.

Nebulizer solution (single-dose units) 1mg/mL, 20 × 2.5mL (2.5mg) = £2; 2mg/mL, 20 × 2.5mL (5mg) = £4; *may be diluted with sterile 0.9% saline.*

Airomir® Autohaler® (Teva)

Breath-actuated inhaler, 100microgram/puff, 28 days @ 200microgram p.r.n. up to q.d.s. = £6.

Easyhaler Salbutamol® (Orion)

Dry powder inhaler 100microgram/inhalation, 200microgram/inhalation, 28 days @ 200microgram p.r.n. up to q.d.s. = £3.50; *contains lactose.*

Ventolin® (GlaxoSmithKline UK)

Dry powder inhaler blisters for use with Accuhaler® device, 200microgram/blister, 28 days @ 200microgram p.r.n. up to q.d.s = £3.50.

Nebulizer solution (multiple-dose bottle for use with a nebulizer or ventilator) 5mg/mL, 20mL = £2.25; *may be diluted with sterile 0.9% saline.*

With **ipratropium bromide**, see p.113.

For spacer devices, see p.110.

Note. See BNF for oral and parenteral formulations.

1 BTS/SIGN (2016) British guideline on the management of asthma. A National Clinical Guideline. Revised edition September 2016. British Thoracic Society and Scottish Intercollegiate Guidelines Network. Available from: www.brit-thoracic.org.uk
2 NICE (2010) Chronic obstructive pulmonary disease in over 16s: diagnosis and management. *Clinical Guideline*. CG101. www.nice.org.uk
3 Sears M (2000) Short-acting inhaled B-agonists: to be taken regularly or as needed? *Lancet*. **355**: 1658–1659.
4 Baxter K and Preston CL. *Stockley's Drug Interactions*. London: Pharmaceutical Press www.medicinescomplete.com (accessed May 2017).

Updated July 2017

INHALED LONG-ACTING β_2 AGONISTS (LABAS)

Class: β_2-Adrenergic receptor agonist (β_2 agonist, sympathomimetic).

Indications: Add-on therapy in asthma (including nocturnal asthma and exercise-induced symptoms) for those treated with inhaled corticosteroids (see Bronchodilators, Box A, p.109). Reversible airways obstruction in COPD in patients requiring long-term regular bronchodilator therapy (see Bronchodilators, Box B, p.111).

Contra-indications: Salmeterol should not be used for the relief of acute asthma because of its slow onset of action.

Pharmacology

The selective LABAs **salmeterol** and **formoterol** have a bronchodilating effect which lasts for 12h. **Indacaterol**, authorized only for COPD, has a duration of action of 24h but is less well established than other LABAs. **Salmeterol** has a relatively slow onset of action; **formoterol** has an onset of action similar to **salbutamol**, and can be used *in addition to maintenance treatment* as a p.r.n. reliever inhaler in certain circumstances (see Dose and use).

In patients with asthma, inhaled LABAs are added when symptoms are inadequately relieved by a regular *low-dose* inhaled corticosteroid (see Bronchodilators, Box A, p.109).[1] The addition of inhaled LABAs to inhaled corticosteroids improves lung function and symptoms, and decreases asthma attacks more effectively than increasing the dose of inhaled corticosteroids alone.[1]

However, safety concerns have been identified when LABAs have been used *without* an inhaled corticosteroid, i.e. increased life-threatening and fatal exacerbations of asthma. *Thus, in patients with asthma inhaled LABAs should not be used without inhaled corticosteroids* (see Cautions).[1]

Combined LABA + corticosteroid inhalers are recommended in asthma guidelines.[1] Although there is no difference in efficacy compared with separate inhalers, combination inhalers ensure that inhaled LABAs are not used without a corticosteroid, and may aid patient adherence.[1]

The safety of LABAs used even with an inhaled corticosteroid remains a controversial issue, with the FDA mandating large trials to compare combined inhaled LABA + corticosteroid vs. corticosteroid alone. The first of these studies found no difference in serious asthma-related events between groups (but a reduction in severe asthma attacks in the combination group).[2] However, patients with a history of life-threatening or unstable asthma were excluded from the trial, thereby limiting the generalizability of the findings.[3]

LABAs can also be used *regularly* to prevent exercise-induced bronchospasm in patients whose asthma is otherwise well-controlled on an inhaled corticosteroid.

In patients with asthma, a long-acting antimuscarinic bronchodilator, e.g. **tiotropium** (p.115), is considered only when the response to adding a LABA to an inhaled corticosteroid is insufficient (see Bronchodilators, Box A, p.109).[1]

In patients with COPD, a LABA can be introduced and used alone when symptoms are unrelieved by the use of p.r.n. short-acting bronchodilators, or as an add-on therapy when other regular long-acting bronchodilator approaches are insufficient (see Bronchodilators, Box B, p.111).[4]

Unlike asthma, the combined use of LABAs with an inhaled corticosteroid is not essential in COPD (unless co-existent asthma), but is recommended for patients with exacerbations or persistent breathlessness and a predicted FEV_1 <50%, or when other approaches are inadequate (see Bronchodilators, Box B, p.111).[4]

Inhaled LABAs and long-acting antimuscarinic bronchodilators, e.g. **tiotropium** (p.115), have similar efficacy in terms of improving lung function, relieving breathlessness, reducing exacerbations and hospitalizations, and improving quality of life. Compared with **salmeterol**, **tiotropium** appears better tolerated.[4,5] The combination of **tiotropium** and a LABA leads to a small improvement in quality of life and spirometry, compared to either drug given alone.[6] For pharmacokinetic details see Table 1.

Table 1 Pharmacokinetics of inhaled LABAs

	Formoterol	*Salmeterol*
Bio-availability	30–50% of the delivered dose reaches the lungs (Turbohaler®)	Approximately 10% of the delivered dose reaches the lungs (aerosol)[7]
Onset of action	1–3min	10–20min
Peak response	5–10min	≤30min[7]
Plasma halflife	≤8h	≤8h (plasma concentration low or undetectable after therapeutic doses)[7]
Duration of action	About 12h	12–16h[7]

Cautions

In asthma, inhaled LABAs should *not* be used without inhaled corticosteroids because of concern over an increase in life-threatening and fatal exacerbations. To ensure safe use, the MHRA/CHM advise that in chronic asthma:[8]

- patients receiving **formoterol** or **salmeterol** should always be prescribed an inhaled corticosteroid
- adherence will be aided by the use of a combination LABA + corticosteroid inhaler.

Hyperthyroidism, cardiovascular disease, arrhythmias, susceptibility to QT prolongation or concurrent use of drugs which prolong the QT interval (see p.731), hypertension, paradoxical bronchoconstriction (discontinue and use alternative treatment), severe liver cirrhosis (**formoterol**), diabetes mellitus (may cause hyperglycaemia; monitor blood glucose).

Drug interactions

Serious drug interaction: increased risk of hypokalaemia with corticosteroids, diuretics, **theophylline**.

Undesirable effects

Common (<10%, >1%): headache, tremor, palpitations, muscle cramps.
Uncommon (<1%, >0.1%): tachycardia.
Rare (<0.1%) or very rare (<0.01%): arrhythmias, e.g. atrial fibrillation, supraventricular tachycardia, QT interval prolongation, paradoxical bronchoconstriction.

Dose and use

The dose varies for **formoterol** and **salmeterol** with formulation and indication (see Table 2).

Asthma

An inhaled LABA should be added *only* if p.r.n. treatment with a short-acting β_2 agonist *and* regular prophylactic therapy with an inhaled corticosteroid is insufficient to control symptoms (see Bronchodilators, Box A, p.109). Use of a combination inhaler will help ensure the concurrent use of a LABA + a corticosteroid (see Table 3).

Because **formoterol** has a fast onset of action, extra doses can be used on a p.r.n. basis *in addition to regular maintenance LABA + corticosteroid treatment* to relieve bronchospasm instead of a short-acting β_2 agonist (see Tables 2 and 3 for authorized products). This approach is generally limited to those patients poorly controlled on an inhaled corticosteroid and LABA (or selected patients on medium-dose inhaled corticosteroid alone) and a history of asthma attacks. However, such use ≥1/day should prompt a treatment review.[3]

Table 2 Adult doses (as puffs) of LABA

Formulation	*Formoterol or Foradil® (DPI)*	*Atimos Modulite® (MDI)*	*Oxis®Turbohaler® (DPI)*		*Salmeterol or Serevent®Evohaler® (MDI)*	*Serevent®Accuhaler® (DPI)*
LABA	Formoterol	Formoterol	Formoterol	Formoterol	Salmeterol	Salmeterol
Labelled strength (microgram)	12	12	6	12	25	50
Asthma[a]						
Starting dose	1 b.d.	1 b.d.	1–2 daily–b.d.	1 daily–b.d	2 b.d.	1 b.d.
Maximum dose	2 b.d.	2 b.d.	4 b.d.[b]	2 b.d.[b]	4 b.d.	2 b.d.
Reliever dose	n/a	n/a	1–2 p.r.n.	1 p.r.n.	n/a	n/a
COPD						
Starting dose	1 b.d.	1 b.d.[c]	2 daily–b.d.	1 daily–b.d	2 b.d.	1 b.d.
Maximum dose	1 b.d.	1 b.d.[c]	2 b.d.[c]	1 b.d.[c]	2 b.d.	1 b.d.
Cost per 60 puffs	£12, £24	£18	£25	£25	£15	£35

DPI = dry powder inhaler; MDI = metered-dose inhaler (pressurized); n/a = not authorized

a. LABA must only be used in patients receiving an inhaled corticosteroid (see Cautions)
b. occasionally higher doses are used; seek specialist advice
c. additional doses above those prescribed for regular therapy may be used for relief of symptoms, see SPC for details.

3

Table 3 Adult doses (as puffs) of LABA and corticosteroid combination inhalers (examples only; see BNF for all available products)

Formulation	*Fostair®* *(MDI)*	*Symbicort® Turbohaler®* *(DPI)*		*Flutiform®* *(MDI)*	*Seretide® Evohaler®* *(MDI)*	*Seretide® Accuhaler®* *(DPI)*
Corticosteroid	Beclometasone	Budesonide	Budesonide	Fluticasone	Fluticasone	Fluticasone
LABA	Formoterol	Formoterol	Formoterol	Formoterol	Salmeterol	Salmeterol
Labelled strengths[a]	100/6	100/6, 200/6	400/12	50/5, 125/5, 250/10	50/25, 125/25, 250/25	100/50, 250/50, 500/50
Asthma maintenance						
Starting dose	1–2 b.d.	1–2 b.d.	1 b.d.	2 b.d.	2 b.d.	1 b.d.
Maximum dose	2 b.d.	4 b.d.	2 b.d.	2 b.d.	2 b.d.	1 b.d.
Asthma maintenance and reliever therapy						
Maintenance dose	1 b.d.	1 b.d. (or 2 daily)[b]	n/a	n/a	n/a	n/a
Reliever dose	1 p.r.n.	1 p.r.n (maximum of 6 per episode)	n/a	n/a	n/a	n/a
Maximum reliever doses/24h	8	8[c]	n/a	n/a	n/a	n/a
COPD when FEV_1 <50% predicted						
Starting dose	2 b.d.	2 b.d.[b]	1 b.d.	n/a	n/a	1 b.d.[d]
Maximum dose	2.b.d.	2 b.d.[b]	1 b.d.	n/a	n/a	1 b.d.[d]
Cost per 60 puffs	£15	£17, £19	£38	£9, £15, £23	£9, £17, £30	£18, £35, £41

DPI = dry powder inhaler; MDI = metered-dose inhaler (pressurized); n/a = not authorized

a. inhaled corticosteroid/LABA dose in microgram/metered inhalation
b. Symbicort® Turbohaler® 200/6 only; authorized to a maximum of 2 puffs b.d.
c. up to 12 puffs/24h for a limited time
d. Seretide 500 Accuhaler® only; authorized for COPD when FEV_1<60% predicted.

COPD

An inhaled LABA is one option when exacerbations or persistent symptoms occur despite short-acting bronchodilators p.r.n. (see Table 2). Combined use with an inhaled corticosteroid is recommended for patients with exacerbations or persistent breathlessness and a predicted FEV_1 <50%, or when other approaches are inadequate (Table 3; also see Bronchodilators, Box B, p.111).

Because **formoterol** has a fast onset of action, extra doses can be used on a p.r.n. basis *in addition to regular maintenance LABA* to relieve bronchospasm, instead of a short-acting β_2 agonist (see Table 2 for authorized products). However, such use ≥1/day should prompt a treatment review.

Supply

See Table 2 and Table 3.

1 BTS/SIGN (2016) British guideline on the management of asthma. A National Clinical Guideline. Revised edition September 2016. British Thoracic Society and Scottish Intercollegiate Guidelines Network. Available from: www.brit-thoracic.org.uk

2 Stempel DA *et al.* (2016) Serious asthma events with fluticasone plus salmeterol versus fluticasone alone. *New England Journal of Medicine.* **374**: 1822–1830.

3 Martinez FD (2016) Safety of fluticasone plus salmeterol in asthma–reassuring data, but no final answer. *New England Journal of Medicine.* **374**: 1887–1888.

4 NICE (2010) Chronic obstructive pulmonary disease in over 16s: diagnosis and management. *Clinical Guideline.* CG101. www.nice.org.uk

5 Chong J *et al.* (2012) Tiotropium versus long-acting beta-agonists for stable chronic obstructive pulmonary disease. *Cochrane Database of Systematic Reviews.* **9**: CD009157. www.thecochranelibrary.com

6 Farne HA and Cates CJ (2015) Long-acting $beta_2$-agonist in addition to tiotropium versus either tiotropium or long-acting $beta_2$-agonist alone for chronic obstructive pulmonary disease. *Cochrane Database of Systematic Reviews.* **10**: CD008989. www.thecochranelibrary.com

7 Cazzola M *et al.* (2002) Clinical pharmacokinetics of salmeterol. *Clinical Pharmacokinetics.* **41**: 19–30.

8 MHRA (2010) Long-acting B2-agonists for asthma: review. *Drug Safety Update.* **4(2)**: www.mhra.gov.uk/safetyinformation

Updated July 2017

THEOPHYLLINE

Class: Methylxanthine.

Indications: Reversible airways obstruction; given by injection as **aminophylline** for severe or life-threatening asthma attacks (see below).

Contra-indications: Uncontrolled arrhythmias, seizure disorders.

Pharmacology

In patients with asthma and COPD, because of its inferior safety and efficacy, theophylline should generally be considered only after the use of an inhaled corticosteroid and one or more inhaled long-acting bronchodilators (see Bronchodilators, Box A, p.109 and Box B, p.111).[1,2]

Theophylline is given by injection as **aminophylline**, a mixture containing ethylenediamine to increase the solubility of theophylline. **Aminophylline** must be given by slow IV injection over 20–30min; it is too irritant for IM use and is a potent gastric irritant PO. **Aminophylline** should be used only with guidance from senior/experienced staff. It is generally reserved for use in severe or life-threatening asthma attacks or an exacerbation of COPD which does not respond to initial therapy (see Bronchodilators, Table 1, p.108 and Box C, p.112).[1,2]

Theophylline shares the actions of the other xanthine alkaloids (e.g. caffeine) on the CNS, myocardium, kidney and smooth muscle. It has a relatively weak CNS effect but a more powerful relaxant effect on bronchial smooth muscle. This is mainly by inhibiting phosphodiesterase 3 (PDE3). This leads to an accumulation of cyclic AMP which through various mechanisms (e.g. reduced intracellular calcium) leads to smooth muscle relaxation.

An anti-inflammatory effect in the airways through inhibition of PDE4 and activation of histone deacetylase-2 has been shown at plasma concentrations as low as 5mg/L.[3] Thus, there is interest in the use of low-dose theophylline alongside inhaled corticosteroids in patients with asthma and COPD, particularly as reduced histone deacetylase-2 activity is associated with corticosteroid resistance and reduced benefit.[3,4] However, in patients with COPD receiving LABA + an inhaled corticosteroid, the addition of low-dose theophylline in a RCT did not increase histone deacetylase-2 levels or reduce the number of exacerbations.[5]

Numerous other effects of theophylline have been described but their benefit in relation to asthma or COPD is unclear. Some require plasma concentrations at the higher end of, or exceeding, the usual therapeutic range.[6] Theophylline is an adenosine receptor antagonist. Plasma adenosine levels are increased in situations where intra-abdominal pressure is pathologically increased, e.g. as a result of bowel obstruction, pancreatitis and peritonitis, resulting in tissue hypoxia. Early work suggests that infusions of theophylline reduce mortality in this situation, possibly by preventing the deleterious effect of adenosine on renal perfusion.[7] This may also explain why theophylline reduces the incidence of radiological contrast-induced acute kidney injury.[8] Conversely, an adenosine antagonist effect may account for some of the more serious undesirable effects of theophylline, e.g. cardiac arrhythmia, seizure.

Although theophylline inhibits proliferation and augments apoptosis of cancer cells, the clinical relevance of this remains to be determined.[9] An anti-inflammatory effect may also explain the benefit seen in an animal model of cancer cachexia.[10]

Theophylline is metabolized by the liver. Its therapeutic index is narrow and some patients experience toxic effects even in the therapeutic range. Plasma concentrations of theophylline are influenced by infection, hypoxia, smoking, various drugs (see below), hepatic impairment, thyroid disorders, and heart failure; all these can make the use of theophylline difficult. Steady-state theophylline levels are attained within 3–4 days of adjusting the dose of a m/r preparation. Blood for theophylline levels should be taken 4–6h after the last dose.

Bio-availability ≥90%; 80% m/r.

Onset of action 40–60min PO; immunomodulation ≤3 weeks.

Plasma halflife 6–12h, but wide interindividual variation.

Duration of action 12h m/r theophylline PO; immunomodulation several days.

Cautions

Elderly, cardiac disease, hypertension, hyperthyroidism and hypothyroidism, peptic ulcer, hepatic impairment, pyrexia.

Drug interactions

Theophylline may potentiate hypokalaemia associated with β_2 agonists, corticosteroids, diuretics and hypoxia.[11,12]

Theophylline is metabolized mainly by CYP1A2, and to some extent by CYP3A4 and CYP2E1. Caution is required with concurrent use of drugs which inhibit or induce these enzymes (see Chapter 19, Table 8, p.725). Reports of interactions where closer monitoring ± dose adjustment are required are listed in Box A.

Theophylline can reduce the plasma levels of **lithium** by 20–30%.

Undesirable effects

Common (<10%, >1%): headache, dyspepsia, nausea, vomiting; risk of seizures and arrhythmias increases as plasma levels increase; hyperpnoea (fast breathing) when given IV.

Dose and use

Because it is not possible to ensure bio-equivalence between different m/r theophylline products, they should be prescribed by brand name and not interchanged.

A m/r formulation should be used.[1] For patients with swallowing difficulties, Slo-phyllin® capsules containing m/r granules can be opened and the contents sprinkled onto soft food and swallowed whole. An unauthorized immediate-release oral liquid is also available for patients who may require it, e.g. those being fed by enteral feeding tube (see Chapter 28, Table 2, p.793). For m/r products:

- starting dose varies between brands; see individual SPCs
- maintain on a single brand because absorption rates vary between products
- titrate dose according to response and plasma theophylline level
- in patients whose symptoms manifest diurnal fluctuation, a larger evening or morning dose is appropriate to ensure maximum therapeutic benefit when symptoms are most severe

Box A Interactions between theophylline and other drugs involving CYP450[12]

Plasma concentrations of theophylline	
Increased by	**Decreased by**
Aciclovir	Smoking
Allopurinol	Heavy alcohol intake
Cimetidine	Carbamazepine
Clarithromycin	Isoprenaline
Diltiazem	Phenobarbital and other barbiturates
Erythromycin	Phenytoin
Fluconazole	Rifampicin
Fluvoxamine[a]	Ritonavir
Mexiletine[b]	St John's wort
Oral contraceptives	Sulfinpyrazone
Quinolone antibacterials (ciprofloxacin, but not ofloxacin)	
Troleandomycin[b] (not UK)	
Verapamil	

a. avoid concurrent use; if unavoidable, reduce the dose of theophylline by 50% and monitor closely
b. reduce the dose of theophylline by 50%.

- samples for drug plasma concentration monitoring should be taken 4–6h after a PO dose of theophylline m/r, and at least 5 days after the dose was started/adjusted
- for bronchodilation, the recommended therapeutic range is 10–20mg/L (55–110micromol/L).

However, some patients may experience unacceptable undesirable effects even within the recommended therapeutic range and for them a lower range may suffice, e.g. 5–15mg/L (28–83micromol/L). This is also considered an appropriate range for the anti-inflammatory effects of theophylline.[3] Ultimately, the clinical response, rather than the plasma level, will determine the need for dose adjustment.

Give IV **aminophylline** in severe asthma attack or exacerbation of COPD only with guidance from senior/experienced staff:[1,2]

- loading dose 250–500mg (maximum 5mg/kg) IV over 20–30min; omit if already on regular PO theophylline and check theophylline levels stat
- maintenance dose 500–700microgram/kg/h CIVI; check blood levels 4–6h after starting CIVI and then daily; adjust dose to achieve a level of 10–20mg/L (55–110micromol/L).

If converting a patient from IV **aminophylline** to PO theophylline, multiply the total daily dose of IV **aminophylline** by 0.8 (salt factor) to give the total daily dose of PO theophylline; this should be halved into a practical b.d. m/r dose and plasma levels monitored as above.[13]

Supply

Modified-release
Uniphyllin Continus® (Napp)
Tablets m/r 200mg, 300mg, 400mg, 28 days @ 200mg b.d. = £3.

Slo-phyllin® (Merk Sorono)
Capsules containing m/r granules 60mg, 125mg, 250mg, 28 days @ 250mg b.d. = £4.50; *capsule contents can be opened, sprinkled on soft food and swallowed whole.*

Immediate-release
Oral liquid 60mg/5mL, 28 days @ 120mg t.d.s. = £294. (Unauthorized, available as a special order from Martindale; see Chapter 24, p.751); *3 month expiry.*

Aminophylline (generic)
Injection 25mg/mL, 10mL amp = £0.75.

1 BTS/SIGN (2016) British guideline on the management of asthma. A National Clinical Guideline. Revised edition September 2016. British Thoracic Society and Scottish Intercollegiate Guidelines Network. Available from: www.brit-thoracic.org.uk
2 NICE (2010) Chronic obstructive pulmonary disease in over 16s: diagnosis and management. *Clinical Guideline*. CG101. www.nice.org.uk
3 Barnes PJ (2013) Theophylline. *American Journal of Respiratory and Critical Care Medicine*. **188**: 901–906.
4 Ford PA *et al.* (2010) Treatment effects of low-dose theophylline combined with an inhaled corticosteroid in COPD. *Chest*. **137**: 1338–1344.
5 Cosio BG *et al.* (2016) Oral low-dose theophylline on top of inhaled fluticasone-salmeterol does not reduce exacerbations in patients with severe COPD. *Chest*. **150**: 123–130.
6 Mokry J and Mokra D (2013) Immunological aspects of phosphodiesterase inhibition in the respiratory system. *Respiratory Physiology and Neurobiology*. **187**: 11–17.
7 Bodnar Z *et al.* (2011) Beneficial effects of theophylline infusions in surgical patients with intra-abdominal hypertension. *Langenbecks Archive of Surgery*. **396**: 793–800.
8 Dai B *et al.* (2012) Effect of theophylline on prevention of contrast-induced acute kidney injury: a meta-analysis of randomized controlled trials. *American Journal of Kidney Disease*. **60**: 360–370.
9 Kapoor S (2016) Theophylline and its direct anti-neoplastic effects. *Respiratory Medicine*. **119**: e1.
10 Olivan M *et al.* (2012) Theophylline is able to partially revert cachexia in tumour-bearing rats. *Nutrition and Metabolism*. **9**: 76.
11 Sweetman S (2011) Martindale: the Complete Drug Reference (online edition). Available from: www.medicinescomplete.com/mc/martindale/current/
12 Baxter K and Preston CL Stockley's Drug Interactions London: Pharmaceutical Press, www.medicinescomplete.com (accessed May 2017).
13 UK Medicines Information (2017) How is an intravenous aminophylline dose converted to an oral aminophylline dose? *Medicines Q&A*. 130.6. www.evidence.nhs.uk

Updated July 2017

INHALED CORTICOSTEROIDS

Indications: Reversible and irreversible airways obstruction, †stridor, †lymphangitis carcinomatosa, †radiation pneumonitis, †cough after insertion of a bronchial stent (see Nebulized drugs, p.835).

Pharmacology

Inhaled corticosteroids reduce airway inflammation. **Fluticasone** is given in a smaller dose because it is twice as potent as **beclometasone** and **budesonide**, which are considered approximately equivalent. However, variations with different formulations can occur. For example, one **beclometasone** formulation (Qvar®), delivers a greater fraction of smaller particles to the lung, approximately doubling its potency compared with other **beclometasone** formulations (see Dose and use, Table 2). This is also true for the combined **beclometasone** + **formoterol** formulations in Fostair® and Fostair® NEXThaler®.[1] **Ciclesonide** and **mometasone** are relatively new and less well-established inhaled corticosteroids.

Inhaled corticosteroids reach the systemic circulation via both the pulmonary circulation and the GI tract. Long-term high-dose inhaled corticosteroids have been associated with adrenal suppression, and deaths from Addisonian crisis (acute adrenal failure) have occurred rarely (see Cautions).[2] Daily doses of **budesonide** ≤1,500microgram or equivalent do not generally lead to adrenal suppression. However, there is significant variation amongst individuals, and formulation and duration of treatment are also important. Accordingly, systemic corticosteroids (see p.513) should be considered to cover stressful periods (e.g. infection, surgery) in patients receiving long-term high-dose inhaled corticosteroids, i.e. **budesonide** >800microgram/day or equivalent.[3]

In patients with asthma, inhaled corticosteroids are the most effective preventer drug and there is a low threshold for their use (see Bronchodilators, Box A, p.109).[4] Improvement in symptoms generally occurs within 3–7 days, but maximal improvement in symptoms and lung function may take 1–2 months. If a low dose fails to improve symptoms, it is recommended that an inhaled long-acting β_2 agonist (LABA), e.g. **salmeterol** or **formoterol** (p.1190), is added before using higher doses of an inhaled corticosteroid (see Bronchodilators, Box A, p.109).[4] If medium- or high-dose inhaled corticosteroids are subsequently used, they should be continued only if they have clear benefit over the lower dose. If there is insufficient response to medium- or high-dose inhaled corticosteroids, alternatives include PO leukotriene-receptor antagonists (**montelukast**, **zafirlukast**), which complement the anti-inflammatory effect of inhaled corticosteroids (see Bronchodilators, Box A, p.109).

In patients with COPD, inhaled corticosteroids are recommended in conjunction with an inhaled LABA for patients with exacerbations or persistent breathlessness and a predicted FEV_1 <50%, or when other approaches are inadequate (see Bronchodilators, Box B, p.111).[5] It should be noted that studies in COPD have generally used high-dose inhaled corticosteroids, e.g. **fluticasone** 1,000microgram/day. Despite this, the overall clinical benefit of inhaled corticosteroids is relatively small.[6] For example, the addition of an inhaled corticosteroid to a LABA reduces the proportion of people experiencing one or more exacerbations from 47% to 42% per annum.[6] Further, inhaled corticosteroids do not modify the long-term decline in FEV_1, nor mortality.[7] This relatively small benefit must be balanced on an individual patient basis against the undesirable effects of using inhaled corticosteroids. If the inhaled corticosteroid is ineffective or poorly tolerated, it can be safely stopped, provided the inhaled LABA is continued.[7]

The only evidence to support the other indications for inhaled or nebulized corticosteroids listed above is clinical experience.

For pharmacokinetic details, see Table 1.

Table 1 Pharmacokinetics of inhaled corticosteroids in asthma

	Beclometasone dipropionate[8-10]	*Budesonide*[a,11]	*Fluticasone propionate*[a,11]
Bio-availability	62%[b] MDI	39% DPI 6% nebulizer solution	30% MDI 14% DPI
Onset of action	Days to weeks	Days to weeks	Days to weeks
Time to peak plasma concentration	30–60min[b] MDI	5–10min DPI 10–30min nebulizer solution	1–2h DPI
Plasma halflife	3h[b] MDI	2–3h	8h

DPI = dry powder inhaler; MDI = metered-dose inhaler (pressurized)

a. data from Micromedex

b. values for beclometasone *17-monopropionate*, the form to which most of the dipropionate is converted before reaching the circulation.

Cautions

Active or quiescent tuberculosis, mycetoma, immunosuppression.

Because of the risk of adrenal suppression, patients receiving the following should be warned not to abruptly stop treatment, and should be given a steroid card (see Systemic corticosteroids, Box G, p.519):[12]

- long-term high-dose inhaled corticosteroids (e.g. doses higher than the authorized maximum, such as **beclometasone** >2,000microgram/24h)
- inhaled corticosteroids with drugs which may inhibit their metabolism by CYP3A4 e.g. azole antifungals, protease inhibitors (see below); patients have also become Cushingoid.

Drug interactions

Increased systemic exposure can occur when co-administered with strong CYP3A4 inhibitors, e.g. **clarithromycin, itraconazole** (see Chapter 19, Table 8, p.725).

Undesirable effects

Oral candidosis, sore throat, hoarse voice, cough, paradoxical bronchospasm, hypersensitivity reactions (e.g. rash), skin bruising. Rarely, psychiatric effects, including psychomotor hyperactivity, sleep disorders, anxiety, depression or aggression.[13]

Inhaled corticosteroids are associated with increased risk of cataract, which is dose and duration related.[14] There is a small increased risk of glaucoma with higher doses (i.e. **beclomethasone** >1,600microgram/day).[15] Increased risk of onset and worsening of diabetes, particularly in patients receiving the equivalent of **fluticasone** ≥1,000microgram/day.[16]

Data on the impact of inhaled corticosteroids on bone mineral density and risk of fracture are mixed; a recent meta-analysis found a small statistically significant, but clinically questionable, increase in risk of fracture.[17]

In COPD, inhaled corticosteroids (**budesonide**, **fluticasone**) are associated with a small increase in the frequency of non-fatal pneumonia (6–18 additional hospital admissions per 1,000 patients treated),[18] and it is recommended that patients are informed of this when inhaled corticosteroids are prescribed.[5] Data are mixed, but the risk appears similar for both **budesonide** and **fluticasone**.[18] An increased risk of infection may also exist in patients with asthma taking inhaled corticosteroids.[19] However, any such risk is far outweighed by their overall benefit in asthma.

Dose and use

Because of their differing potency and doses (see Table 2), inhalers containing **beclometasone** should be prescribed by brand name and not interchanged.[1]

Pressurized metered-dose inhaler (MDI) and Dry powder inhaler

MDIs are most commonly prescribed, alternatives include breath-actuated and dry powder inhalers.

- check the patient's inhaler technique
- use a large-volume spacer device if patient on an MDI, particularly when they:
  - ▷ have a poor inhaler technique
  - ▷ are using a high dose (Table 2)
  - ▷ develop a hoarse voice, sore throat or oral candidosis
- instruct patient to rinse their mouth out after use to reduce systemic availability and oral candidosis
- in asthma, start with a dose appropriate to severity, e.g. **beclometasone** 100–400microgram b.d. or equivalent (Table 2), and titrate to the lowest dose effective against symptoms (see Bronchodilators, Box A, p.109); b.d. dosing is generally preferred (except for **ciclesonide** which is given once daily);[4] however, if subsequently the asthma is controlled on a low dose, e.g. 200–400microgram/day, once daily administration could be considered[4]
- in COPD, inhaled corticosteroids, e.g. **fluticasone** 1,000microgram/day, are recommended in conjunction with an inhaled LABA for patients with a predicted FEV_1 <50%, or when other approaches are inadequate (see Bronchodilators, Box B, p.111).[5]

Nebulizer solution

- **budesonide** 1–2mg b.d.; occasionally more or **fluticasone** 0.5–2mg b.d.
- use a mouthpiece to limit environmental contamination and/or contact with the patient's eyes. However, a mask may be unavoidable in those incapable of using a mouthpiece, e.g. when acutely ill, fatigued or very young.

Supply

Beclometasone (generic)
Dry powder inhaler 200microgram/inhalation, 28 days @ 200microgram b.d. = £6; *available as Beclometasone Easyhaler®*.

Clenil Modulite® (Chiesi)
Pressurized metered-dose inhaler 50microgram, 100microgram, 200microgram, 250microgram/puff, 28 days @ 200microgram b.d. = £4.50.

Qvar® (Teva)
Pressurized metered-dose inhaler 50microgram, 100microgram/puff, 28 days @ 100microgram b.d. = £5; *also available as Qvar Easi-breathe®*.
Breath-actuated inhaler Autohaler®, 50microgram, 100microgram/puff, 28 days @ 100microgram b.d. = £5.
Qvar® is approximately twice as potent as Clenil Modulite®

Budesonide (generic)
Dry powder inhaler 100microgram, 200microgram, 400microgram/inhalation, 28 days @ 200microgram b.d. = £5; *available as Budesonide Easyhaler®*.
Nebulizer solution (single-dose units) Respules®, 250microgram/mL, 20 x 2mL (500microgram) = £25; 500microgram/mL, 20 x 2mL (1,000microgram) = £39.

Table 2 Categorization of doses (in microgram/24h) of inhaled corticosteroids in single or combination inhalers[a] [4]

	Low-dose	*Medium-dose*	*High-dose*[b]
Pressurized metered-dose inhalers			
Beclometasone			
Clenil Modulite®	400	800	1,000
Fostair®, Qvar® (any)	200	400	800
Cicelsonide			
Alvesco®	160	320	
Fluticosone propionate			
Flixotide Evohaler®, Flutiform®, Seretide Evohaler®	200	500	1,000
Dry powder inhalers			
Beclometasone			
Beclometasone Easyhaler®	400	800	
Fostair NEXThaler®	200	400	800
Budesonide			
Budelin Novolizer®, Budesonide Easyhaler®, DuoResp Spiromax®, Pulmicort Turbohaler®, Symbicort Turbohaler®	400	800	1,600
Fluticasone			
Flixotide Accuhaler®, Seretide Accuhaler®	200	500	1,000
Relvar®		92	184
Mometasone			
Asmanex Twisthaler®	400	800	

a. with a LABA (p.119); formoterol: DuoResp Spiromax®, Flutiform®, Fostair® (any), Symbicort Turbohaler®; salmeterol: Seretide® (any); vilanterol: Relvar®

b. in patients with asthma, high doses should be used only after referral to secondary care.

Ciclesonide
Alvesco® (Takeda)
Pressurized metered-dose inhaler 80microgram, 160microgram/puff, 28 days @ 160microgram once daily = £9.

Fluticasone
Flixotide® (A&H)
Pressurized metered-dose inhaler Evohaler®, 50microgram, 125microgram, 250microgram/puff, 28 days @ 100microgram b.d. = £5.
Dry powder inhaler blisters for use with Accuhaler® device, 50microgram, 100microgram, 250microgram, 500microgram/blister, 28 days @ 100microgram b.d. = £9.
Nebulizer solution (single-dose units) Nebules®, 250microgram/mL, 10 x 2mL (500microgram) = £9.50; 1mg/mL, 10 x 2mL (2mg) = £37.

Mometasone
Asmanex® (MSD)
Dry powder inhaler Twisthaler®, 200microgram, 400microgram/inhalation, 28 days @ 400microgram once daily = £18.

For combination products containing inhaled corticosteroids and LABAs, see Inhaled long-acting β_2 agonists (LABAs), p.119.

1 MHRA (2008) Inhaled products that contain corticosteroids. *Drug Safety Update*. **1**: www.mhra.gov.uk/safetyinformation
2 Tattersfield AE *et al.* (2004) Safety of inhaled corticosteroids. *Proceedings of the American Thoracic Society*. **1**: 171–175.
3 DTB (2000) The use of inhaled corticosteroids in adults with asthma. *Drug and Therapeutics Bulletin*. **38**: 5–8.
4 BTS/SIGN (2016) British guideline on the management of asthma. A National Clinical Guideline. Revised edition September 2016. British Thoracic Society and Scottish Intercollegiate Guidelines Network. Available from: www.brit-thoracic.org.uk
5 NICE (2010) Chronic obstructive pulmonary disease in over 16s: diagnosis and management. *Clinical Guideline*. CG101. www.nice.org.uk
6 Nannini LJ *et al.* (2012) Combined corticosteroid and long-acting beta(2)-agonist in one inhaler versus long-acting beta(2)-agonists for chronic obstructive pulmonary disease. *Cochrane Database of Systematic Reviews*. **9**: CD006829. www.thecochranelibrary.com
7 NHLBI/WHO (2017) Global initiative for chronic obstructive lung disease. Global strategy for the diagnosis, management and prevention of chronic obstructive pulmonary disease. www.goldcopd.com
8 Daley-Yates PT *et al.* (2001) Beclomethasone dipropionate: absolute bioavailability, pharmacokinetics and metabolism following intravenous, oral, intranasal and inhaled administration in man. *British Journal of Clinical Pharmacology*. **51**: 400–409.
9 Harrison LI *et al.* (2002) Pharmacokinetics of beclomethasone 17-monopropionate from a beclomethasone dipropionate extrafine aerosol in adults with asthma. *European Journal of Clinical Pharmacology*. **58**: 197–201.
10 Woodcock A *et al.* (2002) Modulite technology: pharmacodynamic and pharmacokinetic implications. *Respiratory Medicine*. **96 (Suppl D)**: S9–15.
11 Harrison TW and Tattersfield AE (2003) Plasma concentrations of fluticasone propionate and budesonide following inhalation from dry powder inhalers by healthy and asthmatic subjects. *Thorax*. **58**: 258–260.
12 CHM (2006) High dose inhaled steroids: new advice on supply of steroid treatment cards. *Current Problems in Pharmacovigilance*. **31 (May)**: 5.
13 MHRA (2010) Inhaled and intranasal corticosteroids: risk of psychological and behavioural side effects. *Drug Safety Update*. **4**: www.mhra.gov.uk/safetyinformation
14 Smeeth L *et al.* (2003) A population based case-control study of cataract and inhaled corticosteroids. *British Journal of Ophthalmology*. **87**: 1247–1251.
15 Carnahan M and Goldstein D (2000) Ocular complications of topical, peri-ocular, and systemic corticosteroids. *Current Opinion in Ophthalmology*. **11**: 478–483.
16 Suissa S *et al.* (2010) Inhaled corticosteroids and the risks of diabetes onset and progression. *American Journal of Medicine*. **123**: 1001–1006.
17 Loke YK *et al.* (2011) Risk of fractures with inhaled corticosteroids in COPD: systematic review and meta-analysis of randomised controlled trials and observational studies. *Thorax*. **66**: 699–708.
18 Kew KM and Seniukovich A (2014) Inhaled steroids and risk of pneumonia for chronic obstructive pulmonary disease. *Cochrane Database of Systematic Reviews*. **3**: CD010115. www.thecochranelibrary.com
19 McKeever T *et al.* (2013) Inhaled corticosteroids and the risk of pneumonia in people with asthma: a case-control study. *Chest*. **144**: 1788–1794.

Updated August 2017

OXYGEN

Oxygen is used to correct hypoxaemia. It should *not* be used to relieve breathlessness unless the patient is hypoxic and/or other treatment options are ineffective.[1,2] It should be prescribed only after careful consideration, particularly if for home use. Used inappropriately, oxygen can have serious effects, or even be fatal (see Cautions and Box A).[3]

Indications: Acute and chronic hypoxaemia; breathlessness unrelieved by other measures in, for example, severe COPD, pulmonary fibrosis, heart failure, or cancer.

Pharmacology

Oxygen is prescribed for *hypoxaemic* patients to increase alveolar oxygen tension and decrease the work of breathing necessary to maintain a given arterial oxygen tension. The appropriate concentration varies with the underlying condition and the dose is generally titrated to achieve normoxaemia/near normoxaemia which is associated with better outcomes than hyperoxaemia.[4]

Medical emergencies involving critically ill patients are an exception, e.g. anaphylaxis, carbon monoxide poisoning, cardiopulmonary resuscitation, sepsis, when high-concentration oxygen should initially be used, 15L/min via a reservoir mask. Examples of established short- and long-term uses include severe asthma attacks and selected patients with COPD (see Prescribing oxygen below).

Despite the widespread use of oxygen to relieve breathlessness, most of the available evidence does *not* support this.[2,4,5] One short-term study in cancer-related breathlessness suggests that oxygen is generally better than medical air in moderate–severe hypoxaemia (SpO_2 <90%).[6] However, short- and long-term (7 days) studies in patients mostly with lesser degrees of hypoxaemia/normoxia have found no additional benefit from oxygen over that seen with medical air delivered by nasal prongs.[7–10] This suggests that a sensation of airflow is an important determinant of benefit.[11–15] Thus, these patients should be encouraged to test the benefit of a cool draught, e.g. open window or electric fan (table or hand-held).[16]

Consequently, national guidelines now recommend that home oxygen should *not* be prescribed for the relief of breathlessness, unless the patient is hypoxaemic ($SpO_2 \leq 92\%$) and/or other treatment options (e.g. opioids, breathing control, hand-held fan) are ineffective.[1,2]

Ideally, patients should undergo a formal assessment, e.g. shuttle walk test, symptom scores/diaries, to examine the benefit of oxygen, e.g. on exercise capacity, breathlessness and quality of life.[5] The assessment should be tailored to the circumstances of each patient. As a minimum, a pulse oximeter will help identify those patients who are hypoxaemic at rest for whom it appears reasonable to give sufficient oxygen to achieve a SpO_2 of 94–98% (or 88–92% for those at risk of hypercapnic respiratory failure). A trial of oxygen therapy can be given for 10–15min and the impact on any breathlessness assessed.

When oxygen is being used in hypoxaemic patients for purely palliative purposes (i.e. to improve breathlessness rather than impact on long-term survival), the degree of symptom relief rather than the SpO_2 should be used to help guide the dose of oxygen given. If benefit is obtained, review again after a longer period of use, e.g. 2–3 days. If the patient has persisted in using the oxygen and has found it useful, it can be continued but, if the patient has any doubts about its benefit, it should be stopped.[10]

High-flow oxygen therapy has been compared with non-invasive ventilation (NIV) in patients with cancer and acute respiratory failure caused by complications of their disease, e.g. bronchial obstruction, lymphangitis.[17] Compared with high-flow oxygen, NIV provided greater relief of breathlessness and reduced opioid requirements, particularly in patients with hypercapnia, although about 10% of patients were unable to tolerate it. The wider clinical relevance of these findings remain to be determined, particularly because NIV is a specialist intervention.[17]

When death is imminent, the findings of one study suggest that in the absence of respiratory distress, even with severe hypoxaemia, oxygen should *not* be routinely given.[18] Further, in 90% of those already receiving oxygen, it was possible to discontinue it without causing distress.[18]

Helium 79%-oxygen 21% mixture (Heliox®) is less dense and viscous than air.[19] Its use helps to reduce the respiratory work required to overcome upper airway obstruction.[20–22] It can be used as a temporary measure in patients breathless at rest while more definitive therapy is arranged. A high concentration non-rebreathing mask must be used for optimal benefit, and the patient's voice will be squeaky. Mixtures containing higher concentrations of oxygen are also available, e.g. **helium** 72%-oxygen 28%. This improves exercise capacity, oxygen saturation and breathlessness in patients with lung cancer.[23] However, this approach is expensive (each cylinder lasts only 2–3h) and limited by the practical difficulties of transporting a large cylinder. Nonetheless, there is interest in the use of **helium**-oxygen mixtures in various settings, e.g. severe asthma attacks or COPD, or to improve exercise capacity in patients with COPD.[24–27] However, in a study of patients with COPD undergoing pulmonary rehabilitation, there was no overall benefit from breathing **helium**-oxygen (or supplemental oxygen) during exercise training.[28]

Cautions

Patients with hypercapnic respiratory failure who are dependent upon hypoxia for their respiratory drive, e.g. some patients with COPD, cystic fibrosis, neuromuscular disease, kyphoscoliosis or morbid obesity. Patients with a prior episode of hypercapnic respiratory failure should have been issued with an oxygen alert card.

Fire risks

Patients and carers must be warned verbally and in writing of the fire risks of oxygen therapy:

- *no smoking near the cylinder*; this also includes e-cigarettes and their chargers
- *no open flames*, including candles, matches and gas stoves
- *keep away from sources of heat*, e.g. radiators and direct sunlight
- *use only water-based skin products* on the face and hands; oil-based emollients and petroleum jelly support combustion in the presence of oxygen.

Patients who smoke should be offered help to stop. The risk of prescribing oxygen when the patient ± carers are smokers should be evaluated on an individual basis, and can be declined on the grounds of safety.

Oxygen cylinders carried in cars should be made secure so as not to move during travel or in the event of an accident.

Patients should notify the fire brigade and their home insurer that they have oxygen at home, and their car insurer if oxygen is carried in the car.

Undesirable effects (Box A)

Box A Undesirable effects of oxygen therapy[5]

Hypercapnic respiratory failure.

Psychological dependence:

- increased anxiety
- increased likelihood of excessive use
- excessive restriction of normal activities
- withdrawal difficult.

Apparatus restricts activities.

Oxygen mask may cause claustrophobia.

Nasal prongs may cause dryness and soreness of the nasal mucosa.

Humidification is noisy and not always effective.

Impaired communication.

Social stigma.

Additional burden on carers.

Cost.

Patients who benefit from oxygen under the care of a home palliative care service report that the advantages outweigh the disadvantages [29]

Equipment

Delivery devices

A high concentration reservoir (non-rebreathe) mask is used in medical emergencies. Otherwise, either constant (e.g. Venturi) or variable performance masks are used.

Venturi masks provide an almost constant supply of oxygen, over a wide range of oxygen flow rates. *Venturi masks should be used when an accurate delivery of oxygen is necessary, i.e. in patients at risk of hypercapnic respiratory failure.* The masks are colour-coded, with the oxygen concentration delivered (24%, 28%, 35%, 40% or 60%) and the minimum recommended flow rate written on each mask. For patients with a respiratory rate >30 breaths/min, the minimum recommended flow rate may be insufficient, and flow rates generally 50–100% higher than the minimum should be used.

With variable performance masks, the concentration of oxygen supplied to the patient varies with the rate of flow of the oxygen (2L/min is recommended and provides 24% oxygen) and with the patient's breathing pattern.

Nasal cannulae permit talking, eating and drinking and are thus better suited to chronic use. However, they are the least accurate, with the concentration of oxygen delivered dependent on factors other than flow rate, e.g. breathing pattern. At 2L/min, oxygen concentrations can vary from 24–35%.[30] Although oxygen concentration continues to increase with flow rates >6L/min (the usual maximum), nasal discomfort and dryness limit tolerability, particularly with flow rates >4L/min.

High flow nasal oxygen delivery devices are now available which deliver humidified oxygen at 40–70L/min and are increasingly used in hospitals outside of intensive care units.[31,32]

Containers

Oxygen can be provided via a cylinder (large for home and small for ambulatory use), oxygen concentrator, or liquid oxygen system. It is more economical to use an oxygen concentrator for long-term oxygen therapy, and other situations where use is likely to exceed 1.5h/day. Modern concentrators are compact, quiet and cheap to run (2p per hour; reimbursed to the patient).

Generally, concentrators deliver flow rates of up to 4L/min, although some high-flow models deliver 8L/min. However, performance tends to decline with increasing flow rates. If necessary, two concentrators can be linked by tubing and a Y-connector to deliver higher flow rates (e.g. 12L/min, using two high flow models set at 6L/min); both concentrators must be set to the same flow rate. A 'back up' oxygen cylinder is provided to all patients using a concentrator. Transportable and portable concentrators are also available.

Liquid oxygen systems make use of the fact that 1L of liquid oxygen produces 860L of gaseous oxygen. Relatively compact base units can provide home oxygen, or be used to fill portable units to provide ambulatory oxygen; these are lighter and last longer than a portable cylinder, e.g. about 8h vs. 2h at 2L/min. Liquid oxygen systems are the most expensive, but are quiet, and require no electric power; the base unit is refilled as required.

Oxygen-conserving devices significantly increase the duration of use of a cylinder or liquid oxygen system, and should be considered for use out of the home. These permit gas flow during inspiration only, generally either as a fixed volume per breath (pulsed devices), or as a variable volume according to the length of inspiration (demand devices). However, they vary in their ability to maintain SaO_2 levels during exertion and some patients have difficulty triggering them.

Home oxygen equipment for ambulatory use can be carried in backpacks, trolleys or wheeled carts.

Prescribing oxygen

Oxygen is generally poorly prescribed and monitored.[33] A specific oxygen prescription chart should be used that includes details of:[4,34,35]

- target SpO_2 range
- name of delivery device
- flow rate/oxygen concentration
- duration of use
- method for monitoring to avoid under- or over-dosing of oxygen.

For domiciliary use, the home oxygen order form (HOOF) requires the prescriber to specify:

- number of hours per day that oxygen will be used
- whether nasal cannulae or a mask
- flow rate
- oxygen concentration (if using a mask)
- need for humidification (only when oxygen given via a tracheostomy).

Completion of a home oxygen record form (HORF) is also recommended to document initial and ongoing assessments. Generally, these will be required unless home oxygen is provided on a palliative basis.

Emergency oxygen therapy

This is primarily used to treat hypoxaemia resulting from acute illness, e.g. severe anaemia, acute heart failure, pleural effusion, pneumonia, pneumothorax, pulmonary embolism and severe asthma attack. Specialty guidelines exist.[4] In brief, for patients not at risk of hypercapnic respiratory failure, initial oxygen therapy is via:

- preferably nasal cannulae at 2–6L/min *or*
- simple face mask at 5–10L/min *or*
- when $SpO_2 < 85\%$, a high concentration reservoir (non-rebreathe) mask at 15L/min.

Avoid flow rates <5L/min with a simple face mask because this may result in carbon dioxide rebreathing. Subsequently the delivery device and flow rate are adjusted to maintain the SpO_2 within 94–98%. Wait at least 5min before assessing the effect of a dose adjustment.

Greater caution is required in patients at risk of hypercapnic respiratory failure (see Cautions); oxygen treatment should commence via:

- preferably a 24% Venturi mask (2–3L/min) *or*
- a 28% Venturi mask (4L/min) *or*
- nasal cannulae (1–2L/min).

Aim for a target SpO_2 of 88–92%, pending urgent blood gas results:

- if $PaCO_2$ normal or low ($\leq$6kPa):
  - ▷ + no risk factor(s) for hypercapnia, adjust oxygen therapy to achieve SpO_2 target of 94–98%
  - ▷ + risk factor(s) for hypercapnia, maintain SpO_2 target of 88–92%
- if $PaCO_2$ raised ($>$6kPa), but pH $\geq$7.35 (or $H^+ \leq$45nmol/L), maintain SpO_2 target of 88–92%
- for all of the above, recheck blood gases after 30–60min
- if at any time $PaCO_2$ raised and pH $<$7.35 (or $H^+ >$45nmol/L), consider non-invasive ventilation (seek experienced help urgently).

A clinical assessment is recommended if the SpO_2 falls $\geq$3% below the target range.

In the emergency setting, humidification is generally reserved for patients:

- with a tracheostomy or artificial airway
- with difficulty clearing viscous airway secretions (nebulized 0.9% saline is an alternative)
- needing high-flow oxygen >24h with upper airway discomfort because of dryness.

Humidification requires the use of a large-volume oxygen humidifier device (essentially a large nebulizer); *bubble bottles should not be used because they are ineffective and pose an infection risk.*

Oxygen can be progressively reduced once a patient is stable and the SpO_2 is either above or has been at the upper end of the target range for ≥4h; it can be discontinued when, with the patient breathing air, the SpO_2 is maintained above or within the target range, or has returned to their usual baseline. A repeat SpO_2 is recommended after 1h, to confirm that it is safe to discontinue oxygen therapy.

Long-term oxygen therapy

Long-term oxygen (≥15h/day) can be considered for use in patients with cancer or other life-threatening diseases who are hypoxaemic (SpO_2 ≤92% or ≤94% when secondary complications are present).[1] More specifically with:

- COPD, cystic fibrosis, heart failure or interstitial lung disease with PaO_2 ≤7.3kPa or ≤8kPa when peripheral oedema, polycythaemia (haematocrit ≥55%) or pulmonary hypertension present
- pulmonary hypertension, without parenchymal lung involvement and PaO_2 ≤8kPa
- obstructive sleep apnoea who remain hypoxic during sleep despite nasal continuous positive airway pressure (CPAP)
- neuromuscular or chest wall disorders causing inspiratory muscle weakness, when hypoxaemia is not corrected by non-invasive ventilation.

The oxygen is used overnight, and for several hours during the day. Evidence of benefit from such use relates mainly to patients with COPD, where correction of severe hypoxaemia improves survival (particularly with use for 20h/day), breathlessness, quality of life and possibly cognitive function.[36,37] The precise mechanism for the improved survival is unknown, but possibilities include a reduction in pulmonary vascular resistance and the subsequent load on the right side of the heart.

When long-term oxygen is considered appropriate (if in doubt, obtain advice from a specialist respiratory physician), a referral should be made to a specialist home oxygen service for further assessment, provision of long-term ± ambulatory oxygen and ongoing review. For example, in patients with COPD, arterial blood gas tensions should be measured before treatment when the patient's condition has been stable for at least 8 weeks to ensure the criteria are met (see first bullet above). Supplemental oxygen is given for 20min to ensure a PaO_2 of >8kPa is achieved without an unacceptable rise in $PaCO_2$ (capillary blood gases are sufficient for titration purposes, unless hypercapnia present at baseline). Arterial blood gas tensions should be measured at the end of titration, and ≥3 weeks later, to confirm the need for long-term therapy.[2] Generally, these measurements should be detailed on the home oxygen record form (see Prescribing oxygen).

A full assessment is not always appropriate when home oxygen is purely palliative in end-of-life care.[1]

Nocturnal oxygen therapy

This is recommended when nocturnal hypoxaemia occurs in patients with:

- COPD, cystic fibrosis, or interstitial lung disease *and* who meet the criteria for long-term oxygen therapy (see above)
- heart failure with evidence of sleep-disordered breathing and daytime symptoms, even when not meeting the criteria for long-term oxygen therapy, provided heart failure treatment has been optimized and other causes excluded, e.g. obstructive sleep apnoea.

When nocturnal hypoxaemia is caused by ventilatory failure, e.g. due to neuromuscular weakness, nocturnal oxygen therapy can be considered as part of non-invasive ventilation support.

Ambulatory oxygen

This can be prescribed in patients who fulfil the criteria for long-term oxygen therapy, are mobile, and wish to leave the home (see above).[2]

Some patients, e.g. with interstitial lung disease, who do not qualify for long-term oxygen therapy but desaturate on exercise (defined as a fall in SpO_2 ≥4% to <90%), can also be considered for ambulatory oxygen provided other treatments have been optimized.[2]

Ambulatory oxygen is also used to enhance participation in pulmonary rehabilitation or exercise programmes for patients who are not hypoxaemic at rest but desaturate on exertion, providing it improves exercise capacity >10% in a formal evaluation, e.g. shuttle walk test.[2]

In some patients, ambulatory oxygen fails to prevent significant desaturation on exertion. Failure varied with different delivery devices, but was as high as 20% in COPD and 40% in interstitial lung disease.[38] This emphasizes the importance of individual evaluation.

A breath-activated conserver can be added into ambulatory oxygen circuits using nasal cannulae to extend the life of the cylinder. However, conservers are unsuitable for patients who mouth breathe.

3

Palliative oxygen therapy

Opioids are more effective than oxygen in reducing breathlessness at rest in patients with advanced disease, with and without hypoxaemia (see p.382).[2,39]

Generally, patients with advanced cancer or end-stage cardiorespiratory disease with intractable breathlessness should *not* be given oxygen unless they meet the long-term oxygen therapy thresholds (SpO_2 ≤92%).[1,2] However, palliative oxygen therapy may be considered when breathlessness is unresponsive to opioids and non-drug approaches, e.g. breathing control, hand-held fan. A formal assessment of benefit and quality of life should be made.[2]

When death is imminent, if severe intractable breathlessness is present, oxygen may be used when hypoxaemia cannot be confirmed without discomfort to the patient (this should be rare given the wide availability of pulse oximeters).[1] Conversely, oxygen can often be discontinued when death is imminent (see Pharmacology).

Short-burst oxygen therapy

This is not recommended in the absence of hypoxaemia. When the underlying cause is irreversible, patients should be assessed for long-term oxygen therapy ± ambulatory oxygen as above.[1,2]

Short-term (intermittent) home oxygen therapy may be required for patients rendered temporarily hypoxaemic, e.g. as a result of a chest infection or episode of heart failure. These patients should also undergo a specialist assessment. For those likely to continue to experience recurrent episodes of hypoxaemia, an intermittent source of home oxygen, probably in the form of cylinders, may be appropriate.[1]

Previously, for exercise-induced breathlessness, some patients used oxygen before the exercise and others afterwards to aid recovery. However, in patients with COPD, most studies fail to show benefit from this strategy. Thus, it is no longer recommended.[2]

Travel by air

Patients with lung conditions and certain other comorbidities who wish to travel by air should be given specific advice (Box B).

In-flight oxygen provision

- generally airlines charge for providing in-flight oxygen (fees and services vary)
- passengers may carry their own small, full oxygen cylinders with them as hand luggage for medical use, provided they have airline approval; a charge may be made for this service, in addition to a charge for in-flight oxygen
- certain types of lightweight battery-operated portable oxygen concentrators may be permitted with airline approval; sufficient batteries are required to cover the flight and possible delays
- the airline must be informed at the time of the booking, and at least one month before the flight
- the airline will issue a Medical Information Form (MEDIF) to be completed by the patient and GP/hospital specialist; the airline's Medical Officer then evaluates the patient's needs; regular flyers can obtain a Frequent Travellers Medical Card from the airline which avoids the need to complete multiple forms
- in-flight oxygen is usually prescribed at a rate of 2–4L/min through nasal cannulae and has to be used in accordance with the airline's instructions
- pulsed dose (breath-actuated) systems are increasingly used by airlines; if there is concern over the patient's suitability for such a system, e.g. the patient is frail or has an irregular or shallow breathing pattern, a trial should be undertaken, and if necessary, an alternative system arranged with the airline.

Box B Fitness to undertake air travel in adults[40]

Air travel exacerbates hypoxaemia in patients with lung disease and may cause compensatory hyperventilation and tachycardia.

Aircraft cabins are pressurized, generally to reflect an altitude of about 8,000ft. This is equivalent to breathing a PO_2 of 15% instead of 21% at sea level. Even in the healthy, blood oxygen levels (PaO_2) will fall to between 8–10kPa (60–75mmHg; SpO_2 89–94%) or more during exercise or sleep.

Contra-indications to commercial air travel

- need for >4L/min of oxygen (at sea level)
- infectious tuberculosis
- pneumothorax
- major haemoptysis.

Evaluation

Undertake a clinical history and examination, ± simple spirometry, to determine if the patient is low or high risk.

Low risk

Patients who can walk 50m on the level at a steady pace without oxygen, breathlessness or needing to stop are unlikely to experience problems with reduced cabin pressure.

High risk

Referral for a more detailed assessment by a specialist respiratory physician is advised when any of the following are present:

- previous air travel intolerance with respiratory symptoms (breathlessness, chest pain, confusion or syncope)
- use of oxygen, continuous positive airway pressure or ventilator support
- severe COPD (FEV_1 <30% predicted) or asthma
- bullous lung disease
- severe (vital capacity <1L) restrictive disease (including chest wall and respiratory muscle disease), particularly with blood gas abnormalities
- cystic fibrosis
- co-morbidity worsened by hypoxaemia (cerebrovascular disease, cardiac disease, pulmonary hypertension)
- pulmonary tuberculosis
- <6 weeks since hospital discharge for acute respiratory illness
- recent pneumothorax (avoid flights for at least 7 days (spontaneous) or 14 days (traumatic) *after* full radiographic resolution)
- risk of VTE or previous VTE (avoid flights for ≥4 weeks, unless no residual symptoms and no hypoxaemia at rest or following exercise)
- other concerns regarding the patient's fitness to fly.

Further assessment can include the hypoxic challenge test where the patient breathes 15% oxygen at sea level for 20min to mimic air cabin conditions:

- if PaO_2 ≥6.6kPa (>50mmHg) or SpO_2 ≥85%, oxygen is not required
- if PaO_2 <6.6kPa (<50mmHg) or SpO_2 <85%, in-flight oxygen required at 2L/min via nasal cannulae.

For guidance on specific diseases, patients oxygen-dependent at sea level, those requiring ventilation and infants and children, see the full guidance.[40]

For guidance on specific diseases, patients oxygen-dependent at sea level, those requiring ventilation, and infants and children, see the full guidance.[40]

General advice

- *medical insurance*, travel with a European Health Insurance Card (if visiting a European Economic Area country) and ensure fully covered for medical costs that may arise related to the lung disease, including the cost of an air ambulance
- *documentation*, have a medical letter on their person detailing condition and medication
- *medication*, take a full supply of all medication as hand luggage, e.g. well-filled reliever and preventer inhalers (also see Taking controlled and prescription drugs to other countries, p.749)
- *equipment*, e.g. portable battery-operated nebulizers may be used at the discretion of the cabin crew, but the airline must be notified in advance (an inhaler + spacer is an alternative)
- *ground transportation*, airports can usually provide transport assistance
- *DVT prophylaxis*, see LMWH, p.95.

Free booklets/fact sheets are also available from various patient organisations, e.g.:

- 'Going on Holiday with a Lung Condition', British Lung Foundation (Tel: 0845 850 5020, www.lunguk.org)
- 'Air travel for those affected by chest heart or stroke conditions' and 'Holiday Information', Chest Heart & Stroke Scotland Advice Line (Tel: 0845 077 6000, www.chss.org.uk).

Supply

Oxygen is classified as a General Sales List (GSL) product and therefore some companies will sell or rent cylinders privately if needed, e.g. for travel outside the UK (see below) or as an emergency back-up supply in a care home.[41]

England and Wales

Any registered health professional can order home oxygen from regional suppliers using a home oxygen order form (HOOF). Patient consent, using the home oxygen consent form (HOCF), must also be obtained to allow their details to be passed on to the supplier and relevant authorities, e.g. the fire service. The following types of oxygen treatment can be ordered:

- emergency oxygen
- short-burst (intermittent) oxygen
- long-term oxygen; unless for palliative care, patients should be referred to the hospital home oxygen service for a full assessment
- ambulatory oxygen.

Standard delivery is generally within 3 days of receipt of order, during working hours. Other delivery services can also be specified but will incur a higher charge:

- urgent response (4-hour delivery)
- next day (clinical assessment services and hospital discharges only).

HOOFs and HOCFs can be downloaded from the NHS Primary Care Commissioning website www.pcc-cic.org.uk.

The completed HOOF should be faxed to the appropriate regional supplier (Table 1) which are available 24h a day, 7 days a week. Copies should be sent to the NHS regional/CCG home oxygen service contract lead or to the patient's GP if appropriate, and placed in the patient's notes.

Table 1 Regional suppliers of home oxygen in England and Wales[42]

Supplier	*Region covered*	*Contact details*
Air Liquide (Homecare)	London East Midlands North West South West	Tel: 0808 1439992 / 1439999 (South West) Fax: 0800 7814610 www.uk.airliquide.com/en/home-healthcare.html
Baywater Healthcare	Yorkshire & Humberside West Midlands Wales	Tel: 0800 373580 Fax: 0800 214709 www.baywater.co.uk
BOC Healthcare	East of England North East	Tel: 0800 136603 Fax: 0800 1699989 www.bochomeoxygen.co.uk
Dolby Vivisol	South East Coast South Central	Tel: 01786 446640 Fax: 0800 7814610 www.dolbyvivisol.com/england

A breath-activated conserver can be added into ambulatory oxygen circuits using nasal cannulae to extend the life of the cylinder. However, conservers are unsuitable for patients who mouth breathe.

The supplier will ensure that the appropriate equipment is provided (cylinder or oxygen concentrator), contact the patient to arrange its delivery, installation and maintenance, payment of patient's electricity costs in relation to use of equipment supplied and train the patient in its use. The supplier will continue the service until a revised order is received, or until notified that the patient no longer requires home oxygen. For more information contact the relevant supplier (Table 1).

Scotland[43]

The Scottish Home Oxygen Order Form (SHOOF) should be completed and e-mailed to Health Facilities Scotland, who work in partnership with Dolby Vivisol to provide the equipment required and arrange installation in the patient's home. The ordering/prescribing of oxygen via the NHS must be by a specialist, generally a respiratory or paediatric consultant, who is specified by the local health authority.

For palliative care patients, each health board should have a local solution developed, e.g. access by palliative care teams to portable concentrators or facilities placed in local cottage hospitals. For further details including the national guidance document see the Health Facilities Scotland website www.hfs.scot.nhs.uk. Alternatively, contact them via Tel: 0131 275 6860; Fax: 0131 314 0724; e-mail: nss.oxycon@nhs.net.

Northern Ireland

Home oxygen is supplied via the Home Oxygen Service Contractor, BOC using the Northern Ireland Health and Social Care HOOF. The prescription form can only be signed by a qualified prescriber listed on the BOC register of authorised oxygen prescribers. In primary care, GPs can also use a HS21 prescription to obtain oxygen cylinders (portable and non-portable) from community pharmacy oxygen contractors. For further details, the HOOF and guidelines, see Home Oxygen Services in the FPS Pharmaceutical Services section of the Business Services Organization website http://www.hscbusiness.hscni.net/services/2359.htm. Alternatively, contact them via Tel: 02890 535613; Fax: 02890 535557.

Note. Community Pharmacy Palliative Care Network (CPPCN) pharmacies all provide oxygen cylinders.

Temporary supplies at other UK addresses

Patients travelling to other parts of the UK, e.g. for holidays, can obtain a temporary supply at the alternative address through reciprocal arrangements between the various UK authorities and oxygen suppliers. This is organized as a holiday order on a HOOF, including Scottish or Northern Irish residents.[43,44] Ideally, at least 2 weeks' notice should be given, but up to 4 weeks may be needed during peak holiday periods in popular tourist destinations or remote areas such as the Scottish Isles. Permission has to be obtained from the householder/hotel to allow oxygen onto the premises.

Patients travelling outside the UK (including the Isle of Man, the Channel Islands, and on cruises which start in the UK) need to arrange a private supply with their local oxygen supplier. Some specialist travel companies can help organize this. Their details can be obtained from the Chest Heart & Stroke Scotland Holiday Information fact sheet (see above).

1 NHS (2011) Service specification: home oxygen service assessment and review. Gateway reference 17874 www.gov.uk (archived).

2 Hardinge M *et al.* (2015) British Thoracic Society guidelines for home oxygen use in adults. *Thorax.* **70 (Suppl 1)**: i1–43.

3 Lamont T *et al.* (2010) Improving the safety of oxygen therapy in hospitals: summary of a safety report from the National Patient Safety Agency. *British Medical Journal.* **340**: C187.

4 O'Driscoll BR *et al.* (2017) BTS guideline for oxygen use in adults in healthcare and emergency settings. *Thorax.* **72**: ii1–90.

5 Booth S *et al.* (2004) The use of oxygen in the palliation of breathlessness. A report of the expert working group of the scientific committee of the association of palliative medicine. *Respiratory Medicine.* **98**: 66–77.

6 Bruera E *et al.* (1993) Effects of oxygen on dyspnoea in hypoxaemic terminal cancer patients. *Lancet.* **342**: 13–14.

7 Uronis HE *et al.* (2008) Oxygen for relief of dyspnoea in mildly- or non-hypoxaemic patients with cancer: a systematic review and meta-analysis. *British Journal of Cancer.* **98**: 294–299.

8 Bruera E *et al.* (2003) A randomized controlled trial of supplemental oxygen versus air in cancer patients with dyspnea. *Palliative Medicine.* **17**: 659–663.

9 Philip J *et al.* (2006) A randomized, double-blind, crossover trial of the effect of oxygen on dyspnea in patients with advanced cancer. *Journal of Pain and Symptom Management.* **32**: 541–550.
10 Abernethy AP *et al.* (2010) Effect of palliative oxygen versus room air in relief of breathlessness in patients with refractory dyspnoea: a double-blind, randomised controlled trial. *Lancet.* **376**: 784–793.
11 Schwartzstein R *et al.* (1987) Cold facial stimulation reduces breathlessness induced in normal subjects. *American Review of Respiratory Disease.* **136**: 58–61.
12 Burgess K and Whitelaw W (1988) Effects of nasal cold receptors on pattern of breathing. *Journal of Applied Physiology.* **64**: 371–376.
13 Freedman S (1988) Cold facial stimulation reduces breathlessness induced in normal subjects. *American Review of Respiratory Diseases.* **137**: 492–493.
14 Kerr D (1989) A bedside fan for terminal dyspnea. *American Journal of Hospice Care.* **89**: 22.
15 Liss H and Grant B (1988) The effect of nasal flow on breathlessness in patients with chronic obstructive pulmonary disease. *American Review of Respiratory Disease.* **137**: 1285–1288.
16 Galbraith S *et al.* (2010) Does the use of a handheld fan improve chronic dyspnea? A randomized, controlled, crossover trial. *Journal of Pain and Symptom Management.* **39**: 831–838.
17 Nava S *et al.* (2013) Palliative use of non-invasive ventilation in end-of-life patients with solid tumours: a randomised feasibility trial. *Lancet Oncology.* **14**: 219–227.
18 Campbell ML *et al.* (2013) Oxygen is nonbeneficial for most patients who are near death. *Journal of Pain and Symptom Management.* **45**: 517–523.
19 Boorstein J *et al.* (1989) Using helium-oxygen mixtures in the emergency management of acute upper airway obstruction. *Annals of Emergency Medicine.* **18**: 688–690.
20 Lu T-S *et al.* (1976) Helium-oxygen in treatment of upper airway obstruction. *Anesthesiology.* **45**: 678–680.
21 Rudow M *et al.* (1986) Helium-oxygen mixtures in airway obstruction due to thyroid carcinoma. *Canadian Anaesthesiology Society Journal.* **33**: 498–501.
22 Khanlou H and Eiger G (2001) Safety and efficacy of heliox as a treatment for upper airway obstruction due to radiation-induced laryngeal dysfunction. *Heart and Lung.* **30**: 146–147.
23 Ahmedzai SH *et al.* (2004) A double-blind, randomised, controlled Phase II trial of Heliox28 gas mixture in lung cancer patients with dyspnoea on exertion. *British Journal of Cancer.* **90**: 366–371.
24 Laude EA and Ahmedzai SH (2007) Oxygen and helium gas mixtures for dyspnoea. *Current Opinion in Supportive and Palliative Care.* **1**: 91–95.
25 Chiappa GR *et al.* (2009) Heliox improves oxygen delivery and utilization during dynamic exercise in patients with chronic obstructive pulmonary disease. *American Journal of Respiratory and Critical Care Medicine.* **179**: 1004–1010.
26 Eves ND *et al.* (2009) Helium-hyperoxia: a novel intervention to improve the benefits of pulmonary rehabilitation for patients with COPD. *Chest.* **135**: 609–618.
27 Hunt T *et al.* (2010) Heliox, dyspnoea and exercise in COPD. *European Respiratory Review.* **19**: 30–38.
28 Scorsone D *et al.* (2010) Does a low-density gas mixture or oxygen supplementation improve exercise training in COPD? *Chest.* **138**: 1133–1139.
29 Jaturapatporn D *et al.* (2010) Patients' experience of oxygen therapy and dyspnea: a qualitative study in home palliative care. *Supportive Care in Cancer.* **18**: 765–770.
30 Bazuaye E *et al.* (1992) Variability of inspired oxygen concentration with nasal cannulas. *Thorax.* **47**: 609–611.
31 Ward JJ (2013) High-flow oxygen administration by nasal cannula for adult and perinatal patients. *Respiratory Care.* **58**: 98–122.
32 Epstein AS *et al.* (2011) Humidified high-flow nasal oxygen utilization in patients with cancer at Memorial Sloan-Kettering Cancer Center. *Journal of Palliative Medicine.* **14**: 835–839.
33 O'Driscoll R (2012) Emergency oxygen use. *British Medical Journal.* **345**: e6856.
34 Bateman NT and Leach RM (1998) ABC of oxygen. Acute oxygen therapy. *British Medical Journal.* **317**: 798–801.
35 Dodd ME *et al.* (2000) Audit of oxygen prescribing before and after the introduction of a prescription chart. *British Medical Journal.* **321**: 864–865.
36 NICE (2010) Chronic obstructive pulmonary disease in over 16s: diagnosis and management. *Clinical Guideline.* CG101. www.nice.org.uk
37 Thakur N *et al.* (2010) COPD and cognitive impairment: the role of hypoxemia and oxygen therapy. *International Journal of Chronic Obstructive Pulmonary Disease.* **5**: 263–269.
38 Marti S *et al.* (2013) Are oxygen-conserving devices effective for correcting exercise hypoxemia? *Respiratory Care.* **58**: 1606–1613.
39 Clemens KE *et al.* (2009) Use of oxygen and opioids in the palliation of dyspnoea in hypoxic and non-hypoxic palliative care patients: a prospective study. *Supportive Care in Cancer.* **17**: 367–377.
40 BTS (2011) Air Travel Working Group. Managing passengers with stable respiratory disease planning air travel: British Thoracic Society recommends. Available from: http://www.britthoracic.org.uk
41 UKMI (2013) Do oxygen cylinders need to be prescribed on an individual patient basis in residential nursing homes? . *Medicines Q&A.* **335.2** www.evidence.nhs.uk
42 NHSBSA (2014) The January 2014 Electronic Drug Tariff. www.nhsbsa.nhs.uk/prescriptions
43 NHS Scotland (2012) Domicillary Oxygen Therapy National Guidance. *National advisory group for respiratory managed clinical networks domicillary oxygen therapy service National guidelines/best practice.* www.hfs.scot.nhs.uk
44 Health and Social Care (2013) Oxygen Services. Business Services Organisation. www.hscbusiness.hscni.net

Updated July 2017

DRUGS FOR COUGH

General strategy

Coughing helps clear the central airways of foreign matter, secretions or pus, and should generally be encouraged.[1] It is pathological when:

- ineffective, e.g. dry or unproductive
- it adversely affects sleep, rest, eating, or social activities
- it causes other symptoms such as muscle strain, rib fracture, vomiting, syncope, headache, or urinary incontinence.

Generally, the primary aim is to identify and treat the cause. However, when this is not possible, a symptomatic approach is appropriate in palliative care. Drugs for cough can be divided into two main categories:

- *protussives:* make coughing more effective and less distressing
- *antitussives:* reduce the intensity and frequency of coughing (Box A).

The choice of drug depends largely on whether the cough is 'wet' or 'dry' (Figure 1).

Box A Examples of drugs for cough (modified from[2,3])

Protussives (expectorants)	Antitussives
Topical mucolytics	*Peripheral*
Nebulized saline (normal 0.9%; hypertonic, e.g. 3–7%)	Simple linctus BP (demulcent)
Chemical inhalations	Benzonatate (not UK)
benzoin tincture, compound, BP (Friars' balsam)	Levocloperastine (not UK)
menthol and eucalyptus BP	Levodropropizine (not UK)
	Local anaesthetics (nebulized)
Irritant mucolytics[a]	Sodium cromoglicate
Ambroxol (not UK)	
Ammonium chloride	*Central*
Bromhexine (not UK)	Anti-epileptics
Capsicum	gabapentin
Guaifenesin[b]	pregabalin
Ipecacuanha[b]	Baclofen
Potassium iodide	Opioids
	codeine[b]
Chemical mucolytics	diamorphine
Acetylcysteine	dihydrocodeine
Carbocisteine	hydrocodone (not UK)
Erdosteine	hydromorphone
	morphine
	methadone
	Opioid derivatives
	dextromethorphan[b]
	pholcodine[b]

a. generally found as constituents in OTC cough products

b. restricted use in children;[4,5] also see mucolytics (p.142) and antitussives (p.144).

The choice and use of antitussives (including demulcents) is discussed on p.144. Nebulized 0.9% saline is generally the protussive of choice but sometimes an irritant mucolytic (e.g. **guaifenesin**) or a chemical mucolytic (e.g. **carbocisteine**, p.142) may be preferable. Nebulized hypertonic 3–7% saline is used in cystic fibrosis and this is extending to other conditions, e.g. bronchiectasis (also see p.835). Further specialist options are authorized for use in cystic fibrosis, e.g. **dornase alpha, mannitol**.

The evidence supporting the use of protussives or antitussives in acute or chronic cough is generally low-level.[6–9] However, recent advances in the understanding of cough and the mechanism of mucin production may lead to more targeted treatments.[10] For example, various receptors important in cough generation have been identified (e.g. P2X purinoceptor 3, several of the transient receptor potential (TRP) class), and specific antagonists are under development.[3,11]

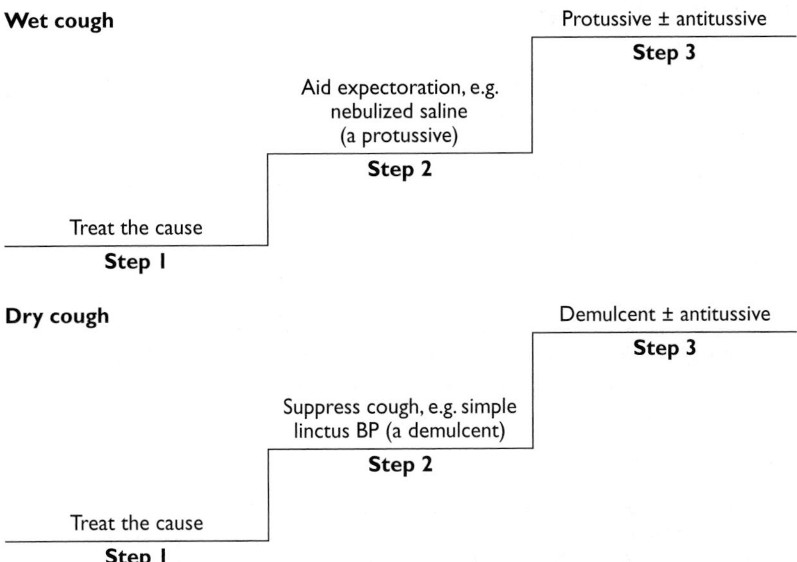

Figure 1 Treatment ladders for cough. Non-drug approaches, generally provided by physiotherapists ± speech and language therapists, should also be considered.

Menthol, long used in OTC cough remedies, is now known to be an agonist at the inhibitory TRP melastin 8 receptor.[12]

Sensitization of the cough reflex, resulting in cough hypersensitivity, appears important in chronic cough of various causes.[3,11] Thus, there are parallels with neuropathic pain:

- paraesthesia ~ laryngeal paraesthesia, abnormal throat sensation or tickle
- hyperalgesia ~ hypertussia, increased cough sensitivity to known tussigens
- allodynia ~ allotussia, cough triggered by non-tussive stimuli, e.g. talking, cold air.

This will see a greater use of drugs which target such sensitization either generally, e.g. **amitriptyline** (p.210), **baclofen** (p.608), **gabapentin** (p.272),[3,9,13,14] or more specifically, e.g. correction of iron deficiency.[15]

Further, some drugs may have a role in specific circumstances, e.g. **thalidomide** (p.558) 100mg PO at bedtime improves cough in idiopathic pulmonary fibrosis (seek specialist advice).[16]

1 Twycross R and Wilcock A (eds) (2016) *Introducing Palliative Care* (5e). palliativedrugs.com, Nottingham, pp 155–162.
2 Homsi J *et al.* (2001) Important drugs for cough in advanced cancer. *Supportive Care in Cancer*. **9**: 565–574.
3 Smith JA and Woodcock A (2016) Chronic Cough. *New England Journal of Medicine*. **375**: 1544–1551.
4 MHRA (2009) Over-the-counter cough and cold medicines for children. *Drug Safety Update*. www.gov.uk/drug-safety-update
5 MHRA (2015) Codeine for cough and cold: restricted use in children. *Drug Safety Update*. www.gov.uk/drug-safety-update
6 Wee B *et al.* (2012) Management of chronic cough in patients receiving palliative care: review of evidence and recommendations by a task group of the Association for Palliative Medicine of Great Britain and Ireland. *Palliative Medicine*. **26**: 780–787.
7 Smith SM *et al.* (2014) Over-the-counter (OTC) medications for acute cough in children and adults in community settings. *Cochrane Database of Systematic Reviews*. **11**: CD001831. www.thecochranelibrary.com
8 Molassiotis M *et al.* (2015) Interventions for cough in cancer. *Cochrane Database of Systematic Reviews*. **5**: CD007881. www.thecochranelibrary.com
9 Gibson P *et al.* (2016) Treatment of unexplained chronic cough: CHEST guideline and expert panel report. *Chest*. **149**: 27–44.
10 Nadel JA (2013) Mucous hypersecretion and relationship to cough. *Pulmonary Pharmacology and Therapeutics*. **26**: 510–513.
11 Chung KF (2017) Advances in mechanisms and management of chronic cough: The Ninth London International Cough Symposium 2016. *Pulmonary Pharmacology and Therapeutics*. (in press).
12 Millqvist E *et al.* (2013) Inhalation of menthol reduces capsaicin cough sensitivity and influences inspiratory flows in chronic cough. *Respiratory Medicine*. **107**: 433–438.

13 Wei W et al. (2016) The efficacy of specific neuromodulators on human refractory chronic cough: a systematic review and meta-analysis. *Journal of Thoracic Diseases*. **8**: 2942–2951.
14 Atreya S et al. (2016) Gabapentin for chronic refractory cancer cough. *Indian Journal of Palliative Care*. **22**: 94–96.
15 Bucca C et al. (2012) Effect of iron supplementation in women with chronic cough and iron deficiency. *International Journal of Clinical Practice*. **66**: 1095–1100.
16 Horton MR et al. (2012) Thalidomide for the treatment of cough in idiopathic pulmonary fibrosis: a randomized trial. *Annals of Internal Medicine*. **157**: 398–406.

Updated July 2017

MUCOLYTICS

Class: Chemical mucolytic.

Indications: Reduction of sputum viscosity.

Contra-indications: Active peptic ulceration. **Erdosteine**: severe hepatic or renal impairment.

Pharmacology

Carbocisteine, **erdosteine** and **acetylcysteine** are thiol compounds used as chemical mucolytics to facilitate expectoration. They reduce the viscosity of bronchial secretions by breaking links between mucin polymers. However, an anti-inflammatory effect is probably also relevant; this includes enhanced clearance of apoptotic neutrophils by alveolar macrophages (also see below).[1]

Erdosteine is authorized only for ≤10 days' use during an exacerbation of COPD. The long-term use of other mucolytics in COPD is controversial; at best they produce a small reduction in frequency of exacerbation (NNT = 8 for 1 less patient with an exacerbation over 10 months) and a small improvement in quality of life of uncertain clinical relevance.[2] UK guidelines recommend that they should be considered for patients with a chronic productive cough, and continued only when there is symptomatic benefit.[3] There is no strong evidence to support routine use of mucolytics in bronchiectasis.[4]

Thiol compounds also have antioxidant, free-radical scavenging and anti-inflammatory properties. For example, IV **acetylcysteine** is well established in the treatment of **paracetamol** overdose when it is given to replenish glutathione, the antioxidant which neutralizes the highly reactive hepatotoxic metabolite N-acetyl-p-benzoquinoneimine (see p.303).

Although the clinical relevance remains to be determined, **acetylcysteine** has also shown benefit in various other conditions. These include idiopathic pulmonary fibrosis, systemic lupus erythematosis, neuropsychiatric disorders (e.g. Alzheimer's and Parkinson's diseases, autism, schizophrenia, depression and bipolar disorder), and animal models of neuropathic pain and ulcerative colitis.[5–8]

Benefit in such disparate neuropsychiatric disorders may be explained through a reduction in oxidative damage and inflammation. For example, in the CNS, toxic free radicals (i.e. reactive oxygen and nitrogen species) are generated as a result of neurotransmitter activity and mitochondrial metabolism, but are neutralized by antioxidants (mainly glutathione). In disease, various mechanisms increase oxidative stress to levels which overwhelm the relatively low levels of antioxidants in the CNS. The unchecked free-radicals cause damage, leading to cell dysfunction and ultimately apoptosis. **Acetylcysteine**, in part by increasing glutathione levels, has several beneficial effects including:

- decreased synaptic glutamate (thereby reducing the production of free radicals from NMDA-receptor-channel activation)
- increased neutralization of free radicals
- decreased mitochondrial dysfunction (thereby reducing the production of free radicals)
- decreased inflammation by reducing cytokine production, e.g. TNF-α and IL-6
- enhanced neurogenesis by increasing levels of neuroprotective and anti-apoptotic proteins.[8]

Such neuroprotective effects of **acetylcysteine** are also evident in peripheral nerve injury, where its ability to protect against oxidative stress-related mitochondrial dysfunction appears key to preventing cell apoptosis.[9] However, the clinical application of these findings remains to be determined.

Carbocisteine, **erdosteine** and **acetylcysteine** are all metabolized in the liver and excreted in the urine as unchanged drug or metabolites. A dose reduction is advised for **erdosteine** in mild–moderate hepatic impairment.

Table 1 Pharmacokinetics of mucolytics

	Carbocisteine	*Erdosteine*	*Acetylcysteine*
Bio-availability	<10%	No data	<10%
Peak plasma concentration	1–3h	1h; 1.5h (active metabolite)	0.5–1h
Plasma halflife	1.5–2.5h	1.5h	6.5h; increased by up to 80% in severe hepatic impairment

Cautions

History of peptic ulcer disease (mucolytics can disrupt the gastric mucosal barrier). **Erdosteine**: hepatic impairment (see below).

Undesirable effects

Occasional dyspepsia, rash.
Rare (<0.1%, ≥0.001%): GI haemorrhage.

Dose and use

Carbocisteine

- start with 750mg PO t.d.s.
- reduce to 750mg b.d. when there is a satisfactory decrease in cough and sputum production.

Erdosteine

- give 300mg PO b.d. for up to 10 days
- limit dose to 300mg/24h in mild–moderate hepatic impairment; avoid in severe hepatic impairment and renal impairment (CrCl <25mL/min) due to a lack of data.

Acetylcysteine

- give 200mg (1 sachet, dissolved in water) PO t.d.s. *or*
- when available 600mg (1 capsule) PO once daily, a cheaper and more convenient regimen.

Supply

Carbocisteine (generic)
Capsules 375mg, 28 days @ 750mg t.d.s. = £16.
Oral liquid 250mg/5mL, 28 days @ 750mg t.d.s. = £35.
Oral liquid sachets 750mg/10mL sachet, 28 days @ 1 sachet t.d.s. = £22.

Erdosteine
Erdotin® (Galen)
Capsules 300mg, 10 days @ 300mg b.d. = £4.25.

Acetylcysteine
Oral powder 200mg sachet, 28 days @ 200mg t.d.s. = £315.
Capsules 600mg, 28 days @ 600mg once daily = £40; availability varies.

1 Inoue M *et al.* (2012) Carbocisteine promotes phagocytosis of apoptotic cells by alveolar macrophages. *European Journal of Pharmacology*. **677**: 173–179.

2 Poole P and Black P (2015) Mucolytic agents versus placebo for chronic bronchitis or chronic obstructive pulmonary disease. *Cochrane Database of Systematic Reviews*. **7**: CD001287. www.thecochranelibrary.com

3 NICE (2010) Chronic obstructive pulmonary disease in over 16s: diagnosis and management. *Clinical Guideline*. CG101. www.nice.org.uk

4 Wilkinson M *et al.* (2014) Mucolytics for bronchiectasis. *Cochrane Database of Systematic Reviews*. **5**: CD001289. www.thecochranelibrary.com
5 Li J *et al.* (2016) N-acetyl-cysteine attenuates neuropathic pain by suppressing matrix metalloproteinases. *Pain*. **157**: 1711–1723.
6 Lai ZW *et al.* (2012) N-acetylcysteine reduces disease activity by blocking mammalian target of rapamycin in T cells from systemic lupus erythematosus patients: a randomized, double-blind, placebo-controlled trial. *Arthritis and Rheumatism*. **64**: 2937–2946.
7 Uraz S *et al.* (2013) N-acetylcysteine expresses powerful anti-inflammatory and antioxidant activities resulting in complete improvement of acetic acid-induced colitis in rats. *Scandinavian Journal of Clinical and Laboratory Investigation*. **73**: 61–66.
8 Deepmala *et al.* (2015) Clinical trials of N-acetylcysteine in psychiatry and neurology: A systematic review. *Neuroscience and Biobehavioral Reviews*. **55**: 294–321.
9 Terenghi G *et al.* (2011) The nerve injury and the dying neurons: diagnosis and prevention. *Journal of Hand Surgery, European Volume*. **36**: 730–734.

Updated July 2017

ANTITUSSIVES

Antitussives can be divided into peripherally-acting and centrally-acting agents. The former include local pharyngeal soothing agents (demulcents) and local anaesthetics and their derivatives.[1] Most centrally-acting antitussives are opioids or opioid derivatives. Generally, the evidence supporting the use of antitussives in acute or chronic cough is low-level.[2–7]

Opioid antitussives are given precedence here because they are more commonly used in palliative care. However, when hypersensitivity of the cough reflex may be contributing, other neuromodulating drugs are increasingly used, e.g. **gabapentin** (see below and p.140).

Demulcents

These contain soothing substances such as syrup or **glycerol**. The high sugar content stimulates the production of saliva and soothes the oropharynx. The associated swallowing may also interfere with the cough reflex. The sweet taste itself may be antitussive by stimulating the release of endogenous opioids in the brain stem, and this may contribute to the large placebo effect seen in RCTs of demulcents.[8] Honey, a traditional remedy, presumably acts in the same way.

However, the antitussive effect of demulcents is generally short-lived and there is no evidence that combination products are better than **simple linctus BP** (5mL t.d.s.–q.d.s.). Thus, if **simple linctus BP** is ineffective, there is little point in trying combination products.

Opioids

Opioids act primarily by suppressing the cough reflex centre in the brain stem. Opioids appear less effective for cough caused by upper airway disorders, e.g. upper respiratory tract infection, possibly because laryngeal cough involves opioid-insensitive central mechanisms and/or reflects a different reflex (i.e. an expiration reflex).[9]

Codeine, **pholcodine** and **dextromethorphan** are common ingredients in combination antitussive products but often in small and probably ineffective doses.[10] Thus, the benefit of combination products may reside mainly in the sugar content (see Demulcents above).[8] The MHRA has advised against the use of OTC cough products containing **codeine** for those under 18 years old (contra-indicated in under 12 years old), and **dextromethorphan** and **pholcodine** for those under 6 years old.[11,12]

For analgesia in palliative care, strong opioids are increasingly preferred over weak opioids. The same rationale can also be applied to cough (see Weak opioids, p.295).[5] For opioid-naïve patients, the initial dose is generally **morphine** 10–20mg/24h (see Drug treatment below). For those already receiving strong opioids, if a p.r.n. dose relieves the cough, continue to use it in this way or increase the regular dose. However, if no benefit is obtained from a p.r.n. dose, there is little point in further regular dose increments. Some patients with cough but no pain benefit from a bedtime dose of **morphine** to prevent cough disturbing sleep.

If a weak opioid is used, **codeine** is preferred to **pholcodine**, which has little analgesic effect. **Pholcodine** has been withdrawn in some countries because of concerns that it may cause IgE-sensitization to neuromuscular blocking agents.[13] However, the EMA concluded that the evidence for this is weak and that the risk:benefit ratio for **pholcodine** remains favourable.[14] If **codeine** or **hydrocodone** (not UK)[15] is ineffective, **morphine** should be prescribed. *If a patient is already receiving a strong opioid for pain relief it is a nonsense to prescribe* ***codeine*** *as well.*

3

Local anaesthetics

Nebulized local anaesthetics have been used as antitussives in patients with chronic cough and also cancer.[16–18] They probably act locally by inhibiting the sensory nerves in the airways involved in the cough reflex but there could be a central effect as well. Their use has not been evaluated in an RCT, and they should be considered only when other measures have failed.

Typical doses are 5mL of either 2% **lidocaine** or 0.25% **bupivacaine** nebulized t.d.s.–q.d.s. In a case series of 100 patients with chronic cough given nebulized **lidocaine**, only about 20% considered their cough much improved and would definitely recommend it to other patients.[17] Undesirable effects include:

- unpleasant taste, irritation of the mouth or throat[17]
- oropharyngeal numbness → reduced gag/cough reflex; patients should be advised not to eat or drink for 1h after treatment to reduce risk of aspiration
- risk of bronchoconstriction → consider pretreatment with **salbutamol** in asthmatic patients[18]
- a short duration of action (10–30min).[10]

Even so, there are anecdotal reports of patients with chronic lung disease, sarcoidosis or cancer, in whom a single treatment with nebulized **lidocaine** 400mg relieved cough for 1–8 weeks.[19–21] Also see Chapter 31, p.835.

Benzonatate

Benzonatate (not UK) is chemically related to the **procaine** class of local anaesthetics. It acts peripherally by inhibiting the stretch receptors in the lower respiratory tract, lungs and pleura. It acts in 15–20min, and the effect lasts 3–8h. It is used PO at some centres in the USA when opioids such as **hydrocodone** fail to relieve a dry irritating cough, or if opioid antitussives are poorly tolerated.[22]

Management strategy

Correct the correctable

If possible, the cause of the cough should be treated specifically, e.g. antibacterials for infection. However, when the cause of the cough is not amenable to specific treatment or is unknown, measures should be taken to suppress the cough (see Drugs for cough, Figure 1, p.141).

Drug treatment

If a locally soothing demulcent (e.g. **simple linctus BP** 5mL t.d.s.–q.d.s.) is inadequate, consider a centrally-acting opioid antitussive (see also Opioids above):

- **codeine** (linctus or tablet) 15–30mg (5–10mL) PO t.d.s.–q.d.s.
- if not effective, switch to **morphine**, starting with:
  - ▷ an *immediate-release* formulation 5–10mg PO q.d.s.–q4h (but 2.5–5mg q.d.s.–q4h if not switching from **codeine**) *or*
  - ▷ a *modified-release* formulation 10–20mg PO b.d. (but 5–10mg b.d. if not switching from **codeine**)
- if necessary, increase the dose until the cough is relieved or until undesirable effects prevent further escalation (see p.375).

If a patient is already receiving a strong opioid for pain relief it is a nonsense to prescribe **codeine** or a second strong opioid for cough suppression.

If opioid antitussives are unsatisfactory, other possible treatments include:

- **sodium cromoglicate** 10mg inhaled q.d.s. improves cough in patients with lung cancer within 36–48h[23]
- **gabapentin** 300–600mg PO t.d.s. is more effective than placebo in idiopathic chronic cough (NNT = 3.6 for a meaningful reduction in Leicester Cough Questionnaire score);[24] case reports have used smaller starting doses, e.g. 100mg PO b.d.[25]
- **diazepam** e.g. 5mg PO once daily/at bedtime is reported to have an effect in intractable cough associated with lung metastases[26]
- **baclofen** 10mg PO t.d.s. or 20mg PO once daily has an antitussive effect in healthy volunteers and in patients with ACE inhibitor cough; maximum effect is seen after 2–4 weeks.[1,27]

Baclofen, **diazepam** and **gabapentin** all have neuro-inhibitory effects. They may act by interfering with the cough reflex and/or central sensitization which leads to cough hypersensitivity, present in most patients with chronic cough.[28] **Baclofen** also inhibits relaxation of the lower oesophageal sphincter and thereby reduces gastro-oesophageal reflux, which is associated with chronic cough in some patients.[29]

Other, non-UK options include:

- **levodropropizine** 75mg PO t.d.s. (not UK) is as effective as **dihydrocodeine** 10mg PO t.d.s. in patients with lung cancer and causes less drowsiness[30]
- **benzonatate** 100mg PO t.d.s. (not UK); if necessary, increase to 200mg t.d.s.

Supply

Simple linctus BP

Oral syrup 28 days @ 5mL q.d.s. = £3.

Codeine linctus BP

Oral solution 15mg/5mL, 28 days @ 15mg q.d.s. = £5.50.
Also see **codeine** (p.349) for other formulations.

All of the above products are available OTC.

Morphine sulfate

Oral solution 2mg/mL (10mg/5mL), 28 days @ 5mg q.d.s. = £6.
Also see **morphine**, p.375 for other formulations.

Morphine solution is available in two strengths, 2mg/mL and a high potency concentrate of 20mg/mL supplied with a calibrated syringe. *Deaths have occurred from accidental overdose with the concentrated solution*, mostly when doses prescribed in *mg* were administered as *mL*, resulting in *20 times* the prescribed dose being given.[31]

Sodium cromoglicate
Intal® (Sanofi)
Aerosol inhalation 5mg/dose, 28 days@ 2 puffs q.d.s. = £36.

Also see **gabapentin** (p.272), **benzodiazepines** (for **diazepam**, p.149) and **baclofen** monographs (p.608).

1 Dicpinigaitis PV (2006) Current and future peripherally-acting antitussives. *Respiratory Physiology and Neurobiology*. **152**: 356–362.
2 Molassiotis A *et al.* (2010) Pharmacological and non-pharmacological interventions for cough in adults with respiratory and non-respiratory diseases: A systematic review of the literature. *Respiratory Medicine*. **104**: 934–944.
3 Molassiotis M *et al.* (2015) Interventions for cough in cancer. *Cochrane Database of Systematic Reviews*. **5**: CD007881. www.thecochranelibrary.com
4 Smith SM *et al.* (2014) Over-the-counter (OTC) medications for acute cough in children and adults in community settings. *Cochrane Database of Systematic Reviews*. **11**: CD001831. www.thecochranelibrary.com
5 Wee B *et al.* (2012) Management of chronic cough in patients receiving palliative care: review of evidence and recommendations by a task group of the Association for Palliative Medicine of Great Britain and Ireland. *Palliative Medicine*. **26**: 780–787.
6 Molassiotis A *et al.* (2017) Symptomatic treatment of cough among adult patients with lung cancer: CHEST guideline and expert panel report. *Chest*. **151**: 861–874.
7 Gibson P *et al.* (2016) Treatment of unexplained chronic cough: CHEST guideline and expert panel report. *Chest*. **149**: 27–44.
8 Eccles R (2006) Mechanisms of the placebo effect of sweet cough syrups. *Respiratory Physiology and Neurobiology*. **152**: 340–348.
9 Bolser DC (2006) Current and future centrally acting antitussives. *Respiratory Physiology and Neurobiology*. **152**: 349–355.
10 Fuller R and Jackson D (1990) Physiology and treatment of cough. *Thorax*. **45**: 425–430.
11 MHRA (2015) Codeine for cough and cold: restricted use in children. *Drug Safety Update*. www.gov.uk/drug-safety-update
12 MHRA (2009) Over-the-counter cough and cold medicines for children. *Drug Safety Update*. www.gov.uk/drug-safety-update
13 Florvaag E and Johansson SG (2012) The pholcodine case. Cough medicines, igE-sensitization, and anaphylaxis: a devious connection. *World Allergy Organ Journal*. **5**: 73–78.
14 EMA (2011) Questions and answers on the review of the marketing authorisations for medicines containing pholcodine. Available from: www.ema.europe.eu
15 Homsi J *et al.* (2002) A phase II study of hydrocodone for cough in advanced cancer. *American Journal of Hospice and Palliative Care*. **19**: 49–56.
16 Truesdale K and Jurdi A (2013) Nebulized lidocaine in the treatment of intractable cough. *American Journal of Hospital Palliative Care*. **30**: 587–589.
17 Lim KG *et al.* (2013) Long-term safety of nebulized lidocaine for adults with difficult-to-control chronic cough: a case series. *Chest*. **143**: 1060–1065.
18 Slaton RM *et al.* (2013) Evidence for therapeutic uses of nebulized lidocaine in the treatment of intractable cough and asthma. *Annals of Pharmacotherpy*. **47**: 578–585.
19 Howard P *et al.* (1977) Lignocaine aerosol and persistent cough. *British Journal of Diseases of the Chest*. **71**: 19–24.
20 Stewart C and Coady T (1977) Suppression of intractable cough. *British Medical Journal*. **1**: 1660–1661.

21 Sanders RV and Kirkpatrick MB (1984) Prolonged suppression of cough after inhalation of lidocaine in a patient with sarcoid. *Journal of the American Medical Association*. **252**: 2456–2457.
22 Doona M and Walsh D (1998) Benzonatate for opioid-resistant cough in advanced cancer. *Palliative Medicine*. **12**: 55–58.
23 Moroni M *et al.* (1996) Inhaled sodium cromoglycate to treat cough in advanced lung cancer patients. *British Journal of Cancer*. **74**: 309–311.
24 Ryan NM *et al.* (2012) Gabapentin for refractory chronic cough: a randomised, double-blind, placebo-controlled trial. *Lancet*. **380**: 1583–1589.
25 Mintz S and Lee JK (2006) Gabapentin in the treatment of intractable idiopathic chronic cough: case reports. *American Journal of Medicine*. **119**: e13–15.
26 Estfan B and Walsh D (2008) The cough from hell: diazepam for intractable cough in a patient with renal cell carcinoma. *Journal of Pain and Symptom Management*. **36**: 553–558.
27 Dicpinigaitis P *et al.* (1998) Inhibition of capsaicin-induced cough by the gamma-aminobutyric acid agonist baclofen. *Journal of Clinical Pharmacology*. **38**: 364–367.
28 Smith JA and Woodcock A (2016) Chronic Cough. *New England Journal of Medicine*. **375**: 1544–1551.
29 Lidums I *et al.* (2000) Control of transient lower esophageal sphincter relaxations and reflux by the GABA(B) agonist baclofen in normal subjects. *Gastroenterology*. **118**: 7–13.
30 Luporini G *et al.* (1998) Efficacy and safety of levodropropizine and dihydrocodeine on nonproductive cough in primary and metastatic lung cancer. *European Respiratory Journal*. **12**: 97–101.
31 FDA (2011) Medwatch safety alert. Morphine sulfate oral solution 100mg per 5mL (20mg/mL): medication use error - reports of accidental overdose. Available from: www.fda.gov/Safety/MedWatch/SafetyInformation (archived).

Updated July 2017

4: CENTRAL NERVOUS SYSTEM

BENZODIAZEPINES AND Z-DRUGS

Class: GABAmimetics; hypnotics (Z-drugs and short acting benzodiazepines); anxiolytics (long acting benzodiazepines).

Indications: Authorized indications vary; see individual SPCs for details. Insomnia; anxiety and panic disorder; seizures; myoclonus; skeletal muscle spasm; alcohol withdrawal; sedation; †terminal agitation; †restless legs syndrome; †drug-induced movement disorders; †neuropathic pain; †spasticity; †nausea and vomiting; †intractable pruritus; †intractable hiccup.

Contra-indications: Unless in the imminently dying: acute severe pulmonary insufficiency, untreated sleep apnoea syndrome, severe hepatic impairment, myasthenia gravis. Also see individual SPCs.

Pharmacology

GABA is the major inhibitory neurotransmitter of the nervous system. Several drug classes enhance its action (GABAmimetics):

- $GABA_A$ modulators: benzodiazepines, Z-drugs (e.g. **zopiclone**), ethanol, barbiturates, some general anaesthetics (e.g. **propofol**), valerian (herbal product)
- $GABA_B$ agonists: **baclofen, sodium oxybate**
- inhibitors of GABA transaminase (e.g. **vigabatrin**) or re-uptake (e.g. **tiagibine**).[1–3]

The $GABA_A$ receptor is a chloride channel formed by 5 subunits comprising varying subtypes (Figure 1). $GABA_A$ modulators bind to sites distinct from GABA itself (allosteric modulation), increasing the receptor's affinity for GABA (benzodiazepines) or prolonging channel opening (barbiturates).[4] The α subunit of the $GABA_A$ receptor, of which there are six subtypes, is the predominant determinant of benzodiazepine affinity and function (Table 1).

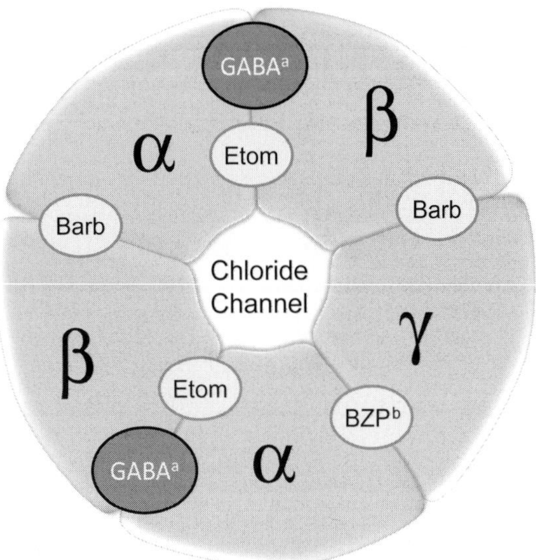

Figure 1 The $GABA_A$ receptor's putative drug binding sites.[2,5–7]

Barb = barbiturates; BZP = benzodiazepines; Etom = etomidate

a. the central chloride channel is opened by the concurrent binding of 2 GABA molecules

b. benzodiazepines bind to the same site as endogenous neurosteroids.

Synaptic channels (α1–3) detect intermittent (phasic) release of GABA within the synapse. GABA is then partly removed by a re-uptake transporter with the remainder diffusing away from the synapse forming a diffuse tonic (i.e. relatively stable) background. The latter is detected by extra-synaptic (α4–6) channels.[8] Synaptic channels are more likely to become desensitized by repeated stimulation than extra-synaptic channels.[9] This partly explains why some actions (e.g. hypnotic and anti-epileptic effects) diminish over time more quickly than others (e.g. undesirable cognitive effects; also see Table 1).[10]

The sedative effects of benzodiazepines and Z-drugs result from α1-$GABA_A$ receptor mediated inhibition of the wakefulness-promoting system (see p.164).[11] Their anxiolytic effects result from α2-$GABA_A$ receptor mediated inhibition of 'fear circuits', which are co-ordinated by the amygdala (Figure 2).[12] The location and α-subunits involved in their anti-epileptic effects vary depending on seizure type.

Selective modulation of α-subunits might improve tolerability by separating desirable from undesirable effects. **Clobazam** and its active N-desmethyl metabolite relatively selectively bind to α2 subunits.[13,14] This may explain the lower incidence of sedation and cognitive impairment compared with other benzodiazepines.[15] More selective α2-modulators are under investigation, e.g. as non-sedating anxiolytics and antihyperalgesics.[14,16] Z-drugs are more α1 selective, but the clinical relevance is questionable because many undesirable effects are direct consequences of sedation. Although indirect comparisons find fewer undesirable effects compared with benzodiazepine hypnotics,[17] this may reflect their shorter halflives rather than subunit selectivity.

Most benzodiazepines and Z-drugs are well absorbed, widely distributed and metabolized before being eliminated. Their receptor profiles are similar (Table 1) but their potency and halflives differ (Table 2). Their varied metabolic pathways affect their pharmacogenetic profiles and drug interactions (see individual SPCs). In high doses, **diazepam** induces hepatic metabolism. **Lorazepam** is sometimes given SL, generally when a rapid onset of effect is required and/or the patient cannot reliably swallow tablets. However, ease of dissolution varies between brands (see 'buccal and sublingual administration', below).

Table 1 $GABA_A$ α-subunit subtypes and relative activity of selected GABAmimetics[1,8–10,13,14,16,18,19]

Location		*GABAergic synapses (phasic response to GABA release)*				*Extra-synaptic (tonic response to background GABA)*	
Alpha subunit subtype		*1*	*2*	*3*	*4*[a]	*5*	*6*[a]
Function of agonists		*Addiction Amnesia Anti-epilepsis*[b] *Sleep*	*Anxiolysis Antihyperalgesia Muscle relaxation*	*Antihyperalgesia Muscle relaxation*		*Amnesia Cognitive impairment Benzodiazepine tolerance*	
Benzodiazepines	Clobazam[c]	+	++	+	-	++	+[c]
	Clonazepam	++	++	++	-	++	-
	Diazepam	++	++	++	-	++	-
	Flunitrazepam	++	++	++	-	++	-
	Midazolam	++		++	-	++	-
Z-drugs	Zaleplon[d]	++	++/+	++/+		++/+	
	Zolpidem[d]	++	+	+	-	-	-
	Zopiclone	++	++	-/+[d]	-	+	-
Other	Ethanol[e]	+	+	+	++	+	+
	Neurosteroids	+	+	+	++	++	++
	Pentobarbital	++	++	++	++	++	

Activity: ++ high, + low, - negligible or none; blank = no data.

a. benzodiazepines do not bind to α4- and α6-subunits, or to receptors lacking a and g subunits (benzodiazepine-insensitive $GABA_A$ receptors)
b. relative importance of subunits varies with different seizure models
c. clobazam and its active N-desmethyl metabolite are α2-selective. The clinical significance of clobazam binding to the (normally benzodiazepine insensitive) α6 channel is unclear
d. subunit affinity varies with different β and γ subunit configurations. Prior to cloning, $GABA_A$ classifications encompassed more than one subunit configuration which may account for earlier conflicting affinity data
e. tonic $\alpha 4(\delta)$ mediated inhibition predominates at lower doses whereas synaptic (α1, 2 and 3) effects are responsible for severe intoxication. Ethanol also enhances release of GABA and GABAmimetic neurosteroids.

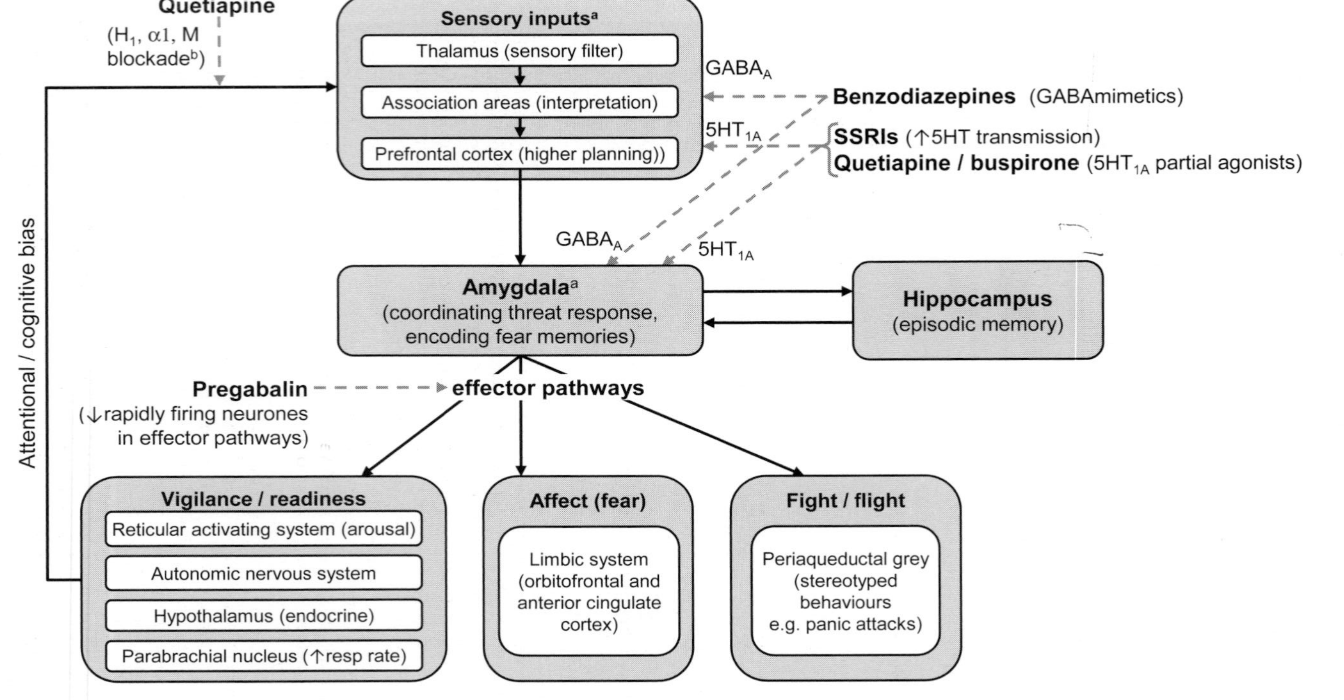

Figure 2 Putative sites of action of anxiolytics on fear circuits[3,12,20]

α_1 = adrenergic type 1 receptor; $GABA_A$ – see text; H_1 = histamine type 1 receptor; 5HT = 5-hydroxytryptamine (serotonin); $5HT_{1A}$ = serotonin type 1A receptor; M = muscarinic acetylcholine receptor

a. $GABA_A$ and $5HT_{1A}$ receptors alter both sensory input and amygdala circuits. Not all antipsychotics are $5HT_{1A}$ agonists and thus their anxiolytic properties vary (see p.171)

b. quetiapine also affects monoamines involved in arousal and attention, but their relative importance to its anxiolytic effects are unclear.

Table 2 Pharmacokinetics of selected benzodiazepines and related drugs; PO unless stated otherwise[21–25]

Drug	*Bio-availability PO (%)*	*Tmax (h)*	*Plasma halflife (h)*	*Metabolism*
Alprazolam	≥90[a]	1–2	12–15	CYP3A4
Clobazam	85	0.5–4	35; (80)[b]	CYP3A4[b]; metabolite inactivated by CYP2C19
Clonazepam	>80	1–4	20–60	Multiple non-P450 pathways[b]
Diazepam	>90 65–85 (PR)	0.5–1.5 ≤0.5 (PR) ≤0.25 (IV) 1–2 (IM)[c]	25–50; (≤200)[b]	Multiple P450 pathways[b]
Lorazepam	90	2.5 2.5 (SL)	10–20	Non-P450 glucuronidation
Midazolam	40 95 (SC) 85 (Buccal)	0.5–1 0.5 (SC) ≤0.5 (Buccal)	1–4[d]; (1)[b]	CYP3A4[b]
Oxazepam	≥90[a]	1–5	6–20	Non-P450 glucuronidation
Temazepam	≥90[a]	1	8–15	Non-P450 glucuronidation
Zaleplon	30[e]	1.5	1	CYP3A4 and non-P450 oxidation
Zolpidem	70	1.5	2	CYP3A4 and CYP1A2
Zopiclone	75	1.5	3.5	CYP3A4[b]

a. estimated

b. active metabolite(s)

c. 1–1.5h for oil-based formulation; 2h for emulsion formulation

d. up to 24h when given by CIVI in critical care

e. well absorbed but undergoes extensive first pass hepatic metabolism.

Cautions

Fatalities from oversedation or cardiorespiratory depression have occurred after concurrent use of **midazolam** with higher than approved doses of parenteral **olanzapine** (not UK) (see p.187).

Benzodiazepines with long halflives accumulate when given repeatedly and undesirable effects may manifest only after several days or weeks. Caution is required in renal impairment (reduce dose; see p.692) and mild–moderate hepatic impairment (see p.712).

Because their central depressant effect can depress respiration, caution is required in chronic respiratory disease or with IV administration. Although mortality was higher amongst recipients of benzodiazepines in two case series (US Veterans; patients with advanced respiratory disease), it is not known whether this is causal and/or confounded (e.g. reflecting higher use in those with more severe illness).[26,27]

It is not known whether benzodiazepines are associated with suicidal thoughts and behaviour; the manufacturer of **clonazepam** advises similar caution to other anti-epileptic drugs (see p.261).

Benzodiazepines and Z-drugs can cause physical and psychological dependence. Patients with a history of substance abuse should be monitored closely. If long-term treatment is discontinued, taper gradually to avoid withdrawal symptoms, e.g. by 5–10% every 2 weeks.[28] Peak-trough variability can be sufficient to cause withdrawal symptoms when tapering short-acting benzodiazepines; consider switching to an alternative with a longer halflife.

Benzodiazepines are generally safer in overdose than barbiturates and tricyclic antidepressants. However, fatal iatrogenic overdoses of IV **midazolam** have occurred during procedural sedation. Thus, regulators recommend that **flumazenil** is available for emergency use wherever **midazolam** is used clinically.[29]

Drug interactions

Additive effects with other CNS depressants, e.g. alcohol, opioids.

The metabolism of Z-drugs and several benzodiazepines is mostly CYP3A4 dependent (Table 2) and plasma concentrations may be decreased or increased to a clinically relevant degree by moderate or potent CYP3A4 inducers (e.g. **carbamazepine**, **phenytoin, rifampicin**) or inhibitors (e.g. antifungal azoles, **clarithromycin**, **diltiazem**, **erythromycin**, protease inhibitors, **verapamil**) respectively (see Chapter 19, Table 8, p.725). Reduce doses, increase monitoring and/or explain the need for increased caution (e.g. the likelihood of increased morning impairment with hypnotics).

Midazolam is a substrate for CYP3A4. Plasma levels of **midazolam** can be eight times higher following the addition of a CYP3A4 inhibitor.[30] Thus ≥50% reduction in the midazolam dose may be required when a moderate or potent inhibitor is used concurrently, particularly for PO **midazolam** (not UK).

Diazepam or **clonazepam** and **phenytoin** have unpredictable effects on each other's plasma concentrations. Monitor the **phenytoin** plasma concentration.

Undesirable effects

Dose-dependent drowsiness, impaired psychomotor skills (e.g. impaired driving ability), reduced independence, fatigue, cognitive impairment, hypotonia (manifesting as unsteadiness/ataxia) with an increased (almost double) risk of femoral fracture in the elderly.[31,32]

Paradoxical arousal, agitation and aggression can occur in <10%; risk factors include high-trait anxiety, borderline personality disorder and alcohol misuse.[33–35]

Less commonly, complex actions while apparently asleep (e.g. driving, eating, cooking, conversations) occur both with benzodiazepines and Z-drugs.[36]

The incidence of dementia is higher among users of benzodiazepines.[37] It is not known whether this is causal and/or confounded (e.g. reflecting their use for the prodromal sleep disturbance and anxiety which commonly precedes a diagnosis of dementia). Results of studies accounting for the latter by examining use over a longer period are conflicting.[37–39]

Results of observational studies comparing the use of benzodiazepines and Z-drugs with the risk of cancer and overall mortality are conflicting and likely to be influenced by confounding factors (e.g. smoking, obesity, alcohol).[40–43]

Diazepam may cause painful thrombophlebitis with given IV. **Clonazepam** has been associated with salivary hypersecretion and drooling in children. **Zopiclone** commonly causes an unpleasant taste.

Toxicity from propylene glycol, an excipient in parenteral **lorazepam** and **phenobarbital** (see p.289), has been reported with prolonged high dose IVI, resulting in confusion, drowsiness, seizures, cardiac arrhythmias and/or renal failure.[44] However, the doses necessary in palliative care are unlikely to approach the mean dose of **lorazepam** (270mg/24h) required to achieve toxic levels of propylene glycol.

Dose and use of benzodiazepines in palliative care

Benzodiazepines are useful in the management of various symptoms encountered in palliative care. Tolerance and dependence are unlikely to be a problem when used for ≤4 weeks.[45] Appropriate caution and monitoring is required, particularly for those at greater risk of drowsiness, falls, and memory and cognitive impairment, e.g. the elderly and frail patients.

Benzodiazepines are included in a new law in England and Wales relating to driving with certain drugs above specified plasma concentrations (see Chapter 22, p.743).

Insomnia

Initial treatment includes:

- correcting contributory factors if possible:[46–48]
  - ▷ pain
  - ▷ delirium
  - ▷ depression, anxiety or rumination
  - ▷ obstructive sleep apnoea
- non-drug measures.[47,49–52]

Where drug treatment is required, use a Z-drug or a short-halflife benzodiazepine, ideally for <4 weeks:

- **zolpidem** (halflife 2h) 10mg PO at bedtime (5mg initially if elderly or frail) *or*
- **zopiclone** (halflife 3.5h) 7.5mg PO at bedtime (3.75mg initially if elderly or frail) *or*
- **midazolam** (halflife 1–4h) 2.5mg SC at bedtime,[53] when PO route unavailable.

Generic Z-drugs are cheaper than **temazepam** (halflife 8–15h). Although the latter is available as an oral solution, it is significantly more expensive. See Chapter 28 for other options for patients with swallowing difficulties or EFT.

A meta-analysis confirmed that, in people >60 years of age, benzodiazepines and Z-drugs had an NNT of 13 but an NNH of 6.[54] The undesirable effects were cognitive impairment, day-time drowsiness, ataxia and falls. Even low doses of short halflife benzodiazepines increase the risk of falls.[55] Alternatives include sedating antidepressants (e.g. **doxepin, mirtazapine, trazodone**; see p.204) and **melatonin** (p.164).[56]

Anxiety and panic disorder

The efficacy of cognitive behavioral and drug therapy is comparable.[57] Choice of drug is largely influenced by likely duration of use.

Benzodiazepines act within hours. They are used to rapidly alleviate symptoms if prognosis is <4 weeks or while awaiting benefit from an SSRI:

- **diazepam** 2–10mg PO at bedtime and p.r.n. *or*
- **lorazepam** 500microgram–1mg PO b.d. and p.r.n. *or*
- **midazolam** 5–10mg/24h CSCI.

Because of dependence and undesirable effects, long term (>4 weeks) use of benzodiazepines is reserved for severe anxiety refractory to other treatments.[45] Tolerance to their anxiolytic effects may not occur.[10]

Pregabalin (p.272) and **quetiapine** (p.191) act within days but are, respectively, more expensive and less well tolerated than alternatives. Thus, they are reserved for second/third-line use or where there are concurrent indications; e.g. neuropathic pain or delirium.

SSRIs (p.212) act within weeks and can exacerbate anxiety initially but are, respectively, more effective and better tolerated than **pregabalin** and **quetiapine**.[58,59]

If anxiety persists, anxiolytics with different sites of action (Figure 2) are combined; e.g. a mono-amine re-uptake inhibitor with either a benzodiazepine or **pregabalin**.

Seizures

Acute treatment

Benzodiazepines are first-line treatments for acute seizures (also see p.264), including status epilepticus:[60]

- **lorazepam** 4mg IV over 2min *or*
- **midazolam** 10mg buccal/SC/IM stat or IV over 2min; the injection formulation can be given buccally in status epilepticus.

If necessary, repeat once after 10–20min.

In children, buccal **midazolam** is more effective than rectal **diazepam**.[61] An authorized oromucosal solution for buccal administration is available for children and adolescents (see below).

In the imminently dying

- manage acute seizures with **midazolam** 10mg buccal/SC/IM stat or IV over 2min; repeat once after 10min p.r.n. For prophylaxis, commence **midazolam** 20–30mg/24h CSCI
- if seizures persist, consider switching to **phenobarbital** (p.289).

Consider alternative SC/CSCI anti-epileptics if it is desirable to avoid sedation, e.g. **lacosamide**,[62] **levetiracetam** (p.287), **valproate** (p.282).

Chronic treatment

Long-term use is limited by the development of tolerance; thus, benzodiazepines are reserved for epilepsy refractory to other measures:

- **clobazam**
  - ▷ start with 20–30mg PO at bedtime
  - ▷ if necessary, increase by 20–30mg every 5–7 days up to 60mg daily

- **clonazepam**
  - ▷ start with 500microgram–1mg PO at bedtime
  - ▷ if necessary, increase by 500microgram every 3–5 days up to 2–4mg, occasionally more
  - ▷ doses above 2mg can be divided, e.g. 2mg at bedtime and 1mg each morning.

Myoclonus

Treat the underlying cause if possible:

- drug-related, e.g. opioids, **gabapentin** or **pregabalin**: consider dose reduction or switching to an alternative
- metabolic disturbance, e.g. hyponatraemia, uraemia.

Otherwise, a benzodiazepine should be used, e.g.:

- **clonazepam** 500microgram PO at bedtime *or*
- **midazolam** 5mg SC stat and 10mg/24h CSCI in moribund patients.

If necessary, give p.r.n. doses and consider increasing the regular dose.

Alcohol withdrawal

Benzodiazepines reduce withdrawal symptoms, particularly seizures.[63] The choice is as for seizures (see above) with dose and route dependent on severity of withdrawal syndrome. **Gabapentin** (p.272) and barbiturates are alternatives if benzodiazepines are insufficient.[64,65]

Terminal agitation

Because this is often a feature of hyperactive delirium, antipsychotics are commonly used first-line to treat agitation in the imminently dying (Box A), either alone or in combination with a benzodiazepine.

When anxiety is prominent and there are no obvious features of a hyperactive delirium, **midazolam** can be used alone, at least initially. In various case series, the average effective dose was 15–60mg/24h (range 5–200mg/24h).[66–75]

Box A Drugs for agitation in the imminently dying

For more information, see respective drug monographs.

First-line drugs

Haloperidol (particularly if delirium present or likely)

- start with 1.5–5mg SC stat and q1h p.r.n. (0.5–2.5mg SC q1h in the elderly)
- maintain with 2.5–10mg/24h CSCI (see p.180).

If the patient fails to settle with 10mg/24h in combination with midazolam, consider levomepromazine.

Midazolam (particularly if anxiety is prominent)

- start with 2.5–5mg SC/IV stat and q1h p.r.n.
- if necessary, increase progressively to 10mg SC/IV q1h p.r.n.
- maintain with 10–60mg/24h CSCI/CIVI.

Although some centres titrate up to 200mg/24h,[30] it is probably better to add in an antipsychotic before increasing above 30mg/24h.

Second-line drugs

Levomepromazine

Note. Some centres use smaller doses first-line, e.g. 12.5mg SC stat and q1h p.r.n. (6.25mg in the elderly).

If given with the intention to reduce a patient's level of consciousness:

- start with 25mg SC stat and q1h p.r.n. (12.5mg in the elderly)
- if necessary, titrate dose according to response
- maintain with 50–200mg/24h CSCI. Alternatively, smaller doses can be given as an SC bolus at bedtime–b.d., and p.r.n. (see p.184).

continued

Box A Continued

Third-line drugs

Specialist use only. For patients who fail to respond to adequate titration and p.r.n. use of the above, e.g. midazolam together with levomepromazine.

Phenobarbital

Because of the irritant nature of the injection and the volume after dilution, stat doses are generally given IM/IV, followed by CSCI (see p.289).

Propofol

Necessitates the use of an IVI and a variable-rate syringe driver (see p.651).[31]

Other drugs

Successful use of dexmedetomidine and sodium oxybate has been reported (parenteral preparation; not UK).[76]

Sedation for massive haemorrhage

Readily available 'crisis' medication is often recommended (e.g. **midazolam**), but unless immediately available, it is of no use in the event of a massive haemorrhage: the patient would be left alone during those final seconds of consciousness while **midazolam** was obtained and administered and/or die before the medication could take effect. Sitting with the patient and holding their hand is the only realistic comfort measure.[77] However, if the patient does not die immediately and is distressed, give **midazolam** 5–10mg buccal/SC/IM/IV.

Breathlessness

Benzodiazepines do not relieve breathlessness *per se*[78] but anxiolytics do have a role when *anxiety* exacerbates breathlessness. Either a benzodiazepine or an SSRI is used depending on prognosis (see above). In an RCT (n=432), **buspirone** 20mg/24h was ineffective for breathlessness and anxiety in cancer.[79]

In the last days of life, for patients with distressing breathlessness at rest, the combined use of an opioid with a benzodiazepine is more effective than either alone.[80]

Restless legs syndrome

Clonazepam is sometimes used when first-line options (e.g. **gabapentin**, **pregabalin**, **ropinirole**, **rotigotine**) are ineffective or inappropriate (see p.272).[81–83]

- **clonazepam** 500microgram PO at bedtime, increased if necessary to 1mg at bedtime.[82]

Drug-induced movement disorders

Acute movement disorders

Reduce or stop the causal drug if possible (see p.739). Otherwise, switch to an alternative with a lower risk of extrapyramidal reactions, e.g. **metoclopramide** → **domperidone**, **haloperidol** → **quetiapine**. If symptoms are causing distress, give an antimuscarinic, e.g. **procyclidine**; if latter ineffective or contra-indicated, RCTs indicate a *possible* role for benzodiazepines in acute akathisia and dystonia:

- **clonazepam** 500microgram–1mg PO at bedtime, increased if necessary to 2.5mg at bedtime[84] *or*
- **diazepam** 5mg IV.[85]

Tardive dyskinesia

Reduce, stop or switch the causal drug as above and seek specialist advice. No symptomatic treatment has been found consistently effective. Small RCTs have found **clonazepam** (mean daily dose 5mg) of modest benefit.[86]

Neuropathic pain

Clonazepam is reported to improve both cancer-related and non-cancer neuropathic pain.[87–90] Anti-hyperalgesic properties have been demonstrated in healthy volunteers.[91] Its anxiolytic and muscle-relaxant properties and the ability to administer it SC in some countries (not UK), has led to its use in selected palliative care patients despite the absence of supporting RCTs.[92]

Spasticity and skeletal muscle spasm

Baclofen is used for the long-term management of spasticity secondary to neurological disorders.[93] **Tizanidine**, **dantrolene** and **botulinum toxin** are alternatives. Benzodiazepines are reserved for spasticity where the above are ineffective or where short-term SC/CSCI administration is desirable (see p.605). Although authorized for refractory spasticity in multiple sclerosis, the cost effectiveness of **cannabinoids** has been questioned (p.229).[94]

Baclofen is also used for pain due to skeletal muscle spasm, e.g. acute low back pain. Benzodiazepines are alternatives, particularly if the anticipated duration of use is ≤4 weeks or parenteral treatment is required:[95]

- **diazepam** 2–5mg PO at bedtime and p.r.n. *or*
- **midazolam** 10mg/24h CSCI.

Nausea and vomiting

Benzodiazepines are effective for chemotherapy-related[96–100] and postoperative[101] nausea and vomiting:

- **lorazepam** 500microgram SL p.r.n. *or*
- **midazolam** 10mg/24h CSCI.

Although a specific role for benzodiazepines in *anticipatory* nausea has been proposed, there is limited evidence to support this over and above their general anti-emetic effect. Alternative approaches to anticipatory nausea include relaxation, hypnosis and other psychological interventions.[102,103]

Pruritus

Benzodiazepines are not consistently effective for pruritus; their role, if any, is limited to patients refractory to other measures (see Chapter 26, p.757).[104–106]

Hiccup

Midazolam is reported to improve hiccup refractory to various other approaches (see Prokinetics, Table 2, p.26), e.g. **metoclopramide**, **haloperidol**, **chlorpromazine**, **simeticone**, **baclofen**, alone or in combination.[107]

Buccal and sublingual administration

Buccal **midazolam** in prefilled buccal syringes may be preferable when a rapid onset of action is required but parenteral injections are impractical, e.g. at home (see Pre-emptive prescribing in the community, p.671). However, it is significantly more expensive.

In some countries, specific SL **lorazepam** tablets are available, *but not in the UK*. Thus, in the UK, proprietary tablets which dissolve easily are often used SL, e.g. the generic tablets made by Genus (the manufacturer's name should be stipulated on the prescription to ensure this). However, although one pharmacokinetic study suggested more rapid absorption SL than PO, others have found no difference.[108–111] Thus, it is likely that the amount of **lorazepam** absorbed SL is variable and formulation-dependent. Tablets will not dissolve SL in patients with a dry mouth; dissolve the tablet in a few drops of warm water, draw up in a 1mL oral syringe and put between the patient's cheek and gum (i.e. given buccally).[112] Alternatively, **lorazepam** *injection* can be given bucally.

Subcutaneous and intravenous administration

Midazolam, **clonazepam** (not UK), **flunitrazepam** (not UK), and **lorazepam** can be given SC or by CSCI. **Diazepam** is strongly irritant and must not be given SC or CSCI. If given IV, the emulsion formulation of **diazepam** is preferred.

The SC and IV routes are generally considered equipotent.[113,114] Because IV acts more rapidly, the minimum interval between p.r.n. doses is typically 10min, compared with 1h if SC, allowing dose titration with smaller more frequent doses.

Clonazepam CSCI should be administered using non-PVC tubing (e.g. IVAC®); up to 50% of infused clonazepam is adsorbed onto PVC tubing.[115] However, because of the long halflife (20–60h) a bolus injection of **clonazepam** at bedtime can be given. **Lorazepam** may also adsorb to PVC, in addition, it is poorly soluble and can precipitate when diluted. The solubilizing agents polyethylene and propylene glycol and preservative benzyl alcohol may cause irritation by SC bolus injection. Accidental intra-arterial administration or extravasation close to an artery has been associated with thrombosis and gangrene. Thus, CSCI **lorazepam** is rarely used.

CSCI compatibility with other drugs:

Midazolam

There are 2-drug compatibility data for midazolam in WFI with **alfentanil**, **diamorphine**, **glycopyrronium**, **haloperidol**, **hydromorphone**, **hyoscine *butylbromide***, **hyoscine *hydrobromide***, **ketamine**, **levomepromazine**, **metoclopramide**, **morphine sulfate**, **octreotide** and **oxycodone**.

Concentration dependent *incompatibility* may occur with **cyclizine**. Midazolam is *incompatible* with **dexamethasone** and **ketorolac**.

Clonazepam

There are 2-drug compatibility data for clonazepam in WFI with **alfentanil**, **diamorphine**, **glycopyrronium**, **haloperidol**, **hyoscine *butylbromide***, **hyoscine *hydrobromide***, **morphine sulfate**, and **oxycodone**.

Concentration dependent *incompatibility* may occur with **cyclizine** or **dexamethasone**.

For more details and 3-drug compatibility data, see Appendix 3 (p.863). Compatibility charts for mixing **midazolam** or **clonazepam** (not UK) with other drugs in 0.9% saline, can be found in the extended appendix of the on-line *PCF* on *www.palliativedrugs.com*. Combinations including **flunitrazepam** (not UK) are included in the on-line syringe driver database.

Switching between benzodiazepines

Dose conversion is not straightforward and switching is best avoided when possible. However, when necessary, use the dose equivalence table to provide a starting point (Table 3). Equivalent doses are always approximations, and appropriate caution and monitoring is required. Particularly when switching at a high dose, it is prudent to use, say, a 30–40% lower dose than predicted and to ensure that both flumazenil and additional benzodiazepine doses are available for p.r.n. use.

Table 3 Approximate equivalent anxiolytic-sedative doses[116–119]

Drug	*Dose (PO)*	*Dose (SC)*
Alprazolam	0.25–0.5mg	
Chlordiazepoxide	12.5–15mg	
Clobazam	10mg	
Clonazepam	250–500microgram	250–500microgram (not UK)
Diazepam	5mg	
Flurazepam	7.5–15mg	
Loprazolam	0.5–1mg	
Lorazepam	500microgram	500microgram
Lormetazepam	0.5–1mg	
Midazolam	5mg (not UK)	2.5mg
Nitrazepam	5mg	
Oxazepam	10–15mg	
Temazepam	10mg	

Supply

Clobazam

All products are Schedule 4 part 1 **CD**.

Tablets 10mg, 28 days @ 20mg at bedtime = £6.50.

Oral suspension 5mg/5mL, 10mg/5mL, 28 days @ 20mg at bedtime = £177.

Clonazepam (generic)

All products are Schedule 4 part 1 **CD**.

Tablets 500microgram, 2mg, 28 days @ 500microgram at bedtime = £8.

Oral solution 500microgram/5mL, 2mg/5mL, 28 days @ 500microgram at bedtime = £65 and £25 respectively; *may contain ethanol and not suitable for children, do not further dilute with water.*
Oral drops 2.5mg/mL, 10mL = £68; unauthorized product, available for special order, price based on Specials tariff in the community (see Chapter 24, p.751).
Injection (concentrate) 1mg/mL, 1mL amp and 1mL amp of solvent = £6; unauthorized product, available to import via IDIS (see Chapter 24, p.751).

Diazepam (generic)
All products are Schedule 4 part 1 **CD**.
Tablets 2mg, 5mg, 10mg, 28 days @ 5mg at bedtime = £0.75.
Oral suspension 2mg/5mL, 5mg/5mL, 28 days @ 5mg at bedtime = £92.
Oral solution 2mg/5mL, 28 days @ 5mg at bedtime = £111.
Injection (oil-based solution) 5mg/mL, 2mL amp = £0.50; *excipients include ethanol and propylene glycol.*
Injection (emulsion) 5mg/mL, 2mL amp = £1.
Rectal solution 2mg/mL, 2.5mg or 5mg (1.25mL or 2.5mL tube) = £1.25; 4mg/mL, 10mg (2.5mL tube) = £1.50.

Midazolam
All products are Schedule 3 **CD**.
Midazolam (generic)
Injection 1mg/mL, 2mL amp, 5mL amp, 50mL vial = £0.50, £0.75 and £10 respectively;
High strength injections 2mg/mL, 5mL amp, and 50mL vial = £0.75 and £10 respectively; 5mg/mL, 2mL, 10mL amp = £0.75 and £2.50 respectively.

Many hospitals restrict the availability of high strength midazolam injections (2mg/mL and 5mg/mL) following fatal dose errors.[120]

Buccolam® (Shire Pharmaceuticals)
Oromucosal solution (prefilled oral syringe) 5mg/mL, 2.5mg, 5mg, 7.5mg and 10mg = £23.

Do not confuse Buccolam 5mg/mL with other *unauthorized* buccal liquids which are 10mg/mL (e.g. Epistatus®; Special products) and still available via special order (see Chapter 24, p.751).[121]

Lorazepam (generic)
All products are Schedule 4 part 1 **CD**.
Tablets 1mg, 2.5mg, 28 days @ 1mg b.d. = £4.25; *tablets manufactured by Genus are scored.*

Ativan
Injection 4mg/mL, 1mL amp = £0.50 ; *excipients include benzyl alcohol and propylene glycol.*

Zopiclone (generic)
Tablets 3.75mg, 7.5mg, 28 days @ 7.5mg at bedtime = £1.25.
Oral solution 3.75mg/5mL, 7.5mg/5mL, 28 days @ 7.5mg at bedtime = £79; unauthorized product, available for special order, price based on Specials tariff in the community (see Chapter 24, p.751).
Oral suspension 3.75mg/5mL, 7.5mg/5mL, 28 days @ 7.5mg at bedtime = £95; unauthorized product, available for special order, price based on Specials tariff in the community (see Chapter 24, p.751).

Zolpidem (generic)
Tablets 5mg, 10mg, 28 days @ 10mg at bedtime = £1.25.

1 Rudolph U and Knoflach F (2011) Beyond classical benzodiazepines: novel therapeutic potential of GABAA receptor subtypes. *Nature Reviews Drug Discovery*. **10**: 685–697.
2 Benke D *et al.* (2009) GABA A receptors as in vivo substrate for the anxiolytic action of valerenic acid, a major constituent of valerian root extracts. *Neuropharmacology*. **56**: 174–181.
3 Stahl SM (2013) Chapter 9: Anxiety disorders and anxiolytics. In: *Essential Psychopharmacology: Neuroscientific Basis and Practical Applications (4e)*. Cambridge University Press, USA. 388–419.
4 Rudolph U and Mohler H (2006) GABA-based therapeutic approaches: GABAA receptor subtype functions. *Current Opinion in Pharmacology*. **6**: 18–23.
5 Chiara DC *et al.* (2013) Specificity of intersubunit general anesthetic-binding sites in the transmembrane domain of the human alpha1beta3gamma2 gamma-aminobutyric acid type A (GABAA) receptor. *Journal of Biological Chemistry*. **288**: 19343–19357.

6 Yip GM *et al.* (2013) A propofol binding site on mammalian GABAA receptors identified by photolabeling. *Nature Chemical Biology*. **9**: 715–720.
7 Howard RJ *et al.* (2014) Seeking structural specificity: direct modulation of pentameric ligand-gated ion channels by alcohols and general anesthetics. *Pharmacological Reviews*. **66**: 396–412.
8 Carver CM and Reddy DS (2013) Neurosteroid interactions with synaptic and extrasynaptic GABA(A) receptors: regulation of subunit plasticity, phasic and tonic inhibition, and neuronal network excitability. *Psychopharmacology* **230**: 151–188.
9 Brickley SG and Mody I (2012) Extrasynaptic GABA(A) receptors: their function in the CNS and implications for disease. *Neuron*. **73**: 23–34.
10 Vinkers CH and Olivier B (2012) Mechanisms underlying tolerance after long-term benzodiazepine use: a future for subtype-selective GABA(A) receptor modulators? *Advances in Pharmacological Sciences*. **2012**: 416864.
11 Idzikowski C (2014) The pharmacology of human sleep, a work in progress? *Current Opinion in Pharmacology*. **14**: 90–96.
12 Dias BG *et al.* (2013) Towards new approaches to disorders of fear and anxiety. *Current Opinion in Neurobiology*. **23**: 346–352.
13 Jensen HS *et al.* (2014) Clobazam and its active metabolite N-desmethylclobazam display significantly greater affinities for alpha(2)- versus alpha(1)-GABA(A)-receptor complexes. *PLoS One*. **9**: e88456.
14 Ralvenius WT *et al.* (2016) The clobazam metabolite N-desmethyl clobazam is an alpha2 preferring benzodiazepine with an improved therapeutic window for antihyperalgesia. *Neuropharmacology*. **109**: 366–375.
15 Sankar R (2012) GABA(A) receptor physiology and its relationship to the mechanism of action of the 1,5-benzodiazepine clobazam. *CNS Drugs*. **26**: 229–244.
16 Mohler H (2011) The rise of a new GABA pharmacology. *Neuropharmacology*. **60**: 1042–1049.
17 Buscemi N *et al.* (2007) The efficacy and safety of drug treatments for chronic insomnia in adults: a meta-analysis of RCTs. *Journal of General Internal Medicine*. **22**: 1335–1350.
18 Hammer H *et al.* (2015) Functional characterization of the 1,5-benzodiazepine clobazam and its major active metabolite N-desmethylclobazam at human GABA(A) receptors expressed in Xenopus laevis oocytes. *PLoS One*. **10**: e0120239.
19 Olsen RW and Sieghart W (2008) International Union of Pharmacology. LXX. Subtypes of gamma-aminobutyric acid(A) receptors: classification on the basis of subunit composition, pharmacology, and function. Update. *Pharmacological Reviews*. **60**: 243–260.
20 Hill JL and Martinowich K (2016) Activity-dependent signaling: influence on plasticity in circuits controlling fear-related behavior. *Current Opinion in Neurobiology*. **36**: 59–65.
21 Riss J *et al.* (2008) Benzodiazepines in epilepsy: pharmacology and pharmacokinetics. *Acta Neurologica Scandinavica*. **118**: 69–86.
22 Drover DR (2004) Comparative pharmacokinetics and pharmacodynamics of short-acting hypnosedatives: zaleplon, zolpidem and zopiclone. *Clinical Pharmacokinetics*. **43**: 227–238.
23 Pecking M *et al.* (2002) Absolute bioavailability of midazolam after subcutaneous administration to healthy volunteers. *British Journal of Clinical Pharmacology*. **54**: 357–362.
24 Scott LJ *et al.* (2012) Oromucosal midazolam: a guide to its use in paediatric patients with prolonged acute convulsive seizures. *CNS Drugs*. **26**: 893–897.
25 Beigmohammadi MT *et al.* (2013) Pharmacokinetics alterations of midazolam infusion versus bolus administration in mechanically ventilated critically ill patients. *Iranian Journal of Pharmaceutical Research*. **12**: 483–488.
26 Park TW *et al.* (2015) Benzodiazepine prescribing patterns and deaths from drug overdose among US veterans receiving opioid analgesics: case-cohort study. *British Medical Journal*. **350**: h2698.
27 Ekstrom MP *et al.* (2014) Safety of benzodiazepines and opioids in very severe respiratory disease: national prospective study. *British Medical Journal*. **348**: g445.
28 NICE (2015) CKS. http://cks.nice.org.uk/benzodiazepine-and-z-drug-withdrawal
Update ref 28 to: NICE (2015) Benzodiazepine and Z-drug withdrawal. *Clinical Knowledge Summaries*. www.nice.org.uk
29 National Patient Safety Agency (2008) Reducing risk of overdose with midazolam injection in adults. *Rapid Response Report*. NPSA/2008/RRR2011: www.nrls.npsa.nhs.uk
30 Kotlinska-Lemieszek A (2013) Should midazolam drug-drug interactions be of concern to palliative care physicians? *Drug Safety*. **36**: 789–790.
31 Grad R (1995) Benzodiazepines for insomnia in community-dwelling elderly: a review of benefit and risk. *Journal of Family Practice*. **41**: 473–481.
32 Petrov ME *et al.* (2014) Benzodiazepine (BZD) use in community-dwelling older adults: Longitudinal associations with mobility, functioning, and pain. *Archives of Gerontology and Geriatrics*. **59**: 331–337.
33 Mancuso CE *et al.* (2004) Paradoxical reactions to benzodiazepines: literature review and treatment options. *Pharmacotherapy*. **24**: 1177–1185.
34 Weinbroum AA *et al.* (2001) The midazolam-induced paradox phenomenon is reversible by flumazenil. Epidemiology, patient characteristics and review of the literature. *European Journal of Anaesthesiology*. **18**: 789–797.
35 Saias T and Gallarda T (2008) Paradoxical aggressive reactions to benzodiazepine use: a review. *Encephale*. **34**: 330–336.
36 Dolder CR and Nelson MH (2008) Hypnosedative-induced complex behaviours : incidence, mechanisms and management. *CNS Drugs*. **22**: 1021–1036.
37 Pariente A *et al.* (2016) The benzodiazepine-dementia disorders link: current state of knowledge. *CNS Drugs*. **30**: 1–7.
38 Gray SL *et al.* (2016) Benzodiazepine use and risk of incident dementia or cognitive decline: prospective population based study. *British Medical Journal*. **352**: i90.
39 Billioti de Gage S *et al.* (2014) Benzodiazepine use and risk of Alzheimer's disease: case-control study. *British Medical Journal*. **349**: g5205.
40 Pottegard A *et al.* (2013) Use of benzodiazepines or benzodiazepine related drugs and the risk of cancer: a population-based case-control study. *British Journal of Clinical Pharmacology*. **75**: 1356–1364.
41 Weich S *et al.* (2014) Effect of anxiolytic and hypnotic drug prescriptions on mortality hazards: retrospective cohort study. *British Medical Journal*. **348**: g1996.
42 Kao CH *et al.* (2012) Relationship of zolpidem and cancer risk: a Taiwanese population-based cohort study. *Mayo Clinic Proceedings*. **87**: 430–436.
43 Kao CH *et al.* (2012) Benzodiazepine use possibly increases cancer risk: a population-based retrospective cohort study in Taiwan. *Journal of Clinical Psychiatry*. **73**: e555–560.
44 Horinek EL *et al.* (2009) Propylene glycol accumulation in critically ill patients receiving continuous intravenous lorazepam infusions. *Annals of Pharmacotherpy*. **43**: 1964–1971.
45 Baldwin DS *et al.* (2013) Benzodiazepines: risks and benefits. A reconsideration. *Journal of Psychopharmacology*. **27**: 967–971.
46 Mercadante S *et al.* (2015) Sleep disturbances in patients with advanced cancer in different palliative care settings. *Journal of Pain and Symptom Management*. **50**: 786–792.
47 Induru RR and Walsh D (2014) Cancer-related insomnia. *American Journal of Hospice and Palliative Care*. **31**: 777–785.

48 Renom-Guiteras A *et al.* (2014) Insomnia among patients with advanced disease during admission in a Palliative Care Unit: a prospective observational study on its frequency and association with psychological, physical and environmental factors. *BMC Palliative Care*. **13**: 40–52.

49 Morin CM *et al.* (1994) Nonpharmacological interventions for insomnia: a meta-analysis of treatment efficacy. *American Journal of Psychiatry*. **151**: 1172–1180.

50 Murtagh DR and Greenwood KM (1995) Identifying effective psychological treatments for insomnia: a meta-analysis. *Journal of Consulting and Clinical Psychology*. **63**: 79–89.

51 Smith MT *et al.* (2002) Comparative meta-analysis of pharmacotherapy and behavior therapy for persistent insomnia. *American Journal of Psychiatry*. **159**: 5–11.

52 Hugel H *et al.* (2004) The prevalence, key causes and management of insomnia in palliative care patients. *Journal of Pain and Symptom Management*. **27**: 316–321.

53 Kaneishi K *et al.* (2015) Single-dose subcutaneous benzodiazepines for insomnia in patients with advanced cancer. *Journal of Pain and Symptom Management*. **49**: e1–2.

54 Glass J *et al.* (2005) Sedative hypnotics in older people with insomnia: meta-analysis of risks and benefits. *British Medical Journal*. **331**: 1169.

55 Wang PS *et al.* (2001) Hazardous benzodiazepine regimens in the elderly: effects of half-life, dosage, and duration on risk of hip fracture. *American Journal of Psychiatry*. **158**: 892–898.

56 Wilson SJ *et al.* (2010) British Association for Psychopharmacology consensus statement on evidence-based treatment of insomnia, parasomnias and circadian rhythm disorders. *Journal of Psychopharmacology*. **24**: 1577–1601.

57 Bandelow B *et al.* (2007) Meta-analysis of randomized controlled comparisons of psychopharmacological and psychological treatments for anxiety disorders. *World Journal of Biological Psychiatry*. **8**: 175–187.

58 Baldwin (2011) Efficacy of drug treatments for generalised anxiety disorder: systemic review and meta-analysis. *British Medical Journal*. **342**: 1199.

59 Baldwin DS *et al.* (2014) Evidence-based pharmacological treatment of anxiety disorders, post-traumatic stress disorder and obsessive-compulsive disorder: a revision of the 2005 guidelines from the British Association for Psychopharmacology. *Journal of Psychopharmacology*. **28**: 403–439.

60 NICE (2012) The epilepsies: the diagnosis and management of the epilepsies in adults and children in primary and secondary care. *Clinical Guideline*. CG137 www.nice.org.uk

61 McKee HR and Abou-Khalil B (2015) Outpatient pharmacotherapy and modes of administration for acute repetitive and prolonged seizures. *CNS Drugs*. **29**: 55–70.

62 Remi C *et al.* (2016) Subcutaneous use of lacosamide. *Journal of Pain Symptom Management*. **51**: e2–4.

63 Amato L *et al.* (2010) Benzodiazepines for alcohol withdrawal. *Cochrane Database of Systematic Reviews*. **3**: CD05063. www.thecochranelibrary.com

64 Hammond CJ *et al.* (2015) Anticonvulsants for the treatment of alcohol withdrawal syndrome and alcohol use disorders. *CNS Drugs*. **29**: 293–311.

65 Martin K and Katz A (2016) The role of barbiturates for alcohol withdrawal syndrome. *Psychosomatics*. **57**: 341–347.

66 Ensor B and Cohen D (2012) Benchmarking benzodiazepines and antipsychotics in the last 24 hours of life. *New Zealand Medical Journal*. **125**: 19–30.

67 Alonso-Babarro A *et al.* (2010) At-home palliative sedation for end-of-life cancer patients. *Palliative Medicine*. **24**: 486–492.

68 Mercadante S *et al.* (2014) Palliative sedation in patients with advanced cancer followed at home: a prospective study. *Journal of Pain Symptom Management*. **47**: 860–866.

69 Muller-Busch HC *et al.* (2003) Sedation in palliative care - a critical analysis of 7 years experience. *BMC Palliative Care*. **2**: 2.

70 Goncalves F *et al.* (2016) A protocol for the control of agitation in palliative care. *American Journal of Hospice and Palliative Care*. **33**: 948–951.

71 Chater S *et al.* (1998) Sedation for intractable distress in the dying – a survey of experts. *Palliative Medicine*. **12**: 255–269.

72 Cowan JD and Walsh D (2001) Terminal sedation in palliative medicine – definition and review of the literature. *Supportive Care in Cancer*. **9**: 403–407.

73 Mercadante S *et al.* (2012) Palliative sedation in advanced cancer patients followed at home: a retrospective analysis. *Journal of Pain Symptom Management*. **43**: 1126–1130.

74 Cherny NI and Radbruch L (2009) European Association for Palliative Care (EAPC) recommended framework for the use of sedation in palliative care. *Palliative Medicine*. **23**: 581–593.

75 Radha Krishna LK *et al.* (2012) The use of midazolam and haloperidol in cancer patients at the end of life. *Singapore Medical Journal*. **53**: 62–66.

76 Ciais JF *et al.* (2015) Using sodium oxybate (gamma hydroxybutyric acid) for deep sedation at the end o flife. *Journal of Palliative Medicine*. **18**: 822.

77 Harris DG *et al.* (2011) The use of crisis medication in the management of terminal haemorrhage due to incurable cancer: a qualitative study. *Palliative Medicine*. **25**: 691–700.

78 Simon ST *et al.* (2016) Benzodiazepines for the relief of breathlessness in advanced malignant and non-malignant diseases in adults. *Cochrane Database of Systematic Reviews*. **10**: CD007354. www.thecochranelibrary.com

79 Peoples AR *et al.* (2016) Buspirone for management of dyspnea in cancer patients receiving chemotherapy: a randomized placebo-controlled URCC CCOP study. *Supportive Care in Cancer*. **24**: 1339–1347.

80 Navigante AH *et al.* (2006) Midazolam as adjunct therapy to morphine in the alleviation of severe dyspnea perception in patients with advanced cancer. *Journal of Pain and Symptom Management*. **31**: 38–47.

81 Mackie S and Winkelman JW (2015) Long-term treatment of restless legs syndrome (RLS): an approach to management of worsening symptoms, loss of efficacy, and augmentation. *CNS Drugs*. **29**: 351–357.

82 Aurora RN *et al.* (2012) The treatment of restless legs syndrome and periodic limb movement disorder in adults – an update for 2012: practice parameters with an evidence-based systematic review and meta-analyses: an American Academy of Sleep Medicine Clinical Practice Guideline. *Sleep*. **35**: 1039–1062.

83 Garcia-Borreguero D *et al.* (2012) European guidelines on management of restless legs syndrome: report of a joint task force by the European Federation of Neurological Societies, the European Neurological Society and the European Sleep Research Society. *European Journal of Neurology*. **19**: 1385–1396.

84 Lima AR *et al.* (2002) Benzodiazepines for neuroleptic-induced acute akathisia. *Cochrane Database of Systematic Reviews*. **1**: CD001950. www.thecochranelibrary.com

85 Gagrat D *et al.* (1978) Intravenous diazepam in the treatment of neuroleptic-induced acute dystonia and akathisia. *American Journal of Psychiatry*. **135**: 1232–1233.
86 Bhidayasiri R *et al.* (2013) Evidence-based guideline: treatment of tardive syndromes: report of the Guideline Development Subcommittee of the American Academy of Neurology. *Neurology*. **81**: 463–469.
87 Swerdlow M and Cundill J (1981) Anticonvulsant drugs used in the treatment of lancinating pain: a comparison. *Anaesthesia*. **36**: 1129–1132.
88 Bouckoms AJ and Litman RE (1985) Clonazepam in the treatment of neuralgic pain syndrome. *Psychosomatics*. **26**: 933–936.
89 Hugel H *et al.* (2003) Clonazepam as an adjuvant analgesic in patients with cancer-related neuropathic pain. *Journal of Pain and Symptom Management*. **26**: 1073–1074.
90 Bartusch S *et al.* (1996) Clonazepam for the treatment of lancinating phantom limb pain. *Clinical Journal of Pain*. **12**: 59–62.
91 Vuilleumier PH *et al.* (2013) Evaluation of anti-hyperalgesic and analgesic effects of two benzodiazepines in human experimental pain: a randomized placebo-controlled study. *PLoS One*. **8**: e43896.
92 Corrigan R *et al.* (2012) Clonazepam for neuropathic pain and fibromyalgia in adults. *Cochrane Database of Systematic Reviews*. **5**: CD009486. www.thecochranelibrary.com
93 Nair KP and Marsden J (2014) The management of spasticity in adults. *British Medical Journal*. **349**: g4737.
94 NICE (2014) Multiple sclerosis in adults: management. *Clinical Guideline*. CG186. www.nice.org.uk
95 Chou R and Huffman LH (2007) Medications for acute and chronic low back pain: a review of the evidence for an American Pain Society/American College of Physicians clinical practice guideline. *Annals of Internal Medicine*. **147**: 505–514.
96 Bishop J *et al.* (1984) Lorazepam: a randomized, double-blind, crossover study of a new antiemetic in patients receiving cytotoxic chemotherapy and prochlorperazine. *Journal of Clinical Oncology*. **2**: 691–695.
97 Tsavaris N *et al.* (1994) Comparison of ondansentron (GR 38032F) versus ondansentron plus alprazolam as antiemetic prophylaxis during cisplatin-containing chemotherapy. *American Journal of Clinical Oncology*. **17**: 516–521.
98 Bauduer F *et al.* (1999) Granisetron plus or minus alprazolam for emesis prevention in chemotherapy of lymphomas: a randomized multicenter trial. Granisetron Trialists Group. *Leukemia and Lymphoma*. **34**: 341–347.
99 Razavi D *et al.* (1993) Prevention of adjustment disorders and anticipatory nausea secondary to adjuvant chemotherapy: a double-blind, placebo-controlled study assessing the usefulness of alprazolam. *Journal of Clinical Oncology*. **11**: 1384–1390.
100 Malik IA *et al.* (1995) Clinical efficacy of lorazepam in prophylaxis of anticipatory, acute, and delayed nausea and vomiting induced by high doses of cisplatin. A prospective randomized trial. *American Journal of Clinical Oncology*. **18**: 170–175.
101 Di Florio T and Goucke CR (1999) The effect of midazolam on persistent postoperative nausea and vomiting. *Anaesthesia and Intensive Care*. **27**: 38–40.
102 Mandala M *et al.* (2005) Midazolam for acute emesis refractory to dexamethasone and granisetron after highly emetogenic chemotherapy: a phase II study. *Supportive Care in Cancer*. **13**: 375–380.
103 Aapro MS *et al.* (2005) Anticipatory nausea and vomiting. *Supportive Care in Cancer*. **13**: 117–121.
104 Hagermark O (1973) Influence of antihistamines, sedatives, and aspirin on experimental itch. *Acta Dermato-Venereologica*. **53**: 363–368.
105 Muston H *et al.* (1979) Differential effect of hypnotics and anxiolytics on itch and scratch. *Journal of Investigative Dermatology*. **72**: 283.
106 Ebata T *et al.* (1998) Effects of nitrazepam on nocturnal scratching in adults with atopic dermatitis: a double-blind placebo-controlled crossover study. *British Journal of Dermatology*. **138**: 631–634.
107 Calsina-Berna A *et al.* (2012) Treatment of chronic hiccups in cancer patients: a systematic review. *Journal of Palliative Medicine*. **15**: 1142–1150.
108 Caille G *et al.* (1983) Pharmacokinetics of two lorazepam formulations, oral and sublingual, after multiple doses. *Biopharmaceutics and Drug Disposition*. **4**: 31–42.
109 Greenblatt DJ *et al.* (1982) Pharmacokinetic comparison of sublingual lorazepam with intravenous, intramuscular, and oral lorazepam. *Journal of Pharmaceutical Sciences*. **71**: 248–252.
110 Spenard J *et al.* (1988) Placebo-controlled comparative study of the anxiolytic activity and of the pharmacokinetics of oral and sublingual lorazepam in generalized anxiety. *Biopharmaceutics and Drug Disposition*. **9**: 457–464.
111 Gram-Hansen P and Schultz A (1988) Plasma concentrations following oral and sublingual administration of lorazepam. *International Journal of Clinical Pharmacology Therapy and Toxicology*. **26**: 323–324.
112 Nicholson A (2007) Lorazepam. In: *Bulletin board*. Palliativedrugs.com Ltd. Available from: www.palliativedrugs.com
113 Nelson KA *et al.* (1997) A prospective within-patient crossover study of continuous intravenous and subcutaneous morphine for chronic cancer pain. *Journal of Pain and Symptom Management*. **13**: 262–267.
114 Moulin D *et al.* (1991) Comparisons of continuous subcutaneous and intravenous hydromorphone infusion for management of cancer pain. *Lancet*. **337**: 465–468.
115 Schneider JJ *et al.* (2006) Effect of tubing on loss of clonazepam administered by continuous subcutaneous infusion. *Journal of Pain and Symptom Management*. **31**: 563–567.
116 Whitwam JG *et al.* (1983) Comparison of midazolam and diazepam in doses of comparable potency during gastroscopy. *British Journal of Anaesthesia*. **55**: 773–777.
117 Cole SG *et al.* (1983) Midazolam, a new more potent benzodiazepine, compared with diazepam: a randomized, double-blind study of preendoscopic sedatives. *Gastrointestinal Endoscopy*. **29**: 219–222.
118 UK Medicines Information (2014) *What are the equivalent doses of oral benzodiazepines? Q&A* 293.3. www.evidence.nhs.uk
119 McEvoy GK. *American Hospital Formulary Service*. Maryland, USA: American Society of Health-System Pharmacists www.medicinescomplete.com (accessed April 2017).
120 Department of Health (2015) Never events list for 2015/2016. www.gov.uk
121 MHRA (2011) Buccal midazolam (Buccolam): new authroised medicine for paediatric use - care needed when transferring from unlicensed formulations. *Drug Safety Update*. **5**: www.mhra.gov.uk/safetyinformation

Updated August 2017

MELATONIN

Class: Melatonin-receptor agonist.

Indications: Primary insomnia in adults >55 years old, †secondary insomnia, †sleep phase disorders.

Pharmacology

Melatonin is a hormone released during darkness by the pineal gland. It is one of several mechanisms through which the central circadian clock synchronises the day/night cycle with numerous physiological rhythms (Figure 1).[1–4] Melatonin also modifies the circadian clock phase through a feedback loop.[5]

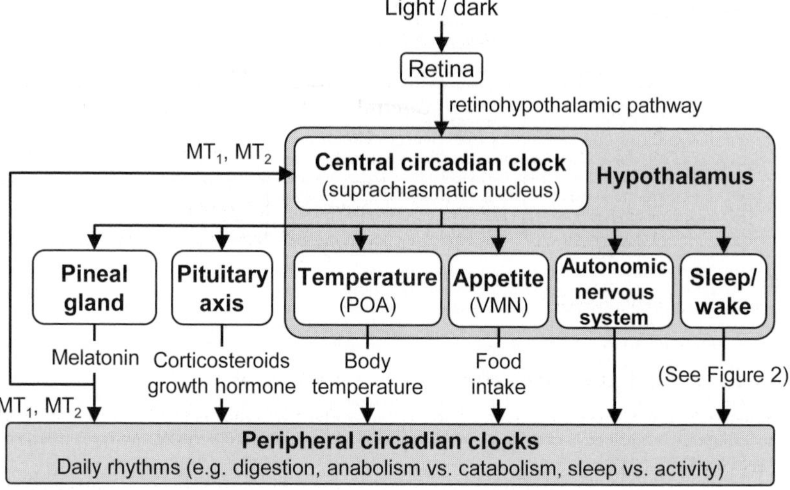

Figure 1 The circadian rhythm.[1–4,6]

Abbreviations: MT_1, MT_2 = melatonin receptor type 1, type 2; POA = pre-optic area; VMN = ventromedial nucleus.

Circadian dysregulation is implicated in sleep disorders,[6] neuropsychiatric disorders, e.g. delirium, dementia, depression, psychosis[7] and metabolic disorders (atherosclerosis, diabetes, hypertension, obesity).[4] The relative importance of melatonin to the above disorders is unclear.

Sleep disorders: Sleep is considered important for learning. New memories, temporarily held in the hippocampus, are reviewed during sleep when underlying patterns are identified, allowing these memories to be moved into long-term storage throughout the neocortex.

The drive to sleep arises from energy depletion, neuroplasticity (synaptic re-modelling) and immune activation. Sleep can be postponed by goal-directed and threat-related drives (Figure 2).[5,8] Melatonin acts indirectly, influencing the circadian clock phase, which alters the bias given to these competing drives.[9,11]

Melatonin and **ramelteon** (a melatonin receptor agonist; not UK) are less effective for insomnia than Z-drugs, reducing sleep latency (the delay in getting to sleep) by 5–10min compared to 20min.[12–14] Head-to-head comparisons found no clinically significant differences between melatonin doses[15] or formulations (immediate-release vs. m/r).[16,17] Reduced melatonin production does not predict response.[18]

Although authorized for primary insomnia (i.e. insomnia not due to a known physiological condition or drug), greater reductions in sleep latency, along with improvements in sleep quality and fragmentation, are seen in specific groups, e.g. patients with autism (40min),[19] intellectual disabilities (35min)[20,21] and those on haemodialysis (30min).[22]

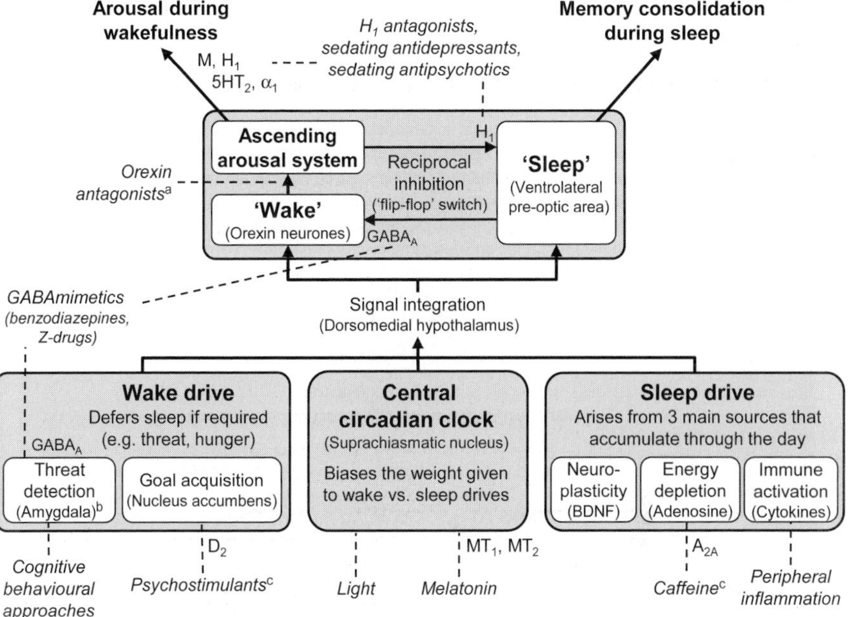

Figure 2 Putative targets of drugs influencing sleep and wakefulness.[3,5,6,8–11]

a. suvorexant (not UK), an orexin receptor antagonist, has recently been authorized for insomnia in the USA
b. the amygdala is implicated in both the hypnotic and anxiolytic properties of GABAergics (also see benzodiazepines, p.149)
c. wake drive is activated by dopamine and inhibited by adenosine. Thus, both dopamimetics (e.g. methylphenidate and modafinil, see p.225) and adenosine antagonists (e.g. caffeine) have wakefulness-promoting properties.

Abbreviations: BDNF = brain derived neurotrophic factor; the remainder refer to receptor types: M = muscarinic acetylcholine; A_{2A} = adenosine type 2_A; α_1 = α_1-adrenergic; D_2 = dopamine type 2; $GABA_A$ = gamma-aminobutyric acid type A; H_1 = histamine type 1; $5HT_2$ = 5-hydroxytriptamine (serotonin) type 2; MT_1, MT_2 = melatonin type 1, type 2.

Modest reductions in sleep latency (≤10min) are seen in patients with Parkinson's disease[23,24] and COPD.[25] A case series found melatonin improved self-reported sleep quality and reduced sleep fragmentation in 32 patients with advanced breast cancer.[26]

Melatonin is not consistently effective for sleep disturbance in dementia.[27]

Neuropsychiatric disorders: Neuropsychiatric disorders are commonly associated with altered sleep/wake rhythms.[28,29] Variations in circadian clock genes predispose to such disorders suggesting a possible *causal* role for circadian dysregulation.[6,30,31]

Melatonin reduces peri-operative anxiety.[32] In depression, melatonin is not consistently effective.[33] The association of depression with circadian dysregulation led to the development of the melatonergic antidepressant, **agomelatine**. Although it is as effective as other antidepressants,[34] the significance, if any, of its affinity for melatonin receptors is unclear because it is also a $5HT_{2C}$ antagonist (c.f. **mirtazapine**).

Melatonin is not consistently effective in preventing delirium in older patients admitted to hospital.[35,36] However, **ramelteon** (not UK), in a small study, reduced the incidence in patients ≥65 years admitted with a range of diagnoses including sepsis, stroke and fractures.[37]

Metabolic disturbance: Many organs use clocks to govern physiological rhythms. These peripheral clocks are synchronized to the central circadian clock by numerous signals (Figure 1).[1,2] If these

signals conflict, peripheral clocks can become desynchronized (e.g. glucose secretion coinciding with daytime food intake rather than overnight fasting, resulting in hyperglycaemia). In animal models, metabolic syndrome can be caused by altering peripheral clock genes or feeding times. Thus, melatonin and peripheral clock genes are of potential therapeutic interest in several common conditions including diabetes, obesity and atherosclerosis.[4]
Cancer and immunity: Some RCTs found a beneficial effect of melatonin on cancer survival.[38] Possible mechanisms include immunomodulation, reduced angiogenesis and direct anti-proliferative effects.[3,39,40] However, RCTs found no effect on cancer-related fatigue, anorexia or weight loss.[41,42]
Pain: Melatonin reduced pain from fibromyalgia, irritable bowel syndrome, chronic low back pain, migraine and cluster headaches.[43] Potential mechanisms include reduced inflammation, altered descending pain modulation, and inhibition of N-type calcium channels (compare with **gabapentin** and **pregabalin** (see p.272)).[43,44] However, sleep also improved which could indirectly lead to benefit.

Oral bio-availability of exogenous melatonin is limited by extensive first pass hepatic metabolism. It is 60% protein bound and is metabolised by CYP1A1 and 1A2 to an inactive sulphatoxy metabolite, which is renally excreted.
Bio-availability 15% (because of first-pass hepatic metabolism).
Time to peak plasma concentration 3h (with food), 45min (empty stomach).
Plasma halflife 3.5–4h.

Cautions

Auto-immune disease (although there are no data in humans, melatonin can cause deleterious immunostimulation in animals with auto-immunity); hepatic impairment (reduced clearance).

Drug interactions

Melatonin may enhance the sedative effect of sedative drugs.

Fluvoxamine (a potent CYP1A2 inhibitor) can increase melatonin plasma concentrations 12-fold and concurrent administration should be avoided. Caution should be taken with other CYP1A2 inhibitors, (e.g. **ciprofloxacin**, see Chapter 19, Table 8, p.725). Melatonin can increase or decrease INR (consider increased monitoring).

Undesirable effects

No undesirable effects occurred in >1% for melatonin m/r (Circadin®). In RCTs and open-label follow-up, rates of undesirable effects are comparable to placebo.[18]
Uncommon (<1%, >0.1%): Restlessness, irritability, abnormal dreams, dizziness, somnolence, constipation, dry mouth, hyperbilirubinaemia.
Rare (<0.1%, >0.01%): Laboratory changes (leukopenia, thrombocytopenia, altered LFTs), rashes, mood alteration, vertigo, blurred vision, nausea and vomiting.

Dose and use

Sleep disturbance is common in palliative care. Management involves the correction of underlying causes (sleep-disturbing symptoms, fears, concurrent depression, delirium), non-drug approaches (e.g. relaxation techniques), as well as sedative drugs.[45–48] The efficacy of both conventional hypnotics (p.149) and melatonin is modest.

The place of melatonin for sleep problems in palliative care remains uncertain. It could be considered when other options have failed or lack of tolerability limits the use of conventional hypnotics. The marketing authorization is restricted to adults ≥55 years old, reflecting the age of trial participants:

- melatonin m/r 2mg PO 1–2h before bedtime.

Supply

Circadin® (Flynn)
Tablets m/r 2mg, 28 days @ 2mg at night = £15.

1 Slominski RM *et al.* (2012) Melatonin membrane receptors in peripheral tissues: distribution and functions. *Molecular and Cellular Endocrinology.* **351**: 152–166.
2 Saper CB (2013) The central circadian timing system. *Current Opinion in Neurobiology.* **23**: 747–751.
3 Westermann J *et al.* (2015) System consolidation during sleep - a common principle underlying psychological and immunological memory formation. *Trends in Neurosciences.* **38**: 585–597.
4 Brown SA (2016) Circadian metabolism: from mechanisms to metabolomics and medicine. *Trends Endocrinology and Metabolism.* **27**: 415–426.
5 Rihel J and Schier AF (2013) Sites of action of sleep and wake drugs: insights from model organisms. *Current Opinion in Neurobiology.* **23**: 831–840.
6 Mattis J and Sehgal A (2016) Circadian rhythms, sleep, and disorders of aging. *Trends in Endocrinology and Metabolism.* **27**: 192–203.
7 Landgraf D *et al.* (2014) Circadian clock and stress interactions in the molecular biology of psychiatric disorders. *Current Psychiatry Reports.* **16**: 483.
8 Porkka-Heiskanen T (2013) Sleep homeostasis. *Current Opinion in Neurobiology.* **23**: 799–805.
9 Idzikowski C (2014) The pharmacology of human sleep, a work in progress? *Current Opinion in Pharmacology.* **14**: 90–96.
10 Kuriyama A and Tabata H (2016) Suvorexant for the treatment of primary insomnia: a systematic review and meta-analysis. *Sleep Medicine Reviews.* (in press).
11 Lazarus M *et al.* (2013) Role of the basal ganglia in the control of sleep and wakefulness. *Current Opinion in Neurobiology.* **23**: 780–785.
12 Ferracioli-Oda E *et al.* (2013) Meta-analysis: melatonin for the treatment of primary sleep disorders. *PLoS One.* **8**: e63773.
13 Kuriyama A *et al.* (2014) Ramelteon for the treatment of insomnia in adults: a systematic review and meta-analysis. *Sleep Medicine.* **15**: 385–392.
14 Huedo-Medina TB *et al.* (2012) Effectiveness of non-benzodiazepine hypnotics in treatment of adult insomnia: meta-analysis of data submitted to the Food and Drug Administration. *British Medical Journal.* **345**: e8343.
15 Zhdanova IV *et al.* (2001) Melatonin treatment for age-related insomnia. *Journal of Clinical Endocrinology and Metabolism.* **86**: 4727–4730.
16 Haimov I *et al.* (1995) Melatonin replacement therapy of elderly insomniacs. *Sleep.* **18**: 598–603.
17 Hughes RJ *et al.* (1998) The role of melatonin and circadian phase in age-related sleep-maintenance insomnia: assessment in a clinical trial of melatonin replacement. *Sleep.* **21**: 52–68.
18 Wade AG *et al.* (2010) Nightly treatment of primary insomnia with prolonged release melatonin for 6 months: a randomized placebo controlled trial on age and endogenous melatonin as predictors of efficacy and safety. *BMC Medicine.* **8**: 51.
19 Rossignol DA and Frye RE (2011) Melatonin in autism spectrum disorders: a systematic review and meta-analysis. *Developmental Medicine and Child Neurology.* **53**: 783–792.
20 Gringras P *et al.* (2012) Melatonin for sleep problems in children with neurodevelopmental disorders: randomised double masked placebo controlled trial. *British Medical Journal.* **345**: e6664.
21 Braam W *et al.* (2009) Exogenous melatonin for sleep problems in individuals with intellectual disability: a meta-analysis. *Developmental Medicine and Child Neurology.* **51**: 340–349.
22 Koch BC *et al.* (2009) The effects of melatonin on sleep-wake rhythm of daytime haemodialysis patients: a randomized, placebo-controlled, cross-over study (EMSCAP study). *British Journal of Clinical Pharmacology.* **67**: 68–75.
23 Dowling GA *et al.* (2005) Melatonin for sleep disturbances in Parkinson's disease. *Sleep Medicine.* **6**: 459–466.
24 Medeiros CA *et al.* (2007) Effect of exogenous melatonin on sleep and motor dysfunction in Parkinson's disease. A randomized, double blind, placebo-controlled study. *Journal of Neurology.* **254**: 459–464.
25 Nunes DM *et al.* (2008) Effect of melatonin administration on subjective sleep quality in chronic obstructive pulmonary disease. *Brazilian Journal of Medical and Biological Research.* **41**: 926–931.
26 Innominato PF *et al.* (2016) The effect of melatonin on sleep and quality of life in patients with advanced breast cancer. *Supportive Care in Cancer.* **24**: 1097–1105.
27 McCleery J *et al.* (2014) Pharmacotherapies for sleep disturbances in Alzheimer's disease. *Cochrane Database of Systematic Reviews.* **3**: CD009178. www.thecochranelibrary.com
28 Fitzgerald JM *et al.* (2013) Delirium: a disturbance of circadian integrity? *Medical Hypotheses.* **81**: 568–576.
29 Yoshitaka S *et al.* (2013) Perioperative plasma melatonin concentration in postoperative critically ill patients: its association with delirium. *Journal of Critical Care.* **28**: 236–242.
30 Jagannath A *et al.* (2013) Sleep and circadian rhythm disruption in neuropsychiatric illness. *Current Opinion in Neurobiology.* **23**: 888–894.
31 Comai S and Gobbi G (2014) Unveiling the role of melatonin MT2 receptors in sleep, anxiety and other neuropsychiatric diseases: a novel target in psychopharmacology. *Journal Psychiatry and Neuroscience.* **39**: 6–21.
32 Hansen MV *et al.* (2015) Melatonin for pre- and postoperative anxiety in adults. *Cochrane Database of Systematic Reviews.* **4**: CD009861. www.thecochranelibrary.com
33 Hansen MV *et al.* (2014) The therapeutic or prophylactic effect of exogenous melatonin against depression and depressive symptoms: a systematic review and meta-analysis. *European Neuropsychopharmacology.* **24**: 1719–1728.
34 Guaiana G *et al.* (2013) Agomelatine versus other antidepressive agents for major depression. *Cochrane Database of Systematic Reviews.* **12**: CD008851. www.thecochranelibrary.com
35 Walker CK and Gales MA (2016) Melatonin receptor agonists for delirium prevention. *Annals of Pharmacotherapy.* **51**: 72–78.
36 Siddiqi N *et al.* (2016) Interventions for preventing delirium in hospitalised non-ICU patients. *Cochrane Database of Systematic Reviews.* **3**: CD005563. www.thecochranelibrary.com
37 Hatta K *et al.* (2014) Preventive effects of ramelteon on delirium: a randomized placebo-controlled trial. *JAMA Psychiatry.* **71**: 397–403.
38 Seely D *et al.* (2012) Melatonin as adjuvant cancer care with and without chemotherapy: a systematic review and meta-analysis of randomized trials. *Integrative Cancer Therapies.* **11**: 293–303.
39 Lin GJ *et al.* (2013) Modulation by melatonin of the pathogenesis of inflammatory autoimmune diseases. *International Journal of Molecular Sciences.* **14**: 11742–11766.
40 Di Bella G *et al.* (2013) Melatonin anticancer effects: review. *International Journal of Molecular Sciences.* **14**: 2410–2430.
41 Lund Rasmussen C *et al.* (2015) Effects of melatonin on physical fatigue and other symptoms in patients with advanced cancer receiving palliative care: A double-blind placebo-controlled crossover trial. *Cancer.* **121**: 3727–3736.
42 Del Fabbro E *et al.* (2013) Effects of melatonin on appetite and other symptoms in patients with advanced cancer and cachexia: a double-blind placebo-controlled trial. *Journal of Clinical Oncology.* **31**: 1271–1276.
43 Danilov A and Kurganova J (2016) Melatonin in chronic pain syndromes. *Pain and Therapy.* **5**: 1–17.
44 Chen WW *et al.* (2016) Pain control by melatonin: Physiological and pharmacological effects. *Experimental and Therapeutics Medicine.* **12**: 1963–1968.
45 Davis MP *et al.* (2014) Insomnia in patients with advanced cancer. *American Journal of Hospice and Palliative Care.* **31**: 365–373.

46 Induru RR and Walsh D (2014) Cancer-related insomnia. *American Journal of Hospice and Palliative Care.* **31**: 777–785.
47 Renom-Guiteras A *et al.* (2014) Insomnia among patients with advanced disease during admission in a Palliative Care Unit: a prospective observational study on its frequency and association with psychological, physical and environmental factors. *BMC Palliative Care.* **13**: 40.
48 Yennurajalingam S *et al.* (2016) Association between daytime activity, fatigue, sleep, anxiety, depression, and symptom burden in advanced cancer patients: a preliminary report. *Journal of Palliative Medicine.* **19**: 849–856.

Updated August 2017

ANTIPSYCHOTICS

Indications: Authorized indications vary between products; consult SPC for details. Psychosis, mania and bipolar disorders, intractable hiccup, †nausea and vomiting, †treatment-resistant anxiety and/or depression, †delirium, †terminal agitation.

Pharmacology

Antipsychotics act predominantly through D_2 receptor antagonism, countering the symptoms of dopamine excess in delirium (Figure 1), psychosis (Figure 2), and nausea related to stimulation of the area postrema. However, *unopposed* D_2 antagonism causes *dopamine depletion* symptoms in other pathways (e.g. the extrapyramidal system) and may worsen 'negative' psychotic symptoms (e.g. apathy, anhedonia).[1,2] Thus the development of antipsychotics has been driven, with partial success, by attempts to reduce extrapyramidal symptoms and improve efficacy for 'negative' psychotic symptoms.

Serotonin receptors and D_2 partial agonists

$5HT_{2A}$ receptors *inhibit*, and $5HT_{1A}$ receptors *stimulate*, dopaminergic neurones. Thus, both $5HT_{2A}$ antagonists and $5HT_{1A}$ partial agonists increase activity in underactive dopaminergic pathways, countering the extrapyramidal impact of D_2 antagonism and improving 'negative' symptoms.[2]

Other antipsychotics (e.g. **aripiprazole**) use *D_2 partial agonism* to reduce the problem of unopposed D_2 antagonism. Such drugs displace dopamine from, but only partially activate, the D_2 receptor. Thus they reduce overall transmission in overactive pathways. However, in *underactive* pathways, the partial D_2 receptor activation is sufficient to *increase* overall transmission. Thus, a D_2 partial agonist antipsychotic can potentially improve both 'positive' (e.g. hallucinations, delusions) and 'negative' symptoms and limit undesirable extrapyramidal effects.[2,3]

Other actions

Some antipsychotics have additional actions that alleviate non-dopaminergic symptoms (e.g. depression, anxiety; see Table 1).[2,4] The beneficial effect of **olanzapine** on cancer-related anorexia may relate to $5HT_{2C}$ and H_1 antagonism.[5] Muscarinic antagonism reduces the risk of acute extrapyramidal symptoms because cholinergic neurones affect dopamine release in the nigrostriatal pathway.[6] Differences in receptor profile result in varying anti-emetic properties (see p.235). Some antipsychotics antagonize sigma receptors (implicated in the pathophysiology of neuropathic and opioid poorly responsive pain).[7,8] Dopamine also modulates pain pathways.[9]

Classification

Antipsychotic classification reflects the varying propensity to cause extrapyramidal symptoms and treat 'negative' psychotic symptoms (in descending order):[2]

- typical ('first generation'):
  - less sedating (butyrophenones; highest extrapyramidal risk), e.g. **haloperidol**
  - more sedating (phenothiazines), e.g. **levomepromazine**, **chlorpromazine**, **prochlorperazine**, **perphenazine**
- atypical ('second generation'):
  - less sedating, e.g. **risperidone**
  - more sedating (lowest extrapyramidal risk), e.g. **olanzapine**, **quetiapine**.

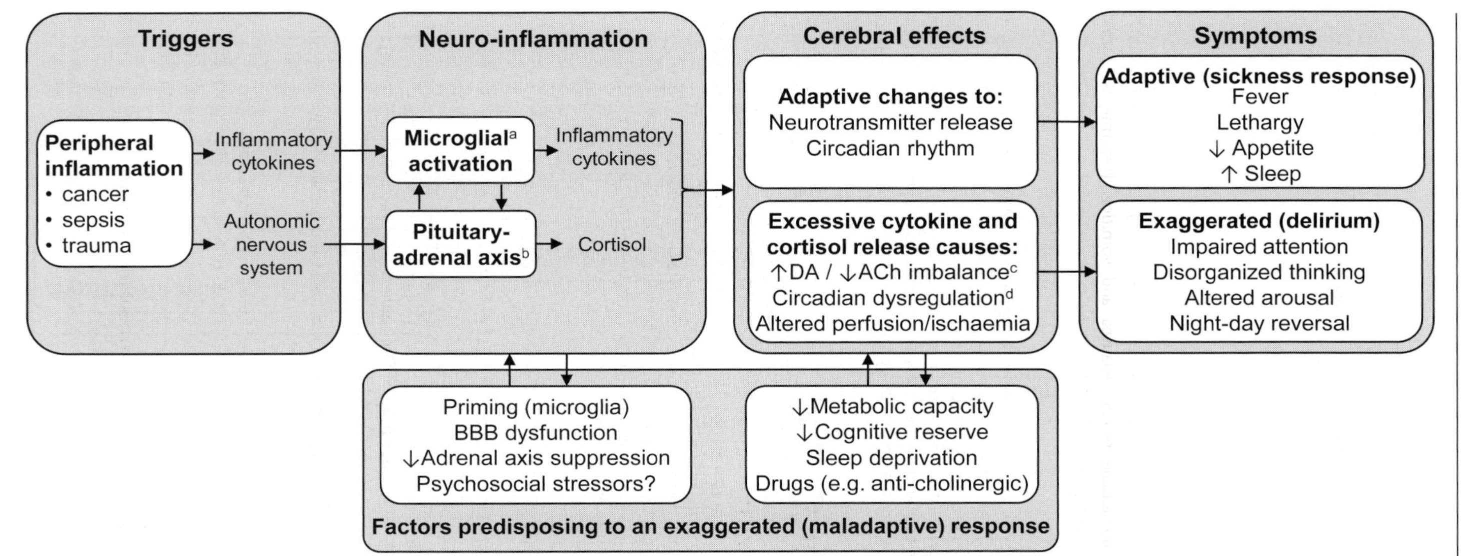

Figure 1 Delirium is a maladaptive exaggeration of symptoms which aid recovery from acute illnesses.[14–18]

Abbreviations: ACh, acetylcholine; BBB, blood brain barrier; COMT, catechol-O-methyl transferase; DA, dopamine.

a. microglia are CNS resident macrophages. On detecting inflammatory cytokines, they release similar cytokines, promoting adaptive responses to sickness. When excessive, the response becomes maladaptive, i.e. delirium. Further, once activated, they respond more strongly to ongoing stimuli, thereby lowering the delirium threshold. They are implicated in other neurodegenerative diseases, e.g. dementia, which may partly explain why delirium and dementia predispose to each other

b. the pituitary-adrenal axis, via cortisol, protects against excessive peripheral inflammation. Conversely, in the CNS, cortisol increases microglial activation, synaptic dysfunction and cerebral hypoperfusion. Thus, impaired negative feedback of the pituitary-adrenal axis, which is common in older age, lowers the delirium threshold

c. in addition to cytokines and cortisol, synaptic function is also changed by hypoperfusion/hypoxia which results in ↑DA and ↓ACh; these further exacerbate neuroinflammation and thereby delirium. This may explain why antipsychotics prevent, and antimuscarinic drugs predispose to, delirium

d. ↓melatonin disinhibits dopaminergic neurones.

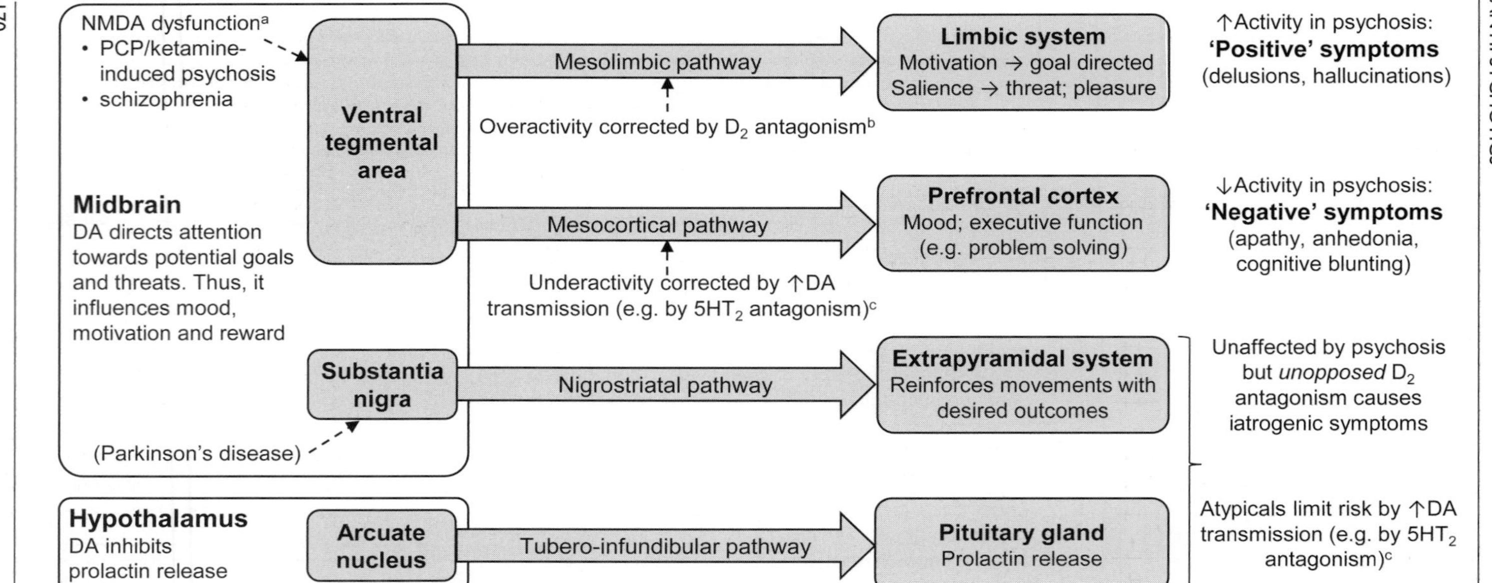

Figure 2 Dopaminergic pathways and the pathophysiology of psychosis.[1,2,6,19,20]

Abbreviations: DA = dopamine; D_2 = dopamine receptor type 2; $5HT_2$ = 5-hydroxytryptamine (serotonin) receptor type 2.

a. NMDA hypofunction causes mesolimbic overactivity and mesocortical underactivity. Schizophrenia may be caused by a localized developmental abnormality in NMDA transmission

b. dopamine overactivity causes stimuli to become associated with an exaggerated sense of relevance (the 'salience hypothesis'). Delusions are an attempt to understand this exaggerated significance by interpreting it as threatening (e.g. paranoid delusions) or pleasurable (e.g. grandiose delusions)

c. *atypical* antipsychotics attempt to reduce the impact of unopposed D_2 antagonism by stimulating underactive dopamine pathways, e.g. via $5HT_{2A}$ antagonism, $5HT_{1A}$ partial agonism and D_2 partial agonism (see text).

Table 1 Beneficial actions and receptor affinities for selected antipsychotics[2,4,7,21,22]

Action[a]	*Reduced 'positive' symptoms*	*Reduced extrapyramidal and 'negative' symptoms*		*Antidepressant effect*[b]			*Anxiolytic effect*[c]			*Analgesia*[d]*?*
Receptor	D_2	$5HT_{1A}$	$5HT_{2A}$	$5HT_{2C}$	$5HT_3$	a_2	α_1	H_1	*M*	*Sigma*
Aripiprazole	+++PA	++PA	++	++	–	++	++	++	–	
Chlorpromazine	++	–	+++	++	–	+	+++	+++	++	–
Clozapine	+	++PA	+++	++	+	+	+++	+++	+++	–
Flupentixol	+++	–	+	+	–	–		+++		
Haloperidol	+++	–	+	–	–	–	+++	–	–	+++
Levomepromazine	++		+++			+	+++	+++	++	
Olanzapine	++	–	+++	++	+	+	++	+++	++	–
Perphenazine	+++	+	+++	+		+	+++	+++	–	++
Prochlorperazine	++	–	++	+	–	–	++	++	+	
Quetiapine	+	+PA	+	+	–	++	+++	+++	–	+
Risperidone	+++	+	+++	++	–	+++	+++	++	–	–

Affinity: +++ high, ++ moderate, + low, – negligible or none; blank = no data.

PA = partial agonist; D = dopamine receptor; 5HT = serotonin receptor; α = adrenoceptor; H = histamine receptor; M = muscarinic acetylcholine receptor

a. anti-emetic actions are associated with several receptors, including D_2, $5HT_2$, $5HT_3$, H_1 and M (also see p.235)

b. other actions implicated in an antidepressant effect include $5HT_{1A}$ and D_2 partial agonism, $5HT_7$ antagonism (quetiapine) and monoamine reuptake inhibition (norquetiapine, an active metabolite of quetiapine)

c. $5HT_{1A}$ partial agonism is also implicated in the anxiolytic effect of some antipsychotics

d. clinical significance unknown.

Although atypical antipsychotics reduce dopamine depletion symptoms, none completely avoids them.[10] Further, non-dopaminergic actions themselves cause undesirable effects (Table 3). Thus, although both desirable and undesirable effects vary, the overall tolerability of antipsychotics is comparable.[10,11] In an RCT, although extrapyramidal effects accounted for more discontinuations of **perphenazine** compared with several atypicals (8% vs. 2–4%), overall discontinuation rates for undesirable effects or lack of efficacy were comparable.[10] Further, all treatment groups experienced some degree of involuntary movement (13–17%), akathisia (5–9%) or extrapyramidal signs (4–8%).

Pharmacokinetics and pharmacogenetics

Pharmacokinetic details of selected antipsychotics are summarized in Table 2. Dopamine and serotonin receptor polymorphisms affect both efficacy and the risk of undesirable effects (e.g. tardive dyskinesia and weight gain).[12,13]

Table 2 Pharmacokinetic details for selected antipsychotics[23,24]

	Oral bio-availability (%)	*Time to peak plasma concentration*	*Halflife (h)*	*Metabolism (predominant P450 isoenzyme)*
Aripiprazole	85–90	3–5h (PO)	75–145[a]	CYP2D6, CYP3A4
Chlorpromazine	10–25	2–4h (PO)	30	CYP2D6
Clozapine	50–60	2h	12	CYP1A2, CYP3A4
Haloperidol	40–85	2–6h (PO) 20–30min (IM)	12–38	CYP2D6, CYP3A4
Levomepromazine	20–50	2–3h (PO) 30–90min (SC)	15–30	CYP3A4[b]
Olanzapine	60	5–8h	34[c] (52[d])	CYP1A2, CYP2D6
Prochlorperazine	6 14 (buccal)	4h (PO) 8h (buccal; 4h with multiple doses)	14–21	Multiple
Quetiapine	≥75	1.5h	7[e] (10–14[d]) (12[b])	CYP3A4
Risperidone	70	1–2h	24[f,g]	CYP2D6, CYP3A4[h]

a. 75h in ultra-rapid metabolizers; 145h in slow metabolizers
b. active metabolite(s)
c. unaffected by hepatic or renal impairment
d. in the elderly
e. clearance reduced by both renal and hepatic impairment
f. for risperidone + active 9-hydroxy metabolite
g. clearance reduced by renal impairment
h. activity of 9-hydroxyrisperidone, the predominant CYP2D6 metabolite, is comparable to risperidone; thus overall clinical effect is not altered by CYP2D6 polymorphisms or inhibitors.

Cautions

Stroke risk and mortality

Meta-analysis of RCTs in the elderly with dementia indicates that the risk of stroke and death with antipsychotics is ≤2 and ≤1.6 times higher compared with placebo, respectively.[25] The mechanism of this association is not known. The risk is greatest within the first month of starting treatment, and with higher doses. It is a class effect.[25–27] An association with myocardial infarction is also reported; this may be due to confounding life-style factors and co-morbidities, rather than a causal association.[28]

Epilepsy

Similar to many other psychotropic medications, antipsychotics cause a dose-dependent reduction in seizure threshold. **Quetiapine**, **olanzapine** and **clozapine** carry a higher risk than other antipsychotics.[29] Use an alternative (e.g. **haloperidol** or **risperidone**) at the lowest effective dose. Avoid depot formulations; they cannot be withdrawn quickly if problems occur.

Parkinsonism and Parkinson's disease

All antipsychotics, through D_2 antagonism, can cause or exacerbate parkinsonism. The risk is lowest with **clozapine** and **quetiapine**. In patients with parkinsonism, alternatives to antipsychotics should be used where possible, e.g. for agitation, consider **trazodone** (see p.223) or a benzodiazepine, for nausea and vomiting consider:

- **domperidone**
- **ondansetron**
- **hyoscine *hydrobromide***, but may cause delirium.

Nonetheless, at the end of life, despite being D_2 antagonists, it may be necessary to prescribe small doses of **levomepromazine** or **quetiapine** if all else fails.

Where delirium or psychotic symptoms occur in the context of Parkinson's disease or Lewy Body dementia, look for potentially reversible causes of delirium, e.g. urinary retention, faecal impaction, sepsis.

If symptoms persist, seek specialist advice. Options include:

- trial reduction of antiparkinsonian medication
- **quetiapine** PO 12.5–25mg/24h (well tolerated, but not consistently effective in RCTs)
- **clozapine** (effective in RCTs, but specialist monitoring required).[30,31]

Cardiovascular disease

All antipsychotics have the potential to predispose to arrhythmias through muscarinic antagonism and QT prolongation. A direct known link between prolonged QT and *torsade de pointes* exists for **haloperidol** and **levomepromazine**; for others the relationship is either possible, or conditional on the presence of other factors, e.g. high doses, drug interactions, hypokalaemia, hypomagnesaemia (see Chapter 20, p.731).

Renal and hepatic impairment

Antipsychotics differ in their potential to cause toxicity when renal or hepatic function is impaired. See Chapter 17, p.691, and Chapter 18, p.703, for general information on the choice of antipsychotic and use in ESRF and severe hepatic impairment, respectively.

Drug interactions

Several pharmacodynamic interactions (additive sedation, hypotension, reduced effect of antiparkinsonian drugs) can be predicted from the receptor profile of antipsychotics (see Table 1).

Antipsychotics are one of several classes of drugs which can prolong the QT interval, and at least theoretically increase the risk of cardiac tachyarrthymias, including potentially fatal *torsade de pointes*. Generally, concurrent prescribing of two drugs which can significantly prolong the QT interval should be avoided (see Chapter 20, p.731).

Potentially serious interactions may result from the concurrent use of antipsychotics with potent inhibitors or inducers of the relevant CYP450 enzyme, resulting in undesirable effects or failure of treatment. See the individual drug monographs and Chapter 19, Table 8, p.725 for more details.

Severe neurotoxic or extrapyramidal adverse effects have been reported with **lithium** and several antipsychotics including **haloperidol, levomepromazine, prochlorperazine or quetiapine** but appear to be uncommon and the mechanism unexplained.

Undesirable effects

These are summarized in Table 3.

Clozapine may be associated with a small increased risk of leukaemia. Animal studies suggest other antipsychotics may also have carcinogenic properties. However, human trials and observational studies have found either no difference or a small *protective* effect on the risk of cancer.[32]

Severe bone pain has been reported with **aripiprazole**.[33]

Acute dopamine depletion syndrome (neuroleptic/antipsychotic malignant syndrome)

Acute dopamine depletion syndrome (Box A) is a potentially life-threatening idiosyncratic reaction to:

- starting, or increasing the dose of, dopamine antagonists, e.g. antipsychotics, **metoclopramide** *or*
- abruptly stopping anti-parkinsonian dopamimetics, e.g. **L-dopa**, dopamine agonists.

The incidence amongst those starting antipsychotics is 0.01%. The higher incidence (<3%) in older series may reflect higher doses, higher risk with 'typical' antipsychotics and/or changes in diagnostic criteria.[38,39] The incidence with dopamimetic withdrawal is unknown.

Table 3 Relative frequency and putative mechanisms of undesirable effects[2,26,27,29,34–37]

Undesirable effect		*Mechanism*	*Relative frequency with selected antipsychotics*							
			aripiprazole	*clozapine*	*haloperidol*	*levomepromazine*	*olanzapine*	*prochlorperazine*	*quetiapine*	*risperidone*
Extrapyramidal		D_2 antagonism	+/++	+	++++	+++	+/++	+++	+	++
Cardiovascular	Postural hypotension	$\alpha 1$-adrenergic antagonism	++	+++	++	+++	++	+++	+++	++
	QT prolongation (see text)	K channel blockade								
	Stroke; mortality[b]	unknown	++	++	++[b]	++[b]	++	++	++[b]	++
	Venous thrombo-embolism	unknown	++	+++	++	+++	+++	+++	++	++
Metabolic	Hyperprolactinaemia (amenorrhoea, gynaecomastia, sexual dysfunction)	D_2 antagonism	+	+	++++	+++	++	+++	+	+++
	Weight gain, dyslipidaemia, type 2 diabetes mellitus	H_1, $5HT_{2C}$ and M_3 antagonism[a]	++	++++	+	++	++++	++	+++	++
Miscellaneous	Agranulocytosis	Immune mediated?	+	++++	+	+	+	+	+	+
	Dry mouth, constipation	M_1 and M_3 antagonism	+	+++	+	++++	++	+++	++	+
	Lowered seizure threshold	unknown	+	++++	+	++	+++	++	++/+++	++
	Sedation	M_1, H_1 and α_1 antagonism	++	++++	+	++++	+++	+++	++++	+

+ = lowest risk; ++++ = highest risk

a. H_1 and $5HT_{2C}$ antagonism increase appetite and weight; M_3 antagonism reduces insulin secretion (thus diabetes can occur rapidly and in the absence of weight gain)

b. confounding may explain the higher and lower risk seen with typicals and quetiapine in observational studies.[26,27]

Box A Acute dopamine depletion syndrome[38,39]

Diagnosis requires 4 features unexplained by other diagnoses or frailty:
- recent dopaminergic medication change (most cases <2 weeks) *and*
- severe muscle rigidity *and*
- pyrexia *and*
- ≥2 additional features:
  - ▷ altered consciousness
  - ▷ dysphagia
  - ▷ incontinence
  - ▷ mutism
  - ▷ sweating
  - ▷ tremor
  - ▷ tachycardia
  - ▷ labile blood pressure
  - ▷ leukocytosis
  - ▷ muscle injury, e.g.
    - myoglobinuria
    - raised creatine phosphokinase.

Treatment
- discontinuation (or re-instatement) of the causal drug
- supportive care, e.g. hydration
- muscle relaxants[a], e.g. benzodiazepine and/or **dantrolene** (causes hepatotoxicity; thus reserved for severe symptoms and withdrawn when symptoms resolve)
- dopamimetics[a] (if caused by dopamine antagonists), e.g. **bromocriptine**; generally continued for 10 days (longer if caused by *depot* antipsychotics).

Prognosis
- resolves in 1–2 weeks (longer if caused by a depot antipsychotic)
- residual extrapyramidal symptoms can occur, particularly if treatment was delayed
- 10% mortality
- 30–50% risk of recurrence if antipsychotic-associated and an alternative is tried.

a. although benefit has not been confirmed in RCTs, mortality is lower in case reports employing such measures (10% vs. 20–30%).

Use of antipsychotics in palliative care

When long term (>months) use of **olanzapine**, **quetiapine** or phenothiazines is anticipated, consider monitoring weight, glucose and lipids at baseline and 3-monthly thereafter.

Doses are described in individual monographs: **haloperidol** (p.180), **levomepromazine** (p.184), **prochlorperazine** (p.183), **olanzapine** (p.187), **risperidone** (p.189) and **quetiapine** (p.191). For terminal agitation, also see Box A, p.156.

Acute mania

Haloperidol, **olanzapine**, **quetiapine** or **risperidone** are used first-line because they act more quickly than 'mood stabilizers'.[40] The latter (e.g. **valproate**, p.282) are added if antipsychotics are insufficient.[41] **Lithium** is *not* generally used for mania caused by drugs or cerebral disease; it requires specific experience and monitoring, and may be less effective than for 'classical' bipolar mania.

Intractable hiccup

The benefit reported with **chlorpromazine** and **haloperidol** remains unconfirmed by RCTs.[42,43] Thus they are used when more specific treatment, e.g. **metoclopramide** (see p.244) ± **simeticone** (an antifoaming agent; see p.4) for gastric distension, or **baclofen** are ineffective (see Prokinetics, Table 2, p.26). Antipsychotics occasionally *cause* hiccup.[44]

Nausea and vomiting

Haloperidol is used where specific D_2 antagonism is required in the area postrema (chemoreceptor trigger zone; see p.235), e.g. most chemical causes of nausea. RCTs find benefit in post-operative and chemotherapy-related nausea and vomiting, and in patients referred to specialist gastro-enterological clinics with multifactorial nausea. Open-label series also suggest benefit in palliative care patients.[45–47]

Many antipsychotics bind to other receptors involved in the transduction of emetic signals and, to a variable extent, are broad-spectrum anti-emetics (see p.235). **Olanzapine** is effective for chemotherapy-related nausea and vomiting (15 RCTs; n=1552).[48–50] Case series report benefit for nausea and vomiting in advanced cancer.[51,52] However, the parenteral preparation is unavailable in the UK. Thus, **levomepromazine** is widely used because it can be administered SC/CSCI, although the benefit reported in case series is unconfirmed in RCTs (p.184).[53–55] The buccal formulation of **prochlorperazine** is a convenient alternative for patients at home (p.183).

Delirium

Delirium is common, distressing and associated with poorer outcomes (including higher mortality).[56–58] Management includes addressing the underlying cause(s) when possible and appropriate, and non-drug approaches, e.g. ensure adequate vision and hearing, presence of a carer to reassure and reorientate. Drug treatment is generally reserved for when there is severe distress or behavioural disturbance, non-drug approaches are inadequate, or safety concerns.

Until recently, there has been a clear consensus that antipsychotics are the drug treatment of choice based on 3 RCTs, numerous open label series and extensive clinical experience in psychiatry, critical care and palliative medicine.[56,59–63] They improve symptoms in 75% of patients, *irrespective of delirium type* (agitated, hypo-active or mixed).[59] The efficacy and tolerability of **haloperidol**, **olanzapine**, **quetiapine** and **risperidone** appear comparable.[59,64–66] Further, *prophylactic* use is associated with better outcomes than *reactive* use (e.g. the proportion of patients discharged home), suggesting that it may be preferable to start antipsychotic treatment earlier, in parallel with cause-specific and non-drug measures.[67,68] **Aripiprazole**, the only parenteral, 'atypical' antipsychotic available in a formulation for acute use in the UK, also appears effective in open label series (n=78) at a mean dose of 20mg/24h IM (range 5–30mg/24h).[69]

A recent RCT in palliative care inpatients has cast doubt on this consensus. Patients with delirium with an expected survival of >1 week were randomized to receive either b.d. PO placebo, **haloperidol** or **risperidone** (both titrated to a maximum of 2–4mg/day, depending on age). After 72h, there was improvement in delirium symptom scores in all groups, which was significantly greater in those receiving placebo, although probably not to a clinically relevant degree. For those receiving an antipsychotic, extrapyramidal symptom scores were higher (probably not to a clinically relevant degree), median survival was shorter (16 vs. 26 days) and the likelihood of death 1.5 times greater (hazard ratio (95%CI) 1.47 (0.2–2.0), p=0.01).[70] This has led to the suggestion that antipsychotics should no longer be used for delirium.[71] However, the study population and methodology used raise questions about its generalizability. Half of the patients had mild delirium (MDAS ≤15; rated only 'a bit worse' by a relative) and in all groups, only 1–2 doses of 'rescue' midazolam 2.5mg SC were required over 72h, and potentially the study included patients that may not have received an antipsychotic in usual clinical practice. Interpretation of the differences between the groups is difficult because of the use of a non-validated primary outcome measure, together with a lack of data on the potential cause(s) of the delirium, and hence likelihood of reversibility vs. progressive worsening. Thus, although this RCT suggests that antipsychotics add little to corrective and non-drug approaches in mild–moderate delirium, it does not definitively exclude potential for benefit from antipsychotics in delirium, particularly when severe and/or occurring in the last days of life.

When antipsychotics alone are insufficient, benzodiazepines (see p.149) or **trazodone** (see p.223) can be added.

Although benzodiazepines can paradoxically worsen agitation, they are preferred for delirium related to alcohol withdrawal, acute dopamine depletion (antipsychotic/neuroleptic malignant) syndrome or Parkinson's disease. Results of RCTs examining prophylactic **melatonin** are conflicting (see p.164). Cholinesterase inhibitors, e.g. **rivastigmine** are not consistently effective and may increase mortality.[67,72]

Terminal agitation

Because it is often associated with hyperactive delirium, **haloperidol** is commonly used first-line to treat agitation in the imminently dying (see p.156). **Midazolam** is an alternative, particularly when anxiety is prominent and there are no obvious features of a hyperactive delirium. **Levomepromazine's** sedative properties are beneficial if **haloperidol** and **midazolam** are ineffective. **Phenobarbital** (p.289) or **propofol** (p.651) are reserved for terminal agitation refractory to **levomepromazine** and **midazolam**.

Challenging behaviours in dementia

Patients with dementia may become agitated for many reasons, including an *appropriate* response to a distressing situation. Possible precipitants should be treated or modified:

- intercurrent infections
- pain and/or other distressing symptoms
- environmental factors.

If carers or the care setting changes, seek information about the patient's daily routine. Consider the use of 'This is me' or a similar tool.[73]

If no cause is found, consider an empirical trial of **paracetamol**. Pain can be difficult to identify.[74] In an RCT, an empirical stepwise trial of analgesia (**paracetamol** → opioid → **pregabalin**) reduced agitation in unselected patients (i.e. without any specific indicator of pain).[75]

Psychotropic medication should be used only where other measures have failed. Training in non-drug management of behavioural disturbance reduces the need for psychotropic medication.[76] The efficacy of antipsychotics for challenging behaviour is marginal and generally outweighed by their undesirable effects (including increased risk of stroke and overall mortality).[77] Antidepressants, benzodiazepines and anti-epileptics are not consistently effective. Where drug treatment is required, consider seeking specialist advice. Options include:

- **haloperidol**
- atypicals, e.g. **risperidone**
- cholinesterase inhibitors (benefit is marginal, but may be better tolerated)
- **trazodone** (50mg at bedtime, where sleep disturbance predominates).[77,78]

Whichever drug is selected, use the lowest effective dose for the shortest possible time; attempt dose reduction every 2–3 months; many patients do not deteriorate when medication is withdrawn.[77]

Treatment-resistant depression

Certain antipsychotics have been used as adjuncts for depression refractory to conventional antidepressants, particularly when switching antidepressants has been unsuccessful. Generally, **aripiprazole** or **quetiapine** is added to an SSRI or **venlafaxine** (see p.203). Alternatives include **risperidone**, **olanzapine** and **mirtazapine**.[79]

Treatment-resistant anxiety

Prochlorperazine is authorized for short term adjunctive treatment. However, most RCTs in treatment-resistant anxiety examined **quetiapine**; which is generally reserved for anxiety refractory to antidepressants ± benzodiazepines ± **pregabalin**.[80]

Anorexia and weight loss

An open-label trial found cancer-related anorexia improved in 65% of people when **olanzapine** was combined with **megestrol** compared to 5% of those receiving **megestrol** alone. Although muscle mass and strength were not measured, there was a greater increase in weight, walking and general activity in the **olanzapine** group.[5]

Olanzapine has not been directly compared with corticosteroids (p.513) or progestogens (p.552). In a case series, **olanzapine** did not reduce weight loss during chemotherapy. Appetite was not assessed.[81]

Pain

Antipsychotics are no longer used as analgesics. RCTs in acute, arthritic, neuropathic and fibromyalgic pain yield conflicting results,[82,83] and alternatives are better tolerated (see p.299).

Switching antipsychotics

Equivalent PO doses of typical antipyschotics have been estimated, predominantly from surveys of psychiatric practice, and provide a starting point if switching PO from one to another (Table 4). However, doses of atypical antipsychotics are less variable, and thus starting doses are generally unaffected by the dose of a previous antipsychotic.

Table 4 Equivalent PO doses of typical antipsychotics used for psychosis[84]

Drug	*Dose (mg)*
Chlorpromazine	100
Flupentixol	2
Haloperidol	2–3
Levomepromazine	50–100
Promazine	100
Perphenazine	5–10
Risperidone	0.5–1
Sulpiride	150–300
Trifluoperazine	3–6

1 Stahl SM (2013) Chapter 4: Psychosis and schizophrenia. In: *Essential Psychopharmacology: Neuroscientific Basis and Practical Applications* (4e). Cambridge University Press, USA. 79–128.

2 Stahl SM (2013) Chapter 5: Antipsychotic agents. In: *Essential Psychopharmacology: Neuroscientific Basis and Practical Applications* (4e). Cambridge University Press, USA. 129–236.

3 Tadori Y *et al.* (2011) In vitro pharmacology of aripiprazole, its metabolite and experimental dopamine partial agonists at human dopamine D2 and D3 receptors. *European Journal of Pharmacology.* **668**: 355–365.

4 Stahl SM *et al.* (2013) Serotonergic drugs for depression and beyond. *Current Drug Targets.* **14**: 578–585.

5 Navari RM and Brenner MC (2010) Treatment of cancer-related anorexia with olanzapine and megestrol acetate: a randomized trial. *Supportive Care in Cancer.* **18**: 951–956.

6 Surmeier DJ *et al.* (2014) Dopaminergic modulation of striatal networks in health and Parkinson's disease. *Current Opinion in Neurobiology.* **29**: 109–117.

7 Cobos EJ and Baeyens JM (2015) Use of very-low-dose methadone and haloperidol for pain control in palliative care patients: are the sigma-1 receptors involved? *Journal of Palliative Medicine.* **18**: 660.

8 Davis MP (2015) Sigma-1 receptors and animal studies centered on pain and analgesia. *Expert Opinion on Drug Discovery.* **10**: 885–900.

9 Abdallah K *et al.* (2015) GABAAergic inhibition or dopamine denervation of the A11 hypothalamic nucleus induces trigeminal analgesia. *Pain.* **156**: 644–655.

10 Lieberman JA *et al.* (2005) Effectiveness of antipsychotic drugs in patients with chronic schizophrenia. *New England Journal of Medicine.* **353**: 1209–1223.

11 Jones PB *et al.* (2006) Randomized controlled trial of the effect on quality of life of second- vs first-generation antipsychotic drugs in schizophrenia: cost utility of the latest antipsychotic drugs in schizophrenia study (CUtLASS 1). *Archives of General Psychiatry.* **63**: 1079–1087.

12 Muller DJ *et al.* (2013) The pharmacogenetics of antipsychotic-induced adverse events. *Current Opinion in Psychiatry.* **26**: 144–150.

13 Arranz MJ *et al.* (2011) Pharmacogenetics of response to antipsychotics in patients with schizophrenia. *CNS Drugs.* **25**: 933–969.

14 Maldonado JR (2013) Neuropathogenesis of delirium: review of current etiologic theories and common pathways. *American Journal of Geriatric Psychiatry.* **21**: 1190–1222.

15 Cerejeira J *et al.* (2012) The cholinergic system and inflammation: common pathways in delirium pathophysiology. *Journal of the American Geriatrics Society.* **60**: 669–675.

16 Fitzgerald JM *et al.* (2013) Delirium: a disturbance of circadian integrity? *Medical Hypotheses.* **81**: 568–576.

17 Cerejeira J *et al.* (2013) The stress response to surgery and postoperative delirium: evidence of hypothalamic-pituitary-adrenal axis hyperresponsiveness and decreased suppression of the GH/IGF-1 Axis. *Journal of Geriatric Psychiatry and Neurology.* **26**: 185–194.

18 Matt SM and Johnson RW (2016) Neuro-immune dysfunction during brain aging: new insights in microglial cell regulation. *Current Opinion in Pharmacology.* **26**: 96–101.

19 Laruelle M (2014) Schizophrenia: from dopaminergic to glutamatergic interventions. *Current Opinion in Pharmacology.* **14**: 97–102.

20 White TP *et al.* (2010) Aberrant salience network (bilateral insula and anterior cingulate cortex) connectivity during information processing in schizophrenia. *Schizophrenia Research.* **123**: 105–115.

21 Lal S *et al.* (1993) Levomepromazine receptor binding profile in human brain-implications for treatment-resistant schizophrenia. *Acta Psychiatrica Scandinavica.* **87**: 380–383.

22 Binding DB (2015) Skaggs School of Pharmacy and Pharmaceutical Sciences Binding Database. Available from: http://bindingdb.org/as/search.html (acessed June 2015).

23 Eiermann B *et al.* (1997) The involvement of CYP1A2 and CYP3A4 in the metabolism of clozapine. *British Journal of Clinical Pharmacology.* **44**: 439–446.

24 Finn A *et al.* (2005) Bioavailability and metabolism of prochlorperazine administered via the buccal and oral delivery route. *Journal of Clinical Pharmacology.* **45**: 1383–1390.

25 Mittal V *et al.* (2011) Risk of cerebrovascular adverse events and death in elderly patients with dementia when treated with antipsychotic medications: a literature review of evidence. *American Journal of Alzheimers Disease and Other Dementias.* **26**: 10–28.

26 Huybrechts KF *et al.* (2012) Differential risk of death in older residents in nursing homes prescribed specific antipsychotic drugs: population based cohort study. *British Medical Journal.* **344**: e977.

27 Murray-Thomas T *et al.* (2013) Risk of mortality (including sudden cardiac death) and major cardiovascular events in atypical and typical antipsychotic users: a study with the general practice research database. *Cardiovascular Psychiatry Neurology.* **2013**: 247486.

28 Brauer R *et al.* (2011) The association between antipsychotic agents and the risk of myocardial infarction: a systematic review. *British Journal of Clinical Pharmacology*. **72**: 871–878.
29 Adachi N *et al.* (2013) Basic treatment principles for psychotic disorders in patients with epilepsy. *Epilepsia*. **54 Suppl 1**: 19–33.
30 Seppi K *et al.* (2011) The movement disorder society evidence-based medicine review update: treatments for the non-motor symptoms of Parkinson's disease. *Movement Disorders*. **26 Suppl 3**: S42–80.
31 Starkstein SE *et al.* (2012) Psychiatric syndromes in Parkinson's disease. *Current Opinion in Psychiatry*. **25**: 468–472.
32 Fond G *et al.* (2012) Antipsychotic drugs: pro-cancer or anti-cancer? A systematic review. *Medical Hypotheses*. **79**: 38–42.
33 Wilson MS, 2nd (2005) Aripiprazole and bone pain. *Psychosomatics*. **46**: 187.
34 Peuskens J *et al.* (2014) The effects of novel and newly approved antipsychotics on serum prolactin levels: a comprehensive review. *CNS Drugs*. **28**: 421–453.
35 Rummel-Kluge C *et al.* (2012) Second-generation antipsychotic drugs and extrapyramidal side effects: a systematic review and meta-analysis of head-to-head comparisons. *Schizophrenia Bulletin*. **38**: 167–177.
36 Rummel-Kluge C *et al.* (2010) Head-to-head comparisons of metabolic side effects of second generation antipsychotics in the treatment of schizophrenia: a systematic review and meta-analysis. *Schizophrenia Research*. **123**: 225–233.
37 Weston-Green K *et al.* (2013) Second generation antipsychotic-induced type 2 diabetes: a role for the muscarinic M3 receptor. *CNS Drugs*. **27**: 1069–1080.
38 Perry PJ and Wilborn CA (2012) Serotonin syndrome vs neuroleptic malignant syndrome: a contrast of causes, diagnoses, and management. *Annals of Clinical Psychiatry*. **24**: 155–162.
39 Berman BD (2011) Neuroleptic malignant syndrome: a review for neurohospitalists. *Neurohospitalist*. **1**: 41–47.
40 NICE (2014) Bipolar disorder: assessment and mangement. *Clinical Guideline*. CG185. www.nice.org.uk
41 Grande I and Vieta E (2015) Pharmacotherapy of acute mania: monotherapy or combination therapy with mood stabilizers and antipsychotics? *CNS Drugs*. **29**: 221–227.
42 Calsina-Berna A *et al.* (2012) Treatment of chronic hiccups in cancer patients: a systematic review. *Journal of Palliative Medicine*. **15**: 1142–1150.
43 Moretto EN *et al.* (2013) Interventions for treating persistent and intractable hiccups in adults. *Cochrane Database of Systematic Reviews*. **1**: CD008768 www.thecochranelibrary.com
44 Silverman MA *et al.* (2014) Aripiprazole-associated hiccups: a case and closer look at the association between hiccups and antipsychotics. *Journal of Pharmacy Practice*. **27**: 587–590.
45 McLean SL *et al.* (2013) Using haloperidol as an antiemetic in palliative care: informing practice through evidence from cancer treatment and postoperative contexts. *Journal of Pain and Palliative Care Pharmacotherpy*. **27**: 132–135.
46 Buttner M *et al.* (2004) Is low-dose haloperidol a useful antiemetic?: A meta-analysis of published and unpublished randomized trials. *Anesthesiology*. **101**: 1454–1463.
47 Digges M *et al.* (2017) Pharmacovigilance in hospice/palliative care: net effect of haloperidol for nausea or vomiting. (In press).
48 Chiu L *et al.* (2016) Efficacy of olanzapine for the prophylaxis and rescue of chemotherapy-induced nausea and vomiting (CINV): a systematic review and meta-analysis. *Supportive Care in Cancer*. **24**: 2381–2392.
49 Nakagaki M *et al.* (2017) A randomized trial of olanzapine versus palonosetron versus infused ondansetron for the treatment of breakthrough chemotherapy-induced nausea and vomiting in patients undergoing hematopoietic stem cell transplantation. *Supportive Care in Cancer*. **25**: 607–613.
50 Mukhopadhyay S *et al.* (2017) Role of olanzapine in chemotherapy-induced nausea and vomiting on platinum-based chemotherapy patients: a randomized controlled study. *Supportive Care in Cancer*. **25**: 145–154.
51 Fonte C *et al.* (2015) A review of olanzapine as an antiemetic in chemotherapy-induced nausea and vomiting and in palliative care patients. *Critical Reviews in Oncology/Hematology*. **95**: 214–221.
52 MacKintosh D (2016) Olanzapine in the management of difficult to control nausea and vomiting in a palliative care population: a case series. *Journal of Palliative Medicine*. **19**: 87–90.
53 Cox L *et al.* (2015) Levomepromazine for nausea and vomiting in palliative care. *Cochrane Database of Systematic Reviews*. **11**: CD009420. www.thecochranelibrary.com
54 Palliativedrugs.com (2017) Levomepromazine for anti-emesis - how do you use it. Palliativedrugs.com survey, April-May 2016.
55 Dietz I *et al.* (2013) Evidence for the use of Levomepromazine for symptom control in the palliative care setting: a systematic review. *BMC Palliative Care*. **12**: 2.
56 Bush SH *et al.* (2014) Treating an established episode of delirium in palliative care: expert opinion and review of the current evidence base with recommendations for future development. *Journal of Pain Symptom and Management*. **48**: 231–248.
57 Rainsford S *et al.* (2014) Delirium in advanced cancer: screening for the incidence on admission to an inpatient hospice unit. *Journal of Palliative Medicine*. **17**: 1045–1048.
58 Hosie A *et al.* (2013) Delirium prevalence, incidence, and implications for screening in specialist palliative care inpatient settings: a systematic review. *Palliative Medicine*. **27**: 486–498.
59 Meagher DJ *et al.* (2013) What do we really know about the treatment of delirium with antipsychotics? Ten key issues for delirium pharmacotherapy. *American Journal of Geriatric Psychiatry*. **21**: 1223–1238.
60 Morandi A *et al.* (2013) Consensus and variations in opinions on delirium care: a survey of European delirium specialists. *International Psychogeriatrics*. **25**: 2067–2075.
61 Kishi T *et al.* (2016) Antipsychotic medications for the treatment of delirium: a systematic review and meta-analysis of randomised controlled trials. *Journal of Neurology Neurosurgery and Psychiatry*. **87**: 767–774.
62 Grassi L *et al.* (2015) Management of delirium in palliative care: a review. *Current Psychiatry Reports*. **17**: 550.
63 NICE (2010) Delirium. *Clinical Guideline*. CG103 www.nice.org.uk
64 Grover S *et al.* (2011) Comparative efficacy study of haloperidol, olanzapine and risperidone in delirium. *Journal of Psychosomatic Research*. **71**: 277–281.
65 Yoon HJ *et al.* (2013) Efficacy and safety of haloperidol versus atypical antipsychotic medications in the treatment of delirium. *BMC Psychiatry*. **13**: 240.
66 Maneeton B *et al.* (2013) Quetiapine versus haloperidol in the treatment of delirium: a double-blind, randomized, controlled trial. *Drug Design, Development and Therapy*. **7**: 657–667.
67 Friedman JI *et al.* (2014) Pharmacological treatments of non-substance-withdrawal delirium: a systematic review of prospective trials. *American Journal of Psychiatry*. **171**: 151–159.
68 Teslyar P *et al.* (2013) Prophylaxis with antipsychotic medication reduces the risk of post-operative delirium in elderly patients: a meta-analysis. *Psychosomatics*. **54**: 124–131.
69 Kirino E (2015) Use of aripiprazole for delirium in the elderly: a short review. *Psychogeriatrics*. **15**: 75–84.

70 Agar MR *et al.* (2017) Efficacy of oral risperidone, haloperidol, or placebo for symptoms of delirium among patients in palliative care: a randomized clinical trial. *JAMA Internal Medicine*. **177**: 34–42.
71 Maust DT and Kales HC (2017) Medicating Distress. *JAMA Internal Medicine*. **177**: 42–43.
72 van Eijk MM *et al.* (2010) Effect of rivastigmine as an adjunct to usual care with haloperidol on duration of delirium and mortality in critically ill patients: a multicentre, double-blind, placebo-controlled randomised trial. *Lancet*. **376**: 1829–1837.
73 Royal College of Nursing and Alzheimer's Society This is me tool. Available from: www.alzheimers.org.uk
74 Achterberg WP *et al.* (2013) Pain management in patients with dementia. *Clinical Interventions in Aging*. **8**: 1471–1482.
75 Husebo BS *et al.* (2011) Efficacy of treating pain to reduce behavioural disturbances in residents of nursing homes with dementia: cluster randomised clinical trial. *British Medical Journal*. **343**: d4065.
76 Fossey J *et al.* (2006) Effect of enhanced psychosocial care on antipsychotic use in nursing home residents with severe dementia: cluster randomised trial. *British Medical Journal*. **332**: 756–761.
77 Rabins PV *et al* (2014) Guideline watch: practice guideline for the treatment of patients with alzheimer's disease and other dementias. *American Psychistric Association*. www.psychiatryonline.org
78 McCleery J *et al.* (2014) Pharmacotherapies for sleep disturbances in Alzheimer's disease. *Cochrane Database of Systematic Reviews*. **3**: CD009178. www.thecochranelibrary.com
79 Cleare A *et al.* (2015) Evidence-based guidelines for treating depressive disorders with antidepressants: A revision of the 2008 British Association for Psychopharmacology guidelines. *Journal of Psychopharmacology*. **29**: 459–525.
80 Baldwin DS *et al.* (2014) Evidence-based pharmacological treatment of anxiety disorders, post-traumatic stress disorder and obsessive-compulsive disorder: a revision of the 2005 guidelines from the British Association for Psychopharmacology. *Journal of Psychopharmacology*. **28**: 403–439.
81 Naing A *et al.* (2015) Olanzapine for cachexia in patients with advanced cancer: an exploratory study of effects on weight and metabolic cytokines. *Supportive Care in Cancer*. **23**: 2649–2654.
82 Seidel (2013) Antipsychotics for acute and chronic pain in adults. *Cochrane Database of Systematic Reviews*. **8**: CD004844. www.thecochranelibrary.com
83 Walitt B *et al.* (2016) Antipsychotics for fibromyalgia in adults. *Cochrane Database of Systematic Reviews*. **6**: CD011804. www.thecochranelibrary.com
84 Cunningham Owens D (2012) Meet the relatives: a reintroduction to the clinical pharmacology of 'typical' antipsychotics (Part 1). *Advances in Psychiatric Treatment*. **18**: 323–336.

Updated September 2017

HALOPERIDOL

Class: Butyrophenone antipsychotic.

Indications: Authorized indications vary between products; consult SPC for details. Psychosis, nausea and vomiting, intractable hiccup, †delirium, †terminal agitation.

Contra-indications: Parkinson's disease (but also see p.173).

Pharmacology

Haloperidol is a D_2, α_1-adrenergic and sigma receptor antagonist. Compared with other antipsychotics, haloperidol causes less drowsiness, antimuscarinic and metabolic effects, but more extrapyramidal symptoms (see Antipsychotics, p168).[1]

Haloperidol is widely used in palliative care for delirium and as an anti-emetic. For delirium, it is as effective as **risperidone**, **olanzapine** and **quetiapine**.[2,3] For nausea and vomiting, RCTs find benefit in post-operative and chemotherapy-related nausea and vomiting, and in patients referred to specialist gastro-enterology clinics with nausea due to various causes. Open-label series also suggest benefit in palliative care patients.[4–6] As a D_2 antagonist, haloperidol might have a gastric prokinetic effect (comparable with **domperidone** and **metoclopramide**); this remains unconfirmed. The benefit reported for hiccup has not been confirmed in RCTs.[7,8]

Haloperidol has variable PO bio-availability, in part due to enterohepatic recycling during first-pass metabolism. It is metabolized in the liver, principally by CYP3A4 and possibly CYP2D6; some metabolites are biologically active.[1]

Bio-availability 40-85% (mean 60%) PO.
Onset of action 10–15min SC; >1h PO.
Time to peak plasma concentration 2–6h PO; 20-30min IM.[1]
Plasma halflife 12–38h.
Duration of action up to 24h, sometimes longer.

Cautions

Dementia (increased mortality and stroke risk (p.172); also see use for challenging behaviours in dementia (p.177)); epilepsy (lowered seizure threshold, although the risk is smaller than for more sedating antipsychotics);[10] renal and hepatic impairment (see Chapter 17, p.687 and Chapter 18, p.712, respectively); cardiac disease (may prolong QT interval, particularly IV or in those with risk factors. Although the manufacturer advises against use in 'significant' cardiac disorders, one series reporting low doses of haloperidol for peri-operative delirium found no effect on QT interval; also see Chapter 20, p.734).[9]

Drug interactions

Use caution with drugs which inhibit or induce CYP3A4 or CYP2D6 (see Chapter 19, Table 8, p.725). In particular, close monitoring ± dosage adjustment are required for:

- **carbamazepine**, **phenobarbital**, **phenytoin** and **rifampicin** (potent CYP3A4 inducers); can decrease haloperidol concentrations ≤50% (≤70% for rifampicin)
- **itraconazole** (potent CYP3A4 inhibitor); can increase the haloperidol plasma concentrations and neurological undesirable effects
- **fluoxetine** (potent CYP2D6 inhibitor); can increase haloperidol plasma concentrations.

Other drugs known to significantly increase haloperidol plasma concentrations, (mechanism of action is unknown), include **fluvoxamine** and **venlafaxine**.

See Antipsychotics, p.173 for class wide interactions, e.g. other QT prolonging drugs, **lithium**.

Undesirable effects

Extrapyramidal effects (see Chapter 21, p.739), hypothermia, sedation, hypotension, endocrine effects, blood disorders, altered LFTs, acute dopamine depletion (neuroleptic/antipsychotic malignant) syndrome (see p.173), prolongation of the QT interval and *torsade de pointes* (see p.731).

Dose and use

The PO bio-availability of haloperidol suggests that when converting from PO to SC a dose reduction of ≤50% may be required. This is unlikely to be problematic when titrating to effect and a 1:1 ratio is convenient. However, monitor for undesirable effects when switching route at higher doses; some patients will require a dose reduction.

Anti-emetic

For chemical/toxic causes of nausea and vomiting:

- start with 500microgram–1.5mg/24h CSCI or PO/SC at bedtime & q2h p.r.n.
- if necessary, titrate dose according to response
- maintain with 500microgram–10mg/24h
- If 5–10mg/24h ineffective, review the cause; consider switching to **levomepromazine** (p.184).

Also see QCG: Nausea and vomiting, p.240 and QCG: Inoperable bowel obstruction, p.242.

Intractable hiccup

Haloperidol is generally used when more specific treatment, e.g. **metoclopramide** (p.244) ± an anti-foaming agent (see **simeticone**, p.4), or **baclofen** (p.608) are ineffective (see Table, p.26):

- give haloperidol 1.5–3mg PO b.d.–t.d.s. (≤5mg t.d.s if severe)
- maintenance dose 500microgram–1mg t.d.s. (≤3mg t.d.s. if severe).

Alternatives include **gabapentin** (p.272) or benzodiazepines (p.149).

Delirium

Also see p.176:

- start with 500microgram/24h CSCI or PO/SC at bedtime and q2h p.r.n.
- if necessary, increase in 0.5–1mg increments
- median effective dose 2.5mg/24h; range 250microgram–10mg/24h[11–13]
- consider a higher starting dose (1.5–3mg PO/SC) when a patient's distress is severe and/or immediate danger to self or others.

If insufficient, consider switching to an alternative antipsychotic (e.g. **olanzapine** (p.187) or **quetiapine** (p.191)) *or* concurrent use of a benzodiazepine (p.149) or **trazodone** (p.223).

Terminal agitation

- start with 1.5–5mg SC stat and q1h p.r.n. (500microgram–2.5mg SC q1h p.r.n. in the elderly)
- median effective dose 2.5–10mg/24h CSCI; range 500microgram–25mg/24h.[14–20]

If the patient fails to settle with 10mg/24h in combination with **midazolam**, consider switching haloperidol to **levomepromazine** (see Box A, p.156).

CSCI compatibility with other drugs: There are 2-drug compatibility data for haloperidol in WFI with **alfentanil, clonazepam, cyclizine, glycopyrronium, hyoscine *butylbromide*, hyoscine *hydrobromide*, metoclopramide, midazolam** and **oxycodone**.

Haloperidol is *incompatible* with **ketorolac**. Concentration-dependent *incompatibility* occurs with **dexamethasone, diamorphine, hydromorphone** and **morphine sulfate**. For more details and 3-drug compatibility data, see Appendix 3 charts and tables (p.863).

Compatibility charts for mixing drugs in 0.9% saline can be found in the extended appendix section of the on-line *PCF* on *www.palliativedrugs.com.* High concentrations of haloperidol (>1mg/mL after mixing) are incompatible if diluted with 0.9% saline (see Chapter 29, p.819).

Supply

Do not confuse haloperidol injection 5mg/mL with haloperidol decanoate depot injection 50mg/mL and 100mg/mL.

Haloperidol (generic)
Tablets 500microgram, 1.5mg, 5mg, 10mg, 20mg, 28 days @ 1.5mg at bedtime = £2.50.
Oral liquid 5mg/5mL, and 10mg/5mL 28 days @ 1.5mg at bedtime = £3.
Injection 5mg/mL, 1mL amp = £3.50.

Serenace® (Teva)
Capsules 500microgram, 28 days @ 1.5mg at bedtime = £3.50.

1 Prommer E (2012) Role of haloperidol in palliative medicine: an update. *American Journal of Hospice Palliative Care.* **29**: 295–301.
2 Grover S *et al.* (2011) Comparative efficacy study of haloperidol, olanzapine and risperidone in delirium. *Journal of Psychosomatic Research.* **71**: 277–281.
3 Maneeton B *et al.* (2013) Quetiapine versus haloperidol in the treatment of delirium: a double-blind, randomized, controlled trial. *Drug Design, Development and Therapy.* **7**: 657–667.
4 McLean SL *et al.* (2013) Using haloperidol as an antiemetic in palliative care: informing practice through evidence from cancer treatment and postoperative contexts. *Journal of Pain and Palliative Care Pharmacotherpy.* **27**: 132–135.
5 Buttner M *et al.* (2004) Is low-dose haloperidol a useful antiemetic?: A meta-analysis of published and unpublished randomized trials. *Anesthesiology.* **101**: 1454–1463.
6 Digges M *et al.* (2017) Pharmacovigilance in hospice/palliative care: net effect of haloperidol for nausea or vomiting. (In press).
7 Calsina-Berna A *et al.* (2012) Treatment of chronic hiccups in cancer patients: a systematic review. *Journal of Palliative Medicine.* **15**: 1142–1150.
8 Moretto EN *et al.* (2013) Interventions for treating persistent and intractable hiccups in adults. *Cochrane Database of Systematic Reviews.* 1: CD008768 www.thecochranelibrary.com
9 Blom MT *et al.* (2015) In-hospital haloperidol use and perioperative changes in QTc-duration. *Journal of Nutrition of Health and Aging.* **19**: 583–589.
10 Adachi N *et al.* (2013) Basic treatment principles for psychotic disorders in patients with epilepsy. *Epilepsia.* **54**: 19–33.
11 Kang JH *et al.* (2013) Comprehensive approaches to managing delirium in patients with advanced cancer. *Cancer Treatment Reviews.* **39**: 105–112.
12 Bush SH *et al.* (2014) Treating an established episode of delirium in palliative care: expert opinion and review of the current evidence base with recommendations for future development. *Journal of Pain Symptom and Management.* **48**: 231–248.
13 Meagher DJ *et al.* (2013) What do we really know about the treatment of delirium with antipsychotics? Ten key issues for delirium pharmacotherapy. *American Journal of Geriatric Psychiatry.* **21**: 1223–1238.
14 Ensor B and Cohen D (2012) Benchmarking benzodiazepines and antipsychotics in the last 24 hours of life. *New Zealand Medical Journal.* **125**: 19–30.
15 Radha Krishna LK *et al.* (2012) The use of midazolam and haloperidol in cancer patients at the end of life. *Singapore Medical Journal.* **53**: 62–66.
16 Mercadante S *et al.* (2014) Palliative sedation in patients with advanced cancer followed at home: a prospective study. *Journal of Pain Symptom Management.* **47**: 860–866.
17 Goncalves F *et al.* (2016) A protocol for the control of agitation in palliative care. *American Journal of Hospice and Palliative Care.* **33**: 948–951.
18 Chater S *et al.* (1998) Sedation for intractable distress in the dying--a survey of experts. *Palliative Medicine.* **12**: 255–269.
19 Cowan JD and Walsh D (2001) Terminal sedation in palliative medicine--definition and review of the literature. *Supportive Care in Cancer.* **9**: 403–407.
20 Mercadante S *et al.* (2012) Palliative sedation in advanced cancer patients followed at home: a retrospective analysis. *Journal of Pain Symptom Management.* **43**: 1126–1130.

Updated September 2017

PROCHLORPERAZINE

Class: Phenothiazine antipsychotic.

Indications: Nausea and vomiting, vertigo in labyrinthine disorders, short-term adjunctive treatment of anxiety.

Contra-indications: Bone marrow depression.

Pharmacology

Prochlorperazine is a D_2, $5HT_{2A}$, $5HT_{2C}$, H_1, α_1 and muscarinic receptor antagonist. It is a broad spectrum anti-emetic.[1,2]

Oral bio-availability is low because of high first-pass hepatic metabolism. Buccal prochlorperazine is about 2.5 times more bio-available and variance is much less, but it is expensive. Prochlorperazine is rapidly metabolized via eight isoforms of cytochrome P450, most extensively by CYP3A4, 2C19 and 2D6. The multiple metabolic pathways suggest that clinically important drug interactions are unlikely.[3]

Bio-availability 6% PO, 14% buccal.[3]
Onset of action 30–40min PO, 10–20min IM, 1h PR.
Time to peak plasma concentration 4h PO, 8h buccal; 4h buccal when given regularly.[3]
Plasma halflife 14–21h.[3]
Duration of action 6–8h PO, PR (possibly longer when taken regularly); 12h buccal, IM.[3,4]

Cautions

Dementia (increased mortality and stroke risk (p.172); also see use for challenging behaviours in dementia (p.177)).

Epilepsy (lowered seizure threshold), Parkinson's disease (exacerbation), renal and hepatic impairment (see Chapter 17, p.687 and Chapter 18, p.712, respectively).

Drug Interactions

Prochlorperazine may increase the plasma concentration of **phenytoin** (mechanism unknown); if given concurrently, monitor **phenytoin** levels.

See Antipsychotics, p.173 for class wide interactions, e.g. other QT prolonging drugs, **lithium**.

Undesirable effects

Very common (>10%): antimuscarinic effects (see p.5).
Frequency not stated: photosensitivity, slate-grey skin pigmentation, extrapyramidal reactions (see p.739), drowsiness, confusion, paradoxical psychotic behaviour and agitation, seizures, acute dopamine depletion (neuroleptic/antipsychotic malignant) syndrome (see p.173), postural hypotension, blood dyscrasias.

Dose and use

Prochlorperazine is irritant: do not give by CSCI; avoid direct contact of the oral solution or injection with the skin.

Because of the risk of photosensitivity, patients should be advised to use high-factor (25–30) sun screen cream and a wide-brimmed hat if going outdoors in sunny weather.

Anti-emetic

Start with:

- buccally, 3–6mg b.d. *or*
- PO, 5–10mg t.d.s.–q.d.s. *or*
- IM, 12.5mg deep IM stat, followed by PO treatment if vomiting subsides *or*
- PR (not UK), 10mg t.d.s.–q.d.s.

The manufacturer recommends PO maximum of 30mg/24h. This approximates to 6mg b.d. buccally. Administration of 10mg †IV stat is reported.[1,2] Higher doses (>500mg/24h CIVI for 1 day only) have been used for chemotherapy-related nausea, but drowsiness was universal and 20% experienced extrapyramidal symptoms.[5]

Labyrinthine disorders

- start with 5mg PO t.d.s.
- if necessary, increase to 10mg t.d.s.
- reduce gradually to 5mg once daily–b.d. after 2–3 weeks.

Short term adjunctive treatment of anxiety

Note. Guidelines advocate †**quetiapine** (p.191) as the antipsychotic of choice for anxiety refractory to antidepressants ± benzodiazepines ± **pregabalin**.[6] However, if prochlorperazine is used:

- start with 5mg PO t.d.s.
- recommended maximum dose 40mg/24h.

Supply

Prochlorperazine (generic)
Tablets *(as maleate)* 5mg, 28 days @ 5mg q.d.s. = £3.75.
Buccal tablets *(as maleate)* 3mg, 28 days @ 3mg b.d. = £48; *place tablet high between upper lip and gum and leave to dissolve.*
Injection *(as mesilate)* 12.5mg/mL, 1mL amp = £0.50.

Stemetil® (Sanofi-Aventis)
Tablets *(as maleate)* 5mg, 28 days @ 5mg q.d.s. = £8.
Oral liquid (syrup) *(as mesilate)* 5mg/5mL, 28 days @ 5mg q.d.s. = £19.
Injection *(as mesilate)* 12.5mg/mL, 1mL amp = £0.50.

1 Furyk JS *et al.* (2015) Drugs for the treatment of nausea and vomiting in adults in the emergency department setting. *Cochrane Database of Systemtic Reviews.* **9**: CD010106. www.thecochranelibrary.com
2 Carlisle JB and Stevenson CA (2006) Drugs for preventing postoperative nausea and vomiting. *Cochrane Database of Systematic Reviews.* **3**: CD004125. www.thecochranelibrary.com
3 Finn A *et al.* (2005) Bioavailability and metabolism of prochlorperazine administered via the buccal and oral delivery route. *Journal of Clinical Pharmacology.* **45**: 1383–1390.
4 Lacy C *et al.* (eds) (2003) Lexi-Comp's Drug Information Handbook. (11e). Lexi-Comp and the American Pharmaceutical Association, Hudson, Ohio.
5 Morgan RJ, Jr. *et al.* (2001) Continuous infusion prochlorperazine: pharmacokinetics, antiemetic efficacy, and feasibility of high-dose therapy. *Cancer Chemotherapy and Pharmacology.* **47**: 327–332.
6 Baldwin DS *et al.* (2014) Evidence-based pharmacological treatment of anxiety disorders, post-traumatic stress disorder and obsessive-compulsive disorder: a revision of the 2005 guidelines from the British Association for Psychopharmacology. *Journal of Psychopharmacology.* **28**: 403–439.

Updated September 2017

LEVOMEPROMAZINE

Class: Phenothiazine antipsychotic.

Indications: Psychosis, pain and agitation in the terminally ill, †nausea and vomiting.

Pharmacology

Levomepromazine is a D_2, $5HT_{2A}$, α_1- and α_2-adrenergic, H_1 and muscarinic antagonist.[1] It is structurally and functionally similar to **chlorpromazine**, but is more widely used in palliative care, in part because it can be administered SC/CSCI.

Despite the absence of RCT evidence,[2,3] levomepromazine is widely used in palliative care in the UK for terminal agitation and as a second-line anti-emetic (see p.235).[2,4] Doses ≥25mg/24h tend to cause drowsiness and postural hypotension. **Olanzapine** (p.187) is an alternative broad-spectrum anti-emetic for those unable to tolerate levomepromazine, although it is not available parenterally in the UK.

Although authorized for pain and accompanying distress in the terminally ill, RCTs for pain are small, results conflicting, and undesirable effects (particularly sedation and extrapyramidal effects) common.[5] Thus, for pain, other adjuvant analgesics, which have more supporting evidence and are better tolerated, should generally be used in preference.

Levomepromazine is largely metabolized by CYP3A4 to desmethyl- and sulfoxide metabolites.[6] It accumulates within brain tissue, particularly the basal ganglia, where it's elimination halflife is 1 week.[7]
Bio-availability 20–50% PO.[8,9]
Onset of action 30min.
Time to peak plasma concentration 2–3h PO; 30–90min SC.
Plasma halflife 15–30h, sometimes longer.[10]
Duration of action 12–24h.

Cautions

Dementia (increased mortality and stroke risk (p.172); also see use for challenging behaviours in dementia (p.177)); cardiac disease (may prolong QT interval, particularly IV or in those with risk factors (see Chapter 20, Box B, p.733); Parkinsonism (exacerbation); postural hypotension; epilepsy (lowered seizure threshold); hypothyroidism; myasthenia gravis; renal and hepatic impairment (see Chapter 17, p.687 and Chapter 18, p.712, respectively).

Drug interactions

Levomepromazine is largely metabolized by CYP3A4; it inhibits CYP2D6 and, to a lesser extent, CYP1A2 and CYP3A4.[11] Although there are no clinically significant reports of interactions with CYP3A4 inhibitors or inducers, nor levomepromazine affecting other drugs via this mechanism, caution is advised with the concurrent use of drugs metabolised by CYP2D6 (see Chapter 19, Table 8, p.725) e.g. TCAs, some beta-blockers, as theoretically levomepromazine may cause plasma concentrations to increase, or reduce conversion of pro-drugs to the active metabolite, e.g. **codeine → morphine**.

See Antipsychotics, p.173 for class wide interactions, e.g. other QT prolonging drugs, **lithium**.

Undesirable effects

Drowsiness, postural hypotension, extrapyramidal and antimuscarinic effects (see p.173). Prolongation of the QT interval and *torsade de pointes* (see p.731). Painful glossitis has been reported.[12]

Dose and use

When long term (>months) use is anticipated, consider monitoring weight, glucose and lipids at baseline and 3-monthly thereafter.

Although the PO bio-availability of levomepromazine suggests that when converting from PO to SC a dose reduction may be required, most centres use the same dose regardless of route.[4]

Anti-emetic

- start with 6.25mg PO/SC at bedtime & q2h p.r.n.
- if necessary, progressively increase to 25mg/24h.

To obtain 6.25mg and 12.5mg doses, quarter or halve a 25mg tablet; a tablet cutter can be requested on the prescription to facilitate this. Although 6mg tablets are available (see Supply), they are more expensive; their use should be reserved for when the splitting of tablets is impractical.

Some centres report benefit with lower starting doses, e.g. 2.5–5mg PO/SC. If drowsiness limits dose titration, switch to **olanzapine** (p.187) or reduce the dose and combine with an anti-emetic of a different profile of action (e.g. **ondansetron**; see Table 2, p.238).[4] Also see QCG: Nausea and vomiting, p.240 and QCG: Inoperable bowel obstruction, p.242.

Terminal agitation

Generally, a second-line treatment (see Box A, p.156), given only if it is intended to reduce a patient's level of consciousness:

- start with 25mg SC stat and q1h p.r.n. (12.5mg in the elderly)
- if necessary, titrate dose according to response
- maintain with 50–200mg/24h CSCI. Alternatively, smaller doses can be given as a SC bolus at bedtime–b.d., and p.r.n.

Some centres use smaller doses first-line, e.g. 12.5mg SC stat and q1h p.r.n. (6.25mg in the elderly).[2]

Analgesic

Seek advice from specialist palliative care or pain teams before such use (see Pharmacology). RCTs started with 12.5–25mg PO/SC and titrated according to response. Reported maximum doses varied widely; typically 75mg/24h.[5]

SC administration

To reduce the likelihood of inflammatory reactions at the skin infusion site, dilute CSCI to the largest practical volume and consider the use of 0.9% saline as the diluent (see p.819). Syringes and lines must be protected from light to prevent degradation of the drug and must be discarded if a yellow/pink/purple colour occurs, see Chapter 29, Box B, p.821.

Alternatively, given its halflife, levomepromazine can be given as a SC bolus at bedtime–b.d. (see Chapter 29, p.818).

CSCI compatibility with other drugs: There are 2-drug compatibility data for levomepromazine in WFI with **alfentanil, diamorphine, glycopyrronium, hydromorphone, hyoscine *butylbromide*, hyoscine *hydrobromide*, midazolam, morphine sulfate** and **oxycodone.**

Levomepromazine is *incompatible* with **ketorolac.** Concentration-dependent *incompatibility* occurs with **dexamethasone, ranitidine** and **octreotide.** For more details and 3-drug compatibility data, see Appendix 3 charts and tables (p.863).

Compatibility charts for mixing drugs in 0.9% saline can be found in the extended appendix section of the on-line *PCF* on *www.palliativedrugs.com.*

Supply

The cost of a 6mg tablet is £2, the equivalent cost of one quarter of a 25mg tablet is £0.06.

Levomepromazine (generic)
Oral solution 2.5mg/5mL, 28 days @ 6.25mg at bedtime = £199 (Unauthorized, price based on community specials tariff, see Chapter 24, p.751).
Tablets 6mg, 28 days @ 6mg at bedtime = £57 (Unauthorized, available as a special order via IDIS see Chapter 24, p.751). *Levinan brand is scored and disperses in water. Note. Not all brands are scored.*
Tablets 100mg, 100 = £62.50 (Unauthorized, available as a special order via IDIS see Chapter 24, p.751).
Injection 25mg/mL, 1mL amp = £2.

Nozinan® (Sanofi-Aventis)
Tablets *(scored)* 25mg, 28 days @ 12.5mg at bedtime = £3.50.
Injection 25mg/mL, 1mL amp = £2.

1 Lal S *et al.* (1993) Levomepromazine receptor binding profile in human brain--implications for treatment-resistant schizophrenia. *Acta Psychiatrica Scandinavica.* **87**: 380–383.
2 Dietz I *et al.* (2013) Evidence for the use of Levomepromazine for symptom control in the palliative care setting: a systematic review. *BMC Palliative Care.* **12**: 2.
3 Cox L *et al.* (2015) Levomepromazine for nausea and vomiting in palliative care. *Cochrane Database of Systematic Reviews.* **11**: CD009420. www.thecochranelibrary.com
4 Palliativedrugs.com (2016) Levomepromazine for anti-emesis - how do you use it? *Latest additions: Survey results (June).* www.palliativedrugs.com
5 Seidel (2013) Antipsychotics for acute and chronic pain in adults. *Cochrane Database of Systematic Reviews.* **8**: CD004844. www.thecochranelibrary.com
6 Wojcikowski J *et al.* (2014) The cytochrome P450-catalyzed metabolism of levomepromazine: a phenothiazine neuroleptic with a wide spectrum of clinical application. *Biochemical Pharmacology.* **90**: 188–195.
7 Kornhuber J *et al.* (2006) Region specific distribution of levomepromazine in the human brain. *Journal of Neural Transmission.* **113**: 387–397.
8 Bagli M *et al.* (1995) Bioequivalence and absolute bioavailability of oblong and coated levomepromazine tablets in CYP2D6 phenotyped subjects. *International Journal of Clinical Pharmacology and Therapeutics.* **33**: 646–652.
9 Dahl SG (1975) Pharmacokinetics of methotrimeprazine after single and multiple doses. *Clinical Pharmacology and Therapeutics.* **19**: 435–442.
10 Dahl SG *et al.* (1977) Pharmacokinetics and relative bioavailability of levomepromazine after repeated administration of tablets and syrup. *European Journal of Clinical Pharmacology.* **11**: 305–310.
11 Basinska-Ziobron A *et al.* (2015) Inhibition of human cytochrome P450 isoenzymes by a phenothiazine neuroleptic levomepromazine: An in vitro study. *Pharmacological Reports.* **67**: 1178–1182.
12 Murray-Brown FL (2012) A case of possible glossitis in a patient with non small cell carcinoma of the lung secondary to levomepromazine. *Palliative Medicine.* **26**: 860–861.

Updated September 2017

OLANZAPINE

Class: Atypical antipsychotic.

Indications: Psychosis, mania and bipolar disorders, †nausea and vomiting, †delirium, †treatment-resistant depression.

Contra-indications: Narrow angle glaucoma.

4

Pharmacology

Olanzapine is a potent D_1, D_2, D_3, D_4, $5HT_{2A}$, $5HT_{2C}$, $5HT_3$, $5HT_6$ and $5HT_7$ antagonist. It also binds to other receptors, including α_1 and α_2-adrenergic, H_1 and muscarinic receptors.[1]

Olanzapine is as effective as **haloperidol**, **quetiapine** and **risperidone** in treating delirium.[2,3] Olanzapine is more effective than placebo, **aprepitant**, **fosaprepitant** and **metoclopramide** for preventing (11 RCTs; n=1182) and treating (4 RCTs; n=370) chemotherapy-related nausea and vomiting despite $5HT_3$ antagonists and **dexamethasone**.[4–6] Case series report benefit for nausea and vomiting in advanced cancer[7,8] and paraneoplastic sweating.[9]

Olanzapine, **quetiapine** and **clozapine** cause fewer drug-induced movement disorders than other antipsychotics.[10] However, other undesirable effects are more common, e.g. drowsiness, weight gain. Thus, overall, tolerability is comparable.[11,12]

Olanzapine is metabolized in the liver by glucuronidation and, to a lesser extent, by oxidation via the cytochrome P450 system (see p.172), primarily via CYP1A2 with a minor contribution via CYP2D6. The major metabolite is the 10-N-glucuronide which does not pass the blood-brain barrier. Elimination of metabolites is both renal (60%) and faecal (30%).[13]

Bio-availability 60%, sometimes >80% PO.

Onset of action hours–days in delirium; days–weeks in psychoses.

Time to peak plasma concentration 5–8h, not affected by food.

Plasma halflife 34h; 52h in the elderly; shorter in smokers; unchanged in hepatic and renal impairment.

Duration of action 12–48h, situation dependent.

Cautions

Injections (not UK): fatalities from oversedation or cardiorespiratory depression have occurred after higher than approved doses or *concurrent use with benzodiazepines*. Monitor blood pressure, heart rate, respiratory rate and level of consciousness for ≥4h after IM olanzapine, and do not give parenteral benzodiazepines within 1h of IM olanzapine.

Dementia (increased mortality and stroke risk (p.172); also see use for challenging behaviours in dementia (p.177)); elderly patients; renal and hepatic impairment (see Chapter 17, p.687 and Chapter 18, p.712, respectively); Parkinson's disease (exacerbation); epilepsy (lowers seizure threshold; consider an alternative, e.g. **haloperidol**, also see p.172).[14] May cause or adversely affect diabetes mellitus; rare reports of keto-acidosis.

Drug interactions

Carbamazepine and tobacco exposure induce CYP1A2 and decrease the plasma concentration of olanzapine; in contrast, **fluvoxamine**, a potent inhibitor of CYP1A2, increases the plasma concentration ≤80% and a lower dose should be considered if concurrent administration cannot be avoided. Caution should be taken with other CYP1A2 inhibitors, (e.g. **ciprofloxacin**, see Chapter 19, Table 8, p.725).

See Antipsychotics, p.173 for class wide interactions, e.g. other QT prolonging drugs, **lithium**.

Undesirable effects

Very common (>10%): drowsiness, weight gain, orthostatic hypotension.

Common (<10%, >1%): extrapyramidal symptoms.

Uncommon (<1%, >0.1%): dry mouth, constipation, agitation, nervousness, dizziness, peripheral oedema.

The incidence and severity of extrapyramidal symptoms are less than with **haloperidol**, but greater than with **quetiapine**.[15]

Dose and use

When long term (>months) use is anticipated, consider monitoring weight, glucose and lipids at baseline and every 3 months thereafter.

Subcutaneous use of parenteral olanzapine (not UK) is reported without evidence of site reactions.[16]

Psychosis or mania

- generally start with 10mg PO at bedtime
- for acute severe mania 15mg
- if necessary, increase to 20mg at bedtime.

Delirium

Also see p.176:
- start with 2.5mg PO at bedtime & p.r.n.
- if necessary, increase → 5mg → 10mg/24h
- mean effective dose 5mg/24h (range 1.25–20mg).[3]

Anti-emetic

- start with 2.5–5mg PO stat & at bedtime
- typical effective dose 5mg/24h, occasionally 10mg/24h.[4–8]

Treatment-resistant depression

As adjunct therapy to mono-amine re-uptake inhibitors (also see p.203):
- start with 5mg PO at bedtime, but 2.5mg if frail
- typical effective dose 10mg at bedtime
- maximum dose 20mg at bedtime.[17]

Supply

Olanzapine (generic)
Tablets 2.5mg, 5mg, 7.5mg, 10mg, 15mg, 20mg, 28 days @ 5mg at bedtime = £1.
Tablets orodispersible 5mg, 10mg, 15mg, 20mg, 28 days @ 5mg at bedtime = £2; *may be placed on the tongue and allowed to dissolve and then swallowed, or dispersed in water, orange juice, apple juice, milk or coffee immediately before administration.*

1 Stahl SM (2013) Chapter 5: Antipsychotic agents. In: Essential Psychopharmacology: Neuroscientific Basis and Practical Applications (4e). Cambridge University Press, USA. 129–236.
2 Yoon HJ *et al.* (2013) Efficacy and safety of haloperidol versus atypical antipsychotic medications in the treatment of delirium. *BMC Psychiatry.* **13**: 240.
3 Meagher DJ *et al.* (2013) What do we really know about the treatment of delirium with antipsychotics? Ten key issues for delirium pharmacotherapy. *American Journal of Geriatric Psychiatry.* **21**: 1223–1238.
4 Chiu L *et al.* (2016) Efficacy of olanzapine for the prophylaxis and rescue of chemotherapy-induced nausea and vomiting (CINV): a systematic review and meta-analysis. *Supportive Care in Cancer.* **24**: 2381–2392.
5 Nakagaki M *et al.* (2017) A randomized trial of olanzapine versus palonosetron versus infused ondansetron for the treatment of breakthrough chemotherapy-induced nausea and vomiting in patients undergoing hematopoietic stem cell transplantation. *Supportive Care in Cancer.* **25**: 607–613.
6 Mukhopadhyay S *et al.* (2017) Role of olanzapine in chemotherapy-induced nausea and vomiting on platinum-based chemotherapy patients: a randomized controlled study. *Supportive Care in Cancer.* **25**: 145–154.
7 Fonte C *et al.* (2015) A review of olanzapine as an antiemetic in chemotherapy-induced nausea and vomiting and in palliative care patients. *Critical Reviews in Oncology/Hematology.* **95**: 214–221.
8 MacKintosh D (2016) Olanzapine in the management of difficult to control nausea and vomiting in a palliative care population: a case series. *Journal of Palliative Medicine.* **19**: 87–90.
9 Zylicz Z and Krajnik M (2003) Flushing and sweating in an advanced breast cancer patient relieved by olanzapine. *Journal of Pain and Symptom Management.* **25**: 494–495.
10 Rummel-Kluge C *et al.* (2012) Second-generation antipsychotic drugs and extrapyramidal side effects: a systematic review and meta-analysis of head-to-head comparisons. *Schizophrenia Bulletin.* **38**: 167–177.
11 Lieberman JA *et al.* (2005) Effectiveness of antipsychotic drugs in patients with chronic schizophrenia. *New England Journal of Medicine.* **353**: 1209–1223.

12 Jones PB *et al.* (2006) Randomized controlled trial of the effect on quality of life of second- vs first-generation antipsychotic drugs in schizophrenia: cost utility of the latest antipsychotic drugs in schizophrenia study (CUtLASS 1). *Archives of General Psychiatry.* **63**: 1079–1087.
13 Prommer E (2013) Olanzapine: palliative medicine update. *American Journal Hospice and Palliative Care.* **30**: 75–82.
14 Adachi N *et al.* (2013) Basic treatment principles for psychotic disorders in patients with epilepsy. *Epilepsia.* **54(Suppl 1)**: 19–33.
15 Rummel-Kluge C *et al.* (2010) Head-to-head comparisons of metabolic side effects of second generation antipsychotics in the treatment of schizophrenia: a systematic review and meta-analysis. *Schizophrenia Research.* **123**: 225–233.
16 Elsayem (2010) Subcutaneous olanzapine for hyperactive or mixed delirium in patients with advanced cancer: a preliminary study. *Journal of Pain and Symptom Management.* **40**: 774–782.
17 Kato M and Chang CM (2013) Augmentation treatments with second-generation antipsychotics to antidepressants in treatment-resistant depression. *CNS Drugs.* **27(Suppl 1)**: S11–19.

4

Updated September 2017

RISPERIDONE

Class: Atypical antipsychotic.

Indications: Psychosis, mania and bipolar disorders, †delirium.

Pharmacology

Risperidone is a potent D_2 and $5HT_{2A}$ antagonist. It also binds to $5HT_{2C}$, H_1, α_1- and α_2-adrenergic, but *not* muscarinic, receptors.[1]

Risperidone is as effective as **haloperidol**, **olanzapine** and **quetiapine** in treating delirium.[2,3] The benefit reported for refractory opioid-induced nausea and vomiting[4] has not been confirmed in RCTs.

The incidence of drug-induced movement disorders is less than with **haloperidol** and phenothiazines but greater than with more sedating atypical antipsychotics (e.g. **olanzapine, quetiapine**; see p.191).[5] Weight gain and appetite stimulation is generally less than with other atypical antipsychotics.[6]

Risperidone is metabolized by CYP2D6 to 9-OH-risperidone (**paliperidone**, which is also commercially available). Both are active; risperidone is less readily removed from the brain by active transport but has a higher affinity for $5HT_2$ receptors (believed to reduce undesirable extrapyramidal effects; see p.168).[7] Their overall activity is similar. Thus, although risperidone's halflife varies (17, 5 and 3h in poor, extensive and ultra-rapid metabolizers, respectively,[8] the effect of CYP2D6 metabolizer status on dose requirements is small.[9] 9-OH-risperidone is renally excreted unchanged (75%) or further metabolized (25%; multiple pathways including CYP 3A4).

Bio-availability 70%.

Time to peak plasma concentration 1–2h, not affected by food.

Onset of action hours–days in delirium; days–weeks in psychoses.

Plasma halflife 24h (for risperidone + 9-OH-risperidone; see text).

Duration of action 12–48h, situation dependent.

Cautions

Dementia (increased mortality and stroke risk (p.172); also see use for challenging behaviours in dementia (p.177); elderly patients; renal and hepatic impairment (see Chapter 17, p.687 and Chapter 18, p.712, respectively);[10] Parkinson's disease (exacerbation); epilepsy (lowers seizure threshold, although the risk is lower than with more sedating atypical antipsychotics).[11]

Drug interactions

Use caution with drugs which inhibit or induce CYP3A4 and possibly CYP2D6 (see Chapter 19, Table 8, p.725). In particular, close monitoring ± dosage adjustment may be required for:

- **carbamazepine** and **rifampicin** (potent CYP3A4 inducers); can decrease risperidone plasma concentrations ($\leq$50% for rifampicin)
- **verapamil** (potent CYP3A4 inhibitor); can increase risperidone plasma concentrations.

Some CYP3A4 and CY2D6 inhibitors may increase the risperidone plasma concentration but not the overall combined active antipsychotic effect of risperidone and its metabolite, unless high doses are used, e.g. **itraconazole**, **paroxetine**.

See Antipsychotics, p.173 for class wide interactions, e.g. other QT prolonging drugs, **lithium**.

Undesirable effects

Very common (>10%): parkinsonism.
Common (<10%, >1%): insomnia, agitation, anxiety, headache, akathisia, dystonia, dyskinesia (see below), drowsiness, weight gain.
Uncommon (<1%, >0.1%): drowsiness, fatigue, dizziness, impaired concentration, seizures, blurred vision, syncope, dyspepsia, nausea and vomiting, constipation, sexual dysfunction (including priapism and erectile dysfunction), urinary incontinence, rhinitis.

Dose and use

Despite being commonly given b.d. there is no advantage in dividing the total daily dose, which can conveniently be given at bedtime.[12] Doses above 10mg/24h generally do not provide added benefit and may increase the risk of drug-induced movement disorders.

Psychosis and mania

- start with 2mg PO at bedtime
- if necessary, increase to 4mg and 6mg at bedtime on successive days
- in elderly patients and those with severe renal or hepatic impairment, the starting dose should be halved to 1mg at bedtime and titration extended over 6 days (see Chapter 17, p.691 and Chapter 18, p.712).

Delirium

Also see p.176:
- start with 0.5–1mg PO at bedtime & p.r.n.
- if necessary, increase by 0.5–1mg after two days
- mean effective dose 1.5mg/24h (range 0.5–3mg).[3]

Supply

Risperidone (generic)
Tablets 500microgram, 1mg, 2mg, 3mg, 4mg, 6mg, 28 days @ 1mg at bedtime = £1.
Tablets orodispersible 500microgram, 1mg, 2mg, 3mg, 4mg, 28 days @ 1mg at bedtime = £21; *tablets should be placed on the tongue, allowed to dissolve, then swallowed.*
Oral solution 1mg/mL, 28 days @ 1mg at bedtime = £1.25; *may be diluted with any non-alcoholic drink except tea.*

1 Stahl SM (2013) Chapter 5: Antipsychotic agents. In: Essential Psychopharmacology: Neuroscientific Basis and Practical Applications (4e). Cambridge University Press, USA. 129–236.
2 Yoon HJ *et al.* (2013) Efficacy and safety of haloperidol versus atypical antipsychotic medications in the treatment of delirium. *BMC Psychiatry*. **13**: 240.
3 Meagher DJ *et al.* (2013) What do we really know about the treatment of delirium with antipsychotics? Ten key issues for delirium pharmacotherapy. *American Journal of Geriatric Psychiatry*. **21**: 1223–1238.
4 Okamoto Y *et al.* (2007) A retrospective chart review of the antiemetic effectiveness of risperidone in refractory opioid-induced nausea and vomiting in advanced cancer patients. *Journal of Pain and Symptom Management*. **34**: 217–222.
5 Rummel-Kluge C *et al.* (2012) Second-generation antipsychotic drugs and extrapyramidal side effects: a systematic review and meta-analysis of head-to-head comparisons. *Schizophrenia Bulletin*. **38**: 167–177.
6 Rummel-Kluge C *et al.* (2010) Head-to-head comparisons of metabolic side effects of second generation antipsychotics in the treatment of schizophrenia: a systematic review and meta-analysis. *Schizophrenia Research*. **123**: 225–233.
7 de Leon J *et al.* (2010) The pharmacokinetics of paliperidone versus risperidone. *Psychosomatics*. **51**: 80–88.
8 Xiang Q *et al.* (2010) Effect of CYP2D6, CYP3A5, and MDR1 genetic polymorphisms on the pharmacokinetics of risperidone and its active moiety. *Journal of Clinical Pharmacology*. **50**: 659–666.
9 Mas S *et al.* (2012) Intuitive pharmacogenetics: spontaneous risperidone dosage is related to CYP2D6, CYP3A5 and ABCB1 genotypes. *Pharmacogenomics Journal*. **12**: 255–259.
10 Snoecke E *et al.* (1995) Influence of age, renal and liver impairment on the pharmacokinetics of risperidone in man. *Psychopharmacology (Berl)*. **122**: 223–229.
11 Adachi N *et al.* (2013) Basic treatment principles for psychotic disorders in patients with epilepsy. *Epilepsia*. **54(Suppl 1_**: 19–33.
12 Nair N (1998) Therapeutic equivalence of risperidone given once daily and twice daily in patients with schizophrenia. The Risperidone Study. *Journal of Clinical Psychopharmacology*. **18**: 10–110.

Updated September 2017

QUETIAPINE

Class: Atypical antipsychotic.

Indications: Psychosis, mania and bipolar disorders, †delirium, †treatment-resistant depression and/or anxiety.

Pharmacology

Quetiapine is an α_1-adrenergic, D_2, D_3, H_1, $5HT_{2A}$ and muscarinic antagonist and a $5HT_{1A}$ partial agonist. Like **mirtazapine** (p.221), it is an α_2 and $5HT_{2C}$ antagonist,[1,2] and an active metabolite, norquetiapine, is a noradrenaline re-uptake inhibitor; all may contribute to quetiapine's antidepressant effect.[3]

For delirium, quetiapine is as effective as **haloperidol**, **olanzapine** and **risperidone**.[4–6] For anxiety, it is generally reserved for symptoms refractory to antidepressants ± benzodiazepines ± **pregabalin**.[7] For depression, it is added when the response to a mono-amine reuptake inhibitor is insufficient (see p.202).

Quetiapine and **clozapine** have the lowest risk of extrapyramidal effects of all antipsychotics (see Chapter 21, p.739).[8] The Movement Disorder Society recommends **clozapine** for Parkinson's-related psychosis, but quetiapine is used more commonly because the former requires specialist haematological monitoring. When directly compared in 2 small RCTs (n=72), their efficacy and tolerability (including worsening of motor symptoms) were comparable (also see p.173).[9–11]

Quetiapine shares the undesirable metabolic effects, and the increased mortality in patients with dementia, of the other atypicals.[12,13] Compared with **olanzapine** and **risperidone**, it causes more antimuscarinic effects. Like **olanzapine**, it is more sedating than **risperidone**.

It is rapidly absorbed after oral administration. Although not known precisely, bio-availability is at least 75% (the proportion of radio-labelled quetiapine excreted in urine).[14] Metabolism is predominantly by CYP3A4. Elimination is both renal (75%) and faecal (25%); <1% of quetiapine is excreted unchanged.[14]

Bio-availability ≥75%.[14]
Onset of action hours–days in delirium; 1–2 weeks in psychoses.
Time to peak plasma concentration 1.5h.
Plasma halflife 7h (10–14h in the elderly).
Duration of action 12h (although serotoninergic activity may persist for much longer).[14]

Cautions

Dementia (increased mortality and stroke risk (p.172); also see use for challenging behaviours in dementia (p.177)); elderly patients; renal and hepatic impairment (see Chapter 17, p.687 and Chapter 18, p.712, respectively); Parkinson's disease (exacerbation, but lower risk than for other antipsychotics (see p.173); epilepsy (lowers seizure threshold; consider an alternative, e.g. **haloperidol**, also see p.172).[15] May cause or adversely affect diabetes mellitus. Possibly an increased risk of neutropenia.

Drug interactions

Plasma quetiapine concentrations can be significantly increased by CYP3A4 inhibitors (e.g. azole antifungals, macrolide antibiotics, see Chapter 19, Table 8, p.725) and concurrent use is contra-indicated by the manufacturer. Quetiapine plasma concentrations can be significantly reduced by enzyme inducers (e.g. **carbamazepine**, **phenytoin**) and concurrent administration should be avoided where possible.

See Antipsychotics, p.173 for class wide interactions, e.g. other QT prolonging drugs, **lithium**.

Undesirable effects

Very common (>10%): drowsiness, dizziness.
Common (<10%, >1%): dry mouth, constipation, leukopenia, tachycardia, orthostatic hypotension, peripheral oedema, altered liver transaminases.

Dose and use

When long term (>months) use is anticipated, consider monitoring weight, glucose and lipids at baseline and 3-monthly thereafter.

Reduce starting dose and rate of titration in the elderly and those with renal or hepatic impairment or Parkinson's disease (also see Chapter 17, p.691 and Chapter 18, p.712, respectively). Doses can be split asymmetrically (e.g. 12.5mg in the morning, 25mg at bedtime) if daytime drowsiness and/or insomnia are present.

Delirium

Also see p.176:
- start with 12.5mg PO b.d. (halve a 25mg tablet)
- if necessary, increase in 12.5–25mg increments
- mean effective dose 75mg/24h (range 25–300mg).[6]

Anxiety, depression and psychosis

- start with 12.5–25mg PO b.d.
- if necessary, increase in 12.5–25mg increments
- can be titrated rapidly over 3–4 days for severe symptoms, e.g. → 50mg b.d. → 100mg b.d. → 150mg b.d.
- typical effective dose:
  - ▷ anxiety 50–150mg/24h; occasionally titrated ≤400mg/24h[16]
  - ▷ depression 150–300mg/24h; occasionally titrated ≤600mg/24h[17]
  - ▷ psychosis 300–450mg/24h.

Bipolar mania

As monotherapy or as adjunct therapy to mood stabilizers:
- start with 50mg PO b.d.
- increase to 100mg b.d. (day 2) → 150mg b.d. (day 3) → 200mg b.d. (day 4)
- typical effective dose 400–800mg/24h.

Supply

Immediate-release
Quetiapine (generic)
Tablets 25mg, 100mg, 150mg, 200mg, 300mg, 28 days @ 100mg b.d.= £1.50.
Oral solution 12.5mg/5mL, 25mg/5mL, 50mg/5mL and 100mg/5mL 28 days @ 100mg b.d.= £81 (unauthorized, available as a special order, see Chapter 24, p.751); *price based on community specials tariff.*

Modified-release
Quetiapine (generic)
Tablets m/r 50mg, 150mg, 200mg, 300mg, 400mg, 28 days @ 200mg once daily = £25.

1 NIMH (National Institute of Mental Health) (2015) Psychoactive Drug Screening Program. University of North Carolina. Available from: https://pdspdb.unc.edu/pdspWeb/ (accessed August 2017)
2 Stahl SM (2013) Chapter 5: Antipsychotic agents. In: Essential Psychopharmacology: Neuroscientific Basis and Practical Applications (4e). Cambridge University Press, USA. 129–236.
3 Stahl SM *et al.* (2013) Serotonergic drugs for depression and beyond. *Current Drug Targets.* **14**: 578–585.
4 Maneeton B *et al.* (2013) Quetiapine versus haloperidol in the treatment of delirium: a double-blind, randomized, controlled trial. *Drug Design, Development Therapy.* **7**: 657–667.
5 Yoon HJ *et al.* (2013) Efficacy and safety of haloperidol versus atypical antipsychotic medications in the treatment of delirium. *BMC Psychiatry.* **13**: 240.
6 Meagher DJ *et al.* (2013) What do we really know about the treatment of delirium with antipsychotics? Ten key issues for delirium pharmacotherapy. *American Journal of Geriatric Psychiatry.* **21**: 1223–1238.
7 Baldwin DS *et al.* (2014) Evidence-based pharmacological treatment of anxiety disorders, post-traumatic stress disorder and obsessive-compulsive disorder: a revision of the 2005 guidelines from the British Association for Psychopharmacology. *Journal of Psychopharmacology.* **28**: 403–439.

8 Rummel-Kluge C *et al.* (2012) Second-generation antipsychotic drugs and extrapyramidal side effects: a systematic review and meta-analysis of head-to-head comparisons. *Schizophrenia Bulletin*. **38**: 167–177.
9 Seppi K *et al.* (2011) The movement disorder society evidence-based medicine review update: treatments for the non-motor symptoms of Parkinson's disease. *Movement Disorders*. **26 Suppl 3**: S42–80.
10 Weintraub D *et al.* (2011) Patterns and trends in antipsychotic prescribing for Parkinson disease psychosis. *Archives of Neurology*. **68**: 899–904.
11 Starkstein SE *et al.* (2012) Psychiatric syndromes in Parkinson's disease. *Current Opinion in Psychiatry*. **25**: 468–472.
12 Rummel-Kluge C *et al.* (2010) Head-to-head comparisons of metabolic side effects of second generation antipsychotics in the treatment of schizophrenia: a systematic review and meta-analysis. *Schizophrenia Research*. **123**: 225–233.
13 Mittal V *et al.* (2011) Risk of cerebrovascular adverse events and death in elderly patients with dementia when treated with antipsychotic medications: a literature review of evidence. *American Journal of Alzheimers Disease and Other Dementias*. **26**: 10–28.
14 DeVane CL and Nemeroff CB (2001) Clinical pharmacokinetics of quetiapine: an atypical antipsychotic. *Clinical Pharmacokinetics*. **40**: 509–522.
15 Adachi N *et al.* (2013) Basic treatment principles for psychotic disorders in patients with epilepsy. *Epilepsia*. **54(Suppl 1)**: 19–33.
16 Hershenberg R *et al.* (2014) Role of atypical antipsychotics in the treatment of generalized anxiety disorder. *CNS Drugs*. **28**: 519–533.
17 Kato M and Chang CM (2013) Augmentation treatments with second-generation antipsychotics to antidepressants in treatment-resistant depression. *CNS Drugs*. **27(Suppl 1)**: S11–19.

Updated September 2017

ANTIDEPRESSANTS

Indications: Authorized indications vary; see individual SPCs for details. Depression, anxiety and panic disorders, neuropathic pain, stress incontinence and urgency, †agitated delirium, †sweating, †hot flushes, †insomnia, †pruritus, †bladder spasm, †pathological laughing and crying, †drooling, †refractory cough.

Pharmacology

Conventional antidepressants enhance mono-amine transmission. Because mono-amines regulate activity in numerous circuits, antidepressants are of benefit in many symptoms:

- pre-frontal cortex → depression (see figure 1)[1]
- fear circuits → anxiety (see Figure 2, p.152)
- descending pain modulation pathways → neuropathic pain (see Figure 1, p.299)
- descending bladder control pathways → urinary incontinence.

Enhanced mono-amine transmission is also believed to underlie their action in hot flushes, pruritus, pathological laughing and crying, and cough, although their site of action is less well characterized.[2–5]

Some have additional actions of relevance to both beneficial and undesirable effects (Table 1), e.g.:

- histamine type 1 receptor antagonism → insomnia
- muscarinic receptor antagonism → bladder spasm, drooling
- sodium channel blockade (tricyclic antidepressants) → neuropathic pain (but in overdose: coma, arrhythmias, seizures).

Classification

Antidepressants are classified according to their mechanism(s) of action (Table 1). However, many have multiple actions and some labels are applied inconsistently. For example, SNRI (serotonin and noradrenaline re-uptake inhibitor) can refer to all SNRIs or be reserved for those without additional receptor binding affinities (e.g. **venlafaxine** and **duloxetine**).

SRIs (serotonin re-uptake inhibitors) with relatively minor additional actions ('selective' SRIs; SSRIs) are generally considered separately from those with more significant additional actions (e.g. **clomipramine**, **trazodone** or **vortioxetine**). However, all SSRIs except **escitalopram** have additional actions and, thus, their differences form a spectrum.

The tricyclic antidepressants (TCAs) are structurally related but functionally variable, encompassing SRIs (e.g. **clomipramine**), SNRIs (e.g. **amitriptyline**) and NRIs (e.g. **lofepramine**, **nortriptyline**). They all inhibit voltage gated sodium channels making them more dangerous in overdose than other antidepressants.

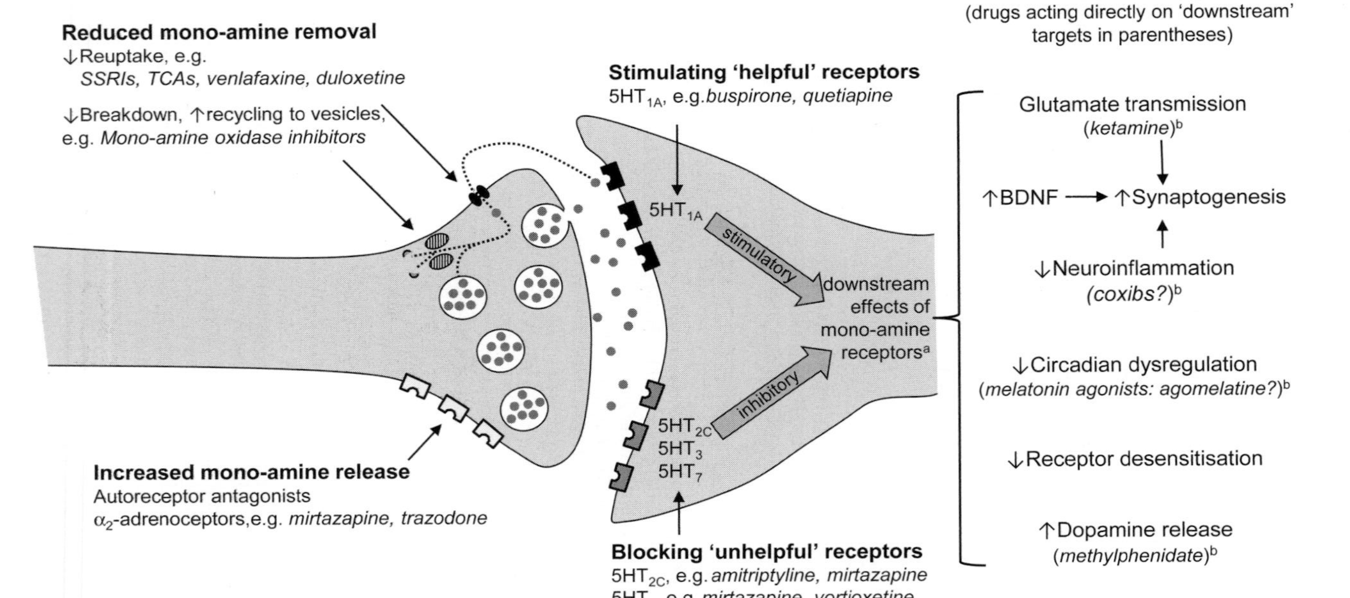

Figure 1. Mechanism of action of antidepressants and related drugs.[1,6–8]

a. mono-amines are not directly mood elevating; they act on depression through a variety of downstream effects (see text); this partly explains the delayed improvement in depression despite antidepressants increasing mono-amine transmission within hours of commencing.

b. drugs acting directly on these downstream effects might act faster (e.g. ketamine, methylphenidate) or improve residual symptoms (e.g. coxibs).

Table 1 Classification and action of selected antidepressants

	Classification	Drug	Re-uptake Transporters			Receptors									Ion channels
			5HT	*NA*[a]	*DA*	$5HT_{1A}$	$5HT_{2A}$	$5HT_{2C}$	$5HT_3$	H_1	α_1	α_2	*M*	*MT*	Na_v
Mono-amine reuptake inhibitors	SRI	Citalopram	+++	-	-	-	-	-	-	+	-	-	-		-
		Clomipramine	+++	+	-	-	+++	++	++	++	++	+	+++		++
		Escitalopram	+++	-	-	-	-	-	-	-	-	-	-		-
		Fluoxetine	+++	-	-	-	+	+	-	-	-	-	-		-
		Paroxetine	+++	+	-	-	-	-	-	-	-	-	+		-
		Sertraline	+++	-	+	-	-	-		-	+	-	-		-
		Trazodone	++	-	-	++[d]	++	+	-	+	++	+	-		-
		Vortioxetine	+++	+	-	++PA	-	-	++	-	-	-	-		-
	SNRI	Amitriptyline	+++	+++[b]	-	+[d]	+++	+++		+++	+++	+	+++		++
		Duloxetine	+++	+++	+	-	-	-		-	-	-	-		-
		Imipramine	+++	++	-	-	+	+	-	+++	++	-	+/+++[e]		++
		Venlafaxine	+++	++[c]	-	-	-	-	-	-	-	-	-		-
	NRI	Lofepramine	+	+++	-	-	-			+	+	-	-/++[e]		++
		Nortriptyline	+	+++	-		+++	+++		+++	++	-	++		++
		Reboxetine	-	+++	-	-	-	-	-		-	-			-
	NDRI	Bupropion	-	+	++	-	-	-			-	-	-		-
Psychostimulants		Methylphenidate	-	-	+++	-	-	-	-		-	-	-		-
Receptor ligands without MARI properties		Agomelatine					-	+	-	-	-		-	++A	-
		Buspirone				+++PA	-	-	-						-
		Mirtazapine	-	-	-	++[d]	++	++	++	+++	-	+++	-		-

Affinity: +++ high, ++ moderate, + low, - negligible or none; blank = no data.

Abbreviations: A = agonist; DA = dopamine; 5HT = 5-hydroxytryptamine (serotonin); MAO = mono-amine oxidase; Na_V = voltage gated sodium channels; NDRIs = noradrenaline (norepinephrine) and dopamine re-uptake inhibitor; NA = noradrenaline; NRI = noradrenaline re-uptake inhibitor; PA = partial agonist; SNRI = serotonin and noradrenaline re-uptake inhibitor ('dual' inhibitor); SRI = serotonin reuptake inhibitor; the remainder refer to receptor types: M = muscarinic acetylcholine; $\alpha_{1/2}$ = α-adrenergic type 1 or 2; H_1 = histamine type 1; $5HT_{1A/2A/2C}$ = 5-hydroxytryptamine (serotonin) type 1A, 2A or 2C; MT = melatonin.

a. the noradrenaline re-uptake transporter also clears dopamine in the prefrontal cortex where dopamine re-uptake transporters are absent
b. amitriptyline's higher affinity for the serotonin re-uptake transporter is offset by it's metabolite, nortriptyline, which has a higher affinity for the noradrenaline re-uptake transporter
c. serotonin re-uptake inhibition predominates at lower doses; noradrenaline re-uptake inhibition occurs at higher doses
d. assay measured *affinity* for $5HT_{1A}$ receptor but not whether the drug bound as an agonist, partial agonist or antagonist
e. varies with different M receptor subtypes.

4

Psychostimulants are generally considered separately because they *reverse*, rather than inhibit, re-uptake transporters (i.e. actively pump neurotransmitters, particularly dopamine, out of the neurone; see p.225).

Only the Mono-Amine Oxidase Inhibitors (MAOIs) form a clear discrete subclass, but their use requires specialist oversight. MAO type A breaks down serotonin, noradrenaline (norepinephrine) and dopamine. Type B breaks down dopamine. Antidepressant-MAOIs are either non-selective or type A selective. Antiparkinsonian MAOIs (e.g. **selegiline**) are Type B selective.

Depression

Conventional antidepressants increase the synaptic concentration of mono-amines within hours. This triggers a cascade of events within the post-synaptic neurone that alter secondary messengers and genes controlling synaptogenesis (e.g. brain derived neurotrophic factor), circadian rhythm (clock genes), inflammation and receptor sensitivity (see Figure 1).[1,6,7,17] Thus, an improvement in symptoms is slower to manifest. Drugs acting directly on these downstream events act faster (e.g. **ketamine, methylphenidate**) and/or improve symptoms refractory to conventional treatment (e.g. coxibs).[13,17,18]

Various mono-amines contribute to different depressive symptoms. For example, reduced serotonin is believed to result in low mood whereas reduced dopamine is believed to result in anhedonia, reduced motivation and inattention.[1] Thus, a second strategy for treating residual depressive symptoms is to increase additional mono-amines (e.g. switching from an SRI to an SNRI).

Not all mono-amine receptors are helpful in depression. Some have regulatory roles that *reduce* the release of mono-amines within the synapse (e.g. type 2 α-adrenergic autoreceptors) or elsewhere (e.g. post-synaptic $5HT_{2C}$ and $5HT_7$ receptors, which inhibit the downstream release of dopamine and serotonin, respectively). Thus, mono-amine re-uptake inhibitors increase transmission at both helpful and unhelpful receptors. A third strategy for refractory depression is to block one or more unhelpful mono-amine receptor (e.g. adding **mirtazapine** to an existing SNRI).

Some mono-amine receptors mediate opposing effects depending on their location. For example, *post-synaptic* $5HT_{1A}$ receptors mediate many helpful effects whereas *pre-synaptic* $5HT_{1A}$ receptors inhibit serotonin release (i.e. are unhelpful autoreceptors). Some antidepressants and antipsychotics use $5HT_{1A}$ *partial* agonism to enable them to stimulate underactive post-synaptic receptors whilst reducing transmission at overstimulated autoreceptors.[16]

St John's wort (hypericum extract) is as effective as conventional antidepressants in treating mild–moderate depression and causes fewer undesirable effects.[19] However, NICE discourages its use because of:

- uncertainty about appropriate doses
- variation in the nature of products
- potential serious interactions with other drugs (including oral contraceptives, anticoagulants and anti-epileptics).[20]

Anxiety and panic disorder

Antidepressants and benzodiazepines inhibit the amygdala's 'fear circuits' through $5HT_{1A}$ and $GABA_A$ receptors, respectively (see Figure 1, p.150).[21,22] The amygdala is a threat sensor which integrates sensory information with contextual information (e.g. interpretations, memories). If a fear response is required, the amygdala's effector pathway activates the relevant circuits (respiratory and cardiovascular centres, pituitary-adrenal axis, sympathetic autonomic nervous system, and fear-related areas of the cerebral cortex).

Pain

The analgesic effect of antidepressants is predominantly due to enhanced noradrenaline transmission in descending pain modulation pathways, acting upon spinal $\alpha 2$-adrenoceptors.[23,24] Noradrenaline also influences pain transmission in the brain (e.g. the limbic system) and possibly also the peripheral nervous system.[25,26]

The effect of serotonin transmission is more variable; it can induce either analgesia or hyperalgesia depending on the context. The latter may explain both the inconsistent analgesic effect of SSRIs and why SNRIs appear no more effective than NRIs.[27]

Duloxetine, and, to a lesser extent, **amitriptyline**, inhibit P2X4 receptors. These purine-gated calcium channels are upregulated on spinal microglia in neuropathic pain.[28] Sodium-channel blockade and NMDA-glutamate-receptor antagonism may also contribute to the analgesic efficacy of some antidepressants,[23] including the modest effect of topical doxepin.[29,30]

Urological symptoms

Antidepressants act through parasympatholytic and sympathomimetic mechanisms. Antimuscarinic-antidepressants (e.g. **amitriptyline**) inhibit detrusor stimulation and thus overactive bladder symptoms. Mono-amine re-uptake inhibitors (e.g. **duloxetine**, and probably **amitriptyline**) enhance mono-amine transmission in descending bladder control pathways, thus stimulating the sympathetic fibres that control sphincter tone. This explains their modest effect on urinary incontinence.[31]

Pharmacokinetics and pharmacogenetics

The pharmacokinetics of antidepressants are summarized in Table 2. The clearance of many antidepressants is significantly affected by CYP2D6 metabolizer phenotype, and to a lesser extent by CYP2C19. Further, serotonin re-uptake transporter polymorphisms may influence SSRI efficacy.[32] However, clinical benefit from genotyping has yet to be demonstrated.[33]

Table 2 Pharmacokinetic details for selected antidepressants[34–42]

	Bio-availability PO (%)	*T_{max} (h)*	*Plasma halflife (h)*	*Metabolism*
Agomelatine	>80	1–2	1–2	CYP1A2[a]
Amitriptyline	45	4	9–25	Multiple pathways[b] (nortriptyline[b])
Bupropion	>87	1.5	21	CYP2B6[b]
Citalopram	80[c]	3	36	Multiple pathways[b]
Duloxetine	90	6	8–17	CYP1A2, CYP2D6
Fluoxetine	90	4–8	1–4 days 7–15 days[b]	Multiple pathways[b]
Imipramine	45	3	21	Multiple pathways[b] (desipramine[b])
Lofepramine		1–2	1.6	Multiple pathways[b] (desipramine[b])
Methylphenidate	30	1–3	2	Non-CYP hepatic carboxylesterase[a]
Mirtazapine	50	2	20–40	CYP1A2, CYP2D6, CYP3A4
Nortriptyline	60	7–8.5	15–39	CYP2D6[a,b]
Paroxetine	50[d]	5	15–20	Multiple pathways
Reboxetine	95	2–4	12	CYP3A4
Sertraline	>44	6–8	26	CYP3A4
Trazodone	65	1	5–13	CYP2D6, CYP3A4[b]
Venlafaxine	13 45[e]	2.5 4.5–7.5[e]	5 11[b]	CYP2D6, CYP3A4[b]

Blank = no data.

a. significant first pass metabolism
b. active metabolite(s); listed in table if can be administered separately
c. tablet product: bio-availability of drops 25% higher
d. increases with multiple dosing
e. m/r product.

Cautions

In patients with a history of mania, antidepressants may precipitate a recurrent episode, particularly if administered without a mood stabilizer.

Suicide risk

The risk of antidepressant-related suicidal ideation needs to be balanced against the greater risk of non-fatal self harm and completed suicide from untreated depression.[43]

In those aged ≤25 years, antidepressants are associated with suicidal ideation and non-fatal self harm (NNH 143). Some studies found a greater risk with SSRIs than TCAs.[44] In adults ≥25 years, there is a smaller increase in risk (NNH around 700) and no association with the type of antidepressant.[44,45] *The risk is present even when an antidepressant is used for non-depressive indications.*[46]

There *is* a clear association between type of antidepressant and the risk of dying from an overdose: TCAs and MAO inhibitors (highest risk); **mirtazapine** and **venlafaxine** (intermediate); SSRIs (lowest risk).[44]

Suicidal ideation should be evaluated when treating depression in all age groups. Consider the safety in overdose of both the antidepressant and concurrent medicines. In both Europe and the USA, regulators have emphasized the need for close monitoring of adherence to treatment, treatment response, and emergence of thoughts of self harm, particularly during the first month after starting or stopping an antidepressant, and to encourage patients to report to their doctor any deterioration in mood or behaviour.[45,47,48]

Cardiovascular disease and QT prolongation

Citalopram, **escitalopram**, **mirtazapine** and TCAs exhibit dose-related QT prolongation.[49] **Fluoxetine**, **paroxetine** and **sertraline** are less affected. The risk is lowest with **paroxetine**, but drug interactions and withdrawal reactions are more common.[50] Compared with other antidepressants, **citalopram** and **mirtazapine** are associated with a small increase in overall mortality in people aged >65 years[51] but not in those aged 24–65 years.[52]

Consider alternatives (e.g. **sertraline**) in those with cardiovascular disease and/or risk factors for QT prolongation (p.731). If **citalopram** or **escitalopram** is required, note the specific precautions and dose limits recommended by Regulatory Authorities (p.212).

Epilepsy

Although all antidepressants cause seizures in *overdose* (and perhaps also in slow metabolizers), only **amoxapine** (not UK), **bupropion**, **clomipramine** and **maprotiline** (not UK) reduce seizure threshold at therapeutic levels.[53] Antidepressants also cause seizures through hyponatraemia or by altering anti-epileptic drug concentrations as a result of a drug–drug interaction.[54]

Citalopram is widely favoured for use in patients with epilepsy because of the lack of significant interactions with anti-epileptic drugs.[53]

Low-dose TCAs for neuropathic pain have not been studied in patients with previous seizures, but the risk is dose-related and animal studies even suggest a possible *anti*-epileptic action at low doses.[55]

Epilepsy is associated with both mood disorders and psychosis. Symptoms may occur in between (inter-ictal), during (ictal), or in the days or weeks after (post-ictal) seizures. Optimization of anti-epileptic medication should be considered alongside antidepressant treatment, particularly for ictal and post-ictal mood-related symptoms.[56] Further, anti-epileptic drugs can *cause* (and treat) mood disorders: seek specialist advice if negative mood changes occur after anti-epileptics are started.

Parkinson's disease

SSRIs can worsen extrapyramidal symptoms because serotonin reduces nigrostriatal dopamine release via inhibitory $5HT_2$ receptors. However, the risk appears small; few RCTs report any worsening.[57] SSRIs are thus still often used in preference to TCAs which can worsen autonomic dysfunction (α blockade) and cognitive impairment (M blockade).

$5HT_2$ antagonist antidepressants might be expected to avoid serotonin-mediated exacerbations. In small pilot RCTs, Parkinsonian symptoms improved with **nefazodone**[58] but not **mirtazapine**.[59]

Antiparkinsonian D_2 agonists can themselves improve mood. In RCTs evaluating **pramipexole** for motor symptoms, mood and motivation also improved.[60] Further, in an RCT, **pramipexole** was more effective than **sertraline** for depression in patients with Parkinson's disease.[61]

Mono-amine oxidase inhibitors (MAOIs)

Included for general information. MAOIs are *not recommended* in palliative care. They can cause serious adverse events when prescribed concurrently with various other drugs. Seek advice from a psychiatrist if caring for a patient already receiving an MAOI; their previous mental illness is likely to have been difficult to treat and switching or adding other psychotropics is difficult and risky.

MAOIs are potentially dangerous because of the risk of serious dietary and drug interactions. Hypertensive crises are mainly associated with the consumption of tyramine-containing foods (Table 3). Typically, the patient experiences severe headache, and may suffer an intracranial haemorrhage. Drug interactions occur with sympathomimetics (e.g. **ephedrine**, **pseudoephedrine**, **dexamfetamine**, **nefopam**), serotoninergics (see below) and **levodopa**.

Toxicity has been reported with serotoninergic opioids (e.g. fentanils, **pethidine**, **tramadol**). Although companies marketing **morphine** and **oxycodone** advise against concurrent use, their affinity for the serotonin re-uptake transporter is negligible,[62] and toxicity has not been reported.[63] Insisting on a 2-week washout before treating pain is unnecessary.

Table 3 Tyramine-containing foods associated with MAOI-related syndrome

Alcohol	Fava beans
red wine (white wine is safe)	Meat (smoked or pickled)
beer	Meat or yeast extracts
Broad bean pods	Pickled herring
Cheese (old)	

Renal and hepatic impairment

Antidepressants differ in their potential to cause toxicity when renal or hepatic function is impaired, see Chapter 17, p.681 and Chapter 18, p.703 for general information on the choice of antidepressant and use in ESRF or severe hepatic impairment respectively.

Drug interactions

MAOIs have numerous clinically significant drug interactions, which may result in hypertensive crises and serotonin toxicity.

Several pharmacodynamic interactions (e.g. serotonin toxicity, see Box A, bleeding risk, antimuscarinic effects, QT prolongation with **citalopram** and **escitalopram**) can be predicted from the mode of action of antidepressants (see Table 1). Different drugs increase serotonin levels to differing degrees; severe serotonin toxicity is generally associated with the combination of two or more serotonergic drugs.[64] Opioids are relatively weak serotonin re-uptake inhibitors and may only cause symptoms in higher doses or susceptible individuals. Fatalities from serotonin toxicity involving opioids have been seen with **dextromethorphan**, **pethidine**, **tramadol**, and possibly **fentanyl**.[62]

In addition, potentially serious interactions may result from induction or inhibition of hepatic metabolism. Some antidepressants inhibit cytochrome P450 enzymes:

- CYP1A2 inhibition by **fluvoxamine**, e.g. **tizanidine** levels increased ≤33 times
- CYP2C19 inhibition by **fluvoxamine**, e.g. **diazepam** clearance reduced by ≤65%
- CYP2D6 inhibition by **duloxetine**, **fluoxetine** and **paroxetine**, e.g. TCA levels increased ≤10 times; **paroxetine** may reduce the efficacy of **tamoxifen** (a pro-drug).[65]

The metabolism of some antidepressants is affected by other potent P450 inhibitors and inducers:

- **duloxetine**, **mirtazapine** by CYP1A2 inducers and/or inhibitors
- most TCAs, **duloxetine** by CYP2D6 inhibitors
- **mirtazapine, trazodone, venlafaxine** by CYP3A4 inducers and/or inhibitors.

See Chapter 19, Table 8 p.725 and individual monographs for more detail.

Box A Serotonin toxicity[62,64,66,67]

Cause

Ingestion of drug(s) which increase brain serotonin in combination and/or high doses (e.g. overdose):

Antidepressants
Mono-amine oxidase inhibitors
Serotonin re-uptake inhibitors
Dual re-uptake inhibitors

Opioids
Dextromethorphan
Dextropropoxyphene
Fentanils
Methadone
Pentazocine
Pethidine
Tramadol
(but *not* other opioids)

Other psychotropic drugs
Anti-emetic $5HT_3$ antagonists (including metoclopramide)
Psychostimulants
Selegiline (antiparkinsonian)
Sibutramine (anorectic)
Triptans ($5HT_1$ agonists)

Miscellaneous
Chlorphenamine, brompheniramine (but not reported with other H_1 antihistamines)
Furazolidone, linezolid (antibacterials)
Lithium
Methylene blue
Procarbazine (antineoplastic)

Clinical features

Diagnosis is based on a triad of neuro-excitatory features in the presence of serotonergic drugs and the absence of alternative explanations (e.g. sepsis). Symptoms can develop rapidly (e.g. after one or two doses) or gradually (e.g. mild symptoms for weeks before the development of severe toxicity):

- *autonomic hyperactivity*; sweating, fever, mydriasis, tachycardia, hypertension, tachypnoea, sialorrhoea, diarrhoea
- *neuromuscular hyperactivity*; tremor, hyperreflexia, hypertonia, myoclonus, clonus
- *altered mental status*; agitation, altered consciousness, hypomania, delirium.

Treatment

In severe cases (e.g. rigidity, rhabdomyolysis, haemodynamic instability, temperature >38.5°C, deteriorating blood gases) seek urgent advice from a critical care specialist: ventilation and paralysis ± inotropic support may be required.

Discontinue causal medication (toxicity generally resolves within 24h).
Provide supportive care, e.g. IV fluids, oxygen.
Symptomatic measures in mild–moderate cases:

- benzodiazepines for agitation, myoclonus and seizures, e.g. midazolam 5–10mg SC p.r.n.
- $5HT_{2A}$ antagonist[a], e.g.:
  - ▷ chlorpromazine 50–100mg IM *or*
  - ▷ olanzapine 10mg IM (not UK) *or*
  - ▷ cyproheptadine 12mg PO stat followed by 8mg q6h and 2mg q2h p.r.n. until symptoms resolve; tablets can be dispersed (or crushed if necessary) and given by enteral feeding tube (see p.785).

a. prevents deaths from hyperpyrexia in animals and probably in humans. Generally give IM; the PO route is suitable only for mild toxicity and, in the case of overdose, in patients who have *not* received oral activated charcoal.[68,69]

Undesirable effects

A synopsis is contained in Table 4. Overall, discontinuation rates are marginally lower with SSRIs than with TCAs.[70]

Table 4 Relative frequency and putative mechanisms of undesirable effects of antidepressants[44,71,72]

Undesirable effect	*Mechanism*	*Relative frequency*													
		SNRI				*NRI*			*SSRI*					*RA*	
		Amitriptyline	*Duloxetine*	*Imipramine*	*Venlafaxine*	*Desipramine*	*Lofepramine*	*Nortriptyline*	*Citalopram*	*Clomipramine*	*Fluoxetine*	*Paroxetine*	*Sertraline*	*Mirtazapine*	*Trazodone*
GI (nausea, diarrhoea)	↑ Serotonin (acting on $5HT_3$)	–	++	–	++	–	–	–	++	+	++	++	++	–	–
CNS (agitation, restlessness, anxiety, insomnia)	↑ Serotonin (acting on $5HT_2$)	–	+	+	+	+	+	+	+	+	+	+	+	–	–
Weight gain	$5HT_2$ and H_1 antagonism	++	–	+	–	–	–	–	–	+	–	–	–	++	+
Sedation	H_1, M and α_1-adrenergic antagonism	++	–	+	–	+	–	+	–	++	–	–	–	++	++
Postural hypotension	α_1-adrenergic antagonism	++	–	++	–	+	+	+	–	++	–	–	–	–	++
QT prolongation	Cardiac potassium channel blockade	+	+	+	+	+	+	+	++	+	+	-	+	++	+
Sexual dysfunction	↑ Serotonin (acting on $5HT_2$)	+	++	+	++	+	+	+	++	++	++	++	++	–	–
Dry mouth, constipation	M antagonism	++	–	++	–	+	+	+	–	++	–	–	–	–	–
SIADH	↑ Serotonin (acting on $5HT_2$); ↑ noradrenaline (norepinephrine) (acting on α_1)	+	+	+	+	+	+	+	++	+	++	++	++	+	+

++ = relatively common or strong; + = may occur or moderately strong; – = absent or rare/weak.

Abbreviations: NRI = noradrenaline (norepinephrine) re-uptake inhibitor; SNRI = serotonin and noradrenaline re-uptake inhibitor; SSRI = selective serotonin re-uptake inhibitor; RA = receptor antagonist; the remainder refer to receptor types: M = muscarinic acetylcholine; $\alpha_{1/2}$ = α-adrenergic type 1 or 2; H_1 = histamine type 1; $5HT_{2/3}$ = 5-hydroxytryptamine (serotonin) type 2 or 3.

GI bleeding and platelet function

SSRIs and SNRIs decrease serotonin uptake from the blood by platelets. Because platelets do not synthesize serotonin, the amount of serotonin in platelets is reduced.[73] This reduces platelet aggregation.[74] After confounding factors have been controlled for, SRIs increase the risk of GI bleeding, and possibly also intracranial haemorrhage, particularly when used in combination with an NSAID.[75–77] If an antidepressant is indicated in high-risk patients, safer alternatives would include an NRI (e.g. **nortriptyline**) or **mirtazapine**.[78]

Fracture risk

A number of observational studies found an increased fracture risk with SSRIs, SNRIs and TCAs.[79,80] The mechanism is uncertain; data regarding both the risk of falls and bone density is conflicting.

Sweating

In an RCT, the α_1-adrenoceptor antagonist, **terazosin**, alleviated SSRI-related sweating within 14 days of starting 1mg at bedtime.[81]

Use of antidepressants in palliative care

See individual monographs for doses and titration.

Depression

Treatment is tailored to the severity of symptoms, their functional impact and patient preference (Figure 2). The efficacy of cognitive behavioural and drug therapy is comparable.[82] First-line drug treatment is generally with **sertraline** or **citalopram**. They have fewer drug interactions, lower risk in overdose, and are marginally better tolerated than alternatives.[20] Efficacy has been confirmed in palliative populations.[83,84] **Mirtazapine** may be preferred if there is concurrent nausea, insomnia or reduced appetite. An SNRI (e.g. **duloxetine**) may be considered if depression and neuropathic pain co-exist.[85] Frequent re-evaluation of response, adherence, and alternative and concurrent sources of distress is required throughout.

Both **methylphenidate** (p.225) and **ketamine** (p.641) act within days and are sometimes used where prognosis is thought to be ≤4 weeks. However, trials are of short duration; conventional antidepressants should be used if the patient has a sufficient prognosis for a response to manifest.

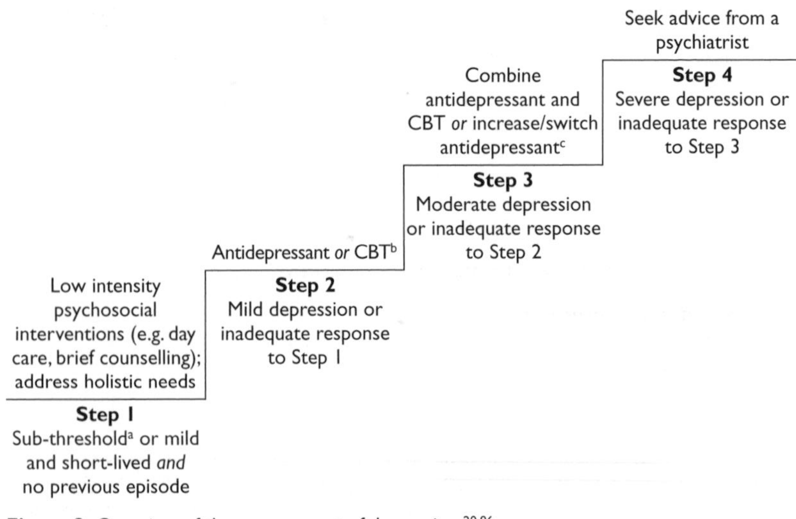

Figure 2 Overview of the management of depression.[20,86]

a. sub-threshold symptoms = patients with <5 DSM IV symptoms required for a diagnosis of depression
b. CBT = cognitive-behavioural therapy
c. see below, managing an inadequate initial response.

Titrating, switching and combining antidepressants

If there is *no* response after 2–4 weeks or only a partial response after 6–8 weeks:

- increase the dose, particularly if there has been a partial response and minimal undesirable effects *or*
- switch antidepressants, particularly if there has been minimal improvement or bothersome undesirable effects *or*
- combine with a second antidepressant or adjuvant psychotropic drug, particularly if a previous switch was unhelpful.[20,44,87]

Dose titration is straightforward but, for SSRIs and **duloxetine**, of uncertain value. A systematic review found dose titration in patients not responding to SSRIs taken for 3–6 weeks no more effective than continuing the dose unaltered.[88] Nonetheless, many guidelines highlight individual variation in effective doses and therefore recommend dose titration if the existing drug is well tolerated.[20,44] A dose-response effect is more clearly established with some TCAs and **venlafaxine**.

The efficacy of second-line antidepressants appears comparable regardless of mode of action.[44,89,90] Options include an alternative SSRI or **mirtazapine**. One SSRI can be directly substituted for another without cross-tapering or a washout period.[44,90] **Mirtazapine** 15mg can be directly substituted for SSRIs at usual doses (**fluoxetine**, **citalopram** or **paroxetine** 20mg; **sertraline** 50mg).[44,91]

Opinion varies on the need to taper higher SSRI doses before switching.[89,91] Switching SSRIs is most effective when the first SSRI is poorly tolerated but benefit is also seen in non-responders,[90] perhaps because of differing additional actions (see p.213). The effect of **mirtazapine** on additional monoamines is theoretically advantageous, and its onset may be faster.[92]

Venlafaxine has a marginally higher response rate compared with switching to a second SSRI[90] but is less well tolerated. Switching to or from TCAs and MAOIs requires additional care because of the potential for clinically significant pharmacokinetic or pharmacodynamic drug interactions, respectively (see above).[93]

A partial response to an antidepressant can be increased ('augmented') by adding a second psychotropic drug to an SSRI or SNRI. This avoids potential loss of the initial improvement but is generally less well tolerated than monotherapy.[20] Options include:[44]

- antipsychotics (e.g. **quetiapine or olanzapine**)
- **mirtazapine**
- a range of options used only by psychiatrists (e.g. **lithium**, **tri-iodothyronine**).

NICE suggests primary care clinicians seek advice before adding a second drug.[20] Palliative care specialists using some of the above for other indications should be aware of their potential benefit when concurrent depression has only partially responded to an antidepressant.

Duration of treatment

Consider stopping treatment 6 months after full remission in those without risk factors for relapse. Risk factors include previous depression and the severity, duration, degree of treatment resistance, and the presence of residual symptoms. Treatment is tapered slowly (see below). Treat those with risk factors for longer:

- 1 year if full remission but one risk factor
- ≥2 years if ≥2 risk factors.[20,44]

In palliative care, the latter is likely to mean lifelong/indefinitely.

Anxiety and panic disorders

The efficacy of cognitive behavioural and drug therapy is comparable.[94] Choice of drug is largely influenced by likely duration of use:

- benzodiazepine, if prognosis is days to weeks
- SSRI (± a benzodiazepine initially), if prognosis is months.

Supporting evidence (and market authorization) for SSRIs varies for different anxiety disorders.[94] **Citalopram** and **sertraline** are authorized for panic disorder, well tolerated, have fewer drug interactions, and are generally more familiar to prescribers. All SSRIs can initially exacerbate anxiety: start low and consider a concurrent benzodiazepine for the first few weeks. If response is inadequate, consider:

- combining with cognitive behavioural therapy
- switching to **venlafaxine** or **duloxetine**
- combining with or switching to **pregabalin** or a benzodiazepine.

In general psychiatry, switching is not advocated within 3 months because benefit from SSRIs can take longer to manifest than in depression.[94,95] However, in patients with a short prognosis, adding **pregabalin** or a benzodiazepine may bring more rapid benefit. **Quetiapine** also acts quickly but is less well tolerated and so is generally reserved for anxiety refractory to antidepressants ± benzodiazepines ± **pregabalin**.[94]

Neuropathic pain

Amitriptyline, **imipramine** and **duloxetine** are commonly used for neuropathic pain.[96] In both direct comparisons and network analyses, their efficacy and tolerability appear to be similar to each other and to **gabapentin/pregabalin**.[27,97–107] Inhibition of noradrenaline re-uptake is important to their analgesic action: SSRIs are not consistently effective.[96] The benefit reported with **mirtazapine**[108] has *not* been confirmed in RCTs.

If the first choice treatment is poorly tolerated, consider switching to an alternative antidepressant (e.g. **amitriptyline** → **duloxetine**). **Nortriptyline** is used less commonly because it is more expensive than alternatives (including **duloxetine**). However, switching is unlikely to improve efficacy unless undesirable effects have prevented dose titration; all predominantly act on noradrenaline transmission; the clinical relevance of their dissimilar actions is unclear (e.g. **amitriptyline** → sodium channels, **duloxetine** → P2X4 receptors, see above).[28]

If the first choice treatment fails, switch to or combine with an anti-epileptic (p.256). The combination of **imipramine** or **nortriptyline** with **gabapentin**, **pregabalin** or **morphine** is superior to any treatment alone.[109–112]

Other pain syndromes

Antidepressants are of benefit for various pain syndromes, including migraine and tension headache (TCAs),[113] chronic low back pain (**duloxetine**),[114] fibromyalgia (**amitriptyline**, **duloxetine**, **milnacipran** (not UK), **mirtazapine**),[115–117] and osteo-arthritis (**duloxetine**).[118]

Agitated delirium

The benefit reported with **trazodone**[119] remains unconfirmed in clinical trials. Treatment of underlying causes, non-drug management (e.g. orientation strategies, correction of sensory deprivation) and prevention of complications are central to delirium management. Antipsychotics are generally used first-line when medication is needed (see p.176).

Agitation and challenging behaviours in dementia

Evidence for antidepressants is insufficient to justify routine use. Although **citalopram** was more effective than placebo, a subgroup of patients appeared to deteriorate more rapidly compared to controls.[120] A small RCT (n=30) found **trazodone** improved sleep disturbance.[121]

Sweating

Like other antimuscarinics, **amitriptyline** is used for paraneoplastic sweating unresponsive to NSAIDs.[122] However, like all mono-amine reuptake inhibitors, it can also *cause* sweating.[123]

Hot flushes

Trials in patients with breast cancer have found benefit from SSRIs (p.212), **venlafaxine** (p.216) and **gabapentin** (see p.272).[124] **Venlafaxine** works faster than **clonidine** (p.77), and participants prefer **venlafaxine** over **gabapentin**.[124] **Venlafaxine** and SSRIs are also reported to improve hot flushes in men resulting from medical or surgical castration.[125–127]

Insomnia

When insomnia co-exists with other indications, sedating antidepressants are often selected (e.g. TCAs, **mirtazapine**, **trazodone**). **Doxepin** 3–6mg PO at bedtime improves both sleep latency and fragmentation in primary insomnia (UK preparation = 25mg and is significantly more expensive than other TCAs). Benefit is sustained for ≥12 weeks without rebound insomnia after discontinuation.[128] **Trazodone** is commonly used, although evidence is limited (see p.223).

Pruritus

Two small RCTs found benefit within a few days from **sertraline** (cholestatic pruritus)[129] and **paroxetine** (pruritus of mixed cause in cancer patients).[130] A slower response to **sertraline** was seen in uraemic pruritus (>2 weeks).[131] Benefit is also reported in pruritus in polycythemia vera (mostly **paroxetine**),[132] pruritus of mixed cause in advanced disease (**mirtazapine**),[133] and carcinoma en cuirasse (**mirtazapine**).[134] H_1 antagonists can be used for histamine-mediated pruritus and/or for night sedation (p.757).

Bladder spasm, stress incontinence and urgency

Antimuscarinic antidepressants (e.g. **amitriptyline**) reduce detrusor contractions associated with urgency, although authorized alternatives have additional direct effects on the detrusor muscle.[135] **Duloxetine** has a limited role in stress incontinence.[136]

Pathological laughter and crying

Frequent brief uncontrollable laughter and/or crying incongruent with external events can complicate numerous neurological disorders, including strokes, Parkinson's disease, cerebral tumours, multiple sclerosis, MND/ALS, and dementia. It can be socially disabling. Functional imaging suggests dysregulation of serotoninergic and other mono-aminergic pathways. The differential diagnosis includes:

- seizures: generally complex partial seizures and thus an alteration of consciousness during/after episodes
- depression or other mood disorders; mood alteration is persistent whereas the emotion which may accompany pathological laughter and crying is short-lived.

Validated assessment tools are available to aid diagnosis.[137] First-line treatment is with **citalopram** or **sertraline**; doses can be lower than those required for depression. Benefit is often seen within days. Second-line options include **amitriptyline, imipramine, nortriptyline** and **levodopa**.[138]

Drooling

Like other antimuscarinics, **amitriptyline** reduces salivation (see p.5).

Refactory cough

Amitriptyline is more effective than **codeine** for cough which persists despite resolution of the initial cause.[139] **Gabapentin** is an alternative (p.272). Benefit probably relates to reducing cough reflex hypersensitivity, which is generally present in this group of patients (see p.140).[2]

Breathlessness

An RCT in cancer found **buspirone** was *ineffective* for breathlessness and secondary anxiety.[140] **Sertraline** is reported to improve breathlessness in COPD (n=7).[141]

Stopping antidepressants

Abrupt cessation of antidepressant therapy (particularly an MAOI) after regular administration for >8 weeks may result in a discontinuation reaction (withdrawal syndrome, Box B).[142] Discontinuation reactions depend on the class of antidepressant, and are more common with drugs with shorter half-lives. Thus, with SSRIs, they are most common with **paroxetine** and least common with **fluoxetine**.

Discontinuation reactions differ from a depressive relapse or a panic disorder. They generally start abruptly within a few days of stopping the antidepressant (*or reducing its dose*). In contrast, a depressive relapse is uncommon in the first week after stopping an antidepressant, and symptoms tend to build up gradually and persist. Discontinuation reactions generally resolve within 24h of re-instating antidepressant therapy, whereas the response is slower with a depressive relapse.

Ideally, antidepressants taken for >8 weeks should be progressively reduced over 4 weeks. If a mild discontinuation reaction is suspected, re-assurance alone may be adequate. If distressing, restart the antidepressant and reduce more gradually.

Some patients experience discontinuation symptoms even during tapering. When this happens, increase the dose and, before continuing with tapering, consider:

- using a liquid formulation and reducing the dose in smaller steps *or*
- switching from **venlafaxine** or a short half-life SSRI to **fluoxetine**.[142]

Box B Antidepressant discontinuation reactions[142]

SSRIs and venlafaxine: '*FINISH*' [143]
Flu-like symptoms (fatigue, lethargy, myalgia, chills)
Insomnia (including vivid dreams)
Nausea
Imbalance (ataxia, vertigo, dizziness)
Sensory disturbances (paraesthesia, sensations of electric shock)
Hyperarousal (restlessness, anxiety, agitation)

TCAs
Flu-like symptoms (fatigue, lethargy, myalgia, chills)
Insomnia (including vivid dreams)
GI disorders (nausea, diarrhoea)
Mood disorders (depression or mania)
Movement disorders (rare: akathisia, parkinsonism)

Trazodone
Flu-like symptoms (fatigue, lethargy, myalgia, chills)
GI disorders (nausea, diarrhoea)
Restlessness
Tremor
Headache

Mirtazapine
Nausea
Dizziness
Hyperarousal (anxiety, agitation)
Headache

MAOIs
Insomnia
Movement disorders (ataxia, athetosis, catatonia, myoclonus)
Mood disorders (lability, depression, agitation, aggression)
Paranoia
Hallucinations
Seizures
Altered speech (pressured, slow)

1 Stahl SM (2013) Chapter 6: Mood disorders. In: *Essential Psychopharmacology: Neuroscientific Basis and Practial Applications* (4e). Cambridge University Press, USA. 237–283.
2 Wei W *et al.* (2016) The efficacy of specific neuromodulators on human refractory chronic cough: a systematic review and meta-analysis. *Journal of Thoracic Diseases*. **8**: 2942–2951.
3 Bassari R and Koea JB (2015) Jaundice associated pruritis: a review of pathophysiology and treatment. *World Journal of Gastroenterology*. **21**: 1404–1413.
4 Archer DF *et al.* (2011) Menopausal hot flushes and night sweats: where are we now? *Climacteric*. **14**: 515–528.
5 Lauterbach EC *et al.* (2013) Toward a more precise, clinically--informed pathophysiology of pathological laughing and crying. *Neuroscience and Biobehavorial Reviews*. **37**: 1893–1916.
6 Miller BR and Hen R (2015) The current state of the neurogenic theory of depression and anxiety. *Current Opinion in Neurobiology*. **30**: 51–58.
7 Duman RS *et al.* (2016) Synaptic plasticity and depression: new insights from stress and rapid-acting antidepressants. *Nature Medicine*. **22**: 238–249.
8 Tynan RJ *et al.* (2012) A comparative examination of the anti-inflammatory effects of SSRI and SNRI antidepressants on LPS stimulated microglia. *Brain Behavior and Immunity*. **26**: 469–479.
9 Stahl SM *et al.* (2004) A Review of the Neuropharmacology of Bupropion, a Dual Norepinephrine and Dopamine Reuptake Inhibitor. *Primary Care Companion Journal of Clinical Psychiatry*. **6**: 159–166.
10 Beique JC *et al.* (1998) Affinities of venlafaxine and various reuptake inhibitors for the serotonin and norepinephrine transporters. *European Journal of Pharmacology*. **349**: 129–132.

11 Hamon M and Bourgoin S (2006) Pharmacological profile of antidepressants: a likely basis for their efficacy and side effects? *European Neuropsychopharmacology*. **16 (Suppl 5)**: s625–s632.
12 Garnock-Jones KP (2014) Vortioxetine: a review of its use in major depressive disorder. *CNS Drugs*. **28**: 855–874.
13 Stahl SM (2013) Chapter 7: Antidepressants. In: *Essential Psychopharmacology: Neuroscientific Basis and Practical Applications* (4e). Cambridge University Press, USA, pp. 284–369.
14 Gillman PK (2007) Tricyclic antidepressant pharmacology and therapeutic drug interactions updated. *British Journal of Pharmacology*. **151**: 737–748.
15 Binding DB (2015) Skaggs School of Pharmacy and Pharmaceutical Sciences Binding Database. Available from: http://bindingdb.org/as/search.html Accessed June 2015
16 Stahl SM *et al.* (2013) Serotonergic drugs for depression and beyond. *Current Drug Targets*. **14**: 578–585.
17 Yirmiya R *et al.* (2015) Depression as a microglial disease. *Trends Neurosciences*. **38**: 637–658.
18 Williams NR and Schatzberg AF (2016) NMDA antagonist treatment of depression. *Current Opinion in Neurobiology*. **36**: 112–117.
19 Linde (2008) St John's wort for major depression. *Cochrane Database of Systematic Reviews*. **4**: CD000448. www.thecochranelibrary.com
20 NICE (2009) Depression. *Clinical Guidelines*. CG90 and CG91. www.nice.org.uk
21 Capogna M (2014) GABAergic cell type diversity in the basolateral amygdala. *Current Opinion in Neurobiology*. **26**: 110–116.
22 Stahl SM (2013) Chapter 9: Anxiety disorders and anxiolytics. In: *Essential Psychopharmacology: Neuroscientific Basis and Practical Applications (4e)*. Cambridge University Press, USA, pp. 388–419.
23 Kremer M *et al.* (2016) Antidepressants and gabapentinoids in neuropathic pain: Mechanistic insights. *Neuroscience*. **338**: 183–206.
24 Llorca-Torralba M *et al.* (2016) Noradrenergic Locus Coeruleus pathways in pain modulation. *Neuroscience*. **338**: 93–113.
25 Bannister K and Dickenson AH (2016) What the brain tells the spinal cord. *Pain*. **157**: 2148–2151.
26 Taylor BK and Westlund KN (2017) The noradrenergic locus coeruleus as a chronic pain generator. *Journal of Neuroscience Research*. **95**: 1336–1346.
27 Watson CP *et al.* (1998) Nortriptyline versus amitriptyline in postherpetic neuralgia: a randomized trial. *Neurology*. **51**: 1166–1171.
28 Yamashita T *et al.* (2016) Duloxetine inhibits microglial P2X4 receptor function and alleviates neuropathic pain after peripheral nerve injury. *PLoS One*. **11**: e0165189.
29 McCleane G (2000) Topical application of doxepin hydrochloride, capsaicin and a combination of both produces analgesia in chronic human neuropathic pain: a randomized, double-blind, placebo-controlled study. *British Journal of Clinical Pharmacology*. **49**: 574–579.
30 McCleane (1999) Topical doxepin hydrochloride reduces neuropathic pain: a randomised, double-blind, placebo-controlled study. *Pain Clinic*. **12**: 47–50.
31 Deepak P and Kumar TN (2011) Duloexetine - pharmacological aspects. *International Journal of Biological and Medical Research*. **2**: 589–592.
32 Porcelli S *et al.* (2012) Meta-analysis of serotonin transporter gene promoter polymorphism (5-HTTLPR) association with antidepressant efficacy. *European Neuropsychopharmacology*. **22**: 239–258.
33 Kirchheiner J and Rodriguez-Antona C (2009) Cytochrome P450 2D6 genotyping: potential role in improving treatment outcomes in psychiatric disorders. *CNS Drugs*. **23**: 181–191.
34 Wen B *et al.* (2008) Detection of novel reactive metabolites of trazodone: evidence for CYP2D6-mediated bioactivation of m-chlorophenylpiperazine. *Drug Metabolism and Disposition*. **36**: 841–850.
35 Jefferson JW *et al.* (2005) Bupropion for major depressive disorder: Pharmacokinetic and formulation considerations. *Clinical Therapeutics*. **27**: 1685–1695.
36 Hiemke (2000) Pharmacokinetics of selective serotonin reuptake inhibitors. *Pharmacology and Therapeutics*. **85**: 11–28.
37 Fleishaker JC (2000) Clinical pharmacokinetics of reboxetine, a selective norepinephrine reuptake inhibitor for the treatment of patients with depression. *Clinical Pharmacokinetics*. **39**: 413–427.
38 Venkatakrishnan K *et al.* (1998) Five distinct human cytochromes mediate amitriptyline N-demethylation in vitro: dominance of CYP 2C19 and 3A4. *Journal of Clinical Pharmacology*. **38**: 112–121.
39 Richelson E (1997) Pharmacokinetic drug interactions of new antidepressants: A review of the effects on the metabolism of other drugs. *Mayo Clinic Proceedings*. **72**: 835–847.
40 Kaye CM *et al.* (1989) A review of the metabolism and pharmacokinetics of paroxetine in man. *Acta Psychiatrica Scandinavica Supplementum*. **350**: 60–75.
41 Schulz P *et al.* (1985) Discrepancies between pharmacokinetic studies of amitriptyline. *Clinical Pharmacokinetics*. **10**: 257–268.
42 Abernethyl DR *et al.* (1984) Absolute bioavailability of imipramine: influence of food. *Psychopharmacology (Berl)*. **83**: 104–106.
43 Lu CY *et al.* (2014) Changes in antidepressant use by young people and suicidal behavior after FDA warnings and media coverage: quasi-experimental study. *British Medical Journal*. **348**: g3596.
44 Cleare A *et al.* (2015) Evidence-based guidelines for treating depressive disorders with antidepressants: A revision of the 2008 British Association for Psychopharmacology guidelines. *Journal of Psychopharmacology*. **29**: 459–525.
45 Coupland C *et al.* (2015) Antidepressant use and risk of suicide and attempted suicide or self harm in people aged 20 to 64: cohort study using a primary care database. *British Medical Journal*. **350**: h517.
46 Pereira A *et al.* (2014) Suicidal ideation and behavior associated with antidepressant medications: Implications for the treatment of chronic pain. *Pain*. **155**: 2471–2475.
47 MHRA (2007) Antidepressants: suicidal behaviour. *Drug Safety Update*. **(1) 1**: www.mhra.gov.uk/safetyinformation
48 Sinyor M and Cheung AH (2015) Antidepressants and risk of suicide. *British Medical Journal*. **350**: h783.
49 Jasiak NM and Bostwick JR (2014) Risk of QT/QTc prolongation among newer non-SSRI antidepressants. *Annals of Pharmacotherpy*. **48**: 1620–1628.
50 Funk KA and Bostwick JR (2013) A comparison of the risk of QT prolongation among SSRIs. *Annals of Pharmacotherapy*. **47**: 1330–1341.
51 Danielsson B *et al.* (2016) Antidepressants and antipsychotics classified with torsades de pointes arrhythmia risk and mortality in older adults - a Swedish nationwide study. *British Journal of Clinical Pharmacology*. **81**: 773–783.
52 Coupland C *et al.* (2016) Antidepressant use and risk of cardiovascular outcomes in people aged 20 to 64: cohort study using primary care database. *British Medical Journal*. **352**: i1350.
53 Kanner AM (2013) The treatment of depressive disorders in epilepsy: what all neurologists should know. *Epilepsia*. **54 (Suppl 1)**: 3–12.
54 Kerr MP *et al.* (2011) International consensus clinical practice statements for the treatment of neuropsychiatric conditions associated with epilepsy. *Epilepsia*. **52**: 2133–2138.
55 Dailey JW and Naritoku DK (1996) Antidepressants and seizures: clinical anecdotes overshadow neuroscience. *Biochemical Pharmacology*. **52**: 1323–1329.

56 Blumer D *et al.* (2004) The interictal dysphoric disorder: recognition, pathogenesis, and treatment of the major psychiatric disorder of epilepsy. *Epilepsy and Behaviour.* **5**: 826–840.

57 Skapinakis P *et al.* (2010) Efficacy and acceptability of selective serotonin reuptake inhibitors for the treatment of depression in Parkinson's disease: a systematic review and meta-analysis of randomized controlled trials. *BMC Neurology.* **10**: 49.

58 Avila A *et al.* (2003) Does nefazodone improve both depression and Parkinson disease? A pilot randomized trial. *Journal of Clinical Psychopharmacology.* **23**: 509–513.

59 Zhang LS *et al.* (2006) Mirtazapine vs fluoxetine in treatng Parkinson's disease with depression and anxiety. *Medical Journal of Chinese People's Health.* DOI: CNKI:SUN:ZMYX.0.2006-2023–2001.

60 Leentjens AF *et al.* (2009) The effect of pramipexole on mood and motivational symptoms in Parkinson's disease: a meta-analysis of placebo-controlled studies. *Clinical Therapeutics.* **31**: 89–98.

61 Barone P *et al.* (2006) Pramipexole versus sertraline in the treatment of depression in Parkinson's disease: a national multicenter parallel-group randomized study. *Journal of Neurology.* **253**: 601–607.

62 Gillman PK (2005) Monoamine oxidase inhibitors, opioid analgesics and serotonin toxicity. *British Journal of Anaesthesia.* **95**: 434–441.

63 Baxter K and Preston CL Stockley's Drug Interactions London: Pharmaceutical Press, www.medicinescomplete.com (accessed May 2017).

64 Werneke U *et al.* (2016) Conundrums in neurology: diagnosing serotonin syndrome - a meta-analysis of cases. *BMC Neurology.* **16**: 97.

65 Kelly CM *et al.* (2010) Selective serotonin reuptake inhibitors and breast cancer mortality in women receiving tamoxifen: a population based cohort study. *British Medical Journal.* **340**: c693.

66 Gillman K (2006) Serotonin toxicity, serotonin syndrome. *Psycho Tropical Research.* www.psychotropical.com (accessed April 2013).

67 Gillman PK (2006) A review of serotonin toxicity data: implications for the mechanisms of antidepressant drug action. *Biological Psychiatry.* **59**: 1046–1051.

68 Gillman PK (1999) The serotonin syndrome and its treatment. *Journal of Psychopharmacology.* **13**: 100–109.

69 Gillman PK (1998) Serotonin syndrome: history and risk. *Fundamental and Clinical Pharmacology.* **12**: 482–491.

70 Anderson IM (2000) Selective serotonin reuptake inhibitors versus tricyclic antidepressants: a meta-analysis of efficacy and tolerability. *Journal of Affective Disorders.* **58**: 19–36.

71 Bhuvaneswar CG *et al.* (2009) Adverse endocrine and metabolic effects of psychotropic drugs: selective clinical review. *CNS Drugs.* **23**: 1003–1021.

72 Jacob S and Spinler SA (2006) Hyponatremia associated with selective serotonin-reuptake inhibitors in older adults. *Annals of Pharmacotherapy.* **40**: 1618–1622.

73 Ross S *et al.* (1980) Inhibition of 5-hydroxytryptamine uptake in human platelets by antidepressant agents in vivo. *Psychopharmacology.* **67**: 1–7.

74 Li N *et al.* (1997) Effects of serotonin on platelet activation in whole blood. *Blood Coagulation Fibrinolysis.* **8**: 517–523.

75 vanWalraven C *et al.* (2001) Inhibition of serotonin reuptake by antidepressants and upper gastrointestinal bleeding in elderly patients: retrospective cohort study. *British Medical Journal.* **323**: 655–657.

76 Paton C and Ferrier IN (2005) SSRIs and gastrointestinal bleeding. *British Medical Journal.* **331**: 529–530.

77 Shin JY *et al.* (2015) Risk of intracranial haemorrhage in antidepressant users with concurrent use of non-steroidal anti-inflammatory drugs: nationwide propensity score matched study. *British Medical Journal.* **351**: h3517.

78 deAbajo FJ and Garcia-Rodriguez LA (2008) Risk of upper gastrointestinal tract bleeding associated with selective serotonin reuptake inhibitors and venlafaxine therapy: interaction with nonsteroidal anti-inflammatory drugs and effect of acid-suppressing agents. *Archives of General Psychiatry.* **65**: 795–803.

79 European Medicines Agency (2010) Pharmacovigilance working party March 2010 plenary meeting report. Available from: www.emea.europa.eu

80 Lanteigne A *et al.* (2015) Serotonin-norepinephrine reuptake inhibitor and selective serotonin reuptake inhibitor use and risk of fractures: a new-user cohort study among US adults aged 50 years and older. *CNS Drugs.* **29**: 245–252.

81 Ghaleiha A *et al.* (2013) Effect of terazosin on sweating in patients with major depressive disorder receiving sertraline: a randomized controlled trial. *International Journal of Psychiatry in Clinical Practice.* **17**: 44–47.

82 Amick HR *et al.* (2015) Comparative benefits and harms of second generation antidepressants and cognitive behavioral therapies in initial treatment of major depressive disorder: systematic review and meta-analysis. *British Medical Journal.* **351**: h6019.

83 Rayner L *et al.* (2011) Antidepressants for the treatment of depression in palliative care: systematic review and meta-analysis. *Palliative Medicine.* **25**: 36–51.

84 Ostuzzi G *et al.* (2015) Efficacy and acceptability of antidepressants on the continuum of depressive experiences in patients with cancer: Systematic review and meta-analysis. *Cancer Treatment Reviews.* **41**: 714–724.

85 Rosenberg L and deLima Thomas J (2016) Pharmacologic management of depression in advanced illness. *Journal of Palliative Medicine.* **19**: 783–784.

86 Rayner L *et al.* (2011) The development of evidence-based European guidelines on the management of depression in palliative cancer care. *European Journal of Cancer.* **47**: 702–712.

87 Kudlow PA *et al.* (2014) Early switching strategies in antidepressant non-responders: current evidence and future research directions. *CNS Drugs.* **28**: 601–609.

88 Adli M *et al.* (2005) Is dose escalation of antidepressants a rational strategy after a medium-dose treatment has failed? A systematic review. *European Archives of Psychiatry and Clinical Neuroscience.* **255**: 387–400.

89 Rush AJ *et al.* (2009) STAR*D: revising conventional wisdom. *CNS Drugs.* **23**: 627–647.

90 Ruhe HG *et al.* (2006) Switching antidepressants after a first selective serotonin reuptake inhibitor in major depressive disorder: a systematic review. *Journal of Clinical Psychiatry.* **67**: 1836–1855.

91 Fava GA and Mangelli L (2001) Assessment of subclinical symptoms and psychological well-being in depression. *European Archives of Psychiatry and Clinical Neuroscience.* **251 (Suppl 2)**: II47–52.

92 Watanabe N *et al.* (2011) Mirtazapine versus other antidepressive agents for depression. *Cochrane Database of Systematic Reviews.* **12**: CD006528. www.thecochranelibrary.com

93 Taylor (2007) *The Maundsley Prescribing Guidelines* (9e). Informa Healthcare, London.

94 Baldwin DS *et al.* (2014) Evidence-based pharmacological treatment of anxiety disorders, post-traumatic stress disorder and obsessive-compulsive disorder: a revision of the 2005 guidelines from the British Association for Psychopharmacology. *Journal of Psychopharmacology.* **28**: 403–439.

95 NICE (2011) Generalised anxiety disorder and panic disorder (with or without agoraphobia) in adults: Management in primary, secondary and community care. *Clinical Guideline.* CG113. www.nice.org.uk

96 Finnerup NB *et al.* (2016) Pharmacotherapy for neuropathic pain in adults: a systematic review and meta-analysis. *Lancet Neurology.* **14**: 162–173.

97 Boyle J *et al.* (2012) Randomized, placebo-controlled comparison of amitriptyline, duloxetine, and pregabalin in patients with chronic diabetic peripheral neuropathic pain: impact on pain, polysomnographic sleep, daytime functioning, and quality of life. *Diabetes Care.* **35**: 2451–2458.
98 Bansal D *et al.* (2009) Amitriptyline vs. pregabalin in painful diabetic neuropathy: a randomized double blind clinical trial. *Diabetic Medicine.* **26**: 1019–1026.
99 Morello C *et al.* (1999) Randomized double-blind study comparing the efficacy of gabapentin with amitriptyline on diabetic peripheral neuropathy pain. *Archives of Internal Medicine.* **159**: 1931–1937.
100 Chandra K *et al.* (2006) Gabapentin versus nortriptyline in post-herpetic neuralgia patients: a randomized, double-blind clinical trial--the GONIP Trial. *International Journal of Clinical Pharmacology and Therapeutics.* **44**: 358–363.
101 Mishra S *et al.* (2012) A comparative efficacy of amitriptyline, gabapentin, and pregabalin in neuropathic cancer pain: a prospective randomized double-blind placebo-controlled study. *American Journal of Hospice and Palliative Care.* **29**: 177–182.
102 Kaur H *et al.* (2011) A comparative evaluation of amitriptyline and duloxetine in painful diabetic neuropathy: a randomized, double-blind, cross-over clinical trial. *Diabetes Care.* **34**: 818–822.
103 Sindrup SH *et al.* (2003) Venlafaxine versus imipramine in painful polyneuropathy: a randomized, controlled trial. *Neurology.* **60**: 1284–1289.
104 Watson CP *et al.* (2011) Nontricyclic antidepressant analgesics and pain: are serotonin norepinephrine reuptake inhibitors (SNRIs) any better? *Pain.* **152**: 2206–2210.
105 Griebeler ML *et al.* (2014) Pharmacologic interventions for painful diabetic neuropathy: An umbrella systematic review and comparative effectiveness network meta-analysis. *Annals of Internal Medicine.* **161**: 639–649.
106 Banerjee M *et al.* (2013) A comparative study of efficacy and safety of gabapentin versus amitriptyline as coanalgesics in patients receiving opioid analgesics for neuropathic pain in malignancy. *Indian Journal of Pharmacology.* **45**: 334–338.
107 NICE (2013) Neuropathic pain - pharmacological management (appendix G). *Clinical Guideline.* CG173. www.nice.org.uk
108 Christodoulou C *et al.* (2010) Effectiveness of mirtazapine in the treatment of postherpetic neuralgia. *Journal of Pain and Symptom Management.* **39**: e3–6.
109 Gilron I *et al.* (2009) Nortriptyline and gabapentin, alone and in combination for neuropathic pain: a double-blind, randomised controlled crossover trial. *Lancet.* **374**: 1252–1261.
110 Holbech JV *et al.* (2015) Imipramine and pregabalin combination for painful polyneuropathy: a randomized controlled trial. *Pain.* **156**: 958–966.
111 Gilron I *et al.* (2015) Combination of morphine with nortriptyline for neuropathic pain. *Pain.* **156**: 1440–1448.
112 Tesfaye S *et al.* (2013) Duloxetine and pregabalin: high-dose monotherapy or their combination? The "COMBO-DN study"--a multinational, randomized, double-blind, parallel-group study in patients with diabetic peripheral neuropathic pain. *Pain.* **154**: 2616–2625.
113 Jackson JL *et al.* (2010) Tricyclic antidepressants and headaches: systematic review and meta-analysis. *British Medical Journal.* **341**: c5222.
114 Moore RA *et al.* (2014) Duloxetine use in chronic painful conditions--individual patient data responder analysis. *European Journal of Pain.* **18**: 67–75.
115 Hauser W *et al.* (2012) The role of antidepressants in the management of fibromyalgia syndrome: a systematic review and meta-analysis. *CNS Drugs.* **26**: 297–307.
116 Lunn MP *et al.* (2014) Duloxetine for treating painful neuropathy, chronic pain or fibromyalgia. *Cochrane Database of Systematic Reviews.* **1**: CD007115. www.thecochranelibrary.com
117 Miki K *et al.* (2016) Efficacy of mirtazapine for the treatment of fibromyalgia without concomitant depression: a randomized, double-blind, placebo-controlled phase IIa study in Japan. *Pain.* **157**: 2089–2096.
118 Citrome L and Weiss-Citrome A (2012) A systematic review of duloxetine for osteoarthritic pain: what is the number needed to treat, number needed to harm, and likelihood to be helped or harmed? *Postgraduate Medicine.* **124**: 83–93.
119 Okamoto Y *et al.* (1999) Trazodone in the treatment of delirium. *Journal of Clinical Psychopharmacology.* **19**: 280–282.
120 Forlenza OV *et al.* (2017) Recent advances in the management of neuropsychiatric symptoms in dementia. *Current Opinion in Psychiatry.* **30**: 151–158.
121 McCleery J *et al.* (2014) Pharmacotherapies for sleep disturbances in Alzheimer's disease. *Cochrane Database of Systematic Reviews.* **3**: CD009178. www.thecochranelibrary.com
122 Twycross R and Wilcock A (eds) (2016) *Introducing Palliative Care* (5e). palliativedrugs.com Ltd, Nottingham, p. 340.
123 Marcy TR and Britton ML (2005) Antidepressant-induced sweating. *Annals of Pharmacotherapy.* **39**: 748–752.
124 Johns C *et al.* (2016) Informing hot flash treatment decisions for breast cancer survivors: a systematic review of randomized trials comparing active interventions. *Breast Cancer Research and Treatment.* **156**: 415–426.
125 Quella S *et al.* (1999) Pilot evaluation of venlafaxine for the treatment of hot flashes in men undergoing androgen ablation therapy for prostate cancer. *Journal of Urology.* **162**: 98–102.
126 Loprinzi CL *et al.* (2011) Nonestrogenic management of hot flashes. *Journal of Clinical Oncology.* **29**: 3842–3846.
127 Roth AJ and Scher HI (1998) Sertraline relieves hot flashes secondary to medical castration as treatment of advanced prostate cancer. *Psychooncology.* **7**: 129–132.
128 Weber J *et al.* (2010) Low-dose doxepin: in the treatment of insomnia. *CNS Drugs.* **24**: 713–720.
129 Mayo MJ *et al.* (2007) Sertraline as a first-line treatment for cholestatic pruritus. *Hepatology.* **45**: 666–674.
130 Zylicz Z *et al.* (2003) Paroxetine in the treatment of severe non-dermatological pruritus: a randomized, controlled trial. *Journal of Pain and Symptom Management.* **26**: 1105–1112.
131 Pakfetrat M *et al.* (2017) Sertraline can reduce the uremic pruritus in hemodialysis patient: A double blind randomized clinical trial from Southern Iran. *Hemodialysis International.* (Epub ahead of print).
132 Tefferi A and Fonseca R (2002) Selective serotonin reuptake inhibitors are effective in the treatment of polycythemia vera-associated pruritus. *Blood.* **99**: 2627.
133 Zylicz Z *et al.* (2004). *Pruritus in Advanced Disease.* Oxford University Press, Oxford.
134 Lee JJ *et al.* (2016) Effective use of mirtazapine for refractory pruritus associated with carcinoma en cuirasse. *BMJ Supportive and Palliative Care.* **6**: 119–121.
135 Twycross R and Wilcock A (eds) (2016) *Introducing Palliative Care* (5e). palliativdrugs.com Ltd., Nottingham, pp. 173–180.
136 NICE (2006) Urinary incontinence: the management of urinary incontinence in women. *Clinical Guideline.* CG40. www.nice.org.uk
137 Chang YD *et al.* (2016) Pseudobulbar affect or depression in dementia? *Journal of Pain and Symptom Management.* **51**: 954–958.
138 Wortzel HS *et al.* (2008) Pathological laughing and crying : epidemiology, pathophysiology and treatment. *CNS Drugs.* **22**: 531–545.
139 Gibson PG and Vertigan AE (2015) Management of chronic refractory cough. *British Medical Journal.* **351**: h5590.
140 Peoples AR *et al.* (2016) Buspirone for management of dyspnea in cancer patients receiving chemotherapy: a randomized placebo-controlled URCC CCOP study. *Supportive Care in Cancer.* **24**: 1339–1347.

141 Smoller J *et al.* (1998) Sertraline effects on dyspnea in patients with obstructive airways disease. *Psychosomatics.* **39**: 24–29.
142 Haddad PM (2001) Antidepressant discontinuation syndromes: Clinical relevance, prevention and management. *Drug Safety.* **24**: 183–197.
143 Berber MJ (1998) FINISH: remembering the discontinuation syndrome. Flu-like symptoms, Insomnia, Nausea, Imbalance, Sensory disturbances, and Hyperarousal (anxiety/agitation). *Journal of Clinical Psychiatry.* **59**: 255.

Updated September 2017

AMITRIPTYLINE

Class: Serotonin and noradrenaline (norepinephrine) re-uptake inhibitor (SNRI), tricyclic antidepressant (TCA).

Indications: Depression, anxiety and panic disorders, nocturnal enuresis, †neuropathic pain, †urgency and urge incontinence, †sweating, †bladder spasm, †pathological laughing and crying, †drooling, †refractory cough.

Contra-indications: Concurrent use with an MAOI or within 2 weeks of its cessation (see Serotonin toxicity, p.200), CHF, coronary artery insufficiency, recent myocardial infarction, arrhythmias (particularly any degree of heart block), mania, severe hepatic impairment.

Pharmacology

Like all tricyclic antidepressants, amitriptyline is a mono-amine re-uptake inhibitor, sodium channel blocker, and a muscarinic, $5HT_{2A}$, $5HT_{2C}$, H_1, and α_1-adrenergic receptor antagonist.[1] Amitriptyline differs from other tricyclic antidepressants in its relative effects on serotonin and noradrenaline re-uptake, risk in overdose, antimuscarinic effects and cost (see Table 1).

Table 1. Differences between selected TCAs[1,2]

	Re-uptake inhibition		*Relative to other TCAs*		
	5HT	*NA*	*Antimuscarinic effects*	*Risk in overdose*[c]	*Cost*[d]
Amitriptyline[a]	+++	+++	+++	++	+
Clomipramine	+++	+	+++	++	+
Desipramine (not UK)	+	+++	+	++	
Dosulepin (dothiepin)[b]	+++	+++	++	+++	+
Doxepin[b]	++	+++	+++	++	+++
Imipramine	+++	++	++	++	+
Lofepramine	+	+++	+	+	++
Nortriptyline[b]	+	+++	+	++	++

+++ high; ++ moderate; + low
Abbreviations: 5HT = 5-hydroxytryptamine (serotonin); NA = noradrenaline (norepinephrine).

a. amitriptyline's higher affinity for the serotonin re-uptake transporter is offset by its metabolite, nortriptyline, which has a higher affinity for the noradrenaline re-uptake transporter
b. use is discouraged in the UK because of higher risk in overdose (dosulepin) or higher cost (doxepin; nortriptyline)
c. all TCAs are more dangerous in overdose than SSRIs, venlafaxine, duloxetine and mirtazapine
d. typical monthly cost of UK tablet preparations: + (<£10); ++ (£10–80); +++ (>£80).

For depression, amitriptyline is marginally more effective than other antidepressants. However, because it is less well tolerated and more dangerous in overdose, it is generally reserved for severe unresponsive depression.[3]

For neuropathic pain, its efficacy and tolerability are comparable with alternatives (see p.204). Noradrenaline re-uptake inhibition is the predominant action. Sodium channel blockade and

NMDA-glutamate receptor antagonism may also contribute.[4] Generally, a dose-response effect is evident with patients benefitting from higher doses. However, for some patients benefit is *lost* at higher doses.[5] One potential explanation for this is that at higher doses pro-nociceptive effects (e.g. serotonin re-uptake inhibition, α_1 antagonism) predominate over anti-nociceptive effects. *Topical* amitriptyline is ineffective.[6]

For cough which persists despite resolution of the initial cause, amitriptyline is more effective than **codeine**.[7] Benefit probably relates to reducing cough reflex hypersensitivity, which is generally present in this group of patients (see p.140).

Bio-availability 45%.[8]
Onset of action 2–4 weeks; <1 week in neuropathic pain.
Time to peak plasma concentration 4h PO; 24–48h IM.
Plasma halflife 9–25h; active metabolite nortriptyline 15–39h.
Duration of action 24h, situation dependent.

Cautions

Suicide risk: the possibility of a suicide attempt is inherent in major depression and persists until remission. Antidepressants may themselves cause suicidal ideation, particularly in those aged ≤25 years (see p.198). If there is concern about suicide, consider alternatives that are safer in overdose (e.g. an SSRI).

Bipolar disorder (can transform into manic phase); epilepsy (may lower seizure threshold); cardiac disease (risk of arrhythmia); renal or hepatic impairment (see Chapter 17, p.685 and Chapter 18, p.712); urinary hesitancy and narrow-angle glaucoma (antimuscarinic).

Drug interactions

Additive pharmacodynamic interactions with other drugs (see p.199), notably serotonin toxicity (see p.200). Concurrent administration with an MAOI or within 2 weeks of its cessation is contra-indicated (see above).

Amitriptyline is metabolized mainly by CYP2D6, and to a lesser degree by CYP1A2 and possibly other hepatic enzymes. Caution should be taken with concurrent use of drugs which inhibit or induce these enzymes, particularly in those who are poor CYP2D6 metabolizers (see p.717).

Specific significant interactions[9]

- TCAs and SSRIs: **fluoxetine**, **paroxetine** (strong CYP2D6 inhibitors) and **fluvoxamine** (strong CYP1A2 inhibitor) have the greatest effect, *increasing* plasma concentrations of TCAs by *≤10 times*. In addition, the plasma concentration of the SSRI may also *increase*. If an SSRI and a TCA are prescribed concurrently, use an alternative SSRI (e.g. **citalopram** or **sertraline**) or reduce the dose of the TCA to 25–33% of the previous dose (and possibly prescribe a relatively low SSRI dose)
- other drugs shown to *increase* the plasma concentrations of amitriptyline are **cimetidine**, **fluconazole**, **quinidine** (strong CYP2D6 inhibitor) and **terbinafine**
- concurrent prescription of **carbamazepine** *decreases* the plasma concentrations of amitriptyline by up to 60%.

Undesirable effects

Antimuscarinic effects (see p.5), sedation, delirium, postural hypotension, hyponatraemia, falls.

Dose and use

Because of the potential for undesirable effects, low doses should be used initially, particularly in the frail elderly.

Amitriptyline can be given as a single dose at bedtime for all indications. If a patient experiences early morning drowsiness, or takes a long time to settle at night, amitriptyline should be taken 2h before bedtime.

Avoid abrupt withdrawal after prolonged use (see Stopping antidepressants, p.205).

A small number of patients are stimulated by amitriptyline and experience insomnia, unpleasant vivid dreams, myoclonus and physical restlessness. In these patients, administer in the morning or change to an alternative.

Neuropathic pain

- start with 10mg PO at bedtime
- if tolerated, increase to 25mg after 3–7 days
- if necessary, increase by 25mg every 1–2 weeks
- if successive increases are well tolerated *and bring additional benefit*, increase up to a maximum of 150mg at bedtime (seldom required)
- if helpful but poorly tolerated, consider switching to **duloxetine** (see p.219)
- if no response, switch to an anti-epileptic (see p.256).

Urgency and urge incontinence, sweating, bladder spasm, drooling

Dose as for neuropathic pain.

Depression, anxiety and panic disorders, †pathological laughing and crying

Amitriptyline is no longer used first-line for depression, panic or anxiety disorders, but might retain a place for depression refractory to other treatments or with co-existent neuropathic pain (see p.204).

Titrate the dose as for neuropathic pain; 75–100mg PO at bedtime is generally as effective as higher doses, and better tolerated.[10] Occasionally, it is necessary to increase the dose to 150–225mg/24h.

Supply

Amitriptyline (generic)
Tablets 10mg, 25mg, 50mg, 28 days @ 50mg at bedtime = £3.50.
Oral solution 10mg/5mL, 25mg/5mL, 50mg/5mL, 28 days @ 50mg at bedtime = £18.

1 Binding DB (2015) Skaggs School of Pharmacy and Pharmaceutical Sciences Binding Database. Available from: http://bindingdb.org/as/search.html (accessed June 2015)
2 Gillman PK (2007) Tricyclic antidepressant pharmacology and therapeutic drug interactions updated. *British Journal of Pharmacology*. **151**: 737–748.
3 Leucht C *et al.* (2012) Amitriptyline versus placebo for major depressive disorder. *Cochrane Database of Systematic Reviews*. **12**: CD009138. www.thecochranelibrary.com
4 Kremer M *et al.* (2016) Antidepressants and gabapentinoids in neuropathic pain: Mechanistic insights. *Neuroscience*. **338**: 183–206.
5 Watson C (1984) Therapeutic window for amitriptyline analgesia. *Canadian Medical Association Journal*. **130**: 105–106.
6 Thompson DF and Brooks KG (2015) Systematic review of topical amitriptyline for the treatment of neuropathic pain. *Journal of Clinical Pharmacy and Therapeutics*. **40**: 496–503.
7 Gibson PG and Vertigan AE (2015) Management of chronic refractory cough. *British Medical Journal*. **351**: h5590.
8 Schulz P *et al.* (1985) Discrepancies between pharmacokinetic studies of amitriptyline. *Clinical Pharmacokinetics*. **10**: 257–268.
9 Baxter K and Preston CL (2011). *Stockley's Drug Interactions*. London:- Pharmaceutical Press www.medicinescomplete.com (accessed June 2013).
10 Furukawa (2009) Low dosage tricyclic antidepressants for depression. *Cochrane Database of Systematic Reviews*. CD003197. www.thecochranelibrary.com

Updated September 2017

SELECTIVE SEROTONIN RE-UPTAKE INHIBITORS

Class: Antidepressant.

Indications: Authorized indications vary; see individual SPCs for details. Depression, anxiety and panic disorders, †hot flushes, †pruritus, †pathological laughing and crying.

Contra-indications: Concurrent use with an MAOI or within 2 weeks of its cessation (see Serotonin toxicity, p.200); known prolonged QT interval or concurrent use with other drugs which prolong the QT interval (**citalopram, escitalopram**), concurrent use with **pimozide**; mania.

Pharmacology

SSRIs inhibit the serotonin re-uptake transporter. They differ in their propensity for causing pharmacokinetic drug interactions, and discontinuation reactions. They also have varying additional actions which may partly explain why some individuals respond when switched to an alternative SSRI (Table 1).

Table 1 Differences between SSRIs[1–6]

Drug	*Additional actions*	*Hepatic enzyme inhibitor*					*Discontinuation reaction risk*[a]
		CYP1A2	*CYP2C9*	*CYP2C19*	*CYP2D6*	*CYP3A4*	
Citalopram	H_1 antagonist (*R*-enantiomer)				+		Low
Escitalopram	None				+		Low
Fluoxetine	$5HT_{2C}$ antagonist[b]		++	++	+++	+	Minimal
Fluvoxamine	Sigma-1 agonist[c]	+++		+++		++	Moderate
Paroxetine	Noradrenaline (norepinephrine) re-uptake inhibitor[b], P2X4 receptor inhibitor[d]				+++		High
Sertraline	Dopamine re-uptake inhibitor[b]				+		Low

+ = weak inhibitor; ++ = moderate inhibitor; +++ = strong inhibitor (also see Chapter 19, p.717).

a. approximates to halflife (see p.197)

b. these actions theoretically contribute to their antidepressant effects (see p.193) but the affinity, and overall contribution of these additional actions is much less than the predominant serotonin re-uptake inhibition

c. the action of sigma-1 receptors is poorly defined, but sigma-1 receptor agonists may have antidepressant, pro-seizure, euphoric and/or dysphoric effects

d. P2X4 receptors are expressed by microglia and implicated in neuro-inflammation and neuropathic pain (see p.196).

In palliative care, **citalopram** or **sertraline** are generally the SSRIs of choice; they combine a low risk of drug interactions and discontinuation reactions. They are first-line treatments for depression (see p.202), anxiety and panic disorders (see p.203), and pathological laughter and crying (see p.205). **Sertraline** is preferred in patients with risk factors for QT interval prolongation (see below).

Two small RCTs suggest benefit in pruritus within a few days from **sertraline** (cholestatic pruritus)[7] and **paroxetine** (pruritus of mixed cause in cancer patients).[8] A slower response to **sertraline** was seen in uraemic pruritus (>2 weeks).[9] Benefit is also reported in pruritus associated with polycythaemia vera.[10]

SSRIs are not consistently effective for neuropathic pain; an SNRI (e.g. **amitriptyline**, **duloxetine**) or an anti-epileptic is preferable (see p.204).

Escitalopram is the *S*-enantiomer of **citalopram**. *R*-citalopram does not inhibit the serotonin re-uptake transporter but may hinder the binding of *S*-citalopram. Some fixed-dose comparisons do find a marginally higher response rate with **escitalopram** 10mg vs. **citalopram** 20mg,[11] but titrating **citalopram** might be expected to achieve the same result.

For pharmacokinetic details, see Table 2.

Table 2 Pharmacokinetic details for selected SSRIs[11–13]

Drug	*Bio-availability PO (%)*	T_{max} *(h)*	*Plasma halflife*	*Metabolism*
Citalopram	80[a]	3	36h	Multiple pathways[b]
Escitalopram	80[c]	4	30h	Multiple pathways[b]
Fluoxetine	90	4–8	1–4 days; 1–2 *weeks*[b]	Multiple pathways[b]
Paroxetine	50[d]	5	15–20h	Multiple pathways
Sertraline	>44	6–8	26h	CYP3A4

a. for tablets; bio-avaiability of drops is nearly 100%
b. active metabolite(s)
c. the bio-availability of tablets and oral solution is comparable
d. increases with multiple dosing.

Cautions

Suicide risk: the possibility of a suicide attempt is inherent in major depression and persists until remission. Antidepressants may themselves cause suicidal ideation, particularly in those aged ≤25 years (see p.198).

Bipolar disorder (can transform into manic phase). Epilepsy (may lower seizure threshold but less than other antidepressants; ***citalopram*** *is generally preferred because it lacks significant interactions with anti-epileptics*).

QT prolongation risk factors (particularly **citalopram** and **escitalopram**; see below and p.731); renal impairment (see Chapter 17, p.685) hepatic impairment (see Chapter 18, p.712); diabetes mellitus (reduced hypoglycaemic awareness); peptic ulceration or bleeding disorders (SSRIs increase the risk of GI bleeding,[14] particularly in those aged >80 years).[15]

Drug interactions

Fluoxetine, **fluvoxamine** and **paroxetine** are strong hepatic enzyme inhibitors (see p.717) and potentially serious interactions can result when used with other drugs that are metabolized by these enzymes.[16]

Citalopram, **escitalopram** and **sertraline** are only weak hepatic enzyme inhibitors and are less likely to affect the metabolism of other drugs.[4,5]

Additive pharmacodynamic interactions with other drugs (see p.199) notably bleeding risk, QT prolongation (**citalopram** and **escitalopram**) and serotonin toxicity (see p.200). Concurrent administration with an MAOI or within 2 weeks of its cessation is contra-indicated (see above).

Sertraline is metabolized mainly by CYP3A4, and to a minor degree by CYP2D6. Caution should be taken with concurrent use of drugs which inhibit or induce these enzymes particularly in those who are poor CYP2D6 metabolizers (see p.719). However, generally **sertraline** rarely requires dose reduction with other enzyme inhibitors; consider only if symptoms of toxicity occur.

Citalopram and **escitalopram** are metabolized by CYP2C19, CYP2D6 and CYP3A4. Although the FDA recommends a reduced dose of **citalopram** when used with **cimetidine**, **omeprazole** or other drugs which inhibit CYP2C19, the effect on plasma citalopram levels is likely to be small.[17]

Undesirable effects

Frequencies based on **sertraline** and **citalopram**.

Very common (>10%): somnolence, insomnia, dizziness, headache, dry mouth, nausea, diarrhoea, sweating.

Common (<10%, >1%): agitation, anxiety, nervousness, confusion, tremor, tinnitus, yawning, fatigue, dizziness, paraesthesia, bruxism (teeth grinding), palpitations, altered taste, decreased appetite, vomiting, sexual dysfunction, myalgia, arthralgia, pruritus.

Uncommon (<1%, >0.1%): aggression, depersonalization, hallucinations, mania.
Rare (<0.01%) or unknown incidence: psychosis, hyponatraemia, seizures, movement disorders (e.g. dyskinesia), hepatitis, haemorrhage, fracture risk (see p.202).

Myocardial infarction

The manufacturer reports myocardial infarction as a rare consequence of taking **sertraline**. However, this would be expected because depression is an independent risk factor for myocardial infarction. Further, case control studies suggest that SSRIs confer a protective effect,[18] possibly because they impact negatively on platelet aggregation (see p.200). **Sertraline** has been used safely in patients with unstable angina, and after myocardial infarction.[19]

QT prolongation

Citalopram and **escitalopram** exhibit dose-related QT prolongation. Regulators recommend correction of hypokalaemia and hypomagnaesemia, advise ECG monitoring in those with cardiac disease, and contra-indication in patients receiving other QT prolonging drugs (see p.733).[20] **Sertraline** and other SSRIs appear safer in this respect.[21] Also see Prolongation of the QT interval in palliative care, p.731.

Dose and use

Treatment should not be discontinued abruptly (see p.205).

Sertraline (depression, anxiety and panic)

- if anxiety/panic symptoms are prominent, start with 25mg PO each morning and increase to 50mg each morning after 1 week
- otherwise, start with 50mg each morning, if necessary, increase the dose to 100mg after 2–4 weeks
- if no response after 4 weeks, or only a partial response after 6–8 weeks, consider further increases to a maximum of 200mg or an alternative (see p.203)
- if effective, continue until the patient has been symptom-free for ≥6 months (see p.203); after this, discontinue over 2–4 weeks.

Citalopram (depression, anxiety and panic)

Because of concerns regarding QT prolongation, do not exceed the maximum dose (also see comments above).[20]

- start with 10mg PO each morning and increase to 20mg each morning after 1 week
- if no response after 4 weeks, or only a partial response after 6–8 weeks, consider further increases to a maximum of 40mg or switch to an alternative (see p.203)
- restrict maximum dose to 20mg in those over 60, hepatic impairment, and consider with patients also taking **cimetidine**, **omeprazole** or other inhibitors of CYP2C19[17,20]
- if effective, continue until the patient has been symptom-free for ≥6 months (see p.203); after this, discontinue over 2–4 weeks.

Other indications

- **cholestatic pruritus**
  - ▷ start with **sertraline** 25mg PO each morning, if necessary, increase in 25mg increments
  - ▷ doses above 100mg rarely gave additional relief.[7]
- **pathological laughter and crying**
  - ▷ often responds to lower doses than required for depression[22]
  - ▷ start with **citalopram** 5mg PO each morning; if necessary, increase in 5–10mg increments to a maximum of 40mg each morning (20mg in those with risk factors, see above) *or*
  - ▷ start with **sertraline** 12.5mg PO each morning; if necessary, increase in 12.5–25mg increments to a maximum of 200mg each morning.

Supply

Citalopram (generic)
Tablets (as *hydrobromide*) 10mg, 20mg, 40mg, 28 days @ 20mg each morning = £1.
Oral liquid drops (as *hydrochloride*) 40mg/mL, 28 days @ 16mg (8 drops) each morning = £3.50; *16mg as drops is equivalent to 20mg as tablets. Mix with water, orange juice or apple juice before taking.*

Sertraline (generic)
Tablets 50mg, 100mg, 28 days @ 50mg each morning = £1.25.
Oral solution 50mg/5mL, 28 days @ 50mg each morning = £48; unauthorized, available as a special order from Rosemont, see p.751). *Note based on specials tariff in community.*

1 Hashimoto K (2009) Sigma-1 receptors and selective serotonin reuptake inhibitors: clinical implications of their relationship. *Central Nervous System Agents in Medicinal Chemistry*. **9**: 197–204.
2 Carrasco JL and Sandner C (2005) Clinical effects of pharmacological variations in selective serotonin reuptake inhibitors: an overview. *International Journal of Clinical Practice*. **59**: 1428–1434.
3 Haddad PM (2001) Antidepressant discontinuation syndromes: Clinical relevance, prevention and management. *Drug Safety*. **24**: 183–197.
4 Preskorn SH (1997) Clinically relevant pharmacology of selective serotonin reuptake inhibitors. An overview with emphasis on pharmacokinetics and effects on oxidative drug metabolism. *Clinical Pharmacokinetics*. **32 (Suppl 1)**: 1–21.
5 Rao N (2007) The clinical pharmacokinetics of escitalopram. *Clinical Pharmacokinetics*. **46**: 281–290.
6 Yamashita T *et al.* (2016) Duloxetine inhibits microglial P2X4 receptor function and alleviates neuropathic pain after peripheral nerve injury. *PLoS One*. **11**: e0165189.
7 Mayo MJ *et al.* (2007) Sertraline as a first-line treatment for cholestatic pruritus. *Hepatology*. **45**: 666–674.
8 Zylicz Z *et al.* (2003) Paroxetine in the treatment of severe non-dermatological pruritus: a randomized, controlled trial. *Journal of Pain and Symptom Management*. **26**: 1105–1112.
9 Pakfetrat M *et al.* (2017) Sertraline can reduce the uremic pruritus in hemodialysis patient:A double blind randomized clinical trial from Southern Iran. *Hemodialysis International*. (Epub ahead of print).
10 Tefferi A and Fonseca R (2002) Selective serotonin reuptake inhibitors are effective in the treatment of polycythemia vera-associated pruritus. *Blood*. **99**: 2627.
11 Garnock-Jones KP and McCormack PL (2010) Escitalopram: a review of its use in the management of major depressive disorder in adults. *CNS Drugs*. **24**: 769–796.
12 Hiemke (2000) Pharmacokinetics of selective serotonin reuptake inhibitors. *Pharmacology and Therapeutics*. **85**: 11–28.
13 Kaye CM *et al.* (1989) A review of the metabolism and pharmacokinetics of paroxetine in man. *Acta Psychiatrica Scandinavica Supplementum*. **350**: 60–75.
14 Paton C and Ferrier IN (2005) SSRIs and gastrointestinal bleeding. *British Medical Journal*. **331**: 529–530.
15 vanWalraven C *et al.* (2001) Inhibition of serotonin reuptake by antidepressants and upper gastrointestinal bleeding in elderly patients: retrospective cohort study. *British Medical Journal*. **323**: 655–657.
16 Baxter K and Preston CL (2011). *Stockley's Drug Interactions*. London:- Pharmaceutical Press www.medicinescomplete.com (accessed June 2013).
17 FDA (2012) Celexa (citalopram hydrobromide) Revised recommendations, potential risk of abnormal heart rhythms. *Drug safety communication*. www.fda.gov/Safety/MedWatch/
18 Sauer WH *et al.* (2001) Selective serotonin reuptake inhibitors and myocardial infarction. *Circulation*. **104**: 1894–1898.
19 Glassman AH *et al.* (2002) Sertraline treatment of major depression in patients with acute MI or unstable angina. *Journal of the American Medical Association*. **288**: 701–709.
20 MHRA (2011) Citalopram and escitalopram: QT interval prolongation - new maximum daily dose restrictions (including in elderly patients), contraindications, and warnings. *Drug Safety Update*. **5**. www.gov.uk/drug-safety-update
21 Funk KA and Bostwick JR (2013) A comparison of the risk of QT prolongation among SSRIs. *Annals of Pharmacotherapy*. **47**: 1330–1341.
22 Wortzel HS *et al.* (2008) Pathological laughing and crying : epidemiology, pathophysiology and treatment. *CNS Drugs*. **22**: 531–545.

Updated September 2017

*VENLAFAXINE

Class: Antidepressant; serotonin and noradrenaline re-uptake inhibitor (SNRI).

Indications: Depression, anxiety and panic disorders, †neuropathic pain, †hot flushes.

Contra-indications: Concurrent use with an MAOI or within 2 weeks of its cessation (see Serotonin toxicity, p.200). Uncontrolled hypertension.

Pharmacology

Like **duloxetine**, venlafaxine inhibits serotonin and noradrenaline (norepinephrine) re-uptake transporters, but lacks the sodium channel blockade and muscarinic, α-adrenergic and H_1-receptor antagonism of **amitriptyline** and other tricyclic SNRIs.[1,2] Inhibition of noradrenaline re-uptake transporters increases with higher doses.[3] Because these also clear dopamine in the prefrontal cortex, which lacks separate dopamine re-uptake transporters, venlafaxine enhances dopamine transmission here too.

For depression, venlafaxine is generally reserved for second-line use where it is marginally more effective than switching to an alternative SSRI, but less well tolerated (see p202).[4,5]

For neuropathic pain, benefit from venlafaxine ≥150mg/24h appears similar to that of **duloxetine**. Lower doses (75mg/24h) were no more effective than placebo.[6] In a comparative trial, venlafaxine 112.5mg/24h was as effective as **imipramine** 75mg/24h.[7] Dry mouth was more common with **imipramine**, and tiredness more common with venlafaxine.

For hot flushes, trials in patients with breast cancer have found benefit from venlafaxine, SSRIs (p.212) and **gabapentin** (see p.272).[8] Venlafaxine works faster than **clonidine** (p.77), and participants prefer venlafaxine to **gabapentin**.[8] Venlafaxine and SSRIs are also reported to improve hot flushes in men resulting from medical or surgical castration.[9-11]

Venlafaxine is metabolized by CYP2D6 to a pharmacologically active metabolite, O-desmethylvenlafaxine (ODV), which has a similar pharmacodynamic profile, and by CYP3A4 to a minor, less active metabolite. Venlafaxine and its metabolites are primarily renally excreted.
Bio-availability 13%; 45% m/r.
Onset of action >2 weeks for depression.
Time to peak plasma concentration about 2.5h; 4.5–7.5h m/r and 6.5–11h ODV m/r.
Plasma halflife 5h; 11h for ODV.
Duration of effect 12–24h, situation dependent.

Cautions

Suicide risk: the possibility of a suicide attempt is inherent in major depression and persists until remission. Antidepressants may themselves cause suicidal ideation, particularly in those aged ≤25 years (see p.198). If there is concern about suicide, MHRA advises that supply should be limited to 2 weeks. The risk in overdose is greater than with SSRIs, similar to **mirtazapine** and less than with TCAs.[5]

Bipolar disorder (can transform into manic phase); epilepsy (lowers seizure threshold); cardiac disease (risk of hypertension and arrhythmia); renal impairment (see Dose and use and Chapter 17, p.685; mild–moderate hepatic impairment (see Dose and use and Chapter 18, p.712); narrow-angle glaucoma (mydriasis reported).

Drug interactions

Additive pharmacodynamic interactions with other drugs (see p.199) notably QT prolongation and serotonin toxicity (see Box A, p.200). Concurrent administration with an MAOI or within 2 weeks of its cessation is contra-indicated (see above).

Venlafaxine is metabolized by CYP2D6 and CYP3A4. Concurrent use with drugs which inhibit these enzymes may result in higher plasma concentrations (see Chapter 19, Table 8, p.725), and should generally be avoided in order to prevent clinically important interactions in poor metabolizers.[12]

Venlafaxine may increase concurrent **haloperidol** plasma concentrations (up to 70% increase in AUC).[13] The mechanism is unknown and the dose of haloperidol may need to be reduced. The dose of **warfarin** may need to be reduced when used concurrently with venlafaxine (reports of increased prothrombin times; unknown mechanism).[13]

Undesirable effects

Very common (>10%): drowsiness, dizziness, insomnia, nervousness, dry mouth, nausea, constipation, sexual dysfunction, asthenia, headache, sweating.
Common (<10%, >1%): abnormal dreams, agitation, confusion, abnormal vision/accommodation, mydriasis, tinnitus, tremor, hypertonia, paraesthesia, dyspnoea, hypertension, palpitations, postural hypotension, vasodilation, anorexia, diarrhoea, dyspepsia, vomiting, abdominal pain, urinary frequency, decreased libido, impotence, menstrual disorders, arthralgia, myalgia, weight gain/loss, chills, pyrexia, pruritus, rash, ecchymosis.
Uncommon (<1%): hallucinations, urinary retention, muscle spasm, hyponatraemia, increased liver enzymes, angioedema, maculopapular eruptions, urticaria.

Dose and use

Remains of m/r tablets may appear in the patient's faeces ('ghost tablets'). These are inert residues, and do not affect the efficacy of the products.

May be taken with or after food to improve tolerability (see p.657). If moderate renal or mild–moderate hepatic impairment, reduce the dose by 50% and give once daily, avoid in ESRF and severe hepatic impairment (see p.685 and p.712).

Check blood pressure before and after starting, and after dose increases; consider dose reduction or discontinuation in those who show a sustained increase.

Avoid abrupt withdrawal after prolonged use (see Stopping antidepressants, p.205). If ≥75mg/day have been taken for >1 week, taper over at least 1 week; if ≥150mg/day have been taken for >6 weeks, taper over at least 2 weeks.

Depression

Because of concerns about its tolerability and safety in overdose, venlafaxine is reserved for depression refractory to other antidepressants (see p.202).

- generally start with 37.5mg PO b.d.
- in frail or elderly patients, start with 37.5mg once daily for 4–7 days
- if necessary, increase by 37.5mg b.d. every 2 weeks
- maximum recommended dose 375mg daily. Specialist supervision required if a dose of ≥300mg is necessary in severely depressed or hospitalized patients
- if effective, continue until the patient has been symptom-free for ≥6 months (see p202); after this, discontinue over 2–4 weeks.

Anxiety and panic

Venlafaxine is reserved for anxiety or panic disorders refractory to other antidepressants (see p.203).

- use as for depression
- maximum recommended dose 225mg PO daily.

Neuropathic pain and hot flushes

Venlafaxine is not a first-line treatment for neuropathic pain (see p.204).[14]

- start with 37.5mg PO once daily
- increase to 37.5mg b.d. after 1 week
- if necessary, increase to 75mg b.d. after a further 2 weeks.

Supply

Venlafaxine (generic)

Tablets 37.5mg, 75mg, 28 days @ 75mg b.d. = £2.25.

Capsules m/r 37.5mg, 75mg, 150mg, 28 days @ 150mg once daily = £17.

Tablets m/r 37.5mg, 75mg, 150mg, 225mg, 28 days @ 150mg once daily = £18.

Oral solution 37.5mg/5mL, 75mg/5mL 28 days @ 150mg once daily = £94; (unauthorized, available as a special order, see p.751). *Note price based on specials tariff in community.*

1 Bymaster FP *et al.* (2001) Comparative affinity of duloxetine and venlafaxine for serotonin and norepinephrine transporters in vitro and in vivo, human serotonin receptor subtypes, and other neuronal receptors. *Neuropsychopharmacology*. **25**: 871–880.

2 Beique JC *et al.* (1998) Affinities of venlafaxine and various reuptake inhibitors for the serotonin and norepinephrine transporters. *European Journal of Pharmacology*. **349**: 129–132.

3 Melichar J *et al.* (2001) Venlafaxine occupation at the noradrenaline reuptake site: in-vivo determination in healthy volunteers. *Journal of Psychopharmacology*. **15**: 9–12.

4 NICE (2009) Depression. *Clinical Guidelines*. CG90 and CG91. www.nice.org.uk

5 Cleare A *et al.* (2015) Evidence-based guidelines for treating depressive disorders with antidepressants: A revision of the 2008 British Association for Psychopharmacology guidelines. *Journal of Psychopharmacology*. **29**: 459–525.

6 Finnerup NB *et al.* (2015) Pharmacotherapy for neuropathic pain in adults: a systematic review and meta-analysis. *Lancet Neurology*. **14**: 162–173.

7 Sindrup SH *et al.* (2003) Venlafaxine versus imipramine in painful polyneuropathy: a randomized, controlled trial. *Neurology*. **60**: 1284–1289.

8 Johns C *et al.* (2016) Informing hot flash treatment decisions for breast cancer survivors: a systematic review of randomized trials comparing active interventions. *Breast Cancer Research and Treatment*. **156**: 415–426.

9 Quella S *et al.* (1999) Pilot evaluation of venlafaxine for the treatment of hot flashes in men undergoing androgen ablation therapy for prostate cancer. *Journal of Urology*. **162**: 98–102.

10 Loprinzi CL *et al.* (2011) Nonestrogenic management of hot flashes. *Journal of Clinical Oncology*. **29**: 3842–3846.

11 Roth AJ and Scher HI (1998) Sertraline relieves hot flashes secondary to medical castration as treatment of advanced prostate cancer. *Psychooncology*. **7**: 129–132.

12 MHRA (2006) Updated prescribing advice for venlafaxine (Efexor/Effexor XL). Letter from the chairman of the Commission on Human Medicines, 31st May 2006. Available from: http://www.mhra.gov.uk/Safetyinformation/

13 Baxter K and Preston CL *Stockley's Drug Interactions*. London: Pharmaceutical Press, www.medicinescomplete.com (accessed May 2017).

14 Gallagher HC *et al.* (2015) Venlafaxine for neuropathic pain in adults. *Cochrane Database of Systematic Reviews*. **8**: CD011109. www.thecochranelibrary.com

Updated September 2017

DULOXETINE

Class: Antidepressant, serotonin and noradrenaline re-uptake inhibitor (SNRI).

Indications: Depression, diabetic neuropathic pain, †other neuropathic pain, generalized anxiety disorder, moderate–severe stress incontinence in women.

Contra-indications: Concurrent use with an MAOI or within 2 weeks of its cessation (see Serotonin toxicity, p.200). Concurrent use with strong CYP1A2 inhibitors, e.g. **fluvoxamine, ciprofloxacin**.[1] Uncontrolled hypertension, hepatic impairment, creatinine clearance <30mL/min.

Pharmacology

Like **venlafaxine**, duloxetine inhibits serotonin and noradrenaline (norepinephrine) re-uptake transporters, but lacks the sodium channel blockade and muscarinic, α-adrenergic and H_1-receptor antagonism of **amitriptyline** and other tricyclic SNRIs.[2] **Duloxetine** also inhibits P2X4 receptors, a subset of purine-gated calcium channels upregulated on microglia in neuropathic pain.[3]

For neuropathic pain, the NNT for a 50% reduction in pain score is 5. The majority of trials examined painful diabetic neuropathy.[4] There is a dose response effect up to 120mg/24h.[5] In two RCTs efficacy was comparable to **amitriptyline**, and undesirable effects were similar; although in one of the RCTs, dry mouth occurred less with duloxetine, and constipation more.[6,7] Duloxetine is also of benefit in fibromyalgia and osteo-arthitic pain.[4,8]

For depression, duloxetine is less well tolerated than **venlafaxine** and SSRIs.[9] For stress incontinence, duloxetine has a limited role;[10] serotonin and noradrenaline increase urethral sphincter tone (see p.193).

Bio-availability 90%.

Onset of action 2 weeks in depression.[11]

Time to peak plasma concentration 6h.

Plasma halflife 8-17h.

Duration of action >24h, situation dependent.

Cautions

Suicide risk: the possibility of a suicide attempt is inherent in major depression and persists until remission. Antidepressants themselves may cause suicidal ideation, particularly in those aged ≤25 years (see p.198).

Bipolar disorder (can transform into manic phase); epilepsy (lowers seizure threshold); cardiac disease (risk of hypertension and arrhythmia); renal impairment (see Dose and use and Chapter 17, p.685); hepatic impairment (see Dose and use and Chapter 18, p.712); urinary hesitancy and narrow-angle glaucoma (may exacerbate).

Drug interactions

Additive pharmacodynamic interactions with other drugs (see p.199), notably serotonin toxicity (see Box A, p.200). Concurrent administration with an MAOI or within 2 weeks of its cessation is contra-indicated.

Duloxetine is metabolized by CYP1A2 and CYP2D6, and also *inhibits* CYP2D6. Caution should be taken with concurrent use of drugs which inhibit or induce these enzymes, particularly in those who are poor CYP2D6 metabolizers (see Chapter 19, Table 8, p.725).

Specific significant interactions[1]

- **fluvoxamine** (strong CYP1A2 inhibitor) *significantly increases* duloxetine plasma concentrations, and **ciprofloxacin** probably does the same; concurrent use of these drugs with duloxetine is contra-indicated
- **fluoxetine**, **paroxetine** and **quinidine** (strong CYP2D6 inhibitors) can increase plasma concentrations
- smoking (CYP1A2 inducer) can *decrease* duloxetine plasma concentration by ≤50%; however, a routine dose increase in smokers is not recommended.

Undesirable effects

Very common (>10%): drowsiness, headache, dry mouth, nausea.
Common (<10%, >1%): dizziness, tremor, paraesthesia, blurred vision, tinnitus, sleep disturbance, agitation, palpitations, hypertension, diarrhoea, constipation, anorexia, rash, sweating, dysuria, sexual dysfunction.
Uncommon (<1%, >0.1%): altered taste, extrapyramidal symptoms, postural hypotension, arrhythmias, urinary hesitancy and retention.
Rare (<0.1%): hypertensive crises.
Like SSRIs and **venlafaxine**, duloxetine increases the risk of bleeding.[12]

Dose and use

The timing of once daily doses is immaterial, although it should be constant. Monitor blood pressure; consider dose reduction or discontinuation if there is a sustained increase.

No dose reduction is required in mild–moderate renal impairment; use is contra-indicated in patients with creatinine clearance <30mL/min) and in hepatic impairment (see p.685 and p.712).

Avoid abrupt withdrawal after prolonged use (see Stopping antidepressants, p.205).

Neuropathic pain

Although authorized for painful *diabetic* neuropathy, duloxetine is commonly advocated as a first-line choice for neuropathic pain of any cause:[13]

- start at 30mg PO once daily and increase to 60mg after 1–2 weeks
- if necessary, increase to 60mg b.d.

Depression

Duloxetine is less effective and less well tolerated than alternatives (see above). It may have a role in depression with concurrent neuropathic pain:

- start at 30mg PO once daily and increase to 60mg after 1–2 weeks.

Although there is no direct evidence of benefit, increasing the dose to 60mg b.d. is one of several options if the response to the starting dose is inadequate (see p.203).[11]

Stress incontinence in women

In physically fit women, management is primarily non-drug, e.g. pelvic floor muscle training (sometimes followed by surgery).[10] If prescribing duloxetine:

- start with 20mg PO b.d.
- if necessary, increase to 40mg b.d. after 2 weeks.

Supply

Duloxetine (generic)
Capsules enclosing e/c pellets 20mg, 30mg, 40mg, 60mg, 28 days @ 60mg once daily = £2.50.

1 Baxter K and Preston CL. *Stockley's Drug Interactions*. London: Pharmaceutical Press www.medicinescomplete.com (accessed May 2017).

2 Bymaster FP *et al.* (2001) Comparative affinity of duloxetine and venlafaxine for serotonin and norepinephrine transporters in vitro and in vivo, human serotonin receptor subtypes, and other neuronal receptors. *Neuropsychopharmacology*. **25**: 871–880.

3 Yamashita T *et al.* (2016) Duloxetine inhibits microglial P2X4 receptor function and alleviates neuropathic pain after peripheral nerve injury. *PLoS One*. **11**: e0165189.

4 Lunn MP *et al.* (2014) Duloxetine for treating painful neuropathy, chronic pain or fibromyalgia. *Cochrane Database of Systematic Reviews*. **1**: CD007115. www.thecochranelibrary.com

5 Goldstein DJ *et al.* (2005) Duloxetine vs. placebo in patients with painful diabetic neuropathy. *Pain.* **116**: 109–118.
6 Kaur H *et al.* (2011) A comparative evaluation of amitriptyline and duloxetine in painful diabetic neuropathy: a randomized, double-blind, cross-over clinical trial. *Diabetes Care.* **34**: 818–822.
7 Boyle J *et al.* (2012) Randomized, placebo-controlled comparison of amitriptyline, duloxetine, and pregabalin in patients with chronic diabetic peripheral neuropathic pain: impact on pain, polysomnographic sleep, daytime functioning, and quality of life. *Diabetes Care.* **35**: 2451–2458.
8 Citrome L and Weiss-Citrome A (2012) A systematic review of duloxetine for osteoarthritic pain: what is the number needed to treat, number needed to harm, and likelihood to be helped or harmed? *Postgraduate Medicine.* **124**: 83–93.
9 Cipriani A *et al.* (2012) Duloxetine versus other anti-depressive agents for depression. *Cochrane Database of Systematic Reviews.* **10**: CD006533. www.thecochranelibrary.com
10 NICE (2013) Urinary incontinence in women: management. *Clinical guideline* CG171. www.nice.org.uk
11 Cleare A *et al.* (2015) Evidence-based guidelines for treating depressive disorders with antidepressants: A revision of the 2008 British Association for Psychopharmacology guidelines. *Journal of Psychopharmacology.* **29**: 459–525.
12 Perahia DG *et al.* (2013) The risk of bleeding with duloxetine treatment in patients who use nonsteroidal anti-inflammatory drugs (NSAIDs): analysis of placebo-controlled trials and post-marketing adverse event reports. *Drug Healthcare and Patient Safety.* **5**: 211–219.
13 Finnerup NB *et al.* (2016) Pharmacotherapy for neuropathic pain in adults: a systematic review and meta-analysis. *Lancet Neurology.* **14**: 162–173.

Updated September 2017

4

MIRTAZAPINE

Class: α_2 Adrenergic and $5HT_{2A/C}$ antagonist antidepressant.

Indications: Depression, †anxiety and panic disorders, †pruritus, †serotonin toxicity.

Contra-indications: Concurrent use with an MAOI or within 2 weeks of its cessation (see Serotonin toxicity, p.200).

Pharmacology

Mirtazapine antagonizes receptors which inhibit mono-amine release:[1]

- pre-synaptic α_2-adrenergic antagonism disinhibits serotonin and noradrenaline (norepinephrine) release
- post-synaptic $5HT_{2A}$, $5HT_{2C}$ and $5HT_3$ antagonism disinhibits noradrenaline and dopamine release.

In addition, H_1 antagonistic activity is responsible for its sedative properties. At lower doses, the sedative antihistaminic effect of mirtazapine predominates. With higher doses, sedation is reduced as noradrenergic and dopaminergic neural transmission increases. It has no significant antimuscarinic activity.

The antidepressant effects of mirtazapine manifest faster than with SSRIs.[2] There are also fewer relapses compared with **amitriptyline**.[3] For refractory depression, mirtazapine can be combined with an SSRI or **venlafaxine**, particularly if a previous switch of antidepressant monotherapy was unhelpful (see p.202). For anxiety disorders, mirtazapine is *not* consistently effective.[4]

Mirtazapine is not associated with cardiovascular toxicity or sexual dysfunction.[3] A blockade of $5HT_2$ and H_1 leads to appetite stimulation. Its anti-emetic properties may be due to H_1, $5HT_2$ and/or $5HT_3$ antagonism.[5,6]

Mirtazapine is effective for fibromyalgia (NNT = 6.8 for >30% reduction in pain).[7] Benefit is also reported for neuropathic pain,[8,9] intractable pruritus,[10] and serotonin toxicity[11] but has not been confirmed in RCTs.

Mirtazapine displays linear pharmacokinetics at usual doses. Food does not affect absorption, binding to plasma proteins is about 85% and steady-state is reached after 5 days. Mirtazapine is extensively metabolized and eliminated via the urine and faeces. It is a racemic mixture of two active enantiomers: the *R*-enantiomer is metabolized by CYP3A4 to the active metabolite, demethylmirtazapine, whereas the *S*-enantiomer is metabolized by CYP2D6 and CYP1A2.[3] Clearance in the elderly may be reduced by ≤40%.

Bio-availability 50% PO.
Onset of action hours–days (off-label indications); 1–2 weeks (antidepressant).
Time to peak plasma concentration 2h.
Plasma halflife 20–40h; often shorter in men (26h) than women (37h) but can extend up to 65h.
Duration of action variable; up to several days.

Cautions

Suicide risk: the possibility of a suicide attempt is inherent in major depression and persists until remission. Antidepressants may themselves cause suicidal ideation, particularly in those aged ≤25 years (see p.198).

Bipolar disorder (can transform into manic phase); epilepsy (seizures occur rarely; risk relative to other antidepressants is uncertain); cardiac disease (manufacturer advises increased monitoring with ischaemic heart disease or risk of arrhythmia); renal impairment (see Dose and use and Chapter 17, p.685); hepatic impairment (see Dose and use and Chapter 18, p.712); diabetes mellitus (may alter glycaemic control); narrow-angle glaucoma (mydriasis reported).

Drug interactions

Additive pharmacodynamic interactions with other drugs (see p.199), notably serotonin toxicity (see Box A, p.200). Concurrent administration with an MAOI or within 2 weeks of its cessation is contra-indicated.

Mirtazapine is metabolized by CYP1A2, CYP2D6, and CYP3A4. Caution should be taken with concurrent use of drugs which inhibit or induce these enzymes, particularly in those who are poor CYP2D6 metabolizers (see Chapter 19, Table 8, p.725).

Specific significant interactions[12]

- **ketoconazole** (strong CYP3A4 inhibitor) can *increase* the plasma concentrations of mirtazapine by ≤40%; other strong CYP3A4 inhibitors (e.g. azole antifungals, HIV-protease inhibitors, and macrolides) will probably have a similar effect; a dose reduction of mirtazapine may be necessary
- **fluvoxamine** (strong CYP1A2 inhibitor can *increase* the plasma concentrations of mirtazapine up to four times and **cimetidine** by 50%
- **carbamazepine and phenytoin** (hepatic enzyme inducers) *decrease* mirtazapine plasma concentrations by up to 40%; other enzyme-inducing drugs (e.g. other anti-epileptic drugs and **rifampicin**) probably have a similar effect.

Undesirable effects

Very common (>10%): increase in appetite and weight gain;[13] drowsiness during the first few weeks of treatment. *Dose reduction reduces the likelihood of an antidepressant effect and does not necessarily alleviate drowsiness.*
Uncommon (<1%, >0.1%): hepatic impairment.
Very rare (<0.01%): agranulocytosis.

Dose and use

In elderly or frail patients and those with hepatic impairment or renal impairment with creatinine clearance <40mL/min, titrate slowly to a maximum dose of 30mg PO at bedtime. In ESRF clearance is halved and mirtazapine should be avoided (see p.685 and p.712).

Depression[3]

- start with 15mg PO at bedtime
- if necessary, increase the dose by 15mg every 2 weeks up to 45mg
- if no response after 4 weeks on 45mg, switch to an alternative antidepressant
- if effective, continue until the patient has been symptom-free for ≥6 months (see p.196); then discontinue over 2–4 weeks.

Intractable itch

Use as for depression; continue indefinitely.[8,10]

Panic and anxiety disorders

As for depression, although mirtazapine is *not* a first-line treatment (see p.196).[4]

Supply

Mirtazapine (generic)
Tablets 15mg, 30mg, 45mg, 28 days @ 30mg at bedtime = £1.50.
Tablets orodispersible 15mg, 30mg, 45mg, 28 days @ 30mg at bedtime = £1.50; *tablets should be placed on the tongue, allowed to disperse, then swallowed.*
Oral solution 15mg/mL, 28 days @ 30mg at bedtime = £42.

1 Stahl SM (2013) Chapter 7: Antidepressants. In: *Essential Psychopharmacology: Neuroscientific Basis and Practical Applications* (4e). Cambridge University Press, USA. 284–369.
2 Watanabe N *et al.* (2011) Mirtazapine versus other antidepressive agents for depression. *Cochrane Database of Systematic Reviews.* **12**: CD006528. www.thecochranelibrary.com
3 Croom KF *et al.* (2009) Mirtazapine: a review of its use in major depression and other psychiatric disorders. *CNS Drugs.* **23**: 427–452.
4 Baldwin DS *et al.* (2014) Evidence-based pharmacological treatment of anxiety disorders, post-traumatic stress disorder and obsessive-compulsive disorder: a revision of the 2005 guidelines from the British Association for Psychopharmacology. *Journal of Psychopharmacology.* **28**: 403–439.
5 Kim SW *et al.* (2008) Effectiveness of mirtazapine for nausea and insomnia in cancer patients with depression. *Psychiatry and Clinical Neurosciences.* **62**: 75–83.
6 Chen CC *et al.* (2008) Premedication with mirtazapine reduces preoperative anxiety and postoperative nausea and vomiting. *Anesthesia and Analgesia.* **106**: 109–113.
7 Miki K *et al.* (2016) Efficacy of mirtazapine for the treatment of fibromyalgia without concomitant depression: a randomized, double-blind, placebo-controlled phase IIa study in Japan. *Pain.* **157**: 2089–2096.
8 Brannon G and Stone K (1999) The use of mirtazapine in a patient with chronic pain. *Journal of Pain and Symptom Management.* **18**: 382–385.
9 Ritzenthaler B and Pearson D (2000) Efficacy and tolerability of mirtazapine in neuropathic pain. *Palliative Medicine.* **14**: 346.
10 Krajnik M and Zylicz Z (2001) Understanding pruritus in systemic disease. *Journal of Pain and Symptom Management.* **21**: 151–168.
11 Hoes M and Zeijpveld J (1996) Mirtazapine as treatment for serotonin syndrome. *Pharmacopsychiatry.* **29**: 81.
12 Baxter K and Preston CL (2011). *Stockley's Drug Interactions.* London: Pharmaceutical Press www.medicinescomplete.com (accessed June 2013).
13 Abed R and Cooper M (1999) Mirtazapine causing hyperphagia. *British Journal of Psychiatry.* **174**: 181–182.

Updated September 2017

TRAZODONE

Class: α-Adrenergic and $5HT_{2A/C}$ antagonist antidepressant; serotonin re-uptake inhibitor.

Indications: Depression, †anxiety and panic disorders, †agitated delirium, †insomnia.

Contra-indications: Concurrent use with an MAOI or within 2 weeks of its cessation (see Serotonin toxicity, p.200). Avoid use in the initial recovery period after an acute myocardial infarction.

Pharmacology

Trazodone is an α_1-adenergic, α_2-adrenergic, H_1, $5HT_{2A}$ and $5HT_{2C}$-receptor antagonist and, at higher doses, a serotonin reuptake inhibitor.[1,2] Its receptor profile accounts for its sedative effect and contributes to its antidepressant action by disinhibiting mono-amine release. It is devoid of antimuscarinic activity. Trazodone has an active metabolite, m-chlorophenylpiperazine. Excretion is almost entirely as free or conjugated metabolites.

Trazodone is *not* a first-line treatment for depression (p.202) or anxiety (p.203). However, adjunctive use of doses lower than those authorized may have a place in selected patients. The benefit reported for insomnia and delirium is unconfirmed in RCTs.[2–4] In dementia, trazodone is *not* effective for challenging behaviours,[5] but *may* improve sleep disturbance.[6] For spinal cord injury pain, an RCT found no benefit, although possibly underpowered (n=19).[7]
Bio-availability 65%.
Onset of action 30–60min for insomnia or agitation; 1–4 weeks as an antidepressant.
Time to peak plasma concentration 1h if taken fasting; 2h if taken after food.
Plasma halflife 5–13h
Duration of action variable, situation dependent.

Cautions

Suicide risk: the possibility of a suicide attempt is inherent in major depression and persists until remission. Antidepressants may themselves cause suicidal ideation, particularly in those aged ≤25 years (see p.198).

Bipolar disorder (can transform into manic phase); epilepsy (lowers seizure threshold); risk factors for QT prolongation (see p.731) and cardiac disease (risk of arrhythmia); renal impairment (see Chapter 17, p.685; severe hepatic impairment (increased drowsiness, see Chapter 18, p.712).

Drug interactions

Additive pharmacodynamic interactions with other drugs (see p.199) notably serotonin toxicity (see p.200). Concurrent administration with an MAOI or within 2 weeks of its cessation is contra-indicated (see above).

Trazodone is metabolized by CYP3A4, and possibly CYP2D6. Caution should be taken with concurrent use of drugs which inhibit or induce these enzymes particularly in those who are poor CYP2D6 metabolizers (see Chapter 19, Table 8, p.725).

Specific significant interactions[8]

- **clarithromycin** and **ritonavir** (strong CYP3A4 inhibitors) can *increase* plasma concentrations of trazodone by one third and double the elimination half-life; thus, strong CYP3A4 inhibitors should be avoided where possible or a lower dose of trazodone used
- **carbamazepine** can *decrease* plasma concentrations of trazodone by ≤75%.

If trazodone is prescribed concurrently, the dose of **warfarin** may need to be *increased*[9] and, because of reports of toxicity, the dose of **digoxin** and **phenytoin** *decreased*; the mechanism for these interactions is unknown.

Undesirable effects

Common: drowsiness, headaches, dizziness, dry mouth.[2]
Other: include agitation, restlessness, myoclonus, altered taste nausea, vomiting, sweating, diarrhoea, constipation, hyponatraemia, postural hypotension, rash
Rare: include hepatic impairment (may be severe), increased libido, priapism, arrhythmias, blood dyscrasias.

Dose and use

Trazodone is not a first-line treatment for any indication. Undesirable effects are minimized by a low starting dose. An oral solution is available but is prohibitively expensive:

- start with 50mg PO at bedtime
- usual effective dose:
  - ▷ insomnia 50mg at bedtime[2,3,6]
  - ▷ anxiety or depression ≤300mg/24h in divided doses
  - ▷ delirium ≤100mg at bedtime (occasionally ≤200mg/24h).[4]

Supply

Trazodone (generic)
Capsules 50mg, 100mg, 28 days @ 100mg at bedtime = £12.
Tablets (scored) 150mg, 28 days @ 150mg at bedtime = £16.
Oral solution (sugar-free) 50mg/5mL, 28 days @ 100mg at bedtime = £353.

1 Stahl SM (2013) Chapter 7: Antidepressants. In: *Essential Psychopharmacology: Neuroscientific Basis and Practical Applications* (4e). Cambridge University Press, USA. 284–369.
2 Fagiolini A *et al.* (2012) Rediscovering trazodone for the treatment of major depressive disorder. *CNS Drugs.* **26**: 1033–1049.
3 Tanimukai H *et al.* (2013) An observational study of insomnia and nightmare treated with trazodone in patients with advanced cancer. *American Journal of Hospice and Palliative Care.* **30**: 359–362.
4 Okamoto Y *et al.* (1999) Trazodone in the treatment of delirium. *Journal of Clinical Psychopharmacology.* **19**: 280–282.
5 Seitz D *et al.* (2011) Antidepressants for agitation and psychosis in dementia. *Cochrane Database of Systematic Reviews.* **2**: CD008191. www.thecochranelibrary.com

6 McCleery J *et al.* (2016) Pharmacotherapies for sleep disturbances in dementia. *Cochrane Database of Systematic Reviews.* **11**: CD009178. www.thecochranelibrary.com
7 Davidoff G *et al.* (1987) Trazodone hydrochloride in the treatment of dysesthetic pain in traumatic myelopathy: a radomized double-blind, placebo controlled study. *Pain.* **29**: 151–161.
8 Baxter K and Preston CL *Stockley's Drug Interactions*. London: Pharmaceutical Press www.medicinescomplete.com (accessed May 2017).
9 Small NL and Giamonna KA (2000) Interaction between warfarin and trazodone. *Annals of Pharmacotherapy.* **34**: 734–736.

Updated September 2017

4

*PSYCHOSTIMULANTS

Indications: Attention deficit hyperactivity disorder (**methylphenidate, dexamfetamine**), daytime drowsiness due to narcolepsy (**modafinil, dexamfetamine**), †obstructive sleep apnoea or chronic shift work-related sleep disorder (discouraged by regulators),[1] †depression when prognosis limited (i.e. ≤4 weeks), †opioid-related drowsiness, †fatigue refractory to correction of underlying contributory factors.

Contra-indications: Severe cardiovascular disease (e.g. uncontrolled hypertension or angina, arrhythmias; also see Cautions), use within the last 2 weeks of a monoamine oxidase inhibitor (MAOI), including **procarbazine** (an antineoplastic drug and a weak MAOI, see p.199).

Manufacturers of **methylphenidate** and **dexamfetamine** also recommend avoiding in glaucoma, phaechromocytoma, thyrotoxicosis and history of severe psychiatric illness.

Pharmacology

The psychostimulants, **dexamfetamine, methylphenidate** and **modafinil**, inhibit or reverse dopamine re-uptake transporters thereby increasing synaptic dopamine.[2,3] Dopamine has a central role in attention, arousal and motivation. It is released in response to stimuli and thoughts perceived as relevant, particularly with regard to 'threat' or 'reward'.[4,5] Thus, psychostimulants can improve alertness, motivation and mood.

Dopaminergic dysfunction in the mesolimbic and mesocortical systems is implicated in several disorders. In attention-deficit hyperactivity disorder, psychostimulants may improve attention by correcting a deficit in dopamine release in response to relevant stimuli.[6] Conversely, in psychoses, dopamine excess increases the importance attached to thoughts and perceptions, e.g. the actions of others gain an enhanced relevance, and are interpreted as evidence of threat (paranoid delusions) or importance (grandiose delusions). This explains the beneficial effects of D_2 antagonists in patients experiencing hallucinations and delusions (see p.168).[4,7]

Dexamfetamine, methylphenidate and **modafinil** have the best evidence base to support use in palliative care,[8] with **methylphenidate** probably the most widely used.[9,10] Although m/r formulations of **dexamfetamine** or **methylphenidate** are available (both generally given once daily), they have more risk of insomnia, particularly if taken later in the day.[11]

Modafinil is sometimes suggested as an alternative where **methylphenidate** is poorly tolerated. However, its undesirable cardiovascular and psychotropic effects appear similar. Further, regulators have recommended withdrawing Marketing Authorizations for all indications except narcolepsy because of concerns about undesirable skin and neuropsychiatric effects and abuse potential.[1]

The milder psychostimulant, **caffeine**, also acts indirectly via dopamine. Adenosine receptors are co-localised with and inhibit D_1 and D_2 receptors and as adenosine accumulates during the daytime, dopamine-mediated arousal is reduced; **caffeine**, which acts as an adenosine receptor antagonist, helps prevent this. Present in some OTC combination analgesics, **caffeine** appears beneficial for headache.[12] Although IV **caffeine** is better than placebo in cancer pain, the degree of benefit is unlikely to be clinically relevant.[13] In Parkinson's Disease, adenosine receptor antagonists prolonged the duration of action of L-Dopa without worsening dyskinesia.[14]

Table 1 contains selected pharmacokinetic data. About half or less of a dose of **dexamfetamine** is excreted renally and largely unchanged; thus there is a theoretical risk of increased toxicity in renal impairment.[9]

Table 1 Pharmacokinetic details for selected psychostimulants.[15–18]

	Oral bio-availability (%)	*Time to peak plasma concentration (h)*	*Halflife (h)*	*Metabolism*
Dexamfetamine	No data	2–4	6–12	Multiple routes; ≤50% renally excreted unchanged
Methylphenidate	30[a]	1–3	2	Non-CYP carboxylesterase[b]
Modafinil	40–65[c]	1.5–3	*d*-modafinil[d] 3; *l*-modafinil[d] 10–16	CYP3A4; non-CYP esterase[b]

a. almost completely absorbed but undergoes extensive first-pass hepatic metabolism
b. metabolites are inactive
c. estimated from urinary recovery of radiolabelled doses; absolute bio-availability unknown because of the lack of an IV preparation
d. enantiomers are equipotent.

Cautions

Psychostimulants may exacerbate cardiovascular disease (e.g. severe hypertension, angina, arrhythmia; manufacturers recommend specialist cardiac evaluation; also see Contra-indications). Psychostimulants may also exacerbate psychiatric illness (e.g. anxiety, agitation, psychosis, addiction disorders), epilepsy (possible lowering of seizure threshold), hyperthyroidism and closed-angle glaucoma (not **modafinil**).

Although rare in adults, serious skin reactions occur with **modafinil** in 1% of children; consider alternatives where possible (e.g. **methylphenidate**).

Drug interactions

Pharmacodynamic interactions include those with sympathomimetics (e.g. MAOIs, see Contra-indications) and antipsychotics (reduced stimulant effect).

Methylphenidate and **modafinil** may increase plasma concentrations of TCAs, **phenytoin** and **warfarin** (check INR at least weekly until stabilized). **Modafinil** may also increase the plasma concentrations of **diazepam**.

Modafinil induces CYP3A4/5 resulting in reduced efficacy of **ciclosporin**, HIV-protease inhibitors, **midazolam**, L-type calcium-channel blockers, statins and hormonal contraception. **Modafinil** also inhibits CYP2C19 and thus may decrease the plasma concentrations of the active metabolites of **clopidogrel**.

Undesirable effects

Undesirable effects have been reported in up to 30% of patients.

Neuropsychiatric: insomnia, agitation and anorexia (generally settle after 2–3 weeks if the drug is continued or resolve after 2–3 days if the drug is discontinued), psychosis, movement disorders.
Cardiovascular: tachyarrhythmias, hypertension, angina (rare).
Other: headache, common and responds to slower dose titration; nausea; *very rarely cerebral arteritis occurs with **methylphenidate***. Mild rashes are common with **modafinil**; serious skin reactions occur in 1% of children.

Use of psychostimulants in palliative care

Depression

Psychostimulants are used where prognosis is thought to be ≤4 weeks. Trials generally show psychostimulants to be well tolerated in the short term but methodological limitations preclude firm conclusions about their efficacy as antidepressants.[8,19,20] Thus, conventional antidepressants should be used if the patient has a prognosis sufficient for a response to manifest.[8,19] Concurrent use of a psychostimulant with a conventional antidepressant may hasten the response compared with the latter alone, particularly in relation to fatigue.[19]

Methylphenidate is probably the most commonly used psychostimulant for depression in palliative care. Although undesirable effects are similar for all psychostimulants, some patients may benefit by switching to an alternative (e.g. **modafinil**) if the first choice is ineffective or poorly tolerated. **Ketamine** (p.641) is an alternative rapid-onset antidepressant.

Fatigue

The use of psychostimulants for fatigue is controversial. Although 2 meta-analyses (n=410,[21] n=498[22]) found **methylphenidate** to be moderately beneficial for cancer-related fatigue, subsequent RCTs found **methylphenidate** (2 RCTs; n=184), **modafinil** (2 RCTs; n=197) and **armodafinil** (n=50) to be no better than placebo.[23–28] Similarly, RCTs examining **armodafinil**, *D*-**methylphenidate** (not UK) and **modafinil** found conflicting results for fatigue related to chemotherapy,[27,29–32] cranial radiotherapy,[33] Parkinson's disease[34–36] and multiple sclerosis.[37,38] **Modafinil** may be beneficial for fatigue related to MND/ALS (n=32)[39] and HIV (n=115).[40]

Many trials found large placebo responses. Psychostimulants were generally well tolerated and some 'negative' RCTs noted clinically meaningful responses in sub-groups (e.g. those with more severe fatigue)[26,30]

Given this uncertainty, psychostimulants should be reserved for fatigue refractory to other measures, such as:

- correction of underlying causal factors, e.g. anaemia, depression, electrolyte disturbance
- modification of daily routine, e.g. exercise, energy conservation, practical help to aid adjustment to changing circumstances.[41–44]

Opioid-related drowsiness

Drowsiness is common when opioids are commenced or the dose is increased; it is generally transient, lasting about 1 week. Persistent drowsiness may indicate opioid toxicity; a trial dose reduction should be made and other drug and non-drug approaches considered to provide adequate analgesia (see p.299). However, some patients experience persistent drowsiness despite adjusting the opioid dose. In this circumstance, switching to an alternative opioid may be of benefit (see Appendix 2, p.855).

Psychostimulants are occasionally used for opioid-related drowsiness refractory to these measures. They may improve psychomotor performance and allow opioid dose escalation to a higher level than would otherwise be possible, including in some instances of difficult to manage break-through pain.[45] However, these reports predated the availability of other potential options, e.g. transmucosal **fentanyl** (see p.419).

Dose

SPCs recommend that heart rate, BP and an ECG (**modafanil**) are assessed at baseline, and subsequently heart rate and BP are monitored at regular intervals (e.g. every 6 months) or after an increase in dose.

Methylphenidate

- start with 2.5–5mg PO b.d. (on waking/breakfast time and noon/lunchtime)
- if necessary, increase by *daily* increments of 2.5–5mg b.d.
- usual maximum 20–40mg/24h
- up to 60mg/24h has been used for depression.[19]

Modafinil

Dose titration is slower:

- start with 100mg PO each morning
- if necessary after *1 week*, increase to 200mg each morning
- maximum dose 400mg/24h.

The manufacturer recommends either a single morning dose or divided doses in the morning and at noon. However, given the relatively long halflife of **modafinil**, the latter may increase the risk of sleep disturbance.

Dexamfetamine

- start with 2.5–5mg PO each morning
- if necessary, increase progressively *every 1–2 days* to 40mg each morning.

Supply

All products are **CD**.

Dexamefetamine

Dexamfetamine sulfate (generic)
Tablets *(scored)* 5mg, 28 days @ 5mg once daily = £25.
Oral solution 5mg/5mL, 28 days @ 5mg once daily = £30.

Amfexa (Flynn)
Tablets *(scored)* 10mg, 20mg, 28 days @ 5mg once daily = £20.

Methylphenidate

Methylphenidate hydrochloride (generic)
Tablets *(scored)* 5mg, 10mg, 20mg, 28 days @ 10mg b.d. = £11.
Oral suspension 5mg/5mL, 28 days @ 10mg b.d. = £180 (unauthorized product, available as a special order, see Chapter 24, p.751). *Price based on the Specials tariff in the community.*
Note. M/r products are available, but are not appropriate as daytime stimulants in palliative care.

Modafinil

Modafinil (generic)
Tablets 100mg, 200mg, 28 days @ 200mg each morning = £16.
Oral suspension 100mg/5mL, 28 days @ 200mg each morning = £391 (unauthorized product, available as a special order, see Chapter 24, p.751). *Price based on the Specials tariff in the community.*

1 MHRA (2010) European Medicines Agency recommends restricting the use of modafinil *Drug Safety Update*. **4**: www.mhra.gov.uk/Safetyinformation
2 Heal DJ *et al.* (2014) Dopamine reuptake transporter (DAT) "inverse agonism"–a novel hypothesis to explain the enigmatic pharmacology of cocaine. *Neuropharmacology*. **87**: 19–40.
3 Schmitt KC *et al.* (2013) Nonclassical pharmacology of the dopamine transporter: atypical inhibitors, allosteric modulators, and partial substrates. *Journal of Pharmacology and Experimental Therapeutics*. **346**: 2–10.
4 Stahl SM (2013) Chapter 4: Psychosis and schizophrenia. In: *Essential Psychopharmacology: Neuroscientific Basis and Practical Applications (4e)*. Cambridge University Press, USA. 79–128.
5 Phillips JM *et al.* (2016) A subcortical pathway for rapid, goal-driven, attentional filtering. *Trends Neurosciences*. **39**: 49–51.
6 del Campo N *et al.* (2013) A positron emission tomography study of nigro-striatal dopaminergic mechanisms underlying attention: implications for ADHD and its treatment. *Brain*. **136**: 3252–3270.
7 Stahl SM (2013) Chapter 5: Antipsychotic agents. In: *Essential Psychopharmacology: Neuroscientific Basis and Practical Applications (4e)*. Cambridge University Press, USA. 129–236.
8 Candy *et al.* (2008) Psychostimulants for depression. *Cochrane Database of Systematic Reviews*. **2**: CD006722. www.thecochranelibrary.com
9 Dein S and George R (2002) A place for psychostimulants in palliative care? *Journal of Palliative Care*. **18**: 196–199.
10 Masand PS and Tesar GE (1996) Use of stimulants in the medically ill. *Psychiatric Clinics of North America*. **19**: 515–547.
11 Burns MM and Eisendrath SJ (1994) Dextroamphetamine treatment for depression in terminally ill patients. *Psychosomatics*. **35**: 80–83.
12 Sawynok J (2011) Caffeine and pain. *Pain*. **152**: 726–729.
13 Suh SY *et al.* (2013) Caffeine as an adjuvant therapy to opioids in cancer pain: a randomized, double-blind, placebo-controlled trial. *Journal of Pain and Symptom Management*. **46**: 474–482.
14 Pinna A (2014) Adenosine A2A receptor antagonists in Parkinson's disease: progress in clinical trials from the newly approved istradefylline to drugs in early development and those already discontinued. *CNS Drugs*. **28**: 455–474.
15 Challman TD and Lipsky JJ (2000) Methylphenidate: its pharmacology and uses. *Mayo Clinic Proceedings*. **75**: 711–721.
16 de la Torre R *et al.* (2004) Clinical pharmacokinetics of amfetamine and related substances: monitoring in conventional and non-conventional matrices. *Clinical Pharmacokinetics*. **43**: 157–185.
17 Connor DF and Steingard RJ (2004) New formulations of stimulants for attention-deficit hyperactivity disorder: therapeutic potential. *CNS Drugs*. **18**: 1011–1030.
18 Robertson P, Jr. and Hellriegel ET (2003) Clinical pharmacokinetic profile of modafinil. *Clinical Pharmacokinetics*. **42**: 123–137.
19 Orr K and Taylor D (2007) Psychostimulants in the treatment of depression : a review of the evidence. *CNS Drugs*. **21**: 239–257.
20 Centeno C *et al.* (2012) Multi-centre, double-blind, randomised placebo-controlled clinical trial on the efficacy of methylphenidate on depressive symptoms in advanced cancer patients. *BMJ Supportive and Palliative Care*. **2**: 328–333.
21 Minton O *et al.* (2010) Drug therapy for the management of cancer-related fatigue. *Cochrane Database of Systematic Reviews*. **7** CD006704. www.thecochranelibrary.com
22 Gong S *et al.* (2014) Effect of methylphenidate in patients with cancer-related fatigue: a systematic review and meta-analysis. *PLoS One*. **9**: e84391.
23 Bruera E *et al.* (2013) Methylphenidate and/or a nursing telephone intervention for fatigue in patients with advanced cancer: a randomized, placebo-controlled, phase II trial. *Journal of Clinical Oncology*. **31**: 2421–2427.
24 Spathis A *et al.* (2014) Modafinil for the treatment of fatigue in lung cancer: results of a placebo-controlled, double-blind, randomized trial. *Journal of Clinical Oncology*. **32**: 1882–1888.
25 Berenson JR *et al.* (2015) A phase 3 trial of armodafinil for the treatment of cancer-related fatigue for patients with multiple myeloma. *Supportive Care in Cancer*. **23**: 1503–1512.

26 Mitchell GK *et al.* (2015) The effect of methylphenidate on fatigue in advanced cancer: an aggregated N-of-1 trial. *Journal of Pain and Symptom Management*. **50**: 289–296.
27 Heckler CE *et al.* (2016) Cognitive behavioral therapy for insomnia, but not armodafinil, improves fatigue in cancer survivors with insomnia: a randomized placebo-controlled trial. *Supportive Care in Cancer*. **24**: 2059–2066.
28 Boele FW *et al.* (2013) The effect of modafinil on fatigue, cognitive functioning, and mood in primary brain tumor patients: a multicenter randomized controlled trial. *Neuro-Oncology*. **15**: 1420–1428.
29 Lower EE *et al.* (2009) Efficacy of dexmethylphenidate for the treatment of fatigue after cancer chemotherapy: a randomized clinical trial. *Journal of Pain and Symptom Management*. **38**: 650–662.
30 Jean-Pierre P *et al.* (2010) A phase 3 randomized, placebo-controlled, double-blind, clinical trial of the effect of modafinil on cancer-related fatigue among 631 patients receiving chemotherapy: a University of Rochester Cancer Center Community Clinical Oncology Program Research base study. *Cancer*. **116**: 3513–3520.
31 Mar Fan HG *et al.* (2008) A randomised, placebo-controlled, double-blind trial of the effects of d-methylphenidate on fatigue and cognitive dysfunction in women undergoing adjuvant chemotherapy for breast cancer. *Supportive Care in Cancer*. **16**: 577–583.
32 Hovey E *et al.* (2014) Phase III, randomized, double-blind, placebo-controlled study of modafinil for fatigue in patients treated with docetaxel-based chemotherapy. *Supportive Care in Cancer*. **22**: 1233–1242.
33 Butler JM, Jr. *et al.* (2007) A phase III, double-blind, placebo-controlled prospective randomized clinical trial of d-threo-methylphenidate HCl in brain tumor patients receiving radiation therapy. *International Journal of Radiation Oncology, Biology, Physics*. **69**: 1496–1501.
34 Lou JS *et al.* (2009) Using modafinil to treat fatigue in Parkinson disease: a double-blind, placebo-controlled pilot study. *Clinical Neuropharmacology*. **32**: 305–310.
35 Mendonca DA *et al.* (2007) Methylphenidate improves fatigue scores in Parkinson disease: a randomized controlled trial. *Movement Disorders*. **22**: 2070–2076.
36 Tyne HL *et al.* (2010) Modafinil for Parkinson's disease fatigue. *Journal of Neurology*. **257**: 452–456.
37 Lange R *et al.* (2009) Modafinil effects in multiple sclerosis patients with fatigue. *Journal of Neurology*. **256**: 645–650.
38 Stankoff B *et al.* (2005) Modafinil for fatigue in MS: a randomized placebo-controlled double-blind study. *Neurology*. **64**: 1139–1143.
39 Rabkin JG *et al.* (2009) Modafinil treatment of fatigue in patients with ALS: a placebo-controlled study. *Muscle and Nerve*. **39**: 297–303.
40 Rabkin JG *et al.* (2010) Modafinil treatment for fatigue in HIV/AIDS: a randomized placebo-controlled study. *Journal of Clinical Psychiatry*. **71**: 707–715.
41 National Comprehensive Care Network (2014) Cancer related fatigue. In: *Clinical practice guidelines in oncology*. www.nccn.org
42 Radbruch L *et al.* (2008) Fatigue in palliative care patients – an EAPC approach. *Palliative Medicine*. **22**: 13–32.
43 Minton O *et al.* (2008) A systematic review and meta-analysis of the pharmacological treatment of cancer-related fatigue. *Journal of the National Cancer Institute*. **100**: 1155–1166.
44 Cramp F and Byron-Daniel J (2012) Exercise for the management of cancer-related fatigue in adults. *Cochrane Database of Systematic Reviews*. **11**: CD006145. www.thecochranelibrary.com
45 Stone P and Minton O (2011) European Palliative Care Research collaborative pain guidelines. Central side-effects management: what is the evidence to support best practice in the management of sedation, cognitive impairment and myoclonus? *Palliative Medicine*. **25**: 431–441.

Updated September 2017

*CANNABINOIDS

Indications: Chemotherapy-induced nausea and vomiting (nabilone); refractory spasticity in multiple sclerosis (Sativex®); †pain unresponsive to standard treatments.

Contra-indications: history (including family history) of psychosis.

Pharmacology

Endocannabinoids have important regulatory roles throughout the nervous system, immune system, and elsewhere, making them a potential therapeutic target for a wide range of disorders, including nausea, pain, cancer, cardiovascular disease, spasticity, epilepsy and immunomodulation.[1–7]

Currently prescribable cannabinoids all contain the psycho-active constituent of *Cannabis sativa*, Δ^9-tetrahydrocannabinol (Δ^9-THC) or a synthetic analogue. They are generally less effective or less well tolerated than alternative drugs and are relatively expensive. Their use as anti-emetics was rapidly eclipsed by the advent of $5HT_3$ antagonists. Although **dronabinol** (not UK) reduced AIDS-related anorexia and weight loss, there was a trend towards more rapid deterioration in performance status.[8] In cancer-related anorexia, cannabinoids were inferior to **megestrol** and no more effective than placebo.[9,10] Their analgesic effect is modest.[11] Further, despite interest in their respiratory effects,[12,13] benefit in breathlessness has *not* been confirmed by RCT.

Although patients report buying cannabidiol (CBD) from on-line suppliers, the MHRA considers these to be medicines and thus, subject to usual authorization processes.[14] Further, trials examining cannabinoids for symptom relief use Δ^9-THC, or a synthetic analogue, ± CBD, and not CBD *alone*.

An improved understanding of the endocannabinoid system and *Cannabis sativa's* many non-psycho-active compounds[1,15] has led to several developments in an attempt to improve effectiveness and tolerability:

- CB_2-selective agonists[16,17]
- peripherally-acting cannabinoids[18]
- inhibitors of endocannabinoid breakdown[19,20]
- combining cannabinoids with different properties, e.g. Δ^9-THC with CBD (see below).[21]

Endocannabinoid system

The endocannabinoid system comprises:[22]

- two known receptors
  - ▷ CB_1, expressed mainly by central and peripheral neurons
  - ▷ CB_2, expressed mainly by immune cells
- endogenous cannabinoids (endocannabinoids), mainly fatty acids derived from arachidonic acid, produced *de novo* as required, and then rapidly removed by hydrolysis. Several have been identified, notably:
  - ▷ anandamide (arachidonylethanolamide)
  - ▷ 2-arachidonyl glycerin (2-AG)[23]
- enzymes and uptake systems involved in endocannabinoid metabolism, including COX-2 and fatty acid amide hydrolase-1.[19,20]

CB_1 (an inhibitory receptor) reduces neuronal excitability and neurotransmitter release by opening potassium channels and blocking N/P/Q-type calcium channels respectively. It is part of a negative feedback loop which regulates neurotransmitter release and thereby the function of various CNS circuits (Figure 1). This partly explains some of the antispasticity, analgesic and other effects of cannabinoids.[22,24]

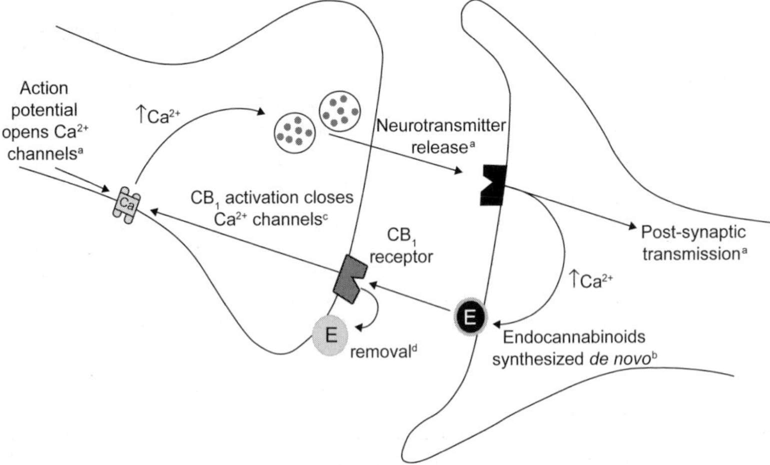

Figure 1 Cannabinoids and neurotransmission. Endocannabinoids are retrograde neurotransmitters, travelling from the post- to the pre-synaptic neurone as part of a negative feedback loop that regulates neurotransmitter release.

a. arriving action potential opens voltage gated calcium channels; increasing *pre-synaptic* intracellular calcium triggers the release of stored neurotransmitter. Post-synaptic events depend on the neurotransmitter but include an increase in intracellular calcium
b. increasing *post-synaptic* intracellular calcium triggers the *de novo* synthesis of endocannabinoids from arachidonic acid
c. activation of CB_1 closes *pre-synaptic* calcium channels preventing further calcium influx, thereby terminating neurotransmitter release. These channels are also targeted by other drugs of analgesic relevance, e.g. gabapentin, pregabalin, ziconotide
d. endocannabinoids removed by hydrolysis, e.g. fatty acid amide hydrolase-1.

Central and peripheral CB_1 receptors also modulate appetite and energy metabolism, respectively. CNS receptors are expressed on hypothalamic and limbic neurones; those in the periphery exist on adipocytes, skeletal muscle cells and hepatocytes. Activation of peripheral CB_1 receptors promotes fat deposition and insulin resistance.[25]

Animal studies suggest that central and peripheral CB_1 receptors also impact on the cardiorespiratory system. In the brainstem, CB_1 stimulation elicits respiratory depression, bradycardia and hypertension.[26] In the lung, the effect is variable, with CB_1 stimulation able to attenuate capsaicin-induced bronchoconstriction but also induce bronchoconstriction in vagotomized animals.[27]

CB_2 is implicated in immune regulation. Located on antigen-presenting cells, it influences their cytokine profile and thereby that of T-helper cells[4] This may partly explain its anti-inflammatory and antihyperalgesic effects. Its expression on microglia is upregulated in the dorsal root ganglia and spinal cord following sciatic nerve injury. It may also be expressed on neurones.[28]

The antihyperalgesic effects of CB_1 and CB_2 activation are distinct and additive, and include:[29]

- peripheral immunomodulation (antigen-presenting cell CB_2; interactions between immune cells and neurones contributes to peripheral sensitization and neuropathic pain)[30]
- central immunomodulation (CB_2 on microglia within the dorsal columns)
- disinhibition of antinociceptive neurones of a descending pain modulatory pathway (CB_1 on the pathway's GABAergic 'brake'; cf. opioids)[16,17,31,32]
- central dissociative effects.[33]

Further, unlike opioid receptors, CB_1 persists in the spinal cord after peripheral nerve injury.[34,35]

Endocannabinoids also act at other receptors, including the capsaicin receptor (TRPV1, involved in pain signalling), and perhaps also G protein-coupled receptors 55 and 119.[36]

Exogenous cannabinoids

Δ^9-THC is a CB_1 and CB_2 partial agonist. Its effects include muscle relaxation, analgesia, anti-emesis, but it can also cause sedation, anxiety and psychosis. **Dronabinol** (not UK) is a synthetic preparation of its (-)-*trans* isomer, the best studied of several isomers present in *Cannabis sativa*; **nabilone** is a synthetic analogue.

The effects of Δ^9-THC are modified by other cannabinoids present in *Cannabis sativa*. For example, cannabidiol (CBD) reduces Δ^9-THC-induced anxiety in healthy volunteers, perhaps by inhibiting the metabolism of Δ^9-THC to a more psycho-active metabolite, 11-hydroxyTHC. CBD is also a CB_1/CB_2 antagonist; its apparently low affinity for both receptors suggesting non-competitive antagonism through a separate binding site. Although a less potent analgesic and anti-emetic, CBD is anxiolytic, antipsychotic and non-sedating.[37,38]

In an attempt to improve the efficacy/tolerability profile of Δ^9-THC, a combined formulation of Δ^9-THC with CBD (**Sativex**®) has been developed; each oromucosal spray contains Δ^9-THC 2.7mg and CBD 2.5mg. It is authorized for refractory spasticity in multiple sclerosis and, in some countries, for pain (e.g. Canada, but not UK). However, results of RCTs in patients with pain comparing Δ^9-THC and CBD in combination with Δ^9-THC alone have been mixed; two RCTs found modest improvements in tolerability and patient preference,[39,40] one found modest improvements in efficacy, but not tolerability,[41] and one found no difference.[42]

The non-psycho-active constituents of *Cannabis sativa* are poorly understood but they may interact with non-CB_1/CB_2 cannabinoid receptors and/or the metabolism of endocannabinoids.[15] However, an RCT examining an inhibitor of endocannabinoid breakdown found no benefit for osteoarthritic pain.[20]

The therapeutic potential of cannabinoid antagonists and inverse agonists has also been investigated. Rimonabant, a CB_1 inverse agonist (i.e. results in a *reduction* in basal activity of the receptor), was approved for appetite suppression in obesity. However, it also caused depression, anxiety and aggression, and has been withdrawn.

The pharmacokinetic profiles of selected cannabinoids are summarized in Table 1. Food increases the absorption of Δ^9-THC and CBD oromucosal spray, suggesting a proportion of the dose is swallowed before absorption.

Cautions

Psychiatric history (mood, cognitive and behavioral changes can occur); severe ischemic heart disease, heart failure or arrhythmias (risk of postural hypotension or reflex tachycardia); renal or hepatic impairment (no data, but active hepatic metabolites undergo biliary and renal clearance); epilepsy (cannabinoids can either lower or raise seizure threshold).

Table 1 Pharmacokinetic profiles of selected cannabinoids[21,43]

	Oral bio-availability (%)	*Time to peak plasma concentration (h)*	*Halflife (h)*	*Metabolism*
Cannabidiol (CBD)	Not known	1–4	5–9	Multiple pathways[a, b]
Nabilone	85	1–4	2 5–10[a]	Multiple pathways[a, b]
Tetrahydrocannabinol (Δ^9-THC)	≥50	1–4	2–5	CYP2C9[c]

a. has active metabolite(s)

b. eliminated by both biliary and renal pathways

c. caffected by combined use: cannabidiol reduces Δ^9-THC-induced anxiety in healthy volunteers, perhaps by inhibiting the metabolism of Δ^9-THC to a more psycho-active metabolite, 11-hydroxyTHC.

Drug interactions

Additive CNS depressant effects with other psychotropics.

The metabolism of **Sativex**® is marginally inhibited by CYP3A4 inhibitors (e.g. **clarithromycin**, **ritonavir**) and may be induced by CYP3A4 inducers, (e.g. **carbamazepine**, **rifampicin**).

Cannabinoids inhibit numerous CYP450 enzymes, although generally not at typical therapeutic concentrations. Caution is advised when substrates for CYP2C19, 2D6 (e.g. **amitriptyline**) and 3A4 (e.g. **alfentanil**, **fentanyl**, **sufentanil**) are used concurrently with **Sativex**®.

Undesirable effects

Box A Undesirable effects of cannabinoids

Psychological[a]
Common (<10%, >1%): depression, euphoria, disorientation, dissociation
Uncommon (<1%, >0.1%): hallucinations, paranoia, delusions, suicidal ideation

Neurological[b]
Very common (>10%): dizziness (**Sativex**®, particularly during titration)
Common: ataxia, amnesia, drowsiness, blurred vision

Gastro-intestinal[c]
Common: appetite (↑ or ↓), nausea
Uncommon: abdominal pain

Cardiovascular
Uncommon: palpitations, tachycardia, syncope, hyper/hypotension

Buccal irritation[d] (**Sativex**® only)
Common: ulceration, pain
Uncommon: discoloration

a. illicit use is a risk factor for schizophrenia[44]

b. tolerance to CNS depressant effects generally develops after a few days

c. delayed onset nausea and vomiting ('cannabinoid hyperemesis') are described with illicit use of *Cannabis sativa*. Symptoms are generally worst in the morning (70%), associated with abdominal colic (86%), and resolve when the cannabinoid is discontinued. Although most patients have used cannabis weekly for at least 2 years before symptom onset, a third have symptoms within one year[45]

d. **Sativex**® contains 50% v/v ethanol and propylene glycol. Two reports of suspected leukoplakia occurred in RCTs.

Use of cannabinoids in palliative care

Food increases the absorption of **Sativex®**, resulting in both an increased C_{max} (some 2–3 times) and AUC (3–5 times). Consistent timing of administration with regard to mealtimes may be important in some patients.

The spray should only be directed beneath the tongue or inside the cheeks. The site of application should be varied and the buccal mucosa inspected regularly for signs of irritation caused by the excipients (ethanol (50%v/v), propylene glycol).

Δ^9-THC is included in a new law in England and Wales relating to driving with certain drugs above specified plasma concentrations (see Chapter 22, p.743).

Chemotherapy-induced nausea and vomiting (nabilone)

Although cannabinoids have some anti-emetic efficacy in *moderately* emetogenic chemotherapy regimens, $5HT_3$ antagonists are more effective and better tolerated and should be generally used instead.[46] The manufacturer advises against the use of **nabilone** for non-chemotherapy related nausea.

Nabilone should be given immediately before, during and for 2 days after each pulse of chemotherapy:

- start with 1mg PO b.d.
- if necessary, increase to 2mg b.d.
- maximum recommended dose 2mg t.d.s.

Dronabinol (not UK) is authorized in the US for this indication for patients who have failed to respond to conventional anti-emetics.

Refractory spasticity in multiple sclerosis (Sativex®)

The place, if any, of cannabinoids is uncertain. RCTs do not show consistent benefit.[11]

- start with 1 oromucosal spray at bedtime (see precautions above)
- increase over 2 weeks to a maximum of 12 sprays/24h given in divided doses, e.g. 1–2 sprays b.d.–3 sprays q.d.s.

Refractory pain (Sativex®, nabilone)

A systematic review found moderate benefit for a variety of non-cancer pains (NNT 3.5–9 for 30% pain reduction). Smoked cannabis, oromucosal cannabis extracts (including **Sativex®**), **nabilone**, and **dronabinol** (not UK) were effective for neuropathic pain, fibromyalgia, and painful spasticity. Undesirable effects were generally mild.[47–49] Most trials were short (<6 weeks) but open-label extension studies found that analgesia was maintained without dose escalation for up to 1.5 years.[50–52]

Two RCTs have examined **Sativex®** for intractable cancer pain with mixed results. In one, it was more effective than placebo or Δ^9-THC alone (NNT 4.5 for 30% pain reduction) but withdrawal due to undesirable effects was three-times higher with **Sativex®** than placebo (17% vs. 5%).[41] The other study found no difference between **Sativex®** and placebo in the primary endpoint of the proportion of patients reporting ≥30% reduction in pain. However, this was a graded dose study, which did not include titration to an optimal effect.[53]

For chemotherapy-related neuropathic pain, a small cross-over study found **Sativex®** no better than placebo.[54]

Sativex® (adapted from the Canadian Product Monograph):

- start with 1 oromucosal spray up to q4h (maximum 4 sprays in the first 24h); see precautions above
- titrate up on a daily basis (but more slowly if dizziness occurs)
- most patients require ≤12 sprays/24h (median dose = 5–8 sprays/24h).

Nabilone:

- start with 0.25mg to 0.5mg PO b.d.
- titrate in 0.5mg increments on a weekly basis
- maximum dose 1mg b.d.[55]

Supply

Nabilone (generic) is a Schedule 2 **CD**

Capsules 250microgram, 20 = £185. (Unauthorized, available as a special order from Creo Pharma; see Chapter 24, p.751).

Capsules 1mg, 20 = £196. (Unauthorized, available as a special order from Creo Pharma; see Chapter 24, p.751).

Sativex® (Bayer) is a Schedule 4 (part 1) **CD**.
Oromucosal spray *Cannabis sativa* extract (dronabinol) 27mg and CBD 25mg/mL each spray = 0.1mL, pack of 3 x 10mL (approx. 90 sprays/bottle) = £375; *the unopened pack should be stored in a refrigerator. Once opened, store at room temperature and use within 6 weeks.*

Records must be kept for 2 years for cannabis-based medicines (1961 UN Convention on Narcotic Drugs); this includes the quantities possessed or destroyed by those authorized to do so (patients and their representatives are exempt). The Home Office strongly recommends using a standard **CD** register for this.

1 Hill AJ *et al.* (2012) Cannabidivarin is anticonvulsant in mouse and rat in vitro and in seizure models. *British Journal of Pharmacology.* **167**: 1629–1642.
2 Preet A *et al.* (2011) Cannabinoid receptors, CB1 and CB2, as novel targets for inhibition of non-small cell lung cancer growth and metastasis. *Cancer Prevention Research.* **4**: 65–75.
3 Torres S *et al.* (2011) A combined preclinical therapy of cannabinoids and temozolomide against glioma. *Molecular Cancer Therapeutics.* **10**: 90–103.
4 Tanasescu R and Constantinescu CS (2010) Cannabinoids and the immune system: an overview. *Immunobiology.* **215**: 588–597.
5 Stanley CP *et al.* (2013) Is the cardiovascular system a therapeutic target for cannabidiol? *British Journal of Clinical Pharmacology.* **75**: 313–322.
6 Scotter EL *et al.* (2010) The endocannabinoid system as a target for the treatment of neurodegenerative disease. *British Journal of Pharmacology.* **160**: 480–498.
7 Castillo PE *et al.* (2012) Endocannabinoid signaling and synaptic function. *Neuron.* **76**: 70–81.
8 Beal JE *et al.* (1995) Dronabinol as a treatment for anorexia associated with weight loss in patients with AIDS. *Journal of Pain and Symptom Management.* **10**: 89–97.
9 Strasser F *et al.* (2006) Comparison of orally administered cannabis extract and delta-9-tetrahydrocannabinol in treating patients with cancer-related anorexia-cachexia syndrome: a multicenter, phase III, randomized, double-blind, placebo-controlled clinical trial from the Cannabis-In-Cachexia-Study-Group. *Journal of Clinical Oncology.* **24**: 3394–3400.
10 Jatoi A *et al.* (2002) Dronabinol versus megestrol acetate versus combination therapy for cancer-associated anorexia: a North Central Cancer Treatment Group study. *Journal of Clinical Oncology.* **20**: 567–573.
11 Farrell M *et al.* (2014) Should doctors prescribe cannabinoids? *British Medical Journal.* **348**: 2737.
12 Ahmedzai S (1988) Respiratory distress in the terminally ill patient. *Respiratory Disease in Practice.* **5**: 21–29.
13 Pickering EE *et al.* (2011) Cannabinoid effects on ventilation and breathlessness: a pilot study of efficacy and safety. *Chronic Respiratory Disease.* **8**: 109–118.
14 MHRA (2016) MHRA statement on products containing Cannabidiol (CBD). Available from: www.gov.uk
15 Izzo AA *et al.* (2009) Non-psychotropic plant cannabinoids: new therapeutic opportunities from an ancient herb. *Trends in Pharmacological Sciences.* **30**: 515–527.
16 Wilkerson JL *et al.* (2012) Intrathecal cannabilactone CB(2)R agonist, AM1710, controls pathological pain and restores basal cytokine levels. *Pain.* **153**: 1091–1106.
17 Gu X *et al.* (2011) Intrathecal administration of the cannabinoid 2 receptor agonist JWH015 can attenuate cancer pain and decrease mRNA expression of the 2B subunit of N-methyl-D-aspartic acid. *Anesthesia and Analgesia.* **113**: 405–411.
18 Yu XH *et al.* (2010) A peripherally restricted cannabinoid receptor agonist produces robust anti-nociceptive effects in rodent models of inflammatory and neuropathic pain. *Pain.* **151**: 337–344.
19 Roques BP *et al.* (2012) Inhibiting the breakdown of endogenous opioids and cannabinoids to alleviate pain. *Nature Reviews Drug Discovery.* **11**: 292–310.
20 Huggins JP *et al.* (2012) An efficient randomised, placebo-controlled clinical trial with the irreversible fatty acid amide hydrolase-1 inhibitor PF-04457845, which modulates endocannabinoids but fails to induce effective analgesia in patients with pain due to osteoarthritis of the knee. *Pain.* **153**: 1837–1846.
21 Barnes MP (2006) Sativex: clinical efficacy and tolerability in the treatment of symptoms of multiple sclerosis and neuropathic pain. *Expert Opinion on Pharmacotherpy.* **7**: 607–615.
22 Rea K *et al.* (2007) Supraspinal modulation of pain by cannabinoids: the role of GABA and glutamate. *British Journal of Pharmacology.* **152**: 633–648.
23 Mechoulam R *et al.* (1998) Endocannabinoids. *European Journal of Pharmacology.* **359**: 1–18.
24 Pryce G and Baker D (2007) Control of spasticity in a multiple sclerosis model is mediated by CB1, not CB2, cannabinoid receptors. *British Journal of Pharmacology.* **150**: 519–525.
25 Tibirica E (2010) The multiple functions of the endocannabinoid system: a focus on the regulation of food intake. *Diabetology and Metabolic Syndrome.* **2**: 5.
26 Pfitzer T *et al.* (2004) Central effects of the cannabinoid receptor agonist WIN55212-2 on respiratory and cardiovascular regulation in anaesthetised rats. *British Journal of Pharmacology.* **142**: 943–952.
27 Calignano A *et al.* (2000) Bidirectional control of airway responsiveness by endogenous cannabinoids. *Nature.* **408**: 96–101.
28 Atwood BK and Mackie K (2010) CB2: a cannabinoid receptor with an identity crisis. *British Journal of Pharmacology.* **160**: 467–479.
29 Gutierrez T *et al.* (2007) Activation of peripheral cannabinoid CB1 and CB2 receptors suppresses the maintenance of inflammatory nociception: a comparative analysis. *British Journal of Pharmacology.* **150**: 153–163.
30 Scholz J and Woolf CJ (2007) The neuropathic pain triad: neurons, immune cells and glia. *Nature Neuroscience.* **10**: 1361–1368.
31 Meng ID *et al.* (1998) An analgesia circuit activated by cannabinoids. *Nature.* **395**: 381–383.
32 Welch SP (2009) Interaction of the cannabinoid and opioid systems in the modulation of nociception. *International Reviews on Psychiatry.* **21**: 143–151.
33 Lee MC *et al.* (2013) Amygdala activity contributes to the dissociative effect of cannabis on pain perception. *Pain.* **154**: 124–134.

34 Farquhar-Smith WP and Rice AS (2001) Administration of endocannabinoids prevents a referred hyperalgesia associated with inflammation of the urinary bladder. *Anesthesiology*. **94**: 507–513; discussion 506A.
35 Hohmann AG and Herkenham M (1998) Regulation of cannabinoid and mu opioid receptors in rat lumbar spinal cord following neonatal capsaicin treatment. *Neuroscience Letters*. **252**: 13–16.
36 Brown AJ (2007) Novel cannabinoid receptors. *British Journal of Pharmacology*. **152**: 567–575.
37 Fusar-Poli P *et al.* (2009) Distinct effects of {delta}9-tetrahydrocannabinol and cannabidiol on neural activation during emotional processing. *Archives of General Psychiatry*. **66**: 95–105.
38 Russo E and Guy GW (2006) A tale of two cannabinoids: the therapeutic rationale for combining tetrahydrocannabinol and cannabidiol. *Medical Hypotheses*. **66**: 234–246.
39 Wade DT *et al.* (2003) A preliminary controlled study to determine whether whole-plant cannabis extracts can improve intractable neurogenic symptoms. *Clinical Rehabilitation*. **17**: 21–29.
40 Notcutt W *et al.* (2004) Initial experiences with medicinal extracts of cannabis for chronic pain: results from 34 'N of 1' studies. *Anaesthesia*. **59**: 440–452.
41 Johnson JR *et al.* (2010) Multicenter, double-blind, randomized, placebo-controlled, parallel-group study of the efficacy, safety, and tolerability of THC:CBD extract and THC extract in patients with intractable cancer-related pain. *Journal of Pain and Symptom Management*. **39**: 167–179.
42 Berman JS *et al.* (2004) Efficacy of two cannabis based medicinal extracts for relief of central neuropathic pain from brachial plexus avulsion: results of a randomised controlled trial. *Pain*. **112**: 299–306.
43 Grotenhermen F (2003) Pharmacokinetics and pharmacodynamics of cannabinoids. *Clinical Pharmacokinetics*. **42**: 327–360.
44 Malone DT *et al.* (2010) Adolescent cannabis use and psychosis: epidemiology and neurodevelopmental models. *British Journal of Pharmacology*. **160**: 511–522.
45 Simonetto DA *et al.* (2012) Cannabinoid hyperemesis: a case series of 98 patients. *Mayo Clinic Proceedings*. **87**: 114–119.
46 Davis MP (2008) Oral nabilone capsules in the treatment of chemotherapy-induced nausea and vomiting and pain. *Expert Opinion Investigational Drugs*. **17**: 85–95.
47 Lynch ME and Campbell F (2011) Cannabinoids for treatment of chronic non-cancer pain; a systematic review of randomized trials. *British Journal of Clinical Pharmacology*. **72**: 735–744.
48 Toth C *et al.* (2012) An enriched-enrolment, randomized withdrawal, flexible-dose, double-blind, placebo-controlled, parallel assignment efficacy study of nabilone as adjuvant in the treatment of diabetic peripheral neuropathic pain. *Pain*. **153**: 2073–2082.
49 Langford RM *et al.* (2013) A double-blind, randomized, placebo-controlled, parallel-group study of THC/CBD oromucosal spray in combination with the existing treatment regimen, in the relief of central neuropathic pain in patients with multiple sclerosis. *Journal of Neurology*. **260**: 984–997.
50 Wade DT *et al.* (2006) Long-term use of a cannabis-based medicine in the treatment of spasticity and other symptoms in multiple sclerosis. *Multiple Sclerosis*. **12**: 639–645.
51 Nurmikko TJ *et al.* (2007) Sativex successfully treats neuropathic pain characterised by allodynia: a randomised, double-blind, placebo-controlled clinical trial. *Pain*. **133**: 210–220.
52 Johnson JR *et al.* (2013) An open-label extension study to investigate the long-term safety and tolerability of THC/CBD oromucosal spray and oromucosal THC spray in patients with terminal cancer-related pain refractory to strong opioid analgesics. *Journal of Pain and Symptom Management*. **46**: 207–218.
53 Portenoy RK *et al.* (2012) Nabiximols for opioid-treated cancer patients with poorly-controlled chronic pain: a randomized, placebo-controlled, graded-dose trial. *Journal of Pain*. **13**: 438–449.
54 Lynch ME *et al.* (2014) A double-blind, placebo-controlled, crossover pilot trial with extension using an oral mucosal cannabinoid extract for treatment of chemotherapy-induced neuropathic pain. *Journal of Pain and Symptom Management*. **47**: 166–173.
55 CADTH (2011) Nabilone for chronic pain management: a review of clinical efectiveness, safety and guidelines. In: *Canadian Agency for Drugs and Technologies in Health; Rapid Response Report: summary with critical appraisal* Available from: www.cadth.ca

Updated September 2017

ANTI-EMETICS

Indications: Authorized indications vary between products; consult SPC for details. Nausea and vomiting, †delayed gastric emptying, †hiccup, †pruritus, †diarrhoea associated with carcinoid syndrome.

Pharmacology

Anti-emetics are a functionally diverse group of drugs acting on one or more sites implicated in nausea and/or vomiting (Figure 1). Because there is little direct RCT evidence to guide drug selection in palliative care,[1–3] choice of anti-emetic is guided by the probable mechanism by which the drug acts (Table 1). This 'mechanistic approach' is successful in most patients.[4,5] Other factors to consider include the response to anti-emetics already given and the undesirable effects, cost and available routes of alternatives (see individual monographs).

The model underlying this approach is extrapolated from experimental data, RCTs in postoperative and chemotherapy-related nausea and vomiting, and neuro-imaging.[6–11] For example, whilst **droperidol** reduces *nausea* more successfully than vomiting, $5HT_3$ antagonists are more effective for *vomiting*; thus, they might be expected to act in the effector pathways responsible for these respective symptoms (see Figure 1).[6] Neuro-imaging confirms that D_2 and $5HT_3$ receptors, respectively, *are* present in these locations.

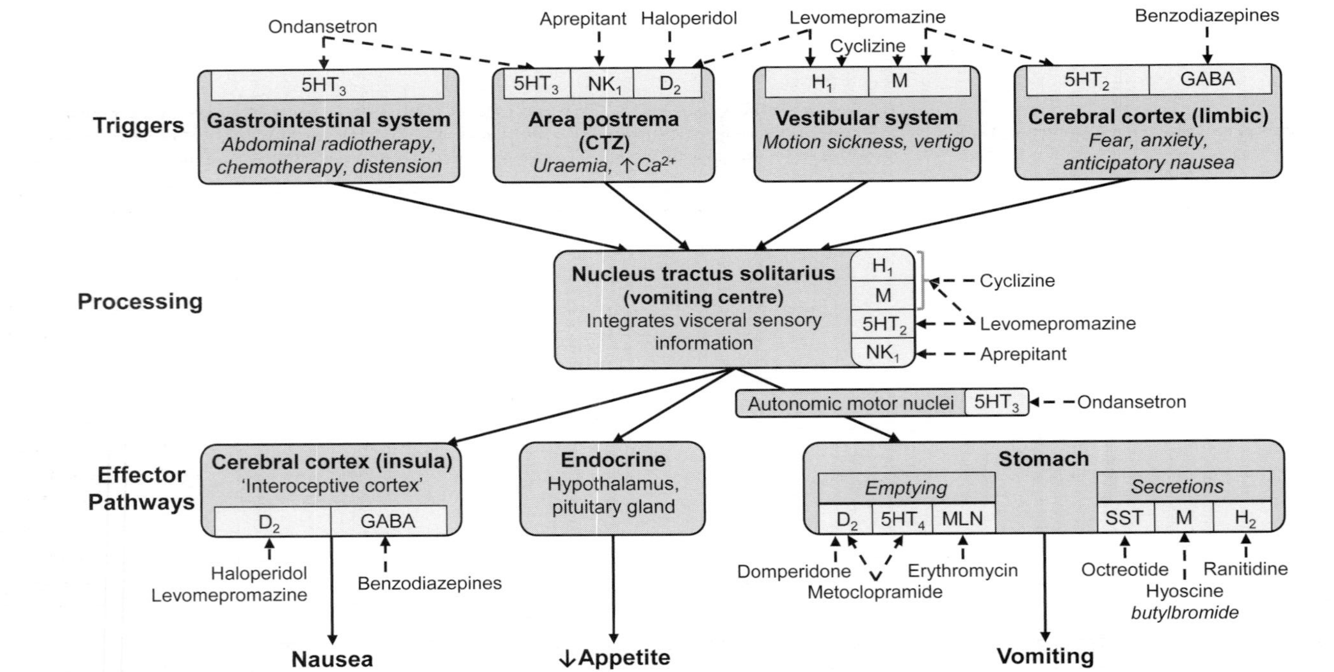

Figure 1 Putative peripheral and central sites of action of selected anti-emetics. Also see individual drug monographs.[6–11]

Ca^{2+} = Calcium; CTZ = Chemoreceptor Trigger Zone. Other abbreviations refer to receptor types: M = muscarinic cholinergic; D_2 = dopamine type 2; $5HT_2$, $5HT_3$ = 5-hydroxytriptamine (serotonin) type 2, type 3; H_1, H_2 = histamine type 1, type 2; NK_1 = neurokinin 1. Anti-emetics act as *antagonists* at these receptors, whereas the effects on $5HT_4$ (5-hydroxytriptamine type 4), MLN (Motilin), SST (Somatostatin) and GABA (gamma-aminobutyric acid) are *agonistic*.

Table 1 Receptor site affinities of selected anti-emetics[12–16]

	D_2 antagonist	*H_1 antagonist*	*Muscarinic antagonist*	*$5HT_2$ antagonist*	*$5HT_3$ antagonist*	*NK_1 antagonist*	*$5HT_4$ agonist*	*CB_1 agonist*	*GABAmimetic*
Aprepitant	–	–	–	–	–	+++	–	–	–
Chlorpromazine	+++	+++	++	++	–	–	–	–	–
Cyclizine	–	++	++	–	–	–	–	–	–
Domperidone	++[a]	–	–	–	–	–	–	–	–
Haloperidol, droperidol	+++	–	–	–	+/–	–	–	–	–
Hyoscine *hydrobromide*[b]	–	–	+++	–	–	–	–	–	–
Levomepromazine	++	+++	++	+++	–	–	–	–	–
Lorazepam	–	–	–	–	–	–	–	–	+++
Metoclopramide	++	–	–	–	+	–	++	–	–
Nabilone	–	–	–	–	–	–	–	+++	–
Ondansetron, granisetron	–	–	–	–	+++	–	–	–	–
Olanzapine	++	+	++	++	+	–	–	–	–
Prochlorperazine	+++	++	+	+/++	–	–	–	–	–
Promethazine	+/++	++	++	–	–	–	–	–	–

Pharmacological activity: +++ = marked; ++ = moderate; + = slight; – = none or insignificant.

a. domperidone does not normally cross the blood-brain barrier; thus the risk of extrapyramidal effects is negligible (see p.247)

b. hyoscine *butylbromide* and glycopyrronium also act on muscarinic receptors in the periphery (GI tract antisecretory effect). However, because they do not cross the blood brain barrier, they do not act in the vestibular system (or cause the undesirable CNS effects associated with hyoscine *hydrobromide*).

The model is also based on clinical experience. Thus, H_1 receptors were hypothesized to exist in the vestibular system because H_1 antagonists appear effective for nausea related to vestibular irritation. Although neuro-imaging is starting to corroborate these locations, there are knowledge-gaps in the 'mechanistic approach'.

Cautions

For information on the use of anti-emetics in renal and hepatic impairment, see p.687 and p.711.

Use in palliative care

Nausea and vomiting

Also see QCG: Nausea and vomiting (p.240), and QCG: Inoperable bowel obstruction (p.242).

First-line anti-emetics

Generally, in palliative care, the initial choice depends upon the cause:

- for vestibular irritation or raised intracranial pressure → anti-emetic acting principally in the vestibular system and vomiting centre, e.g. **cyclizine** (p.249)
- for most chemical causes of vomiting, e.g. **morphine**, hypercalcaemia, renal failure → anti-emetic acting principally in chemoreceptor trigger zone, e.g. **haloperidol** (p.180)
- for gastritis, gastric stasis or functional bowel obstruction (peristaltic failure) → a prokinetic, e.g. **domperidone** (p.247) or **metoclopramide** (p.244).

Drug-induced nausea and vomiting can be caused by several different mechanisms (Table 2), each of which requires a distinct therapeutic response.

Table 2 Causes of drug-induced nausea and vomiting

Mechanism	*Drugs*
Gastric irritation	Antibacterials Corticosteroids Iron supplements Misoprostol NSAIDs Spironolactone Tranexamic acid
Gastric stasis	Antimuscarinics (e.g. TCAs) Opioids
Area postrema stimulation (chemoreceptor trigger zone)	Antibacterials Cytotoxics Digoxin Imidazoles Opioids
$5HT_3$-receptor stimulation	Antibacterials Cytotoxics SSRIs

Second-line anti-emetics

If symptoms persist, consider an alternative first-line anti-emetic or switch to a broader spectrum drug, e.g. **levomepromazine** (p.184) and **olanzapine** (p.187); these have affinity at many receptors and may be as effective as, and easier for patients to handle than, two or more different anti-emetics simultaneously.

Third-line anti-emetics

If **levomepromazine** or **olanzapine** fail to relieve nausea and vomiting, they can be *combined* with an anti-emetic with different receptor affinities, typically a $5HT_3$ antagonist (p.253).

Alternatives include **dexamethasone** (p.760) and benzodiazepines (p.149). Although a specific role for benzodiazepines in *anticipatory* nausea has been proposed, there is limited evidence to support this over and above their general anti-emetic effect (see p.149).

Although **aprepitant**, a neurokinin 1 (NK_1) antagonist, and **nabilone** (p.229), a cannabinoid, also act at distinct sites, their place, if any, in the palliative care setting is unclear. Both are expensive. Further, **aprepitant** is a CYP 3A4 inhibitor (see p.725). A parenteral pro-drug, **fosaprepitant**, is available for IV use.

Hiccup and delayed gastric emptying

In palliative care, prokinetics (p.24) are used for hiccup, early satiety and other symptoms of delayed gastric emptying. First-line options include **domperidone** (p.247) and **metoclopramide** (p.244). Alternatives include **clonidine** (p.77) and **erythromycin** (p.24). All are unauthorized and have important safety considerations (see individual monographs).

4

Carcinoid-related diarrhoea

Ondansetron is reported to be beneficial for diarrhoea refractory to **octreotide** (see p.253).

Pruritus

Ondansetron relieves pruritus related to spinal **morphine** but not cholestatic or uraemic pruritus (p.253, also see Chapter 26, p.757).

Aprepitant is reported to improve pruritus due to Sezary syndrome,[17] mycosis fungoides,[18] chemotherapy (mainly **cetuximab** or **erlotinib**)[19] and chronic pruritus of mixed cause (including uraemic, diabetic and idiopathic pruritus).[20] Most used 80mg once daily; benefit was often seen ≤2 days. It is expensive and a CYP 3A4 inhibitor (p.725).

1 Davis MP *et al.* (2010) A systematic review of the treatment of nausea and/or vomiting in cancer unrelated to chemotherapy or radiation. *Journal of Pain and Symptom Management.* **39**: 756–767.
2 Glare P *et al.* (2011) Treating nausea and vomiting in palliative care: a review. *Clinical Interventions in Aging.* **6**: 243–259.
3 Glare P *et al.* (2004) Systematic review of the efficacy of antiemetics in the treatment of nausea in patients with far-advanced cancer. *Support Care Cancer.* **12**: 432–440.
4 Bentley A and Boyd K (2001) Use of clinical pictures in the management of nausea and vomiting: a prospective audit. *Palliative Medicine.* **15**: 247–253.
5 Stephenson J and Davies A (2006) An assessment of aetiology-based guidelines for the management of nausea and vomiting in patients with advanced cancer. *Supportive Care in Cancer.* **14**: 348–353.
6 Stern RM (2011) Section II: Physiology of Nausea. In: *Nausea mechanisms and management.* Oxofrd University Press, USA, 39–167.
7 Santana TA *et al.* (2015) Meta-analysis of adjunctive non-NK1 receptor antagonist medications for the control of acute and delayed chemotherapy-induced nausea and vomiting. *Supportive Care in Cancer.* **23**: 213–222.
8 Saulin A *et al.* (2012) Serotonin and molecular neuroimaging in humans using PET. *Amino Acids.* **42**: 2039–2057.
9 Farmer AD *et al.* (2015) Visually induced nausea causes characteristic changes in cerebral, autonomic and endocrine function in humans. *Journal of Physiology.* **593**: 1183–1196.
10 Napadow V *et al.* (2013) The brain circuitry underlying the temporal evolution of nausea in humans. *Cerebral Cortex.* **23**: 806–813.
11 Becker DE (2010) Nausea, vomiting, and hiccups: a review of mechanisms and treatment. *Anesthesia Progress.* **57**: 150–156.
12 Peroutka SJ and Snyder SH (1982) Antiemetics: neurotransmitter receptor binding predicts therapeutic actions. *Lancet.* **1**: 658–659.
13 Fleming M and Hawkins C (2005) Use of atypical antipsychotic olanzapine as an anti-emetic. *European Journal of Palliative Care.* **12**: 144–146.
14 Saito R *et al.* (2003) Roles of substance P and NK(1) receptor in the brainstem in the development of emesis. *Journal of Pharmacology Science.* **91**: 87–94.
15 Aapro MS *et al.* (2005) Anticipatory nausea and vomiting. *Supportive Care in Cancer.* **13**: 117–121.
16 Davis M *et al.* (2007) The emerging role of cannabinoid neuromodulators in symptom management. *Supportive Care in Cancer.* **15**: 63–71.
17 Torres T *et al.* (2012) Aprepitant: Evidence of its effectiveness in patients with refractory pruritus continues. *Journal of the American Academy of Dermatology.* **66**: e14–15.
18 Jimenez Gallo D *et al.* (2014) Treatment of pruritus in early-stage hypopigmented mycosis fungoides with aprepitant. *Dermatologic Therapy.* **27**: 178–182.
19 Santini D *et al.* (2012) Aprepitant for management of severe pruritus related to biological cancer treatments: a pilot study. *Lancet Oncology.* **13**: 1020-1024.
20 Stander S *et al.* (2010) Targeting the neurokinin receptor 1 with aprepitant: a novel antipruritic strategy. *PLoS One.* **5**: e10968.

Updated September 2017

Quick Clinical Guide: Nausea and vomiting

1 From the patient's history and physical examination, decide what is the most likely cause (or causes) of the nausea and vomiting. Take a blood sample if biochemical derangement is suspected. For bowel obstruction, see QCG: Inoperable bowel obstruction.

2 Correct correctable causes/exacerbating factors, e.g. drugs, severe pain, cough, infection, hypercalcaemia. *(Remember: antibacterial treatment and correction of hypercalcaemia are not always appropriate in a dying patient).*

3 Prescribe the most appropriate anti-emetic regularly and p.r.n.

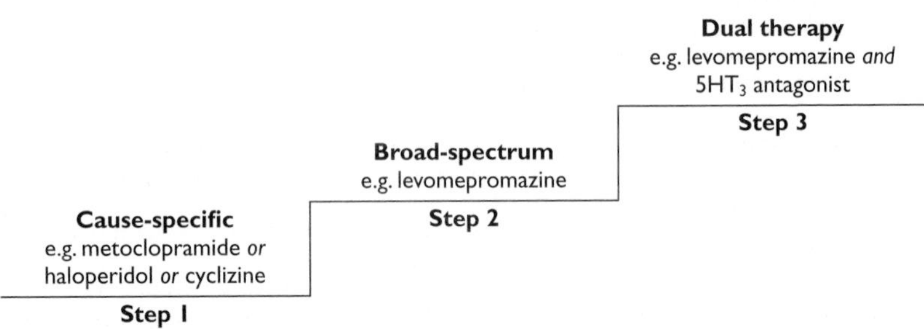

Commonly used Step 1 (cause-specific) anti-emetics

For gastritis, gastric stasis, functional bowel obstruction (peristaltic failure)

Prokinetic anti-emetic:

- metoclopramide
  - ▷ PO 10mg t.d.s.–q.d.s. & 10mg q2h p.r.n.
  - ▷ CSCI 30–40mg/24h & 10mg SC q2h p.r.n.
  - ▷ PO/CSCI usual maximum 100mg/24h
- domperidone
  - ▷ PO 10mg b.d.–t.d.s.

For most chemical causes of vomiting, e.g. morphine, hypercalcaemia, renal failure

Anti-emetic acting principally in chemoreceptor trigger zone:

- haloperidol
  - ▷ PO 500microgram–1.5mg at bedtime & q2h p.r.n.
  - ▷ SC/CSCI 2.5–5mg/24h & 1mg SC q2h p.r.n
  - ▷ PO/SC/CSCI usual maximum 10mg/24h.

Metoclopramide also has a central action.

For raised intracranial pressure (in conjunction with dexamethasone) and/or vestibular symptoms

Anti-emetic acting principally in the vestibular system and vomiting centre:

- cyclizine
  - ▷ PO 50mg b.d.–t.d.s. & 50mg p.r.n.
  - ▷ CSCI 100–150mg/24h & 50mg SC p.r.n.
  - ▷ PO/CSCI usual maximum 200mg/24h.

4 Give by SC injection or CSCI if continuous nausea or frequent vomiting.

5 Start with a stat p.r.n. dose to cover the period before the first regular dose or the delay in reaching therapeutic levels by CSCI.

6 Initially, review anti-emetic dose each day; take note of p.r.n. use, and adjust the regular dose accordingly.

7 If little benefit despite upward titration of the dose, reconsider the likely cause(s), and review the choice of anti-emetic and route of administration. Sometimes it is necessary to convert to a broad-spectrum anti-emetic, and occasionally dual therapy will be needed.

Commonly used Step 2 and 3 anti-emetics

Step 2: Broad-spectrum

- levomepromazine
  - ▷ PO/SC: 6.25mg at bedtime & q2h p.r.n.
  - ▷ usual maximum 25mg/24h
  - ▷ at home, consider CSCI if a bedtime SC injection is impractical.

Step 3: Dual therapy (combining anti-emetics with different mechanisms)

- levomepromazine + a $5HT_3$ antagonist, e.g. granisetron 1–2mg SC once daily or CSCI, or ondansetron 16mg/24h CSCI
- levomepromazine + a benzodiazepine, e.g. lorazepam 0.5–1mg SL b.d. or midazolam 10mg/24h CSCI, *particularly when anxiety or anticipatory nausea*
- levomepromazine + dexamethasone 8–16mg PO/SC stat & once daily *when all else fails*; stop dexamethasone if no benefit after one week; otherwise taper by 2mg/week to the minimum effective dose.

8 Prokinetics act through a cholinergic system which is competitively antagonized by antimuscarinics; concurrent use is best avoided.

9 Seizures occasionally present as nausea (e.g. with meningeal carcinomatosis); this responds to anti-epileptic drugs or benzodiazepines.

10 Continue the anti-emetic(s) unless the cause is self-limiting. Except in mechanical bowel obstruction (see QCG: Inoperable bowel obstruction), consider changing to PO after 3 days of good control with CSCI.

11 With successful dual therapy, it may be possible to simplify the regimen after 1–2 weeks by tapering the dose of one of the two anti-emetics.

Updated September 2017

Quick Clinical Guide: Inoperable bowel obstruction

Initial management

1 Resting the GI tract for several days may allow an obstruction to settle spontaneously:
- restrict PO intake to sips of fluid to keep the mouth comfortable, and hydrate IV/SC, e.g. 10–20mL/Kg/24h
- a nasogastric (NG) tube can be reserved for patients experiencing large volume vomits more than 2–3 times/24h
- correct electrolyte imbalances which may contribute to peristaltic failure, e.g. low potassium, low magnesium
- a combination of analgesics (opioids and antispasmodics), anti-emetics and antisecretory drugs should be used to manage abdominal pain, colic, and nausea and vomiting (see below)
- some centres add dexamethasone, e.g. 6.6mg once daily SC for 5–7 days (evidence suggests only a trend towards benefit) with ranitidine 50mg t.d.s.–q.d.s. IV/SC or 150–200mg/24h CSCI as antacid cover; ranitidine, unlike PPIs, reduces gastric secretions and can be combined with many other drugs used in a syringe driver.

Ongoing management (≥1 week)

2 If the obstruction does not settle with the above measures, the aim (*although not always achieved*) is to:
- control pain and nausea *and*
- minimize vomiting so as to avoid the need for a nasogastric tube *and*
- permit sufficient oral fluids to maintain hydration.

Symptom management

3 For constant background cancer pain, morphine should be given regularly by the clock and p.r.n. For those with colic, an antispasmodic antisecretory anti-emetic should be given (see below).

4 Drugs for inoperable bowel obstruction are best given by CSCI (for more information on anti-emetic doses, see QCG: Nausea and vomiting), but some, e.g. dexamethasone, levomepromazine, can be given as a single SC daily dose.

5 The ladder shows a general approach; dose titration over several days may be necessary before optimum relief is achieved:
- start on Step 1 if *no* colic: probable functional obstruction (i.e. peristaltic failure):
  - ▷ metoclopramide 30–40mg/24h CSCI & 10mg SC q2h p.r.n.
  - ▷ if beneficial, optimize the dose up to 100mg/24h
- start on Step 2 if colic: probable mechanical obstruction:
  - ▷ hyoscine *butylbromide* 60–120mg/24h CSCI & 20mg SC q1h p.r.n.
  - ▷ maximum reported dose 300mg/24h.

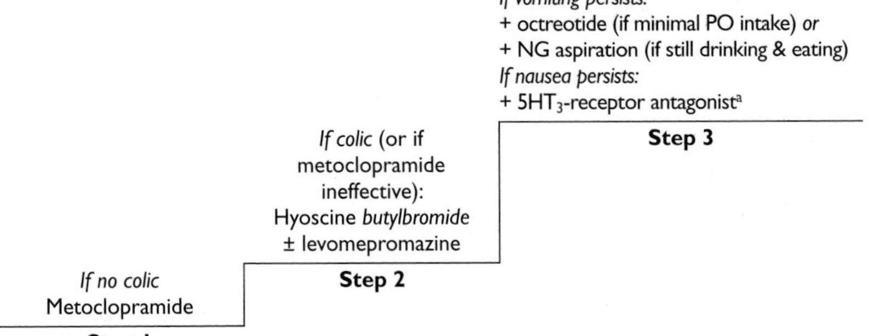

± Dexamethasone[b]

a. e.g. granisetron 1–2mg SC once daily, ondansetron 16mg/24h CSCI
b. see point 1 above.

6 Instead of levomepromazine, some centres use:
- cyclizine 100–150mg/24h CSCI & 50mg SC p.r.n. (maximum 200mg/24h) *or*
- haloperidol 1.5–5mg/24h CSCI & 1mg SC q2h p.r.n. (maximum 10mg/24h).

Note. Cyclizine mixed with hyoscine *butylbromide* may be incompatible.

7 If levomepromazine is too sedative, consider as alternatives:
- cyclizine and haloperidol combined, *or*
- olanzapine 1.25–2.5mg SC (not UK) at bedtime.

8 If heartburn/acid reflux occurs, start/continue ranitidine (see point 1).

9 If hyoscine *butylbromide* is inadequate to control vomiting, or to obtain more rapid relief, consider octreotide (a somatostatin analogue and antisecretory agent):
- if colic, add to hyoscine *butylbromide*
- if no colic, substitute or use instead of hyoscine *butylbromide:*
  - ▷ octreotide 100microgram SC stat
  - ▷ CSCI 500microgram/24h
  - ▷ usual maximum 750microgram/24h, occasionally higher.

10 If vomiting persists, review the patient's oral intake. Antisecretory drugs cannot fully alleviate the vomiting of ingested fluid and food; consider NG tube or venting gastrostomy.

11 In partial obstruction, there may be passage of flatus and faeces. When a laxative is required, use a stool softener that does not distend the bowel, i.e. sodium docusate 100–200mg PO b.d.

Nutrition

12 Some patients and carers are concerned about a restricted oral caloric intake, and need sensitive counselling. Note:
- with a distal obstruction a patient may still manage and absorb small amounts of oral fibre-free nutritional supplements and/or readily digestible food
- sometimes a patient chooses a long-term nasogastric tube or considers a venting gastrostomy to permit unrestricted oral intake
- parenteral nutrition generally has no role in patients with limited options for anti-cancer treatment or poor performance status.

Updated September 2017

METOCLOPRAMIDE

Class: Prokinetic anti-emetic.

Indications: Nausea and vomiting caused by surgery, chemotherapy (delayed, not acute), radiation therapy or migraine. All other uses are unauthorized, e.g. †delayed gastric emptying, †dysmotility dyspepsia, †gastric irritation, †heartburn, †hiccups.

Contra-indications: Children <1 year old. Phaeochromocytoma (may induce an acute hypertensive response). GI haemorrhage or perforation. Use within <4 days of GI surgery (vigorous contractions may impair healing).

Pharmacology

Metoclopramide is a D_2 antagonist which acts both centrally in the area postrema (chemoreceptor trigger zone) and peripherally in the upper GI tract, where it blocks the 'dopamine brake' on gastric emptying induced by stress, anxiety and nausea. Further, as a $5HT_4$ agonist, it has a direct excitatory effect in the upper GI tract. Although $5HT_3$ antagonism occurs at higher doses (e.g. 2–4mg/kg IV), the use of high-dose metoclopramide for chemotherapy-related nausea and vomiting has been superseded by specific $5HT_3$-receptor antagonists (see p.253).

For gastroparesis, its efficacy is comparable to **domperidone** (p.247).[1] However, it causes more frequent and more severe undesirable effects including drowsiness, loss of mental acuity, and extrapyramidal symptoms.[2]

Metoclopramide is metabolized in the liver, with CYP2D6 the main CYP450 enzyme involved. It is eliminated mainly via the kidney, either as conjugated metabolites or unchanged (20–30%). Both hepatic and renal impairment reduce the clearance of metoclopramide, resulting in higher plasma levels and a prolonged halflife and the SPC advises a reduced dose. Thus, in patients with moderate–severe renal impairment or ESRF or severe cirrhosis, reduce the usual starting dose and monitor carefully (see Chapter 17, p.681 and Chapter 18, p.703).[3]

Metoclopramide is a commonly used anti-emetic in palliative care. In RCTs, cancer-related nausea and vomiting resolves in about ≤33% and ≤50%, respectively.[4,5] Although metoclopramide often has immediate effect, benefit may increase throughout the first week of use.[6–8]

Bio-availability 50–80% PO.
Onset of action 10–15min IM; 15–60min PO.
Time to peak plasma concentration 1–2.5h PO.
Plasma halflife 2.5–5h.
Duration of action 1–2h (data for single dose and relating to gastric emptying).

Cautions

Cardiac disease; enhanced effects of catecholamines in patients with essential hypertension[9,10] (also see Undesirable effects); epilepsy (lowers seizure threshold); Parkinson's disease; mechanical GI obstruction (but is commonly used in palliative care to restore peristalsis in functional GI obstruction).[11,12]

Moderate–severe renal impairment or ESRF, severe hepatic impairment, (see pharmacology and Chapter 17, p.681 and Chapter 18, p.703).

Drug interactions

Serious drug interaction: a combination of IV metoclopramide and IV **ondansetron** occasionally causes cardiac arrhythmias.[13] $5HT_3$-receptors influence various aspects of cardiac function, including inotropy, chronotropy and coronary arterial tone,[14] effects which are mediated by both the parasympathetic and the sympathetic nervous systems. Thus, in any given patient, blockade of $5HT_3$-receptors will produce effects dependent on the pre-existing serotoninergic activity in both arms of the autonomic nervous system.

Risk of serotonin toxicity when used in combination with other serotoninergic drugs, e.g. SSRIs, see Antidepressants, Box A, p.200.

Because antimuscarinics competitively block the final common (cholinergic) pathway through which prokinetics act, concurrent prescription with metoclopramide should be avoided if possible. Opioids may also impede this action.

Undesirable effects

Because of concerns about tardive dyskinesia, the EMA have reduced the authorized indications for metoclopramide and limited the maximum daily dose and duration of use to 30mg (0.5mg/kg) for 5 days. High-dose formulations have been withdrawn.[15] The FDA has issued similar restrictions.[16] Use of metoclopramide has subsequently declined.[17] However, the EMA recognizes that the risk:benefit ratio may be different in populations where off-label use is accepted practice, e.g. palliative care.[18]

Also see Drug-induced movement disorders, p.739. The risk of extrapyramidal effects is dose-related and increased by the co-administration of other drugs known to cause extrapyramidal effects, e.g. antipsychotics, $5HT_3$ antagonists and antidepressants. Other risk factors include female gender, age (<20 and >80 years), past psychiatric history, Parkinson's disease, diabetes mellitus and renal or hepatic failure.[19]

Acute dystonic reactions occur in <5% of patients receiving metoclopramide, and are more common in the young, particularly girls and young women. They generally occur ≤5 days of starting treatment, and subside within 24h of stopping the drug. When possible, use alternatives in patients 1–20 years old.

Acute akathisia occurs in 10–15% of patients receiving a single dose of metoclopramide 20mg IV, and is severe enough to require treatment in 1–3%.[20] In a small series of palliative care patients, 10% exhibited acute akathisia after two weeks of metoclopramide, median dose 30mg/24h (range 10–60mg).[21] Acute akathisia is easily missed; patients may not spontaneously volunteer the symptoms, or clinicians misinterpret them as anxiety-related or another psychiatric condition.[22] Paradoxically, this can result in the use of neuroleptic drugs which, via their dopamine antagonist effects, exacerbates the situation.

Drug-induced parkinsonism generally develops <3 months after starting metoclopramide. The exact incidence is unknown. In one series, 30% of patients had signs of parkinsonism after ≥3 months of use.[19] In another series, tremor was present in 5% after two weeks of use.[21]

The overall incidence of tardive dyskinesia is probably <1%.[23] The risk increases with duration of treatment and total cumulative dose. Onset is generally after months of use; in one series after a median of 14 months (range 4–44 months).[24] However, about 20% of palliative care clinicians report seeing tardive dyskinesia in their patients, sometimes after only 2 weeks of use.[25] Further, it has occurred in a 16 year old male after only two days of 30mg/24h PO.[26] A possible mechanism is a direct neurotoxic effect of metoclopramide.[27] The likelihood of recovery is inversely related to age, probably reflecting capacity for CNS repair.

Patients experiencing extrapyramidal effects should be counselled against future use and the reaction clearly documented in their medical records.

Other undesirable effects include neuroleptic (antipsychotic) malignant syndrome (see p.173), drowsiness, depression, diarrhoea. Very rarely: hypotension, cardiac arrhythmia and cardiac arrest; mainly with IV use in at risk patients.

Dose and use

Avoid metoclopramide in patients in whom it has previously caused extrapyramidal effects.

If a long-term prokinetic is necessary, consider **domperidone** instead (see p.247). When this is not possible (e.g. because of contra-indications or the need for parenteral administration), review the use of metoclopramide frequently (e.g. at least every week) and discontinue if an optimal dose fails to provide benefit.

With long-term use, continue to monitor the patient regularly, particularly when higher than usual doses are being used, and discontinue metoclopramide if extrapyramidal signs or symptoms develop.

Nausea and vomiting, delayed gastric emptying or peristaltic failure

Also see QCG: Nausea and vomiting, p.240 and QCG: Inoperable bowel obstruction, p.242.

- start 10mg PO t.d.s. or 30mg/24h CSCI and 10mg PO/SC q2h p.r.n.
- titrate if necessary to a maximum dose of 20mg PO q.d.s. or 100mg/24h CSCI.

Gastric irritation

- as above; also consider an appropriate gastroprotective drug and, if possible, discontinue causal drug/substance.

Hiccup

If caused by delayed gastric emptying, gastric distension, or acid reflux:
- as above, ± an antifoaming agent (see Prokinetics, Table 2, p.26)
- if no response to PO treatment, consider stat dose of 10–20mg IV; give over ≥3min.[15]

Note. Increasing IV administration time to 15min reduced the incidence of acute akathisia in one study, but not another.[20,28]

For CSCI, dilute with WFI or 0.9% saline.

CSCI compatibility with other drugs: There are 2-drug compatibility data for metoclopramide in WFI with **alfentanil**, **diamorphine**, **glycopyrronium**, **haloperidol**, **hydromorphone**, **ketamine**, **midazolam**, **morphine sulfate**, **octreotide** and **oxycodone**. For more details and 3-drug compatibility charts, see Appendix 3, p.863.

Compatibility charts for mixing drugs in 0.9% saline can be found in the extended appendix section of the on-line *PCF* on *www.palliativedrugs.com*.

Supply

Metoclopramide (generic)
Tablets 10mg, 28 days @ 10mg q.d.s. = £3.
Oral solution 5mg/5mL, 28 days @ 10mg q.d.s. = £148.
Injection 5mg/mL, 2mL and 20mL amp = £0.50 and £2.50 respectively.

1 Barone J (1999) Domperidone: a peripherally acting dopamine$_2$-receptor antagonist. *Annals of Pharmacotherapy*. **33**: 429–440.
2 Patterson D *et al.* (1999) A double-blind multicenter comparison of domperidone and metoclopramide in the treatment of diabetic patients with symptoms of gastroparesis. *American Journal of Gastroenterology*. **94**: 1230–1234.
3 Magueur E *et al.* (1991) Pharmacokinetics of metoclopramide in patients with liver cirrhosis. *British Journal of Clinical Pharmacology*. **31**: 185–187.
4 Davis MP *et al.* (2010) A systematic review of the treatment of nausea and/or vomiting in cancer unrelated to chemotherapy or radiation. *Journal of Pain and Symptom Management*. **39**: 756–767.
5 Glare P *et al.* (2004) Systematic review of the efficacy of antiemetics in the treatment of nausea in patients with far-advanced cancer. *Support Care Cancer*. **12**: 432–440.
6 Bruera E *et al.* (2004) Dexamethasone in addition to metoclopramide for chronic nausea in patients with advanced cancer: a randomized controlled trial. *Journal of Pain and Symptom Management*. **28**: 381–388.
7 Bruera E *et al.* (1996) Chronic nausea in advanced cancer patients: a retrospective assessment of a metoclopramide-based antiemetic regimen. *Journal of Pain and Symptom Management*. **11**: 147–153.
8 Bruera E *et al.* (2000) A double-blind, crossover study of controlled-release metoclopramide and placebo for the chronic nausea and dyspepsia of advanced cancer. *Journal of Pain and Symptom Management*. **19**: 427–435.
9 Kuchel O *et al.* (1985) Effect of metoclopramide on plasma catecholamine release in essential hypertension. *Clinical Pharmacology and Therapeutics*. **37**: 372–375.
10 Agabiti-Rosei E (1995) Hypertensive crises in patients with phaeochromocytoma given metoclopramide. *Annals of Pharmacology*. **29**: 381–383.
11 Twycross RG and Back I (1998) Nausea and vomiting in advanced cancer. *European Journal of Palliative Care*. **5**: 39–45.
12 Ripamonti C *et al.* (2001) Clinical-practice recommendations for the management of bowel obstruction in patients with end-stage cancer. *Supportive Care in Cancer*. **9**: 223–233.
13 Baguley W *et al.* (1997) Cardiac dysrhythmias associated with the intravenous administration of ondansetron and metoclopramide. *Anesthesia and Analgesia*. **84**: 1380–1381.
14 Saxena P and Villalon C (1991) 5-Hydroxytryptamine: a chameleon in the heart. *Trends in Pharmacological Sciences*. **12**: 223–227.
15 MHRA (2013) Metoclopramide: risk of neurological adverse effects - restricted dose and duration of use. *Drug Safety Update*. **7**: www.mhra.gov.uk/safetyinformation
16 FDA (2009) Summary of warnings for metoclopramide containing products. *Medwatch*. www.fda.gov/Safety/MedWatch/SafetyInformation/
17 Ehrenpreis ED *et al.* (2013) The metoclopramide black box warning for tardive dyskinesia: effect on clinical practice, adverse event reporting, and prescription drug lawsuits. *American Journal of Gastroenterology*. **108**: 866–872.
18 EMA (2013) Personal communication.
19 Ganzini L *et al.* (1993) The prevalence of metoclopramide-induced tardive dyskinesia and acute extrapyramidal movement disorders. *Archives of Internal Medicine*. **153**: 1469–1475.
20 Egerton-Warburton D and Povey K (2013) Administration of metoclopramide by infusion or bolus does not affect the incidence of drug-induced akathisia. *Emergency Medicine Australasia*. **25**: 207–212.
21 Currow DC *et al.* (2012) Pharmacovigilance in hospice/palliative care: rapid report of net clinical effect of metoclopramide. *Journal of Palliative Medicine*. **15**: 1071–1075.

22 Akagi H and Kumar TM (2002) Lesson of the week: Akathisia: overlooked at a cost. *British Medical Journal*. **324**: 1506–1507.
23 Rao A and Camilleri M (2009) Review article: metoclopramide and tardive dyskinesia. *Alimentary Pharmacology and Therapeutics*. **31**: 11–19.
24 Wiholm BE *et al.* (1984) Tardive dyskinesia associated with metoclopramide. *British Medical Journal*. **288**: 545–547.
25 Palliativedrugs.com (2014) Metoclopramide - What is your experience? Survey November-December 2013. www.palliativedrugs.com
26 Karimi Khaledi M *et al.* (2012) Tardive dyskinesia after short-term treatment with oral metoclopramide in an adolescent. *International Journal of Clinical Pharmacy*. **34**: 822–824.
27 Lai TK *et al.* (2012) Cell membrane lytic action of metoclopramide and its relation to tardive dyskinesia. *Synapse*. **66**: 273–276.
28 Tura P *et al.* (2012) Slow infusion metoclopramide does not affect the improvement rate of nausea while reducing akathisia and sedation incidence. *Emergency Medical Journal*. **29**: 108–112.

Updated September 2017

DOMPERIDONE

Class: Prokinetic anti-emetic.

Indications: Nausea and vomiting. All other uses are unauthorized, e.g. †symptoms associated with upper GI dysmotility (post-prandial epigastric discomfort, bloating and belching); †gastro-oesophageal reflux.

Contra-indications: Prolactinoma; conditions where cardiac conduction is, or could be, impaired, e.g. prolonged QT interval (congenital or acquired); underlying cardiac disease, e.g. CHF; concurrent use with potent CYP3A4 inhibitors or other drugs known to prolong QT interval; GI haemorrhage or perforation, mechanical GI obstruction; moderate–severe hepatic impairment.

Pharmacology

Like **metoclopramide**, domperidone antagonizes D_2-receptors in:

- the chemoreceptor trigger zone (CTZ) in the area postrema
- the gastro-oesophageal and gastroduodenal junctions, counteracting the gastric 'dopamine brake' associated with nausea from any cause.[1]

Unlike **metoclopramide**, domperidone's blood-brain barrier penetration is negligible; thus it causes less frequent and less severe undesirable effects including drowsiness, loss of mental acuity,[2] and extrapyramidal symptoms. It is the anti-emetic of choice for nausea related to anti-Parkinsonian dopamimetics.[3]

However, the usefulness of domperidone is limited by the absence of a parenteral formulation and concern about QT prolongation. Epidemiological studies found domperidone was associated with an increased risk of serious ventricular arrhythmia/sudden cardiac death of ≤60%.[4] The risk was higher in those >60 years old, receiving doses >30mg/24h, and/or receiving a CYP3A4 inhibitor or drug known to cause QT prolongation.[4–6] Although some consider that the risk has been overstated,[7,8] regulators have restricted its Marketing Authorization to nausea and vomiting for ≤1 week and added new contra-indications (see above).[9] Further, the maximum authorized dose is now 30mg/24h and many studies found benefit only with 40–80mg/24h.[10]

For gastroparesis, the efficacy of domperidone and **metoclopramide** are similar, despite the latter's additional prokinetic $5HT_4$ agonist action (see Table 1, Prokinetics, p.24).[11] Domperidone may be effective even when there is no response to **metoclopramide**.[12,13] In diabetic patients, the prokinetic effect for solids attenuates after 1–2 months, although the effect on liquid emptying persists.[14,15]

Although almost completely absorbed from the GI tract, bio-availability is relatively poor because of extensive first-pass metabolism in the wall of the GI tract and the liver. Bio-availability in healthy volunteers is nearly doubled if taken *after* a meal.[16] Maximal absorption requires an acid environment; H_2 antagonists, PPIs and antacids all reduce absorption. PO and PR bio-availability are almost the same, but suppositories are not available in the UK.

Domperidone is metabolized in the liver to inactive compounds, principally via CYP3A4. Because of safety concerns regarding high plasma levels of domperidone (see Undesirable effects), the manufacturer suggests moderate–severe hepatic impairment is a contra-indication to its use. However, domperidone has previously been used in this setting and is the anti-emetic of choice in many liver centres; thus, if it is considered necessary, a reduction in dose and careful monitoring is recommended (see Chapter 18, p.703).

Renal clearance is a minor route of elimination (<1% unchanged). In renal failure although the plasma halflife is increased by up to three times, plasma concentration does not increase (possibly because of an altered volume of distribution).[17] However, most sources recommend limiting the maximum daily dose in severe renal impairment/ESRF (see Chapter 17, p.681).
Bio-availability 12–18% PO (fasting), 24% PO (after food).
Onset of action 30min.
Time to peak plasma concentration 0.5–2h PO.
Plasma halflife 7–16h; increasing up to 21h in severe renal impairment.[12]
Duration of action 12–24h (estimate based on halflife).

Cautions

Underlying cardiac disease and other risk factors for prolonged QT, e.g. electrolyte disturbances (also see Chapter 20, p.731). Severe renal impairment or ESRF, hepatic impairment (see Pharmacology, Chapter 17, p.681 and Chapter 18, p.703).

Drug interactions

Avoid concurrent use with drugs known to:

- increase the QT interval (see Chapter 20, p.731)
- inhibit the metabolism of domperidone, i.e. CYP3A4 inhibitors. These may increase the domperidone plasma concentration, increasing the risk of QT prolongation and thus *torsade de pointes*.

Examples of strong CYP3A4 inhibitors include **aprepitant**, azoles (**fluconazole**, **itraconazole**) grapefruit juice, macrolide antibiotics (**clarithromycin**, **erythromycin**), protease inhibitors (**ritonavir**), SSRIs (**fluvoxamine, fluoxetine**). Also see Chapter 19, Table 8, p.725.

Because antimuscarinics competitively block the final common (cholinergic) pathway through which prokinetics act, concurrent prescription with domperidone should be avoided if possible. Opioids may also impede this action.

H_2 antagonists, PPIs and antacids reduce absorption and bio-availability.

Undesirable effects

Very rare (<0.01%): transient colic, gynaecomastia, galactorrhoea, amenorrhoea (secondary to increased prolactin secretion), reduced libido, cramp, pruritus, rash;[12] headache, extrapyramidal effects (acute dystonias), which resolve rapidly and completely once domperidone is stopped.[18] In two women with polycystic ovaries, hyperoestrogenism may have been a predisposing factor.[12]

Paradoxical vomiting has been reported in children with severe brain injury requiring tube feeding. Inhibition of pyloric relaxation was considered the likely cause, due to the D_2 antagonist effect of domperidone in the presence of a severe reduction in vagal tone.[19]
Unknown frequency: QT prolongation, see p.731.

Dose and use

In 2014, because of a small increased risk of serious ventricular arrhythmia, particularly in those >60 years old, receiving >30mg/24h, and/or receiving a CYP3A4 inhibitor or drug known to cause QT prolongation, regulators concluded that the risk:benefit ratio was only acceptable for nausea and vomiting, and recommended restricting dose and duration of use to 10mg t.d.s and ≤1 week, respectively. Further, they added new contra-indications related to cardiovascular disease and drug interactions (see above).

However, the risk:benefit balance should be determined on an individual patient basis, taking circumstances and other options into account. For example, if a patient with end-stage CHF requires a long-term anti-emetic, domperidone may be preferable to **cyclizine** (also pro-arrhythmic) or **metoclopramide** (risk of extrapyramidal effects).

Advise patients to seek prompt medical attention should symptoms such as syncope or cardiac arrhythmias occur.

The manufacturer recommends giving domperidone t.d.s. (previously up to q.d.s. 15–30min before meals in patients with upper GI dysmotility). However, given its halflife, b.d. may suffice and its bio-availability is higher if taken after food:

- start with 10mg PO b.d
- increase to 10mg t.d.s., the *authorized* maximum dose
- If symptoms persist, consider increasing to 20mg b.d. → 20mg t.d.s. → 20mg q.d.s. (the *previous* authorized maximum dose, used in many trials).[10]

Alternative options to higher dose domperidone are **metoclopramide** (p.244) and **erythromycin** (p.24).

Also see QCG: Nausea and vomiting, p.240.

Supply

Domperidone (generic)

Tablets 10mg, 28 days @ 10mg q.d.s. = £2.75.

Oral suspension 5mg/5mL, 28 days @ 10mg q.d.s. = £75.

1 Barone J (1999) Domperidone: a peripherally acting dopamine$_2$-receptor antagonist. *Annals of Pharmacotherapy*. **33**: 429–440.
2 Patterson D *et al.* (1999) A double-blind multicenter comparison of domperidone and metoclopramide in the treatment of diabetic patients with symptoms of gastroparesis. *American Journal of Gastroenterology*. **94**: 1230–1234.
3 Langdon N *et al.* (1986) Comparison of levodopa with carbidopa, and levodopa with domperidone in Parkinson's disease. *Clinical Neuropharmacology*. **9**: 440–447.
4 Johannes CB *et al.* (2010) Risk of serious ventricular arrhythmia and sudden cardiac death in a cohort of users of domperidone: a nested case-control study. *Pharmacoepidemiology and Drug Safety*. **19**: 881–888.
5 van Noord C *et al.* (2010) Domperidone and ventricular arrhythmia or sudden cardiac death: a population-based case-control study in the Netherlands. *Drug Safety*. **33**: 1003–1014.
6 Leelakanok A (2016) Domperidone and risk of ventricular arrhythmia and cardiac death: a systematic review and meta-analysis. *Clinical Drug Investigation*. **36**: 97–107.
7 Buffery PJ (2015) Domperidone safety: a mini-review of the science of QT prolongation and clinical implications of recent global regulatory recommendations. *New Zealand Medical Journal*. **128**: 66–74.
8 Ortiz A (2015) Cardiovascular safety profile and clinical experience with high-dose domperidone therapy for nausea and vomiting. *American Journal of Medical Sciences*. **349**: 421–424.
9 MHRA (2014) Domperidone: risks of cardiac side effects - indicatiion restricted to nausea and vomiting, new contraindications, and reduced dose and duration of use. *Drug Safety Update*. **7**: www.mhra.gov.uk/safetyinformation
10 Reddymasu SC *et al.* (2007) Domperidone: review of pharmacology and clinical applications in gastroenterology. *American Journal of Gastroenterology*. **102**: 2036–2045.
11 Sturm A *et al.* (1999) Prokinetics in patients with gastroparesis: a systematic analysis. *Digestion*. **60**: 422–427.
12 Prakash A and Wagstaff AJ (1998) Domperidone. A review of its use in diabetic gastropathy. *Drugs*. **56**: 429–445.
13 Dumitrascu D and Weinbeck M (2000) Domperidone versus metoclopramide in the treatment of diabetic gastroparesis. *American Journal of Gastroenterology*. **95**: 316–317.
14 Horowitz M *et al.* (1985) Acute and chronic effects of domperidone on gastric emptying in diabetic autonomic neuropathy. *Dig Dis Sci*. **30**: 1–9.
15 Koch KL *et al.* (1989) Gastric emptying and gastric myoelectrical activity in patients with diabetic gastroparesis: effect of long-term domperidone treatment. *American Journal of Gastroenterology*. **84**: 1069–1075.
16 Heykants J *et al.* (1981) On the pharmacokinetics of domperidone in animals and man. IV. The pharmacokinetics of intravenous domperidone and its bioavailability in man following intramuscular, oral and rectal administration. *European Journal of Drug Metabolism and Pharmacokinetics*. **6**: 61–70.
17 Brogden RN *et al.* (1982) Domperidone. A review of its pharmacological activity, pharmacokinetics and therapeutic efficacy in the symptomatic treatment of chronic dyspepsia and as an antiemetic. *Drugs*. **24**: 360–400.
18 Casteels-Van Daele M *et al.* (1984) Refusal of further cancer chemotherapy due to antiemetic drug. *Lancet*. **1**: 57.
19 Pozzi M *et al.* (2013) Case series: paradoxical action of domperidone leads to increased vomiting. *European Journal of Clinical Pharmacology*. **69**: 289–290.

Updated September 2017

ANTIHISTAMINIC ANTIMUSCARINIC ANTI-EMETICS

Indications: Prevention of motion sickness, nausea and vomiting, vertigo and labyrinthine disorders (**cyclizine, promethazine**), pruritus (**hydroxyzine**), insomnia (**promethazine**).

Contra-indications: *Promethazine:* intra-arterial or SC injection (is a chemical irritant and may cause local necrosis).

Pharmacology

Antihistaminic antimuscarinic anti-emetics embrace several chemical classes including some phenothiazines (e.g. **promethazine**), piperazines (e.g. **buclizine**, **cyclizine**, **meclozine**, **hydroxyzine**) and mono-ethanolamines (e.g. **diphenhydramine**, **dimenhydrinate**). Antihistaminic anti-emetics decrease excitability of the inner ear labyrinth and block conduction in the vestibular-cerebellar pathways, as well as acting directly on the vomiting centre in the brain stem (see p.236). However, there is considerable overlap between their receptor site affinity and that of the antipsychotic phenothiazines (see Antipsychotics, Table 1, p.171).

Antihistaminic anti-emetics are effective in many causes of vomiting, including opioid-induced.[1,2] However, in practice **metoclopramide** (see p.244) and **haloperidol** (see p.180) are often used in preference, sometimes because of more specific indications or to avoid drowsiness and antimuscarinic effects. Metabolism is mainly hepatic, and the inactive metabolites are excreted in the urine.

Hydroxyzine is principally used as an anxiolytic-sedative and antipruritic. Unlike other anthistaminic drugs, **hydroxyzine** inhibits apomorphine-induced vomiting, suggesting that some of its anti-emetic effect is mediated via the chemoreceptor trigger zone. In postoperative patients, **hydroxyzine** 100mg IM (not UK) has analgesic activity approaching that of **morphine** 8mg,[3] and **morphine** 5mg and **hydroxyzine** 100mg gave comparable relief to **morphine** 10mg alone.[4] The sedative effect of the combination was not significantly different from **morphine** alone. For pharmacokinetic details, see Table 1.

Table 1 Pharmacokinetic details[5]

	Cyclizine	*Hydroxyzine*	*Promethazine*
Bio-availability	No data	No data	25% PO
Onset of action	30–60min	15–30min	~20min IM, 3–5min IV
Time to peak plasma concentration	2h PO	~2h	4.5h PO (syrup), 6–9h PR
Plasma halflife	13h	3–7h	7–14h
Duration of effect	4–6h	4–6h	2–6h

Cautions

Renal and hepatic impairment (see Chapter 17, p.687 and Chapter 18, p.711); epilepsy; can precipitate or exacerbate narrow-angle glaucoma; urinary tract obstruction (see Antimuscarinics, p.5). Elderly patients are more susceptible to sedative and central antimuscarinic effects, e.g. postural hypotension, memory impairment, extrapyramidal reactions.

Cyclizine: severe heart failure (antimuscarinic effect → tachycardia).

Hydroxyzine: asthma, COPD, hepatic impairment (restrict to once daily), moderate–severe renal impairment (reduce dose by 50%). When injected IV (not UK), if there is extravasation into the SC tissues, can cause a sterile abscess and tissue induration. Give well diluted as a 15–30min IVI only if strictly necessary.

Undesirable effects

Dry mouth and other antimuscarinic effects (see Antimuscarinics, Box C, p.7), drowsiness, headache, fatigue, nervousness, dizziness, thickening of bronchial secretions.

Severe movement disorders are reported (e.g. 'locked in syndrome'; also see p.739).[6]

Dose and use

Nausea and vomiting

Because of their antimuscarinic properties, the use of this group of drugs tends to be restricted to situations where **metoclopramide** and/or other more specific anti-emetics (e.g. **haloperidol**, $5HT_3$ antagonists) have failed to relieve, e.g. some patients with mechanical bowel obstruction, or as the anti-emetic of choice for raised intracranial pressure.

In the UK, **cyclizine** is generally the antihistaminic antimuscarinic anti-emetic of choice. Depending on circumstances, **cyclizine** is generally given PO or SC:

- start 50mg PO b.d.–t.d.s. or 100–150mg/24h CSCI & 50mg p.r.n.
- usual maximum daily dose 200mg PO and CSCI.

Also see QCG: Nausea and vomiting, p.240 and QCG: Inoperable bowel obstruction, p.242.

For CSCI dilute **cyclizine** with WFI or 5% glucose; **cyclizine** is *incompatible* with 0.9% saline and will precipitate, see Chapter 29, p.819.

CSCI compatibility with other drugs: There are 2-drug compatibility data for cyclizine in WFI with **haloperidol**, **hyoscine *hydrobromide***, **morphine sulfate**, and **morphine tartrate** (not UK).

Concentration-dependent *incompatibility* occurs with **alfentanil**, **dexamethasone**, **diamorphine** and **oxycodone**. *Incompatibility* has also been reported with **clonazepam**, **hydromorphone**, **hyoscine *butylbromide***, **ketorolac**, **midazolam** and **octreotide**. For more details and 3-drug compatibility data, see Appendix 3 (p.863).

Doses of **promethazine** are 25mg PO t.d.s–q.d.s. **Promethazine** is generally not recommended CSCI due to its irritant properties and must *not* be given SC, see Chapter 29, Box F, p.825.

Vertigo

Antihistaminic antimuscarinic anti-emetics are used as a non-specific treatment for vertigo (see QCG: Vertigo, p.252).[7–9]

Supply

Oral products

Cyclizine *hydrochloride* (generic)

Tablets 50mg, 28 days @ 50mg t.d.s. = £6.

Promethazine *hydrochloride*

Phenergan® (Sanofi-Aventis)

Tablets 10mg, 25mg, 28 days @ 25mg t.d.s. = £7.

Oral solution 5mg/5mL, 28 days @ 25mg t.d.s. = £60.

Promethazine *teoclate*

Avomine® (Manx)

Tablets 25mg, 28 days @ 25mg t.d.s. = £9.50. *Also available OTC.*

Parenteral products

Cyclizine *lactate* (generic)

Injection 50mg/mL, 1mL amp = £1.

Promethazine *hydrochloride*

Phenergan® (Sanofi-Aventis)

Injection 25mg/mL, 1mL amp = £1. *For deep IM injection.*

1 Dundee J and Jones P (1968) The prevention of analgesic-induced nausea and vomiting by cyclizine. *British Journal of Clinical Practice*. **22**: 379–382.

2 Walder A and Aitkenhead A (1995) A comparison of droperidol and cyclizine in the prevention of postoperative nausea and vomiting associated with patient-controlled analgesia. *Anaesthesia*. **50**: 654–656.

3 Beaver WT and Feise G (1976) Comparison of analgesic effects of morphine sulphate, hydroxyzine and their combination in patients with postoperative pain. In: JJ Bonica and D Albe-Fessard (eds) *Advances in Pain Research and Therapy* Vol 1. Raven Press, New York, pp. 553–557.

4 Hupert C *et al.* (1980) Effect of hydroxyzine on morphine analgesia for the treatment of postoperative pain. *Anesthesia and Analgesia*. **59**: 690–696.

5 Vella-Brincat JW *et al.* (2012) The pharmacokinetics and pharmacogenetics of the antiemetic cyclizine in palliative care patients. *Journal of Pain and Symptom Management*. **43**: 540–548.

6 Lee P (2013) Locked-in syndrome as a result of cyclizine administration. *Journal of Pain and Symptom Management*. **45**: e5–7.

7 Brandt T (2005) Vertigo and Dizziness: Common Complaints. Second Edition. Springer, London.

8 Bisdorff A *et al.* (2013) The epidemiology of vertigo, dizziness, and unsteadiness and its links to co-morbidities. *Frontiers in Neurology*. **4**: 29.

9 Karatas M (2008) Central vertigo and dizziness: epidemiology, differential diagnosis, and common causes. *Neurologist*. **14**: 355–364.

Updated September 2017

Quick Clinical Guide: Vertigo

Vertigo is an unpleasant spinning sensation generally related to dysfunction of the vestibular system, and is often associated with nausea and vomiting, and difficulties with standing or walking. It is distinct from dizziness, which (in Europe) is widely regarded as a synonym for non-rotational light-headedness. Vertigo can be continuous or paroxysmal, with episodes ranging from seconds/minutes–days/weeks.

In the general population, the main causes are excessive alcohol, benign paroxysmal positional vertigo, Ménière's disease, vestibular neuritis, and labyrinthitis. Vertigo may also be caused by brain tumours (primary or secondary), stroke and neurodegenerative disorders, e.g. Parkinson's disease, multiple sclerosis.

Clinical evaluation

Vertigo needs to be differentiated from non-rotational light-headedness:

'Does everything spin like a top?', 'Is it like being on a merry-go-round?'
'Or is it more a feeling of light-headedness?'

Precipitating factors

- after drugs/alcohol?
- when moving (e.g. walking, turning the head) or when resting/lying down?
- when stressed?

Associated symptoms

- nausea, vomiting?
- difficulties with standing or walking?
- aural symptoms, e.g. tinnitus, impaired hearing?
- headache?
- visual disturbances, e.g. oscillopsia, diplopia?
- anxiety?

Differential diagnosis

The main differential diagnosis is light-headedness, most cases of which are associated with orthostatic (postural) hypotension (Box A). However, some are psychosomatic, e.g. hyperventilation syndrome, panic attack, phobic postural vertigo, agoraphobia.

Box A Common somatic causes of light-headedness

Cardiogenic
- orthostatic hypotension
- presyncope (near-faint)
- vasovagal syncope
- cardiac arrhythmia

Hypoglycaemia

Exogenous substances
- alcohol
- drugs (see Box B)

Box B Drugs and orthostatic hypotension[a]

Cardiac

ACE inhibitors
Alpha blockers (e.g. prazosin, tamsulosin)
Beta blockers (e.g. carvedilol, labetalol)
Clonidine
Diuretics (e.g. furosemide)
Nitrates (e.g. glyceryl trinitrate)

Central nervous system

Antidepressants (e.g. TCAs, trazodone)
Antiparkinsonian drugs (e.g. bromocriptine, levodopa)
Antipsychotics (e.g. chlorpromazine, clozapine)
Opioids
Skeletal muscle relaxants (e.g. baclofen, tizanidine)

Urological

Phosphodiesterase type-5 inhibitors (e.g. sildenafil)
Urinary anticholinergics (e.g. oxybutynin)

a. there may be additive effects with polypharmacy (the norm in palliative care).

Management

Correct the correctable

The cause of the vertigo should be determined and specific treatment considered; *seek specialist advice if necessary*.

When drug-induced orthostatic hypotension is the cause, discontinue or reduce the dose of potential causal drugs.

Non-drug treatment

Particularly in benign paroxysmal positional vertigo, certain manoeuvres can reduce the impact of the vertigo but need to be used appropriately and taught correctly; obtain advice from an otologist.

Drug treatment

Specific: e.g. Ménière's disease, betahistine initially 16mg t.d.s.

Symptomatic relief of acute episodes:

- if vertigo related to a brain tumour (primary or secondary), give a benzodiazepine, e.g. lorazepam 1mg PO or midazolam 2.5mg SC/IV, and repeat 30–60min p.r.n.; combine with an anti-emetic if necessary (see below)
- for vestibular causes:
  - ▷ first-line anti-emetic: antihistaminic antimuscarinic, e.g. cyclizine 50mg PO/SC/IV, dimenhydrinate 50–100mg PO or 62–186mg IV (not UK)
  - ▷ alternative anti-emetic: prokinetic, metoclopramide 10mg PO/SC/IV.

Antimuscarinic drugs should be avoided long-term because they may inhibit compensatory mechanisms; for the management of prolonged continuous vertigo seek advice from an otologist.

Updated September 2017

$5HT_3$ ANTAGONISTS

Indications: Nausea and vomiting after surgery, chemotherapy and radiotherapy, †intractable vomiting due to chemical, abdominal and cerebral causes when usual approaches have failed, †diarrhoea associated with carcinoid syndrome,[1] †opioid-induced pruritus.[2,3]

Contra-indications: Congenital long QT syndrome (**ondansetron**).

Pharmacology

$5HT_3$ antagonists were developed specifically to control emesis associated with highly emetogenic chemotherapy, e.g. **cisplatin**. They block the effect of excess 5HT on vagal nerve fibres, and are thus of particular value in situations when excessive amounts of 5HT are released from the body's stores, i.e. from enterochromaffin cells after chemotherapy or radiation-induced damage of the GI mucosa, or because of intestinal distension, or from leaky platelets when there is severe renal impairment.

A TD **granisetron** patch is authorized for the *prevention* of nausea and vomiting associated with moderately or highly emetogenic chemotherapy. It has a slow onset of action and must be applied 24–48h before chemotherapy. It can be worn ≤7 days if required and is removed ≥24h after completion of chemotherapy. Because it is no more effective than PO **granisetron**, its use is limited to situations where the PO route is not available.[4]

In an open RCT, **tropisetron** (not UK) was shown to be of benefit in patients with far-advanced cancer and nausea and vomiting of indeterminate cause when given either as a sole agent or with a second anti-emetic, particularly **dexamethasone**.[5] $5HT_3$ antagonists also relieve nausea and vomiting associated with head injury, brain stem radiotherapy,[6,7] gastro-enteritis,[8] and in multiple sclerosis with brain stem disease.[9]

Ondansetron relieves pruritus related to spinal **morphine** but not cholestatic or uraemic pruritus (also see Chapter 26, p.757).[2,10]

In carcinoid syndrome, benefit is reported for diarrhoea refractory to **octreotide**. In a case series (n=6), **ondansetron** 8mg b.d. provided satisfactory control within 2–3 days. Subsequently, the dose was reduced to the minimum effective maintenance dose (4–8mg daily).[1]

For pharmacokinetic details see Table 1.

Table 1 Pharmacokinetic details of 5HT$_3$ antagonists

		Ondansetron	*Granisetron*	*Palonosetron*
Bio-availability	PO	56–71% (60% PR)	60%	n/a
Onset of action	PO	<30min	<30min	n/a
	IV	<5min	<15min	
Plasma halflife		3–5h (6h PR)	10–11h	40h
Time to peak plasma concentration	PO	1.5h	No data	n/a
	IM	10min		n/a
	PR	6h		n/a
Duration of action		12h	24h	>24h[11]

Cautions

Risk factors for QT prolongation (particularly ondansetron, see p.731); moderate-severe hepatic impairment (**ondansetron**; see Dose and use and Chapter 18, p.711); reduced colonic motility (can cause or worsen constipation).

Drug interactions

Serious drug interaction: a combination of IV **metoclopramide** and IV **ondansetron** occasionally causes cardiac arrhythmias (see p.244).

Additive effects with other drugs that cause QT interval prolongation (see p.731) and serotonin toxicity (e.g. SSRIs, see Antidepressants, Box A, p.200).

There are mixed reports of the analgesic effect of **tramadol** (p.354) and **paracetamol** (p.303) being reduced by 5HT$_3$ antagonists, possibly by blocking the action of serotonin at presynaptic 5HT$_3$-receptors on primary afferent nociceptive neurones in the spinal dorsal horn.

Undesirable effects

Very common (>10%): headache.[12]
Common (<10%, >1%): lightheadedness, dizziness, nervousness, tremor, ataxia, asthenia, drowsiness, fever, sensation of warmth or flushing (particularly when given IV), thirst, constipation or diarrhoea.
Uncommon (<1%, >0.1%): **ondansetron**: dystonic reactions, arrhythmia, hypotension, raised LFTs.
Rare (<0.1%, >0.01%): hiccup.
Very rare (<0.01%): **ondansetron**: transient blindness during IV administration (sight generally returns within 20min).

Dose and use

Although commonly used first-line in chemotherapy-related and post-operative nausea and vomiting, first-line use is rarely appropriate in palliative care. They are typically *added* to an antipsychotic with affinity for multiple receptors (e.g. **levomepromazine**, **olanzapine**) if the latter is ineffective alone (see p.235).

Granisetron can be given once daily whereas **ondansetron** is given b.d.–t.d.s. 5HT$_3$ antagonists are equally effective PO, by injection or TD.[4,13–15]

Regimens include:

- **granisetron** 1–2mg PO/SC once daily for 3 days *or*
- **ondansetron** 4–8mg PO/SC b.d.–t.d.s. (or 16–24mg/24h CSCI) for 3 days
- if clearly of benefit, continue indefinitely unless the cause is self-limiting
- some patients benefit from higher doses, occasionally as high as **granisetron** 9mg daily[16]
- in patients with moderate–severe hepatic impairment, the dose of **ondansetron** should be limited to 8mg daily, whereas no dose reduction is necessary for **granisetron** (in renal impairment, no dose reduction is necessary with either drug).

Also see QCG: Nausea and vomiting, p.240 and QCG: Inoperable bowel obstruction, p.242. For use in pruritus associated with spinally administered **morphine** or for diarrhoea in carcinoid syndrome, see Pharmacology.

For CSCI dilute with WFI, 0.9% saline or 5% glucose.

CSCI compatibility with other drugs: There are 2-drug compatibility data for **ondansetron** in WFI with **alfentanil, diamorphine**, and **octreotide**. For more details and 3-drug compatibility data, see Appendix 3 (p.863).

Compatibility charts for mixing drugs in 0.9% saline can be found in the extended appendix of the on-line *PCF* on *www.palliativedrugs.com*.

To control nausea and vomiting caused by severely emetogenic chemotherapy, **granisetron** (or other $5HT_3$ antagonist) is used with other anti-emetics, typically **dexamethasone** and **metoclopramide**.[17]

For IV **ondansetron** in chemotherapy-induced nausea and vomiting only, MHRA has placed restrictions on the maximum single IV dose and administration details for patients >65years, based on the risk of dose dependent QT interval prolongation.[18]

Supply

Granisetron (generic)

Tablets 1mg, 2mg, 28 days @ 1mg once daily = £115.

Injection 1mg/mL, for dilution and use as an injection or infusion, 1mL amp = £1.50, 3mL amp = £4.75.

Sancuso® (ProStrakan)

Transdermal Patches (for up to 7 days) 3.1mg/24h, 1 = £56. *Similar considerations apply as for other medical transdermal products, e.g. skin hair should be clipped rather than shaved, fold plasters in half and dispose of safely, remove before MRI scans (see p.831).*

Ondansetron (generic)

Tablets 4mg, 8mg, 28 days @ 8mg b.d. = £11.

Orodispersible tablet 4mg, 8mg, 28 days @ 8mg b.d. = £403.

Oral solution 4mg/5mL, 28 days @ 8mg b.d. = £436.

Injection 2mg/mL, 2mL amp = £1, 4mL amp = £12.

Zofran® (GlaxoSmithKline)

Suppositories 16mg, 1 = £14.

1 Kiesewetter B and Raderer M (2013) Ondansetron for diarrhea associated with neuroendocrine tumors. *New England Journal Medicine*. **368**: 1947–1948.

2 Borgeat A and Stimemann H-R (1999) Ondansetron is effective to treat spinal or epidural morphine-induced pruritus. *Anesthesiology*. **90**: 432–436.

3 Kyriakides K *et al.* (1999) Management of opioid-induced pruritus: a role for 5HT antagonists? *British Journal of Anaesthesia*. **82**: 439–441.

4 Boccia RV *et al.* (2011) Efficacy and tolerability of transdermal granisetron for the control of chemotherapy-induced nausea and vomiting associated with moderately and highly emetogenic multi-day chemotherapy: a randomized, double-blind, phase III study. *Supportive Care in Cancer*. **19**: 1609–1617.

5 Mystakidou K *et al.* (1998) Comparison of the efficacy and safety of tropisetron, metoclopramide, and chlorpromazine in the treatment of emesis associated with far advanced cancer. *Cancer*. **83**: 1214–1223.

6 Kleinerman K *et al.* (1993) Use of ondansetron for control of projectile vomiting in patients with neurosurgical trauma: two case reports. *Annals of Pharmacotherapy*. **27**: 566–568.

7 Bodis S *et al.* (1994) The prevention of radiosurgery-induced nausea and vomiting by ondansetron: evidence of a direct effect on the central nervous system chemoreceptor trigger zone. *Surgery and Neurology*. **42**: 249–252.

8 Cubeddu L *et al.* (1997) Antiemetic activity of ondansetron in acute gastroenteritis. *Alimentary Pharmacology and Therapeutics*. **11**: 185–191.

9 Rice G and Ebers G (1995) Ondansetron for intractable vertigo complicating acute brainstem disorders. *Lancet*. **345**: 1182–1183.

10 To TH *et al.* (2012) The role of ondansetron in the management of cholestatic or uremic pruritus--a systematic review. *Journal of Pain and Symptom Management*. **44**: 725–730.

11 Saito M *et al.* (2009) Palonosetron plus dexamethasone versus granisetron plus dexamethasone for prevention of nausea and vomiting during chemotherapy: a double-blind, double-dummy, randomised, comparative phase III trial. *Lancet Oncology*. **10**: 115–124.

12 Goodin S and Cunningham R (2002) 5-HT3-receptor antagonists for the treatment of nausea and vomiting: a reappraisal of their side-effect profile. *The Oncologist*. **7**: 424–436.

13 Perez EA *et al.* (1997) Efficacy and safety of different doses of granisetron for the prophylaxis of cisplatin-induced emesis. *Support Care Cancer*. **5**: 31–37.
14 Perez E *et al.* (1997) Efficacy and safety of oral granisetron versus IV ondansetron in prevention of moderately emetogenic chemotherapy-induced nausea and vomiting. *Proceedings of the American Society of Clinical Oncology*. **16**: 149.
15 Gralla R *et al.* (1997) Can an oral antiemetic regimen be as effective as intravenous treatment against cisplatin: results of a 1054 patient randomized study of oral granisetron versus IV ondansetron. *Proceedings of the American Society of Clinical Oncology*. **16**: 178.
16 Minami M (2003) Granisetron: is there a dose-response effect on nausea and vomiting? *Cancer Chemotherapy and Pharmacology*. **52**: 89–98.
17 Kris MG *et al.* (2006) American Society of Clinical Oncology guideline for antiemetics in oncology: update 2006. *Journal of Clinical Oncology*. **24**: 2932–2947.
18 MHRA (2013) Ondansetron for intravenous use: dose dependent QT interval prolongation - new posology. *Drug Safety Update*. **6**. www.mhra.gov.uk/safetyinformation

Updated September 2017

ANTI-EPILEPTICS

Indications: (Authorized indications vary between products; consult SPC for details). Neuropathic pain, epilepsy, mania, anxiety, †agitated delirium, †terminal agitation, †sweats and hot flushes, †refractory hiccup, †restless legs syndrome, †refractory cough, †nausea and vomiting, †pruritus, †alcohol withdrawal.

Pharmacology

Anti-epileptic drugs inhibit rapidly firing neurones and can thereby impact on symptoms arising from excessive neuronal activity in any part of the nervous system. They are structurally and functionally diverse. Some influence action potential generation or consequent neurotransmitter release or action. Others act indirectly, increasing the GABA-mediated inhibition of rapidly firing neurones (see Table 1 and Figure 1).

The relationship between clinical activity and mode of action is not fully understood. Further, clinically relevant differences exist between anti-epileptics acting in similar ways, and additional actions contribute to the beneficial and/or undesirable effects of some. Thus, choice of drug remains partly empirical.[1]

Membrane stabilizers reduce excitability by blocking sodium channels and/or opening potassium channels. The normal transport of sodium channels is disrupted by nerve injury; they accumulate creating foci of ectopic action potential generation. Several classes of drug bind to sodium channels during or after opening; thus, repetitive firing results in an increasing proportion of blocked channels ('use-dependent block'):[12]

- some anti-epileptics, e.g. **carbamazepine** (p.278), **oxcarbazepine** (p.280), **phenytoin**, **lamotrigine** and **lacosamide**
- local anaesthetics, e.g. **lidocaine** (p.71)
- class I anti-arrhythmics, e.g. **flecainide** (p.71).

All have been shown to have antinociceptive and/or anti-neuropathic pain effects.[13–16] However, the duration of blockade before the drug dissociates from the channel varies. This, and effects on targets other than sodium channels, creates important clinical differences between such drugs.

Potential future directions for sodium channel blockers in pain management include reduced blood-brain barrier penetration (reducing undesirable central effects by targeting ectopic foci on damaged peripheral neurones)[12] or subtype-selective blockers (inherited abnormalities of one subtype, $Na_v1.7$, cause congenital insensitivity to pain while leaving other senses unaffected).[17,18]

The opening of potassium channels also has a membrane-stabilizing effect by hyperpolarizing the cell membrane, and is thought to account for the effect of the analgesic **flupirtine** (not UK)[10] and the anti-epileptic, **retigabine**.[9]

Neurotransmitter release is affected by both $\alpha2\delta$ and SV2A ligands. The $\alpha2\delta$ ligands, **gabapentin** and **pregabalin**, block N, P and Q-type calcium-channels. This reduces the calcium influx required to trigger neurotransmitter release (see p.272). Thus, in neuropathic pain, they counteract the excessive release of glutamate in the spinal dorsal horn (reducing pain transmission) and GABA in the brainstem locus coeruleus (restoring descending pain inhibitory pathways).[19] Spinal calcium channels are also targeted by **lamotrigine**, **topiramate** and **ziconotide** (an analgesic given IT). **Levetiracetam** binds SV2A, a protein involved in modulating neurotransmitter vesicle release (see p.287).[20]

	Membrane stabilizers		↓Neurotransmitter release			Neurotransmitter receptor antagonist		GABAmimetics		↓Thalamic burst firing
	Na channel blocker	K channel activator	Ca channel blocker (N, P/Q type)	Ca channel blocker (R type)	↓vesicle release (SV2A)	AMPA	NMDA	$GABA_A$ receptor modulation	Altered GABA synthesis and reuptake	Ca channel blocker (T type)
Benzodiazepines								++		
Carbamazepine	++									
Eslicarbazepine	++									
Ethosuximide										++
Gabapentin		+	++							
Lacosamide	++					+				
Lamotrigine	++		++	++						
Levetiracetam					++					
Oxcarbazepine	++	+								
Perampanel						++				
Phenobarbital								++		
Phenytoin	++									
Pregabalin			++							
Retigabine		++						+		
Rufinamide	++									
Tiagabine									++[a]	
Topiramate	++			++				++		
Valproate	+[b]	+					+[b]		+[a,b]	+[b]
Vigabatrin									++[a]	
Zonisamide	++		++							++

++ = predominant action, + = putative or non-predominant action.

a. tiagabine and vigabatrin inhibit GABA reuptake and breakdown (via GABA transaminase) respectively. Valproate affects both synthesis and re-uptake/breakdown of GABA in selected brain regions

b. although many anti-epileptics have more than one mode of action, valproate in particular is thought to have no predominant mode of action, helping to explain its broad spectrum of activity (see p.282).

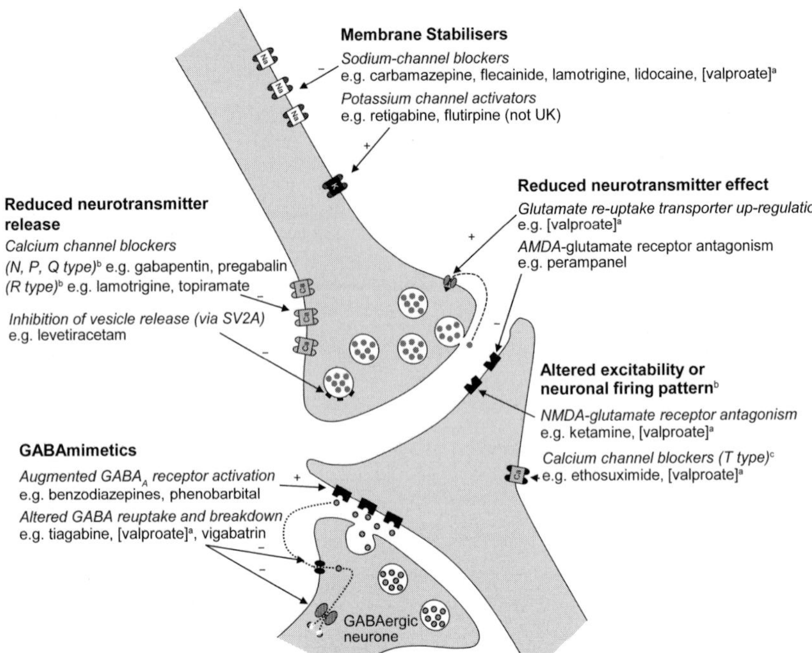

Figure 1 Mechanisms of action of anti-epileptics and related drugs.[1–8,10,11] Squared parentheses indicate a contributory, but not predominant, action of the anti-epileptic.

a. although many anti-epileptics have more than one mode of action, valproate in particular is thought to have no single predominant action (see p.282)
b. arriving action potentials open pre-synaptic N, P, Q and R type calcium channels. The resulting calcium influx triggers neurotransmitter release (see p.272)
c. both NMDA-glutamate receptors and T-type calcium channels affect neuronal excitability and threshold setting. T-type calcium channels also affect neuronal firing patterns, e.g. tonic or burst firing, in nociceptive neurones and the thalamus (burst firing in the latter is implicated in absence seizures).

GABAmimetics affect GABA metabolism or $GABA_A$ receptors. **Tiagabine** and **vigabatrin** inhibit GABA re-uptake transporters and GABA transaminase, the enzyme responsible for GABA breakdown, respectively. **Valproate** probably also affects GABA metabolism. Barbiturates and benzodiazepines affect $GABA_A$ receptors, binding at sites distinct from GABA itself (allosteric modulation). Benzodiazepines increase the receptors affinity for GABA; barbiturates prolong channel opening (see p.149, p.290 and Table 1).[21]

The broad spectrum of efficacy of **valproate** is explained by its multiple actions including blockade of sodium channels and T-type calcium channels. The latter are implicated in neuropathic pain,[22] the burst firing responsible for absence seizures and in regulating pain excitation thresholds in a 'T-rich' subset of peripheral nociceptors.[23]

The endocannabinoid system is another important inhibitory neurotransmitter system; cannabinoids have been proposed as potential future anti-epileptics.[24]

Genetic variations in anti-epileptic targets have been identified (e.g. sodium and potassium channels, the $GABA_A$ receptor complex). Some cause inherited epilepsy, but there is no straightforward link between the affected channel/receptor and either the epilepsy type or optimal choice of anti-epileptic.[25,26] A polymorphism in the gene (SCN1A) encoding the sodium channel α-subunit has been linked to **carbamazepine**-resistant epilepsy.[27]

Genetic factors also affect both pharmacokinetics and the risk of undesirable effects. Two poor metabolizer CYP2C9 alleles (which occur in 10–20% of Caucasians, 10% of Japanese, and 1–5% of Asians and Africans) reduce the mean effective daily **phenytoin** dose by 20–40%.[26] Human leukocyte antigen (HLA) genes are associated with the risk of Stevens-Johnson syndrome in patients taking **carbamazepine**, **eslicarbazepine**, **oxcarbazepine** or **phenytoin** (see p.278).[28,29] The UK MHRA recommends testing HLA B*1502 status before **carbamazepine** is started in people of Han Chinese, Hong Kong Chinese or Thai origin.[30]

The pharmacokinetics of anti-epileptics are summarized in Table 2. Whereas absorption is generally unaffected by increasing age, the volume of distribution may change (reduced albumin, total body water and lean:fat mass ratio) and elimination rates slow (altered metabolism, renal function and volume of distribution).[30,31]

Cautions

Safety concerns with **vigabatrin** (visual field deficits) and **felbamate** (not UK; aplastic anaemia and hepatic failure) limit their use to refractory epilepsy under specialist supervision when all other measures have failed.

Driving

In the UK, patients suffering from epilepsy must notify the DVLA. Generally, a seizure-free period of one year is required before driving can resume (longer for heavy goods vehicles), although this varies (e.g. where a seizure was due to a transient illness).[41]

Skin rashes and cross-reactive hypersensitivity

In relation to skin rashes, cross-reactive hypersensitivity may occur with various anti-epileptics:[42]

- **carbamazepine**: increased risk if rash occurred with a previous anti-epileptic (particularly **phenytoin**, **phenobarbital** or **oxcarbazepine**) or TCA; use alternative if possible
- **phenytoin**: increased risk of skin rash if rash has occurred with a previous anti-epileptic (particularly **carbamazepine** or **phenobarbital**); use alternative if possible
- **oxcarbazepine**: 25–30% risk of cross-reactivity if previous reaction to **carbamazepine**
- **zonisamide**: avoid if hypersensitive to sulfonamides
- **lamotrigine**: increased risk of rash if rash has occurred with a previous anti-epileptic, rapidly titrated and/or receiving concurrent **valproate**.

Hepatic impairment

With the exception of **gabapentin**, **pregabalin,** and **vigabatrin**, the manufacturers advise caution with all the anti-epileptics listed in Table 2 (lower initial doses, slower titration and careful monitoring). Additional advice is given in the individual monographs and summarized in Chapter 18, Hepatic impairment, p.703. Previous or concurrent hepatic disease increases the risk of **valproate** and **carbamazepine**-related hepatic failure. However, no specific information is available about the risks with hepatic metastases, which do not generally affect the hepatic metabolism of drugs unless there is severe hepatic impairment/cirrhosis.[43,44]

Renal impairment

Caution should be taken with all the anti-epileptics listed in Table 2 (i.e. lower initial doses, slower titration and careful monitoring); anti-epileptics differ in their potential to cause toxicity when renal function is impaired (see Chapter 17, p.688). Specific advice on dose adjustment in all stages of renal impairment is available in the individual monographs for **gabapentin** (see Table 3, p.275), **levetiracetam** (see Table 1, p.288) and **pregabalin** (see Table 4, p.275). Further, there are occasional reports of renal failure with **gabapentin** and **pregabalin**.

Females of child-bearing age

Consider teratogenicity when choosing an anti-epileptic. Enquire about oral contraceptive if using an enzyme-inducing anti-epileptic.

Table 2 Pharmacokinetic details of anti-epileptics[9,31–40]

Drug	Bio-availability PO (%)	T_{max} (h)	Plasma protein binding (%)	Plasma halflife (h)	Fate
Carbamazepine	80	4–8	75	8–24	CYP3A4, CYP2C8[a]
Clonazepam	≥80	1–4	80–90	30–40	CYP3A
Diazepam	≥80	1–3	95–98	24–48, 48–120[b]	CYP2C19, CYP3A4[a]
Gabapentin	30–75[c]	2–3	0	5–7	Excreted unchanged
Lamotrigine	98	1–4	55	15–30, 8–20[d], 30–90[e]	Glucuronidation
Levetiracetam	≥95	1–2	<10	6–8	Non-hepatic hydrolysis (70% excreted unchanged)
Oxcarbazepine[f]	≥95	1–3, 3–8[f]	65, 40[f]	1–5, 7–20[f]	Cytosolic keto-reduction to MHD[f], which then undergoes glucuronidation[a]
Perampanel		1	95	53–136	CYP3A4, CYP3A5
Phenobarbital	≥90	2–12	50	72–144	CYP2C9 (25% excreted unchanged)
Phenytoin	90–95	4–8	90	10–70[c]	CYP2C9
Pregabalin	>90	1	0	5–9[g]	Excreted unchanged
Retigabine	60	1–1.5	80	8	Glucuronidation and N-acetylation[a]
Rufinamide	85	5–6	25–35	8–12	Hepatic hydrolysis and oxidation
Tiagabine	≥90	1–2	96	4–13, 2–5[d]	CYP3A4
Topiramate	≥80	1–4	13	20–30, 8–15[d]	Multiple pathways (>60% excreted unchanged)
Valproate	95	1–2[h]	90	9–18, 5–12[d]	Multiple pathways[a] (see p.282)
Vigabatrin	80–90	1–2	0	6	Excreted unchanged
Zonisamide	≥50	1–4	50	50–70, 25–35[d]	CYP3A4 (15–30% excreted unchanged)

a. biologically active metabolites
b. nordiazepam, active metabolite
c. dose or plasma concentration dependent
d. with concurrent enzyme-inducers
e. with concurrent valproate
f. monohydroxycarbazepine, active metabolite of oxcarbazepine (a pro-drug)
g. >2 days in severe renal impairment and haemodialysis patients
h. 3–5h for e/c tablets, 5–10h for m/r tablets.

Suicide

Overall, anti-epileptic drugs are associated with suicidal thoughts or behaviour in 1/500 patients from the start of treatment onwards. The effect appears to differ between drugs, with some even conferring a small protective effect. Nonetheless, all patients should be monitored for suicidal ideation, and advised to report any mood disturbance or suicidal thoughts to a health professional.[45–48]

Additional cautions with specific anti-epileptics

- atrioventricular block: **carbamazepine** and **oxcarbazepine** may cause complete block
- previous bone marrow suppression: **carbamazepine**, possible increased risk
- heart failure: **oxcarbazepine** and **pregabalin**, fluid retention can exacerbate; monitor weight and plasma sodium
- patients at high risk of drug abuse: **gabapentin** and **pregabalin**.[49–51]

Drug interactions

Interactions are described in individual drug monographs:

- **gabapentin** (p.272), **levetiracetam** (p.287) and **pregabalin** (p.272) have no clinically significant pharmacokinetic interactions
- **carbamazepine** (p.278), **phenobarbital** (p.289) and **phenytoin** (Table 3) cause numerous interactions through hepatic enzyme induction.

Table 3 Clinically significant cytochrome P450 interactions with phenytoin resulting in changed drug plasma concentrations

Phenytoin plasma concentration		*Drug plasma concentration*	
increased by	*decreased by*	*increased by phenytoin*	*decreased by phenytoin*
Amiodarone	Antiretrovirals[a]	Phenobarbital	Amiodarone
Antifungal azoles[a]	Benzodiazepines[a]		Antifungal and anthelmintic azoles[a]
Azapropazone	Carbamazepine		Antiretrovirals[a]
Benzodiazepines[a]	Chlorpromazine		Aprepitant
Carbamazepine	Dexamethasone		Benzodiazepines[a]
Celecoxib	Phenobarbital		Calcium-channel blockers[a]
Chlorpromazine	Rifampicin		Carbamazepine
Cimetidine	St John's wort		Clozapine
Dexamethasone	Thioridazine		Corticosteroids
Diltiazem	Valproate		Disopyramide
Ethosuximide	Vigabatrin		Doxycycline
Fluoxetine			Ethosuximide
Fluvoxamine			Fentanyl
Oxcarbazepine			Haloperidol
Phenobarbital			Hormonal contraceptives
Prochlorperazine			Lamotrigine
Stiripentol			Methadone
Thioridazine			Mexiletine
Ticlopidine			Mirtazapine
Topiramate			Primidone
Valproate			Sertindole
			Theophylline
			Tiagabine
			Topiramate
			Tramadol
			Valproate

a. effect not seen with all drug class members.

Undesirable effects

Despite their diverse actions and structures, anti-epileptics share many undesirable effects. Their relative incidence is often similar.[52,53]

All anti-epileptics cause psychotropic and CNS depressant effects including drowsiness, ataxia, cognitive impairment, agitation, diplopia and dizziness. Psychiatric effects (e.g. depression, psychosis, irritability, or lability) are commonest with **levetiracetam**, **perampanel**, **phenobarbital**, **tiagabine**, **topiramate**, **vigabatrin** and **zonisamide**.[47,54] Cognitive impairment is worst with **phenobarbital** and least with newer anti-epileptics and **valproate**.[35,55] Ataxia is commonest with **phenytoin** and **carbamazepine**.[56] In an RCT, **levetiracetam** was better tolerated than **lamotrigine** and m/r **carbamazepine**; discontinuation rates for undesirable effects were 17%, 26% and 32% respectively.[57] Anti-epileptics cause suicidal ideation in 1/500 patients (see Cautions).

Most cause haematological derangements. These are often asymptomatic and may not require stopping the drug (see SPCs for advice). Severe derangement (e.g. aplastic anaemia, agranulocytosis) is reported particularly with **felbamate** (limiting use) and **carbamazepine** (monitor blood counts), and with many newer anti-epileptics. Folate deficiency occurs with enzyme-inducers, e.g. **phenytoin**.

Biochemical derangements (particularly of LFTs) are also common but are generally asymptomatic. Albeit rarely, hepatic failure is seen with many anti-epileptics, again particularly with **felbamate** (not UK; also limiting its use) and **carbamazepine** (where symptoms of hepatic disease and LFTs should be monitored), as well as with newer anti-epileptics. The incidence compared with **carbamazepine** is unknown. Pancreatitis affects 1:3,000 users of **valproate**.[58] It also occurs with many newer anti-epileptics but the incidence compared with **valproate** is unknown. Hyponatraemia is commonest with **carbamazepine** and **oxcarbazepine**.[59] Transient rashes are particularly associated with **lamotrigine**, **carbamazepine** and **oxcarbazepine**. Risk factors include rashes with previous anti-epileptics, higher starting doses and rapid titration (and, with **lamotrigine**, childhood and concurrent **valproate**). Severe rashes such as Stevens-Johnson syndrome are reported with all anti-epileptics, but most commonly with **lamotrigine** (affecting 1:1,000 adults). An HLA type is known to predispose specific groups to **carbamazepine**- and **phenytoin**-related Stevens-Johnson syndrome (see above).

Undesirable effects seen with particular anti-epileptics include: urolithiasis (**topiramate** and **zonisamide**); vitamin deficiencies (hepatic enzyme inducers);[59] hyperammonaemic encephalopathy (**valproate**); and coarse facies, acne, hirsutism and gingival hypertrophy (**phenytoin**). **Phenytoin** also exhibits distinct undesirable effects at supra-therapeutic levels (Box A) or after rapid high-dose IV infusion (purple glove syndrome, a painful discolouration seen distal to the infusion site in <6% of patients).[60]

Use of anti-epileptics in palliative care

Particularly when prescribing more than one anti-epileptic, it is important to consider:

- pharmacokinetic drug–drug interactions
- seizure type (particularly in long-standing epilepsy; generalized seizures may be precipitated by **carbamazepine**, **oxcarbazepine**, **gabapentin**, **tiagabine** and **vigabatrin**)
- additive cognitive impairment.

Switching between formulations

The MHRA recommends *not* switching between brands of anti-epileptics *when used for epilepsy*, except for **ethosuximide**, **gabapentin**, **lacosamide**, **levetiracetam**, **pregabalin**, **tiagabine** and **vigabatrin**.[63]

Switching between different manufacturers products or brands should be avoided if possible because bio-availability and duration of action may differ. Both loss of effect and new undesirable effects have been reported after switching.[63] However, if there is a delay in obtaining the patient's usual brand, *it is better to give a different brand than to miss a dose.*

Phenytoin 300mg as capsules is equivalent to 270mg as oral solution.

Neuropathic pain

Gabapentin and **pregabalin** are commonly used for neuropathic pain.[64] In both direct comparisons and 2 large network analyses, the efficacy and tolerability of **gabapentin**, **pregabalin** and antidepressants are similar.[65–76]

Box A Phenytoin toxicity[61]

Clinical features

Phenytoin toxicity generally manifests as a syndrome of cerebellar, vestibular and ocular effects, including some or all of the following:

- nystagmus:
  - ▷ on lateral gaze only (early sign)
  - ▷ spontaneous (more severe toxicity)
- blurred vision/diplopia
- slurred speech
- ataxia.

These may be accompanied by lethargy and/or delirium. Some patients experience break-through seizures (or an increase in the frequency of seizures) when the free phenytoin plasma concentration increases to toxic levels.

Evaluation

If phenytoin toxicity is suspected, check the plasma phenytoin concentration (and plasma albumin) just before the next dose is due. The normal therapeutic range is 40–80micromol/L (10–20microgram/mL). Because phenytoin is highly protein-bound, it is important to correct the observed concentration in patients with a low albumin:

$$\text{Corrected total phenytoin concentration (normal renal function)} = \frac{\text{observed concentration}}{(0.02 \times \text{albumin [g/L]}) + 0.1}$$

$$\text{Corrected total phenytoin concentration (in end-stage renal failure)} = \frac{\text{observed concentration}}{(0.01 \times \text{albumin [g/L]}) + 0.1}$$

Note. The units for albumin must be g/L; however, the formulae can be used for whatever units the phenytoin concentration is reported in.

Phenytoin toxicity can be present despite being within the therapeutic range; if necessary, make the diagnosis on clinical features alone and act accordingly.

Management

There is no specific antidote to phenytoin. If the patient has clinical features suggestive of toxicity, omit one or more doses, depending on severity of symptoms, and reduce subsequent doses to a previous non-toxic level. Generally, symptoms resolve when the plasma phenytoin concentration falls.[62]

Treat break-through seizures with benzodiazepines (see p.149) because other anti-epileptic drugs may exacerbate toxicity. If the frequency of seizures increases as the phenytoin toxicity drops, obtain advice from a neurologist.

Gabapentin is a first-line choice because benefit has been confirmed for a range of causes of neuropathic pain,[64,76] it has few drug interactions, and Marketing authorizations include peripheral neuropathic pain. **Gabapentin** is effective for cancer-related neuropathic pain, although benefit in a RCT was small (see p.272).[77]

Pregabalin's twice daily administration is an advantage for selected patients. However, **gabapentin** can also be administered twice daily for some patients, particularly the elderly and those with renal impairment (see p.272). Marketing authorizations for **pregabalin** include central and peripheral neuropathic pain.

Carbamazepine is an authorized first-line treatment for trigeminal neuralgia. It has long been used off-label for other neuropathic pains. However, RCTs are small, short (mostly <4 weeks) and use outcome measures of uncertain clinical significance.[15] Further, it requires slow titration and particular care with regard to drug interactions (see p.278). Although results of RCTs of **oxcarbazepine** in diabetic neuropathy show inconsistent benefit *overall*, clinical examination may identify subgroups who *are* likely to benefit (see p.280). Of other membrane stabilizers, in diabetic neuropathy, **lamotrigine** appears ineffective[78] and **lacosamide** less effective than gabapentin/pregabalin (NNT 10–12 vs. 6).[79]

Valproate is used in some centres when a smaller tablet load, once daily regimen, or CSCI is required. Benefit is reported for cancer-related neuropathic pain,[80,81] but the results of RCTs in non-cancer pain are conflicting (see p.282),[82] and international guidelines do not recommend its use.[64,83]

It appears to be well tolerated with lower rates of discontinuation because of undesirable effects (<5%)[82] compared with **gabapentin** (10%)[76] and **pregabalin** (20–30%)[75] in similar populations.

Clonazepam is reported to improve both cancer-related and non-cancer neuropathic pain (see p.149). It has anxiolytic and muscle-relaxant properties and can be given SC (not UK), leading to its use in selected palliative care patients despite the absence of supporting RCTs.[84]

Topiramate is as effective as **carbamazepine** for trigeminal neuralgia.[85] It is also reported to improve cancer-related neuropathic pain; most patients had already tried **gabapentin**, a tricyclic antidepressant and **methadone**.[86] In a cross-over RCT in multiple sclerosis, more patients preferred **topiramate** than placebo (12 versus 2; n=32).[87] However, results of RCTs in non-cancer neuropathic pain (diabetic neuropathy, lumbar radicular pain) do not show consistent benefit.[88] Slow titration and adequate hydration are required to minimize undesirable CNS effects and the risk of urolithiasis, respectively. Studies often gave **topiramate** in divided doses, but because the halflife is 20–30h, this is unlikely to be necessary:

- start with 25mg PO at bedtime
- if necessary, increase in 25mg increments every 1–2 weeks
- typical effective dose ≤200mg/24h.[85–87]

Levetiracetam and **zonisamide** are ineffective for neuropathic pain (see p.287).[89,90]

Few studies have compared **gabapentin/pregabalin** with anti-epileptics with different mechanisms of action. Although an RCT found **pregabalin** to be superior to **carbamazepine** and **venlafaxine**, doses were fixed not titrated.[91]

Switching vs. combining anti-epileptics for neuropathic pain

If the first choice treatment fails, switch to a drug with a different mechanism of action. (e.g. an antidepressant, p.193). For example, **duloxetine** is more effective than **pregabalin** for pain unresponsive to **gabapentin**.[92]

They are often used in combination (p.299), particularly if the first choice treatment is partially successful. The combination of **gabapentin** or **pregabalin** with **morphine**, **imipramine** or **nortriptyline** is superior to any treatment alone.[93–97] An open-label trial in cancer pain with a neuropathic component also found combined treatment with **gabapentin** to be superior to **morphine** alone.[98]

Combinations of ≥2 anti-epileptics are used less commonly. Undesirable effects may be increased and alternative options are often more appropriate (e.g. antidepressants, opioids, **ketamine** and interventional anaesthesia, also see p.299). Where a second anti-epileptic drug is added, the first is generally withdrawn, although examples of combined use are reported. Improvements in efficacy and tolerability have been described in 11 patients with multiple sclerosis whose trigeminal neuralgia had been unsatisfactorily controlled by **carbamazepine** or **lamotrigine**. The addition of **gabapentin** brought relief in 10 patients. The former were reduced to the minimal effective dose, with improved overall tolerability, but could not be withdrawn completely in any patient, suggesting that both anti-epileptics were contributing to overall relief.[99]

Doses are described in individual monographs: **carbamazepine** (p.278), **clonazepam** (p.149), **gabapentin** and **pregabalin** (p.272), **oxcarbazepine** (p.280) and **valproate** (p.282).

Epilepsy

Overtreatment with anti-epileptic drugs is common. Seek specialist advice where the diagnosis of seizures or the dose or choice of anti-epileptic drug is in doubt.

When to start treatment

Anti-epileptic drugs are generally commenced after a first seizure when there is an irreversible underlying focal lesion, e.g. cerebral tumour, multiple sclerosis, which makes further seizures probable. In the absence of a focal lesion, the risk is lower and an anti-epileptic is generally withheld unless a second seizure occurs.[100]

Anti-epileptics should *not* be used *prophylactically* in the absence of a history of seizures; in RCTs, they do not reduce the risk.[101] Peri-neurosurgical use is a possible exception, but results are conflicting.[102] If used for this indication, anti-epileptics should generally be slowly tapered after one week (see stopping anti-epileptics below).[103]

Choice of drug

Seizures caused by focal brain lesions are, by definition, focal onset, even if this is obscured by rapid secondary generalization. Thus, generally in palliative care, factors other than seizure classification influence the choice of anti-epileptic; e.g. the potential for drug interactions, co-morbidities, route and the simplicity of the regimen.[101] Common first-line choices include **levetiracetam**, **oxcarbazepine** and **valproate** (see Box B). In 2 small open-label RCTs, **levetiracetam** was as effective as, but better tolerated than, **phenytoin**.[104] Compared with **pregabalin**, fewer patients using **levetiracetam** required additional anti-epileptic drugs.[105]

4

Because they can interfere with chemotherapy and other medications, many advocate avoiding enzyme-inducing anti-epileptics.[106] Post-hoc analysis of an RCT revealed a possible survival advantage in glioma patients treated with valproate.[106] Because of the risk of teratogenicity with some anti-epileptics, obtain specialist advice when treating women of childbearing age.

Anti-epileptics are better tolerated if commenced at lower than recommended doses.[107] Doses can be increased if seizures persist, but less additional benefit is seen when increasing higher doses. In one study, 90% of those responding to a first-line anti-epileptic required:

- **valproate** ≤1,500mg/24h
- **lamotrigine** ≤300mg/24h
- **carbamazepine** ≤800mg/24h.[108]

Few patients responded to increases above these doses.[108] In non-responders, a change of anti-epileptic is indicated.

For doses, see individual monographs for **valproate** (p.282), **carbamazepine** (p.278), **oxcarbazepine** (p.280), **gabapentin** and **pregabalin** (p.272), **levetiracetam** (p.287), or the manufacturer's SPC.

Box B Anti-epileptics for seizures in palliative care[101,104–106,109,110]

Levetiracetam[a]

Can be titrated rapidly, IV or SC if necessary (see p.287); no clinically significant drug interactions

Oxcarbazepine[a]

Fewer drug interactions than carbamazepine and phenytoin; effective doses achieved more quickly than with lamotrigine and carbamazepine; may have a role in neuropathic pain (see p.280)

Valproate[a,b]

Can be titrated rapidly, IV or SC if necessary; may have a role in agitation and neuropathic pain (see p.282)

Last days of life

Midazolam

Generally first-line because of familiarity, availability, benefit in concurrent symptoms and compatibility with other drugs CSCI

Phenobarbital

Generally second-line where seizures are unresponsive to midazolam (see p.289)

a. In addition to the above, NICE also recommend carbamazepine and lamotrigine as first-line options for focal seizures.[111] However, both require gradual titration over many weeks. Thus, in the palliative care setting, levetiracetam, oxcarbazepine or valproate are generally preferable

b. despite abnormal *in vitro* haemostasis, valproate has not been shown to increase neurosurgical bleeding complications,[112] but some surgeons advise caution; discuss with surgeons before starting if neurosurgery is planned.

Switching vs. combining anti-epileptics for epilepsy

If the first choice treatment fails, add a second anti-epileptic (Box B). When the second one is at an adequate or maximally tolerated dose, the first one is slowly withdrawn (see below).[111] Long-term combination therapy is generally avoided unless two trials of monotherapy have proved ineffective because:

- there is an increased likelihood of drug interactions
- toxicity may be enhanced
- evidence of benefit compared with monotherapy is limited.[107,113]

Combinations are guided by the same considerations as those for choosing first- and second-line anti-epileptics. Many successful combinations have been reported,[113,114] but the relative benefits of such combinations have not been established. Studies of older anti-epileptics indicate probable benefit in combining GABAmimetics with sodium channel blockers or possibly with other GABAmimetics, but not in using two sodium channel blockers together.[115] Despite this, combinations of sodium channel blockers are among those used by epileptologists.[113] Combining **valproate** and **lamotrigine** increases the risk of skin reactions; combining **valproate** with **topiramate** or hepatic enzyme inducers increases the risk of hyperammonaemia.

Do not combine three or more anti-epileptics except on specialist advice; additional benefit is rare.[107]

Convulsive status epilepticus

Figure 2 is modified from NICE guidance.[111] Hypoglycaemia should be excluded in all patients. If alcoholism or severely impaired nutrition is suspected, give **thiamine** 250mg IV. **Phenobarbital** and **midazolam** have been given preference over **phenytoin** and **lorazepam** because they are more likely to be immediately available in many palliative care units.

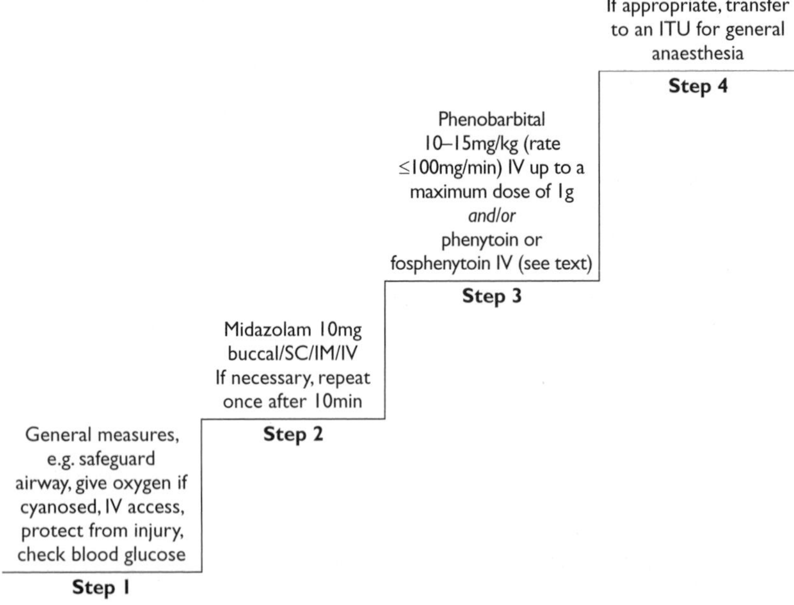

Figure 2 Management of status epilepticus in adults. See text for more detail.

Although IV **lorazepam** is generally recommended for the control of status epilepticus, IM **midazolam** is as effective (see p.155).[116] **Midazolam** 10mg †buccally or **diazepam** 10–20mg PR are alternatives (see p.155).

Phenobarbital injection is diluted 1 in 10 with WFI or 0.9% saline for IV administration. It can also be given IM or CSCI (see p.289).

Fosphenytoin and **phenytoin** are alternatives. **Fosphenytoin** can be given IV more rapidly than **phenytoin**. Both have narrow therapeutic ranges and require careful monitoring and safeguards to avoid toxicity;[117] see SPCs for details. **Levetiracetam** and **valproate** also appear effective, but their place relative to established treatments for status epilepticus is uncertain.[116]

Non-convulsive status epilepticus (NCSE)

NCSE is characterised by seizure activity on an EEG but without associated tonic-clonic activity. Presentations include delirium or coma.[118] In one report, NCSE was diagnosed in 5% of patients admitted to a palliative care unit; of these, half responded to treatment with anti-epileptics.[119] If an EEG is not possible, consider a trial of treatment (see Box B).

Mania

Valproate is generally added when the response to an antipsychotic is inadequate, but is an alternative first-line therapy particularly when it has been effective previously. **Lamotrigine** can also be used.[120]

Anxiety

Pregabalin (see p.272) is authorized for generalized anxiety disorder. It is generally used second- or third-line when the response to an SSRI and/or SNRI is inadequate. It can be combined with an SSRI or SNRI, particularly if there has been a partial response to the latter (also see p.196).[121] Its efficacy is similar to **lorazepam, alprazolam** and **venlafaxine**. It has a faster rate of onset than **venlafaxine**, and causes less nausea. It has a similar rate of onset to **quetiapine**, **lorazepam** and **alprazolam**, and causes less drowsiness but more dizziness.[122] RCTs also show some benefit with **gabapentin**,[123–125] **tiagabine**[126] and **lamotrigine**.[127]

Agitated delirium

Although unconfirmed in clinical trials, case series report benefit with **valproate** (p.282) for distressing symptoms refractory to antipsychotics and/or benzodiazepines.[128,129]

Terminal agitation

Phenobarbital (p.289) is used for terminal agitation refractory to **midazolam** and **levomepromazine** (also see p.156).

Sweats and hot flushes

Gabapentin is effective for hot flushes associated with prostate cancer, breast cancer or the menopause.[130–132] Benefit is also reported in idiopathic sweating in cancer (see p.272).[133]

Refractory hiccup

Gabapentin is reported to be effective for hiccup (see p.272).

Restless legs syndrome

Correct the correctable: treat iron deficiency; if taking antipsychotics or **metoclopramide**, reduce or switch to alternatives (see akathisia, p.739).[134] For symptomatic treatment, guidelines recommend:

- **gabapentin** or **pregabalin** first-line
- dopamimetics (e.g. **rotigotine**, **ropinirole**) second-line
- **opioids** third-line.[135]

Dopamimetics are not recommended first-line because they can exacerbate symptoms in the longer term (≥months). However, in palliative care, choice will be modified by prognosis and concurrent indications (e.g. pain).

Refractory cough

Gabapentin and **pregabalin** improve cough that persists despite resolution of the initial cause.[136] Benefit probably relates to reducing cough reflex hypersensitivity, which is generally present in this group of patients (see p.140).

Nausea and vomiting

Nausea and vomiting in those with CNS lesions (e.g. meningeal carcinomatosis)[137,138] or focal seizures[139] are reported to respond to **carbamazepine**, **valproate** or **levetiracetam**.

Given prophylactically, **gabapentin** reduces both post-operative and chemotherapy-induced nausea and vomiting (CINV)[140,141] Although a second RCT found no benefit, this may reflect good control of CINV in both the placebo and gabapentin groups; most received a long acting $5HT_3$ antagonist.[142]

Pruritus

Gabapentin is effective for uraemic and neuropathic pruritus. **Pregabalin** is reported to be beneficial (see p.272).

Alcohol withdrawal

Benzodiazepines (p.149) reduce withdrawal symptoms, particularly seizures. **Gabapentin** (p.272) and **phenobarbital** (p.289) are alternatives if benzodiazepines are insufficient.[143,144]

Stopping anti-epileptics

Abrupt cessation of long-term anti-epileptic therapy should be avoided because rebound seizures may be precipitated, even if use is for indications other than epilepsy. If treatment is to be discontinued, particularly barbiturates and benzodiazepines, this is best done *slowly over several months* (Table 4). However, both **gabapentin** and **pregabalin** can be stopped progressively over 1–2 weeks.

Table 4 Recommended monthly reductions of selected anti-epileptics[145]

Drug[a]	*Reduction*
Carbamazepine	100mg
Clobazam	10mg
Clonazepam	0.5mg
Ethosuximide	250mg
Lamotrigine	25mg
Levetiracetam	1,000mg[b]
Phenobarbital	15mg
Phenytoin	50mg
Topiramate	25mg
Valproate	250mg
Vigabatrin	500mg

a. gabapentin and pregabalin can be stopped progressively over 1–2 weeks
b. data from SPC.

In adults, the risk of relapse of pre-existing epilepsy on stopping treatment is 40–50%.[146] Caution should also be exercised when switching to an alternative anti-epileptic drug. In contrast to switching opioids (see p.370), the first drug should *not* be withdrawn until the new drug has been titrated up to an anticipated effective dose.

For patients who are unable to swallow PO medication, consider substituting a SC alternative. In the last days of life, generally **midazolam** is used (see Box B). However, remember that some anti-epileptics have a long halflife (see Table 2) and, in a moribund patient, might continue to be effective for 2–3 days after the last PO dose. When patients are not imminently dying, a less sedative alternative to **midazolam** is more appropriate, e.g. **levetiracetam**, **valproate** (see Box B).

1 Perucca E (2011) The pharmacology of new antiepileptic drugs: does a novel mechanism of action really matter? *CNS Drugs*. **25**: 907–912.
2 Kay HY *et al.* (2015) M-current preservation contributes to anticonvulsant effects of valproic acid. *Journal of Clinical Investigation*. **125**: 3904–3914.

3 Loscher W (2002) Basic pharmacology of valproate: a review after 35 years of clinical use for the treatment of epilepsy. *CNS Drugs*. **16**: 669–694.
4 Holtkamp D *et al.* (2017) Activity of the anticonvulsant lacosamide in experimental and human epilepsy via selective effects on slow Na+ channel inactivation. *Epilepsia*. **58**: 27–41.
5 Klitgaard H *et al.* (2016) Brivaracetam: rationale for discovery and preclinical profile of a selective SV2A ligand for epilepsy treatment. *Epilepsia*. **57**: 538–548.
6 Kremer M *et al.* (2016) Antidepressants and gabapentinoids in neuropathic pain: Mechanistic insights. *Neuroscience*. **338**: 183–206.
7 Bourinet E *et al.* (2016) T-type calcium channels in neuropathic pain. *Pain*. **157 (Suppl 1)**: S15–22.
8 Wormuth C *et al.* (2016) Review: Cav2.3 R-type voltage-gated Ca2+ channels - functional implications in convulsive and non-convulsive seizure activity. *Open Neurology Journal*. **10**: 99–126.
9 Stephen LJ and Brodie MJ (2011) Pharmacotherapy of epilepsy: newly approved and developmental agents. *CNS Drugs*. **25**: 89–107.
10 Devulder J (2010) Flupirtine in pain management: pharmacological properties and clinical use. *CNS Drugs*. **24**: 867–881.
11 Hobo (2012) Valproate upregulates glutamate transporters in rat spinal cord after peripheral nerve injury. *Journal of Pain*. **13 (Suppl 1)**: s62.
12 Devor M (2006) Sodium channels and mechanisms of neuropathic pain. *Journal of Pain*. **7**: S3–S12.
13 Sun Y *et al.* (2012) Perioperative systemic lidocaine for postoperative analgesia and recovery after abdominal surgery: a meta-analysis of randomized controlled trials. *Diseases of the Colon and Rectum*. **55**: 1183–1194.
14 Zhou M *et al.* (2013) Oxcarbazepine for neuropathic pain. *Cochrane Database of Systematic Reviews*. **3**: CD007963. www.thecochranelibrary.com
15 Wiffen PJ *et al.* (2014) Carbamazepine for chronic neuropathic pain and fibromyalgia in adults. *Cochrane Database of Systematic Reviews*. **4**: CD005451. www.thecochranelibrary.com
16 von Gunten CF *et al.* (2007) Flecainide for the treatment of chronic neuropathic pain: a Phase II trial. *Palliative Medicine*. **21**: 667–672.
17 Goldberg YP *et al.* (2012) Treatment of Na(v)1.7-mediated pain in inherited erythromelalgia using a novel sodium channel blocker. *Pain*. **153**: 80–85.
18 Zakrzewska JM *et al.* (2017) Safety and efficacy of a Nav1.7 selective sodium channel blocker in patients with trigeminal neuralgia: a double-blind, placebo-controlled, randomised withdrawal phase 2a trial. *Lancet Neurology*. **16**: 291–300.
19 Kukkar A *et al.* (2013) Implications and mechanism of action of gabapentin in neuropathic pain. *Archives of Pharmacal Research*. **36**: 237–251.
20 Lynch BA (2004) The synaptic vesicle protein SV2A is the binding site for the antiepileptic drug levetiracetam. *Proceedings of the National Academy of Sciences of the United States of America*. **101**: 9861–9866.
21 Rudolph U and Mohler H (2006) GABA-based therapeutic approaches: GABAA receptor subtype functions. *Current Opinion in Pharmacology*. **6**: 18–23.
22 Takahashi T *et al.* (2010) Upregulation of Ca(v)3.2 T-type calcium channels targeted by endogenous hydrogen sulfide contributes to maintenance of neuropathic pain. *Pain*. **150**: 183–191.
23 Francois A *et al.* (2013) State-dependent properties of a new T-type calcium channel blocker enhance Ca(V)3.2 selectivity and support analgesic effects. *Pain*. **154**: 283–293.
24 Hill AJ *et al.* (2012) Cannabidivarin is anticonvulsant in mouse and rat in vitro and in seizure models. *British Journal of Pharmacology*. **167**: 1629–1642.
25 Mann MW and Pons G (2007) Various pharmacogenetic aspects of antiepileptic drug therapy: a review. *CNS Drugs*. **21**: 143–164.
26 Loscher W *et al.* (2009) The clinical impact of pharmacogenetics on the treatment of epilepsy. *Epilepsia*. **50**: 1–23.
27 Abe T *et al.* (2008) Association between SCN1A polymorphism and carbamazepine-resistant epilepsy. *British Journal of Clinical Pharmacology*. **66**: 304–307.
28 Locharernkul C *et al.* (2008) Carbamazepine and phenytoin induced Stevens-Johnson syndrome is associated with HLA-B*1502 allele in Thai population. *Epilepsia*. **49**: 2087–2091.
29 Kulkantrakorn K *et al.* (2012) HLA-B*1502 strongly predicts carbamazepine-induced Stevens-Johnson syndrome and toxic epidermal necrolysis in Thai patients with neuropathic pain. *Pain Practice*. **12**: 202–208.
30 MHRA (2008) Carbamazepine: genetic testing in some Asian populations. *Drug Safety Update*. **1**. www.mhra.gov.uk/safetyinformation
31 Perucca E (2006) Clinical pharmacokinetics of new-generation antiepileptic drugs at the extremes of age. *Clinical Pharmacokinetics*. **45**: 351–363.
32 Perucca E (1999) The clinical pharmacokinetics of the new antiepileptic drugs. *Epilepsia*. **40 (Suppl 9)**: S7–13.
33 Garnett WR (2000) Clinical pharmacology of topiramate: a review. *Epilepsia*. **41 (Suppl 1)**: S61–65.
34 Anderson *et al.* (2002) *Handbook of clinical drug data*. (10e). McGraw Hill.
35 Perucca E (2002) Pharmacological and therapeutic properties of valproate: a summary after 35 years of clinical experience. *CNS Drugs*. **16**: 695–714.
36 May TW *et al.* (2003) Clinical pharmacokinetics of oxcarbazepine. *Clinical Pharmacokinetics*. **42**: 1023–1042.
37 Bang LM and Goa KL (2004) Spotlight on oxcarbazepine in epilepsy. *CNS Drugs*. **18**: 57–61.
38 Kwan P and Brodie MJ (2004) Phenobarbital for the treatment of epilepsy in the 21st century: a critical review. *Epilepsia*. **45**: 1141–1149.
39 Patsalos PN and Patsalos PN (2004) Clinical pharmacokinetics of levetiracetam. *Clinical Pharmacokinetics*. **43**: 707–724.
40 Rogawski MA and Hanada T (2013) Preclinical pharmacology of perampanel, a selective non-competitive AMPA receptor antagonist. *Acta Neurologica Scandinavica Supplementum*. **197**: 19–24.
41 Carter T (2006) *Fitness to Drive: A Guide for Health Professionals*. Royal Society of Medicine Press, London.
42 Hirsch LJ *et al.* (2008) Cross-sensitivity of skin rashes with antiepileptic drug use. *Neurology*. **71**: 1527–1534.
43 Morgan DJ and McLean AJ (1995) Clinical pharmacokinetic and pharmacodynamic considerations in patients with liver disease. An update. *Clinical Pharmacokinetics*. **29**: 370–391.
44 Ford-Dunn S (2005) Managing patients with cancer and advanced liver disease. *Palliative Medicine*. **19**: 563–565.
45 FDA (2008) Safety information. Antiepileptic drugs. www.fda.gov/Safety/MedWatch (archived).
46 Pereira A *et al.* (2013) Suicidality associated with antiepileptic drugs: implications for the treatment of neuropathic pain and fibromyalgia. *Pain*. **154**: 345–349.
47 Mula M *et al.* (2013) Antiepileptic drugs and suicidality: an expert consensus statement from the Task Force on Therapeutic Strategies of the ILAE Commission on Neuropsychobiology. *Epilepsia*. **54**: 199–203.
48 MHRA (2008) Antiepileptics: risk of suicidal thoughts and behavior. *Drug Safety Update*. **2**. www.mhra.gov.uk/safetyinformation
49 PHE (2014) Advice for prescribers on the risk of the misuse of pregabalin and gabapentin. *Letter from Public Health England and NHS England*. www.gov.uk

50 Chiappini S and Schifano F (2016) A decade of gabapentinoid misuse: an analysis of the european medicines agency's 'Suspected Adverse Drug Reactions' database. *CNS Drugs.* **30**: 647–654.

51 Schjerning O *et al.* (2016) Abuse potential of pregabalin: a systematic review. *CNS Drugs.* **30**: 9–25.

52 Marson AG *et al.* (2007) The SANAD study of effectiveness of valproate, lamotrigine, or topiramate for generalised and unclassifiable epilepsy: an unblinded randomised controlled trial. *Lancet.* **369**: 1016–1026.

53 Marson AG *et al.* (2007) The SANAD study of effectiveness of carbamazepine, gabapentin, lamotrigine, oxcarbazepine, or topiramate for treatment of partial epilepsy: an unblinded randomised controlled trial. *Lancet.* **369**: 1000–1015.

54 Ettinger AB *et al.* (2015) Psychiatric and behavioral adverse events in randomized clinical studies of the noncompetitive AMPA receptor antagonist perampanel. *Epilepsia.* **56**: 1252–1263.

55 Kwan P and Brodie MJ (2001) Neuropsychological effects of epilepsy and antiepileptic drugs. *Lancet.* **357**: 216–222.

56 van Gaalen J *et al.* (2014) Drug-induced cerebellar ataxia: a systematic review. *CNS Drugs.* **28**: 1139–1153.

57 Werhahn KJ *et al.* (2015) A randomized, double-blind comparison of antiepileptic drug treatment in the elderly with new-onset focal epilepsy. *Epilepsia.* **56**: 450–459.

58 French JA (2007) First-choice drug for newly diagnosed epilepsy. *Lancet.* **369**: 970–971.

59 Gaitatzis A and Sander JW (2013) The long-term safety of antiepileptic drugs. *CNS Drugs.* **27**: 435–455.

60 Lalla R *et al.* (2012) Purple glove syndrome: a dreadful complication of intravenous phenytoin administration. *BMJ Case Reports.* **2012**.

61 Wu MF and Lim WH (2013) Phenytoin: a guide to therapeutic drug monitoring. *Proceedings of Singapore Healthcare.* **22**: 198–203.

62 Perkin GD (2004) Ch. 24:53. Epilepsy in later childhood and adults. In: DA Warrell *et al.* (eds) *Oxford Textbook of Medicine* (5e). Oxford University Press, Oxford.

63 MHRA (2013) Antiepileptic drugs: new advice on switching between different manufacturers' products for a particular drug. *Drug Safety Update.* **7**:A1.

64 Finnerup NB *et al.* (2016) Pharmacotherapy for neuropathic pain in adults: a systematic review and meta-analysis. *Lancet Neurology.* **14**: 162–173.

65 Bansal D *et al.* (2009) Amitriptyline vs. pregabalin in painful diabetic neuropathy: a randomized double blind clinical trial. *Diabetic Medicine.* **26**: 1019–1026.

66 Boyle J *et al.* (2012) Randomized, placebo-controlled comparison of amitriptyline, duloxetine, and pregabalin in patients with chronic diabetic peripheral neuropathic pain: impact on pain, polysomnographic sleep, daytime functioning, and quality of life. *Diabetes Care.* **35**: 2451–2458.

67 Morello C *et al.* (1999) Randomized double-blind study comparing the efficacy of gabapentin with amitriptyline on diabetic peripheral neuropathy pain. *Archives of Internal Medicine.* **159**: 1931–1937.

68 Chandra K *et al.* (2006) Gabapentin versus nortriptyline in post-herpetic neuralgia patients: a randomized, double-blind clinical trial--the GONIP Trial. *International Journal of Clinical Pharmacology and Therapeutics.* **44**: 358–363.

69 Mishra S *et al.* (2012) A comparative efficacy of amitriptyline, gabapentin, and pregabalin in neuropathic cancer pain: a prospective randomized double-blind placebo-controlled study. *American Journal of Hospice and Palliative Care.* **29**: 177–182.

70 Banerjee M *et al.* (2013) A comparative study of efficacy and safety of gabapentin versus amitriptyline as coanalgesics in patients receiving opioid analgesics for neuropathic pain in malignancy. *Indian Journal of Pharmacology.* **45**: 334–338.

71 Griebeler ML *et al.* (2014) Pharmacologic interventions for painful diabetic neuropathy: An umbrella systematic review and comparative effectiveness network meta-analysis. *Annals of Internal Medicine.* **161**: 639–649.

72 Kaydok E and Levendoglu F (2014) Comparison of the efficacy of gabapentin and pregabalin for neuropathic pain in patients with spinal cord injury: a crossover study. *Acta Medica Mediterranea.* **30**: 1343–1348.

73 Kelle B (2012) The efficacy of gabapentin and pregabalin in the treatment of neuropathic pain due to nerve injury. *Journal of Musculoskeletal Pain.* **20**: 300–305.

74 NICE (2013) Neuropathic pain. *Clinical Guideline* CG173 (appendix G). www.nice.org.uk

75 Moore RA *et al.* (2009) Pregabalin for acute and chronic pain in adults. *Cochrane Database of Systematic Reviews.* **3**: CD007076. www.thecochranelibrary.com

76 Moore RA *et al.* (2014) Gabapentin for chronic neuropathic pain and fibromyalgia in adults. *Cochrane Database of Systematic Reviews.* **4**: CD007938. www.thecochranelibrary.com

77 Caraceni A *et al.* (2004) Gabapentin for neuropathic cancer pain: a randomized controlled trial from the Gabapentin Cancer Pain Study Group. *Journal of Clinical Oncology.* **22**: 2909–2917.

78 Wiffen PJ *et al.* (2013) Lamotrigine for chronic neuropathic pain and fibromyalgia in adults. *Cochrane Database of Systematic Reviews.* **12**: CD006044. www.thecochranelibrary.com

79 Hearn L *et al.* (2012) Lacosamide for neuropathic pain and fibromyalgia in adults. *Cochrane Database of Systematic Reviews.* **2:** CD009318. www.thecochranelibrary.com

80 Hardy J *et al.* (2001) A phase II study to establish the efficacy and toxicity of sodium valproate in patients with cancer-related neuropathic pain. *Journal of Pain and Symptom Management.* **21**: 204–209.

81 Snare AJ (1993) Sodium Valproate. Retrospective analysis of neuropathic pain control in patients with advanced cancer. *Journal of Pharmacy Technology.* **9**: 114–117.

82 Gill D *et al.* (2011) Valproic acid and sodium valproate for neuropathic pain and fibromyalgia in adults. *Cochrane Database of Systematic Reviews.* **10**: CD009183. www.thecochranelibrary.com

83 Attal N *et al.* (2010) EFNS guidelines on the pharmacological treatment of neuropathic pain: 2010 revision. *European Journal of Neurology.* **17**: 1113–e1188.

84 Corrigan R *et al.* (2012) Clonazepam for neuropathic pain and fibromyalgia in adults. *Cochrane Database of Systematic Reviews.* **5**: CD009486. www.thecochranelibrary.com

85 Wang QP and Bai M (2011) Topiramate versus carbamazepine for the treatment of classical trigeminal neuralgia: a meta-analysis. *CNS Drugs.* **25**: 847–857.

86 Bendaly EA *et al.* (2007) Topiramate in the treatment of neuropathic pain in patients with cancer. *Supportive Cancer Therapy.* **4**: 241–246.

87 Rog (2003) Double blind, randomised placebo controlled, crossover trial of topiramate in central neuropathic pain due to multiple sclerosis. *Journal of Neurology Neurosurgery and Psychiatry.* **74**: 1457.

88 Wiffen PJ *et al.* (2013) Topiramate for neuropathic pain and fibromyalgia in adults. *Cochrane Database of Systematic Reviews.* **8**: CD008314. www.thecochranelibrary.com

89 Moore RA *et al.* (2015) Zonisamide for neuropathic pain in adults. *Cochrane Database of Systematic Reviews.* **1**: CD011241. www.thecochranelibrary.com

90 Wiffen PJ *et al.* (2014) Levetiracetam for neuropathic pain in adults. *Cochrane Database of Systematic Reviews.* **7**: CD010943. www.thecochranelibrary.com

91 Razazian N *et al.* (2014) Evaluation of the efficacy and safety of pregabalin, venlafaxine, and carbamazepine in patients with painful diabetic peripheral neuropathy. A randomized, double-blind trial. *Neurosciences (Riyadh)*. **19**: 192–198.
92 Tanenberg RJ *et al.* (2014) Duloxetine compared with pregabalin for diabetic peripheral neuropathic pain management in patients with suboptimal pain response to gabapentin and treated with or without antidepressants: a post hoc analysis. *Pain Practice*. **14**: 640–648.
93 Gilron I *et al.* (2015) Combination of morphine with nortriptyline for neuropathic pain. *Pain*. **156**: 1440–1448.
94 Tesfaye S *et al.* (2013) Duloxetine and pregabalin: high-dose monotherapy or their combination? The "COMBO-DN study"--a multinational, randomized, double-blind, parallel-group study in patients with diabetic peripheral neuropathic pain. *Pain*. **154**: 2616–2625.
95 Gilron I *et al.* (2009) Nortriptyline and gabapentin, alone and in combination for neuropathic pain: a double-blind, randomised controlled crossover trial. *Lancet*. **374**: 1252–1261.
96 Gilron I *et al.* (2005) Morphine, gabapentin, or their combination for neuropathic pain. *New England Journal of Medicine*. **352**: 1324–1334.
97 Holbech JV *et al.* (2015) Imipramine and pregabalin combination for painful polyneuropathy: a randomized controlled trial. *Pain*. **156**: 958–966.
98 Keskinbora K *et al.* (2007) Gabapentin and an opioid combination versus opioid alone for the management of neuropathic cancer pain: a randomized open trial. *Journal of Pain and Symptom Management*. **34**: 183–189.
99 Solaro C *et al.* (2000) Low-dose gabapentin combined with either lamotrigine or carbamazepine can be useful therapies for trigeminal neuralgia in multiple sclerosis. *European Neurology*. **44**: 45–48.
100 Angus-Leppan H (2014) First seizures in adults. *British Medical Journal*. **348**: g2470.
101 Guerrini R *et al.* (2013) The medical and surgical treatment of tumoral seizures: current and future perspectives. *Epilepsia*. **54 (Suppl 9)**: 84–90.
102 Pulman J *et al.* (2013) Antiepileptic drugs as prophylaxis for post-craniotomy seizures. *Cochrane Database of Systematic Reviews*. **2**: CD007286. wwwthecochranelibrary.com.
103 Glantz MJ *et al.* (2000) Practice parameter: anticonvulsant prophylaxis in patients with newly diagnosed brain tumors. Report of the Quality Standards Subcommittee of the American Academy of Neurology. *Neurology*. **54**: 1886–1893.
104 Lim DA *et al.* (2009) Safety and feasibility of switching from phenytoin to levetiracetam monotherapy for glioma-related seizure control following craniotomy: a randomized phase II pilot study. *Journal of Neuro-oncology*. **93**: 349–354.
105 Rossetti AO *et al.* (2014) Levetiracetam and pregabalin for antiepileptic monotherapy in patients with primary brain tumors. A phase II randomized study. *Neuro-oncology*. **16**: 584–588.
106 Perucca E (2013) Optimizing antiepileptic drug treatment in tumoral epilepsy. *Epilepsia*. **54 (Suppl 9)**: 97–104.
107 Perucca E and Kwan P (2005) Overtreatment in epilepsy: how it occurs and how it can be avoided. *CNS Drugs*. **19**: 897–908.
108 Kwan P and Brodie MJ (2001) Effectiveness of first antiepileptic drug. *Epilepsia*. **42**: 1255–1260.
109 Koekkoek JAF (2014) Epilepsy in the end of life phase of brain tumor patients: a systematic review. *Neuro-Oncology Practice*. **1**: 134–140.
110 Kerrigan S and Grant R (2011) Antiepileptic drugs for treating seizures in adults with brain tumours. *Cochrane Database of Systematic Reviews*. **8**: CD008586. www.thecochranelibrary.com
111 NICE (2012) The epilepsies: the diagnosis and management of the epilepsies in adults and children in primary and secondary care. *Clinical Guideline*. CG137 www.nice.org.uk
112 Zighetti ML *et al.* (2015) Effects of chronic administration of valproic acid to epileptic patients on coagulation tests and primary hemostasis. *Epilepsia*. **56**: e49–52.
113 Karceski S *et al.* (2005) Treatment of epilepsy in adults: expert opinion. *Epilepsy and Behavior*. **7 (Suppl 1)**: S1–64.
114 Stephen LJ and Brodie MJ (2002) Seizure freedom with more than one antiepileptic drug. *Seizure*. **11**: 349–351.
115 Deckers CL *et al.* (2000) Selection of antiepileptic drug polytherapy based on mechanisms of action: the evidence reviewed. *Epilepsia*. **41**: 1364–1374.
116 Prasad M *et al.* (2014) Anticonvulsant therapy for status epilepticus. *Cochrane Database of Systematic Reviews*. **9**: CD003723. www.thecochranelibrary.com
117 NHS Improvement (2016) Risk of death and severe harm from error with injectable phenytoin. *Patient Safety Alert*. NHS/PSA/W/2016/2010. www.improvement.nhs.uk/resources/patient-safety-alerts
118 Twycross R and Wilcock A (eds) (2016) *Introducing Palliative Care* (5e). palliativedrugs.com Ltd, Nottingham, pp. 206.
119 Lorenzl S *et al.* (2010) Nonconvulsive status epilepticus in palliative care patients. *Journal of Pain and Symptom Management*. **40**: 460–465.
120 NICE (2014) Bipolar disorder: assessment and mangement. *Clinical Guideline*. CG185. www.nice.org.uk
121 Baldwin DS *et al.* (2014) Evidence-based pharmacological treatment of anxiety disorders, post-traumatic stress disorder and obsessive-compulsive disorder: a revision of the 2005 guidelines from the British Association for Psychopharmacology. *Journal of Psychopharmacology*. **28**: 403–439.
122 Frampton JE (2014) Pregabalin: a review of its use in adults with generalized anxiety disorder. *CNS Drugs*. **28**: 835–854.
123 Pande AC *et al.* (1999) Treatment of social phobia with gabapentin: a placebo-controlled study. *Journal of Clinical Psychopharmacology*. **19**: 341–348.
124 Pande AC *et al.* (2000) Placebo-controlled study of gabapentin treatment of panic disorder. *Journal of Clinical Psychopharmacology*. **20**: 467–471.
125 Lavigne JE *et al.* (2012) A randomized, controlled, double-blinded clinical trial of gabapentin 300 versus 900 mg versus placebo for anxiety symptoms in breast cancer survivors. *Breast Cancer Research and Treatment*. **136**: 479–486.
126 Pollack MH *et al.* (2005) The selective GABA reuptake inhibitor tiagabine for the treatment of generalized anxiety disorder: results of a placebo-controlled study. *Journal of Clinical Psychiatry*. **66**: 1401–1408.
127 Hertzberg MA *et al.* (1999) A preliminary study of lamotrigine for the treatment of posttraumatic stress disorder. *Biological Psychiatry*. **45**: 1226–1229.
128 Bourgeois JA *et al.* (2005) Adjunctive valproic acid for delirium and/or agitation on a consultation-liaison service: a report of six cases. *Journal of Neuropsychiatry and Clinical Neurosciences*. **17**: 232–238.
129 Gagnon DJ *et al.* (2017) Valproate for agitation in critically ill patients: a retrospective study. *Journal of Critical Care*. **37**: 119–125.
130 Pandya KJ *et al.* (2005) Gabapentin for hot flashes in 420 women with breast cancer: a randomised double-blind placebo-controlled trial. *Lancet*. **366**: 818–824.
131 Nelson HD *et al.* (2006) Nonhormonal therapies for menopausal hot flashes: systematic review and meta-analysis. *Journal of the American Medical Association*. **295**: 2057–2071.
132 Loprinzi CL *et al.* (2009) A phase III randomized, double-blind, placebo-controlled trial of gabapentin in the management of hot flashes in men (N00CB). *Annals of Oncology*. **20**: 542–549.

133 Porzio G *et al.* (2006) Gabapentin in the treatment of severe sweating experienced by advanced cancer patients. *Supportive Care in Cancer*. **14**: 389–391.
134 Garcia-Borreguero D and Cano-Pumarega I (2017) New concepts in the management of restless legs syndrome. *British Medical Journal*. **356**: j104.
135 Garcia-Borreguero D *et al.* (2016) Guidelines for the first-line treatment of restless legs syndrome/Willis-Ekbom disease, prevention and treatment of dopaminergic augmentation: a combined task force of the IRLSSG, EURLSSG, and the RLS-foundation. *Sleep Medicine*. **21**: 1–11.
136 Gibson PG and Vertigan AE (2015) Management of chronic refractory cough. *British Medical Journal*. **351**: h5590.
137 Strohscheer I and Borasio GD (2006) Carbamazepine-responsive paroxysmal nausea and vomiting in a patient with meningeal carcinomatosis. *Palliative Medicine*. **20**: 549–550.
138 Lee JW *et al.* (2008) Emesis responsive to levetiracetam. *Journal of Neurology, Neurosurgery and Psychiatry*. **79**: 847–849.
139 Yukselen V *et al.* (2003) Partial seizure: an unusual cause of recurrent vomiting. *Internartional Journal of Clinical Practice*. **57**: 742–743.
140 Pandey CK *et al.* (2006) Prophylactic gabapentin for prevention of postoperative nausea and vomiting in patients undergoing laparoscopic cholecystectomy: a randomized, double-blind, placebo-controlled study. *Journal of Postgraduate Medicine*. **52**: 97–100.
141 Cruz FM *et al.* (2012) Gabapentin for the prevention of chemotherapy- induced nausea and vomiting: a pilot study. *Supportive Care in Cancer*. **20**: 601–606.
142 Barton DL *et al.* (2014) Phase III double-blind, placebo-controlled study of gabapentin for the prevention of delayed chemotherapy-induced nausea and vomiting in patients receiving highly emetogenic chemotherapy, NCCTG N08C3 (Alliance). *Cancer*. **120**: 3575–3583.
143 Hammond CJ *et al.* (2015) Anticonvulsants for the treatment of alcohol withdrawal syndrome and alcohol use disorders. *CNS Drugs*. **29**: 293–311.
144 Martin K and Katz A (2016) The role of barbiturates for alcohol withdrawal syndrome. *Psychosomatics*. **57**: 341–347.
145 Chadwick D (1995) The withdrawal of antiepileptic drugs. In: A Hopkins *et al.* (eds) *Epilepsy* (2e). Chapman and Hall, London, pp. 215–220.
146 Hopkins A and Shorvon S (1995) Definitions and epidemiology of epilepsy. In: A Hopkins *et al.* (eds) *Epilepsy* (2e). Chapman and Hall, London, pp. 1–24.

Updated September 2017

GABAPENTIN AND PREGABALIN

Class: Anti-epileptic (pre-synaptic calcium channel blocker).

Indications: Partial seizures, neuropathic pain, anxiety (**pregabalin**), †pruritus, †hot flushes, †sweating, †refractory hiccup, †restless legs syndrome, †refractory cough, †alcohol withdrawal.

Pharmacology

Gabapentin and pregabalin reduce the calcium influx responsible for triggering neurotransmitter release. By binding to the $\alpha 2\delta$ subunit responsible for channel trafficking, they remove pre-synaptic (N, P/Q-type) voltage-gated calcium channels from the cell surface.[1] This counteracts the upregulation of $\alpha 2\delta$ subunits seen in inflammation and neuropathic pain,[2] and thus the excessive release of:

- glutamate in the spinal dorsal horn (reducing pain transmission)
- GABA in the brainstem locus coeruleus (restoring descending pain inhibitory pathways; see p.299).[3,4]

Gabapentin may also inhibit the NMDA-glutamate receptor and microglia (neuro-inflammatory cells), either directly or via the above actions.

Despite being GABA analogues, neither gabapentin nor pregabalin is GABAmimetic.[1,4] They are unrelated to L-type calcium channel blockers, e.g. **diltiazem** (see Table 1).

For pharmacokinetic details, see Table 2.

Gabapentin is a first-line choice for neuropathic pain because benefit has been confirmed for a range of causes;[6,7] it has few drug interactions and peripheral neuropathic pain is included in the Marketing authorizations.

Pregabalin's twice daily administration is an advantage for selected patients; Marketing authorizations include peripheral and central neuropathic pain.

In network analyses, the efficacy and tolerability of gabapentin and pregabalin are comparable across a range of measures.[8,9] Two small direct comparisons in peripheral nerve injury (n=30)[10] and spinal cord injury (n=28)[11] also found similar outcomes. Pain relief was similar in a larger (n=120) RCT in cancer-related neuropathic pain; the greater reduction in **morphine** use with pregabalin compared with gabapentin may reflect the relatively higher doses used (600mg/day and 1800mg/day, respectively).[12] Pregabalin acts within days.[13] In one RCT, gabapentin's onset of action

Table 1 Classification of calcium channels[1,5]

Type	*Location (function)*	*Blocked by*
L-type (Ca_v1.1–1.4)	Cardiovascular and GI tissues (smooth muscle tone, conductivity); neurones (function unknown)	Diltiazem, nifedipine (see p.85), verapamil
N, P/Q-type (Ca_v2.1–2.2)	Pre-synaptic neurones (calcium influx triggers neurotransmitter release; over-expressed in neuropathic pain)	Gabapentin and pregabalin (N and P/Q-type), ziconotide (N-type)
R-type (Ca_v2.3)	Pre-synaptic neurones (calcium influx triggers neurotransmitter release)	Lamotrigine, topiramate
T-type (Ca_v3.1–3.3)	Nociceptive neurones (excitability/threshold setting, pacemaker activity/firing pattern); thalamic neurones (dysregulation responsible for absence seizures)	Ethosuximide, valproate (see p.282)

Table 2 Pharmacokinetic details

Drug	*Gabapentin*	*Pregabalin*
Bioavailability PO (%)	Dose-dependent[a]	≥90%[a]
T_{max} (h)	2–3	1
Protein-bound	No	No
Plasma halflife (h)	5–7	5–9
Elimination	Renally excreted unchanged	Renally excreted unchanged

a. both gabapentin and pregabalin are absorbed through amino acid transporters. At higher doses, gabapentin saturates the available transporters causing a dose-dependent reduction in bio-availability, i.e.: 100mg (74%), 300mg (60%), 600mg (49%), 1,200mg (33%). The absorption of pregabalin is unaffected by dose.

was slower, but drowsiness was twice as common with pregabalin suggesting the difference may relate to the rate of titration.[11]

If the first choice treatment fails, add or switch to a drug with a different mechanism of action, e.g. an antidepressant (p.193). For example, **duloxetine** is more effective than pregabalin for pain unresponsive to gabapentin.[14] Switching to pregabalin has been reported to improve pain unresponsive to gabapentin.[15] Although benefit has *not* been confirmed in an RCT, a difference in response is possible because of their varied absorption at higher doses and binding affinity.

Gabapentin and pregabalin are effective for other pains with suspected neuropathic and/or central sensitization mechanisms including burns,[16] fibromyalgia,[17] chronic masticatory myalgia,[18] and possibly also break-through pain due to bone metastases.[19] One RCT found benefit for pancreatitis pain was predicted by altered sensation in the associated dermatome.[20] However, 'routine' use in *unselected* cancer pain is no better than opioids alone.[21] Results of two small RCTs in painful radiation-induced mucositis are mixed.[22,23]

Pregabalin is authorized for generalized anxiety disorder. It is as effective as **lorazepam**, **alprazolam** and **venlafaxine**. Compared with **venlafaxine**, pregabalin has a faster rate of onset and causes less nausea; it has a similar rate of onset to **quetiapine**, **lorazapam** and **alprazolam** and causes less drowsiness but more dizziness.[24–27] Gabapentin is also effective.[28–30]

Neuronal dysregulation (e.g. CNS sensitization as in neuropathic pain) is implicated in a number of other symptoms. This may part explain the benefit of gabapentin and/or pregabalin in a wide range of settings, including chronic refractory cough due to cough reflex hyperexcitability;[31] neuropathic, idiopathic and uraemic pruritus;[32–35] idiopathic sweating in cancer;[36] hot flushes associated with prostate cancer, breast cancer or the menopause;[37–39] and chemotherapy-related nausea and vomiting.[40]

For refractory hiccup, gabapentin was generally commenced at 100mg t.d.s. and titrated to effect. However, in one series, 'burst gabapentin' relieved persistent hiccup in patients with a history of brain stem stroke. Patients received 400mg t.d.s. for 3 days, 400mg once daily for 3 days, and then stopped. Only 1/15 patients needed a second treatment.[41]

Gabapentin has also been used in spasticity.[42,43] Gabapentin and pregabalin are first-line options for restless legs syndrome and gabapentin is used for this indication in ESRF (see p.267 and p.688).[44,45]

Gabapentin and **phenobarbital** (p.289) are options for alcohol withdrawal when benzodiazepines are ineffective. Regimens vary but typically gabapentin is started at 1,200mg/24h and tapered over a week. Lower doses are described for milder symptoms in the outpatient setting.[46]

Cautions

Absence seizures (may worsen), psychotic illness (may precipitate or exacerbate psychotic episodes), patients at high risk of drug abuse (evidence of possible misuse),[47–49] renal impairment (see Dose and use and Chapter 17, p.681; renal failure reported with pregabalin which resolved on discontinuation), CHF (exacerbation reported).

Gabapentin is reported to cause false positive readings for urinary protein with Ames N-Multistix SG®.

Drug interactions

Clinically significant pharmacokinetic interactions are unlikely.

Aluminium and **magnesium**-containing compounds reduce gabapentin's bio-availability by ≤24%; **morphine** and **naproxen** may increase gabapentin levels. High doses of gabapentin may decrease **hydrocodone** (not UK) levels; mechanism unknown.

Undesirable effects

Undesirable effects are generally similar:

Very common (>10%): drowsiness, dizziness, ataxia.

Common (<10%, >1%): amnesia, confusion, visual disturbance, dysarthria, tremor, arthralgia, myalgia, peripheral oedema, dry mouth, vomiting, constipation.

Uncommon (<1%, >0.1%): suicidal ideation 0.2% (1/500; advise patients to report mood or thought disturbance), impotence, gynaecomastia.

Rare (<0.1%): rhabdomyolysis, pancreatitis, acute renal failure, Stevens Johnson Syndrome.

Donepezil is reported to reduce gabapentin-related drowsiness allowing further titration and thus improve analgesia.[50]

The frequencies of some symptoms differ between SPCs. It is uncertain whether this reflects a difference in incidence or detection. For example, leukopenia and arthralgia occur commonly with gabapentin, but not pregabalin.[51] Similarly, pregabalin is associated with cardiac conduction disturbance, QT prolongation and exacerbation of CHF, but gabapentin less so.[52,53]

Dose and use

Gabapentin

See below for short term use in hiccup and alcohol withdrawal. For most indications:

- start with 300mg PO at night
- if necessary, increase by 300mg/24h every 2–3 days, e.g.:
  - ▷ *Day 3* give 300mg b.d.
  - ▷ *Day 5* give 300mg t.d.s.
  - ▷ *Day 8* give 300mg, 300mg, 600mg
  - ▷ *Day 11* give 600mg, 300mg, 600mg
  - ▷ *Day 14* give 600mg t.d.s.
- in debilitated patients, slower titration is advisable, e.g. 100mg at night, increased if necessary by 100mg/24h every 2–3 days
- typical effective doses
  - ▷ neuropathic pain: 600mg t.d.s.[54]
  - ▷ hot flushes: 300mg t.d.s.[39]
  - ▷ uraemic itch: note the dose adjustment required in renal impairment (below)
  - ▷ hiccup: consider short term use (below)
- maximum recommended dose 1,200mg t.d.s.

The starting and maximum doses of gabapentin should be reduced in adults with renal impairment (Table 3) and those on haemodialysis (HD) (see below and Chapter 17, p.688).

Table 3 Gabapentin dose adjustments in renal impairment, modified from SPC

Creatinine clearance (mL/min)	*Starting dose*[a, b]	*Maximum dose*
50–79	300mg at bedtime	600mg t.d.s.
30–49	300mg at bedtime	300mg t.d.s.
15–29	100mg at bedtime	300mg b.d.[b]
<15 (non-dialysis or peritoneal dialysis only)	100mg on alternate nights	300mg at bedtime[b]

a. starting doses are lower than those recommended by the SPC; a further reduction is advisable in elderly patients and those receiving other CNS-depressant drugs-

b. the SPC recommends the daily dose be administered in three divided doses, but the prolonged halflife in renal impairment permits b.d. or once daily dosing as indicated.

For HD patients with a urine output >100mL/24h:

- start with 100mg PO at bedtime; consider either a supplementary dose after each HD session or timing the daily dose post HD.

For anuric HD patients:

- start with 100mg PO stat and 100mg after every HD session; a regular maintenance dose is generally not required.

Gabapentin (short term use: hiccup; alcohol withdrawal)

- in relatively robust patients, consider a 6-day 'burst' of gabapentin' PO, e.g.:
  - ▷ start with 300–400mg t.d.s. for 3 days
  - ▷ then give 300–400mg once daily for 3 days
  - ▷ if necessary, re-treat long-term if symptoms recur after a 'burst'.
- in frail elderly patients, proceed slowly as for neuropathic pain:
  - ▷ start with a low dose, e.g. 100mg t.d.s.
  - ▷ if necessary, titrate upwards
  - ▷ if successful, consider reducing/stopping gabapentin
  - ▷ if necessary, re-treat long-term if hiccup recurs after a 'burst'.

Pregabalin

- start with 75mg PO b.d.
- if necessary, at intervals of 3–7 days, increase to 150mg b.d. → 225mg b.d. → 300mg b.d. (maximum recommended dose)
- in debilitated patients
  - ▷ start with 25–50mg b.d.
  - ▷ if necessary, increase the dose correspondingly cautiously
- Typical effective dose: 150–300mg b.d.[55]

Dose reduction is necessary in renal impairment (Table 4). For patients on haemodialysis, the regular dose should be adjusted according to the creatinine clearance and a supplementary single dose given after each dialysis (Table 5); alternatively, some centres time the daily dose post haemodialysis session (see Chapter 17, p.688).

Table 4 Pregabalin dose adjustments in renal impairment, modified from SPC

Creatinine clearance (mL/min)	*Starting dose*	*Maximum dose*
>60	75mg b.d.	300mg b.d.
31–60	25mg t.d.s.[a]	150mg b.d.
15–30	25–50mg once daily	150mg once daily
<15	25mg once daily	75mg once daily

a. 37.5mg capsules not available, necessitating t.d.s. regimen.

Table 5 Post-haemodialysis supplementary doses of pregabalin

Daily dose	*Supplementary single dose after every 4h of haemodialysis*
25mg	25–50mg
50mg	50–75mg
75mg	100mg

Stopping gabapentin and pregabalin

To avoid precipitating pain or seizures, withdraw gradually over several weeks.

Supply

Gabapentin (generic)
Capsules 100mg, 300mg, 400mg, 28 days @ 300mg t.d.s. = £6.
Tablets 600mg, 800mg, 28 days @ 600mg t.d.s. = £7.
Oral solution 50mg/mL, 28 days @ 300mg t.d.s. = £464.

The authorized gabapentin oral solution available (Rosemont) contains propylene glycol and other excipients which, in high doses, may exceed WHO daily intake limits. Alternatively, for patients with swallowing difficulties, gabapentin capsules can be opened and the contents mixed with water, fruit juice or apple sauce.[56]

Pregablin (generic)
Capsules 25mg, 50mg, 75mg, 100mg, 150mg, 200mg, 225mg, 300mg, 28 days @ any strength of single capsule b.d. = £20.
Oral solution 20mg/mL, 28 days@ 225mg b.d. = £133.

1 Kremer M *et al.* (2016) Antidepressants and gabapentinoids in neuropathic pain: Mechanistic insights. *Neuroscience*. **338**: 183–206.
2 Lu (2010) Persistent inflammation alters the density and distribution of voltage activated calcium channels in subpopulations of rat cutaneous DRG neurons. *Pain*. **151**: 633–643.
3 Bee LA and Dickenson AH (2008) Descending facilitation from the brainstem determines behavioural and neuronal hypersensitivity following nerve injury and efficacy of pregabalin. *Pain*. **140**: 209–223.
4 Kukkar A *et al.* (2013) Implications and mechanism of action of gabapentin in neuropathic pain. *Archives of Pharmacal Research*. **36**: 237–251.
5 Wormuth C *et al.* (2016) Review: Cav2.3 R-type voltage-gated Ca2+ channels - functional implications in convulsive and non-convulsive seizure activity. *Open Neurology Journal*. **10**: 99–126.
6 Moore RA *et al.* (2009) Pregabalin for acute and chronic pain in adults. *Cochrane Database of Systematic Reviews*. **3**: CD007076. www.thecochranelibrary.com
7 Moore RA *et al.* (2014) Gabapentin for chronic neuropathic pain and fibromyalgia in adults. *Cochrane Database of Systematic Reviews*. **4**: CD007938. www.thecochranelibrary.com
8 Griebeler ML *et al.* (2014) Pharmacologic interventions for painful diabetic neuropathy: An umbrella systematic review and comparative effectiveness network meta-analysis. *Annals of Internal Medicine*. **161**: 639–649.
9 NICE (2013) Neuropathic pain - pharmacological management (appendix G). *Clinical Guideline*. CG173. www.nice.org.uk
10 Kelle B (2012) The efficacy of gabapentin and pregabalin in the treatment of neuropathic pain due to nerve injury. *Journal of Musculoskeletal Pain*. **20**: 300–305.
11 Kaydok E and Levendoglu F (2014) Comparison of the efficacy of gabapentin and pregabalin for neuropathic pain in patients with spinal cord injury: a crossover study. *Acta Medica Mediterranea*. **30**: 1343–1348.
12 Mishra S *et al.* (2012) A comparative efficacy of amitriptyline, gabapentin, and pregabalin in neuropathic cancer pain: a prospective randomized double-blind placebo-controlled study. *American Journal of Hospice and Palliative Care*. **29**: 177–182.
13 Cardenas DD *et al.* (2015) Examining the time to therapeutic effect of pregabalin in spinal cord injury patients with neuropathic pain. *Clinical Therapeutics*. **37**: 1081–1090.
14 Tanenberg RJ *et al.* (2014) Duloxetine compared with pregabalin for diabetic peripheral neuropathic pain management in patients with suboptimal pain response to gabapentin and treated with or without antidepressants: a post hoc analysis. *Pain Practice*. **14**: 640–648.
15 Saldana MT *et al.* (2012) Pain alleviation and patient-reported health outcomes following switching to pregabalin in individuals with gabapentin-refractory neuropathic pain in routine medical practice. *Clinical Drug Investigation*. **32**: 401–412.
16 Gray P *et al.* (2011) Pregabalin in severe burn injury pain: a double-blind, randomised placebo-controlled trial. *Pain*. **152**: 1279–1288.
17 Hauser W *et al.* (2009) Treatment of fibromyalgia syndrome with gabapentin and pregabalin--a meta-analysis of randomized controlled trials. *Pain*. **145**: 69–81.
18 Kimos P *et al.* (2007) Analgesic action of gabapentin on chronic pain in the masticatory muscles: a randomized controlled trial. *Pain*. **127**: 151–160.
19 Caraceni A *et al.* (2008) Gabapentin for breakthrough pain due to bone metastases. *Palliative Medicine*. **22**: 392–393.
20 Olesen SS *et al.* (2013) Quantitative sensory testing predicts pregabalin efficacy in painful chronic pancreatitis. *PLoS One*. **8**: e57963.

21 Mercadante S *et al.* (2013) The effects of low doses of pregabalin on morphine analgesia in advanced cancer patients. *Clinical Journal of Pain*. **29**: 15–19.
22 Starmer HM *et al.* (2014) Effect of gabapentin on swallowing during and after chemoradiation for oropharyngeal squamous cell cancer. *Dysphagia*. **29**: 396–402.
23 Kataoka T *et al.* (2016) Randomized trial of standard pain control with or without gabapentin for pain related to radiation-induced mucositis in head and neck cancer. *Auris Nasus Larynx*. **43**: 677–684.
24 Feltner DE *et al.* (2003) A randomized, double-blind, placebo-controlled, fixed-dose, multicenter study of pregabalin in patients with generalized anxiety disorder. *Journal of Clinical Psychopharmacology*. **23**: 240–249.
25 Pande AC *et al.* (2003) Pregabalin in generalized anxiety disorder: a placebo-controlled trial. *American Journal of Psychiatry*. **160**: 533–540.
26 Rickels K *et al.* (2005) Pregabalin for treatment of generalized anxiety disorder: a 4-week, multicenter, double-blind, placebo-controlled trial of pregabalin and alprazolam. *Archives of General Psychiatry*. **62**: 1022–1030.
27 Montgomery SA *et al.* (2006) Efficacy and safety of pregabalin in the treatment of generalized anxiety disorder: a 6-week, multicenter, randomized, double-blind, placebo-controlled comparison of pregabalin and venlafaxine. *Journal of Clinical Psychiatry*. **67**: 771–782.
28 Lavigne JE *et al.* (2012) A randomized, controlled, double-blinded clinical trial of gabapentin 300 versus 900 mg versus placebo for anxiety symptoms in breast cancer survivors. *Breast Cancer Research and Treatment*. **136**: 479–486.
29 Pande AC *et al.* (1999) Treatment of social phobia with gabapentin: a placebo-controlled study. *Journal of Clinical Psychopharmacology*. **19**: 341–348.
30 Pande AC *et al.* (2000) Placebo-controlled study of gabapentin treatment of panic disorder. *Journal of Clinical Psychopharmacology*. **20**: 467–471.
31 Gibson PG and Vertigan AE (2015) Management of chronic refractory cough. *British Medical Journal*. **351**: h5590.
32 Kanitakis J (2006) Brachioradial pruritus: report of a new case responding to gabapentin. *European Journal of Dermatology*. **16**: 311–312.
33 Yesudian PD and Wilson NJ (2005) Efficacy of gabapentin in the management of pruritus of unknown origin. *Archives of Dermatology*. **141**: 1507–1509.
34 Shavit L *et al.* (2013) Use of pregabalin in the management of chronic uremic pruritus. *Journal of Pain and Symptom Management*. **45**: 776–781.
35 Siemens W *et al.* (2016) Pharmacological interventions for pruritus in adult palliative care patients. *Cochrane Database of Systematic Reviews*. **11**: CD008320. www.thecochranelibrary.com
36 Porzio G *et al.* (2006) Gabapentin in the treatment of severe sweating experienced by advanced cancer patients. *Supportive Care in Cancer*. **14**: 389–391.
37 Loprinzi CL *et al.* (2009) A phase III randomized, double-blind, placebo-controlled trial of gabapentin in the management of hot flashes in men (N00CB). *Annals of Oncology*. **20**: 542–549.
38 Nelson HD *et al.* (2006) Nonhormonal therapies for menopausal hot flashes: systematic review and meta-analysis. *Journal of the American Medical Association*. **295**: 2057–2071.
39 Pandya KJ *et al.* (2005) Gabapentin for hot flashes in 420 women with breast cancer: a randomised double-blind placebo-controlled trial. *Lancet*. **366**: 818–824.
40 Cruz FM *et al.* (2012) Gabapentin for the prevention of chemotherapy- induced nausea and vomiting: a pilot study. *Supportive Care in Cancer*. **20**: 601–606.
41 Thompson DF and Brooks KG (2013) Gabapentin therapy of hiccups. *Annals of Pharmacotherapy*. **47**: 897–903.
42 Paisley S *et al.* (2002) Clinical effectiveness of oral treatments for spasticity in multiple sclerosis: a systematic review. *Multiple Sclerosis*. **8**: 319–329.
43 Cutter NC *et al.* (2000) Gabapentin effect on spasticity in multiple sclerosis: a placebo-controlled, randomized trial. *Archives of Physical Medicine and Rehabilitation*. **81**: 164–169.
44 Mackie S and Winkelman JW (2015) Long-term treatment of restless legs syndrome (RLS): an approach to management of worsening symptoms, loss of efficacy, and augmentation. *CNS Drugs*. **29**: 351–357.
45 Garcia-Borreguero D *et al.* (2012) European guidelines on management of restless legs syndrome: report of a joint task force by the European Federation of Neurological Societies, the European Neurological Society and the European Sleep Research Society. *European Journal of Neurology*. **19**: 1385–1396.
46 Hammond CJ *et al.* (2015) Anticonvulsants for the treatment of alcohol withdrawal syndrome and alcohol use disorders. *CNS Drugs*. **29**: 293–311.
47 PHE (2014) Advice for prescribers on the risk of the misuse of pregabalin and gabapentin. *Letter from Public Health England and NHS England*. www.gov.uk
48 Chiappini S and Schifano F (2016) A decade of gabapentinoid misuse: an analysis of the european medicines agency's 'Suspected Adverse Drug Reactions' database. *CNS Drugs*. **30**: 647–654.
49 Schjerning O *et al.* (2016) Abuse potential of pregabalin: a systematic review. *CNS Drugs*. **30**: 9–25.
50 Kogure T *et al.* (2017) Donepezil, an acetylcholinesterase inhibitor, can attenuate gabapentinoid-induced somnolence in patients with neuropathic pain: a retrospective chart review. *Journal of Pain and Palliative Care Pharmacotherpy*. **31**: 4–9.
51 Zaccara G *et al.* (2011) The adverse event profile of pregabalin: a systematic review and meta-analysis of randomized controlled trials. *Epilepsia*. **52**: 826–836.
52 Feldman AE and Gidal BE (2013) QTc prolongation by antiepileptic drugs and the risk of torsade de pointes in patients with epilepsy. *Epilepsy and Behavior*. **26**: 421–426.
53 MHRA Yellow card reports for gabapentin and pregabalin. *Drug Analysis Prints*. www.mhra.gov.uk/Safetyinformation (accessed May 2013).
54 Tremont-Lukats IW *et al.* (2000) Anticonvulsants for neuropathic pain syndromes: mechanisms of action and place in therapy. *Drugs*. **60**: 1029–1052.
55 Freynhagen R *et al.* (2005) Efficacy of pregabalin in neuropathic pain evaluated in a 12-week, randomised, double-blind, multicentre, placebo-controlled trial of flexible- and fixed-dose regimens. *Pain*. **115**: 254–263.
56 Gidal B *et al.* (1998) Gabapentin absorption: effect of mixing with foods of varying macronutrient composition. *Annals of Pharmacotherapy*. **32**: 405–409.

Updated September 2017

CARBAMAZEPINE

Class: Anti-epileptic (sodium channel blocker).

Indications: Focal seizures, trigeminal neuralgia, †neuropathic pain, mania.

Contra-indications: AV block, previous bone marrow depression, concurrent MAOI, hypersensitivity to TCAs (structurally related).

Pharmacology

Carbamazepine is a sodium channel blocker. These channels accumulate at sites of neuronal injury creating ectopic foci of action potential generation (see p.256). Additional actions of uncertain significance include potassium channel activation, L-type calcium-channel blockade, and antagonism of the NMDA-receptor-channel complex.[1]

Absorption is affected by formulation; slower rates reduce the incidence of undesirable CNS effects.[2] Carbamazepine is mainly metabolized by CYP3A4 to a pharmacologically active epoxide metabolite; this is subsequently inactivated to several renally excreted metabolites. The halflife decreases over the first 1–2 weeks as a result of hepatic enzyme auto-induction.

Carbamazepine is a first-line drug for focal seizures and trigeminal neuralgia. Because it requires slow titration and particular care with regard to drug interactions (see Table 1), its use in other neuropathic pains is limited to those failing to respond to authorized alternatives (see p.272). In painful diabetic neuropathy, trigeminal neuralgia and central post stroke pain, carbamazepine appears superior to placebo and comparable to antidepressants. However, RCTs were small, short (mostly <4 weeks) and used outcome measures of uncertain clinical significance.[3] Benefit is also reported for paroxysmal nausea associated with meningeal carcinomatosis[4] and pruritus associated with haematological malignancy.[5]

A polymorphism in the gene (SCN1A) encoding the sodium channel α-subunit has been linked to carbamazepine-resistant epilepsy.[6] Human leukocyte antigen (HLA) genes, known to influence susceptibility to various infections and auto-immune diseases, are closely associated with the risk of carbamazepine-induced skin reactions. In Han Chinese, HLA B*1502 was found in 100% of 44 individuals with Stevens-Johnson syndrome compared with 3% of unaffected carbamazepine-treated individuals.[7] The MHRA recommends testing HLA B*1502 status before carbamazepine is started in people of Han Chinese, Hong Kong Chinese or Thai origin. In Europeans, HLA-A*3101 increased the risk of less severe skin reactions from 5% to 26%.[8,9]

Bio-availability ≥85%.

Onset of action generally delayed by the need for slow titration, but anti-epileptic response is sometimes seen as early as 2 days.

Time to peak plasma concentration 4–8h (immediate-release tablets), 12–26h (m/r tablets), 0.5–3h (oral liquid).

Plasma halflife 36h initially, 8–24h after multiple dosing (hepatic auto-induction).

Duration of action No specific data.

Cautions

Renal and hepatic impairment (also see Chapter 17, p.681 and Chapter 18, p.703); cardiac disease; absence seizures (may worsen); previous skin reaction to other anti-epileptic drugs or TCAs. Mild skin reactions are common and transient; monitor closely and discontinue carbamazepine if reactions worsen, or if features of Stevens-Johnson syndrome or toxic epidermal necrolysis develop.

Agranulocytosis and aplastic anaemia affect about 5 and 2 patients/million/year respectively. Severe hepatic reactions are rare. Mild leukopenia, thrombocytopenia, or cholestatic abnormalities in LFTs should be monitored, and carbamazepine should be discontinued if severe or symptomatic derangement occurs.

Drug interactions

Carbamazepine is a hepatic enzyme inducer with numerous drug interactions (see Table 1).

Table 1 Clinically significant cytochrome P450 interactions with carbamazepine resulting in changed drug plasma concentrations

Carbamazepine[a] plasma concentration		*Drug plasma concentration*	
increased by	*decreased by*	*increased by carbamazepine*	*decreased by carbamazepine*
Antipsychotics[b]	Efavirenz	Phenytoin	Antipsychotics[b]
Antiretrovirals[b]	Phenobarbital[c]		Antiretrovirals[b]
Azole antifungals[b]	Phenytoin[c]		Azole antifungals[b]
Clarithromycin	Valproate[c]		Benzodiazepines[b]
Dextropropoxyphene			Calcium-channel blockers[b]
Diltiazem			Clozapine
Erythromycin			Corticosteroids[b]
Fluoxetine			Coumarin anticoagulants
Fluvoxamine			Ethosuximide
Haloperidol			Fentanyl
Isoniazid			Haloperidol
Lamotrigine			Indinavir
Valproate			Lamotrigine
Verapamil			Levothyroxine
			Methadone
			Oestrogens, progestogens
			Phenytoin
			Primidone
			SSRIs[b]
			TCAs[b]
			Tiagabine
			Topiramate
			Tramadol
			Valproate

a. or active metabolite

b. effect not seen with all drug class members

c. increase in active metabolite of carbamazepine.

Undesirable effects

Very common (>10%): dizziness, ataxia, drowsiness, fatigue, nausea, mild LFT derangement (see above), urticaria, leukopenia.

Common (<10%, >1%): headache, diplopia, blurred vision, oedema, dry mouth, thrombocytopenia, eosinophilia, hyponatraemia, rectal irritation (with suppositories).

Uncommon (<1%, >0.1%): include suicidal ideation 0.2% (1/500; advise patients to report mood or thought disturbance).

Rare (<0.1%): aseptic meningitis, movement disorders, neuroleptic (antipsychotic) malignant syndrome, arrhythmias and cardiac conduction disorders, pancreatitis, hepatitis, jaundice, renal failure, interstitial nephritis, a delayed-onset multi-organ vasculitic hypersensitivity disorder, severe skin reactions (see above).

Dose and use

MHRA advises that the products available in the UK may differ in bio-availability, and that to avoid changes in effectiveness or increased risk of undesirable effects, it is best to avoid switching between formulations (see also p.262).

Starting dose and titration rate will depend on seizure or pain severity. Undesirable effects are minimized by a low starting dose, slow upward titration, and the use of m/r products.

- check:
  - ▷ baseline FBC, U+E, LFTs, and repeat every 2–3 months
  - ▷ HLA B*1502 status in people of Han Chinese, Hong Kong Chinese or Thai origin[8]
- start with 50–100mg PO b.d. (use m/r product for doses ≥100mg)
- if necessary, increase in 50–100mg increments every 1–2 weeks
- in epilepsy, 90% require ≤800mg/24h[10]
- in neuropathic pain, participants in most RCTs received ≤600mg/24h[3]
- maximum daily dose 2g.

Suppositories are available for short-term use when the PO route is not possible, 100mg PO is approximately equal to 125mg PR, however they are very expensive.

Supply

Immediate-release products *(m/r products are generally preferred, see Dose and use)*
Carbamazepine (generic)
Tablets *(scored)* 100mg, 200mg, 400mg, 28 days @ 200mg b.d. = £2.50.
Oral suspension (sugar-free) 100mg/5mL, 28 days @ 200mg b.d. = £12.
Suppositories 125mg, pack of 5 = £120; 250mg, pack of 5 = £140.

Modified-release products

M/r carbamazepine tablets in the UK are scored to permit splitting into halves; however they should not be crushed or chewed, see Chapter 28, p.788.

Carbamazepine (generic)
Tablets m/r *(scored)* 200mg, 400mg, 28 days @ 200mg b.d. = £5.

1 Schmidt D and Elger CE (2004) What is the evidence that oxcarbazepine and carbamazepine are distinctly different antiepileptic drugs? *Epilepsy and Behaviour.* **5**: 627–635.
2 Tothfalusi L *et al.* (2008) Exposure-response analysis reveals that clinically important toxicity difference can exist between bioequivalent carbamazepine tablets. *British Journal of Clinical Pharmacology.* **65**: 110–122.
3 Wiffen PJ *et al.* (2014) Carbamazepine for chronic neuropathic pain and fibromyalgia in adults. *Cochrane Database of Systematic Reviews.* **4**: CD005451. www.thecochranelibrary.com
4 Strohscheer I and Borasio GD (2006) Carbamazepine-responsive paroxysmal nausea and vomiting in a patient with meningeal carcinomatosis. *Palliative Medicine.* **20**: 549–550.
5 Korfitis C and Trafalis DT (2008) Carbamazepine can be effective in alleviating tormenting pruritus in patients with hematologic malignancy. *Journal of Pain and Symptom Management.* **35**: 571–572.
6 Abe T *et al.* (2008) Association between SCN1A polymorphism and carbamazepine-resistant epilepsy. *British Journal of Clinical Pharmacology.* **66**: 304–307.
7 Chung WH *et al.* (2004) Medical genetics: a marker for Stevens-Johnson syndrome. *Nature.* **428**: 486.
8 MHRA (2008) Carbamazepine: genetic testing in some Asian populations. *Drug Safety Update.* www.gov.uk/drug-safety-update
9 MHRA (2012) Carbamazepine, oxcarbazepine and eslicarbazepine: potential risk of serious skin reactions associated with the HLA-A*3101 allele. *Drug Safety Update.* www.gov.uk/drug-safety-update
10 Kwan P and Brodie MJ (2001) Effectiveness of first antiepileptic drug. *Epilepsia.* **42**: 1255–1260.

Updated September 2017

OXCARBAZEPINE

Class: Anti-epileptic (sodium channel blocker).

Indications: Focal seizures, †neuropathic pain.

Pharmacology

Oxcarbazepine is structurally related to **carbamazepine**. Both act through sodium channel blockade (see p.278 and p.256) but differ in tolerability and propensity for drug interactions.

Additional actions of uncertain significance include potassium channel activation, N, P and R-type calcium channel blockade and antagonism of the NMDA-receptor-channel complex.[1]

Oxcarbazepine is a pro-drug which is activated by reduction to its monohydroxy derivative. This is inactivated by glucuronidation and oxidation, and the metabolites are renally excreted.[2] Oxcarbazepine has fewer drug interactions than **carbamazepine** because it is a weaker inducer of hepatic enzymes.

In RCTs for epilepsy, oxcarbazepine causes less drowsiness, fewer skin reactions, but more nausea, than **carbamazepine**; overall, efficacy and rates of withdrawal due to undesirable effects are similar.[3,4]

In RCTs for neuropathic pain (predominantly diabetic), two found benefit (NNT=6.6 for 50% reduction in pain severity; n=229); one was equivocal (NNT=12 for global assessment of improvement; n=247); and one found no benefit (n=141).[5,6] Certain clinical findings (allodynia, hyperalgesia, normal temperature sensation) may predict a greater response (NNT 3.9 versus 13).[6] Oxcarbazepine is also reported to improve trigeminal neuralgia unresponsive to **carbamazepine**, and post-herpetic neuralgia unresponsive to **carbamazepine** + **gabapentin**.[7,8]

Bio-availability ≥95%.

Onset of action pain improved ≤1 week, maximum response ≤4 weeks.

Time to peak plasma concentration 1–3h.

Plasma halflife 1–5h; 7–20h monohydroxy derivative.

Duration of action no specific data.

Cautions

Hepatic impairment (reduced bio-transformation to the active metabolite reducing effect, see Chapter 18, p.714). Renal impairment (see Dose and use and also Chapter 17, p.688); HLA predisposition or previous hypersensitivity to **carbamazepine** (25–30% cross-reactivity, also see p.278), predisposition to hyponatraemia, cardiac insufficiency (fluid retention), abnormal cardiac conduction (arrhythmias and AV block occur rarely).

Drug interactions

Oxcarbazepine can induce CYP3A4 and inhibit CYP2C19 but not often to a clinically significant extent. Oral hormonal contraception may become ineffective. **Lamotrigine** and **phenytoin** may require dose adjustment.

Undesirable effects

Very common (>10%): drowsiness, dizziness, fatigue, headache, diplopia, nausea and vomiting.

Common (<10%, >1%): confusion, agitation, amnesia, altered mood, vertigo, ataxia, tremor, nystagmus, reduced attention, diarrhoea, constipation, abdominal pain, rash, alopecia, acne, asymptomatic hyponatraemia.

Uncommon (<1%, >0.1%): include suicidal ideation 0.2% (1/500; advise patients to report mood or thought disturbance).

Rare (<0.1%): AV block, arrhythmia, pancreatitis, hepatitis, multi-organ hypersensitivity, systemic lupus erythematosus, angioedema, Stevens-Johnson syndrome, toxic epidermal necrolysis, bone marrow depression.

Dose and use

MHRA advises that the products available in the UK may differ in bio-availability, and that to avoid changes in effectiveness or increased risk of undesirable effects, it is best to avoid switching between formulations (see also p.262).

Many palliative care patients have risk factors for hyponatraemia; monitor sodium at baseline, after 2 weeks, then monthly for 3 months. Doses lower than recommended by the manufacturer have been proposed:[2]

- start with 150mg b.d. (75mg b.d. in elderly, frail or in severe renal impairment (creatinine clearance ≤30mL/min))
- increase the dose in 75–150mg increments weekly
- if necessary, increase to a maximum of 1,200mg b.d.

Supply

Oxcarbazepine (generic)
Tablets 150mg, 300mg, 600mg, 28 days @ 300mg b.d. = £8.

Trileptal® (Novartis)
Tablets *(scored)* 150mg, 300mg, 600mg, 28 days @ 300mg b.d. = £27.
Oral suspension (sugar-free) 300mg/5mL, 28 days @ 300mg b.d. = £55; *may contain propylene glycol.*

1 Schmidt D and Elger CE (2004) What is the evidence that oxcarbazepine and carbamazepine are distinctly different antiepileptic drugs? *Epilepsy and Behaviour.* **5**: 627–635.
2 May TW *et al.* (2003) Clinical pharmacokinetics of oxcarbazepine. *Clinical Pharmacokinetics.* **42**: 1023–1042.
3 Marson AG *et al.* (2007) The SANAD study of effectiveness of carbamazepine, gabapentin, lamotrigine, oxcarbazepine, or topiramate for treatment of partial epilepsy: an unblinded randomised controlled trial. *Lancet.* **369**: 1000–1015.
4 Koch MW and Polman SK (2009) Oxcarbazepine versus carbamazepine monotherapy for partial onset seizures. *Cochrane Database of Systematic Reviews.* **4**: CD006453. www.thecochranelibrary.com
5 Zhou M *et al.* (2013) Oxcarbazepine for neuropathic pain. *Cochrane Database of Systematic Reviews.* **3**: CD007963. www.thecochranelibrary.com
6 Demant DT *et al.* (2014) The effect of oxcarbazepine in peripheral neuropathic pain depends on pain phenotype: a randomised, double-blind, placebo-controlled phenotype-stratified study. *Pain.* **155**: 2263–2273.
7 Gomez-Arguelles JM *et al.* (2008) Oxcarbazepine monotherapy in carbamazepine-unresponsive trigeminal neuralgia. *Journal of Clinical Neuroscience.* **15**: 516–519.
8 Criscuolo S *et al.* (2005) Oxcarbazepine monotherapy in postherpetic neuralgia unresponsive to carbamazepine and gabapentin. *Acta Neurologica Scandinavica.* **111**: 229–232.

Updated September 2017

VALPROATE

Class: Anti-epileptic (multimodal action).

Indications: Epilepsy (see SPC for details), mania associated with bipolar disorder, †neuropathic pain, †migraine prophylaxis, †agitated delirium.

Contra-indications: Manufacturer advises against use in 'active hepatic disease' or past or family history of severe hepatic impairment (particularly drug-related). See Chapter 18, p.703.

Pharmacology

Valproate is a sodium channel blocker, an NMDA-receptor-channel blocker, it increases potassium conductance and the secondary messenger PIP_3, and alters glutamate, GABA, dopamine and serotonin transmission.[1–3] The relative significance of these actions in epilepsy is unclear. Actions of possible relevance in neuropathic pain also include correcting the down-regulation of glutamate re-uptake transporters[4,5] and T-type calcium channel blockade;[6] these channels may be involved in regulating pain excitation thresholds in a 'T-rich' subset of peripheral nociceptors.[7,8]

Valproate is well absorbed orally. It is ≥90% plasma protein-bound, and crosses the blood-brain barrier and neuronal membranes via active transporters. It is metabolized by direct microsomal UDP-mediated glucuronidation (50%), mitochondrial β-oxidation (40%) and cytochrome P450-mediated oxidation (10%: CYP2A6, 2B6, 2C9 and 2C19). Some metabolites are active, but their cerebral concentrations are too low to contribute to valproate's overall effect. Metabolites may be responsible for idiosyncratic hepatic toxicity. CYP enzyme inducers, inhibitors and polymorphisms affect the proportion of cytochrome P450 metabolites, perhaps altering this risk.[9,10]

Compared with immediate-release and enteric-coated preparations, m/r preparations halve the initial peak plasma level without reducing overall bio-availability. Further, plasma levels at 24h are 50% higher and thus peak to trough variability is significantly decreased.[11,12]

Valproate remains a first-line treatment for generalized seizures, its efficacy and tolerability comparing favourably to those of newer anti-epileptics.[13,14] It is effective for status epilepticus.[15,16]

Benefit has been reported for cancer-related neuropathic pain.[17,18] However, because results of RCTs in non-cancer pain are mixed, international guidelines do not recommend its use.[19–21]

Valproate was well tolerated in all 6 studies, with fewer patients (≤5%) discontinuing because of undesirable effects compared with **gabapentin** (10%) and **pregabalin** (20–30%) in similar populations (see p.262). Valproate is used in some centres if **gabapentin** or **pregabalin** are insufficient, particularly when a smaller tablet load, once daily regimen, or CSCI is required.

Two case series reported benefit with valproate for agitated delirium refractory to antipsychotics and/or benzodiazepines.[22,23]

Valproate exhibits anti-cancer properties in pre-clinical studies. It inhibits histone deacetylase, an enzyme involved in aberrant gene expression.[24,25] Post-hoc analysis of an RCT revealed a possible survival advantage in glioma patients treated with valproate.[26]

Bio-availability 95% PO.

Onset of action often within 24h (for neuropathic pain).[17]

Time to peak plasma concentration 1–2h (3–5h for e/c, 5–10h for m/r).

Plasma halflife 9–18h (5–12h with concurrent enzyme inducers).

Duration of action 12–24h.[10]

4

Cautions

Liver disease (see Table 1 and Chapter 18, p.714);[27,28] renal impairment (dose reduction may be required; see Chapter 17, p.688); females of child-bearing age (teratogenicity; seek specialist advice).

Harmless ketone metabolites, detected by bedside urinalysis, may cause diagnostic confusion in diabetic patients.

Drug Interactions

The clearance of valproate is increased by hepatic enzyme inducers such as **carbamazepine**, **phenytoin**, **phenobarbital** and **rifampicin**.[10] Its clearance is inhibited by **isoniazid**.

Valproate inhibits the metabolism of **carbamazepine**'s active epoxide metabolite (increasing undesirable effects), **ethosuximide**, **phenytoin**, **phenobarbital**, **lamotrigine** and some antiretrovirals.

Concurrent administration with carbapenem antibacterials can decrease the plasma concentration of valproate dramatically by 85–90% through the combined impact on intestinal absorption, distribution and metabolism, with consequential loss of therapeutic effect.[29] Because increasing the dose may not overcome this drug–drug interaction, alternative antibacterials should be considered for patients taking valproate.

Undesirable effects

Common problems include gastric intolerance (particularly nausea; reduced by e/c formulations or taking with food), hair loss (transient; dose-related), drowsiness and postural tremor (a rarer flapping tremor is seen with hyperammonaemia), although the incidence varies markedly between individual studies.

Hyperammonaemic encephalopathy and hepatic failure (Table 1), teratogenicity and pancreatitis are the most important idiosyncratic effects.[10,30] Other rare effects include severe skin reactions (e.g. Stevens-Johnson syndrome), reversible parkinsonism and dementia. Whether serious idiosyncratic reactions are any less common with newer anti-epileptics is unknown.

Table 1 Valproate-induced encephalopathy.[27,28,31–33]

	Hyperammonaemic encephalopathy	*Hepatic failure ± encephalopathy*
Prevalence	≤1%	≤1/3,000
Clinical features	Nausea and vomiting Drowsiness → coma Fatigue Ataxia	Nausea and vomiting Drowsiness → coma Fatigue Jaundice
Risk factors	Concurrent hepatic enzyme inducers, topiramate or antipsychotics	Pre-existing liver disease and/or deranged LFTs
Investigation findings	↑Blood ammonia	Deranged LFTs, coagulopathy

continued

Table 1 Continued

	Hyperammonaemic encephalopathy	*Hepatic failure ± encephalopathy*
Management	*Asymptomatic mild hyperammonaemia* is common, does not require discontinuation but monitor closely *Mild symptoms*: reduce dose and monitor closely *Severe or worsening symptoms*: stop valproate and seek specialist advice	*Asymptomatic mildly deranged LFTs* with normal coagulation does not require discontinuation but monitor closely *Coagulopathy, severely deranged LFTs and/or symptoms* in the absence of an alternative explanation: stop valproate and seek specialist advice

Dose and use

The manufacturer recommends that LFTs, prothrombin time (PT) and FBC be checked before and during the first 6 months of treatment, although this may not improve the early detection of hepatotoxicity.

Epilepsy

MHRA advises that the products available in the UK may differ in bio-availability, and that to avoid changes in effectiveness or increased risk of undesirable effects, it is best to avoid switching between formulations (see also p.262).

Valproate is a commonly used first or second-line treatment in palliative care. In the last days of life, **midazolam** is generally preferred (see Anti-epileptics, Box B, p.265):

- start with valproate 150–200mg m/r PO b.d.
- if necessary, increase by 150–200mg b.d. every 3 days
- approximately 90% require ≤1.5g/24h[34]
- maximum recommended dose 2.5g/24h.

When the PO route cannot be used, valproate can be given IV:

- if already on PO treatment, give the same daily dose by continuous or intermittent (over 3–5min) infusions
- if starting *de novo*, give 500–800mg (maximum 10mg/kg), followed by continuous or intermittent infusions of ≤2.5g/24h.

Higher doses have been used for status epilepticus.[15]
For unauthorized SC use, see below.

Neuropathic pain

Valproate is *not* a first-line choice (see text):

- start with valproate 150–200mg m/r PO at bedtime
- if necessary, increase by 150–200mg/24h every 2–3 days; give as a b.d. dose
- maximum used in 'positive' RCTs was ≤1.2g/24h;[20] higher doses are reported in case series (<2g/24h).[17,18]

Mania

Not all marketed products are authorized for mania, but they appear to be clinically equivalent:

- start with valproate 300mg m/r PO b.d.
- increase as rapidly as possible to achieve the optimal response, to a maximum of 60mg/kg/24h
- most patients respond to doses <2g/24h.[35,36]

Agitated delirium

Valproate is *not* a first-line choice (see p.176). Dose as for mania. In two case series, the median effective dose was 1,000 and 1,800mg/24h (range 500–2,000mg/24h).[22,23]

Subcutaneous use

Valproate has been used successfully †CSCI, using a PO:SC dose ratio of 1:1.[37,38] A total of 10 patients (9 with seizures, one with neuropathic pain) received a median dose of 1,000mg/24h

CSCI (range 400–1,800mg). Duration of use ranged 2–39 days, with only one patient experiencing mild erythema at the infusion site. In one report, the valproate was diluted with 30mL of WFI.

Alternative SC/CSCI anti-epileptics include **lacosamide**,[39] **levetiracetam** (p.184), **midazolam** (p.149) and **phenobarbital** (p.289).

CSCI compatibility with other drugs: Because there are no reports of combined use, valproate should be administered via a separate syringe driver (see Chapter 29, p.822).

Supply

Valproate is the UK generic term for valproic acid and its salts and esters, including sodium valproate. The pharmacokinetics, efficacy, and tolerability of valproic acid and sodium valproate are similar; sodium valproate 579mg is equivalent to valproic acid 500mg,[40] and the manufacturer of valproic acid (Convulex®) advises that it is equipotent with products containing sodium valproate.

Immediate-release oral products (*m/r products are generally preferred,* see Pharmacology)
Sodium valproate (generic)
Tablets e/c 200mg, 500mg, 28 days @ 200mg b.d. = £2.50.
Oral solution 200mg/5mL, 28 days @ 200mg b.d. = £4.75.

Epilim® (Sanofi)
Tablets crushable *(scored)* 100mg, 28 days @ 200mg b.d. = £6.50.
Tablets e/c 200mg, 500mg, 28 days @ 200mg b.d. = £4.25.
Oral solution (sugar-free) 200mg/5mL, 28 days @ 200mg b.d. = £7.50.
Oral syrup 200mg/5mL, 28 days @ 200mg b.d. = £9.

Modified-release oral products
Epilim Chrono® (Sanofi)
Tablets m/r (*sodium valproate and valproic acid*) equivalent to sodium valproate 200mg, 300mg, 500mg, 28 days @ 200mg b.d. = £6.50.
Oral granules m/r Epilim Chronosphere® (*sodium valproate and valproic acid*) equivalent to sodium valproate 50mg, 100mg, 250mg, 500mg, 750mg, 1g/sachet, 28 days @ 500mg at bedtime = £28; *the granules may be mixed with soft food or a drink which is cold or at room temperature, and swallowed immediately without chewing.*

Episenta® (Desitin)
Capsules enclosing m/r granules sodium valproate 150mg, 300mg, 28 days @ 150mg b.d. = £4.
Oral granules m/r sodium valproate 500mg, 1g/sachet, 28 days @ 500mg at bedtime = £6.
The granules or contents of the capsules may be mixed with cold food or drink, and swallowed immediately without chewing.

Epival CR® (Chanelle Medical)
Tablets m/r *(scored)* 300mg, 500mg, 28 days @ 150mg b.d. = £3.50; *the tablets may be halved but not crushed or chewed.*

Parenteral products
Sodium valproate (generic)
Injection 100mg/mL, 3mL amp = £7, 4mL amp = £11.50.
Injection (powder for reconstitution) 400mg vial = £12; supplied with a 4mL amp of WFI for reconstitution.

Valproic acid
Convulex® (Pharmacia)
Capsules e/c 150mg, 300mg, 500mg, 28 days @ 150mg b.d. = £2.

Depakote® (Sanofi)
Tablets e/c (semisodium valproate) equivalent to valproic acid 250mg, 500mg, 28 days @ 250mg t.d.s. = £16; *semisodium valproate is a mixture of equimolar amounts of valproic acid and sodium valproate, and is authorized for mania.*

1 Loscher W (2002) Basic pharmacology of valproate: a review after 35 years of clinical use for the treatment of epilepsy. *CNS Drugs*. **16**: 669–694.
2 Chang P *et al.* (2014) Seizure-induced reduction in PIP3 levels contributes to seizure-activity and is rescued by valproic acid. *Neurobiology of Disease*. **62**: 296–306.
3 Kay HY *et al.* (2015) M-current preservation contributes to anticonvulsant effects of valproic acid. *Journal of Clinical Investigation*. **125**: 3904–3914.
4 Hobo (2012) Valproate upregulates glutamate transporters in rat spinal cord after peripheral nerve injury. *Journal of Pain*. **13 (Suppl 1)**: s62.
5 Inquimbert P *et al.* (2012) Peripheral nerve injury produces a sustained shift in the balance between glutamate release and uptake in the dorsal horn of the spinal cord. *Pain*. **153**: 2422–2431.
6 Takahashi T *et al.* (2010) Upregulation of Ca(v)3.2 T-type calcium channels targeted by endogenous hydrogen sulfide contributes to maintenance of neuropathic pain. *Pain*. **150**: 183–191.
7 Jevtovic-Todorovic V *et al.* (2006) The role of peripheral T-type calcium channels in pain transmission. *Cell Calcium*. **40**: 197–203.
8 Francois A *et al.* (2013) State-dependent properties of a new T-type calcium channel blocker enhance Ca(V)3.2 selectivity and support analgesic effects. *Pain*. **154**: 283–293.
9 Mann MW and Pons G (2007) Various pharmacogenetic aspects of antiepileptic drug therapy: a review. *CNS Drugs*. **21**: 143–164.
10 Perucca E (2002) Pharmacological and therapeutic properties of valproate: a summary after 35 years of clinical experience. *CNS Drugs*. **16**: 695–714.
11 Wangemann M *et al.* (1999) Pharmacokinetic characteristics of a new multiple unit sustained release formulation of sodium valproate. *International Journal of Clinical Pharmacology and Therapeutics*. **37**: 100–108.
12 Genton P (2005) Progress in pharmaceutical development presentation with improved pharmacokinetics: a new formulation for valproate. *Acta Neurologica Scandinavica Supplementum*. **182**: 26–32.
13 Marson AG *et al.* (2007) The SANAD study of effectiveness of valproate, lamotrigine, or topiramate for generalised and unclassifiable epilepsy: an unblinded randomised controlled trial. *Lancet*. **369**: 1016–1026.
14 Karceski S *et al.* (2005) Treatment of epilepsy in adults: expert opinion. *Epilepsy and Behavior*. **7 (Suppl 1)**: S1–64.
15 Trinka E *et al.* (2014) Efficacy and safety of intravenous valproate for status epilepticus: a systematic review. *CNS Drugs*. **28**: 623–639.
16 Yasiry Z and Shorvon SD (2014) The relative effectiveness of five antiepileptic drugs in treatment of benzodiazepine-resistant convulsive status epilepticus: a meta-analysis of published studies. *Seizure*. **23**: 167–174.
17 Snare AJ (1993) Sodium Valproate. Retrospective analysis of neuropathic pain control in patients with advanced cancer. *Journal of Pharmacy Technology*. **9**: 114–117.
18 Hardy J *et al.* (2001) A phase II study to establish the efficacy and toxicity of sodium valproate in patients with cancer-related neuropathic pain. *Journal of Pain and Symptom Management*. **21**: 204–209.
19 Attal N *et al.* (2010) EFNS guidelines on the pharmacological treatment of neuropathic pain: 2010 revision. *European Journal of Neurology*. **17**: e1113–1188.
20 Finnerup NB *et al.* (2016) Pharmacotherapy for neuropathic pain in adults: a systematic review and meta-analysis. *Lancet Neurology*. **14**: 162–173.
21 Gill D *et al.* (2011) Valproic acid and sodium valproate for neuropathic pain and fibromyalgia in adults. *Cochrane Database of Systematic Reviews*. **10**: CD009183. www.thecochranelibrary.com
22 Bourgeois JA *et al.* (2005) Adjunctive valproic acid for delirium and/or agitation on a consultation-liaison service: a report of six cases. *Journal of Neuropsychiatry and Clinical Neurosciences*. **17**: 232–238.
23 Gagnon DJ *et al.* (2017) Valproate for agitation in critically ill patients: a retrospective study. *Journal of Critical Care*. **37**: 119–125.
24 Gavrilov V *et al.* (2014) Sodium valproate, a histone deacetylase inhibitor, enhances the efficacy of vinorelbine-cisplatin-based chemoradiation in non-small cell lung cancer cells. *Anticancer Research*. **34**: 6565–6572.
25 Jafary H *et al.* (2014) The enhanced apoptosis and antiproliferative response to combined treatment with valproate and nicotinamide in MCF-7 breast cancer cells. *Tumour Biology*. **35**: 2701–2710.
26 Perucca E (2013) Optimizing antiepileptic drug treatment in tumoral epilepsy. *Epilepsia*. **54 (Suppl 9)**: 97–104.
27 Konig SA *et al.* (1994) Severe hepatotoxicity during valproate therapy: an update and report of eight new fatalities. *Epilepsia*. **35**: 1005–1015.
28 Koenig SA *et al.* (2006) Valproic acid-induced hepatopathy: nine new fatalities in Germany from 1994 to 2003. *Epilepsia*. **47**: 2027–2031.
29 Mancl EE and Gidal BE (2009) The effect of carbapenem antibiotics on plasma concentrations of valproic acid. *Annals of Pharmacotherapy*. **43**: 2082–2087.
30 French JA (2007) First-choice drug for newly diagnosed epilepsy. *Lancet*. **369**: 970–971.
31 Chopra A *et al.* (2012) Valproate-induced hyperammonemic encephalopathy: an update on risk factors, clinical correlates and management. *General Hospital Psychiatry*. **34**: 290–298.
32 Yamamoto Y *et al.* (2012) Risk factors for hyperammonemia associated with valproic acid therapy in adult epilepsy patients. *Epilepsy Research*. **101**: 202–209.
33 Tseng YL *et al.* (2014) Risk factors of hyperammonemia in patients with epilepsy under valproic acid therapy. *Medicine*. **93**: e66.
34 Kwan P and Brodie MJ (2001) Effectiveness of first antiepileptic drug. *Epilepsia*. **42**: 1255–1260.
35 Keck PE, Jr. *et al.* (1993) Valproate oral loading in the treatment of acute mania. *Journal of Clinical Psychiatry*. **54**: 305–308.
36 Macritchie K *et al.* (2003) Valproate for acute mood episodes in bipolar disorder. *Cochrane Database of Systematic Reviews*. **1**: CD004052. www.thecochranelibrary.com
37 O'Connor MN (2014) The use of sodium valproate in a continuous infusion (CSCI) as an anticonvulsant at the end of life - a case series. *Palliative Medicine*. **28**: 740–741.
38 McKenna M (2013) Personal communication.
39 Remi C *et al.* (2016) Subcutaneous use of lacosamide. *Journal of Pain Symptom Management*. **51**: e2–4.
40 Fisher (2003) Sodium valproate or valproate semisodium: is there a difference in the treatment of bipolar disorder? *Psychiatric Bulletin*. **27**: 446–448.

Updated September 2017

LEVETIRACETAM

Class: Anti-epileptic (SV2A ligand).

Indications: Focal seizures, adjunctive therapy of generalized myoclonic and tonic-clonic seizures, †monotherapy of generalized seizures (see text).

Pharmacology

Levetiracetam binds to synaptic vesicle protein SV2A, interfering with the release of the neurotransmitter stored within the vesicle. Because it gains access after the initial release, as the vesicles are recycled in preparation for repeated release, it selectively inhibits rapidly firing neurons.[1]

Food affects the rate but not the extent of its absorption. It does not bind to plasma proteins. It readily crosses the blood-brain barrier and its CSF halflife is 3 times longer than that for plasma.[2] A third is metabolized predominantly by non-hepatic hydrolysis; the remainder is excreted by the kidneys unchanged.

Levetiracetam is effective for a broad range of seizure types. Its efficacy and tolerability compare favourably to other anti-epileptic drugs in both cancer-related and non-cancer-related seizures.[3–6] It is commonly used first- or second-line (see p.264), particularly when the seizure type is unclear (also see **Valproate**, p.282) or when other anti-epileptics are contra-indicated because of co-morbidities.[7] Prophylactic levetiracetam is more effective than **phenytoin** at reducing the incidence of seizures following craniotomy (0% vs. 16%).[8]

Levetiracetam is *not* effective for neuropathic pain.[9] Benefit for bipolar disorder and hot flushes is reported.[3,10,11]

Bio-availability ≥95% PO.
Onset of action anti-epileptic effect generally evident <3 days of starting treatment.
Time to peak plasma concentration 1–2h.
Plasma halflife 6–8h.
Duration of action 24h.

Cautions

Renal impairment (see Dose and use and also Chapter 17, p.688); look for secondary renal impairment in those with hepatic impairment.

Drug interactions

Although the manufacturer advises caution when **carbamazepine** or **phenytoin** are used in combination with levetiracetam, a clinically significant interaction is unlikely.[12]

Undesirable effects

Very common (>10%): fatigue, drowsiness.
Common (<10%, >1%): ataxia, hyperkinesis, tremor, dizziness, headache, diplopia, blurred vision, amnesia, abnormal thinking, attention disturbance, behavioural disturbances (emotional lability, irritability, agitation, hostility/aggression, personality disorders), depression, insomnia, anorexia, abdominal pain, diarrhoea, dyspepsia, nausea, vomiting, myalgia, rash, pruritus, thrombocytopenia.

Behavioural disturbances occur in 3–4% of patients with epilepsy but only 0.5% of those being treated for other conditions. Risk factors include a history of aggression or psychiatric disturbance.[13,14]
Uncommon (<1%, >0.1%): include suicidal ideation 0.2% (1/500; advise patients to report mood or thought disturbance).
Rare (<0.1%): psychosis, pancreatitis, hepatic failure, bone marrow suppression, hyponatraemia.

Dose and use

In epilepsy, the PO and IV dose are identical:

- start with 250–500mg b.d.
- if starting with 250mg b.d., increase automatically after 2 weeks to 500mg b.d. (the minimum effective dose in most people)
- if necessary, increase by 250–500mg b.d. every 2 weeks
- maximum dose 1.5g b.d.

For IV use, dilute the dose in ≥100mL 0.9% saline and infuse over 15min.

Subcutaneous administration

Levetiracetam can be given by †CSCI using a PO:SC dose ratio of 1:1, diluted with either WFI or sodium chloride 0.9% when necessary.[15–18]

Levetiracetam can also be given †SC b.d., diluted in 100mL sodium chloride 0.9% and infused over 30min.[19]

Alternative SC/CSCI anti-epileptics include **lacosamide**,[20] **midazolam** (p.158), **phenobarbital** (p.289) and **valproate** (p.282).

CSCI compatibility with other drugs: limited clinical experience suggests that levetiracetam is compatible with **haloperidol**, **hyoscine** ***butylbromide***, **levomepromazine**, **methadone**, **metoclopramide**, **midazolam**, **morphine sulfate**, **oxycodone** and **ranitidine**, using sodium chloride 0.9% as diluent.[21–23] (Also see Chapter 29, p.822.)

Renal impairment

Because levetiracetam is largely excreted unchanged by the kidneys, the dose should be reduced in patients with renal impairment (Table 1).

Table 1 Dose adjustment for levetiracetam in renal impairment[a]

Creatinine clearance (mL/min/1.73m²)[b]	*Usual maintenance dose (mg)*
>80	500–1,500 b.d.
50–79	500–1,000 b.d.
30–49	250–750 b.d.
<30	250–500 b.d.

a. for patients weighing <50kg, dose on a mg/kg basis, see the SPC

b. based on the Cockroft-Gault formula adjusted for body surface area (see Chapter 17, p.683).

If on peritoneal dialysis or haemodialysis:

- start with 750mg loading dose followed by 500mg–1,000mg *once daily* PO/IV
- consider giving a 250–500mg supplementary dose immediately after each haemodialysis session or timing the daily dose after the dialysis session.

Hepatic impairment

Because metabolism is non-hepatic and the drug is not protein-bound, there is generally no need to reduce the dose in hepatic impairment. However, renal impairment is a common concomitant of severe hepatic impairment, and the dose should be reduced if the creatinine clearance is decreased (Table 1 above).

Stopping levetiracetam

Reduce by a maximum of 500mg b.d. every 2–4 weeks to avoid rebound seizures.

Supply

Levetiracetam (generic)

Tablets 250mg, 500mg, 750mg, 1g, 28 days @ 750mg b.d. = £4.

Granules 250mg, 500mg and 1g sachet, 28 days @ 750mg b.d. = £62.

Oral solution (sugar-free) 100mg/mL, 28 days @ 750mg = £7.50.

Injection (concentrate for dilution and use as an intravenous infusion) 100mg/mL, 5mL vial = £13.

1 Klitgaard H *et al.* (2016) Brivaracetam: rationale for discovery and preclinical profile of a selective SV2A ligand for epilepsy treatment. *Epilepsia*. **57**: 538–548.

2 Patsalos PN and Patsalos PN (2004) Clinical pharmacokinetics of levetiracetam. *Clinical Pharmacokinetics*. **43**: 707–724.

3 Zaccara G *et al.* (2006) Comparison of the efficacy and tolerability of new antiepileptic drugs: what can we learn from long-term studies? *Acta Neurologica Scandinavica*. **114**: 157–168.

4 Lim DA *et al.* (2009) Safety and feasibility of switching from phenytoin to levetiracetam monotherapy for glioma-related seizure control following craniotomy: a randomized phase II pilot study. *Journal of Neuro-oncology*. **93**: 349–354.

5 Rossetti AO *et al.* (2014) Levetiracetam and pregabalin for antiepileptic monotherapy in patients with primary brain tumors. A phase II randomized study. *Neuro-oncology*. **16**: 584–588.
6 Werhahn KJ *et al.* (2015) A randomized, double-blind comparison of antiepileptic drug treatment in the elderly with new-onset focal epilepsy. *Epilepsia*. **56**: 450–459.
7 Karceski S *et al.* (2005) Treatment of epilepsy in adults: expert opinion. *Epilepsy and Behavior*. **7 (Suppl 1)**: S1–64.
8 Fuller KL *et al.* (2013) Tolerability, safety, and side effects of levetiracetam versus phenytoin in intravenous and total prophylactic regimen among craniotomy patients: a prospective randomized study. *Epilepsia*. **54**: 45–57.
9 Wiffen PJ *et al.* (2014) Levetiracetam for neuropathic pain in adults. *Cochrane Database of Systematic Reviews*. **7**: CD010943. www.thecochranelibrary.com
10 Dunteman ED (2005) Levetiracetam as an adjunctive analgesic in neoplastic plexopathies: case series and commentary. *Journal of Pain and Palliative Care Pharmacotherapy*. **19**: 35–43.
11 Thompson S *et al.* (2008) Levetiracetam for the treatment of hot flashes: a phase II study. *Supportive Care in Cancer*. **16**: 75–82.
12 Baxter K and Preston CL. *Stockley's Drug Interactions*. London: Pharmaceutical Press www.medicinescomplete.com (accessed April 2017).
13 Dinkelacker V *et al.* (2003) Aggressive behavior of epilepsy patients in the course of levetiracetam add-on therapy: report of 33 mild to severe cases. *Epilepsy Behaviour*. **4**: 537–547.
14 Cramer JA *et al.* (2003) A systematic review of the behavioral effects of levetiracetam in adults with epilepsy, cognitive disorders, or an anxiety disorder during clinical trials. *Epilepsy Behaviour*. **4**: 124–132.
15 Remi C *et al.* (2014) Continuous subcutaneous use of levetiracetam: a retrospective review of tolerability and clinical effects. *Journal of Pain and Palliative Care Pharmacotherpy*. **28**: 371–377.
16 Sutherland AE *et al.* (2017) Subcutaneous levetiracetam for the management of seizures at the end of life. *British Medical Journal Supportive & Palliative Care*. [Epub ahead of print].
17 Ryan S (2016) The use of additional antiepileptic drugs with subcutaneous levetiracetam for the management of seizures at the end of life: a case series. *Palliative Medicine* **30**: NP262.
18 Wells GH *et al.* (2016) Continuous subcutaneous levetiracetam in the management of seizures at the end of life: a case report. *Age and Ageing*. **45**: 321–322.
19 Lopez-Saca JM *et al.* (2013) Repeated use of subcutaneous levetiracetam in a palliative care patient. *Journal of Pain and Symptom Management*. **45**: e7–8.
20 Remi C *et al.* (2016) Subcutaneous use of lacosamide. *Journal of Pain Symptom Management*. **51**: e2–4.
21 Munich (2017) Munich University syring driver compatability database. Available from: www.pall-iv.de/
22 EMH (2017) Earl Mountbatten Hospice syringe driver compatability guidelines. Available from: www.iwhospice.org/
23 Murray-Brown FL and Stewart A (2016) Remember Keppra: seizure control with subcutaneous levetiracetam infusion. *BMJ Supportive and Palliative Care*. **6**: 12–13.

Updated September 2017

*PHENOBARBITAL

Class: Anti-epileptic (GABAmimetic).

Indications: Epilepsy (except absence seizures), status epilepticus, †terminal agitation, †alcohol withdrawal.

Contra-indications: Unless in the imminently dying: severe renal or hepatic impairment (see Chapter 17, p.681 and Chapter 18, p.703).

Pharmacology

Phenobarbital enhances the post-synaptic inhibitory action of GABA by prolonging the opening of the chloride channel in the GABA receptor-channel complex (see Anti-epileptics, Figure 1, p.258).[1] Phenobarbital is also an AMPA-glutamate receptor antagonist. These actions depress CNS activity, and high doses result in general anaesthesia.

There is considerable interindividual variation in the pharmacokinetics of phenobarbital. Peak CNS concentrations occur some 15–20min after peak plasma concentrations. About 25% is excreted unchanged by the kidney; the rest is converted in the liver, mainly to inactive oxidative metabolites via several enzymes including CYP2C9. Phenobarbital is a strong inducer of CYP3A and glucuronidation, thus reducing plasma concentrations of many concurrently administered drugs.[1,2]

Phenobarbital's efficacy in epilepsy is comparable to alternatives but concerns about its cognitive and behavioural effects have led to a decline in its use, other than for status epilepticus (see p.256).[1]

Phenobarbital is used at some centres for terminal agitation which fails to respond to the combined use of **midazolam** and an antipsychotic (see p.156).

Bio-availability >90% PO and PR.[2,3]

Onset of action 5min IV, maximum effect achieved within 30min, onset after SC or IM administration is slightly slower; 2–3 *weeks* PO (= the time to achieve a therapeutic anti-seizure plasma concentration with a once daily dose of 100–200mg).[4]

Time to peak plasma concentration 2–4h IM;[5] 2h PO (some authorities report up to 12h);[4–7] 2–4h PR (using oral tablets dissolved in water).[8]
Plasma halflife 2–6 *days*; 1–3 *days* in children.
Duration of action situation dependent; chronic administration >24h.

Cautions

Elderly, children, debilitated, respiratory depression, renal impairment (see Chapter 17, p.681), hepatic impairment (see Chapter 18, p.703). Avoid sudden withdrawal (see below).

Drug interactions

Phenobarbital induces various enzymes involved in drug metabolism, including CYP1A2, CYP2C9, CYP2C19 and CYP3A4 (manufacturer's data), and thus reduces plasma concentrations of many drugs.[9] Table 1 lists selected drugs which have clinically important interactions with phenobarbital.

Table 1 Clinically significant cytochrome P450 interactions with phenobarbital resulting in changed drug plasma concentrations[9]

Phenobarbital plasma concentration		*Drug plasma concentration*	
increased by	*decreased by*	*increased by phenobarbital*	*decreased by phenobarbital*
Felbamate (not UK) Influenza vaccine Phenytoin[a] Stiripentol Valproate[a]	Carbamazepine[a] Chlorpromazine Folic acid St John's wort	Hepatotoxic metabolites of paracetamol (possibly) Phenytoin (sometimes)[a]	Some azole antifungals (itraconazole) Some calcium-channel blockers (felodipine, nifedipine, nimodipine, verapamil) Carbamazepine[a] Chlorpromazine Clonazepam Corticosteroids (dexamethasone, methylprednisolone, prednisolone) Coumarins (oral anticoagulants) Ciclosporin Disopyramide Doxycycline Ethosuximide (sometimes)[a] IV fentanyl (significance not known for TD) Haloperidol Lamotrigine Methadone Metronidazole Oral contraceptives Paracetamol Phenytoin (generally)[a] Quinidine (not UK) Rifampicin TCAs Theophylline Tiagabine Valproate

a. interactions between anti-epileptic drugs are complex and unpredictable; plasma concentrations may be increased, decreased or unchanged.

Undesirable effects

Respiratory depression (high doses), drowsiness, lethargy, ataxia, skin reactions (<3%). Paradoxical excitement, irritability, restlessness/hyperactivity and delirium, particularly in the elderly and children.

Long-term treatment is occasionally complicated by folate-responsive megaloblastic anaemia or by osteomalacia.

Toxicity from propylene glycol, an excipient in the injection, has been reported with prolonged high dose IVI, resulting in confusion, drowsiness, seizures, cardiac arrhythmias or renal failure.[10] However, the dose of phenobarbital required to achieve toxic levels of propylene glycol (~14g/24h) is unlikely to be necessary in palliative care (~3,000mg/24h, using 200mg/mL UK injection).

Dose and use

Route of administration

IV infusion: The injection is very alkaline (pH >9.2) and has a high osmolality. Consequently, it has been recommended to dilute with 10 times its own volume with WFI or 0.9% saline to reduce the risk of venous pain and phlebitis.[11]

IM injection: Phenobarbital can be given undiluted.

CSCI: Although a 10:1 dilution has been advocated,[12] this is probably unnecessary; many centres administer phenobarbital ≤1600mg/24h diluted to 17mL with WFI or 0.9% saline when using a 20mL syringe and a T34 syringe driver.[13]

SC bolus injection *is avoided in the UK* because there are reports of tissue necrosis. Although the North American preparation appears well tolerated by SC bolus,[14] it is unclear whether the formulations differ or tissue necrosis is a rare effect.

PR: Phenobarbital tablets have been dissolved in 6mL tap water and given PR.[8]

PO: rarely used in palliative care patients unless already taking under specialist neurological treatment.

CSCI compatibility with other drugs: Phenobarbital should be administered via a separate syringe driver. Due to its alkaline pH, it is likely to be *incompatible* with most palliative care drugs (see Chapter 29, p.822).

Alternative SC/CSCI anti-epileptics include **lacosamide**,[15] **levetiracetam** (p.287), **midazolam** (p.158) and **valproate** (p.282).

Epilepsy

MHRA advises that the oral products available in the UK may differ in bio-availability, and that to avoid changes in effectiveness or increased risk of undesirable effects, it is best to avoid switching between formulations (see also p.262).

Status epilepticus

Phenobarbital is used for the emergency treatment of seizures refractory to benzodiazepines (see Anti-epileptics, Figure 2, p.266):

- give a stat dose of 10–15mg/kg (up to a maximum dose of 1g[16])
  - ▷ IV (each 1mL ampoule diluted with 10mL WFI or 0.9% saline; rate 100mg/min) *or*
  - ▷ IM *undiluted* (if the IV route is not available). Larger doses may be split between ≥2 sites. IM absorption is significantly slower than IV
- if seizures persist:
  - ▷ if ITU is appropriate, transfer for general anaesthesia
  - ▷ if imminently dying, give further p.r.n. doses and commence a CSCI (dose as for terminal agitation).

Maintenance anti-epileptic in patients unable to swallow

Phenobarbital is a second-line alternative to **midazolam**, **valproate** or **levetiracetam** (see p.265):

- give a stat dose of 100mg (0.5mL of a 200mg/mL ampoule) IM (*undiluted*) or IV (diluted with 5mL WFI or 0.9% saline, over 2min)
- then 100mg/24h CSCI
- if seizures occur, give a second stat dose of 100mg IM/IV and titrate the maintenance dose (maximum of 400mg/24h CSCI)
- if seizures persist, treat as for status epileptics (see above; taking account of the phenobarbital already given) or, in the imminently dying, terminal agitation (see below).

Terminal agitation

Phenobarbital is generally used third-line for patients who fail to respond to the combined use of **midazolam** and an antipsychotic (see p.156):

- give a stat dose of 200mg (1mL of a 200mg/mL ampoule) IM (*undiluted*) or IV (diluted with 10mL WFI or 0.9% saline, over 2min)
- if the patient remains unsettled, give 1 or 2 further doses p.r.n. of 200mg IM/IV 30min apart (the median loading dose reported in case series is 600mg)
- if still unsettled or agitation recurs, give further doses of 200mg IM/IV q1h p.r.n.
- maintain with 800mg/24h CSCI; or more if total initial 'settling' dose was ≥600mg
- if necessary, increase the dose progressively, i.e. 800 → 1,200 → 1,600mg/24h
- a typical dose is 800–1,200mg/24h but can range 200–3,800mg/24h.[17–20]

Some centres infuse loading doses SC in 100ml sodium chloride 0.9% over 30min. Other centres use **propofol** (see p.651) or **dexmedetomidine** instead.[21–23]

Alcohol withdrawal

Phenobarbital is reserved for symptoms refractory to benzodiazepines. Regimens vary widely, but typically start with 200mg IV stat, repeated p.r.n. (sometimes at a lower dose) until symptoms settle. All were from settings equipped to manage airways and respiratory depression.[24] **Gabapentin** is an alternative (p.272).

Stopping phenobarbital

Abrupt cessation of long-term PO anti-epileptic therapy, particularly barbiturates and benzodiazepines, should be avoided because rebound seizures may be precipitated. If it is decided to discontinue anti-epileptic therapy, it should be done *slowly over 6 months or more*. For phenobarbital, the recommended monthly reduction in dose is *15mg*.[25]

In adults the risk of relapse on stopping treatment is 40–50%.[26] Substituting one anti-epileptic drug regimen for another should also be done cautiously, withdrawing the first drug only when the new regimen has been introduced.

Supply

All products are Schedule 3 **CD**.

Phenobarbital sodium (generic)

Tablets 15mg, 30mg, 60mg, 28 days @ 60mg at night = £6.

Oral solution 15mg/5mL; 28 days @ 60mg at night = £93; *may contain significant amounts of ethanol.*

Injection 15mg/mL, 30mg/mL, 60mg/mL and 200mg/mL, 1mL amp = £7; *vehicle contains propylene glycol 90%. Must be diluted with ten times it's volume before IV use.*

1 Kwan P and Brodie MJ (2004) Phenobarbital for the treatment of epilepsy in the 21st century: a critical review. *Epilepsia*. **45**: 1141–1149.

2 Dollery C (1999) Phenobarbital. In: C Dollery (ed) *Therapeutic Drugs Release 1*. Harcourt Brace Company.

3 Leppik IE and Patel SI (2015) Intramuscular and rectal therapies of acute seizures. *Epilepsy and Behavior*. **49**: 307–312.

4 McEvoy GK. *American Hospital Formulary Service*. Maryland, USA: American Society of Health-System Pharmacists www.medicinescomplete.com (accessed April 2017).

5 Sweetman SC (2012). *Martindale: The Complete Drug Reference*. London: Pharmaceutical Press www.medicinescomplete.com

6 Stirling LC *et al.* (1999) The use of phenobarbitone in the management of agitation and seizures at the end of life. *Journal of Pain and Symptom Management*. **17**: 363–368.

7 Holford N (ed) (1998) Clinical pharmacokinetics: drug data handbook. (3e). Adis International, Auckland.

8 Lam YW *et al.* (2016) Pharmacokinetics of phenobarbital in microenema via macy catheter versus suppository. *Journal of Pain and Symptom Management*. **51**: 994–1001.

9 Baxter K and Preston CL. *Stockley's Drug Interactions*. London: Pharmaceutical Press www.medicinescomplete.com (accessed April 2017).

10 Pillai U *et al.* (2014) Severe propylene glycol toxicity secondary to use of anti-epileptics. *American Journal of Therapeutics*. **21**: e106–109.

11 Medusa (2016) Phenobarbital monograph. NHS injectable medicines guide. www.injguide.nhs.uk

12 Dickman A and Schneider J (2016) *The Syringe Driver: Continuous Subcutaneous Infusions in Palliative Care* (4e). Oxford University Press, Oxford.

13 Palliativedrugs.com Ltd Phenobarbital CSCI - How do you dilute it? *Latest additions: Survey results (September 2015)*. www.palliativedrugs.com

14 Hosgood JR *et al.* (2016) Evaluation of subcutaneous phenobarbital administration in hospice patients. *American Journal of Hospice and Palliative Care.* **33**: 209–213.

15 Remi C *et al.* (2016) Subcutaneous use of lacosamide. *Journal of Pain Symptom Management.* **51**: e2–4.

16 NICE (2012) The epilepsies: the diagnosis and management of the epilepsies in adults and children in primary and secondary care. *Clinical Guideline.* CG137 www.nice.org.uk

17 de Graeff A and Dean M (2007) Palliative sedation therapy in the last weeks of life: a literature review and recommendations for standards. *Journal of Palliative Medicine.* **10**: 67–85.

18 Gillon S *et al.* (2010) Review of phenobarbitone use for deep terminal sedation in a UK hospice. *Palliative Medicine.* **24**: 100–101.

19 Chater S *et al.* (1998) Sedation for intractable distress in the dying - a survey of experts. *Palliative Medicine.* **12**: 255–269.

20 Cowan J and Walsh D (2001) Terminal sedation in palliative medicine - definition and review of the literature. *Supportive Care in Cancer.* **9**: 403–407.

21 Gertler R *et al.* (2001) Dexmedetomidine: a novel sedative-analgesic agent. *Proceedings (Baylor University Medical Center).* **14**: 13–21.

22 Soares L *et al.* (2002) Dexmedetomidine: a new option for intractable distress in the dying. *Journal of Pain and Symptom Management.* **24**: 6–8.

23 Jackson KC, 3rd *et al.* (2006) Dexmedetomidine: a novel analgesic with palliative medicine potential. *Journal of Pain and Palliative Care Pharmacotherapy.* **20**: 23–27.

24 Martin K and Katz A (2016) The role of barbiturates for alcohol withdrawal syndrome. *Psychosomatics.* **57**: 341–347.

25 Chadwick D (1995) The withdrawal of antiepileptic drugs. In: A Hopkins *et al.* (eds) *Epilepsy* (2e). Chapman and Hall, London, pp. 215–220.

26 Hopkins A and Shorvon S (1995) Definitions and epidemiology of epilepsy. In: A Hopkins *et al.* (eds) *Epilepsy* (2e). Chapman and Hall, London, pp. 1–24.

Updated September 2017

5: ANALGESICS

PRINCIPLES OF USE OF ANALGESICS

Analgesics can be divided into three classes:

- non-opioid
- opioid
- adjuvant (Figure 1).

Drugs from different classes are used alone or in combination according to the type of pain and response to treatment in conjunction with non-drug measures.

Because cancer pain typically has an inflammatory component, it is generally appropriate to optimize treatment with an NSAID and an opioid before introducing adjuvant analgesics. However, with treatment-related pains (e.g. chemotherapy-induced neuropathic pain, chronic postoperative scar pain) and pains unrelated to cancer (e.g. post-herpetic neuralgia, muscle spasm pain), an adjuvant may be an appropriate first-line treatment. For example, an antidepressant or an anti-epileptic for neuropathic pain, or a benzodiazepine or **baclofen** for muscle spasm (also see p.299).

The main broad principles governing analgesic use for persistent cancer pain can be summarized as:

- administer at regular intervals ('by the clock')
- when feasible, use PO route ('by the mouth')
- titrate the dose against individual need ('by the individual')
- back up with doses for break-through pain ('as required')
- monitor benefit
- treat undesirable effects('attention to detail').[3]

The WHO recommends a 3-step analgesic ladder for cancer pain in adults (Figure 2). However, there is no pharmacological need for Step 2.[4] Indeed, compared to a weak opioid, benefit from

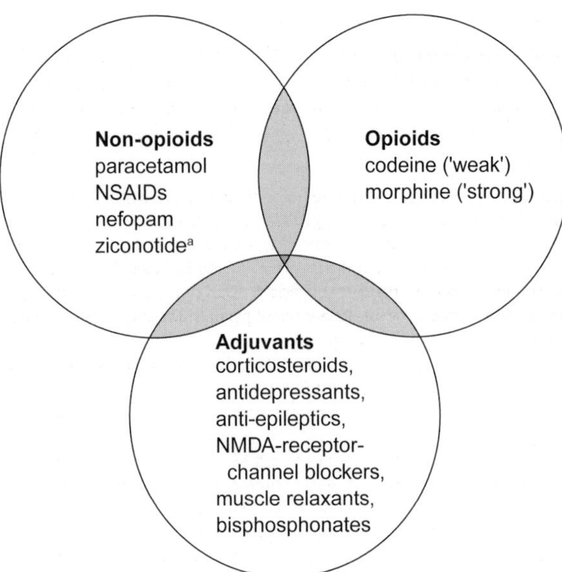

Figure 1 Broad-spectrum analgesia; drugs from different categories are used alone or in combination according to the type of pain and response to treatment.

a. ziconotide is an N-type calcium-channel blocker, the first of a new type of non-opioid. Its place in palliative care remains to be determined.[1,2]

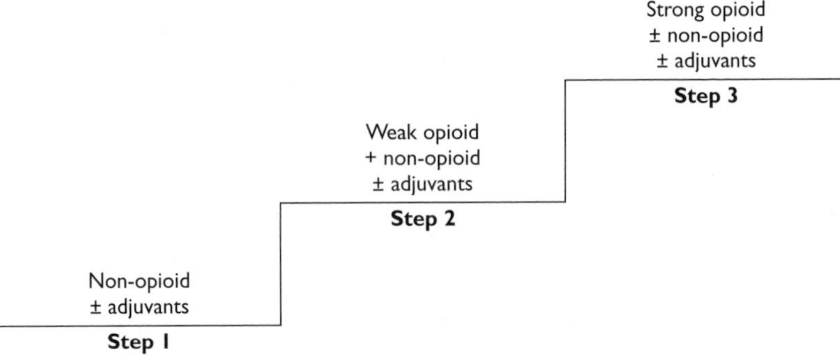

Figure 2 The World Health Organization 3-step analgesic ladder.[3] Step 2 is omitted in children and is unnecessary in countries where morphine is readily available (see text).

low-dose **morphine** (20–30mg/24h PO) is greater and more rapid.[5] Step 2 exists because in many countries accessing strong opioids is difficult (e.g. available only for inpatients, and then sparingly by injection) and sometimes impossible.

Analgesic use in children is comparable with adults. However, because **codeine** (p.855) is no longer recommended in children, the WHO analgesic ladder for children with pain due to medical illness progresses straight from a non-opioid to a strong opioid (see Chapter 16, p.375).[6]

Thus, in countries where **morphine** is readily available, by-passing a weak opioid is likely to also become standard practice in adults.

Note. Patients who have received a regular weak opioid generally start on a higher dose of **morphine** 60mg/24h PO (or the equivalent dose of an alternative strong opioid), also see p.376.

Break-through pain

Several definitions of break-through pain exist.[7,8] Episodic pain, previously synonymous with break-through pain, has also been proposed as a broader overarching concept that encompasses all significant transient pain exacerbations, including those occurring in patients without background pain or requiring regular analgesia.[9] The focus in *PCF* is on break-through pain as defined below.

Break-through pain is a term used to describe a transient exacerbation of pain which occurs either spontaneously or in relation to a specific trigger despite relatively stable and adequately controlled background pain. It may or may not be at the same location as the background (controlled) pain.[10]

Patients with poorly relieved background pain are excluded because this suggests overall poor pain relief which requires an increase in regular analgesia. Similarly, pain recurring shortly before the next dose of a regular analgesic is due ('end-of-dose-interval pain') is not true break-through pain.

There are two main types of break-through pain:

- *predictable (incident) pain*, an exacerbation of pain caused by weight-bearing and/or activity (including swallowing, defaecation, coughing, nursing/medical procedures)
- *unpredictable (spontaneous) pain*, unrelated to movement or activity, e.g. colic, stabbing pain associated with nerve injury.

Break-through pain is common in cancer patients (≤80%) receiving opioid medication for persistent pain.[7] In a large survey, the median number of episodes per day was 3 (range 0–24). These were generally moderate–severe in intensity and interfered with aspects of daily living, in particular, incident pain with walking and normal work, and spontaneous pain with sleep and mood.[11]

Break-through pain is often a resurgence of the background pain, and may be either functional (e.g. tension headache) or pathological, and either nociceptive (associated with tissue distortion or injury) or neuropathic (associated with nerve compression or injury). Patients may experience more than one break-through pain, and these may have different causes. Various strategies reduce the impact of break-through pain (Figure 3).[12] Commonly used non-drug measures include rest, change of position and local heat.[11]

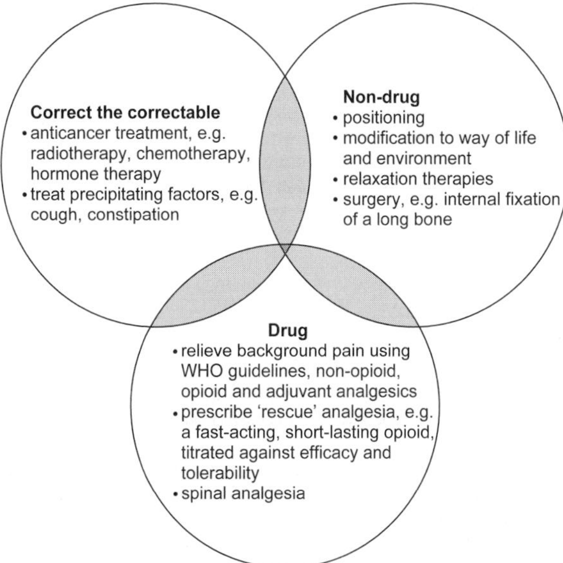

Figure 3 A multimodal approach to managing break-through pain.

Break-through cancer pain is commonly treated by giving an extra dose of the regular analgesic, e.g. a p.r.n. dose of immediate-release **morphine** for patients taking **morphine** regularly round-the-clock.[11] A traditional practice, dating from before m/r opioid products were available, was to give an extra dose of the regular q4h dose of oral **morphine** (i.e. one sixth of the total daily dose). However, many break-through pains are short-lived and this approach effectively doubles the patient's opioid intake for the next 4h.

Accordingly, many centres now recommend that the patient initially takes, as an immediate-release formulation, 10% of the total daily regular dose as the p.r.n. dose.[13,14] However, a standard fixed-dose is unlikely to suit all patients and all pains, particularly because the intensity and the impact of break-through pain vary considerably. Thus, when patients are encouraged to optimize their rescue dose, it varies from 5–20% of the total daily dose.[15,16] When prescribing a p.r.n. dose, it is recommended that:

- a maximum daily amount or frequency is stated
- an individual entry is used for each route, e.g. PO, SC
- patients/carers are taught how to use the formulation correctly
- the amount used is reviewed regularly and where necessary, the background analgesia increased.[17]

Break-through cancer pain generally has a relatively rapid onset (median 5–10min) and short duration (45–60min), but ranging from <1min to 4–6h.[11] By comparison, oral **morphine**, on average, takes about 15–30min (solution quicker than tablet, see p.422) to achieve meaningful pain relief and has a longer duration of effect (3–6h).[18] This helps to explain why many patients choose *not* to take a rescue dose of PO opioid with every episode of break-through pain, particularly when predictable, mild in intensity, and of relatively short duration.[11]

Strategies to circumvent the mismatch between break-through pain duration and drug effect latency include:

- timing a predictable painful activity or procedure to coincide with the peak plasma concentration after a regular or rescue PO dose of **morphine** (1–2h) or other strong opioid
- using routes of administration, e.g. buccal, intranasal, SL, which permit more rapid absorption of some (lipophilic) opioids, e.g. **fentanyl**.[19,20]

Transmucosal **fentanyl** products cost substantially more than short-acting PO opioids and generally their use is reserved for when the latter are unsatisfactory (see p.419); experience with them indicates:[21]

- there is little or no correlation between the dose of the regularly administered strong opioid and the satisfactory rescue dose
- that the rescue dose needs to be individually titrated
- that different products will not be bio-equivalent and cannot be substituted for one another (the formulation and route of administration differ)
- serious adverse events and deaths can occur with inappropriate:
  - ▷ patient selection, e.g. opioid non-tolerant, transient pain (postoperative, migraine)
  - ▷ product use, e.g. exceeding recommended frequency of administration, dose-for-dose substitution of one product with another, e.g. Actiq® for Effentora®.

Another option is SL **alfentanil** (see p.390).

1 Prommer EE (2005) Ziconotide: can we use it in palliative care? *American Journal of Hospice and Palliative Care.* **22**: 369–374.
2 Narayana AK (2005) Elan: ziconotide review focused on off-label uses. *American Journal of Hospice and Palliative Care.* **22**: 408.
3 WHO (1986). *Cancer Pain Relief.* World Health Organization, Geneva.
4 Caraceni A *et al.* (2012) Use of opioid analgesics in the treatment of cancer pain: evidence-based recommendations from the EAPC. *Lancet Oncology.* **13**: e58–68.
5 Bandieri E *et al.* (2016) Randomized trial of low-dose morphine versus weak opioids in moderate cancer pain. *Journal of Clinical Oncology.* **34**: 436–442.
6 WHO (2012) Persisting pain in children package: WHO guidelines on the pharmacological treatment of persisiting pain in children with medical illness. World Health Organisation, Geneva. Available from: www.who.int/publications
7 Mercadante S *et al.* (2016) Breakthrough pain and its treatment: critical review and recommendations of IOPS (Italian Oncologic Pain Survey) expert group. *Supportive Care in Cancer.* **24**: 961–968.
8 Mercadante S and Portenoy RK (2016) Breakthrough cancer pain: twenty-five years of study. *Pain.* **157**: 2657–2663.
9 Lohre ET *et al.* (2016) From "breakthrough" to "episodic" cancer pain? A European Association for Palliative Care Research Network Expert Delphi survey toward a common terminology and classification of transient cancer pain exacerbations. *Journal of Pain and Symptom Management.* **51**: 1013–1019.
10 Davies AN *et al.* (2009) The management of cancer-related breakthrough pain: recommendations of a task group of the Science Committee of the Association for Palliative Medicine of Great Britain and Ireland. *European Journal of Pain.* **13**: 331–338.
11 Davies A *et al.* (2013) Breakthrough cancer pain: an observational study of 1000 European oncology patients. *Journal of Pain and Symptom Management.* **46**: 619–628.
12 Zeppetella G and Ribeiro MD (2002) Episodic pain in patients with advanced cancer. *American Journal of Hospice and Palliative Care.* **19**: 267–276.

13 Davis MP *et al.* (2005) Controversies in pharmacotherapy of pain management. *Lancet Oncology*. **6**: 696–704.
14 Davis MP (2003) Guidelines for breakthrough pain dosing. *American Journal of Hospice and Palliative Care*. **20**: 334.
15 Portenoy K and Hagen N (1990) Breakthrough pain: definition, prevalence and characteristics. *Pain*. **41**: 273–281.
16 Mercadante S *et al.* (2002) Episodic (breakthrough) pain: consensus conference of an expert working group of the EAPC. *Cancer*. **94**: 832–839.
17 NICE (2016) Controlled drugs: safe use and management. *Clinical Guideline* NG46. www.nice.org.uk
18 Zeppetella G (2008) Opioids for cancer breakthrough pain: a pilot study reporting patient assessment of time to meaningful pain relief. *Journal of Pain and Symptom Management*. **35**: 563–567.
19 Davies A *et al.* (2011) Multi-centre European study of breakthrough cancer pain: Pain characteristics and patient perceptions of current and potential management strategies. *European Journal of Pain*. **15**: 756–763.
20 Zeppetella G and Ribeiro MD (2006) Opioids for the management of breakthrough (episodic) pain in cancer patients. *Cochrane Database of Systematic Reviews*. CD004311. www.thecochranelibrary.com
21 Christie J *et al.* (1998) Dose-titration, multicenter study of oral transmucosal fentanyl citrate for the treatment of breakthrough pain in cancer patients using transdermal fentanyl for persistent pain. *Journal of Clinical Oncology*. **16**: 3238–3248.

Updated September 2017

ADJUVANT ANALGESICS

Adjuvant analgesics are drugs whose effect on pain is *circumstance-specific*. Some reduce the painful stimulus directly:

- cancer-related bone pain (bisphosphonates)
- skeletal muscle spasm (skeletal muscle relaxants)
- smooth muscle spasm (antispasmodics)
- cancer-related oedema (corticosteroids).

Others correct changes in pain transmission caused by persistent severe pain and/or damage to the nervous system:

- peripheral sensitization (NSAIDs, corticosteroids)
- ectopic foci caused by nerve damage (e.g. some anti-epileptics)
- central sensitization (e.g. NMDA-receptor-channel blockers, some anti-epileptics)
- altered descending pain modulation (some antidepressants).

Many act in more than one way (Figure 1). Most are marketed for indications other than pain.

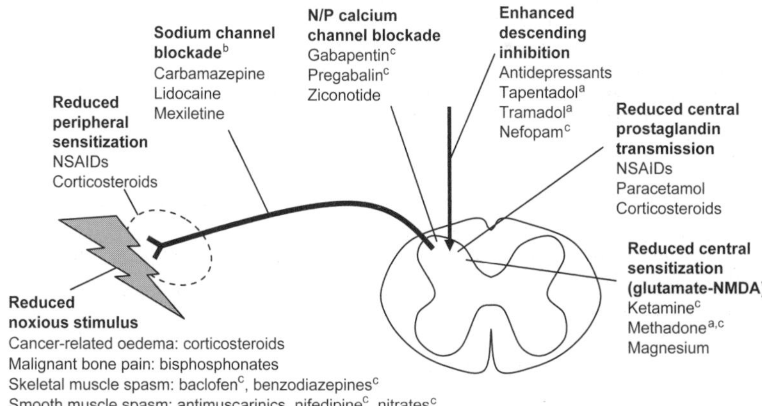

Figure 1 Overview of the peripheral and spinal non-opioid sites of action of analgesics

a. also act as μ-opioid receptor agonists
b. reduces ectopic nerve signal transmission by damaged neurones (see p.256); the higher concentrations of lidocaine used in local/regional anaesthesia completely inhibit nerve signal transmission
c. additional actions (see individual monographs).

Some adjuvant analgesics take longer to act than standard analgesics, and complete pain relief is not always possible. Undesirable effects are often a limiting factor, particularly in frail patients.[1] As with any analgesic, it is important to discuss with the patient desired outcomes, potential problems and the likely timing of benefits.

Low-dose combined treatment may be preferable if a single drug (appropriately titrated) does not provide adequate relief. For example, when used together for neuropathic pain, **nortriptyline** and **gabapentin** were more effective than either drug alone.[2]

Use relative to other measures

Because cancer pain typically has an inflammatory component, it is generally appropriate to optimize treatment with an NSAID and an opioid before introducing adjuvant analgesics. Subsequently, adjuvant analgesics are added to:

- relieve those pains which fail to respond *and/or*
- reduce undesirable effects, e.g. by reducing opioid dose requirements.

However, with treatment-related pains (e.g. chemotherapy-induced neuropathic pain, chronic postoperative scar pain) and pains unrelated to cancer (e.g. post-herpetic neuralgia, muscle spasm pain), an adjuvant may be an appropriate first-line treatment.

Antidepressants and anti-epileptics

First-line choices for neuropathic pain include **amitriptyline** (p.210) and **gabapentin** (p.272). Both direct comparisons[3–9] and a large network analysis[10] found their efficacy and tolerability to be comparable with alternatives: **pregabalin** (p.272), **duloxetine** (p.219) and **nortriptyline**. Choice is thus influenced by cost and individual circumstances (Table 1). There is increasing interest in relating certain patterns of sensory findings (sensory phenotypic profiling) to likelihood of response to a particular class of drug.[11]

Drugs which act via different mechanisms can be combined if patients do not respond to a single drug (Figure 2).[2] Opioids have been shown in RCTs to at least partly relieve neuropathic pain.[12,13]

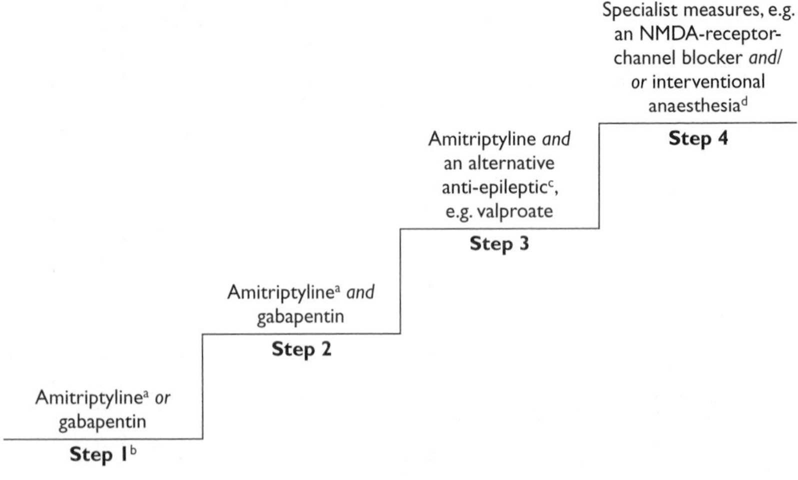

Figure 2 Suggested adjuvant analgesics for neuropathic pain.

a. consider duloxetine if amitriptyline is poorly tolerated, but *not* if it is ineffective because their mechanism of action is similar (see p.204)
b. systemic corticosteroids are an alternative for *cancer-related* neuropathic pain, particularly if pain is associated with limb weakness or awaiting benefit from another treatment, e.g. radiotherapy
c. it is unknown if patients with an inadequate response to gabapentin are best switched to pregabalin (p.272) or to an anti-epileptic which differs in its mechanism of action, e.g. valproate (p.282). Gabapentin can be switched directly to pregabalin; for all others, generally, the gabapentin is withdrawn once the new anti-epileptic has been titrated to an effective dose (see p.262)
d. e.g. spinal analgesia, nerve block.

Table 1 Some considerations when selecting an adjuvant analgesic for neuropathic pain.[14–18]

Drug	*Supporting evidence*[a]	*Ease of administration*			*Propensity for drug interactions*	*Cautions (see also individual monographs)*			*Approximate typical monthly cost*[b]	*Examples of concurrent indications in palliative care*
		Once daily	*Oral solution*	*Parenteral*		*Cardiac disease*	*Renal impairment*	*Seizure threshold*		
First-line treatments for neuropathic pain										
†Amitriptyline	High	Yes	Yes	No	Moderate	Arrhythmias, CHF, HB, IHD	Yes	↓	+	Depression, anxiety, bladder spasms, urgency
Duloxetine	Moderate	Yes	No	No	Moderate	Arrhythmias, CHF, HT, IHD	Avoid if GFR<30	↓	+	Depression, anxiety, stress incontinence
Gabapentin	High	No	Yes[c]	No	Low	No	↓Dose		++	Spasticity, seizures
†Nortriptyline	Moderate	Yes	No	No	Moderate	Arrhythmias, CHF, HB, IHD	Yes	↓	+++	Depression
Pregabalin	High	No	Yes	No	Low	CHF	↓Dose		+++	Anxiety, seizures
Treatments generally reserved for use second-line or in specific situations										
Lidocaine 5% plaster[d]	Moderate	Yes	Topical		Low	Limited systemic absorption			++++	
Carbamazepine[e]	Low	No	Yes	No	High	HB	Yes		+++	Seizures
†Clonazepam	Very low	Yes	Yes[f]	No	Moderate	No	Yes		+++	Spasticity, seizures, anxiety
†Oxcarbazepine	Low	No	Yes	No	Moderate	CCF, HB	↓Dose		+++	Seizures
†Valproate	Low	Yes	Yes	Yes (†CSCI)	Moderate	No	Yes		+++	Seizures
†Venlafaxine	High	Yes (m/r)	No[f]	No	Moderate	Arrhythmias, CHF, HT, IHD	Avoid if GFR<30	↓	+++	Depression, anxiety

Key: CHF = congestive heart failure; HB = heart block; HT = hypertension; IHD = ischaemic heart disease.
Monthly cost: + = ≤£2.50; ++ = £2.50–5; +++ = £5–25; ++++ = >£25.

a. based on RCTs vs. case reports, methodological quality, consistency within and between studies, and applicability to palliative care population. Although few RCTs have been conducted in palliative care patients, generalizability was considered more likely if benefit demonstrated in ≥2 neuropathic pain types
b. oral solutions are generally considerably more expensive
c. capsules can be opened and sprinkled on food (unauthorized use), also see Chapter 28, Table 2, p.793
d. authorized for post-herpetic neuralgia only
e. first-line choice (and authorized) for trigeminal neuralgia
f. disperses in 5min (unauthorized use), also see Chapter 28, Table 2, p.793.

Bisphosphonates

Bisphosphonates (see p.501) are osteoclast inhibitors used to prevent pain and other complications from bone metastases. They may also relieve metastatic bone pain which persists despite analgesics and radiation therapy ± orthopaedic surgery. Although published data relate mainly to breast cancer and myeloma, benefit is also seen with other cancers.

Corticosteroids

Systemic corticosteroids are used for various types of pain (see Box A, Systemic corticosteroids, p.513) particularly for those associated with:

- nerve root/nerve trunk compression
- spinal cord compression
- raised intracranial pressure.

Systemic corticosteroids do not help in pure non-cancer nerve injury pain, e.g. chronic postoperative scar pain, post-herpetic neuralgia. However, in cancer-related nerve injury pain, a 5–7 day trial of **dexamethasone** may be beneficial.

Epidural depot corticosteroids are sometimes used to relieve radicular pain associated with a spinal metastasis (see p.599).

NMDA-receptor-channel blockers

NMDA-receptor-channel blockers are most commonly used when neuropathic pain does not respond well to standard analgesics together with an antidepressant and an anti-epileptic. They have also been used in ischaemic pain,[19] bone pain,[20] and severe mucositis.[21] NMDA-receptor-channel blockers include:

- **ketamine** (see p.641)
- **methadone** (see p.437)
- **magnesium** (see p.588).

Despite promising case reports/series, **ketamine** is *not* consistently beneficial in RCTs (nor are **amantadine, memantine**).[22]

Skeletal muscle relaxants

These include **baclofen**, **diazepam**, and **tizanidine** (see p.605). Although non-drug treatment is generally preferable for painful skeletal muscle spasm (cramp) and myofascial pain, e.g. physical therapy (local heat, massage),[23] some patients also benefit from relaxation therapy ± **diazepam** (see p.158). Myofascial trigger points often benefit from acupuncture or direct injection of local anaesthetic.[24] *However severe,* ***morphine*** *is ineffective for the relief of cramp and trigger point pains.*

Smooth muscle relaxants (antispasmodics)

This is a heterogeneous group of drugs encompassing antimuscarinics, **glyceryl trinitrate** (see p.81), and L-type calcium-channel blockers (e.g. **nifedipine**; see p.85). Antimuscarinics are used to relieve visceral distension pain and colic. In advanced cancer, there is little place for 'weak' antispasmodics, e.g. **dicycloverine**.

Hyoscine *butylbromide* (see p.16) and **glycopyrronium** (see p.13) are quaternary drugs which do not cross the blood-brain barrier, and are widely regarded as the antispasmodics of choice. Although **atropine** and **hyoscine *hydrobromide*** have comparable peripheral effects, they also have central effects, either stimulatory or sedative, and may precipitate delirium (see p.5).

Glyceryl trinitrate and L-type calcium-channel blockers can be used for the same range of indications, but tend to be reserved for painful spasm of the oesophagus, rectum and anus (see p.81).

1 Bennett MI (2011) Effectiveness of antiepileptic or antidepressant drugs when added to opioids for cancer pain: systematic review. *Palliative Medicine*. **25**: 553–559.

2 Gilron I *et al.* (2009) Nortriptyline and gabapentin, alone and in combination for neuropathic pain: a double-blind, randomised controlled crossover trial. *Lancet*. **374**: 1252–1261.

3 Boyle J *et al.* (2012) Randomized, placebo-controlled comparison of amitriptyline, duloxetine, and pregabalin in patients with chronic diabetic peripheral neuropathic pain: impact on pain, polysomnographic sleep, daytime functioning, and quality of life. *Diabetes Care*. **35**: 2451–2458.

4 Bansal D *et al.* (2009) Amitriptyline vs. pregabalin in painful diabetic neuropathy: a randomized double blind clinical trial. *Diabetic Medicine*. **26**: 1019–1026.
5 Morello CM *et al.* (1999) Randomized double-blind study comparing the efficacy of gabapentin with amitriptyline on diabetic peripheral neuropathy pain. *Archives of Internal Medicine*. **159**: 1931–1937.
6 Chandra K *et al.* (2006) Gabapentin versus nortriptyline in post-herpetic neuralgia patients: a randomized, double-blind clinical trial--the GONIP Trial. *International Journal of Clinical Pharmacology and Therapeutics*. **44**: 358–363.
7 Mishra S *et al.* (2012) A comparative efficacy of amitriptyline, gabapentin, and pregabalin in neuropathic cancer pain: a prospective randomized double-blind placebo-controlled study. *American Journal of Hospice and Palliative Care*. **29**: 177–182.
8 Banerjee M *et al.* (2013) A comparative study of efficacy and safety of gabapentin versus amitriptyline as coanalgesics in patients receiving opioid analgesics for neuropathic pain in malignancy. *Indian Journal of Pharmacology*. **45**: 334–338.
9 Kelle B (2012) The efficacy of gabapentin and pregabalin in the treatment of neuropathic pain due to peripheral nerve injury. *Journal of Musculoskeletal Pain*. **20**: 300–305.
10 NICE (2013) Neuropathic pain - pharmacological management. *Clinical Guideline*. CG173: (appendix G) www.nice.org.uk
11 Baron R *et al.* (2017) Peripheral neuropathic pain: a mechanism-related organizing principle based on sensory profiles. *Pain*. **158**: 261–272.
12 Eisenberg E *et al.* (2006) Efficacy of mu-opioid agonists in the treatment of evoked neuropathic pain: Systematic review of randomized controlled trials. *European Journal of Pain*. **10**: 667–676.
13 Eisenberg E *et al.* (2005) Efficacy and safety of opioid agonists in the treatment of neuropathic pain of nonmalignant origin: systematic review and meta-analysis of randomized controlled trials. *Journal of the American Medical Association*. **293**: 3043–3052.
14 Wiffen PJ *et al.* (2010) Anitconvulsant drugs for acute and chronic pain. *Cochrane Database of Systematic Reviews*. **1**: CD0011133. www.thecochranelibrary.com
15 Saarto T and Wiffen PJ (2007) Antidepressants for neuropathic pain. *Cochrane Database of Systematic Reviews*. **4**: CD005454. www.thecochranelibrary.com
16 Attal N *et al.* (2010) EFNS guidelines on the pharmacological treatment of neuropathic pain: 2010 revision. *European Journal of Neurology*. **17**: 1113–e1188.
17 Dworkin RH *et al.* (2010) Recommendations for the pharmacological management of neuropathic pain: an overview and literature update. *Mayo Clinic Proceedings*. **85**: S3–14.
18 Finnerup NB *et al.* (2016) Pharmacotherapy for neuropathic pain in adults: a systematic review and meta-analysis. *Lancet Neurology*. **14**: 162–173.
19 Mitchell AC and Fallon MT (2002) A single infusion of intravenous ketamine improves pain relief in patients with critical limb ischaemia: results of a double blind randomised controlled trial. *Pain*. **97**: 275–281.
20 Mercadante S *et al.* (2009) Opioid switching and burst ketamine to improve the opioid response in patients with movement-related pain due to bone metastases. *Clinical Journal of Pain*. **25**: 648–649.
21 Jackson K *et al.* (2001) 'Burst' ketamine for refractory cancer pain: an open-label audit of 39 patients. *Journal of Pain and Symptom Management*. **22**: 834–842.
22 Collins S *et al.* (2010) NMDA receptor antagonists for the treatment of neuropathic pain. *Pain Medicine*. **11**: 1726–1742.
23 Twycross R and Wilcock A (eds) (2016) *Introducing Palliative Care* (5e), Palliativedrugs.com, Nottingham, pp. 207–209.
24 Sola A and Bonica J (1990) Myofascial pain syndromes. In: J Bonica (ed) *The Management of Pain* (2e). Lea and Febiger, Philadelphia, pp. 352–367.

Updated September 2017

PARACETAMOL

Unintentional overdose of paracetamol (acetaminophen USAN) resulting in hepatotoxicity, sometimes fatal, can occur. To reduce this risk, the dose of paracetamol should *not* exceed the maximum recommended dose, be appropriate for the weight of the patient, and reduced when risk factors for hepatotoxicity exist (see Box A below).

Class: Non-opioid analgesic.

Indications: mild–moderate pain, pyrexia.

Contra-indications: ***IV*** severe hepatic impairment or severe active liver disease.

Pharmacology

Paracetamol is a synthetic non-opioid analgesic and antipyretic. It acts mainly in the CNS, where it has several effects. It is a weak inhibitor of cyclo-oxygenase (COX)-2, an effect that lasts a short time (≤2h) after a dose,[1,2] but can also be anti-inflammatory through inhibition of peroxidase regeneration. The latter action, which prevents the oxidation of inactive COX to active COX, can be significant where peroxidase levels are low, e.g. in intact cells in the CNS, but not where peroxidase levels are much higher, e.g. with tissue damage and/or inflammation in the periphery.[3] In addition, paracetamol:

- interacts with L-arginine-nitric oxide, opioid and cannabinoid systems[4,5]
- activates descending serotoninergic inhibitory pain pathways.[6,7]

The analgesic effect of paracetamol probably depends on synergy between these mechanisms.[8] Further, evidence of synergy between paracetamol and NSAIDs suggests distinct analgesic mechanisms.[9]

Single doses of IV paracetamol provide dose-dependent analgesia in doses up to 2g.[10] Higher peak plasma concentrations lead to earlier and increased concentrations of paracetamol in the CSF. These lead to an earlier onset of action, a longer duration of action, and a greater overall analgesic effect.[11] In patients undergoing molar dental extraction, compared with 1g, 2g of paracetamol gave 50% more relief for 50% longer (5h vs. 3.2h).[12] Thus, there may be a place for an initial loading dose when prescribing paracetamol.

Less than 10% of a therapeutic dose of paracetamol is excreted unchanged in the urine; the remainder is metabolized mainly by the liver. At therapeutic doses, ≤90% of paracetamol is metabolized to inactive glucuronide and sulfate conjugates. About 5–15% is oxidized by hepatic CYP450 enzymes to a highly reactive hepatotoxic metabolite, N-acetyl-p-benzoquinoneimine (NAPQI; Figure 1). With typical therapeutic doses (≤1g q.d.s.), this is normally inactivated sufficiently rapidly not to cause liver damage.

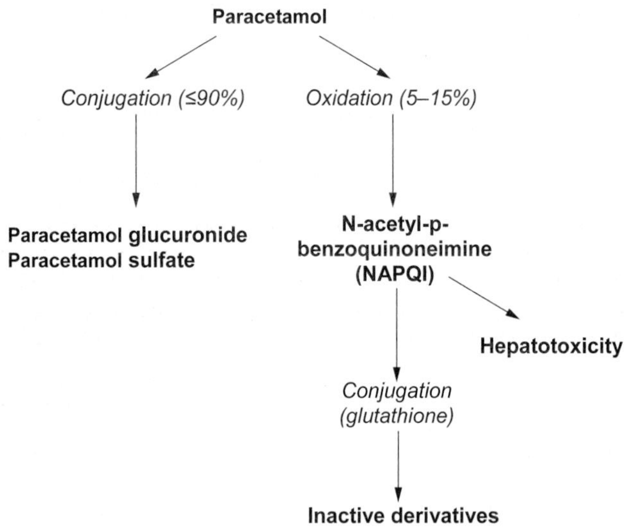

Figure 1 Metabolism of paracetamol.

CYP2E1 is responsible for ≤80% of paracetamol's oxidative metabolism to NAPQI. Up to 25% is oxidized via CYP3A4 (particularly at lower doses) and CYP2D6 (particularly at higher doses).[13] There are also genetic variations.[14] For example, those with CYP2D6 gene duplication (ultra-rapid metabolizers) have a greater susceptibility to hepatotoxicity because of the increased production of NAPQI.[15]

The metabolism of paracetamol is also gender-dependent (women eliminate the drug more slowly[16]) and age-dependent (increased risk of hepatotoxicity in the elderly[17]). *After a dose of IV paracetamol, an 80 year-old may well be exposed to a 50% increase in the amount of NAPQI compared with a 20 year-old* (Box A).[17]

Box A Risk factors for paracetamol hepatotoxicity[13,18,19]	
Old age Poor nutritional status Fasting/anorexia	lower glutathione stores
Weight <50kg	
Chronic alcohol use	

Although it has been suggested that co-administration with inhibitors of glucuronidation and/or CYP2E1-inducers may increase the risk of hepatotoxicity, there is no hard evidence of a significant clinical impact from concurrent use.[20] Indeed, co-administration with **isoniazid** (which is both a CYP2E1 inhibitor and inducer) results in *reduced* conversion to NAPQI.[20]

Unintentional and deliberate overdose and NAPQI-induced hepatotoxicity

An overdose of paracetamol overwhelms normal metabolism, shifting more paracetamol into the NAPQI pathway. NAPQI is normally inactivated by conjugation with glutathione but, in overdose, the body's glutathione store becomes exhausted and the accumulation of NAPQI leads to liver cell death.

Although overdose is typically associated with the deliberate ingestion of a large single dose of paracetamol, unintentional overdose can occur from analgesic use.[21,22] A man aged 43 with Crohn's colitis and weighing 30kg died of hepatic failure after taking 4g/24h for only 4 days.[23] Further, in elderly patients without any obvious risk factors, fatal toxicity has been reported with 4g/24h after a few weeks.[24]

There are also numerous reports of hepatotoxicity associated with chronic use of 5–7.5g/24h.[25] Thus, the dose of paracetamol must always be appropriate for the weight and circumstances of the patient, and the maximum recommended dose should not be exceeded.

Repeated suprathreshold ingestion over a time period of >8h ('staggered overdose') produces a higher risk of liver and multi-organ failure, and a lower unassisted survival rate, than single time point overdose. About two-thirds of staggered overdoses relate to medicinal use rather than attempted suicide.[26] The likelihood of an unintentional/staggered overdose is greater in patients with one or more risk factors for paracetamol hepatotoxicity (see Box A).

A single time point overdose of paracetamol below 125mg/kg (7.5g or 15 tablets in a 60kg person) is unlikely to result in liver damage. At twice this dose, the probability of liver damage is around 50%, but the individual may remain well. A dose of 500mg/kg (30g or 60 tablets in a 60kg person) is almost certain to produce life-threatening liver damage. Paracetamol overdose can also lead to acute renal failure, although this is often reversible without the need for dialysis.[27]

With IV paracetamol poisoning, contact the UK National Poisons Information Service for advice (0844 892 0111).

Overdose can be treated with a glutathione precursor, e.g. IVI **acetylcysteine** (Box B)[28–30] or PO **methionine** (not UK).[31] If given within 15h of the overdose, acetylcysteine prevents NAPQI from reacting with liver cell proteins. Further, because it has a protective effect against apoptosis (programmed cell death), **acetylcysteine** can help to a lesser extent if given for ≤3 days after the overdose.

Box B IVI acetylcysteine[29]

Three separate consecutive IVI totalling 300mg/kg are given in 5% glucose over 21h.
For those weighing 41–100kg:

- *first (loading) IVI:* 150mg/kg diluted in 200mL over 1h
- *second IVI:* 50mg/kg diluted in 500mL over 4h
- *third IVI:* 100mg/kg diluted in 1,000mL over 16h.

For those weighing 21–40kg, use half the volume.
For patients whose weight falls outside of these ranges, see SPC.
Saline 0.9% can be used as an alternative diluent.

Acute alcohol intake does *not* increase the risk of hepatotoxicity. Indeed, because alcohol and paracetamol compete for the same oxidative enzymes, acute alcohol consumption at the time of a paracetamol overdose may be protective. However, because alcohol consumption induces the production of the relevant enzymes, if *chronic* alcohol use suddenly stops, paracetamol will be metabolized more rapidly, and could lead to hepatotoxicity.[32] In any case, some alcoholics are more susceptible to paracetamol toxicity, possibly because of their poor nutritional status.[33]

In the USA, to reduce the chance of unintentional overdose, the FDA has:[34,35]

- reduced the amount of paracetamol in prescription combination products to a maximum of 325mg per dosage unit
- added a boxed warning highlighting the potential for severe liver injury
- recommended that the maximum single dose is lowered to 650mg and patients should not exceed a total daily dose of 4g.

'Extra strength' single ingredient products containing 500mg/dose unit remain available. However, over-the-counter products now recommend a maximum dose of 2.6–3g/24h, which patients should not exceed unless directed by a doctor.

Although the liver remains the main concern in relation to paracetamol toxicity, there is *in vitro* evidence of glutathione-independent renal toxicity.[36] A direct toxic effect on the brain has also been reported, possibly mediated by brain CYP2E1.[37] On the other hand, *in vitro* studies suggest that low doses may be protective.[37]

Bio-availability 60% after 500mg PO, 90% after 1g PO; PR is about two-thirds of PO, but is higher with two 500mg suppositories than with one 1g suppository.

Onset of action 15–30min PO; 5–10min IV (pain relief), 30min IV (antipyretic effect).

Time to peak plasma concentration widely variable PO, e.g. 20min in fasting state but 1–2h if delayed gastric emptying;[38] 15min IVI (i.e. synchronous with the end of a 15min infusion).

Plasma half-life 1–4h PO; 2–3h IV.

Duration of action 4–6h PO and IV.

Cautions

Severe hepatic impairment or severe active liver disease (*IV use contra-indicated in this setting*), particularly if associated with old age, chronic alcohol use, low weight, malnutrition, and/or anorexia (also see Chapter 18, p.709).[39] Renal impairment (see Dose and use and Chapter 17, p.695).

Most *dispersible* and *effervescent* paracetamol-containing tablets (alone or combined with an opioid) have a Na^+ content of ≥14mmol/tablet. Thus, a dose of 8 tablets/24h would exceed the recommended maximum daily dietary Na^+ intake of 100mmol (6g of sodium chloride). Dispersible or effervescent formulations should thus be avoided in patients with hypertension or renal impairment, particularly if already on a salt-restricted diet. In contrast, non-soluble formulations contain negligible Na^+.[40]

Paracetamol can be taken by at least two thirds of patients who are hypersensitive to **aspirin** or other NSAID.[41,42] In people with a history of **aspirin**/NSAID-induced asthma, give a test dose of 250mg (half a tablet) and observe for 2–3h. If no undesirable effects occur, paracetamol can safely be used in standard doses.[43]

Drug interactions

When given to patients taking **warfarin**, the concurrent use of regular paracetamol is associated with a significant dose-dependent increase in the INR.[44] In some individuals, the INR rises to >6 in just a few days.[45,46] Thus, in **warfarin**-treated patients who take ≥2 g/day of paracetamol for ≥3 consecutive days, the INR should be tested 3–5 days after the first dose of paracetamol.[47] However, a total *weekly* dose of paracetamol of ≤2g has no effect.[45] The underlying mechanism possibly relates to interference with the hepatic synthesis of various clotting factors. A post-mortem study found that concurrent paracetamol approximately triples the risk of a bleed with **warfarin**.[48]

Paracetamol 1g q.d.s. decreases **lamotrigine** plasma concentrations by about 20%, possibly by inducing glucuronidation; this may be clinically relevant for patients with **lamotrigine** concentrations at the lower end of the therapeutic range.[49]

There are conflicting reports about the impact of $5HT_3$ antagonists on the analgesic effect of paracetamol. Some report a reduction in analgesia[8] but others an increase,[50] and some no effect.[51]

Undesirable effects

Very common (>10%): dyspepsia, elevated liver enzymes (Box C).

Rare (<0.1%, >0.01%): PO cholestatic jaundice,[52,53] acute pancreatitis, thrombocytopenia, agranulocytosis, serious skin reactions,[54] anaphylaxis.[55,56] ***IV*** malaise, hypotension.

Chronic paracetamol use increases the risk of renal impairment 2.5 times; and the risk is related to dose and cumulative exposure over a lifetime.[59,60] The risk is higher in diabetics, and when renal impairment is associated with systemic vasculitis.

A recent systematic review of eight observational studies suggests that there is a dose-response in relation to adverse events with paracetamol (myocardial infarction, CVA, hypertension, GI haemorrhage, decrease in GFR), with an increase in overall mortality compared with non-use.[61]

Box C Paracetamol and elevated liver enzymes[57,58]

The plasma concentrations of liver enzymes (alanine aminotransferase (ALT), aspartate aminotransferase, γ-glutamyl transferase) can increase with normal doses of paracetamol.

For example, ALT increased >3 times the upper limit of normal in 40% of young healthy volunteers receiving 4g/day, with the highest increase 14–16 times greater. The rise was evident after 72h, and persisted for a median of one week after discontinuation.

These changes are probably unimportant in the absence of functional or synthetic liver impairment (e.g. indicated by an increase in plasma bilirubin or a reduction in clotting factors respectively) and possibly improve with ongoing use, although this is poorly documented.

Awareness of this phenomenon aids interpretation of abnormal LFTs, and help to avoid the erroneous assumption that rapidly worsening LFTs must indicate worsening disease within the liver, e.g. from liver metastases.

However, the results probably suffer from confounding by indication and channelling bias in that paracetamol tends to be prescribed preferentially to frailer patients whose prognosis is likely to be relatively poor. Even so, despite concern, paracetamol can still generally be regarded as a safe drug for most people.[62] Although as indicated above, when analgesic benefit is uncertain, more careful consideration is required as to its continued use.

The use of paracetamol in pregnancy and early childhood increases the risk of a child developing asthma.[63] However, there is no hard evidence that paracetamol precipitates asthma in established asthmatics.[43,64]

Dose and use

Paracetamol is widely used for acute musculoskeletal pains and acute headache. However, a systematic review of paracetamol indicates that paracetamol is of little or no value in the management of osteo-arthritic hip or knee pain.[65] Doubt has also been cast over its value in acute low-back pain.[66]

For patients without risk factors for paracetamol hepatotoxicity (Box A), the standard regimen is 1g PO q.d.s. However, in palliative care patients with more than one hepatic risk factor, a smaller dose, e.g. 500mg q.d.s. (maximum 3g/24h) is advisable.

Similar dose reductions are necessary in patients with renal impairment. With severe impairment (creatinine clearance <30mL/min), the dose interval should be ≥6h. In ESRF, start with 500mg q8h−q6h (maximum 3g/24h).

Despite lower PR bio-availability, the same dose is generally used both PR and PO.

Combining with opioids

When used in combination with an opioid to treat *postoperative pain*, IV paracetamol has an 'opioid-sparing' effect, and improves overall analgesia.[67] However, evidence of efficacy when combined with an opioid in *cancer pain* is mixed, perhaps because the RCTs suggesting no benefit were underpowered.[68–70] A further RCT showed a small but clinically important additive effect in about one-third of patients despite half the patients already taking an NSAID or a corticosteroid.[71]

Given that paracetamol 1g PO q.d.s. is a significant tablet burden, a pragmatic solution might be:

- to limit the long-term use of paracetamol to patients in whom definite benefit is seen within 2 days of starting it
- if already taking paracetamol with definite past benefit and increasing pain necessitates the *addition* of an opioid, the ongoing need for paracetamol should be determined by stopping it after 3–4 days of satisfactory pain relief with both drugs, and restarting paracetamol only if the pain returns.

IV

IV paracetamol (1g in 100mL) is given by infusion over 15min. There have been case reports of massive inadvertent iatrogenic IV overdose leading to hepatic failure, sometimes fatal, particularly in children.[72] The available IV solution contains *10mg/mL*. When written up just as mg, it has occasionally been misread and given as mL, with the result that the patient has received *10 times* the prescribed dose. To minimize the chance of this happening, a prescription for IV paracetamol should be written in terms of *both* mg *and* mL, not just as mg.

IV paracetamol can be used when administration PO or PR is not possible. The dose depends on body weight and the presence/absence of risk factors for paracetamol hepatotoxicity:

- adults and children >50kg, 1g up to q4h, maximum recommended dose 4g/24h
- adults and children >50kg *plus any risk factors*, restrict maximum dose to 3g/24h
- adults and children 10–50kg, 15mg/kg up to q4h, maximum recommended dose 60mg/kg/24h.

For patients with severe renal impairment, (creatinine clearance <30mL/min) the minimum interval must be ≥q6h.

Parenteral **propacetamol** (not UK) is an inactive pro-drug of paracetamol; 2g yields paracetamol 1g.[73,74] Because of a risk of sensitization, the manufacturer's protocol must be adhered to.

Supply

PO paracetamol is available OTC alone and in several combination products with weak opioids (see **Codeine**, p.855; **Dihydrocodeine**, p.352; and **Tramadol**, p.354).

Paracetamol (generic)
Tablets and caplets 500mg, 28 days @ 1g q.d.s. = £5.
Tablets soluble and dispersible 120mg, 500mg, 28 days @ 1g q.d.s. = £20; *may contain Na^+ up to 20mmol/tablet.*
Tablets orodispersible 250mg, 28 days @ 1g q.d.s. = £67.
Capsules 500mg, 28 days @ 1g q.d.s. = £6.50.
Oral solution 120mg/5mL, 500mg/5mL, 28 days @ 1g q.d.s. = £101.
Oral suspension 120mg/5mL, 250mg/5mL, 28 days @ 1g q.d.s. = £26; *available sugar free. A 500mg/5mL oral suspension is available but is almost 8 times the cost.*
Suppositories 60mg, 80mg, 120mg, 125mg, 240mg, 250mg, 500mg, 1g, 28 days @ 1g q.d.s. = £817.
Injection (for IV infusion) 10mg/mL, 50mL (500mg) or 100mL (1g) vial = £1.25.

1 Hinz B *et al.* (2008) Acetaminophen (paracetamol) is a selective cyclooxygenase-2 inhibitor in man. *FASEB J.* **22**: 383–390.
2 Hinz B and Brune K (2012) Paracetamol and cyclooxygenase inhibition: is there a cause for concern? *Annals of the Rheumatic Diseases.* **71**: 20–25.
3 Mattia A and Coluzzi F (2009) What anesthesiologists should know about paracetamol (acetaminophen). *Minerva Anestesiologica.* **75**: 644–653.
4 Bjorkman R *et al.* (1994) Acetaminophen (paracetamol) blocks spinal hyperalgesia induced by NMDA and substance P. *Pain.* **57**: 259–264.
5 Pini L *et al.* (1997) Naloxone-reversible antinociception by paracetamol in the rat. *Journal of Pharmacology and Experimental Therapeutics.* **280**: 934–940.
6 Mallet C *et al.* (2008) Endocannabinoid and serotonergic systems are needed for acetaminophen-induced analgesia. *Pain.* **139**: 190–200.
7 Dogrul A *et al.* (2012) Systemic paracetamol-induced analgesic and antihyperalgesic effects through activation of descending serotonergic pathways involving spinal 5-HT(7) receptors. *European Journal of Pharmacology.* **677**: 93–101.
8 Pickering G *et al.* (2008) Acetaminophen reinforces descending inhibitory pain pathways. *Clinical Pharmacology and Therapeutics.* **84**: 47–51.
9 Ong CK *et al.* (2010) Combining paracetamol (acetaminophen) with nonsteroidal antiinflammatory drugs: a qualitative systematic review of analgesic efficacy for acute postoperative pain. *Anesthesia and Analgesia.* **110**: 1170–1179.
10 Piguet V *et al.* (1998) Lack of acetaminophen ceiling effect on R-III nociceptive flexion reflex. *European Journal of Clinical Pharmacology.* **53**: 321–324.
11 Jarde O and Boccard E (1997) Parenteral versus oral route increases paracetamol efficacy. *Clinical Drug Investigations.* **14**: 474–481.
12 Juhl GI *et al.* (2006) Analgesic efficacy and safety of intravenous paracetamol (acetaminophen) administered as a 2g starting dose following third molar surgery. *European Journal of Pain.* **10**: 371–377.
13 Kalsi S and Wood DM (2011) Does cytochrome P450 liver isoenzyme induction increase the risk of liver toxicity after paracetamol overdose? *Open Access Emergency Medicine.* **3**: 69–76.
14 Zhao L and Pickering G (2011) Paracetamol metabolism and related genetic differences. *Drug Metabolism Reviews.* **43**: 41–52.

15 Dong H *et al.* (2000) Involvement of human cytochrome P450 2D6 in the bioactivation of acetaminophen. *Drug Metabolism and Disposition.* **28**: 1397–1400.
16 Liukas A *et al.* (2011) Pharmacokinetics of intravenous paracetamol in elderly patients. *Clinical Pharmacokinetics.* **50**: 121–129.
17 Mitchell SJ *et al.* (2011) Age-related changes in the hepatic pharmacology and toxicology of paracetamol. *Current Gerontology and Geriatrics Research* **624156**:Available from www.hindawi.com
18 Zimmerman H and Maddrey W (1995) Acetaminophen (paracetamol) hepatotoxicity with regular intake of alcohol: analysis of instances of therapeutic misadventure. *Hepatology.* **22**: 767–773.
19 Horsmans Y *et al.* (1998) Paracetamol-induced liver toxicity after intravenous administration. *Liver.* **18**: 294–295.
20 Toes MJ *et al.* (2005) Drug interactions with paracetamol. *American Journal of Therapeutics.* **12**: 56–66.
21 MHRA (2010) Intravenous paracetamol (Perfalgan): risk of accidental overdose especially in infants and neonates. *Drug Safety Update.* www.gov.uk/drug-safety-update
22 Larson AM *et al.* (2005) Acetaminophen-induced acute liver failure: results of a United States multicenter, prospective study. *Hepatology.* **42**: 1364–1372.
23 Claridge LC *et al.* (2010) Acute liver failure after administration of paracetamol at the maximum recommended daily dose in adults. *British Medical Journal.* **341**: c6764.
24 Ging P *et al.* (2016) Unexpected paracetamol (acetaminophen) hepatotoxicity at standard dosage in two older patients: time to rethink 1g four times daily? *Age and Ageing.* **45**: 566–567.
25 Krenzelok EP (2009) The FDA Acetaminophen Advisory Committee Meeting - what is the future of acetaminophen in the United States? The perspective of a committee member. *Clinical Toxicology.* **47**: 784–789.
26 Craig DG *et al.* (2012) Staggered overdose pattern and delay to hospital presentation are associated with adverse outcomes following paracetamol-induced hepatotoxicity. *British Journal of Clinical Pharmacology.* **73**: 285–294.
27 von Mach MA *et al.* (2005) Experiences of a poison center network with renal insufficiency in acetaminophen overdose: an analysis of 17 cases. *Clinical Toxicology.* **43**: 31–37.
28 MHRA (2012) Paracetamol overdose: new guidance on treatment with intravenous acetylcysteine. *Drug Safety Update.* www.gov.uk/drug-safety-update
29 British National Formulary *Emergency treatment of poisoning.* London: BMJ Group and Pharmaceutical Press www.medicinescomplete.com (accessed March 2014).
30 Antoine DJ and Dear JW (2016) How to treat paracetamol overdose and when to do it. *Expert Review of Clinical Pharmacology.* **9**: 633–635.
31 Buckley NA *et al.* (2016) Treatments for paracetamol poisoning. *British Medical Journal.* **353**: i2579.
32 Gomez-Moreno G *et al.* (2008) Interaction of paracetamol in chronic alcoholic patients. Importance for odontologists. *Medicina Oral, Patologia Oral Y Cirugia Bucal.* **13**: E235–238.
33 Riordan SM and Williams R (2002) Alcohol exposure and paracetamol-induced hepatotoxicity. *Addiction Biology.* **7**: 191–206.
34 FDA (2009) Liver injury related to the use of acetaminophen in both over-the-counter and prescription products. Advisory Committe Meeting (transcript). www.fda.gov/Drugs/DrugSafety
35 FDA (2014) All manufacturers of prescription combination drug products with more than 325mg of acetaminophen have discontinued marketing. Drug Safety and Availability www.fda.gov/Drugs/DrugSafety
36 Vrbova M *et al.* (2016) Characterization of acetaminophen toxicity in human kidney HK-2 cells. *Physiological Research.* **65**: 627–635.
37 Ghanem CI *et al.* (2016) Acetaminophen from liver to brain: New insights into drug pharmacological action and toxicity. *Pharmacological Research.* **109**: 119–131.
38 Prescott LF (1996) *Paracetamol (Acetaminophen) A Critical Bibliographic Review.* Taylor & Francis, London.
39 Hayward KL *et al.* (2016) Can paracetamol (acetaminophen) be administered to patients with liver impairment? *British Journal of Clinical Pharmacology.* **81**: 210–222.
40 UK Medicines Information (2012) What is the sodium content of medicines? *Q&As.* **145.4**: www.evidence.nhs.uk
41 Szczeklik A (1986) Analgesics, allergy and asthma. *Drugs.* **32**: 148–163.
42 Settipane R *et al.* (1995) Prevalence of cross-sensitivity with acetaminophen in aspirin-sensitive asthmatic subjects. *Journal of Allergy and Clinical Immunology.* **96**: 480–485.
43 Shin G *et al.* (2000) Paracetamol and asthma. *Thorax.* **55**: 882–884.
44 Caldeira D *et al.* (2015) How safe is acetaminophen use in patients treated with vitamin K antagonists? A systematic review and meta-analysis. *Thrombosis Research.* **135**: 58–61.
45 Hylek EM *et al.* (1998) Acetaminophen and other risk factors for excessive warfarin anticoagulation. *Journal of the American Medical Association.* **279**: 657–662.
46 Gebauer MG *et al.* (2003) Warfarin and acetaminophen interaction. *Pharmacotherapy.* **23**: 109–112.
47 Lopes RD *et al.* (2011) Warfarin and acetaminophen interaction: a summary of the evidence and biologic plausibility. *Blood.* **118**: 6269–6273.
48 Launiainen T *et al.* (2010) Adverse interaction of warfarin and paracetamol: evidence from a post-mortem study. *European Journal of Clinical Pharmacology.* **66**: 97–103.
49 Gastrup S *et al.* (2016) Paracetamol decreases steady-state exposure to lamotrigine by induction of glucuronidation in healthy subjects. *British Journal of Clinical Pharmacology.* **81**: 735–741.
50 Bhosale UA *et al.* (2015) Randomized, double-blind, placebo-controlled study to investigate the pharmacodynamic interaction of 5-HT3 antagonist ondansetron and paracetamol in postoperative patients operated in an ENT department under local anesthesia. *Journal of Basic and Clinical Physiology and Pharmacology.* **26**: 217–222.
51 Jokela R *et al.* (2010) The influence of ondansetron on the analgesic effect of acetaminophen after laparoscopic hysterectomy. *Clinical Pharmacology and Therapeutics.* **87**: 672–678.
52 Waldum H *et al.* (1992) Can NSAIDs cause acute biliary pain and cholestasis? *Journal of Clinical Gastroenterology.* **14**: 328–330.
53 Wong V *et al.* (1993) Paracetamol and acute biliary pain with cholestasis. *Lancet.* **342**: 869.
54 Watanabe H *et al.* (2016) Toxic epidermal necrolysis caused by acetaminophen featuring almost 100% skin detachment: Acetaminophen is associated with a risk of severe cutaneous adverse reactions. *Journal of Dermatology.* **43**: 321–324.
55 Leung R *et al.* (1992) Paracetamol anaphylaxis. *Clinical and Experimental Allergy.* **22**: 831–833.
56 Morgan S and Dorman S (2004) Paracetamol (acetaminophen) allergy. *Journal of Pain and Symptom Management.* **27**: 99–101.
57 Watkins PB *et al.* (2006) Aminotransferase elevations in healthy adults receiving 4 grams of acetaminophen daily: a randomized controlled trial. *Journal of the American Medical Association.* **296**: 87–93.
58 Dart RC and Bailey E (2007) Does therapeutic use of acetaminophen cause acute liver failure? *Pharmacotherapy.* **27**: 1219–1230.
59 D'Arcy P (1997) Paracetamol. *Adverse Drug Reaction Toxicology Review.* **16**: 9–14.

60 Fored CM *et al.* (2001) Acetaminophen, aspirin, and chronic renal failure. *New England Journal of Medicine.* **345**: 1801–1808.
61 Roberts E *et al.* (2016) Paracetamol: not as safe as we thought? A systematic literature review of observational studies. *Annals of Rheumatic Diseases.* **75**: 552–559.
62 Battagia A *et al.* (2016) Paracetamol: probably still a safe drug. *Annals of Rheumatic Diseases.* **10**: 1136.
63 Holgate ST (2011) The acetaminophen enigma in asthma. *American Journal of Respiratory Critical Care Medicine.* **183**: 147–148.
64 Shaheen S *et al.* (2000) Frequent paracetamol use and asthma in adults. *Thorax.* **55**: 266–270.
65 Ennis ZN *et al.* (2016) Acetaminophen for chronic pain: a systematic review on efficacy. *Basic and Clinical Pharmacology and Toxicology.* **118**: 184–189.
66 Williams CM *et al.* (2014) Efficacy of paracetamol for acute low-back pain: a double-blind, randomised controlled trial. *Lancet.* **384**: 1586–1596.
67 Tzortzopoulou A *et al.* (2011) Single dose intravenous propacetamol or intravenous paracetamol for postoperative pain. *Cochrane Database of Systematic Reviews.* **10**: CD007126. www.thecochranelibrary.com
68 Axelsson B and Christensen S (2003) Is there an additive analgesic effect of paracetamol at step 3? A double-blind randomized controlled study. *Palliative Medicine.* **17**: 724–725.
69 Israel FJ *et al.* (2010) Lack of benefit from paracetamol (acetaminophen) for palliative cancer patients requiring high-dose strong opioids: a randomized, double-blind, placebo-controlled, crossover trial. *Journal of Pain and Symptom Management.* **39**: 548–554.
70 Formby FT (2010) Re: lack of benefit from paracetamol (acetaminophen) for palliative cancer patients. *Journal of Pain and Symptom Management.* **40**: e6.
71 Stockler M *et al.* (2004) Acetaminophen (paracetamol) improves pain and well-being in people with advanced cancer already receiving a strong opioid regimen: a randomized, double-blind, placebo-controlled cross-over trial. *Journal of Clinical Oncology.* **22**: 3389–3394.
72 Dart RC and Rumack BH (2012) Intravenous acetaminophen in the United States: iatrogenic dosing errors. *Pediatrics.* **129**: 349–353.
73 Flouvat B *et al.* (2004) Bioequivalence study comparing a new paracetamol solution for injection and propacetamol after single intravenous infusion in healthy subjects. *International Journal of Clinical Pharmacology and Therapeutics.* **42**: 50–57.
74 Peduto VA *et al.* (1998) Efficacy of propacetamol in the treatment of postoperative pain. Morphine-sparing effect in orthopedic surgery. Italian Collaborative Group on Propacetamol. *Acta anaesthesiologica Scandinavica.* **42**: 293–298.

Updated September 2017

NEFOPAM

Class: Non-opioid analgesic, benzoxazocine.

Indications: Pain.

Contra-indications: Concurrent use of an MAOI, epilepsy.

Pharmacology

Nefopam is a centrally-acting synthetic analgesic. Its dominant mode of action is uncertain. Its effects are *not* reversed by **naloxone**. Nefopam does *not* inhibit cyclo-oxygenase (COX) or affect platelet function,[1] thereby making it a possible alternative if NSAIDs are contra-indicated. However, its acquisition cost is likely to limit use (see below).

Serotonin and noradrenaline (norepinephrine) re-uptake inhibition may explain its effect on descending pain modulatory pathways.[2] However, there are no reports of nefopam alone causing serotonin toxicity or with other serotoninergic drugs.[3] Nefopam also blocks voltage-gated sodium and calcium channels associated with glutamic acid, an excitatory neurotransmitter.[4,5] Antimuscarinic and sympathomimetic properties may account for some of its undesirable effects.

Nefopam is metabolized in the liver to an active metabolite, desmethylnefopam, which is renally eliminated.[6] In ESRF, clearance is reduced by 1/3–1/2, and peak plasma concentrations are increased 2–4 times, possibly because of secondary hepatic impairment.[7] Post-operatively, single parenteral doses provided analgesia for ≤5h.[8,9] However, pharmacological effects were seen for ≤12h after oral doses in healthy volunteers,[6] possibly reflecting the longer halflife of desmethylnefopam.

Nefopam is as effective as NSAIDs in cancer pain[10] and osteo-arthritis, but less well tolerated.[11] Given peri-operatively, nefopam reduces acute postoperative pain, including neuropathic pain, and the incidence of chronic postoperative pain.[12,13] In postoperative pain, IV or IM nefopam 20mg (equivalent to 60mg PO) is:

- comparable with NSAIDs, reducing **morphine** requirements in the first 24h by 10–15mg[14,15]
- comparable with **ketamine** 10mg[16]
- superior to **propacetamol** 2g.[17]

Nefopam does not consistently improve analgesia or reduce opioid requirements when combined with an NSAID ± **ketamine**.[18–21] Nefopam is reported to control refractory hiccup.[22,23]

Bio-availability 36%.
Onset of action <1h.
Time to peak plasma concentration 1–3h PO, 1.5h IM.
Plasma halflife 4–5h; desmethylnefopam 10–15h.[6]
Duration of action ≤12h PO; ≤5h IV.

Cautions

Hepatic and renal impairment (see Chapter 17, p.695); prostatism; closed angle glaucoma (antimuscarinic). Exacerbates the undesirable effects of concurrently administered antimuscarinic (see Antimuscarinics, Box C, p.7) or sympathomimetic agents.

Undesirable effects

Most common: nausea and vomiting, drowsiness, hypotension, epigastric pain.[10] In critical care, tachycardia and sweating was reported in ≤30% and ≤20% of patients respectively.[24] Sweating was also common in patients with rheumatoid arthritis.[25] However, in an RCT in cancer patients, tachycardia was noted in only 3%.[10]
Less common: diarrhoea, confusion and hallucinations (particularly in the elderly), tremor, paraesthesia, dizziness, syncope, seizures, palpitations, dry mouth, urinary retention.
Infrequent: blurred vision, insomnia, headache, pink discolouration of the urine.

Dose and use

- start with 60mg PO t.d.s. but 30mg PO t.d.s. in the elderly or ESRF (also see Chapter 17, p.695)[7] or 20mg IM q6h (not UK)
- if necessary, increase to 90mg PO t.d.s.
- for patients with swallowing difficulties, see Chapter 28, p.785.

Supply

Nefopam (generic)
Tablets 30mg, 28 days @ 60mg t.d.s. = £123.
Injection 10mg/mL, 2mL amp = £4. (Unauthorized, available to import, see Chapter 24, p.751); minimum order 30 amps.

---

1 Dordoni PL *et al.* (1994) Effect of ketorolac, ketoprofen and nefopam on platelet function. *Anaesthesia.* **49**: 1046–1049.
2 Gregori-Puigjane E *et al.* (2012) Identifying mechanism-of-action targets for drugs and probes. *Proceedings of the National Academy of Sciences of the United States of America.* **109**: 11178–11183.
3 Gillman K (2007) *Personal communication.*
4 Novelli A *et al.* (2005) Nefopam inhibits calcium influx, cGMP formation, and NMDA receptor-dependent neurotoxicity following activation of voltage sensitive calcium channels. *Amino Acids.* **28**: 183–191.
5 Verleye M *et al.* (2004) Nefopam blocks voltage-sensitive sodium channels and modulates glutamatergic transmission in rodents. *Brain Research Reviews.* **1013**: 249–255.
6 Aymard G *et al.* (2003) Comparative pharmacokinetics and pharmacodynamics of intravenous and oral nefopam in healthy volunteers. *Pharmacology and Toxicology.* **92**: 279–286.
7 Mimoz O *et al.* (2010) Nefopam pharmacokinetics in patients with end-stage renal disease. *Anaesthesia and Analgesia.* **111**: 1146–1153.
8 Beaver WT and Feise GA (1977) A comparison of the analgetic effect of intramuscular nefopam and morphine in patients with postoperative pain. *Journal of Clinical Pharmacology.* **17**: 579–591.
9 Phillips G and Vickers MD (1979) Nefopam in postoperative pain. *British Journal of Anaesthesia.* **51**: 961–965.
10 Minotti V *et al.* (1989) Double-blind evaluation of analgesic efficacy of orally administered diclofenac, nefopam, and acetylsalicylic acid (ASA) plus codeine in chronic cancer pain. *Pain.* **36**: 177–183.
11 Stamp J *et al.* (1989) A comparison of nefopam and flurbiprofen in the treatment of osteoarthrosis. *British Journal of Clinical Practice.* **43**: 24–26.
12 Ok YM *et al.* (2016) Nefopam reduces dysesthesia after percutaneous endoscopic lumbar discectomy. *Korean Journal of Pain.* **29**: 40–47.
13 Na HS *et al.* (2016) Preventive analgesic efficacy of nefopam in acute and chronic pain after breast cancer surgery: a prospective, double-blind, and randomized trial. *Medicine.* **95**: e3705.
14 Evans MS *et al.* (2008) Nefopam for the prevention of postoperative pain: quantitative systematic review. *British Journal of Anaesthesia.* **101**: 610–617.
15 Cindea I *et al.* (2012) Effect of intraoperative nefopam on acute pain management after major abdomnal surgery. *European Journal of Anaesthesiology.* **29**: 204.
16 Kapfer B *et al.* (2005) Nefopam and ketamine comparably enhance postoperative analgesia. *Anesthesia and Analgesia.* **100**: 169–174.
17 Mimoz O *et al.* (2001) Analgesic efficacy and safety of nefopam vs. propacetamol following hepatic resection. *Anaesthesia.* **56**: 520–525.
18 Delage N *et al.* (2005) Median effective dose (ED50) of nefopam and ketoprofen in postoperative patients: a study of interaction using sequential analysis and isobolographic analysis. *Anesthesiology.* **102**: 1211–1216.

19 Remerand F *et al.* (2013) Nefopam after total hip arthroplasty: role in multimodal analgesia. *Orthopaedics and Traumatology, Surgery and Research.* **99**: 169–174.
20 Moustafa F *et al.* (2013) Usefulness of nefopam in treating pain of severe uncomplicated renal colics in adults admitted to emergency units: a randomised double-blind controlled trial. The 'INCoNU' study. *Emergency Medicine Journal.* **30**: 143–148.
21 Moffat AC *et al.* (1990) Postoperative nefopam and diclofenac. Evaluation of their morphine-sparing effect after upper abdominal surgery. *Anaesthesia.* **45**: 302–305.
22 Bilotta F and Rosa G (2000) Nefopam for severe hiccups. *New England Journal of Medicine.* **343**: 1973–1974.
23 Bilotta F *et al.* (2001) Nefopam for refractory postoperative hiccups. *Anesthesia and Analgesia.* **93**: 1358–1360.
24 Chanques G *et al.* (2011) Analgesic efficacy and haemodynamic effects of nefopam in critically ill patients. *British Journal of Anaesthesia.* **106**: 336–343.
25 Emery P and Gibson T (1986) A double-blind study of the simple analgesic nefopam in rheumatoid arthritis. *British Journal of Rheumatology.* **25**: 72–76.

Updated September 2017

NON-STEROIDAL ANTI-INFLAMMATORY DRUGS (NSAIDS)

NSAIDs are essential drugs for cancer pain management. They are particularly useful when there is an inflammatory component, as is the case with most cancer pains.[1,2] The use of NSAIDs to relieve cancer pain is unauthorized.

Non-steroidal anti-inflammatory drugs (NSAIDs) prevent or reverse inflammation-induced hyperalgesia locally and in the CNS, thereby reducing pain.[3] There is also evidence from several RCTs that NSAIDs may be of benefit in *pure* (non-inflammatory) neuropathic pain.[4] However, because neuropathic pain in cancer is typically *mixed* nociceptive-neuropathic, benefit is more likely.

NSAIDs also have a major role in postoperative pain.[5,6] However, there is little high level evidence for benefit in some chronic pains, e.g. low back.[7]

All NSAIDs are antipyretic.[8] It is generally accepted that inhibition of cyclo-oxygenase (COX) is their main shared mechanism of action.[9]

Cyclo-oxygenase

There are two distinct cyclo-oxygenase (COX) isoforms.[10] COX-1 is mainly 'constitutive', i.e. physiological, with near constant levels and activity in most tissues, including the CNS. COX-2 is constitutive in parts of the CNS, renal cortex, stomach, uterus, cartilage, bone and seminal vesicles, and is massively inducible within a few hours by inflammation, dehydration or trauma (Figure 1).

COX-1 also plays an indispensable role in inflammation; and COX-2, although initially producing pro-inflammatory prostaglandins, later induces anti-inflammatory PGD_2.[11] Both peptic ulcer and bone healing require COX-2.[12,13]

Cyclo-oxygenase inhibition

Inflammation is associated with increased PG production both in the peripheral tissues and in the CNS.[14] The peripheral free nerve endings responsive to noxious stimuli become hypersensitive in the presence of inflammatory substances, increasing transduction and resulting in increased pain (*peripheral* sensitization).

Increased production of PGs in the CNS in response to a noxious stimulus leads to *central* sensitization of neurones in the dorsal horn, with further magnification of the noxious stimulus and more severe pain.[15–17] COX-2 plays a key role in central hyperalgesia.[18]

By inhibiting the production of COX, NSAIDs block the synthesis of PGs both peripherally in the tissues and in the CNS. The relative peripheral and central contributions to the total analgesic effect depends, among other things, on the NSAID in question, its pharmacokinetic characteristics, and the route of administration.[9]

NSAIDs also modify the endocannabinoid system. Endocannabinoids, like PGs, are produced *de novo* from arachidonic acid and are broken down by COX-2 (see p.229). Some NSAIDs (e.g. **ibuprofen**) inhibit other enzymes involved in endocannabinoid metabolism (e.g. fatty acid amide hydroxylase). The relative contribution of PG[19] and endocannabinoid systems to the analgesic effect of NSAIDs is uncertain.[20]

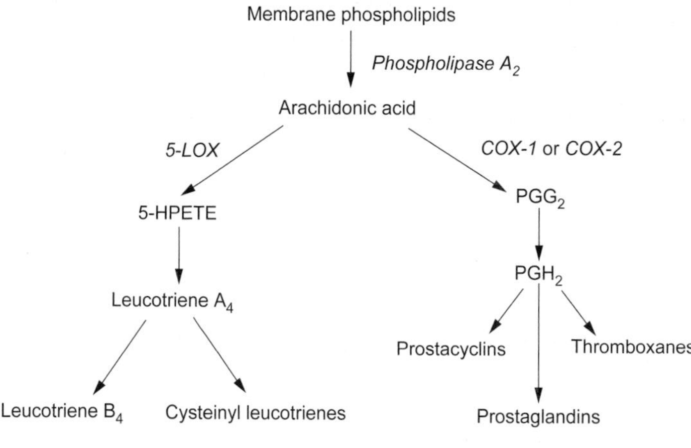

Figure 1 Products of arachidonic acid metabolism involved in inflammation.

COX = cyclo-oxygenase; 5-HPETE = hydroperoxyeicosatetrenoic acid; LOX = lipoxygenase; PG = prostaglandin.

Classification

NSAIDs are now generally classified on the basis of their relative ability to inhibit COX-1 and COX-2. The degree of COX-2 selectivity varies according to the assay used,[21,22] and whether the result is expressed in terms of 50 or 80% inhibition of the enzyme.[23,24] Although 80% inhibition is theoretically a better comparator, most studies use 50% (Table 1). However, the results of *in vitro* assays may not reliably reflect *in vivo* reality.[25] This is certainly the case in relation to **celecoxib**. Despite its relatively modest ranking (Table 1), no significant COX-1 inhibition is seen in volunteers taking 400mg b.d.[26] Dose and inter-patient variation are the main determinants of COX-2 selectivity *in vivo*.[27]

Table 1 COX-2 selectivity ratio of IC_{50} COX-1/COX-2 (human whole blood assays)[24]

Drug	*COX-2 selectivity ratio*
Etoricoxib	106
Celecoxib	7.6
Nimesulide[a]	7.3
Diclofenac	3.0
Etodolac	2.4
Meloxicam	2.0
Indometacin	0.4
Ibuprofen	0.2
Piroxicam	0.08

a. not UK.

Although it is more correct to think of a spectrum of selectivity,[21,23] it is customary to divide NSAIDs into several seemingly disparate categories (Table 2). Inevitably, there will be differences of opinion as to where the cut off between categories should come, particularly because selectivity is partly dose-dependent.[21] For example, with **meloxicam** 7.5mg/day, there is 70%

COX-2 and 7% COX-1 inhibition but, with 15mg/day, there is 80% COX-2 and 25% COX-1 inhibition.[28] Further, thromboxane B_2 production is reduced 66% by **meloxicam** 15mg/day, the result of COX-1 inhibition.[29]

Table 2 Classification of NSAIDS

Preferential COX-1 inhibitors	*Non-selective COX inhibitors*	*Preferential COX-2 inhibitors*	*Selective COX-2 inhibitors*
Flurbiprofen	Aspirin	Diclofenac	Celecoxib
Indometacin	Fenamates	Etodolac	Etoricoxib
Ketoprofen	Ibuprofen	Meloxicam	Parecoxib
Ketorolac	Nabumetone	Nimesulide (not UK)	
	Naproxen		
	Salicylates		

Additional sites of action

The anti-inflammatory properties of an NSAID are *not* predictive of its analgesic effect, suggesting that other mechanisms must be involved.[30] COX-independent actions are not all class effects, but include interactions with:

- synthesis and regulation of activity of dorsal horn neurotransmitters and modulators[31]
- modulation of pain transduction through spinal serotoninergic, adrenergic and cholinergic systems
- endocannabinoids
- nitric oxide production
- interleukin release
- caspase inhibition[32]
- matrix metalloproteinases.[30]

The matrix metalloproteinases (MMPs) are a family of enzymes which cleave the various components of the extracellular matrix. MMPs are activated by tissue plasminogen activator/plasmin, and are inactivated by endogenous tissue inhibitors of metalloproteinases (TIMPs). The dynamic interaction between MMPs and TIMPs determine their overall activity. MMPs can be both pro-inflammatory and anti-inflammatory, and the same MMP might have opposite roles in different circumstances.

PGs are involved in the regulation of MMP pathways. NSAIDs have different effects on MMPs and TIMPs in different inflammatory models. It is likely that the effects of NSAIDs on MMPs are both PG dependent and independent.[30]

NSAIDs also affect brain concentrations of kynurenic acid, an endogenous antagonist which acts on the glycine recognition site of the NMDA-receptor-channel complex.[33] **Diclofenac** (preferential COX-2 inhibitor) and **indometacin** (preferential COX-1 inhibitor) increase brain kynurenic acid concentrations, whereas **meloxicam** and **parecoxib** (preferential and selective COX-2 inhibitors respectively) cause a decrease. It is possible that at least some NSAIDs tonically modulate kynurenic acid metabolism, and thereby impact on central nociceptive mechanisms.

Clinically, non-selective and selective COX-2 inhibitors are equally effective.[34] On the other hand, in dental pain, there is a tendency for weak COX inhibitors to be superior to **aspirin** and for strong inhibitors to be inferior, emphasizing the importance of not adopting too simplistic a view of the mode of action of these drugs (Table 3).

Table 3 Analgesic efficacy of oral NSAIDs in dental pain compared with aspirin 650mg[35]

Significantly superior	*Not significantly different*	*Significantly inferior*
Azapropazone (3)[a,b]	Diclofenac (1)	Fenbufen (1)[b]
Diflunisal (3)[b]	Etodolac (1)	Nabumetone (1)
Flurbiprofen (1)	Sulindac (1)	Ketoprofen (2)
Ketorolac (3)[b]	Naproxen (3)	Tolmetin (3)[b]

a. numbers indicate capacity to inhibit PG synthesis: 1 = strong; 2 = moderate; 3 = weak

b. PO formulation no longer available in the UK.

NSAIDs and pyrexia

All NSAIDs are antipyretic.[8,36] Paraneoplastic fever responds to all NSAIDs, not just to **naproxen** as initially thought.[37] Although the antipyretic effect tends to wear off after a few months, further benefit may be obtained by switching to an alternative NSAID. However, the duration of benefit with second- and third-line drugs is generally shorter. For other options, see Chapter 1, Antimuscarinics, Box D (p.10).

NSAIDs and cancer

For many years, it has been suggested that cancer-associated symptoms such as anorexia, weight loss and cachexia are manifestations of a chronic systemic inflammatory response (see p.552).[38] However, evidence of benefit is not robust enough to recommend the routine use of NSAIDs in these circumstances.[39]

On the other hand, tumour-promoting inflammation is considered one of the enabling characteristics of cancer progression.[40] COX-2 is detectable in 40–50% of adenomas and in >80% of adenocarcinomas.[41,42] It is expressed within tumour vasculature as well as in colon, breast, prostate, and lung cancer cells.[43] COX-2-derived PGs contribute to tumour growth by inducing blood vessel formation (angiogenesis) which sustain tumour cell viability and growth.[43] NSAIDs suppress the production of these PGs, and thus inhibit tumour development. Epidemiological data suggest that NSAIDs, particularly coxibs, may *prevent* the development of certain cancers, including colorectal, oesophageal and lung.[44,45]

As a potential *treatment* for established cancer, a meta-analysis of 11 RCTs encompassing >2,500 patients with advanced cancer showed a significant increase in overall response rate to anticancer treatments in those prescribed 'add-on' celecoxib, although 1-year survival was unchanged.[46] A more recent RCT in >300 patients with non-small cell lung cancer (stage IIIB or IV) and moderate–high COX-2 expression also failed to show a survival benefit.[47] Almost all the trials used 400mg b.d., i.e. 2–4 times more than typical analgesic doses in arthritis.

Interestingly, the pro-apoptotic (cell death) effect of **celecoxib** does *not* rely on COX-2 inhibition.[48] **Celecoxib** induces cell death mainly by activation of an intrinsic mitochondria-dependent apoptosis pathway, independent of COX-2 inhibition.[48] With increased understanding of the specific mechanisms which regulate cancer-associated inflammation and apoptosis, it should become increasingly possible to alter the course of cancer with selective and targeted anti-inflammatory treatment without increasing the risk of CVS events.[49,50]

NSAIDs and platelet function

Platelets contain COX-1 but not COX-2. Thus, NSAIDs differ in their effect on platelet function and bleeding time (Table 4; also see p.319).

Table 4 NSAIDs, platelet function and bleeding time

Drug	*Comment*
Aspirin	Irreversible platelet dysfunction and prolonged bleeding time as a result of acetylation of platelet COX-1
Non-acetylated salicylates e.g. choline magnesium trisalicylate[a], salsalate[a]	No effect on platelet function or bleeding time at recommended doses
Classical NSAIDs (except diclofenac), e.g. flurbiprofen, ibuprofen, ketorolac, naproxen	Reversible platelet dysfunction and prolonged bleeding time
Diclofenac	Reversible inhibition of platelet aggregation in 2/3 of subjects.[52] IV diclofenac has a measurable effect on bleeding time, but most subjects remain within normal limits
Etodolac	No data
Meloxicam[54] Nabumetone Nimesulide[a,55] Coxibs[28]	No effect on platelet function or bleeding time

a. not UK.

Bleeding time is affected by various technical and clinical factors, is difficult to standardize,[51] and is a poor predictor of bleeding in invasive procedures.[52] Although there are other methods for measuring platelet function,[53] these have not completely clarified our understanding about the differing effects of NSAIDs on bleeding. However, COX-2 inhibitors, because they do not affect the COX-1 in platelets and because of their associated low risk of GI bleeding, are likely to be the safest NSAIDs in people with low platelet counts.

NSAIDs and depression

Clinical depression is a complex disorder characterized biochemically by increased levels of CRP and pro-inflammatory cytokines, including IL-6 and TNFα.[56] Further, in the rat, **rofecoxib** has been shown to increase serotonin in the frontal and temporoparietal cortex.[57] Thus, it is not surprising that it is claimed that NSAIDs, notably **celecoxib**, are of benefit in depression (and early schizophrenia) as 'add-on' medication.[58] However, the RCTs which have shown benefit in depressed subjects have typically been small numbers and short-term (e.g. 6 weeks), with significant risks of confounding and bias.[59,60]

It is possible that NSAIDs may decrease the risk of cognitive decline in the elderly.[61]

Undesirable effects

NSAIDs differ in their propensity to cause a range of undesirable effects. For convenience, these have been categorized as type A and type B. Generally, type A effects are mostly dose-dependent and partly predictable, whereas type B effects are mostly dose-independent and unpredictable (Table 5 and Table 6).

Quantitatively, the most serious undesirable effects are GI and CVS toxicity. *All* NSAIDs (both non-selective and COX-2 selective) increase the risk of both upper GI ulceration and major CVS events (non-fatal and fatal myocardial infarction or stroke), albeit to a varying degree.[62] However, particularly in advanced progressive disease, the benefit associated with greater comfort generally far outweighs the potential harm from GI or CVS complications.

NSAIDs and the GI tract

From studies in patients with mainly rheumatoid- and osteo-arthritis taking an NSAID (including **aspirin**) ± gastroprotection, for >2 *months*, the risk of a bleeding ulcer or perforation is about 1 in 500, and the risk of dying from gastroduodenal complications about 1 in 1,200 patients.[65] Given the higher risk in patients with rheumatoid arthritis, and the ability of gastroprotective drugs to reduce serious ulcer complications,[66] these figures probably *overestimate* the risks in cancer and other advanced disease.

Although all NSAIDs increase the risk of GI complications, their propensity varies. The most GI toxic NSAIDs are **azapropazone** (not UK), **ketorolac** (see p.340) and **piroxicam**.[67] Although prescription may be justifiable in specific circumstances (see Routes of administration, p.325), they should generally *not* be used.

A meta-analysis of several hundred RCTs indicates that, compared with placebo, the risk is less than doubled with **celecoxib** and **diclofenac**, but quadrupled with *high dose* **ibuprofen** (2,400mg/24h) and *high dose* **naproxen** (1,000mg/24h).[62]

Indeed, **celecoxib** carries a significantly *lower* risk of clinically important GI events *throughout the entire GI tract*.[68] **Nabumetone** is also low risk (see p.345).[69] Combining thromboprotective **aspirin** with **celecoxib** increases the GI risk, although less than combining with a non-selective NSAID.[70]

Stomach and duodenum

The relative risk of gastric ulcer when taking an NSAID is 5–6.[71] For duodenal ulceration, the relative risk is only 1.1, although a recent population-based nested case-control study suggested it is higher.[72]

Various factors affect gastroduodenal toxicity (Box A). How much of the benefit relates to COX-2 selectivity is uncertain.

In patients who are *H.pylori* positive, the risk of developing an NSAID-related ulcer is almost doubled, and the risk of bleeding trebled.[74] The explanation for this lies in the *H.pylori*-associated chronic atrophic gastritis (mainly affecting the antrum) and makes the extracellular matrix in that part of the stomach wall vulnerable to the back-diffusion of acid. Ionized NSAID molecules, circulating in the plasma, are transported passively through leaky capillary walls into the inflamed matrix where they become unionized in the acidic environment. In this state, the molecules are

Table 5 Type A ('predictable') reactions to NSAIDs[63]

Organ/system	*Clinical reaction*
Blood	Decreased platelet aggregation, prolonged bleeding time (see Table 4)
GI tract	Dyspepsia Peptic ulceration, bleeding, perforation Small bowel stricture, bleeding, perforation Exacerbation of inflammatory bowel disease Protein-losing enteropathy
Kidney	Salt and water retention
Cardiovascular	Thrombosis, e.g. myocardial infarction, stroke
Lung	Bronchospasm (asthma)

Table 6 Type B ('unpredictable') reactions to NSAIDs[63]

Organ/system	*Clinical reaction*	*Most likely NSAIDs*
Immunological	Anaphylaxis	Most NSAIDs
Skin	Morbilliform rash Angioedema	Fenbufen Ibuprofen Azapropazone Piroxicam
Blood	Thrombocytopenia	Diclofenac Ibuprofen Piroxicam
	Haemolytic anaemia	Mefenamic acid Diclofenac
GI tract	Diarrhoea	Fenamates, e.g. mefenamic acid
Kidney	Interstitial nephritis	Fenoprofen[64]
Liver	Reye's syndrome (in children) Hepatotoxicity	Aspirin Diclofenac Sulindac
CNS	Aseptic meningitis	Ibuprofen

Box A Factors intrinsic to NSAIDs which result in low gastroduodenal toxicity[73]

Competitive masking of COX-1 by inactive forms, e.g. *R*-ibuprofen, *R*-etodolac.

Weak/no uncoupling of oxidative phosphorylation
Low disruption of phospholipids in protective mucus and mucous membranes } non-acidic compounds, e.g. nabumetone, coxibs.

High protein-binding (less available).

Weak/no inhibition of platelet aggregation, e.g. non-acetylated salicylates, coxibs, meloxicam, and diclofenac sometimes.

lipid-soluble and they move freely into the mucosal cells where, at a higher pH, the molecules become ionized again and consequently trapped. The local high concentration of NSAID leads to inhibition of the production of gastroprotective COX-1 in the stomach mucosa.

Eradication of *H. pylori* infection will correct the atrophic gastritis and end the sequence of events initiated by acid back-diffusion. Thus, eradication of *H. pylori* makes all COX-1-inhibiting NSAIDs safer to use, halving the incidence of peptic ulcer disease.[74] However, when trying to prevent ulcer recurrence in patients on NSAIDs, *H.pylori* eradication is less effective than a PPI.[75]

Risk factors for an NSAID-related upper GI complication (i.e. ulceration, bleeding, perforation) are listed in Box B. For example, concurrent administration of a non-selective NSAID and **warfarin** increases the risk of bleeding >10 times. This is nearly 4 times that of **warfarin** alone or with a coxib.[76]

In rheumatoid arthritis, the risk of hospitalization and/or death increases progressively from 50 years.[71] Thus, compared with those under 50, the risk is twice as great in patients aged 50–65 years, 6 times greater in patients aged 65–75, and some 14 times greater in the over 75s. However, in rheumatoid arthritis there may well be other interacting risk factors. Thus, 65 years is widely considered to be the appropriate point for regarding age as a risk factor in other situations.

Box B Risk factors for NSAID-related upper GI complications[71,77]

Age >65 years (see text).

Peptic ulcer ± GI bleeding in the last year confirmed by endoscopy, or strong clinical suspicion, e.g. haematemesis, melaena.

Long-term use of maximum recommended doses of an NSAID.

Serious morbidity, e.g. cancer, diabetes mellitus, hypertension, CVS disease, hepatic impairment, renal impairment.

Concurrent use of a
- second GI irritant (e.g. corticosteroid)
- anticoagulant
- antiplatelet drug (e.g. aspirin, SSRI; see drug interactions).

Platelets <50 x 10^9/L.

Acid dyspepsia with an NSAID despite concurrent use of a gastroprotective drug.

Gastric infection with *H. pylori*.

Major reviews give the same ranking for GI protection:
- best = combination of a coxib plus PPI
- second best = coxib alone
- third best = nonselective NSAID plus PPI
- fourth best (because tolerability is poorer) = nonselective NSAID plus **misoprostol**.[78,79]

The difference between the latter three options is relatively small. One systematic review has suggested that an H_2 receptor antagonist may *not* offer significant gastroprotection.[79]

PPIs enable ulcer healing even if the NSAID is continued.[80] However, patients who develop an NSAID-related peptic ulcer should generally be switched to **celecoxib** (plus a PPI).[81]

Small bowel

NSAIDs can also cause small bowel ulceration, bleeding, and perforation. In addition, they can cause protein-losing enteropathy and thin annular strictures which may eventually reduce the bowel lumen to a pinhole.[82]

NSAID effects on the small bowel may be as important as NSAID gastropathy. In a capsule endoscopy study, macroscopic changes were found in more than two thirds of volunteers on a 2-week course of **diclofenac**. Used long-term (>3 months), similar numbers were seen with both non-selective COX and selective COX-2 inhibitors,[83] although the latter are probably safer in the short-term.[84,85] Other studies have given comparable results.[86–89]

Concurrent use of a PPI or H_2 antagonist is a risk factor (relative risk for PPIs = 2.7).[89] Thus, *although gastric acid-reducing drugs reduce the risk of gastroduodenal damage, they increase enteropathy.* As more is learned about the balance between gastroduodenal and small bowel risk, the prophylactic use of PPIs in patients prescribed an NSAID may come under scrutiny.

Changes in bowel permeability may be the root cause of NSAID enteropathy.[90] Prostaglandin deficiency (*not* achieved via COX inhibition) is important.[91,92] NSAIDs which undergo enterohepatic circulation (e.g. **diclofenac**, **indomethacin**, **piroxicam**) are significantly more likely to damage the bowel than NSAIDs which are not (**aspirin**, **nabumetone**, **sulindac**).[93]

Compared with non-selective NSAIDs, **celecoxib** is associated with a significantly lower risk of clinically important GI events *throughout the entire GI tract.*[68]

It is postulated that contact by the NSAID with the bowel wall damages the phosphatidylcholine in the mucosal cell membrane. Mitochondrial and endoplasmic reticulum damage decouples oxidative phosphorylation, leads to release of calcium, and the production of free radicals. The resulting leakiness of bowel mucosal membranes leads to an ingress of Gram negative bacteria, bile acids and proteolytic enzymes. The inflammation produced is mediated by neutrophils, and causes both local and distant damage.[94] It has been suggested that this is related to the shift in intestinal microflora seen when acid is suppressed.

Prevention of intestinal damage is still in its infancy. Agents being investigated include:

- **misoprostol**[95]
- isogladine,[96] a phosphodiesterase inhibitor
- lubiprostone,[97] suppresses the expression of inflammatory mediators via EP4 receptors
- rebamipide,[98] a free radical scavenger
- lactoferrin, a food constituent[99]
- *Lactobacillus.*

Large bowel

Non-selective NSAIDs can cause clinical relapse of inflammatory bowel disease (IBD, i.e. Crohn's disease and ulcerative colitis) within 7–10 days of taking the drugs in about 20% of patients with IBD.[100] The mechanism of the NSAID-induced relapse appears to involve dual inhibition of COX-1 and 2, similar to the mechanism underlying NSAID damage in the small bowel.[100] In relation to IBD, **celecoxib** and **etoricoxib** do not differ from placebo, and thus are first choice NSAIDs for patients with quiescent IBD.[101]

Women who use NSAIDs (but not aspirin) for >15 days a month for six years have an increased risk of developing inflammatory bowel disease *de novo.*[102] NSAIDs can also cause a colitis directly, and increase the risk of complications from diverticular disease.[103]

NSAIDs and the CVS system

All NSAIDs increase CVS risk, particularly in patients who are hypertensive, have had a previous myocardial infarction, or have undergone recent cardiac surgery.[104] The risk manifests in the first few weeks or months of use, but appears *not* to increase long-term.[105,106]

The focus for the last 10–15 years has been on selective COX-2 inhibitors. It was reported that, with coxibs, the number of additional major CVS events would be about 3/1,000 *per year of use*; and about 8/1,000 *per year of use* in high-risk patients, of which two would be fatal.[62] However, the analysis on which these figures were based included patients taking **rofecoxib**, withdrawn in 2004 because of an undisputed higher CVS risk.[107] Thus, these figures *overestimate* the risk with **celecoxib**. Indeed, it now appears that the risk with **celecoxib** is no higher, and may be lower, than with traditional non-selective NSAIDs.[106,107]

Further, another meta-analysis suggests that, in patients with an elevated CRP, *all* NSAIDs (*including* **celecoxib**) may *reduce* all-cause mortality and the risk of first myocardial infarction.[105]

Hypertension and heart failure

Except for **aspirin**, all NSAIDs raise blood pressure by a mean of 5–6mm Hg; this needs to be monitored in hypertensive patients.[108] The use of NSAIDs in heart failure carries a dose-dependent risk of death.[109]

NSAIDs increase the risk of heart failure necessitating hospital admission by up to 100%.[62,110] In a nested case-control study, high-dose **diclofenac** and high-dose **ibuprofen** doubled the odds, and the risk with high-dose **naproxen** was only slightly lower.[111] However, *no* increase was seen with **celecoxib** at commonly used doses (≤400mg/24h), although data are not available for high doses.[111] Thus, high-dose NSAIDs should generally be avoided in patients with chronic heart failure (CHF).

Major cardiac events (non-fatal and fatal myocardial infarction)

All NSAIDs carry a dose-dependent risk of acute myocardial infarction.[62, 112–114] However, three recent meta-analyses have radically altered our understanding of the relative risk.[105–107] Thus, despite the conclusions of the CNT meta-analysis,[62] it now appears that **celecoxib** carries *no* greater risk of acute myocardial infarction than non-selective NSAIDs

Of interest is the Danish nationwide review which indicated that **diclofenac** and **ibuprofen** (but *not* COX-2 inhibitors or **naproxen**) were associated with an increased risk of out-of-hospital cardiac arrest.[115] Further, although it has been generally considered that high-dose **naproxen** (500mg b.d.) was safer than other non-selective NSAIDs,[62] it now seems that the risk is essentially the same for **celecoxib**, **diclofenac**, **ibuprofen** and **naproxen**.[106]

Major cerebrovascular events (non-fatal and fatal stroke)

A systematic review of case-control and cohort studies indicates that the risk of haemorrhagic stroke is significant only for **diclofenac** and **meloxicam.**[116] However, the thromboprotective effect of low-dose **aspirin** for stroke is neutralized by NSAIDs other than **celecoxib**[117] and **naproxen.**[62] Thus, in someone taking **aspirin** thromboprophylaxis, these are the NSAIDs of choice.

NSAIDs and the kidneys

All NSAIDs cause an increase in Cl^- resorption from the proximal tubules, and enhance ADH activity, leading to sodium (Na^+) and water retention. Thus, NSAIDs antagonize the action of diuretics, and can exacerbate existing hypertension or lead to new onset hypertension.[118]

All NSAIDs can cause acute or acute-on-chronic renal failure (Box C).[119] The risk of a first ever episode of acute renal failure in NSAID users is three times that in non-users.[120] Sporadic cases of interstitial nephritis (± nephrotic syndrome or ± papillary necrosis) have been reported with most NSAIDs. The renal risks of different NSAIDs, including coxibs, are similar and thus are not a factor in determining choice.[121]

Box C Risk factors for NSAID-induced renal toxicity[122]

Age >60 years with co-morbidities.

Hypertension

Congestive heart failure

Dehydration, hypovolaemia

Multiple myeloma with Bence-Jones proteinuria[123,124]

Chronic and/or multiple NSAID use.

Concurrent use of diuretics and ACE inhibitors

Hyponatraemia

Cirrhosis, ascites

Nephrotic syndrome.

In hypovolaemia, the plasma concentrations of vasoconstrictor substances such as angiotensin II, noradrenaline (norepinephrine) and vasopressin increase. This would normally lead to increased vasodilator prostaglandin secretion in the kidneys to maintain renal perfusion. However, the inhibition of renal PG production by NSAIDs prevents this, thereby precipitating renal failure.[120,125]

Particularly in elderly patients with underlying chronic kidney disease, the concurrent use of diuretics, an ACE inhibitor or angiotensin receptor antagonist (ARA) and an NSAID ('triple whammy' medication) is a recognized cause of acute kidney injury (AKI).[126] Associated hypotension (e.g. intra-operative) dramatically increases the risk of AKI, and has been termed 'the quadruple whammy'.[127]

Thus, except in patients expected to die in a few days, dehydrated patients should be rehydrated when starting treatment with an NSAID, or an NSAID should not be used. AKI caused by NSAIDs is generally reversible if the drug is stopped promptly, but not always: it can be fatal.

In ESRF, NSAIDs should be avoided because of nephrotoxicity. However, in anuric patients on dialysis, they can be used in normal doses (see Chapter 17, p.695).

NSAIDs and the liver

Non-selective NSAIDs, but *not* **celecoxib,**[128] double the risk of bleeding from oesophageal varices because of their impact on platelet function (see p.315).[128]

Hepatotoxicity is a rare unpredictable effect seen with most NSAIDs, including coxibs. **Diclofenac** and **sulindac** may have the highest risk, and **ibuprofen** the least.[129]

Cholestasis may reduce the elimination of NSAIDs excreted in bile (**indometacin, sulindac**), and may reduce or delay absorption of fat-soluble NSAIDs, e.g. **ibuprofen.**[129]

Patients with hepatic impairment are more susceptible to NSAID-related renal impairment. Thus, most SPCs for NSAIDs include active liver disease or moderate–severe hepatic impairment as a contra-indication.[130]

For doses in hepatic impairment, see Chapter 18, Table 2, p.709.

5

NSAIDs and bronchospasm

Some patients, with or without a history of atopic asthma, give a history of **aspirin**- or NSAID-induced asthma. The prevalence, derived from oral provocation testing studies, is about 20% in the general adult population, and 5% in children.[131] Chronic non-aspirin NSAID users have almost double the risk of developing adult onset asthma.[132]

Genetic polymorphisms in prostanoid receptor genes[133] and leukotriene synthase genes[134] have been described in **aspirin**-induced asthmatics, suggesting that the asthma is caused by an **aspirin**-induced (COX-1 inhibitory) imbalance between bronchodilator PGE_2 and bronchoconstrictor leukotrienes, and is not immunologically mediated (as in atopic asthmatics).[135,136]

Aspirin-induced asthma typically occurs 30min–3h after ingestion of **aspirin**. Half of those affected react to even low-dose **aspirin** (80mg). Cross-sensitivity with other NSAIDs is normal, e.g. **diclofenac** (93%), **ibuprofen** (98%), **naproxen** (100%).[131] A history of allergic-type reactions (asthma, acute rhinitis, nasal polyps, angioedema, urticaria) with **aspirin** or other NSAID calls for extreme caution in prescribing a further NSAID (Table 7). Coxibs rarely induce asthma, and the cause is probably isolated idiosyncratic allergy and *not* cross-reactivity with **aspirin** or other NSAID.[137]

Table 7 Use of NSAIDs in asthmatic patients

Patient characteristics	*Recommendations*
Anyone who has ever had an asthmatic reaction to aspirin or a non-coxib NSAID; or anyone with high risk features of aspirin-induced asthma (severe asthma, nasal polyps, urticaria, or chronic rhinitis)	Avoid all products containing aspirin or a non-coxib NSAID; use paracetamol instead unless also contra-indicated. *Coxibs are almost always safe*, but give the first dose under medical supervision[138]
All other asthmatic patients	Any NSAID, including aspirin, may be considered but, if any respiratory reaction occurs, stop the NSAID and manage as above

Bronchospasm has not been observed with **choline salicylate** (available only as a dental gel and ear drops in the UK), **sodium salicylate** and **azapropazone** (both not UK); it is rare with **benzydamine** (available only as a mouthwash and throat spray in the UK).[139]

The incidence of cross-sensitivity to **paracetamol** is only 7%, and <2% of asthmatic patients are sensitive to both **aspirin** and **paracetamol.**[140] Further, reactions to **paracetamol** are generally less severe. Thus, **paracetamol** should always be the initial non-opioid of choice for asthmatic patients.

Management of NSAID-induced asthma is the same as for other acute asthma attacks (see p.107). Leukotriene receptor inhibitors, e.g. **montelukast**, should be considered.[141] **Omalizumab**, an anti-IgE monoclonal antibody, may also be of benefit.[142]

Some patients may have been treated by **aspirin** desensitization.[143] Such patients will be on daily **aspirin** and can safely take an NSAID without provoking an attack. It is essential *not* to stop the **aspirin** in such patients or sensitization may return.

NSAIDs and bone healing

Some NSAIDs (**indometacin**, **diclofenac**, **tenoxicam**) delay bone healing in animals, but this has not been seen in others (**ibuprofen**, **ketorolac**, **piroxicam**).[144] The clinical impact of this is uncertain, and human data are very limited. However, there is evidence that long-term NSAID use is associated with an increased risk of non-union of fractures.[145] Further, even when used for only 2–5 days, NSAIDs decrease heterotopic (ectopic) bone formation, commonly seen after major hip surgery.[145,146]

Some orthopaedic departments prohibit the use of NSAIDs, including coxibs, for up to 6 weeks postoperatively. There is evidence for impairment in healing with high doses of both non-selective and selective NSAIDs.[144] Thus, when using NSAIDs after fracture or orthopaedic surgery, it would be sensible to use the lowest effective dose for as short a time as necessary. For example, limit the use of an NSAID to ≤10 days, and then discontinue until healing is complete. However, in patients with other risk factors for delayed union or non-union (e.g. smoking, diabetes mellitus, corticosteroids), use **paracetamol** instead.[144] On the other hand, if pain relief is inadequate when using both **paracetamol** and an opioid, an NSAID should be prescribed (instead of the **paracetamol**) despite its potential negative impact.

Contra-indications for NSAIDs

Although the SPCs are not completely consistent in this respect, the following is a general list of contra-indications for NSAIDs:

- hypersensitivity to **aspirin** or other NSAID (urticaria, rhinitis, asthma, angioedema)
- active GI ulceration, bleeding, perforation or inflammation
- severe heart failure
- active liver disease or moderate–severe hepatic impairment
- severe renal impairment (creatinine clearance <30mL/min), deteriorating renal function, hyperkalemia (>5mmol/L).

These contra-indications are not necessarily absolute. There may well be occasions when 'contra-indication' means 'use with great caution in the absence of a safer alternative'. **Diclofenac** and **celecoxib** are both contra-indicated in patients with established CVS disease.

Important drug–drug interactions

Pharmacodynamic

Many pharmacodynamic interactions can be predicted from the mode of action and undesirable effects of NSAIDs:

- increased risk of renal toxicity with other renally toxic drugs, e.g. aminoglycosides, **ciclosporin**
- increased risk of bleeding due to anti-platelet or anti-clotting effects, e.g. SNRIs, SSRIs, LMWH, **warfarin**
- increased risk of upper GI complications e.g. concurrent prescription of low-dose **aspirin**, corticosteroids or **warfarin**
- antagonistic effect of NSAIDs due to Na^+ and fluid retention, e.g. antihypertensives and diuretics
- antagonistic effect of some NSAIDs with thromboprotective effect of low-dose **aspirin** (see individual NSAID monographs)
- antagonistic effect of NSAIDs with the uricosuric drug **probenecid**.

Compared with an SSRI alone *in low risk patients*, concurrent use of an NSAID and an SSRI quadruples the incidence of upper GI bleeding (NNH >600),[147] and perhaps also intracranial haemorrhage.[148]

However, in those with additional risk factors (including many palliative care patients; see Box B, p.318), the NNH is <200. Consider using a non-serotoninergic antidepressant when possible (e.g. **mirtazapine**, **nortriptyline**).[149]

Pharmacokinetic

Pharmacokinetic interactions are summarized in Tables 8 and 9 (also see p.717). Topical NSAIDs are unlikely to reach sufficient plasma concentrations to interact with other drugs.

NSAIDs can significantly affect the plasma concentrations of renally excreted drugs by causing reduced renal function and/or reduced tubular excretion. Of particular importance is the risk of toxic plasma concentrations of aminoglycosides, **ciclosporin**, **digoxin**, **lithium**, and **methotrexate** (see Table 8).

Table 8 Pharmacokinetic interactions: NSAIDs affecting other drugs[150,154]

Drug affected	*Effect of NSAIDs*	*Clinical implications*
Aminoglycosides	May reduce renal function in susceptible individuals, thus reducing aminoglycoside clearance and increasing plasma concentration	Monitor aminoglycoside plasma concentration and renal function; adjust dose accordingly
Ciclosporin	May inhibit the renal prostacyclin synthesis needed to maintain glomerular filtration and renal blood flow. Increased and decreased ciclosporin plasma concentration reported	Monitor ciclosporin plasma concentration and renal function; adjust dose accordingly
Digoxin	May precipitate renal failure, particularly in those with heart failure, thus reducing digoxin excretion and increasing digoxin plasma concentration	Increased risk of digoxin toxicity. Monitor digoxin plasma concentration and renal function; adjust dose accordingly
Lithium	May inhibit renal excretion of lithium, increasing plasma lithium concentration	Increased risk of lithium toxicity. Avoid NSAID if possible; alternatively halve dose of lithium and monitor lithium plasma concentration. *Ketorolac is contra-indicated*
Methotrexate	Competitively inhibit the tubular excretion of methotrexate and inhibit PGE_2 synthesis, reducing renal perfusion; both increase methotrexate plasma concentration. Effect varies between NSAIDs and individuals	Increased risk of methotrexate toxicity. *Fatalities have occurred* (see text). Avoid aspirin and other salicylates during chemotherapy; probably safe between pulses. Use other NSAIDs with caution. Much lower risk with low-dose chronic methotrexate therapy used in psoriasis or rheumatoid arthritis and if no pre-existing renal impairment. Monitor methotrexate dose and its haematological effects
Phenytoin	May displace phenytoin from plasma proteins. May inhibit liver enzymes responsible for phenytoin metabolism	Clinical significance uncertain because the excess free phenytoin may be metabolized by the liver. However, phenytoin toxicity can develop even when the plasma concentration is still within the therapeutic range
Sulfonylureas	May inhibit renal tubular excretion, increasing sulfonylurea plasma concentration and hypoglycaemic effect	Reduce sulfonylurea dose if necessary
Valproate	May displace valproate from plasma proteins, inhibit valproate metabolism and increase plasma concentration	Avoid aspirin. Importance of interaction with other NSAIDs unclear; reduce the dose of valproate if toxicity suspected
Warfarin	May inhibit metabolism of warfarin and increase INR	Isolated cases reported with most NSAIDs (including coxibs); check INR closely during the first week after starting an NSAID and weekly for the next 3–4 weeks, increases of up to 60% have been reported; reduce dose of warfarin if necessary; *ketorolac is contra-indicated*
Zidovudine	May increase the risk of haematological toxicity, particularly in haemophiliacs treated with ibuprofen	Monitor blood count

Table 9 Pharmacokinetic interactions: other drugs affecting NSAIDs[150,154]

Drug implicated	*NSAIDs affected*	*Effect*	*Clinical implications*
Antacids	All e/c NSAIDs	Destruction of enteric coating	Administer at different times
Antacids	?All NSAIDs except celecoxib and diclofenac	Variable. Aluminum-containing antacids can *reduce* rate and/or extent of absorption of fenamates, diflunisal, indometacin and naproxen Magnesium hydroxide alone can *increase* the absorption of ibuprofen and flurbiprofen; also increases gastric toxicity of ibuprofen Sodium bicarbonate *increases* naproxen absorption	Avoid aluminium-containing antacids or use an alternative NSAID
Ciclosporin	Diclofenac	*Increased* plasma concentration of diclofenac due to reduced first-pass metabolism	Halve the dose of diclofenac
Colestyramine	All NSAIDs	Anion exchange resin binds NSAIDs in the GI tract, reducing and/or delaying absorption Binding in GI tract prevents enterohepatic recycling and increases faecal loss, even if NSAID administered IV (meloxicam, piroxicam, tenoxicam, sulindac)	Separate administration of PO NSAIDs by 4h. Colestyramine may be used to speed removal of NSAID after overdose
Fluconazole	Celecoxib Flurbiprofen Ibuprofen	*Increased* plasma concentration due to CYP2C9 inhibition by fluconazole	Halve the dose of celecoxib. Lower doses of flurbiprofen and ibuprofen may be necessary
Probenecid	?All NSAIDs	Reduced metabolism and renal clearance of NSAIDs and glucuronide metabolite which are hydrolyzed back to parent drug; NSAIDs also reduce the uricosuric effect of probenecid	Increased toxicity seen with indometacin, particularly if renal function impaired. Consider a reduction in NSAID dose but could be used therapeutically to increase the response. *Ketorolac is contra-indicated with probenecid*
Rifampicin	Celecoxib Diclofenac	*Decreased* plasma concentration due to CYP3A4 induction by rifampicin	Consider alternative NSAID if pain returns
Ritonavir	Piroxicam ?Other NSAIDs	*Increased* plasma concentration of piroxicam with increased risk of toxicity	Manufacturer of ritonavir advises against concurrent use with prioxicam
Voriconazole	Diclofenac Flurbiprofen Ibuprofen	*Increased* plasma concentration due to CYP2C9 inhibition and reduced clearance by voriconazole	Lower doses of NSAID may be necessary

Fatalities or severe renal failure have occurred when **methotrexate** has been prescribed concurrently with an NSAID, e.g. **aspirin**, **ibuprofen**, **indometacin**, **ketoprofen**, **naproxen**, and life-threatening neutropenia has been reported with several NSAIDs.[150] However, a systematic review has suggested that, apart from anti-inflammatory doses of **aspirin**, concurrent use is generally safe, although monitoring is recommended.[151]

NSAIDs can interact with **warfarin**, resulting in an increased INR; increases of up to 60% have been reported.[152,153] Patients should have their INR closely monitored during the first week after starting an NSAID and weekly for the next 3–4 weeks. The interaction may be due to CYP2C9 inhibition or competitive metabolism and may be more significant in those who are poor CYP2C9 metabolizers (see p.720).

There are few clinically significant interactions of drugs affecting the pharmacokinetics of NSAIDs (see Table 9).

Choice of PO NSAID

NSAIDs are essential drugs for cancer pain management. As with all drugs, it is important to reduce risk as much as possible. Thus, for each patient, select the safest drug and, when indicated, prescribe gastroprotection.

It is unclear if some cancer patients obtain more benefit from one particular NSAID, as is anecdotally reported in rheumatoid arthritis, or whether any apparent differences simply relate to a relative increase in inhibition of PG synthesis.

In practice, the choice of NSAID will depend on factors such as availability, safety, cost, and local guidelines. The renal risks of different NSAIDs, including coxibs, are similar and are *not* a factor in determining choice.[121]

Celecoxib

As already noted, recent reviews of CVS risk indicate that **celecoxib** ≤400mg/24h is *not* more cardiotoxic than non-selective NSAIDs (see p.319). Thus, given its undisputed low risk of upper GI complications, **celecoxib** 100–200mg b.d. is now probably *the overall NSAID of choice in palliative care* (see p.330). Generic **celecoxib** is available, and only high GI risk patients need a PPI concurrently (see p.316).

Celecoxib also has no effect on bleeding time, and is thus a good choice in patients with thrombocytopenia (see p.315).

Other NSAIDs

Other frequently used NSAIDs include **ibuprofen** (p.337), **diclofenac** (p.332) and **naproxen** (p.343).

For high GI risk patients, gastroprotection, e.g. a PPI, should be prescribed concurrently (see p.316).

Although traditionally advised to take NSAIDs with food, there is no evidence that this reduces the risk of GI complications. Further, food may delay the absorption of an NSAID, which could be relevant when treating acute pain (see p.658).

Route of administration

In patients expected to die within 1–2 days, it is generally possible to discontinue NSAID use without a resurgence of pain. However, SC or PR administration can be used if an NSAID is required and the PO route is not feasible

SC Injection

Some centres use **diclofenac** CSCI (p.332), **parecoxib** 40mg SC once daily or **parecoxib** 40–80mg/24h CSCI when the PO route is not feasible.[155–157]

By CSCI, **parecoxib** is given alone and diluted to a volume of 22mL using 0.9% normal saline to reduce the risk of a site reaction; p.r.n. SC doses of 10–20mg are allowed as long as the maximum daily dose is not exceeded. When used for longer periods, most patients are prescribed gastroprotection, although this may be unnecessary.[156]

Although its GI risk is significantly higher, **ketorolac** (p.340) is also used for this purpose.[155] Further, anecdotal experience suggests that CSCI **ketorolac** may be more effective than a PO NSAID in some patients, notably (but not always) for bone pain.[158] Gastro-protection is essential.

Rectal suppositories

The rectal route is used less than in the past, but remains an option:

- **diclofenac** suppositories 50mg t.d.s.
- **indometacin** suppositories 100mg b.d.

Supply

Parecoxib

Dynastat® (Pfizer)

Injection (powder for reconstitution) 40mg, 1 vial = £5.50.

1 McNicol E *et al.* (2004) Nonsteroidal anti-inflammatory drugs, alone or combined with opioids, for cancer pain: a systematic review. *Journal of Clinical Oncology*. **22**: 1975–1992.

2 Shah S and Hardy J (2001) Non-steroidal anti-inflammatory drugs in cancer pain: a review of the literature as relevant to palliative care. *Progress in Palliative Care*. **9**: 3–7.

3 Guindon J and Beaulieu P (2006) Antihyperalgesic effects of local injections of anandamide, ibuprofen, rofecoxib and their combinations in a model of neuropathic pain. *Neuropharmacology*. **50**: 814–823.

4 Vo T *et al.* (2009) Non-steroidal anti-inflammatory drugs for neuropathic pain: how do we explain continued widespread use? *Pain*. **143**: 169–171.

5 Jirarattanaphochai K and Jung S (2008) Nonsteroidal antiinflammatory drugs for postoperative pain management after lumbar spine surgery: a meta-analysis of randomized controlled trials. *Journal of Neurosurgery Spine*. **9**: 22–31.

6 Derry C *et al.* (2009) Single dose oral ibuprofen for acute postoperative pain in adults. *Cochrane Database of Systematic Reviews*. **3**: CD001548. www.thecochranelibrary.com

7 Enthoven WT *et al.* (2016) Non-steroidal anti-inflammatory drugs for chronic low back pain. *Cochrane Database of Systematic Reviews*. **2**: CD012087. www.thecochranelibrary.com

8 Simmons DL *et al.* (2000) Nonsteroidal anti-inflammatory drugs, acetaminophen, cyclooxygenase 2, and fever. *Clinical Infectious Diseases*. **31 (Suppl 5)**: S211–218.

9 Burian M and Geisslinger G (2005) COX-dependent mechanisms involved in the antinociceptive action of NSAIDs at central and peripheral sites. *Pharmacology and Therepeutics*. **107**: 139–154.

10 Simmons DL *et al.* (2004) Cyclooxygenase isozymes: the biology of prostaglandin synthesis and inhibition. *Pharmacological Reviews*. **56**: 387–437.

11 Kapoor M *et al.* (2005) Possible anti-inflammatory role of COX-2-derived prostaglandins: implications for inflammation research. *Current Opinion in Investigational Drugs*. **6**: 461–466.

12 Gerstenfeld LC and Einhorn TA (2004) COX inhibitors and their effects on bone healing. *Expert Opinion on Drug Safety*. **3**: 131–136.

13 Peskar BM (2005) Role of cyclooxygenase isoforms in gastric mucosal defense and ulcer healing. *Inflammopharmacology*. **13**: 15–26.

14 Schwab JM and Schluesener HJ (2003) Cyclooxygenases and central nervous system inflammation: conceptual neglect of cyclooxygenase 1. *Archives of Neurology*. **60**: 630–632.

15 Baba H *et al.* (2001) Direct activation of rat spinal dorsal horn neurons by prostaglandin E2. *Journal of Neuroscience*. **21**: 1750–1756.

16 Samad T *et al.* (2001) Interleukin-1B-mediated induction of COX-2 in the CNS contributes to inflammatory pain hypersensitivity. *Nature*. **410**: 471–475.

17 Farooqui M *et al.* (2007) COX-2 inhibitor celecoxib prevents chronic morphine-induced promotion of angiogenesis, tumour growth, metastasis and mortality, without compromising analgesia. *British Journal of Cancer*. **97**: 1523–1531.

18 Jain NK *et al.* (2008) COX-2 expression and function in the hyperalgesic response to paw inflammation in mice. *Prostaglandins Leukotrienes and Essential Fatty Acids*. **79**: 183–190.

19 Severine Vandevoorde (2008) Overview of the chemical families of fatty acid amide hydrolase and monoacylglycerol lipase inhibitors. *Current Topics in Medicinal Chemistry*. **8**: 247–267.

20 Telleria-Diaz A *et al.* (2010) Spinal antinociceptive effects of cyclooxygenase inhibition during inflammation: Involvement of prostaglandins and endocannabinoids. *Pain*. **148**: 26–35.

21 Churchill L *et al.* (1996) Selective inhibition of human cyclo-oxygenase-2 by meloxicam. *Inflammopharmacology*. **4**: 125–135.

22 Brooks P *et al.* (1999) Interpreting the clinical significance of the differential inhibition of cyclooxygenase-1 and cyclooxygenase-2. *Rheumatology*. **38**: 779–788.

23 Warner T *et al.* (1999) Nonsteroidal drug selectivities for cyclo-oxygenase-1 rather than cyclo-oxygenase-2 are associated with human gastrointestinal toxicity: a full in vitro analysis. *Proceedings of the National Academy of Science USA*. **96**: 7563–7568.

24 Riendeau D *et al.* (2001) Etoricoxib (MK-0663): Preclinical profile and comparison with other agents that selectively inhibit cyclooxygenase-2. *Journal of Pharmacology and Experimental Therapeutics*. **296**: 558–566.

25 Blain H *et al.* (2002) Limitation of the in vitro whole blood assay for predicting the COX selectivity of NSAIDs in clinical use. *British Journal of Clinical Pharmacology*. **53**: 255–265.

26 Fries S *et al.* (2006) Marked interindividual variability in the response to selective inhibitors of cyclooxygenase-2. *Gastroenterology*. **130**: 55–64.

27 Capone ML *et al.* (2007) Pharmacodynamic of cyclooxygenase inhibitors in humans. *Prostaglandins Other Lipid Mediators*. **82**: 85–94.

28 vanHecken A *et al.* (2000) Comparative inhibitory activity of rofecoxib, meloxicam, diclofenac, ibuprofen and naproxen on COX-2 versus COX-1 in healthy volunteers. *Journal of Clinical Pharmacology*. **40**: 1109–1120.

29 deMeijer A *et al.* (1999) Meloxicam, 15mg/day, spares platelet function in healthy volunteers. *Clinical Pharmacology and Therapeutics*. **66**: 425–430.

30 Hamza M and Dionne RA (2009) Mechanisms of non-opioid analgesics beyond cyclooxygenase enzyme inhibition. *Current Molecular Pharmacology*. **2**: 1–14.

31 McCormack K (1994) Nonsteroidal anti-inflammatory drugs and spinal nociceptive processing. *Pain*. **59**: 9–43.

32 Smith CE *et al.* (2017) Non-steroidal Anti-inflammatory Drugs Are Caspase Inhibitors. *Cell Chemical Biology*. **24**: 281–292.

33 Schwieler L *et al.* (2005) Prostaglandin-mediated control of rat brain kynurenic acid synthesis - opposite actions by COX-1 and COX-2 isoforms. *Journal of Neural Transmission*. **112**: 863–872.

34 Dougados M *et al.* (2001) Evaluation of the structure-modifying effects of diacerein in hip osteoarthritis: ECHODIAH, a three-year, placebo-controlled trial. Evaluation of the Chondromodulating Effect of Diacerein in OA of the Hip. *Arthritis and Rheumatism*. **44**: 2539–2547.

35 McCormack K and Brune K (1991) Dissociation between the antinociceptive and anti-inflammatory effects of the nonsteroidal anti-inflammatory drugs: a survey of their analgesic efficacy. *Drugs*. **41**: 533–547.

36 Kathula SK *et al.* (2003) Cyclo-oxygenase II inhibitors in the treatment of neoplastic fever. *Supportive Care in Cancer*. **11**: 258–259.

37 Tsavaris N *et al.* (1990) A randomized trial of the effect of three nonsteroidal anti-inflammatory agents in ameliorating cancer-induced fever. *Journal of Internal Medicine*. **228**: 451–455.

38 Roxburgh CS and McMillan DC (2014) Cancer and systemic inflammation: treat the tumour and treat the host. *British Journal of Cancer*. **110**: 1409–1412.

39 Reid J *et al.* (2013) Non-steroidal anti-inflammatory drugs for the treatment of cancer cachexia: a systematic review. *Palliative Medicine*. **27**: 295–303.

40 Diakos CI *et al.* (2014) Cancer-related inflammation and treatment effectiveness. *Lancet Oncology*. **15**: e493–503.

41 Eberhart CE *et al.* (1994) Up-regulation of cyclooxygenase 2 gene expression in human colorectal adenomas and adenocarcinomas. *Gastroenterology*. **107**: 1183–1188.

42 Koki AT *et al.* (1999) Potential utility of COX-2 inhibitors in chemoprevention and chemotherapy. *Expert Opinion on Investigational Drugs*. **8**: 1623–1638.

43 Masferrer JL *et al.* (2000) Antiangiogenic and antitumor activities of cyclooxygenase-2 inhibitors. *Cancer Research*. **60**: 1306–1311.

44 Liao X *et al.* (2012) Aspirin use, tumor PIK3CA mutation, and colorectal-cancer survival. *New England Journal of Medicine*. **367**: 1596–1606.

45 Liao Z *et al.* (2007) Cyclo-oxygenase-2 and its inhibition in cancer: is there a role? *Drugs*. **67**: 821–845.

46 Chen J *et al.* (2014) Efficacy and safety profile of celecoxib for treating advanced cancers: a meta-analysis of 11 randomized clinical trials. *Clinical Therapeutics*. **36**: 1253–1263.

47 Edelman MJ *et al.* (2017) Phase III Randomized, Placebo-Controlled, Double-Blind Trial of Celecoxib in Addition to Standard Chemotherapy for Advanced Non-Small-Cell Lung Cancer With Cyclooxygenase-2 Overexpression: CALGB 30801 (Alliance). *Journal of Clinical Oncology*. **35**: 2184–2192.

48 Jendrossek V (2013) Targeting apoptosis pathways by Celecoxib in cancer. *Cancer Letters*. **332**: 313–324.

49 Chavez C and Hoffman MA (2013) Complete remission of ALK-negative plasma cell granuloma (inflammatory myofibroblastic tumor) of the lung induced by celecoxib: A case report and review of the literature. *Oncol Letters*. **5**: 1672–1676.

50 Mercurio S *et al.* (2013) Evidence for new targets and synergistic effect of metronomic celecoxib/fluvastatin combination in pilocytic astrocytoma. *Acta Neuropathologica Communications*. **1**: 17.

51 Peterson P *et al.* (1998) The preoperative bleeding time test lacks clinical benefit: College of American Pathologists' and American Society of Clinical Pathologists' position article. *Archives of Surgery*. **133**: 134–139.

52 Ng KF *et al.* (2008) Comprehensive preoperative evaluation of platelet function in total knee arthroplasty patients taking diclofenac. *Journal of Arthroplasty*. **23**: 424–430.

53 Brass L (2010) Understanding and evaluating platelet function. *Hematology/ the Education Program of the American Society of Hematology Education Program*. **2010**: 387–396.

54 Guth B *et al.* (1996) Therapeutic doses of meloxicam do not inhibit platelet aggregation in man. *Rheumatology in Europe*. **25**: Abstract 443.

55 Cullen L *et al.* (1997) Selective suppression of cyclooxygenase-2 during chronic administration of nimesulide in man. In: *Fourth International Congress on essential fatty acids and eicosanoids*; Edinburgh.

56 Maes M (2012) Targeting cyclooxygenase-2 in depression is not a viable therapeutic approach and may even aggravate the pathophysiology underpinning depression. *Metabolic Brain Disease*. **27**: 405–413.

57 Sandrini M *et al.* (2002) Effect of rofecoxib on nociception and the serotonin system in the rat brain. *Inflammation Research*. **51**: 154–159.

58 Muller N (2013) The role of anti-inflammatory treatment in psychiatric disorders. *Psychiatria Danubina*. **25**: 292–298.

59 Kohler O *et al.* (2014) Effect of anti-inflammatory treatment on depression, depressive symptoms, and adverse effects: a systematic review and meta-analysis of randomized clinical trials. *JAMA Psychiatry*. **71**: 1381–1391.

60 Eyre HA *et al.* (2015) A critical review of the efficacy of non-steroidal anti-inflammatory drugs in depression. *Progress in Neuropsychopharmacology and Biological Psychiatry*. **57**: 11–16.

61 Wang W *et al.* (2016) Association between non-steroidal anti-inflammatory drug use and cognitive decline: a systematic review and meta-analysis of prospective cohort studies. *Drugs and Aging*. **33**: 501–509.

62 CNT Collaboration (2013) Vascular and upper gastrointestinal effects of non-steroidal anti-inflammatory drugs: meta-analyses of individual participant data from randomised trials. *Lancet*. **382**: 769–779.

63 Rawlins M (1997) Non-opioid analgesics. In: D Doyle *et al.* (eds) *Oxford Textbook of Palliative Medicine* (2e). Oxford University Press, Oxford, pp. 355–361.

64 Rossert J (2001) Drug-induced acute interstitial nephritis. *Kidney International*. **60**: 804–817.

65 Tramer M *et al.* (2000) Quantitative estimation of rare adverse events which follow a biological progression: a new model applied to chronic NSAID use. *Pain*. **85**: 169–182.

66 Silverstein FE *et al.* (1995) Misoprostol reduces serious gastrointestinal complications in patients with rheumatoid arthritis receiving nonsteroidal anti-inflammatory drugs. *Annals of Internal Medicine*. **123**: 241–249.

67 Castellsague J *et al.* (2012) Individual NSAIDs and upper gastrointestinal complications: a systematic review and meta-analysis of observational studies (the SOS project). *Drug Safety*. **35**: 1127–1146.

68 Moore A *et al.* (2013) Patient-level pooled analysis of adjudicated gastrointestinal outcomes in celecoxib clinical trials: meta-analysis of 51,000 patients enrolled in 52 randomized trials. *Arthritis Research and Therapy*. **15**: R6.

69 Bannwarth B (2008) Safety of the nonselective NSAID nabumetone : focus on gastrointestinal tolerability. *Drug Safety*. **31**: 485–503.

70 Strand V (2007) Are COX-2 inhibitors preferable to non-selective non-steroidal anti-inflammatory drugs in patients with risk of cardiovascular events taking low-dose aspirin? *Lancet*. **370**: 2138–2151.

71 Fries J *et al.* (1991) Nonsteroidal anti-inflammatory drug-associated gastropathy: incidence and risk factor models. *American Journal of Medicine.* **91**: 213–222.
72 Garcia Rodriguez LA and Hernandez-Diaz S (2004) Risk of uncomplicated peptic ulcer among users of aspirin and nonaspirin nonsteroidal antiinflammatory drugs. *American Journal of Epidemiology.* **159**: 23–31.
73 Rainsford K (1999) Profile and mechanisms of gastrointestinal and other side effects of nonsteroidal anti-inflammatory drugs (NsAIDs). *American Journal of Medicine.* **107 (Suppl 6A)**: 27s–36s.
74 Tang CL *et al.* (2012) Eradication of Helicobacter pylori infection reduces the incidence of peptic ulcer disease in patients using nonsteroidal anti-inflammatory drugs: a meta-analysis. *Helicobacter.* **17**: 286–296.
75 Malfertheiner P *et al.* (2007) Current concepts in the management of Helicobacter pylori infection: the Maastricht III Consensus Report. *Gut.* **56**: 772–781.
76 Cheetham TC *et al.* (2009) Gastrointestinal safety of nonsteroidal antiinflammatory drugs and selective cyclooxygenase-2 inhibitors in patients on warfarin. *Annals of Pharmacotherapy.* **43**: 1765–1773.
77 Hawkins C and Hanks G (2000) The gastroduodenal toxicity of nonsteroidal anti-inflammatory drugs. A review of the literature. *Journal of Pain and Symptom Management.* **20**: 140–151.
78 Targownik LE *et al.* (2008) The relative efficacies of gastroprotective strategies in chronic users of nonsteroidal anti-inflammatory drugs. *Gastroenterology.* **134**: 937–944.
79 Yuan JQ *et al.* (2016) Systematic review with network meta-analysis: comparative effectiveness and safety of strategies for preventing NSAID-associated gastrointestinal toxicity. *Alimentary Pharmacology and Therapeutics.* **43**: 1262–1275.
80 Hawkey C *et al.* (1998) Omeprazole compared with misoprostol for ulcers associated with nonsteroidal anti-inflammatory drugs. *New England Journal of Medicine.* **338**: 727–734.
81 NICE (2014) Dyspepsia and gastro-oesophageal reflux disease. *Clinical Guideline.* CG184. www.nice.org.uk
82 Adebayo D and Bjarnason I (2006) Is non-steroidal anti-inflammaory drug (NSAID) enteropathy clinically more important than NSAID gastropathy? *Postgraduate Medical Journal.* **82**: 186–191.
83 Maiden L (2009) Capsule endoscopic diagnosis of nonsteroidal antiinflammatory drug-induced enteropathy. *Journal of Gastroenterology.* **44 (Suppl 19)**: 64–71.
84 Smecuol E *et al.* (2001) Acute gastrointestinal permeability responses to different non-steroidal anti-inflammatory drugs. *Gut.* **49**: 650–655.
85 Goldstein JL *et al.* (2005) Video capsule endoscopy to prospectively assess small bowel injury with celecoxib, naproxen plus omeprazole, and placebo. *Clinical Gastroenterology and Hepatology.* **3**: 133–141.
86 Maiden L *et al.* (2005) A quantitative analysis of NSAID-induced small bowel pathology by capsule enteroscopy. *Gastroenterology.* **128**: 1172–1178.
87 Fujimori S *et al.* (2010) Distribution of small intestinal mucosal injuries as a result of NSAID administration. *European Journal of Clinical Investigations.* **40**: 504–510.
88 Graham DY *et al.* (2005) Visible small-intestinal mucosal injury in chronic NSAID users. *Clinical Gastroenterology and Hepatology.* **3**: 55–59.
89 Washio E *et al.* (2016) Proton pump inhibitors increase incidence of nonsteroidal anti-inflammatory drug-induced small bowel injury: a randomized, placebo-controlled trial. *Clinical Gastroenterology and Hepatology.* **14**: 809–815.e801.
90 Bjarnason I and Takeuchi K (2009) Intestinal permeability in the pathogenesis of NSAID-induced enteropathy. *Journal of Gastroenterology.* **44 (Suppl 19)**: 23–29.
91 Wallace JL (2012) NSAID gastropathy and enteropathy: distinct pathogenesis likely necessitates distinct prevention strategies. *British Journal of Pharmacology.* **165**: 67–74.
92 Adler DH *et al.* (2009) The enteropathy of prostaglandin deficiency. *Journal of Gastroenterology.* **44 (Suppl 19)**: 1–7.
93 Hedner T *et al.* (2004) Nabumetone: Therapeutic use and safety profile in the management of osteoarthritis and rheumatoid arthritis. *Drugs.* **64**: 2315–2343; discussion 2344–2345.
94 Boelsterli UA *et al.* (2013) Multiple NSAID-induced hits injure the small intestine: underlying mechanisms and novel strategies. *Toxicol Sci.* **131**: 654–667.
95 Satoh H *et al.* (2014) Mucosal protective agents prevent exacerbation of NSAID-induced small intestinal lesions caused by antisecretory drugs in rats. *Journal of Pharmacology and Experimental Therapeutics.* **348**: 227–235.
96 Kojima Y *et al.* (2015) Effect of long-term proton pump inhibitor therapy and healing effect of irsogladine on nonsteroidal anti-inflammatory drug-induced small-intestinal lesions in healthy volunteers. *Journal of Clinical Biochemistry and Nutrition.* **57**: 60–65.
97 Hayashi S *et al.* (2014) Lubiprostone prevents nonsteroidal anti-inflammatory drug-induced small intestinal damage by suppressing the expression of inflammatory mediators via EP4 receptors. *Journal of Pharmacology Experimental Therapeutics.* **349**: 470–479.
98 Zhang S *et al.* (2013) Rebamipide helps defend against nonsteroidal anti-inflammatory drugs induced gastroenteropathy: a systematic review and meta-analysis. *Digestive Diseases and Sciences.* **58**: 1991–2000.
99 Satoh H and Takeuchi K (2012) Management of NSAID/aspirin-induced small intestinal damage by GI-sparing NSAIDs, anti-ulcer drugs and food constituents. *Current Medicinal Chemistry.* **19**: 82–89.
100 Takeuchi K *et al.* (2006) Prevalence and mechanism of nonsteroidal anti-inflammatory drug-induced clinical relapse in patients with inflammatory bowel disease. *Clinical Gastroenterology and Hepatology.* **4**: 196–202.
101 Ribaldone DG *et al.* (2015) Coxib's safety in patients with inflammatory bowel diseases: a meta-analysis. *Pain Physician.* **18**: 599–607.
102 Ananthakrishnan AN *et al.* (2012) Aspirin, nonsteroidal anti-inflammatory drug use, and risk for Crohn disease and ulcerative colitis: a cohort study. *Annals of Internal Medicine.* **156**: 350–359.
103 Ballinger A (2008) Adverse effects of nonsteroidal anti-inflammatory drugs on the colon. *Current Gastroenterology Reports.* **10**: 485–489.
104 Schmidt M *et al.* (2016) Cardiovascular safety of non-aspirin non-steroidal anti-inflammatory drugs: review and position paper by the working group for Cardiovascular Pharmacotherapy of the European Society of Cardiology. *European Heart Journal.* **37**: 1015–1023.
105 Zingler G *et al.* (2016) Cardiovascular adverse events by non-steroidal anti-inflammatory drugs: when the benefits outweigh the risks. *Expert Review of Clinical Pharmacology.* **8**: 1–14.
106 Bally M *et al.* (2017) Risk of acute myocardial infarction with NSAIDs in real world use: bayesian meta-analysis of individual patient data. *British Medical Journal.* **357**: 1909.
107 Gunter BR *et al.* (2017) Non-steroidal anti-inflammatory drug-induced cardiovascular adverse events: a meta-analysis. *Journal of Clinical Pharmacy and Therapeutics.* **42**: 27–38.
108 White WB (2007) Cardiovascular risk, hypertension, and NSAIDs. *Current Pain and Headache Reports.* **11**: 428–435.
109 Gislason GH *et al.* (2009) Increased mortality and cardiovascular morbidity associated with use of nonsteroidal anti-inflammatory drugs in chronic heart failure. *Archives of Internal Medicine.* **169**: 141–149.
110 Huerta C *et al.* (2006) Non-steroidal anti-inflammatory drugs and risk of first hospital admission for heart failure in the general population. *Heart.* **92**: 1610–1615.

111 Arfe A *et al.* (2016) Non-steroidal anti-inflammatory drugs and risk of heart failure in four European countries: nested case-control study. *British Medical Journal*. **354**: i4857.
112 Nissen SE *et al.* (2016) Cardiovascular safety of celecoxib, naproxen, or ibuprofen for arthritis. *New England Journal of Medicine*. **375**: 2519–2529.
113 Solomon SD *et al.* (2008) Cardiovascular risk of celecoxib in 6 randomized placebo-controlled trials: the cross trial safety analysis. *Circulation*. **117**: 2104–2113.
114 Trelle S *et al.* (2011) Cardiovascular safety of non-steroidal anti-inflammatory drugs: network meta-analysis. *British Medical Journal*. **342**: c7086.
115 Sondergaard KB *et al.* (2017) Non-steroidal anti-inflammatory drug use is associated with increased risk of out-of-hospital cardiac arrest: a nationwide case-time-control study. *European Heart Journal Cardiovascular Pharmacotherpy*. **3**: 100–107.
116 Ungprasert P *et al.* (2016) Nonaspirin Nonsteroidal Anti-Inflammatory Drugs and Risk of Hemorrhagic Stroke: A Systematic Review and Meta-Analysis of Observational Studies. *Stroke*. **47**: 356–364.
117 Lee W *et al.* (2010) Celecoxib does not attenuate the antiplatelet effects of aspirin and clopidogrel in healthy volunteers. *Korean Circulation Journal*. **40**: 321–327.
118 Cheng HF and Harris RC (2004) Cyclooxygenases, the kidney, and hypertension. *Hypertension*. **43**: 525–530.
119 Griffin M *et al.* (2000) Nonsteroidal antiinflammatory drugs and acute renal failure in elderly persons. *American Journal of Epidemiology*. **151**: 488–496.
120 Huerta C *et al.* (2005) Nonsteroidal anti-inflammatory drugs and risk of ARF in the general population. *American Journal of Kidney Disease*. **45**: 531–539.
121 Schneider V *et al.* (2006) Association of selective and conventional nonsteroidal antiinflammatory drugs with acute renal failure: A population-based, nested case-control analysis. *American Journal of Epidemiology*. **164**: 881–889.
122 Curiel RV and Katz JD (2013) Mitigating the cardiovascular and renal effects of NSAIDs. *Pain Medicine*. **14 (Suppl 1)**: S23–28.
123 Winearls C (1995) Acute myeloma kidney. *Kidney International*. **48**: 1347–1361.
124 Irish AB *et al.* (1997) Presentation and survival of patients with severe renal failure and myeloma. *QJM: monthly journal of the Association of Physicians*. **90**: 773–780.
125 Harirforoosh S and Jamali F (2009) Renal adverse effects of nonsteroidal anti-inflammatory drugs. *Expert Opinion on Drug Safety*. **8**: 669–681.
126 Loboz KK and Shenfield GM (2005) Drug combinations and impaired renal function -- the 'triple whammy'. *British Journal of Clinical Pharmacology*. **59**: 239–243.
127 Onuigbo MA and Agbasi N (2015) Intraoperative hypotension - a neglected causative factor in hospital-acquired acute kidney injury; a Mayo Clinic Health System experience revisited. *Journal of Renal Injury Prevention*. **4**: 61–67.
128 Lee YC *et al.* (2012) Non-steroidal anti-inflammatory drugs use and risk of upper gastrointestinal adverse events in cirrhotic patients. *Liver International*. **32**: 859–866.
129 North-Lewis P (ed) (2008) *Drugs and the Liver*. Pharmaceutical Press, London, pp. 178–187.
130 Delco F *et al.* (2005) Dose adjustment in patients with liver disease. *Drug Safety*. **28**: 529–545.
131 Jenkins C *et al.* (2004) Systematic review of prevalence of aspirin induced asthma and its implications for clinical practice. *British Medical Journal*. **328**: 434.
132 Thomsen SF *et al.* (2009) Regular use of non-steroidal anti-inflammatory drugs increases the risk of adult-onset asthma: a population-based follow-up study. *Clinical Respiratory Journal*. **3**: 82–84.
133 Kim SH *et al.* (2007) Association between polymorphisms in prostanoid receptor genes and aspirin-intolerant asthma. *Pharmacogenet Genomics*. **17**: 295–304.
134 Sanak M and Szczeklik A (2001) Leukotriene C4 synthase polymorphism and aspirin-induced asthma. *Journal of Allergy and Clinical Immunology*. **107**: 561–562.
135 Mastalerz L *et al.* (2008) Prostaglandin E2 systemic production in patients with asthma with and without aspirin hypersensitivity. *Thorax*. **63**: 27–34.
136 Taniguchi M *et al.* (2008) Hyperleukotrieneuria in patients with allergic and inflammatory disease. *Allergology International*. **57**: 313–320.
137 Morales DR *et al.* (2014) Safety risks for patients with aspirin-exacerbated respiratory disease after acute exposure to selective nonsteroidal anti-inflammatory drugs and COX-2 inhibitors: Meta-analysis of controlled clinical trials. *Journal of Allergy and Clinical Immunology*. **134**: 40–45.
138 Celik GE *et al.* (2013) Are drug provocation tests still necessary to test the safety of COX-2 inhibitors in patients with cross-reactive NSAID hypersensitivity? *Allergologia et Immunopathologia (Madr)*. **41**: 181–188.
139 Dicpinigaitis P (2001) Effect of the cyclooxygenase-2 inhibitor celecoxib on bronchial responsiveness and cough reflex sensitivity in asthmatics. *Pulmonary Pharmacology and Therapeutics*. **14**: 93–97.
140 Settipane R *et al.* (1995) Prevalence of cross-sensitivity with acetaminophen in aspirin-sensitive asthmatic subjects. *Journal of Allergy and Clinical Immunology*. **96**: 480–485.
141 Dahlen SE *et al.* (2002) Improvement of aspirin-intolerant asthma by montelukast, a leukotriene antagonist: a randomized, double-blind, placebo-controlled trial. *American Journal Respiratory Critical Care Medicine*. **165**: 9–14.
142 Kennedy JL *et al.* (2016) Aspirin-exacerbated respiratory disease: Prevalence, diagnosis, treatment, and considerations for the future. *American Journal of Rhinology and Allergy*. **30**: 407–413.
143 Stevenson DD (2009) Aspirin sensitivity and desensitization for asthma and sinusitis. *Current Allergy and Asthma Reports*. **9**: 155–163.
144 Boursinos LA *et al.* (2009) Do steroids, conventional non-steroidal anti-inflammatory drugs and selective Cox-2 inhibitors adversely affect fracture healing? *Journal of Musculoskeletal Neuronal Interactions*. **9**: 44–52.
145 Pountos I *et al.* (2008) Pharmacological agents and impairment of fracture healing: what is the evidence? *Injury*. **39**: 384–394.
146 Vuolteenaho K *et al.* (2008) Non-steroidal anti-inflammatory drugs, cyclooxygenase-2 and the bone healing process. *Basic & Clinical Pharmacology and Toxicology*. **102**: 10–14.
147 Anglin R *et al.* (2014) Risk of upper gastrointestinal bleeding with selective serotonin reuptake inhibitors with or without concurrent nonsteroidal anti-inflammatory use: a systematic review and meta-analysis. *American Journal of Gastroenterology*. **109**: 811–819.
148 Shin JY *et al.* (2015) Risk of intracranial haemorrhage in antidepressant users with concurrent use of non-steroidal anti-inflammatory drugs: nationwide propensity score matched study. *British Medical Journal*. **351**: h3517.
149 de Abajo FJ and Garcia-Rodriguez LA (2008) Risk of upper gastrointestinal tract bleeding associated with selective serotonin reuptake inhibitors and venlafaxine therapy: interaction with nonsteroidal anti-inflammatory drugs and effect of acid-suppressing agents. *Archives of General Psychiatry*. **65**: 795–803.
150 Baxter K and Preston CL. *Stockley's Drug Interactions*. London: Pharmaceutical Press www.medicinescomplete.com (accessed May 2017).

151 Colebatch AN *et al.* (2012) Safety of nonsteroidal antiinflammatory drugs and/or paracetamol in people receiving methotrexate for inflammatory arthritis: a Cochrane systematic review. *Journal of Rheumatology.* **90**: 62–73.
152 Brown A *et al.* (2003) An interaction between warfarin and COX-2 inhibitors: two case studies. *The Pharmaceutical Journal.* **271**: 782.
153 Verrico M *et al.* (2003) Adverse drug events involving COX-2 inhibitors. *Annals of Pharmacotherapy.* **37**: 1203–1213.
154 Tonkin A and Wing L (1988) Interactions of nonsteroidal anti-inflammatory drugs. In: P Brooks (ed) *Bailliere's Clinical Rheumatology Anti-rheumatic drugs* Vol 2. Bailliere Tindall, London, pp. 455–483.
155 Palliativedrugs.com (2016) Parenteral NSAIDs - which one do you use? *Latest additions: Survey results (August).* www.palliativedrug.com
156 Armstrong P (2017) The use of parecoxib by continuous subcutaneous infusion for cancer pain in a hospice population. *BMJ Supportive and Palliative Care.* [Epub ahead of print].
157 Kenner DJ *et al.* (2015) Daily subcutaneous parecoxib injection for cancer pain: an open label pilot study. *Journal of Palliative Medicine.* **18**: 366–372.
158 Vacha ME *et al.* (2015) The role of subcutaneous ketorolac for pain management. *Hospital Pharmacy.* **50**: 108–112.

Updated September 2017

CELECOXIB

Class: Non-opioid analgesic, NSAID, selective COX-2 inhibitor.

Indications: Pain in osteoarthritis, rheumatoid arthritis and ankylosing spondylitis, †acute pain, †cancer pain.

Contra-indications: Hypersensitivity to **aspirin** or other NSAID (urticaria, rhinitis, asthma, angioedema), *hypersensitivity to sulfonamides*, active GI ulceration, established ischaemic heart disease, peripheral arterial disease, cerebrovascular disease, severe heart failure, severe hepatic impairment, severe renal impairment, deteriorating renal function, inflammatory bowel disease.

Pharmacology

Celecoxib, a sulphonamide derivative, is a selective COX-2 inhibitor. Despite only modest selectivity when tested *in vitro*,[1–3] 800mg/24h causes no significant COX-1 inhibition in healthy volunteers.[4] Non-COX-2 inhibitory properties may account for some of its activity, e.g. inhibition of endoplasmic reticulum Ca^{2+} ATPase[5] and inhibition of phosphodiesterase-5 activity.[6] The capacity to interact with non-COX-2 targets may be enhanced by accumulation of celecoxib within cells.[7] Central endogenous opioid and cannabinoid systems may also be involved.[8]

Celecoxib is the *PCF NSAID of choice in palliative care.* The risk of gastrointestinal ulceration is lower than non-selective NSAIDs (see p.316). In all except the highest GI risk patients, celecoxib avoids the need for gastro-protection and its consequent risks (p.30). The risk of cardiovascular events and renal impairment is comparable to non-selective NSAIDs, including **naproxen** (see p.319).

Celecoxib is metabolized mainly via CYP2C9. *Slow (poor) metabolizers are at increased risk of undesirable effects.* In people of European ancestry, the CYP2C9*3 variant is particularly important, slowing methylhydroxylation *in vitro* by 90% and more than doubling the AUC in single dose studies.[9] In the UK, the SPC suggests that known or suspected slow metabolizers should be treated with caution.[10] In contrast, the USA PI recommends that the dose should be *halved* in such individuals.[11]

In osteoarthritis, meta-analyses showed celecoxib to be superior to placebo but not to **paracetamol** (perhaps because the dose is restricted to 200mg/24h in this condition in the USA)[12] and inferior to **diclofenac** 150mg/24h.[13] Whereas in two RCTs in rheumatoid arthritis, celecoxib ≥200mg/24h, was as effective as **naproxen** 500mg b.d.,[14] and 400mg/24h was as effective as **diclofenac** 150mg/24h.[15]

Celecoxib is effective in postoperative pain[16] and dysmenorrhoea,[17] but *not* in renal colic.[18] There is a lack of data relating to cancer pain. Unlike opioids, celecoxib failed to control pain in mice with bone tumours.[19,20]

Celecoxib has no effect on platelet function.[21] The thromboprotective effect of low-dose **aspirin** for stroke is neutralized by NSAIDs other than **celecoxib**[22] and **naproxen**.[23] Thus, in someone taking **aspirin** thromboprophylaxis and an NSAID is needed for pain relief, these are the NSAIDs of choice.

Possible roles for celecoxib in cancer-related cachexia (see Progestogens, p.552), psychiatry and dementia are being explored (see p.316). Although animal studies suggest a beneficial effect

on angiogenesis, tumour growth, and metastasis, in humans, the addition of celecoxib to cancer chemotherapy does *not* improve survival.[24,25]
Bio-availability No human data; 22–40% in dogs;[26] increased by 20% after high fat meal.
Onset of action 60min.[27]
Time to peak plasma concentration 3h; high fat meals delay peak by 1–2 hours; aluminium- and magnesium-containing antacids reduce peak concentration.
Plasma halflife. 11h.
Duration of action 5h in single-dose post-dental extraction pain;[27] but given that recommended frequency of administration is once daily–b.d., presumably longer when given regularly.

Cautions

Cardiovascular disease including hypertension and heart failure (risk of exacerbation, though risk may be lower than other NSAIDs;[28–30] renal and hepatic impairment (see p.681 and p.703). Correct hyperkalaemia before use. As with all NSAIDs, concurrent administration with an SSRI is associated with an increased risk of GI bleeding.

Drug interactions

For general interactions between NSAIDs and other drugs, see Tables 8 and 9 (p.323 and p.324). Of particular importance is the risk of toxic plasma levels of **digoxin**, **lithium** and **methotrexate** caused by reduced renal function and/or reduced tubular excretion. If an NSAID is prescribed, monitor the plasma drug concentration or haematological effect of these drugs as appropriate and reduce doses as necessary (see p.322).

Because they cause sodium and fluid retention, all NSAIDs can decrease the effect of diuretics, ACE inhibitors and antihypertensives.

Because an increase in INR occasionally occurs when celecoxib is prescribed for a patient already taking **warfarin**, monitor the INR weekly for 3–4 weeks and adjust the dose of **warfarin** if necessary.[31]

CYP2C9 inhibitors (see Chapter 19, Table 8, p.725) may increase plasma concentrations of celecoxib. The manufacturer recommends halving the celecoxib dose if **fluconazole** is taken concurrently.[31] In known CYP2C9 slow metabolizers, avoid concurrent administration of CYP2C9 inhibitors and celecoxib. Conversely, CYP2C9 inducers (e.g. **carbamazepine**, **phenobarbital**, **rifampicin**) may reduce plasma concentrations of celecoxib.

Celecoxib is an inhibitor of CYP2D6 and theoretically may increase the plasma concentrations of other drugs metabolised by this enzyme (see Chapter 19, Table 8, p.725) if given concurrently.

Undesirable effects

Also see NSAIDs, p.312.
Common (<10%, >1%): dyspepsia, abdominal pain, flatulence, diarrhoea (but all same as or less than other NSAIDs), pharyngitis, rhinitis, allergy, pruritus, insomnia, dizziness, hypertonia, rash, flu-like symptoms, peripheral oedema, fluid retention.
Very rare (<0.01%): aseptic meningitis in patients with SLE.

Dose and use

Gastroprotection, e.g. a PPI (see p.30), need be prescribed only for patients at *high* risk of NSAID-related upper GI complications (see Box B, p.318).

Celecoxib is the *PCF* NSAID of choice:

- start with 100mg PO b.d.
- if necessary, increase to 200mg b.d.

For patients with swallowing difficulties, the capsules can be opened and the contents sprinkled on a small amount of soft food, e.g. yoghurt, applesauce (see p.793). **Diclofenac** CSCI (p.332) or **parecoxib** SC or CSCI (p.325), or **ketorolac** (p.340) are alternatives if the PO route is unavailable.

Supply

Celecoxib (generic)
Capsules 100mg, 200mg, 28 days @ 200mg b.d. = £3.

1 Warner TD and Mitchell JA (2008) COX-2 selectivity alone does not define the cardiovascular risks associated with non-steroidal anti-inflammatory drugs. *Lancet.* **371**: 270–273.
2 Riendeau D *et al.* (2001) Etoricoxib (MK-0663): Preclinical profile and comparison with other agents that selectively inhibit cyclooxygenase-2. *Journal of Pharmacology and Experimental Therapeutics.* **296**: 558–566.
3 Schwartz JI *et al.* (2008) Comparative inhibitory activity of etoricoxib, celecoxib, and diclofenac on COX-2 versus COX-1 in healthy subjects. *Journal of Clinical Pharmacology.* **48**: 745–754.
4 Fries S *et al.* (2006) Marked interindividual variability in the response to selective inhibitors of cyclooxygenase-2. *Gastroenterology.* **130**: 55–64.
5 Alloza I *et al.* (2006) Celecoxib inhibits interleukin-12 alphabeta and beta2 folding and secretion by a novel COX2-independent mechanism involving chaperones of the endoplasmic reticulum. *Molecular Pharmacology.* **69**: 1579–1587.
6 Klein T *et al.* (2007) Celecoxib dilates guinea-pig coronaries and rat aortic rings and amplifies NO/cGMP signaling by PDE5 inhibition. *Cardiovascular Research.* **75**: 390–397.
7 Maier TJ *et al.* (2009) Cellular membranes function as a storage compartment for celecoxib. *Journal of Molecular Medicine.* **87**: 981–993.
8 Rezende RM *et al.* (2012) Endogenous opioid and cannabinoid mechanisms are involved in the analgesic effects of celecoxib in the central nervous system. *Pharmacology.* **89**: 127–136.
9 Gong L *et al.* (2012) Celecoxib pathways: pharmacokinetics and pharmacodynamics. *Pharmacogenetics and Genomics.* **22**: 310–318.
10 Pfizer (2011) Celebrex 100mg & 200mg capsules. *SPC.* www.medicines.org.uk.
11 Pfizer (2012) Celebrex capsules. *US Prescribing Information.* www.accessdata.fda.gov/scripts/cder/drugsatfda/index/cfm
12 Bannuru RR *et al.* (2015) Comparative effectiveness of pharmacologic interventions for knee osteoarthritis: a systematic review and network meta-analysis. *Annals of Internal Medicine.* **162**: 46–54.
13 da Costa BR *et al.* (2016) Effectiveness of non-steroidal anti-inflammatory drugs for the treatment of pain in knee and hip osteoarthritis: a network meta-analysis. *Lancet.* **387**: 2093–2105.
14 Simon LS *et al.* (1999) Anti-inflammatory and upper gastrointestinal effects of celecoxib in rheumatoid arthritis: a randomized controlled trial. *Journal of the American Medical Association.* **282**: 1921–1928.
15 Emery P *et al.* (1999) Celecoxib versus diclofenac in long-term management of rheumatoid arthritis: randomised double-blind comparison. *Lancet.* **354**: 2106–2111.
16 Derry S (2009) Single dose oral celecoxib for acute postoperative pain in adults. *Cochrane Database of Systematic Reviews.* **4**: CD004234. wwwthecochranelibrary.com.
17 Daniels S *et al.* (2009) Celecoxib in the treatment of primary dysmenorrhea: results from two randomized, double-blind, active- and placebo-controlled, crossover studies. *Clinical Therapeutics.* **31**: 1192–1208.
18 Phillips E *et al.* (2009) Celecoxib in the management of acute renal colic: a randomized controlled clinical trial. *Urology.* **74**: 994–999.
19 Saito O *et al.* (2005) Analgesic effects of nonsteroidal antiinflammatory drugs, acetaminophen, and morphine in a mouse model of bone cancer pain. *Journal of Anesthesia.* **19**: 218–224.
20 Mouedden ME and Meert TF (2007) Pharmacological evaluation of opioid and non-opioid analgesics in a murine bone cancer model of pain. *Pharmacology, Biochemistry, and Behavior.* **86**: 458–467.
21 Graff J *et al.* (2007) Effects of selective COX-2 inhibition on prostanoids and platelet physiology in young healthy volunteers. *Journal of Thrombosis and Haemostasis.* **5**: 2376–2385.
22 Lee W *et al.* (2010) Celecoxib does not attenuate the antiplatelet effects of aspirin and clopidogrel in healthy volunteers. *Korean Circulation Journal.* **40**: 321–327.
23 CNT Collaboration (2013) Vascular and upper gastrointestinal effects of non-steroidal anti-inflammatory drugs: meta-analyses of individual participant data from randomised trials. *Lancet.* **382**: 769–779.
24 Chen J *et al.* (2014) Efficacy and safety profile of celecoxib for treating advanced cancers: a meta-analysis of 11 randomized clinical trials. *Clinical Therapeutics.* **36**: 1253–1263.
25 Edelman MJ *et al.* (2017) Phase III Randomized, Placebo-Controlled, Double-Blind Trial of Celecoxib in Addition to Standard Chemotherapy for Advanced Non-Small-Cell Lung Cancer With Cyclooxygenase-2 Overexpression: CALGB 30801 (Alliance). *Journal of Clinical Oncology.* **35**: 2184–2192.
26 Paulson S *et al.* (2001) Pharmacokinetics of celecoxib after oral administration in dogs and humans: effects of food and site absorption. *Journal of Pharmacology and Experimental Therapeutics.* **297**: 638–645.
27 Malmstrom K *et al.* (1999) Comparison of rofecoxib and celecoxib, two cyclooxygenase-2 inhibitors, in postoperative dental pain: a randomised, placebo- and active-comparator-controlled clinical trial. *Clinical Therapeutics.* **21**: 1653–1663.
28 Chan CC *et al.* (2009) Do COX-2 inhibitors raise blood pressure more than nonselective NSAIDs and placebo? An updated meta-analysis. *Journal of Hypertension.* **27**: 2332–2341.
29 Solomon DH *et al.* (2004) Relationship between COX-2 specific inhibitors and hypertension. *Hypertension.* **44**: 140–145.
30 Arfe A *et al.* (2016) Non-steroidal anti-inflammatory drugs and risk of heart failure in four European countries: nested case-control study. *British Medical Journal.* **354**: i4857.
31 Baxter K and Preston CL. *Stockley's Drug Interactions.* London: Pharmaceutical Press www.medicinescomplete.com (accessed May 2017).

Updated September 2017

DICLOFENAC SODIUM

Class: Non-opioid analgesic, NSAID, preferential COX-2 inhibitor.

Indications: Pain in arthritis and other musculoskeletal disorders, postoperative pain, †dysmenorrhoea, acute gout, †cancer pain, †neoplastic fever.

Contra-indications: Hypersensitivity to **aspirin** or other NSAID (urticaria, rhinitis, asthma, angioedema), active GI ulceration, history of two or more distinct episodes of proven ulceration or bleeding, cerebrovascular bleeding or other bleeding disorders, ischaemic heart disease, peripheral arterial disease, cerebrovascular disease, congestive heart failure (New York Heart Association [NYHA] classification II–IV), active liver disease or severe hepatic impairment, severe renal impairment, deteriorating renal function.

Pharmacology

Diclofenac is a preferential COX-2 inhibitor (see Table 1, p.313 and Table 2, p.314).[1,2] The analgesic effect of diclofenac has been shown in animals to be both peripheral and central.[3–5] In addition to inhibiting COX, diclofenac:

- activates the nitric oxide-cGMP nociceptive pathway[6]
- impacts on central nociception by increasing brain concentrations of kynurenic acid, an endogenous antagonist on the glycine recognition site of the NMDA-receptor-channel complex[7]
- is a 'membrane stabilizer' (through the opening of KCNQ2/3 potassium channels, see p.256).[8,9]

It is possible that diclofenac is more broad-spectrum in its central effects than other NSAIDs.[10] Diclofenac causes platelet dysfunction in only two thirds of healthy volunteers.[11]

In terms of effectiveness for osteoarthritis, diclofenac is non-inferior to other NSAIDs.[12] About 10–15% of patients experience undesirable effects (mainly gastric intolerance). These are generally mild and transient; diclofenac needs to be withdrawn in only 2%.

Age[13] and renal and hepatic impairment do not have a significant effect on plasma concentrations of diclofenac. Metabolite concentrations increase in severe renal impairment but the principal metabolite, hydroxydiclofenac, possesses little anti-inflammatory effect. However, because of a greater likelihood of (unpredictable) hepatotoxicity compared with other NSAIDs, it may be best *not* to use diclofenac in severe hepatic impairment.[14]

A meta-analysis of several hundred RCTs indicates that, compared with placebo, the risk of upper GI complications with diclofenac and coxibs is relatively low (about double that seen with placebo), and half that seen with high-dose **ibuprofen** and high-dose **naproxen**.[15]

Diclofenac carries a higher CVS risk than non-selective NSAIDs,[15] and is *contra-indicated* in individuals with CVS disease.[16] In a nationwide review in Denmark, diclofenac and **ibuprofen** (but *not* COX-2 inhibitors or **naproxen**) were associated with an increased risk of out-of-hospital cardiac arrest.[17] The risk of renal failure is comparable with other NSAIDs.[18]

Severe local necrosis has been described anecdotally after IM and SC use.[19] Diclofenac is available as the *sodium* and *potassium* salts; diclofenac *potassium* is absorbed more quickly and peak plasma concentration is reached sooner. It is theoretically a better alternative in patients troubled by Na^+ and water retention. However, it is much more expensive.

Bio-availability 50% PO (both immediate-release and m/r products); suppositories about 33%.
Onset of action 20–30min.
Time to peak plasma concentration diclofenac *sodium:* 2.5h e/c (fasting), 6h e/c (taken with food), ≥4h m/r, 1h suppositories; diclofenac *potassium* PO 20–60min (not significantly affected by food).
Plasma halflife 1–2h.
Duration of action 8h.

Cautions

Renal and hepatic impairment (see p.681 and p.703). Avoid in patients with significant CVS risk factors (hypertension, hyperlipidaemia, diabetes mellitus, smoking). Correct hyperkalaemia before use.

Because of an increased risk of bleeding (from decreased platelet aggregation), avoid concurrent prescription with **warfarin**. As with all NSAIDs, concurrent administration with an SSRI is associated with an increased risk of GI bleeding.

The thromboprotective effect of **aspirin** for stroke is compromised in people taking diclofenac concurrently.[20] Thus, people taking low-dose **aspirin** for thromboprotection should *not* take diclofenac. Instead, prescribe **celecoxib** (with **aspirin**) or **naproxen** alone (see p.343).

Drug interactions

For general interactions between NSAIDs and other drugs, see Tables 8 and 9 (p.323 and p.324). Of particular importance is the risk of toxic plasma levels of **digoxin**, **lithium**, and **methotrexate** caused by reduced renal function and/or reduced tubular excretion. If diclofenac is prescribed, monitor the plasma drug concentration or haematological effect of these drugs as appropriate and reduce doses as necessary (see p.322).

Because they cause sodium and fluid retention, all NSAIDs can decrease the effect of diuretics, ACE inhibitors and antihypertensives.

In addition to the effect on platelet function (see Cautions), an increase in INR may occur when diclofenac is prescribed for a patient already taking **warfarin**; monitor the INR weekly for 3–4 weeks and adjust the dose of **warfarin** if necessary.[21]

Concurrent use of diclofenac with **ciclosporin** may increase the plasma concentration of diclofenac (up to double), and decrease the plasma concentration of **ciclosporin**. If given concurrently, the manufacturer advises halving the dose of diclofenac.

Diclofenac plasma concentration may be *increased* by **voriconazole**. This may relate to inhibition by CYP2C9; lower doses of diclofenac may be necessary. Conversely, **rifampicin** may *decrease* diclofenac plasma concentration due to CYP3A4 enzyme induction; consider an alternative NSAID if pain returns. Caution should be taken with concurrent use of other drugs which inhibit or induce these enzymes (see Chapter 19, Table 8, p.725).

Undesirable effects

Also see NSAIDs, p.312.

Common (<10%, >1%): headache, dizziness, oedema, indigestion, abdominal discomfort, nausea, constipation or diarrhoea, pruritus, rash, ecchymosis.

Very rare (<0.01%): aseptic meningitis in patients with SLE.

Dose and use

Although traditionally advised to take NSAIDs with food, there is no evidence that this reduces the risk of GI complications.

Gastroprotection, e.g. a PPI (see p.30), should be prescribed concurrently for patients at high risk of NSAID-related upper GI complications (see Box B, p.318) or **celecoxib** ± PPI prescribed instead (see p.316).

PCF prefers **celecoxib** (p.330). However, diclofenac sodium is a frequently used NSAID; typical regimens are:

- immediate-release 50mg PO b.d.–t.d.s.
- m/r 75mg PO b.d. or 100mg once daily
- suppositories 50mg PR b.d.–t.d.s.

Anecdotally, some patients obtain greater benefit from 200mg/24h, e.g. m/r 100mg b.d. However, doses >150mg/24h are unauthorized.

Parenteral administration

Diclofenac is available as an injection, primarily for use in biliary and renal colic (75mg IM p.r.n., maximum 150mg/24h).[22] Injection site pain/reaction is common.

In palliative care, it is sometimes given by CSCI when the PO route is no longer possible (unauthorized use). Because PO bio-availability is 50%, a typical regimen is 75mg/24h CSCI, diluted with 0.9% saline to minimize the risk of injection site reactions. Diclofenac must be given alone via a separate syringe driver because its alkalinity makes it incompatible with other drugs (see p.822).

Alternative SC/CSCI NSAIDs include **parecoxib** (p.325) and **ketorolac** (p.340).

For topical use, see p.601.

Supply

Diclofenac *sodium* (generic)

Tablets e/c 25mg, 50mg, 28 days @ 50mg t.d.s. = £8.50.

Suppositories 100mg, 10 = £4.

Voltarol® (Novartis)
Injection 25mg/mL, 3mL amp = £1.
Suppositories 12.5mg, 25mg, 50mg, 100mg; 50mg, 10 = £2; 100mg, 10 = £3.50.

Modified-release
Diclofenac *sodium* (generic)
Tablets m/r 75mg, 100mg, 28 days @ 75mg b.d. or 100mg once daily = £11 and £8.
Capsules m/r 75mg, 100mg, 28 days @ 75mg b.d. or 100mg once daily = £10 and £7.

Motifen® 75mg (Daiichi Sankyo)
Capsules (containing e/c pellets 25mg and m/r pellets 50mg) 75mg, 28 days @ 75mg b.d. = £8.

5

1 John V (1979) The pharmacokinetics and metabolism of diclofenac sodium (Voltarol) in animals and man. *Rheumatology and Rehabilitation.* **(suppl 2)**: 22–37.
2 Schwartz JI *et al.* (2008) Comparative inhibitory activity of etoricoxib, celecoxib, and diclofenac on COX-2 versus COX-1 in healthy subjects. *Journal of Clinical Pharmacology.* **48**: 745–754.
3 McCormack K (1994) Nonsteroidal anti-inflammatory drugs and spinal nociceptive processing. *Pain.* **59**: 9–43.
4 Svensson CI and Yaksh TL (2002) The spinal phospholipase-cyclooxygenase-prostanoid cascade in nociceptive processing. *Annual Review of Pharmacology and Toxicology.* **42**: 553–583.
5 Ortiz MI *et al.* (2008) Additive interaction between peripheral and central mechanisms involved in the antinociceptive effect of diclofenac in the formalin test in rats. *Pharmacology, Biochemistry and Behavior.* **91**: 32–37.
6 Ortiz MI *et al.* (2003) The NO-cGMP-K+ channel pathway participates in the antinociceptive effect of diclofenac, but not of indomethacin. *Pharmacology, Biochemistry and Behavior.* **76**: 187–195.
7 Schwieler L *et al.* (2005) Prostaglandin-mediated control of rat brain kynurenic acid synthesis - opposite actions by COX-1 and COX-2 isoforms. *Journal of Neural Transmission.* **112**: 863–872.
8 Peretz A *et al.* (2005) Meclofenamic acid and diclofenac, novel templates of KCNQ2/Q3 potassium channel openers, depress cortical neuron activity and exhibit anticonvulsant properties. *Molecular Pharmacology.* **67**: 1053–1066.
9 Gan TJ (2010) Diclofenac: an update on its mechanism of action and safety profile. *Current Medical Research Opinion.* **26**: 1715–1731.
10 McCormack K and Twycross RG (2001) Are COX-2 selective inhibitors effective analgesics. *Pain Review.* **8**: 13–26.
11 Ng KF *et al.* (2008) Comprehensive preoperative evaluation of platelet function in total knee arthroplasty patients taking diclofenac. *Journal of Arthroplasty.* **23**: 424–430.
12 Pavelka K (2012) A comparison of the therapeutic efficacy of diclofenac in osteoarthritis: a systematic review of randomised controlled trials. *Current Medical Research Opinion.* **28**: 163–178.
13 Willis JV and Kendall MJ (1978) Pharmacokinetic studies on diclofenac sodium in young and old volunteers. *Scandinavian Journal of Rheumatology.* **Suppl**: 36–41.
14 Gupta NK and Lewis JH (2008) Review article: The use of potentially hepatotoxic drugs in patients with liver disease. *Alimentary Pharmacology and Therapeutics.* **28**: 1021–1041.
15 CNT Collaboration (2013) Vascular and upper gastrointestinal effects of non-steroidal anti-inflammatory drugs: meta-analyses of individual participant data from randomised trials. *Lancet.* **382**: 769–779.
16 MHRA (2013) Diclofenac: new contraindications and warnings after a Europe-wide review of cardiovascular safety. *Drug Safety Update.* www.gov.uk/drug-safety-update
17 Sondergaard KB *et al.* (2017) Non-steroidal anti-inflammatory drug use is associated with increased risk of out-of-hospital cardiac arrest: a nationwide case-time-control study. *European Heart Journal Cardiovascular Pharmacotherpy.* **3**: 100–107.
18 Schneider V *et al.* (2006) Association of selective and conventional nonsteroidal antiinflammatory drugs with acute renal failure: A population-based, nested case-control analysis. *American Journal of Epidemiology.* **164**: 881–889.
19 Kirkpatrick G (2003) SC diclofenac. In: *Bulletin board discussion.* Palliativedrugs.com. Available from: www.palliativedrugs.com/bulletin-board.html
20 Gladding PA *et al.* (2008) The antiplatelet effect of six non-steroidal anti-inflammatory drugs and their pharmacodynamic interaction with aspirin in healthy volunteers. *American Journal of Cardiology.* **101**: 1060–1063.
21 Baxter K and Preston CL *Stockley's Drug Interactions.* London: Pharmaceutical Press www.medicinescomplete.com (accessed May 2017).
22 Lundstam SOA *et al.* (1982) Prostaglandin-synthetase inhibition with diclofenac sodium in treatment of renal colic: comparison with use of a narcotic analgesic. *Lancet.* **1**: 1096–1097.

Updated September 2017

FLURBIPROFEN

Class: Non-opioid analgesic, NSAID, preferential COX-1 inhibitor.

Indications: Pain and inflammation in arthritic conditions, musculoskeletal disorders and trauma, dental pain, dysmenorrhoea, migraine, postoperative analgesia, sore throat (lozenges, see p.619), †cancer pain, †neoplastic fever, †detrusor instability.[1]

Contra-indications: Hypersensitivity to **aspirin** or other NSAID (urticaria, rhinitis, asthma, angioedema), active GI ulceration, history of two or more distinct episodes of proven ulceration or bleeding, cerebrovascular bleeding or other bleeding disorders, severe heart failure, active liver disease or severe hepatic impairment, severe renal impairment, deteriorating renal function.

Pharmacology

Flurbiprofen is a propionic acid derivative and a highly potent COX inhibitor. It inhibits both COX-1 and COX-2 but, along with **indometacin, ketoprofen** and **ketorolac**, has higher COX-1 selectivity than many NSAIDs.[2] The molar potency for 50% inhibition of PGE_2 synthesis *in vitro* is >5,000 times that of **aspirin**, 250 times that of **ibuprofen**, and 125 times that of **naproxen**.[3] In animals, mg for mg, it is 8–20 times more potent than **aspirin**. Flurbiprofen is excreted in the urine both as unchanged drug and several hydroxylated metabolites.

Flurbiprofen has been used for many years by some palliative care services as the NSAID of choice (without routine gastroprotection). However, a recent case-crossover study ranked the risk of myocardial infarction for oral flurbiprofen second only to ketorolac.[4]

In addition to its analgesic use, flurbiprofen has been used to relieve frequency caused by instability of the detrusor muscle of the bladder. Animal studies show that PGs are produced by the detrusor (bladder muscle) and that they increase tone and bladder contractile activity. In humans, frequency, urgency, and urge incontinence are all significantly decreased by flurbiprofen 50mg t.d.s.[1]

Bio-availability >85% PO.
Onset of action 30–60min.
Time to peak plasma concentration 1–2h PO; 4–6h m/r.
Plasma halflife 3–6h.
Duration of action 8–16h.[5]

Cautions

Renal and hepatic impairment (see p.681 and p.703); CVS impairment, see p.319. Correct hyperkalaemia before use. To minimize the potential for serious undesirable effects, use the lowest effective dose for the shortest treatment duration possible. Risk of aseptic meningitis in patients with SLE (very rare).

Because of the increased risk of bleeding (from decreased platelet aggregation) try to avoid concurrent prescription of flurbiprofen and **warfarin**. As with all NSAIDs, concurrent administration with an SSRI is associated with an increased risk of GI bleeding.

The thromboprotective effect of **aspirin** for stroke is compromised in people taking certain NSAIDs concurrently.[6] Although the study did not include flurbiprofen, given its association with an increased risk of myocardial infarction, people taking low-dose **aspirin** for thromboprotection are probably best *not* prescribed flurbiprofen. Instead, prescribe **celecoxib** (with **aspirin**) or **naproxen** alone (see p.320).

Drug interactions

For general interactions between NSAIDs and other drugs, see Tables 8 and 9 (p.323 and p.324). Of particular importance is the risk of toxic plasma levels of **digoxin, lithium**, and **methotrexate** caused by reduced renal function and/or reduced tubular excretion. If flurbiprofen is prescribed, monitor the plasma drug concentration or haematological effect of these drugs as appropriate and reduce doses as necessary (see p.322).

Because they cause sodium and fluid retention, all NSAIDs can decrease the effect of diuretics, ACE inhibitors and antihypertensives.

In addition to the effect on platelet function (see Cautions), an increase in INR occasionally occurs when flurbiprofen is prescribed for a patient already taking **warfarin**; monitor the INR weekly for 3–4 weeks and adjust the dose of **warfarin** if necessary.[7]

Flurbiprofen is metabolized by CYP2C9. Caution should be taken with concurrent use of drugs which inhibit or induce this enzyme, particularly in those who are poor CYP2C9 metabolizers (see p.726). **Fluconazole** and possibly **voriconazole** (strong CYP2C9 inhibitors) increase flurbiprofen plasma concentration, and lower doses may be necessary.

5

Undesirable effects

Also see NSAIDs, p.312.

Common (<10%, >1%): headache, dizziness, oedema, indigestion, abdominal discomfort, nausea, constipation or diarrhoea, pruritus, rash, ecchymosis.

Dose and use

Although traditionally advised to take NSAIDs with food, there is no evidence that this reduces the risk of GI complications.

Gastroprotection, e.g. a PPI (see p.30), should be prescribed concurrently for patients at high risk of NSAID-related upper GI complications (see Box B, p.318) or **celecoxib** ± PPI prescribed instead (see p.316).

PCF prefers **celecoxib** (p.330). Typical regimens for flurbiprofen in cancer pain are:

- start with 100mg PO b.d.
- if necessary, increase to 100mg t.d.s.
- in very elderly or debilitated:
  - ▷ start with 50mg b.d.
  - ▷ if necessary, increase to 100mg b.d.

For sore throat, see p.619.

Supply

Flurbiprofen (generic)

Tablets 50mg, 100mg, 28 days @ 100mg b.d. = £36.

1 Cardozo L *et al.* (1980) Evaluation of flurbiprofen in detrusor instability. *British Medical Journal.* **280**: 281–282.

2 Uzan A (2005) The unexpected side effects of new nonsteroidal anti-inflammatory drugs. *Expert Opinion on Emerging Drugs.* **10**: 687–688.

3 Crook D *et al.* (1976) Effect of aspirin-like drug therapy. Prostaglandin synthetase activity from human rheumatoid synovial microsomes. *Annals of the Rheumatic Diseases.* **35**: 327–332.

4 Shau WY *et al.* (2012) Risk of new acute myocardial infarction hospitalization associated with use of oral and parenteral non-steroidal anti-inflammation drugs (NSAIDS): a case crossover study of Taiwan's National health Insurance claims database and review of current evidence. Available from: www.biomedcentral.com/1471-2261/12/4

5 Kowanko I *et al.* (1981) Circadian variations in the signs and symptoms of rheumatoid arthritis and in the therapeutic effectiveness of flurbiprofen at different times of day. *British Journal of Clinical Pharmacology.* **11**: 477–484.

6 Gladding PA *et al.* (2008) The antiplatelet effect of six non-steroidal anti-inflammatory drugs and their pharmacodynamic interaction with aspirin in healthy volunteers. *American Journal of Cardiology.* **101**: 1060–1063.

7 Baxter K and Preston CL *Stockley's Drug Interactions.* London: Pharmaceutical Press www.medicinescomplete.com (accessed December 2012).

Updated (minor change) September 2017

IBUPROFEN

Class: Non-opioid analgesic, NSAID, non-selective COX inhibitor.

Indications: Pain in arthritic conditions and other musculoskeletal disorders, postoperative pain, dental pain, dysmenorrhoea, headache, migraine, fever, †cancer pain.

Contra-indications: Hypersensitivity to **aspirin** or other NSAID (urticaria, rhinitis, asthma, angioedema), active GI ulceration, history of two or more distinct episodes of proven ulceration or bleeding, cerebrovascular bleeding or other bleeding disorders, severe heart failure, active liver disease or severe hepatic impairment, severe renal impairment, deteriorating renal function.

Pharmacology

Ibuprofen is a non-selective COX inhibitor (see Table 1, p.313 and Table 2, p.314). Like **naproxen**, it is a propionic acid derivative. The analgesic and antipyretic effects of ibuprofen are mediated by both COX inhibition and non-COX mechanisms (see p.314).[1,2] Ibuprofen is three times more potent than **aspirin**, i.e. 200mg is equivalent to 600mg of **aspirin**. Higher doses of ibuprofen have a greater analgesic effect than standard doses of **aspirin**.

Ibuprofen is a chiral NSAID, i.e. it is a mixture of roughly equal amounts of *S*− and *R*−enantiomers, mirror-image molecules.[3,4] The anti-inflammatory activity resides mostly in the *S*−enantiomer, but about half the *R*−enantiomer is converted to the *S*− form in the GI tract and liver.[1,5] The *S*−enantiomer reaches higher levels and persists for longer in the elderly.[6] Both enantiomers are metabolized via CYP450.

Inversion takes time, and the time frame for single doses in acute situations is too short for inversion to play an important part.[7] Even so, a single dose of ibuprofen 200–400mg PO for acute postoperative pain is highly effective, with an NNT of around 2.5.[8] In arthritis, ibuprofen is concentrated at sites of inflammation, e.g. the joint synovium.[9] Doses of 200–400mg are as effective as **paracetamol** 1g, and efficacy increases as the dose increases.[10]

Low-dose ibuprofen (≤1,200mg/24h) has a relatively *low* propensity for causing upper GI complications[11,12] but, with *high dose* ibuprofen (2,400mg/24h), the risk is quadrupled (comparable with high-dose **naproxen**; also see p.316).[13] Concern has been expressed that OTC ibuprofen may occasionally cause small bowel damage.[14]

Cardiovascular risk is dose related; the risk with high-dose ibuprofen (2,400mg/24h) is comparable to, or perhaps even higher than, other NSAIDs (see p.319) The risk of renal failure with ibuprofen is also comparable with other NSAIDs.[17] It is safe in overdose; few deaths attributable to ibuprofen alone have been reported, involving overdoses of 36–200g.[18–22] Ibuprofen may be of benefit in cancer-related cachexia (see Progestogens, p.552).

Ibuprofen can be used topically (as a locally prepared preparation), particularly for sprains, strains and arthritis.[23] Although application to the skin produces plasma concentrations which are only 5% of those obtained with oral administration, the underlying muscle and fascial concentrations are 25 times greater.[24,25]

Topical and PO ibuprofen have been shown to be equally effective for chronic knee pain in patients aged ≥50 years, although those with more severe or widespread pain preferred PO treatment.[27] The incidence of major undesirable effects were similar, but topical treatment led to fewer minor undesirable effects and less treatment discontinuation. Systemic undesirable effects with topical ibuprofen for acute pain are uncommon, and even local effects are not significantly different from placebo.[28]

Because it has a more rapid onset of action, IV ibuprofen (not UK) has a potential role in the management of acute pain.[29]

Bio-availability 90% PO.
Onset of action 20–30min.
Time to peak plasma concentration 1–2h.
Plasma halflife 2–3h.[1]
Duration of action 4–6h.

Cautions

Renal and hepatic impairment (see p.681 and p.703). Restrict dose to ≤1,800mg/24h in patients with significant CVS risk factors (hypertension, hyperlipidaemia, diabetes mellitus, smoking). Correct hyperkalaemia before use.

Because of the increased risk of bleeding (from decreased platelet aggregation) avoid concurrent prescription with **warfarin**. As with all NSAIDs, concurrent administration with an SSRI is associated with an increased risk of GI bleeding.

The thromboprotective effect of **aspirin** for stroke is compromised in people taking ibuprofen concurrently.[30–32] Thus, people taking low-dose **aspirin** for thromboprotection should *not* take ibuprofen. Instead, prescribe **celecoxib** (with **aspirin**) or **naproxen** alone (see p.343).

Drug interactions

For general interactions between NSAIDs and other drugs, see Tables 8 and 9 (p.323 and p.324). Of particular importance is the risk of toxic plasma levels of **digoxin**, **lithium**, and **methotrexate** caused by reduced renal function and/or reduced tubular excretion. If ibuprofen is prescribed, monitor the plasma drug concentration or haematological effect of these drugs as appropriate and reduce doses as necessary (see p.322).

Because they cause sodium and fluid retention, all NSAIDs can decrease the effect of diuretics, ACE inhibitors and antihypertensives.

In addition to the effect on platelet function (see Cautions), an increase in INR occasionally occurs when ibuprofen is prescribed for a patient already taking **warfarin**; monitor the INR weekly for 3–4 weeks and adjust the dose of **warfarin** if necessary.[33]

Ibuprofen is metabolized by CYP2C9. **Fluconazole** and **voriconazole** (strong CYP2C9 inhibitors) increase ibuprofen plasma concentration, and lower doses may be necessary. Caution should be taken with concurrent use of other drugs which inhibit or induce this enzyme (see Chapter 19, Table 8, p.725).

Undesirable effects

Also see NSAIDs, p.312.

Common (<10%, >1%): headache, dizziness, oedema, indigestion, abdominal discomfort, nausea, constipation or diarrhoea, pruritus, rash, ecchymosis.

Very rare (<0.01%): aseptic meningitis in patients with SLE.

Dose and use

Although traditionally advised to take NSAIDs with food, there is no evidence that this reduces the risk of GI complications.

Gastroprotection, e.g. a PPI (see p.000), should be prescribed concurrently for patients at high risk of NSAID-related upper GI complications (see Box B, p.318) or **celecoxib** ± PPI prescribed instead (see p.316).

PCF prefers **celecoxib** (p.330). However, ibuprofen is a frequently used NSAID:

- typical dose 400mg PO t.d.s. or 200mg PO t.d.s in the frail elderly
- higher doses are associated with greater CVS risk (possibly with 600mg PO t.d.s. and definitely with 800mg PO t.d.s.).

For topical use, see p.601.

Supply

Ibuprofen tablets and capsules 200mg and 400mg, orodispersible tablets and oral suspension are available OTC.

Ibuprofen (generic)
Tablets 200mg, 400mg, 600mg, 28 days @ 400mg t.d.s. = £3.
Oral suspension 100mg/5mL, 28 Days @ 400mg t.d.s. = £21; *sugar free suspension also available.*

Nurofen Meltlets® (Reckitt Benckiser)
Orodispersible tablets 200mg, 28 days @ 400mg t.d.s. = £31.

Brufen® (Mylan)
Granules 600mg/sachet, 28 days @ 600mg b.d. = £19 *(contains 6.5mmol Na^+/sachet).*

Modified-release
Brufen Retard® (Mylan)
Tablets m/r 800mg, 28 days @1,600mg once daily. = £7.

1 Rainsford KD (2009) Ibuprofen: pharmacology, efficacy and safety. Inflammopharmacology. 17: 275–342.

2 Soares DM *et al.* (2011) Cyclooxygenase-independent mechanism of ibuprofen-induced antipyresis: the role of central vasopressin V(1) receptors. *Fundamental and Clinical Pharmacology.* **25**: 670–681.

3 Rudy AC *et al.* (1991) Stereoselective metabolism of ibuprofen in humans: administration of R-, S- and racemic ibuprofen. *Journal of Pharmacology and Experimental Therapeutics.* **259**: 1133–1139.

4 Jamali F *et al.* (1992) Human pharmacokinetics of ibuprofen enantiomers following different doses and formulations: intestinal chiral inversion. *Journal of Pharmaceutical Sciences.* **81**: 221–225.

5 Ding G *et al.* (2007) Effect of absorption rate on pharmacokinetics of ibuprofen in relation to chiral inversion in humans. *Journal of Pharmacy and Pharmacology.* **59**: 1509–1513.

6 Tan SC *et al.* (2003) Influence of age on the enantiomeric disposition of ibuprofen in healthy volunteers. *British Journal of Clinical Pharmacology.* **55**: 579–587.

7 Evans AM (2001) Comparative pharmacology of S(+)-ibuprofen and (RS)-ibuprofen. *Clinical Rheumatology.* **20 Suppl 1**: S9–14.

8 Derry C *et al.* (2009) Single dose oral ibuprofen for acute postoperative pain in adults. *Cochrane Database of Systematic Reviews*. **3**: CD001548. www.thecochranelibrary.com
9 Glass RC and Swannell AJ (1978) Concentrations of ibuprofen in serum and synovial fluid from patients with arthritis [proceedings]. *British Journal of Clinical Pharmacology*. **6**: 453P–454P.
10 McQuay HJ and Moore RA (2007) Dose-response in direct comparisons of different doses of aspirin, ibuprofen and paracetamol (acetaminophen) in analgesic studies. *British Journal of Clinical Pharmacology*. **63**: 271–278.
11 Masso Gonzalez EL *et al.* (2010) Variability among nonsteroidal antiinflammatory drugs in risk of upper gastrointestinal bleeding. *Arthritis and Rheumatism*. **62**: 1592–1601.
12 Michels SL *et al.* (2012) Over-the-counter ibuprofen and risk of gastrointestinal bleeding complications: a systematic literature review. *Current Medical Research Opinion*. **28**: 89–99.
13 CNT Collaboration (2013) Vascular and upper gastrointestinal effects of non-steroidal anti-inflammatory drugs: meta-analyses of individual participant data from randomised trials. *Lancet*. **382**: 769–779.
14 Sidhu R *et al.* (2010) Undisclosed use of nonsteroidal anti-inflammatory drugs may underlie small-bowel injury observed by capsule endoscopy. *Clinical Gastroenterology and Hepatology*. **8**: 992–995.
15 McGettigan P and Henry D (2011) Cardiovascular risk with non-steroidal anti-inflammatory drugs: systematic review of population-based controlled observational studies. *PLoS Med*. **8**: e1001098.
16 Sondergaard KB *et al.* (2017) Non-steroidal anti-inflammatory drug use is associated with increased risk of out-of-hospital cardiac arrest: a nationwide case-time-control study. *European Heart Journal Cardiovascular Pharmacotherpy*. **3**: 100–107.
17 Schneider V *et al.* (2006) Association of selective and conventional nonsteroidal antiinflammatory drugs with acute renal failure: A population-based, nested case-control analysis. *American Journal of Epidemiology*. **164**: 881–889.
18 Wood DM *et al.* (2006) Fatality after deliberate ingestion of sustained-release ibuprofen: a case report. *Critical Care*. **10**: R44.
19 Krenova M and Pelclova D (2005) Fatal poisoning with ibuprofen. *Clinical Toxicology*. **43**: 537.
20 Volans G *et al.* (2003) Ibuprofen overdose. *International Journal of Clinical Practice Supplement*. 54–60.
21 Holubek W *et al.* (2007) A report of two deaths from massive ibuprofen ingestion. *Journal of Medical Toxicology*. **3**: 52–55.
22 Lodise M *et al.* (2012) Acute Ibuprofen intoxication: report on a case and review of the literature. *American Journal of Forensic Medicine and Pathology*. **33**: 242–246.
23 Chlud K and Wagener H (1987) Percutaneous nonsteroidal anti-inflammatory drug (NSAID) therapy with particular reference to pharmacokinetic factors. *EULAR Bulletin*. **2**: 40–43.
24 Mondino A *et al.* (1983) Kinetic studies of ibuprofen on humans. Comparative study for the determination of blood concentrations and metabolites following local and oral administration. *Medizinische Welt*. **34**: 1052–1054.
25 Kageyama T (1987) A double blind placebo controlled multicenter study of piroxicam 0.5% gel in osteoarthritis of the knee. *European Journal of Rheumatology and Inflammation*. **8**: 114–115.
26 Peters H *et al.* (1987) Percutaneous kinetics of ibuprofen (German). *Aktuelle Rheumatologie*. **12**: 208–211.
27 Underwood M *et al.* (2008) Topical or oral ibuprofen for chronic knee pain in older people. The TOIB study. Available from: www.hta.ac.uk/project/1302.asp
28 Massey T *et al.* (2010) Topical NSAIDS for acute pain in adults. *Cochrane Database of Systematic Reviews*. **6**: CD007402. www.thecochranelibrary.com
29 Smith HS and Voss B (2012) Pharmacokinetics of intravenous ibuprofen: implications of time of infusion in the treatment of pain and fever. *Drugs*. **72**: 327–337.
30 Awa K *et al.* (2012) Prediction of time-dependent interaction of aspirin with ibuprofen using a pharmacokinetic/pharmacodynamic model. *Journal of Clinical Pharmacy and Therapeutics*. **37**: 469–474.
31 Gladding PA *et al.* (2008) The antiplatelet effect of six non-steroidal anti-inflammatory drugs and their pharmacodynamic interaction with aspirin in healthy volunteers. *American Journal of Cardiology*. **101**: 1060–1063.
32 Gengo FM *et al.* (2008) Effects of ibuprofen on the magnitude and duration of aspirin's inhibition of platelet aggregation: clinical consequences in stroke prophylaxis. *Journal of Clinical Pharmacology*. **48**: 117–122.
33 Baxter K and Preston CL. *Stockley's Drug Interactions*. London: Pharmaceutical Press www.medicinescomplete.com (accessed May 2017).

Updated September 2017

*KETOROLAC TROMETAMOL

Class: Non-opioid analgesic, NSAID, preferential COX-1 inhibitor.

Indications: Short-term management of moderate–severe acute postoperative pain, †intractable cancer pain, unresponsive to usual measures.

Contra-indications: Hypersensitivity to **aspirin** or other NSAID (urticaria, rhinitis, asthma, angioedema), syndrome of nasal polyps, angioedema and bronchospasm, history of asthma, history of or active GI ulceration, cerebrovascular bleeding or other bleeding disorders, severe heart failure, severe hepatic impairment, moderate or severe renal impairment (eGFR <60mL/min/1.73m^2), deteriorating renal function.

Concurrent prescription with **warfarin**, **heparin**, **aspirin**, other NSAID, **pentoxifylline** (increased risk of bleeding), **lithium** (increased plasma concentration and toxicity), and **probenecid** (increased ketorolac plasma concentration and halflife).

Pharmacology

Ketorolac is a cyclic propionate structurally related to the acetate NSAIDs, **tolmetin** and **indometacin**.[1] It inhibits both COX-1 and COX-2 but has higher COX-1 selectivity than many NSAIDs. Other mechanisms include the activation, in the periphery, of the NO-cyclic GMP pathway.[2] This may help to explain why ketorolac's analgesic effect is far greater than the anti-inflammatory and antipyretic properties: in animal studies, ketorolac is about 350 times more potent than **aspirin** as an analgesic but only 20 times more potent as an antipyretic.[1] As an anti-inflammatory, ketorolac is about half as potent as **indometacin** and twice as potent as **naproxen**. Like most COX-1 inhibitors, ketorolac inhibits platelet aggregation.

Ketorolac trometamol is more water-soluble than the parent substance. Over 99% of the oral dose is absorbed and about 75% of a dose is excreted in the urine within 7h, and over 90% within 2 days, over half as unmodified ketorolac.[3] The rest is excreted in the faeces. The analgesic and anti-inflammatory activity of ketorolac resides mainly in the S-enantiomer, which is cleared more rapidly than the less active R-enantiomer.

Of all the NSAIDs, ketorolac (PO or parenteral) carries the highest risk for gastritis and duodenitis, and upper GI complications (ulceration, bleeding, perforation).[4] A meta-analysis calculated a 15 times increase in risk with ketorolac, which is several times the risk of non-selective NSAIDs generally.[5]

Likewise, ketorolac (PO or parenteral) possibly carries the highest risk of acute myocardial infarction of any NSAID.[6] A retrospective case-crossover study of 38,000 people with strokes found PO ketorolac to be associated with only a moderate increase in the risk of stroke (odds ratio 1.9) but parenterally the risk of ischaemic or haemorrhagic stroke was increased 4–6 times.[7]

However, other postoperative studies indicate that, compared with opioids, the *short-term* use of ketorolac is associated with only a small increased risk of GI and operative site bleeding.[8,9] The risk increases with age and a treatment duration >1 week.[8,10] Thus, authorization for ketorolac is restricted to short-term (≤2 days) postoperative use. In some countries, authorization has been withdrawn, e.g. France and Germany.

Although individual doses ≤30mg are recommended in acute pain, in a study in patients attending an Emergency Department with moderate–severe pain (mean score 7–8/10), no difference was detected after 2h between doses of 10mg, 15mg and 30mg (mean scores 5/10).[12] Further, in cancer pain, in a week-long RCT, *PO* ketorolac 10mg q.d.s. was no better than **paracetamol** 600mg + **codeine** 60mg q.d.s.[13] It was also found to be no better than PO **diclofenac**.[14]

However, anecdotal palliative care reports suggests that CSCI ketorolac may be effective in some patients who fail to obtain satisfactory relief with a PO NSAID (plus opioid), mostly in bone pain but also neuropathic pain.[14] It has been used for periods of up to eight months,[15] but always with a gastroprotective drug. Some centres use CSCI **parecoxib** instead in comparable situations, generally in doses of 40–80mg/24h (see p.325).[16]

Bio-availability >99% PO.
Onset of action 30min PO, 10–30min IM/IV.
Time to peak plasma concentration 30–45min PO
Plasma halflife 5h; 7h in the elderly;[17] 6–19h with renal impairment.[10]
Duration of action 6h PO, 4–6h IM.

Cautions

Renal and hepatic impairment (see p.681 and p.703). Avoid in patients with significant CVS risk factors (hypertension, hyperlipidaemia, diabetes mellitus, smoking). Correct hyperkalaemia before use.

Aspirin thromboprotection should be discontinued. Concurrent administration with an SSRI is associated with an increased risk of GI bleeding.

Drug interactions

For general interactions between NSAIDs and other drugs, see Tables 8 and 9 (p.323 and p.324). Of particular importance is the risk of toxic plasma levels of **digoxin**, **lithium**, and **methotrexate** caused by reduced renal function and/or reduced tubular excretion (see p.322). See above for drugs contra-indicated with ketorolac.

Because they cause sodium and fluid retention, all NSAIDs can decrease the effect of diuretics, ACE inhibitors and antihypertensives.

Undesirable effects

Also see NSAIDs, p.312.
Very common (>10%): headache, dyspepsia, nausea, abdominal pain.
Common (<10%, >1%): dizziness, drowsiness, tinnitus, oedema, hypertension, anaemia, stomatitis, vomiting, bloating, flatulence, GI ulceration, diarrhoea, constipation, abnormal renal function, pruritus, purpura, rash, bleeding and pain at injection site (less with CSCI).
Very rare (<0.01%): aseptic meningitis in patients with SLE.

Dose and use

Because ketorolac carries the highest risk of upper GI ulceration, bleeding, and perforation, generally, its use is reserved for patients unresponsive to usual measures, including a PO NSAID. Gastroprotection, e.g. a PPI, must always be given (see p.30).

CSCI: because ketorolac is irritant, dilute to the largest volume possible, and preferably use 0.9% saline as the diluent (see p.819).

Use is generally *short-term* while arranging and awaiting benefit from more definitive therapy, e.g. radiotherapy. However, in the absence of other options, ketorolac has been used for extended periods without causing serious GI events.[18]

Although only authorized for IV or IM use, ketorolac can be given by intermittent injections 15–30mg SC t.d.s. Because these can be uncomfortable, for regular use it is better given by CSCI:

- start with ketorolac 60mg/24h by CSCI; *this is also the recommended maximum dose in people >65 years or <50kg*
- if necessary, increase in 15mg/24h increments to 90mg/24h (authorized maximum dose)
- occasionally, 120mg/24h is used.[18]

During titration, some centres also allow p.r.n. doses of 15mg SC as long as the permitted maximum 24h dose is not exceeded (e.g. a patient <65 years permitted a maximum of 90mg/24h but receiving 60mg/24h CSCI would be allowed up to two p.r.n. doses of 15mg SC/24h). If using for an extended period, maintain on the lowest effective dose.

Alternative SC/CSCI NSAIDs include **diclofenac** (p.332) and **parecoxib** (p.325).

CSCI compatibility with other drugs: Ketorolac is alkaline in solution and there is a high risk of *incompatibility* when mixed with acidic drugs. There are 2-drug compatibility data for ketorolac in 0.9% saline with **diamorphine** and **oxycodone**.[19]

Incompatibility has been reported with **cyclizine**, **glycopyrronium**, **haloperidol**, **hydromorphone**, **levomepromazine**, **midazolam**, and **morphine** (see, p.818).

For more details, 3-drug compatibility data, and compatibility data for mixing drugs in WFI see Appendix 3, p.863 and *www.palliativedrugs.com* Syringe Driver Survey Database (SDSD).

Supply

There is no PO ketorolac product available in the UK.

Ketorolac trometamol (generic)
Injection 30mg/mL, 1mL amp = £1, *vehicle contains alcohol.*

1 Gillis J and Brogden R (1997) Ketorolac: A reappraisal of its pharmacodynamic and pharmacokinetic properties and therapeutic use in pain management. *Drugs*. **53**: 139–188.

2 Lazaro-Ibanez GG *et al.* (2001) Participation of the nitric oxide-cyclic GMP-ATP-sensitive K(+) channel pathway in the antinociceptive action of ketorolac. *European Journal of Pharmacology*. **426**: 39–44.

3 Litvak K and McEvoy G (1990) Ketorolac: an injectable nonnarcotic analgesic. *Clinical Pharmacy*. **9**: 921–935.

4 Chang CH *et al.* (2011) Risk of hospitalization for upper gastrointestinal adverse events associated with nonsteroidal anti-inflammatory drugs: a nationwide case-crossover study in Taiwan. *Pharmacoepidemiology and Drug Safety*. **20**: 763–771.

5 Masso Gonzalez EL *et al.* (2010) Variability among nonsteroidal antiinflammatory drugs in risk of upper gastrointestinal bleeding. *Arthritis and Rheumatism*. **62**: 1592–1601.

6 Shau WY *et al.* (2012) Risk of new acute myocardial infarction hospitalization associated with use of oral and parenteral non-steroidal anti-inflammation drugs (NSAIDS): a case crossover study of Taiwan's National health Insurance claims database and review of current evidence. Available from: www.biomedcentral.com/1471-2261/12/4

7 Chang CH *et al.* (2010) Increased risk of stroke associated with nonsteroidal anti-inflammatory drugs: a nationwide case-crossover study. *Stroke*. **41**: 1884–1890.

8 Strom B *et al.* (1996) Parenteral ketorolac and risk of gastrointestinal and operative site bleeding. A postmarketing surveillance study. *Journal of the American Medical Assocation.* **275**: 376–382.
9 Rainer T *et al.* (2000) Cost effectiveness analysis of intravenous ketorolac and morphine for treating pain after limb injury: double blind randomised controlled trial. *British Medical Journal.* **321**: 1247–1251.
10 Reinhart D (2000) Minimising the adverse effects of ketorolac. *Drug Safety.* **22**: 487–497.
11 Li Q *et al.* (2010) High-dose ketorolac affects adult spinal fusion: a meta-analysis of the effect of perioperative nonsteroidal anti-inflammatory drugs on spinal fusion. *Spine* **36**: E461–E468.
12 Motov S *et al.* (2016) Comparison of intravenous ketorolac at three single-dose regimens for treating acute pain in the emergency department: a randomized controlled trial. *Annals of Emergency Medicine.*
13 Carlson RW *et al.* (1990) A multiinstitutional evaluation of the analgesic efficacy and safety of ketorolac tromethamine, acetaminophen plus codeine, and placebo in cancer pain. *Pharmacotherapy.* **10**: 211–216.
14 Pannuti F *et al.* (1999) A double-blind evaluation of the analgesic efficacy and toxicity of oral ketorolac and diclofenac in cancer pain. The TD/10 recordati Protocol Study Group. *Tumori.* **85**: 96–100.
15 Vacha ME *et al.* (2015) The role of subcutaneous ketorolac for pain management. *Hospital Pharmacy.* **50**: 108–112.
16 Armstrong P (2017) The use of parecoxib by continuous subcutaneous infusion for cancer pain in a hospice population. *BMJ Supportive and Palliative Care.* (in press).
17 Greenwald R (1992) Ketorolac: an innovative nonsteroidal analgesic. *Drugs of Today.* **28**: 41–61.
18 Gaines M *et al.* (2015) Long-term continuous subcutaneous infusion of ketorolac in hospice patients. *Journal of Palliative Medicine.* **18**: 317.
19 Dickman A and Schneider J (2016) *The Syringe Driver: Continuous Subcutaneous Infusions in Palliative Care* (4e). Oxford University Press, Oxford.

Updated September 2017

NAPROXEN

Class: Non-opioid analgesic, NSAID, non-selective COX inhibitor.

Indications: Pain in arthritic conditions and other musculoskeletal disorders, dysmenorrhoea, acute gout, †cancer pain, †fever.

Contra-indications: Hypersensitivity to **aspirin** or other NSAID (urticaria, rhinitis, asthma, angioedema), active GI ulceration, history of ≥2 distinct episodes of proven ulceration or bleeding, cerebrovascular bleeding or other bleeding disorders, severe heart failure, active liver disease or severe hepatic impairment, severe renal impairment, deteriorating renal function.

Pharmacology

Naproxen is a non-selective COX inhibitor. It is a propionic acid derivative (like **ibuprofen**). Absorption is not affected by food or antacids. A steady-state is achieved after 4–5 days of b.d. administration. It is extensively metabolized in the liver to 6-*O*-desmethylnaproxen, and then conjugated. Excretion is almost entirely urinary (95%), with <1% unchanged drug. Plasma concentrations do not increase with doses >500mg b.d. because of rapid urinary excretion.[1]

A meta-analysis of several hundred RCTs indicates that, compared with placebo, the risk the risk of upper GI complications is quadrupled with high-dose naproxen (500mg b.d.), comparable with high-dose **ibuprofen** (2,400mg/24h).[2]

Like other NSAIDs, naproxen increases the risk of CVS events (see p.319).

Naproxen increases the mean arterial pressure by 5–6 mmHg in patients with established hypertension.[3] As with all NSAIDs, naproxen should be avoided in severe heart failure.[4] Naproxen carries a similar risk of inducing acute renal failure as other NSAIDs.[5]

Although generally given b.d., a single dose of naproxen 500mg at bedtime was equal in efficacy to 250mg b.d. in patients with osteo-arthritis[6] and with rheumatoid arthritis.[7]

Naproxen *sodium* 275mg (not UK) is equivalent to 250mg naproxen. It is more rapidly absorbed, resulting in plasma concentrations about 1.5–2 times higher than those of naproxen over the first hour, and better analgesia from 4h onwards.[8]

Bio-availability 95% PO.
Onset of action 20–30min.
Time to peak plasma concentration 1.5–5h depending on dose and formulation.[9,10]
Plasma halflife 12–15h.
Duration of action 6–8h single dose; >12h multiple doses.

Cautions

Renal and hepatic impairment (see p.681 and p.703). Correct hyperkalaemia before use.

Because of an increased risk of bleeding (from decreased platelet aggregation), avoid concurrent prescription with **warfarin**. As with all NSAIDs, concurrent administration with an SSRI is associated with an increased risk of GI bleeding.

Drug interactions

For general interactions between NSAIDs and other drugs, see Tables 8 and 9 (p.323 and p.324). Of particular importance is the risk of toxic plasma levels of **digoxin**, **lithium**, and **methotrexate** caused by reduced renal function and/or reduced tubular excretion. If naproxen is prescribed, monitor the plasma drug concentration or haematological effect of these drugs as appropriate and reduce doses as necessary (see p.322).

Naproxen plasma concentrations are increased by **probenecid**.

Because they cause sodium and fluid retention, all NSAIDs can decrease the effect of diuretics, ACE inhibitors and antihypertensives.

In addition to the effect on platelet function (see Cautions), an increase in INR occasionally occurs when naproxen is prescribed for a patient already taking **warfarin**; monitor the INR weekly for 3–4 weeks and adjust the dose of **warfarin** if necessary.[11]

Undesirable effects

Also see NSAIDs, p.312.

Common (<10%, >1%): confusion, dizziness, drowsiness, fatigue, headache, visual disturbance, tinnitus, oedema, indigestion, abdominal discomfort, nausea, constipation or diarrhoea, pruritus, rash, ecchymosis.

Dose and use

Although traditionally advised to take NSAIDs with food, there is no evidence that this reduces the risk of GI complications.

Ideally, naproxen should *not* be used in patients at high risk of NSAID-related upper GI complications (see Box B, p.318). If unavoidable, gastroprotection, e.g. a PPI (see p.30), should be prescribed concurrently or **celecoxib** ± PPI prescribed instead (see p.330).

PCF prefers **celecoxib** (p.330). However, naproxen is a frequently used NSAID:

- typically 250–500mg PO b.d.
- can be taken as a single daily dose, either each morning or each evening
- occasionally, with careful monitoring, it may be worth titrating up to a total daily dose of 1.5g (e.g. 500mg t.d.s.); this is higher than the manufacturer's recommended maximum daily doses of 1–1.25g (depending on indication) and should normally be done for only a limited period. This is comparable to doses used for severe rheumatoid arthritis.

Supply

Naproxen 250mg tablets are available OTC for dysmenorrhoea.

Naproxen (generic)
Tablets 250mg, 500mg, 28 days @ 500mg b.d. = £4.
Tablets e/c 250mg, 375mg, 500mg, 28 days @ 500mg b.d. = £7.
Oral suspension (sugar-free) 125mg/5mL, 28 days @ 500mg b.d. = £1,232.

Stirlescent® (Stirling)
Tablets effervescent 250mg, 28 days @ 500mg b.d. = £44.

With **esomeprazole**
Tablets m/r naproxen 500mg e/c + **esomeprazole** 20mg, 28 days @ 1 tablet b.d. = £15.

1 Simon L and Mills J (1980) Nonsteroidal anti-inflammatory drugs. Part 2. *New England Journal of Medicine*. **302**: 1237–1243.
2 CNT Collaboration (2013) Vascular and upper gastrointestinal effects of non-steroidal anti-inflammatory drugs: meta-analyses of individual participant data from randomised trials. *Lancet*. **382**: 769–779.
3 Johnson AG *et al.* (1994) Do nonsteroidal anti-inflammatory drugs affect blood pressure? A meta-analysis. *Annals of Internal Medicine*. **121**: 289–300.

4 Gislason GH *et al.* (2009) Increased mortality and cardiovascular morbidity associated with use of nonsteroidal anti-inflammatory drugs in chronic heart failure. *Archives of Internal Medicine*. **169**: 141–149.

5 Schneider V *et al.* (2006) Association of selective and conventional nonsteroidal antiinflammatory drugs with acute renal failure: A population-based, nested case-control analysis. *American Journal of Epidemiology*. **164**: 881–889.

6 Mendelsohn S (1991) Clinical efficacy and tolerability of naproxen in osteoarthritis patients using twice-daily and once-daily regimens. *Clinical Therapy*. **13 (Suppl A)**: 8–15.

7 Graziano F (1991) Once-daily or twice-daily administration of naproxen in patients with rheumatoid arthritis. *Clinical Therapy*. **13 (Suppl A)**: 20–25.

8 Sevelius H *et al.* (1980) Bioavailability of naproxen sodium and its relationship to clinical analgesic effects. *British Journal of Clinical Pharmacology*. **10**: 259–263.

9 Kelly J *et al.* (1989) Pharmacokinetic properties and clinical efficacy of once-daily sustained-release naproxen. *European Journal of Clinical Pharmacology*. **36**: 383–388.

10 Davies N and Anderson K (1997) Clinical pharmacokinetics of naproxen. *Clinical Pharmacokinetics*. **32**: 268–293.

11 Baxter K and Preston CL. *Stockley's Drug Interactions*. London: Pharmaceutical Press www.medicinescomplete.com (accessed May 2017).

5

Updated September 2017

NABUMETONE

Class: Non-opioid analgesic, NSAID, non-selective COX inhibitor.

Indications: Pain in osteo-arthritis and rheumatoid arthritis, †cancer pain.

Contra-indications: Hypersensitivity to **aspirin** or other NSAID (urticaria, rhinitis, asthma, angioedema), active GI ulceration, history of two or more distinct episodes of proven ulceration or bleeding, cerebrovascular bleeding or other bleeding disorders, severe heart failure, active liver disease or severe hepatic impairment, severe renal impairment, deteriorating renal function.

Pharmacology

Although not widely used in UK palliative care, nabumetone possesses several noteworthy characteristics. It is unique in being both a pro-drug and non-acidic.[1] This may explain its low risk for GI toxicity, despite it being a non-selective COX inhibitor.[2,3] Nabumetone has no effect on platelet aggregation.[2,4]

Absorption is mainly unaffected by food, and is increased if taken with milk.[1] It undergoes rapid and extensive first-pass metabolism in the liver to mainly 6-methoxy-2-naphthylacetic acid (6-MNA), which is further metabolized by O-methylation and conjugation to inactive compounds.[5] Less than 1% is excreted as 6-MNA. Steady-state plasma concentrations of 6-MNA are not altered in patients with renal impairment even though the renal excretion of 6-MNA is reduced.[1] This could relate to non-linear protein-binding, changes in apparent volume of distribution[6] or increased excretion by other routes.

A systematic review of *single-dose* nabumetone in postoperative pain failed to find any study showing significant benefit.[7] However, nabumetome is as effective as other NSAIDs when given regularly 1g/24h in rheumatoid and osteo-arthritis and after acute soft tissue injury.[8–10]

In patients with osteo-arthritis, nabumetone is significantly less gastrotoxic than **diclofenac** and **piroxicam**; the incidence of serious GI events (ulceration, bleeding, perforation) over 6 months is 1.1% vs. 4.3%, and no hospitalizations vs. 1.4%.[11] Nabumetone produced fewer endoscopic ulcers over 12 weeks than **ibuprofen**, and was comparable to **ibuprofen** 2,400mg/24h + **misoprostol** 800microgram/24h.[12] It is less gastrotoxic than **naproxen** (endosopic monitoring for 5 years).[13] This low level of ulcer formation is unique to nabumetone; most NSAIDs have a significant level of risk when started, which then diminishes but remains above the baseline even after 5 years.

Meta-analysis of 13 studies incorporating some 50,000 patients showed that serious GI events were 10–36 times less likely than with the comparator NSAIDs.[14] However, it should be noted that the confidence intervals for this were extremely wide, approximately 5–760. Hospitalization for NSAID-related events was also less frequent (odds ratio 3.7, 95% CI 1–11).[14] A more recent review supports these conclusions.[15] Thus, except when there is a very high risk of gastrotoxicity, there is *no* need to prescribe a gastroprotective drug with nabumetone.

The low level upper GI toxicity is at least partly explained by the following characteristics:

- *it is non-acidic:* it does not damage phosphatidylcholine in the mucous layer, is not subject to acid-trapping (see p.316), and it has only a weak uncoupling effect on oxidative phosphorylation, and thus causes little disruption of the tight junctions which control mucosal permeability to acid

- *it is a pro-drug:* it is activated in the liver, and causes little direct damage to the stomach and duodenum.[16]

In addition, there is no enterohepatic recirculation of the active metabolite.[17] This may explain why nabumetone (like **aspirin** but unlike other NSAIDs) does not increase *small bowel* permeability and cause small bowel enteritis.[18] Not prescribing a PPI concurrently will further reduce the risk of small bowel damage (see p.318).

The relative risk of major CVS events with nabumetone is unclear.[19,20] Unlike several other non-selective NSAIDs, it has not been scrutinized in this respect.[21] In patients with treated hypertension, compared with **ibuprofen**, fewer taking nabumetone had a significant increase in blood pressure (17% vs. 6%).[22]

The higher cost (vs. **diclofenac**, **ibuprofen** and **naproxen**) is largely offset by generally *not* needing to prescribe concurrent gastroprotection. In most patients, once daily administration is satisfactory.

Bio-availability *of 6-MNA* 38% (increased by administration with milk).[1,23]
Onset of action 1–2h.
Time to peak plasma concentration *for 6-MNA* 3–6h.[5]
Plasma halflife *of 6-MNA* about 24h.
Duration of action >24h.

Cautions

Renal and hepatic impairment, and CHF (see p.320, p.321, p.319). Correct hyperkalaemia before use. As with all NSAIDs, concurrent administration with an SSRI is associated with an increased risk of GI bleeding.

The thromboprotective effect of **aspirin** for stroke is compromised in people taking certain NSAIDs concurrently.[24] Nabumetone has *no* effect on platelet function and thus should *not* interfere with **aspirin**-thromboprotection.

Drug interactions

For general interactions between NSAIDs and other drugs, see Tables 8 and 9 (p.323 and p.324). Of particular importance is the risk of toxic plasma levels of **digoxin**, **lithium**, and **methotrexate** caused by reduced renal function and/or reduced tubular excretion. If an NSAID is prescribed, monitor the plasma drug concentration or haematological effect of these drugs as appropriate and reduce doses as necessary (see p.322).

Because they cause sodium and fluid retention, all NSAIDs can decrease the effect of diuretics, ACE inhibitors and antihypertensives.

Although nabumetone does not affect the INR in anticoagulated patients, there is an isolated report of haemarthrosis and raised INR in a patient taking **warfarin** concurrently.[25] Thus, if nabumetone is prescribed for a patient already taking **warfarin**, monitor the INR weekly for 3–4 weeks and adjust the dose of **warfarin** if necessary.[26]

6-MNA is highly protein-bound and theoretically may displace other highly bound drugs from plasma proteins, e.g. **phenytoin**, sulfonylureas, the clinical relevance of this is unknown. The main enzyme involved in metabolism of 6-MNA is CYP2C9, which has implications for possible drug interactions (see Chapter 19, p.717).[27]

Undesirable effects

Also see NSAIDs, p.312.
Common (<10%, >1%): tinnitus, dyspepsia, nausea, abdominal pain, diarrhoea, constipation, rash, pruritus, oedema.
Very rare (<0.01%): aseptic meningitis in patients with SLE.

Dose and use

Although traditionally advised to take NSAIDs with food, there is no evidence that this reduces the risk of GI complications.

Generally, there is no need for gastroprotection with nabumetone. However, for patients at *very* high risk of NSAID-related upper GI complications (see Box B, p.318), consider switching to **celecoxib** ± PPI instead (see p.316).

PCF prefers **celecoxib** (p.330). However, if nabumetone is used:
- start with 1g PO each evening
- if necessary, increase to 500mg each morning and 1g each evening
- if necessary, increase further to 1g b.d.
- in very elderly (80+ years) frail patients, start with 500mg, and limit to 1g once daily.

Dose reduction is not necessary in patients with mild–moderate renal impairment.[1]

Supply

Nabumetone (generic)
Tablets 500mg, 28 days @ 1g daily = £7.50.

1 Hedner T *et al.* (2004) Nabumetone: Therapeutic use and safety profile in the management of osteoarthritis and rheumatoid arthritis. *Drugs*. **64**: 2315–2343; discussion 2344–2345.
2 Cipollone F *et al.* (1995) Effects of nabumetone on prostanoid biosynthesis in humans. *Clin Pharmacol Ther.* **58**: 335–341.
3 van Kraaij DJ *et al.* (2002) A comparison of the effects of nabumetone vs meloxicam on serum thromboxane B2 and platelet function in healthy volunteers. *British Journal of Clinical Pharmacology*. **53**: 644–647.
4 Jennings MB *et al.* (2009) A double-blind study of the effect on hemostasis of nabumetone (Relafen) compared to placebo. *Journal of Foot and Ankle Surgery*. **39**: 168–173.
5 Davies NM (1997) Clinical pharmacokinetics of nabumetone. The dawn of selective cyclo-oxygenase-2 inhibition? *Clinical Pharmacokinetics*. **33**: 404–416.
6 Brier ME *et al.* (1995) Population pharmacokinetics of the active metabolite of nabumetone in renal dysfunction. *Clinical Pharmacology and Therapeutics*. **57**: 622–627.
7 Moore RA *et al.* (2009) Single dose oral nabumetone for acute postoperative pain in adults. *Cochrane Database of Systematic Reviews*. **4**: CD007548. www.thecochranelibrary.com
8 Friedel HA *et al.* (1993) Nabumetone. A reappraisal of its pharmacology and therapeutic use in rheumatic diseases. *Drugs*. **45**: 131–156.
9 Lister BJ *et al.* (1993) Efficacy of nabumetone versus diclofenac, naproxen, ibuprofen, and piroxicam in osteoarthritis and rheumatoid arthritis. *American Journal of Medicine*. **(Suppl 2A)**: 2S–9S.
10 Morgan GJ *et al.* (1993) Efficacy and safety of nabumetone versus diclofenac, naproxen, ibuprofen, and piroxicam in the elderly. *American Journal of Medicine*. **(Suppl 2A)**: 19S–27S.
11 Scott DL and Palmer RH (2000) Safety and efficacy of nabumetone in osteoarthritis: emphasis on gastrointestinal safety. *Alimentary Pharmacology and Therapeutics*. **14**: 443–452.
12 Roth SH *et al.* (1993) A controlled study comparing the effects of nabumetone, ibuprofen, and ibuprofen plus misoprostol on the upper gastrointestinal tract mucosa. *Archives of Internal Medicine*. **153**: 2565–2571.
13 Roth SH *et al.* (1994) A longterm endoscopic evaluation of patients with arthritis treated with nabumetone vs naproxen. *Journal of Rheumatology*. **21**: 1118–1123.
14 Huang JQ *et al.* (1999) Gastrointestinal safety profile of nabumetone: a meta-analysis. *American Journal of Medicine*. **(Suppl 6A)**: 55S–61S; discussion 61S–64S.
15 Bannwarth B (2008) Safety of the nonselective NSAID nabumetone : focus on gastrointestinal tolerability. *Drug Safety*. **31**: 485–503.
16 Jeremy JY *et al.* (1990) The effect of nabumetone and its principal active metabolite on in vitro human gastric mucosal prostanoid synthesis and platelet function. *British Journal of Rheumatology*. **29**: 116–119.
17 Reuter BK *et al.* (1997) Nonsteroidal anti-inflammatory drug enteropathy in rats: role of permeability, bacteria, and enterohepatic circulation. *Gastroenterology*. **112**: 109–117.
18 Sigthorsson G *et al.* (1998) Intestinal permeability and inflammation in patients on NSAIDs. *Gut*. **43**: 506–511.
19 Helin-Salmivaara A *et al.* (2006) NSAID use and the risk of hospitalization for first myocardial infarction in the general population: a nationwide case-control study from Finland. *European Heart Journal*. **27**: 1657–1663.
20 Huang WF *et al.* (2006) CVS events associated with the use of four nonselective NSAIDs (etodolac, nabumetone, ibuprofen, or naproxen) versus a cyclooxygenase-2 inhibitor (celecoxib): a population-based analysis in Taiwanese adults. *Clinical Therapeutics*. **28**: 1827–1836.
21 CNT Collaboration (2013) Vascular and upper gastrointestinal effects of non-steroidal anti-inflammatory drugs: meta-analyses of individual participant data from randomised trials. *Lancet*. **382**: 769–779.
22 Palmer R *et al.* (2003) Effects of nabumetone, celecoxib, and ibuprofen on blood pressure control in hypertensive patients on angiotensin converting enzyme inhibitors. *American Journal of Hypertension*. **16**: 135–139.
23 Dollery C (1999) *Therapeutic Drugs*. (2e). Churchill Livingstone, Edinburgh.
24 Gladding PA *et al.* (2008) The antiplatelet effect of six non-steroidal anti-inflammatory drugs and their pharmacodynamic interaction with aspirin in healthy volunteers. *American Journal of Cardiology*. **101**: 1060–1063.
25 Dennis VC *et al.* (2000) Potentiation of oral anticoagulation and hemarthrosis associated with nabumetone. *Pharmacotherapy*. **20**: 234–239.
26 Baxter K and Preston CL. *Stockley's Drug Interactions*. London: Pharmaceutical Press www.medicinescomplete.com (accessed May 2017).
27 Matsumoto K *et al.* (2011) In vitro characterization of the cytochrome P450 isoforms involved in the metabolism of 6-methoxy-2-napthylacetic acid, an active metabolite of the prodrug nabumetone. *Biological and Pharmaceutical Bulletin*. **34**: 734–739.

Updated September 2017

WEAK OPIOIDS

There is no pharmacological need for weak opioids in cancer pain (see p.295). Low doses of **morphine** (or an alternative strong opioid) generally provide quicker and better relief from cancer pain than a weak opioid.[1,2] Moving directly from a non-opioid to a strong opioid is increasingly preferred in adults, and is the norm in children, in whom weak opioids are no longer recommended.[3] However, in some countries, weak opioids remain a practical necessity because of the restricted availability (or non-availability) of oral **morphine** and other strong opioids.

Codeine is the archetypical weak opioid (and **morphine** the archetypical strong opioid).[4] However, the division of opioids into 'weak' and 'strong' is to a certain extent arbitrary. In reality, opioids manifest a range of strengths which is not fully reflected in two discrete categories. **Dihydrocodeine** and **tramadol** can be considered as equipotent to **codeine**, and are also generally classified as weak opioids (Table 1).

Table 1 Weak opioids. Dihydrocodeine and tramadol can be considered equipotent to codeine

Drug	*PO bio-availability (%)*	*Time to peak plasma concentration (h)*	*Plasma halflife (h)*	*Duration of analgesia (h)[a]*
Codeine	40 (12–84)	1–2	2.5–3.5	4–6
Dihydrocodeine	20	1.6–1.8	3.5–4.5	3–6
Tramadol	75[b]	2	6[c]	4–9

a. when used in typical doses for mild–moderate pain
b. multiple doses >90%
c. active metabolite (M1) 7.5h; both figures double in cirrhosis and severe renal failure.

By IM injection, weak opioids can all provide analgesia equivalent, or almost equivalent, to **morphine** 10mg IM. High-dose **codeine** (or alternative) is comparable to low-dose **morphine** (or alternative), and vice versa.

Weak opioids are said to have a 'ceiling' effect for analgesia. This is an oversimplification; although mixed agonist-antagonists (e.g. **pentazocine**) have a true ceiling effect, the maximum effective dose of weak opioid agonists is arbitrary. At higher doses, there are progressively more undesirable effects, e.g. nausea and vomiting, which outweigh any additional analgesic effect. Other dose-limiting factors are the number of tablets which patients will readily accept and, in some combination products, the dose of the non-opioid, e.g. **paracetamol**.

There is little to choose between **codeine** and its alternatives in terms of efficacy[5] but there is no consensus about which is the weak opioid of choice. The following should be noted:

- **codeine** has little or no analgesic effect until metabolized to **morphine**, mainly via CYP2D6. Thus, in poor metabolizers, it is essentially ineffective. In contrast, in ultra-rapid metabolizers, it is potentially toxic; in children this has led to rare postoperative deaths, leading to restrictions in its use (see p.349)
- **dihydrocodeine**, like **codeine**, is a substrate for CYP2D6 and its partial metabolism is limited in poor metabolizers and is blocked by CYP2D6 inhibitors. However, unlike **codeine**, there is no evidence that such inhibition reduces its analgesic effect, i.e. **dihydrocodeine** is an active substance, not a pro-drug like **codeine** (see p.352)
- **tramadol** is less constipating than **codeine** and **dihydrocodeine**, but causes more vomiting, dizziness and anorexia. Further, if used with another drug which affects serotonin metabolism or availability, it can lead to serotonin toxicity, particularly in the elderly. It lowers seizure threshold. Unless metabolized to O-desmethyltramadol (M1) via CYP2D6, **tramadol** has a much reduced analgesic effect; it is thus practically ineffective in poor metabolizers. In contrast, in ultra-rapid metabolizers, it is potentially toxic and similar restrictions exist on its use in children as for **codeine** (see p.354)
- **pentazocine** should *not* be used; it often causes psychotomimetic effects (dysphoria, depersonalization, frightening dreams, hallucinations).[6]

Weak opioids differ in their potential to cause toxicity when renal function is impaired, see Chapter 17, p.693. All weak opioids should be avoided in severe hepatic impairment, see Chapter 18, p.709.

Whichever weak opioid is used, the following general rules should be observed:

- a weak opioid should be added to, not substituted for, a non-opioid analgesic
- it is generally inappropriate to switch from one weak opioid to another weak opioid
- if a weak opioid is inadequate when given regularly, change to **morphine** (or an alternative strong opioid).

As with all opioids, patients must be monitored for undesirable effects (see Strong opioids, Box B, p.365), particularly nausea and vomiting, and constipation. Depending on individual circumstances, an anti-emetic should be prescribed for regular or p.r.n. use (see QCG: Nausea and vomiting, p.240) and, routinely, a laxative prescribed (see QCG: Opioid-induced constipation, p.42).

Opioids can impair driving ability and patients should be counselled accordingly (see p.743).

1 Caraceni A *et al.* (2012) Use of opioid analgesics in the treatment of cancer pain: evidence-based recommendations from the EAPC. *Lancet Oncology*. **13**: e58–68.
2 Bandieri E *et al.* (2016) Randomized trial of low-dose morphine versus weak opioids in moderate cancer pain. *Journal of Clinical Oncology*. **34**: 436–442.
3 WHO (2012) Persisting pain in children package: WHO guidelines on the pharmacological treatment of persisiting pain in children with medical illness. World Health Organisation, Geneva. Available from: www.who.int/publications
4 WHO (1986). *Cancer Pain Relief.* World Health Organization, Geneva.
5 Moore RA and McQuay HJ (1997) Single-patient data meta-analysis of 3453 postoperative patients: oral tramadol versus placebo, codeine and combination analgesics. *Pain*. **69**: 287–294.
6 Woods A *et al.* (1974) Medicines evaluation and monitoring group: central nervous system effects of pentazocine. *British Medical Journal*. **1**: 305–307.

Updated September 2017

CODEINE PHOSPHATE

Class: Opioid analgesic.

Indications: Mild–moderate pain, cough, diarrhoea.

There is no pharmacological need for weak opioids in cancer pain (see p.295). Low doses of **morphine** (or an alternative strong opioid) generally provide quicker and better relief from cancer pain than a weak opioid.[1,2] Moving directly from a non-opioid to a strong opioid is increasingly preferred in adults, and is the norm in children, in whom weak opioids are no longer recommended.[3] However, in some countries, weak opioids remain a practical necessity because of the restricted availability (or non-availability) of oral **morphine** and other strong opioids.

Contra-indications: None absolute if titrated carefully to effect. Avoid use in children and adolescents (see below).[4–6]

Pharmacology

Codeine (methylmorphine) is an opium alkaloid, about one tenth as potent as **morphine**. An increasing analgesic response has been reported with IM doses up to 360mg.[7] However, in practice, codeine is generally used PO in doses of 15–60mg, often in combination with a non-opioid. Although widely prescribed, there is a lack of RCT data on the efficacy and tolerability of fixed-dose **paracetamol**-codeine combinations in cancer pain.

Codeine is metabolized mainly (80%) by conjugation to codeine-6-glucuronide which may contribute to its analgesic effect.[8,9] However, most of its analgesic effect results from the ≤10% of codeine which is converted to **morphine** by O-demethylation via CYP2D6.[10,11] If this pathway is blocked by CYP2D6 inhibitors (see Chapter 19, Table 8, p.725), codeine lacks significant analgesic activity. However, because of genetic polymorphism (see Chapter 19, Table 3, p.721), there is wide interindividual variation in the production of **morphine**, which results in a wide range of responses to codeine.[12–16]

Compared with the general population (extensive metabolizers), poor metabolizers produce little or no **morphine**, and obtain little or no pain relief from codeine. On the other hand, undesirable effects are comparable in both groups.[15,17] In contrast, ultra-rapid metabolizers produce more **morphine**, which can lead to opioid intoxication. Rarely, in children, this has been fatal, and has led to severe restrictions on its use in children (see Cautions).[4,18–21]

Like **morphine**, codeine is antitussive and also slows GI transit.[22] Given that opioids can cause pruritus, it is noteworthy that a patient with primary biliary cirrhosis obtained relief with regular PO codeine (also see Chapter 26, p.757).[23] Because of constipation, codeine was stopped and the pruritus returned. When codeine was restarted, together with a laxative, the patient again obtained relief.

Bio-availability 40% (12–84%) PO.[10]
Onset of action 30–60min for analgesia; 1–2h for antitussive effect.
Time to peak plasma concentration 1–2h.
Plasma halflife 2.5–3.5h.[10]
Duration of action 4–6h.

Cautions

Codeine use in children and adolescents is *contra-indicated* in those:
- <12 years for pain, cough or diarrhoea
- <18 years for pain after surgery to remove tonsils and/or adenoids.

Further, the MHRA advise that codeine:[5,6]
- is not recommended in those 12–18 years whose breathing might be compromised, e.g. by neuromuscular disorders, severe cardiac or respiratory conditions, chest infection, multiple trauma, extensive surgical procedures
- should only be used in children >12 years for acute moderate pain if **paracetamol** or **ibuprofen** alone are ineffective and that:
  - ▷ the maximum total daily dose is ≤240mg/24h given in divided doses ≥q6h
  - ▷ the duration of treatment is ≤3 days and stopped if ineffective
  - ▷ information on recognizing **morphine** toxicity is given to caregivers.

Although not specifically covered by the MHRA advice, similar cautions can be applied to the use of codeine for diarrhoea in those 12–18 years old.

Codeine is *contra-indicated* in adults and children who are *known* CYP2D6 ultra-rapid metabolizers. Although generally unknown in routine clinical practice, the prevalence is higher in some ethnic populations, see Chapter 19, Table 3, p.721.

Driving ability may be impaired by a dose of 50mg, see Chapter 22, p.743.[24,25] Like **morphine** and **dihydrocodeine**, codeine is more toxic in severe renal impairment and should be avoided. This is because of accumulation of **morphine** and other active metabolites (see Chapter 17, p.693).

Codeine is generally best not used in patients with moderate–severe hepatic impairment; reduced metabolism could result in less being transformed into **morphine**, thereby reducing its analgesic effect (see Chapter 18, p.709).[26]

Drug interactions

CYP2D6 inhibitors (e.g. **fluoxetine**, **paroxetine**, **quinidine**) block the biotransformation of codeine to **morphine**, and will render codeine ineffective as an analgesic; see Chapter 19, Table 8, p.725 for more details.

Undesirable effects

Codeine can produce the whole range of opioid undesirable effects (see Strong opioids, Box B, p.365).

Dose and use

Note. Low-dose PO **morphine** (20–30mg/24h) generally provides quicker and better relief from cancer pain than codeine.[2]

As with all opioids, patients must be monitored for undesirable effects, particularly nausea and vomiting, and constipation. Depending on individual circumstances, an anti-emetic should be prescribed for regular or p.r.n. use, (see QCG: Nausea and vomiting, p.240) and, routinely, a laxative prescribed (see QCG: Opioid-induced constipation, p.42).

It is bad practice to prescribe codeine to patients already taking ***morphine*** *or any other strong opioid; if a greater effect is needed, the regular and p.r.n. doses of* ***morphine*** *(or other strong opioid) should be increased.*

5

Pain relief

Codeine is often given PO in a combination product with a non-opioid. Prices can vary significantly between different combination products, codeine content and the individual formulations, i.e. tablets vs capsules or dispersible tablets (see Supply). The codeine content of these products is generally 8mg, 15mg, or 30mg (lower strengths, e.g. 8–12mg, are present in some OTC combination products containing **aspirin**, **ibuprofen** or **paracetamol**). Thus, patients with inadequate relief may benefit by changing to a higher strength product. When given alone, the dose is generally 30–60mg PO q4h. Higher doses can be given but equivalent analgesic PO doses of **morphine** (one tenth of the dose of codeine) may be less constipating.

Cough

Codeine is effective as an antitussive by any route. The dose is tailored to the patient's need, e.g. 15–30mg PO p.r.n., up to q4h. Administration as an oral linctus or solution/syrup is *not* necessary, see Antitussives, p.144.

Diarrhoea

To control diarrhoea, a dose of 30–60mg PO is used both p.r.n. and regularly up to q4h. However, **loperamide** may be preferable (see p.35).

Supply

Codeine phosphate (generic)
Tablets 15mg, 30mg, 60mg, 28 days @ 30mg q.d.s. = £4.50.
Oral linctus 15mg/5mL, 28 days @ 30mg q.d.s. = £9; *sugar-free formulations are available.*
Oral solution 25mg/5mL, 28 days @ 25mg q.d.s. = £7.50
Injections 60mg/mL, 1mL amp = £2.50. Schedule 2 **CD**.

With **aspirin**
Co-codaprin (generic)
Tablets dispersible codeine phosphate 8mg, **aspirin** 400mg, 28 days @ 2 q.d.s. = £183.
Tablets dispersible codeine phosphate 8mg, **aspirin** 500mg, 28 days @ 2 q.d.s. = £23.

With **paracetamol**
Co-codamol 8/500 (generic)
Capsules codeine phosphate 8mg, **paracetamol** 500mg, 28 days @ 2 q.d.s. = £28.
Tablets codeine phosphate 8mg, **paracetamol** 500mg, 28 days @ 2 q.d.s. = £6.
Tablets dispersible codeine phosphate 8mg, **paracetamol** 500mg, 28 days @ 2 q.d.s. = £15.

Co-codamol 15/500
Capsules codeine phosphate 15mg, **paracetamol** 500mg, 28 days @ 2 q.d.s. = £16.
Tablets codeine phosphate 15mg, **paracetamol** 500mg, 28 days @ 2 q.d.s. = £21.
Tablets dispersible codeine phosphate 15mg, **paracetamol** 500mg, 28 days @ 2 q.d.s. = £18.

Co-codamol 30/500 (generic)
Capsules codeine phosphate 30mg, **paracetamol** 500mg, 28 days @ 2 q.d.s. = £8.
Tablets codeine phosphate 30mg, **paracetamol** 500mg, 28 days @ 2 q.d.s. = £8.
Tablets effervescent codeine phosphate 30mg, **paracetamol** 500mg, 28 days @ 2 q.d.s. = £19.

This is not a complete list; see BNF for more information.

Note. Dispersible or effervescent formulations may contain Na^+ up to 20mmol/tablet or sachet. Check individual brand SPC and avoid high Na^+ formulations in renal impairment.

1 Caraceni A *et al.* (2012) Use of opioid analgesics in the treatment of cancer pain: evidence-based recommendations from the EAPC. *Lancet Oncology*. **13**: e58–68.
2 Bandieri E *et al.* (2016) Randomized trial of low-dose morphine versus weak opioids in moderate cancer pain. *Journal of Clinical Oncology*. **34**: 436–442.
3 WHO (2012) Persisting pain in children package: WHO guidelines on the pharmacological treatment of persisiting pain in children with medical illness. World Health Organisation, Geneva. Available from: www.who.int/publications
4 Racoosin JA *et al.* (2013) New evidence about an old drug - risk with codeine after adenotonsillectomy. *New England Journal of Medicine*. **368**: 2155–2157.
5 MHRA (2013) Codeine: restricted use as an analgesic in children and adolescents after European safety review. *Drug Safety Update*. www.gov.uk/drug-safety-update
6 MHRA (2015) Codeine for cough and cold: restricted use in children. *Drug Safety Update*. www.gov.uk/drug-safety-update
7 Beaver W (1966) Mild analgesics: a review of their clinical pharmacology (Part II). *American Journal of Medical Science*. **251**: 576–599.
8 Lotsch J *et al.* (2006) Evidence for morphine-independent central nervous opioid effects after administration of codeine: contribution of other codeine metabolites. *Clinical Pharmacology and Therapeutics*. **79**: 35–48.
9 Vree TB *et al.* (2000) Codeine analgesia is due to codeine-6-glucuronide, not morphine. *International Journal of Clinical Practice*. **54**: 395–398.
10 Persson K *et al.* (1992) The postoperative pharmacokinetics of codeine. *European Journal of Clinical Pharmacology*. **42**: 663–666.
11 Findlay JWA *et al.* (1978) Plasma codeine and morphine concentrations after therapeutic oral doses of codeine-containing analgesics. *Clinical Pharmacology and Therapeutics*. **24**: 60–68.
12 Sindrup SH and Brosen K (1995) The pharmacogenetics of codeine hypoalgesia. *Pharmacogenetics*. **5**: 335–346.
13 Caraco Y *et al.* (1996) Pharmacogenetic determination of the effects of codeine and prediction of drug interactions. *Journal of Pharmacology and Experimental Therapeutics*. **278**: 1165–1174.
14 Lurcott G (1999) The effects of the genetic absence and inhibition of CYP2D6 on the metabolism of codeine and its derivatives, hydrocodone and oxycodone. *Anesthesia Progress*. **45**: 154–156.
15 Eckhardt K *et al.* (1998) Same incidence of adverse drug events after codeine administration irrespective of the genetically determined differences in morphine formation. *Pain*. **76**: 27–33.
16 Lotsch J *et al.* (2004) Genetic predictors of the clinical response to opioid analgesics: clinical utility and future perspectives. *Clinical Pharmacokinetics*. **43**: 983–1013.
17 Susce MT *et al.* (2006) Response to hydrocodone, codeine and oxycodone in a CYP2D6 poor metabolizer. *Progress in Neuropsychopharmacology and Biological Psychiatry*. **30**: 1356–1358.
18 Gasche Y *et al.* (2004) Codeine intoxication associated with ultrarapid CYP2D6 metabolism. *New England Journal of Medicine*. **351**: 2827–2831.
19 Koren G *et al.* (2006) Pharmacogenetics of morphine poisoning in a breastfed neonate of a codeine-prescribed mother. *Lancet*. **368**: 704.
20 Kirchheiner J *et al.* (2007) Pharmacokinetics of codeine and its metabolite morphine in ultra-rapid metabolizers due to CYP2D6 duplication. *Pharmacogenomics Journal*. **7**: 257–265.
21 Williams DG *et al.* (2002) Pharmacogenetics of codeine metabolism in an urban population of children and its implications for analgesic reliability. *British Journal of Anaesthesia*. **89**: 839–845.
22 Anonymous (1989) Drugs in the management of acute diarrhoea in infants and young children. *Bulletin of the World Health Organization*. **67**: 94–96.
23 Zylicz Z and Krajnik M (1999) Codeine for pruritus in primary biliary cirrhosis. *Lancet*. **353**: 813.
24 Linnoila M and Hakkinen S (1974) Effects of diazepam and codeine, alone and in combination with alcohol, on simulated driving. *Clinical Pharmacology and Therapeutics*. **15**: 368–373.
25 Linnoila M and Mattila MJ (1973) Proceedings: Drug interaction on driving skills as evaluated by laboratory tests and by a driving simulator. *Pharmakopsychiatric Neuropsychopharmakologie*. **6**: 127–132.
26 Tegeder I *et al.* (1999) Pharmacokinetics of opioids in liver disease. *Clinical Pharmacokinetics*. **37**: 17–40.

Updated September 2017

DIHYDROCODEINE TARTRATE

Class: Opioid analgesic.

Indications: Moderate–severe pain.

There is no pharmacological need for weak opioids in cancer pain (see p.295). Low doses of **morphine** (or an alternative strong opioid) generally provide quicker and better relief from cancer pain than a weak opioid.[1,2] Moving directly from a non-opioid to a strong opioid is increasingly preferred in adults, and is the norm in children, in whom weak opioids are no longer recommended.[3] However, in some countries, weak opioids remain a practical necessity because of the restricted availability (or non-availability) of oral **morphine** and other strong opioids.

Contra-indications: None absolute if titrated carefully to effect.

Pharmacology

Dihydrocodeine is a semisynthetic analogue of **codeine**. It relieves pain and cough,[4,5] and causes constipation.[6] Like **codeine**, dihydrocodeine is a substrate for CYP2D6. Its partial metabolism to dihydromorphine is limited in poor metabolizers, and is blocked by CYP2D6 inhibitors (see Chapter 19, Table 8, p.725).[7] However, unlike **codeine**, there is no evidence that inhibition reduces the analgesic effect of dihydrocodeine.[8] In other words, dihydrocodeine is an active substance, not a pro-drug like **codeine**.[9,10]

By injection dihydrocodeine 60mg IM is comparable to **morphine** 10mg IM.[11,12] Dihydrocodeine is about twice as potent as **codeine** by injection but, because its oral bio-availability is low, the two drugs are essentially equipotent by mouth.[13]

5

Bio-availability 20% PO.
Onset of action 30min.
Time to peak plasma concentration 1.7h.
Plasma halflife 3.5–4.5h.
Duration of action 4h.

Cautions

May impair the ability to perform skilled tasks, e.g. driving, see Chapter 22, p.743. Prolonged erections have occurred when **sildenafil** was taken concurrently with dihydrocodeine, possibly because abnormally high concentrations of cyclic guanosine monophosphate were produced in peripheral nerve endings.[14]

Like **morphine** and **codeine**, dihydrocodeine is more toxic in severe renal impairment, probably because of accumulation of an active glucuronide, and should be avoided (also see p.693).[15] Dihydrocodeine is best avoided in moderate–severe hepatic impairment (see p.709).

Undesirable effects

Common (<10%, >1%): sedation, dizziness, disturbed dreams, headache, vertigo, nausea and vomiting, constipation, pruritus, rash.
Uncommon (<1%): hallucinations, paralytic ileus, urinary retention.

Dose and use

Note. Low-dose PO **morphine** (20–30mg/24h) generally provides quicker and better relief from cancer pain than a Step 2 analgesic.[1]

As with all opioids, patients must be monitored for undesirable effects (see Strong opioids, Box B, p.365), particularly nausea and vomiting, and constipation. Depending on individual circumstances, an anti-emetic should be prescribed for regular or p.r.n. use (see QCG: Nausea and vomiting, p.240) and, routinely, a laxative prescribed (see QCG: Opioid-induced constipation, p.42).

*It is bad practice to prescribe dihydrocodeine to patients already taking **morphine** or any other strong opioid; if a greater effect is needed, the regular and p.r.n. doses of **morphine** (or other strong opioid) should be increased.*

As a single agent:

- start with 30mg PO q6h–q4h
- if necessary, increase to 60mg q6h–q4h.

The higher dose is associated with a significant increase in undesirable effects.[16]

Supply

Dihydrocodeine tartrate (generic)
Tablets 30mg, 28 days @ 30mg q.d.s. = £4.50.
Oral solution 10mg/5mL, 28 days @ 30mg q.d.s. = £85.
Injection 50mg/mL, 1mL amp = £10. Schedule 2 **CD**.

DF118 Forte® (Martindale)
Tablets 40mg, 28 days @ 40mg t.d.s. = £10.

Modified-release

As for all m/r opioids, brand prescribing is recommended to reduce the risk of confusion and error in dispensing and administration (see p.xvii).

Modified-release 12-hourly oral products
DHC Continus® (Napp)
Tablets m/r 60mg, 90mg, 120mg, 28 days @ 60mg b.d. = £5.

With **paracetamol**
Co-dydramol 10/500 (generic)
Tablets dihydrocodeine tartrate 10mg, **paracetamol** 500mg, 28 days @ 2 q.d.s. = £8.

1 Bandieri E *et al.* (2015) Randomized trial of low-dose morphine versus weak opioids in moderate cancer pain. *Journal of Clinical Oncology.* **34**: 436–442.
2 Caraceni A *et al.* (2012) Use of opioid analgesics in the treatment of cancer pain: evidence-based recommendations from the EAPC. *Lancet Oncology.* **13**: e58–68.
3 WHO (2012) Persisting pain in children package: WHO guidelines on the pharmacological treatment of persisiting pain in children with medical illness. World Health Organisation, Geneva. Available from: www.who.int/publications
4 Weiss B (1959) Dihydrocodeine. A pharmacologic review. *American Journal of Pharmacy.* **August**: 286–301.
5 Luporini G *et al.* (1998) Efficacy and safety of levodropropizine and dihydrocodeine on nonproductive cough in primary and metastatic lung cancer. *European Respiratory Journal.* **12**: 97–101.
6 Freye E *et al.* (2001) Dose-related effects of controlled release dihydrocodeine on oro-cecal transit and pupillary light reflex. A study in human volunteers. *Arzneimittelforschung.* **51**: 60–66.
7 Fromm M *et al.* (1995) Dihydrocodeine: A new opioid substrate for the polymorphic CYP2D6 in humans. *Clinical Pharmacology and Therapeutics.* **58**: 374–382.
8 Wilder-Smith CH *et al.* (1998) The visceral and somatic antinociceptive effects of dihydrocodeine and its metabolite, dihydromorphine. A cross-over study with extensive and quinidine-induced poor metabolizers. *British Journal of Clinical Pharmacology.* **45**: 575–581.
9 Webb JA *et al.* (2001) Contribution of dihydrocodeine and dihydromorphine to analgesia following dihydrocodeine administration in man: a PK-PD modelling analysis. *British Journal of Clinical Pharmacology.* **52**: 35–43.
10 Schmidt H *et al.* (2003) The role of active metabolites in dihydrocodeine effects. *International Journal of Clinical Pharmacology and Therapeutics.* **41**: 95–106.
11 Seed JC *et al.* (1958) A comparison of the analgesic and respiratory effects of dihydrocodeine and morphine in main. *Archives Internationales de Pharmacodynamie et de Therapie.* **116**: 293–339.
12 Palmer RN *et al.* (1966) Incidence of unwanted effects of dihydrocodeine bitartrate in healthy volunteers. *Lancet.* **2**: 620–621.
13 Anonymous (1991) Dihydrocodeine (tartrate). In: C Dollery (ed) *Therapeutic Drugs.* Churchill Livingstone, Edinburgh, pp. 133–136.
14 Goldmeier D and Lamba H (2002) Prolonged erections produced by dihydrocodeine and sildenafil. *British Medical Journal.* **324**: 1555.
15 Barnes J *et al.* (1985) Dihydrocodeine in renal failure: further evidence for an important role in the kidney in the handling of opioid drugs. *British Medical Journal.* **290**: 740–742.
16 McQuay H *et al.* (1993) A multiple dose comparison of ibuprofen and dihydrocodeine after third molar surgery. *British Journal of Oral and Maxillofacial Surgery.* **31**: 95–100.

Updated September 2017

TRAMADOL

Class: Opioid analgesic (but see below).

Indications: Moderate–severe pain.

There is no pharmacological need for weak opioids in cancer pain (see p.295). Low doses of **morphine** (or an alternative strong opioid), generally provides quicker and better relief from cancer pain than a weak opioid.[1,2] Moving directly from a non-opioid to a strong opioid is increasingly preferred in adults, and is the norm in children in whom weak opioids are no longer recommended.[3] However, in some countries, weak opioids remain a practical necessity because of the restricted availability (or non-availability) of oral **morphine** and other strong opioids.

Contra-indications: Use of MAOIs concurrently or within 14 days, severe hepatic impairment, ESRF (creatinine clearance <10mL/min), uncontrolled epilepsy. Avoid use in children (see below).

Pharmacology

Tramadol, like **tapentadol** (p.453), is a synthetic centrally-acting analgesic with both non-opioid and opioid properties.[4,5] Its efficacy is comparable to **codeine** (p.349), and it is often used in preference.[6–8]

Tramadol is derived from **codeine** (p.349) and is structurally similar to **venlafaxine** (p.216). It exists as a racemic mixture and stimulates neuronal serotonin and noradrenaline (norepinephrine) release. It also inhibits presynaptic re-uptake: serotonin mainly via (+) tramadol and noradrenaline mainly via (–) tramadol. This enhances the impact of the descending inhibitory pathways associated with pain transmission, acting synergistically with tramadol's weak opioid effect (Table 1 and Table 2).[5] In animal models, tramadol also has an anti-inflammatory effect independent of PG inhibition.[9]

Table 1 μ-opioid receptor affinities: K_i (micromol) values[a,10]

	Receptor affinity
Morphine	0.009
Tapentadol	0.16
Tramadol[b]	2.4

a. the lower the K_i value, the greater the receptor affinity
b. much lower for (+) M1, i.e. 0.003.

Table 2 Inhibition of mono-amine uptake: K_i (micromol) values[a,10]

	Noradrenaline	*Serotonin*
Morphine	>100	>100
Tapentadol	0.48	2.4
Tramadol	0.59[b]	0.87[c]

a. the lower the Ki value, the greater the functional uptake inhibition
b. (–) tramadol
c. (+) tramadol.

Tramadol is converted in the liver, mainly via CYP2D6, to the active metabolite O-desmethyltramadol (M1) which is several times more potent than tramadol itself. Thus, tramadol can be considered a pro-drug. Further biotransformation of M1 results in inactive metabolites which are excreted by the kidneys.

Although **naloxone** can only partially reverse the effects of tramadol, in a series of 11 patients with a tramadol overdose, seven had a good response to **naloxone**, and only one had no response.[11]

Changes in CYP2D6 activity, both acquired (e.g. drug-induced) and constitutional (≤10% of Caucasians are either CYP2D6 poor or ultra-rapid metabolizers)[12] can affect the response to tramadol. Decreased CYP2D6 activity will result in decreased response/higher dose requirements. Conversely, increased CYP2D6 has resulted in life-threatening respiratory depression in a child (see Cautions and Drug interactions below, and Chapter 19, p.717).[13–17]

In placebo-controlled trials, tramadol significantly relieves neuropathic pain (e.g. diabetic neuropathy, post-herpetic neuralgia, polyneuropathy), with an NNT of 3.8.[18] This is comparable with several anti-epileptics, but not as good as TCAs (NNT = 2.3, see p.300) or as **oxycodone** in post-herpetic neuralgia (NNT of 2.5).[19]

Tramadol is as effective as **codeine** as a cough suppressant.[20,21] Postoperatively, it causes less respiratory depression than equi-analgesic doses of **morphine**.[22] It also causes less constipation than **codeine**, **dihydrocodeine** and **morphine**;[23–25] but more vomiting, dizziness and anorexia than **codeine** and **dihydrocodeine**.[26] In contrast to **morphine**, tramadol reduces the basal pressure in the sphincter of Oddi (for <20min after IM administration) and does not increase the pressure in the common bile duct.[27]

Although the risk of dependence and misuse is less compared with **morphine** and other opioids,[28] tramadol is a Schedule 3 **CD**. Like other opioids, tramadol is associated with the development of physical dependence (see Dose and use below)[29] and, in overdose, CNS depression, respiratory depression and death.[30] There are also case reports of possible opioid-induced hyperalgesia (also see p.368).

By injection, tramadol is generally regarded as one tenth as potent as **morphine** injection (i.e. tramadol 100mg IV is equivalent to **morphine** 10mg IV).[31] In fact, various pre- and postoperative studies give a range between one tenth and one twentieth as potent as **morphine**.[32,33] Thus, the figure of one tenth is more of a 'convenient to remember' number than a scientifically precise one. Some of the postoperative studies also suggest that, to produce adequate analgesia, tramadol needs to be administered more frequently than **morphine** over the first few hours (by IV PCA), after which doses become less frequent. The need for the equivalent of a loading dose with tramadol may reflect its different mode of action from **morphine**. A delayed maximum effect has also been reported in an RCT of oral tramadol and **morphine**.[34]

By mouth, RCTs indicate tramadol is one fifth to one quarter as potent as **morphine** (i.e. tramadol 100mg PO = **morphine** 20–25mg PO).[35,36] However, extensive clinical experience has led many physicians to regard PO tramadol as one tenth as potent as PO **morphine** (i.e. tramadol 100mg PO = **morphine** 10mg PO), i.e. the same as by injection.[37–39]

When converting between PO and SC/IM/IV, generally the same dose can be used.

Bio-availability 65–75% PO; 90% with multiple doses;[40] 77% PR.[41,42]
Onset of action 30min–1h.
Time to peak plasma concentration 2h; 4–8h m/r.
Plasma halflife 6h; active metabolite 7.4h; these more than double in cirrhosis and severe renal failure.
Duration of action 4–9h.

Cautions

Like **codeine**, genetic polymorphism in CYP2D6 affects the metabolism of tramadol. In 2017, following a safety review, the FDA placed similar restrictions on the use of tramadol in children and adolescents as for **codeine** (see p.350).[43] In the UK, a similar review has not been undertaken but tramadol is not recommended nor authorized for use in children <12 years.[3] If tramadol is unavoidable in children 12–18 years, apply the same contra-indications and cautions as for **codeine** (see p.350).

Renal and hepatic impairment (see Dose and use, and also Chapter 17, p.693 and Chapter 18, p.709).

Tramadol has been associated with seizures, notably when the total daily dose exceeds 400mg or when tramadol is used concurrently with other medications which lower the seizure threshold, e.g. TCAs, SSRIs, antipsychotics, and other opioids.[11,44,45] Seizures have also been reported in patients after rapid IV injection of tramadol. Treat with standard measures, i.e. IV benzodiazepines (see p.149). Resolution generally occurs in <1 day.[11] Fatalities resulting from tramadol-induced seizures are rare.[46] Use with caution in controlled epilepsy, head trauma or raised intracranial pressure.

Serotonin toxicity has occasionally occurred when tramadol has been taken concurrently with a second drug which also interferes with presynaptic serotonin re-uptake (see p.200). Risk factors include the use of higher doses, old age, the second drug being a CYP2D6 inhibitor, CYP2D6 poor metabolizer status, and hepatic impairment.[47]

A large population cohort study found that tramadol is significantly associated with an increased risk of hospitalization for hypoglycemia (mostly within 10 days of starting and more frequent in the elderly).[48]

The FDA has warned of an increased risk of suicide in emotionally unstable patients taking tramadol, particularly if they are also taking antidepressants or tranquillizers.

May impair the ability to perform skilled tasks, e.g. driving, see Chapter 22, p.743.

Drug interactions

Because of the increased risk of seizures and serotonin toxicity, concurrent use of tramadol with an MAOI is contra-indicated, and its use with other antidepressants, particularly SSRIs or TCAs, requires caution (see Cautions and below).[47,49]

Carbamazepine and **rifampicin**[50] increase the metabolism of tramadol and M1, and thus may decrease analgesia (see Chapter 19, p.717). CYP2D6 inhibitors, e.g. **fluoxetine**, **paroxetine**, **quinidine**, and **ritonavir**, inhibit the conversion of tramadol to M1 and may decrease analgesia while increasing the risk of serotonin toxicity.[47,51]

Tramadol occasionally prolongs the INR of patients taking **warfarin**.[52,53] Monitor the INR closely for 3–4 weeks if tramadol is prescribed for a patient already taking **warfarin**.

There are mixed reports of the analgesic effect of tramadol being reduced by **ondansetron** (possibly by blocking the action of serotonin at presynaptic $5HT_3$-receptors on primary afferent nociceptive neurones in the spinal dorsal horn).[54] In one postoperative pain study, the dose of tramadol needed by IV PCA was 2–3 times greater in patients receiving **ondansetron**,[55] but was unaffected in another.[56]

5

Undesirable effects

Incidence and nature of undesirable effects (monoamine reuptake inhibition vs. opioid) may vary with activity of CYP2D6 (see Pharmacology). Urinary incontinence, recovering fully on cessation of tramadol, has been reported.[57]
Very common (>10%): dizziness, nausea, vomiting.
Common (<10%, >1%): headache, drowsiness, fatigue, sweating, dry mouth, constipation.
Rare (<0.1%): seizures (dose-dependent, see Cautions above).

Dose and use

Note. Low-dose PO **morphine** (20–30mg/24h) generally provides quicker and better relief from cancer pain than tramadol.[2]

As with all opioids, patients must be monitored for undesirable effects (see Strong opioids, Box B, p.365), particularly nausea and vomiting, and constipation. Depending on individual circumstances, an anti-emetic should be prescribed for regular or p.r.n. use, (see QCG: Nausea and vomiting, p.240) and, routinely, a laxative prescribed (see QCG: Opioid-induced constipation, p.42).

Most cancer patients prescribed tramadol will already be taking a non-opioid:
- start with 50mg PO q.d.s *or* an equivalent daily dose using a q12h or once daily m/r product (see supply); for very frail patients, dose as in renal impairment (see below)
- if necessary, increase the dose in stages to a maximum recommended total daily dose of 400mg
- higher doses have been given, e.g. 600mg/24h, and sometimes more[37,38]
- for break-through pain when taking m/r tramadol, consider immediate-release tramadol or immediate-release **morphine** (p.375).

Renal or hepatic impairment

In severe renal impairment, because of impaired metabolism or elimination:
- *halve* the starting dose by reducing the frequency to 50mg PO q12h using immediate-release products; likewise in very frail patients[4]
- if necessary, increase the dose in stages to a maximum recommended total daily dose of 200mg.

Despite ESRF (creatinine clearance <10mL/min) being a contra-indication, some centres have successfully used tramadol in this setting (see p.681).[58]

Tramadol is contra-indicated in severe hepatic impairment. In moderate hepatic impairment, because of impaired metabolism to the active metabolite, tramadol is best avoided; if unavoidable, dose as in severe renal impairment (see p.703).

Stopping tramadol

Abruptly stopping tramadol, even after only a few days of use, can result in typical symptoms of opioid withdrawal (e.g. anxiety, restlessness, abdominal cramps, diarrhoea, goose flesh, sweating) and tapering the dose over several days is recommended.

However, opioid withdrawal should not occur when tramadol is being substituted by another μ-opioid agonist, e.g. **morphine**. Nonetheless, abruptly stopping tramadol has also sometimes resulted in symptoms *not* typical of opioid withdrawal (e.g. severe anxiety/panic attacks, delirium, paranoia, hallucinations, paraesthesia), particularly with doses >400mg/24h.[59,60] This suggests the potential for a discontinuation reaction similar to that seen with antidepressants (see p.205)[59] and is another reason why tapering the dose over several days is recommended.

Supply

All products are now Schedule 3 **CD** (with storage exemption).

Tramadol (generic)
Capsules 50mg, 28 days @ 100mg q.d.s. = £6.50.
Orodispersible tablets 50mg, 28 days @ 100mg q.d.s. = £27.
Oral drops 100mg/mL (2.5mg/drop), 10mL, 28 days @100mg (40 drops) q.d.s. = £42. *Mix with water before taking.*
Injection 50mg/mL, 2mL amp = £1.

Modified-release

A large number of tramadol m/r products are available, administered either q12h or once daily and prescribers should clearly specify which one they require. As for all m/r opioids, brand prescribing is recommended to reduce the risk of confusion and error in dispensing and administration (see p.xvii).

Modified-release 12-hourly oral products
Zydol® SR (Grunenthal)
Tablets m/r 50mg, 100mg, 150mg, 200mg, 28 days @ 200mg b.d. = £34.
Other brands include Tilodol® SR, Tramulief® SR, Zeridame® SR; not all have the full range of strengths available.

Zamadol® SR (Meda)
Capsules m/r 50mg, 100mg, 150mg, 200mg, 28 days @ 200mg b.d. = £27.
Other brands include Maxitram® SR, Tramquel® SR.

Modified-release 24-hourly oral products
Zydol® XL
Tablets m/r 100mg, 150mg, 200mg, 300mg, 400mg, 28 days @ 400mg once daily = £30.
Other brands include Tradorec® XL, Zamadol® 24h; not all have the full range of strengths available.

With **paracetamol**
Tramacet® (Grünenthal)
Tablets tramadol hydrochloride 37.5mg, **paracetamol** 325mg, 28 days @ 2 q.d.s. = £36.
Tablets soluble tramadol hydrochloride 37.5mg, **paracetamol** 325mg, 28 days @ 2 q.d.s. = £36.

1 Caraceni A *et al.* (2012) Use of opioid analgesics in the treatment of cancer pain: evidence-based recommendations from the EAPC. *Lancet Oncology.* **13**: e58–68.
2 Bandieri E *et al.* (2016) Randomized trial of low-dose morphine versus weak opioids in moderate cancer pain. *Journal of Clinical Oncology.* **34**: 436–442.
3 WHO (2012) Persisting pain in children package: WHO guidelines on the pharmacological treatment of persisiting pain in children with medical illness. World Health Organisation, Geneva. Available from: www.who.int/publications
4 Grond S and Sablotzki A (2004) Clinical pharmacology of tramadol. *Clinical Pharmacokinetics.* **43**: 879–923.
5 Dickman A (2007) Tramadol: a review of this atypical opioid. *European Journal of Palliative Care.* **14**: 181–185.
6 Jadad AR and Browman GP (1995) The WHO analgesic ladder for cancer pain management. *Journal of the American Medical Association.* **274**: 1870–1873.
7 Tassinari D *et al.* (2011) The second step of the analgesic ladder and oral tramadol in the treatment of mild to moderate cancer pain: a systematic review. *Palliative Medicine.* **25**: 410–423.
8 Goncalves JA *et al.* (2015) Does tramadol have a role in pain control in palliative care? *American Journal of Hospice and Palliative Care.* **32**: 631–633.
9 Buccellati C *et al.* (2000) Tramadol anti-inflammatory activity is not related to a direct inhibitory action on prostaglandin endoperoxide synthases. *European Journal of Pain.* **4**: 413–415.
10 Tzschentke TM *et al.* (2014) The Mu-Opioid Receptor Agonist/Noradrenaline Reuptake Inhibition (MOR-NRI) concept in analgesia: The case of tapentadol. *CNS Drugs.* **28**: 319–329.
11 Marquardt KA *et al.* (2005) Tramadol exposures reported to statewide poison control system. *Annals of Pharmacotherapy.* **39**: 1039–1044.
12 Sachse C *et al.* (1997) Cytochrome P450 2D6 variants in a Caucasian population: allele frequencies and phenotypic consequences. *American Journal of Human Genetics.* **60**: 284–295.
13 Stamer UM *et al.* (2003) Impact of CYP2D6 genotype on postoperative tramadol analgesia. *Pain.* **105**: 231–238.
14 Poulsen L *et al.* (1996) The hypoalgesic effect of tramadol in relation to CYP2D6. *Clinical Pharmacology and Therapeutics.* **60**: 636–644.
15 Kim E *et al.* (2010) Adverse events in analgesic treatment with tramadol associated with CYP2D6 extensive-metaboliser and OPRM1 high-expression variants. *Annals of the Rheumatic Diseases.* **69**: 1889–1890.

16 Elkalioubie A *et al.* (2011) Near-fatal tramadol cardiotoxicity in a CYP2D6 ultrarapid metabolizer. *European Journal of Clinical Pharmacology.* **67**: 855–858.
17 Orliaguet G *et al.* (2015) A case of respiratory depression in a child with ultrarapid CYP2D6 metabolism after tramadol. *Pediatrics.* **135**: e753–755.
18 Duehmke RM (2006) tramadol for neuropathic pain. *Cochrane Database of Systematic Reviews.* **3**: CD003726. www.thecochranelibrary.com
19 Watson C and Babul N (1998) Efficacy of oxycodone in neuropathic pain: a randomized trial in postherpetic neuralgia. *Neurology.* **50**: 1837–1841.
20 Szekely SM and Vickers MD (1992) A comparison of the effects of codeine and tramadol on laryngeal reactivity. *European Journal of Anaesthesiology.* **9**: 111–120.
21 Louly PG *et al.* (2009) N-of-1 double-blind, randomized controlled trial of tramadol to treat chronic cough. *Clinical Therapeutics.* **31**: 1007–1013.
22 Houmes R *et al.* (1992) Efficacy and safety of tramadol versus morphine for moderate and severe postoperative pain with special regard to respiratory depression. *Anesthesia and Analgesia.* **74**: 510–514.
23 Wilder-Smith C and Bettiga A (1997) The analgesic tramadol has minimal effect on gastrointestinal motor function. *British Journal of Clinical Pharmacology.* **43**: 71–75.
24 Wilder-Smith CH *et al.* (1999) Effect of tramadol and morphine on pain and gastrointestinal motor function in patients with chronic pancreatitis. *Digestive Diseases and Sciences.* **44**: 1107–1116.
25 Wilder-Smith C *et al.* (2001) Treatment of severe pain from osteoarthritis with slow-release tramadol or dihydrocodeine in combination with NSAID's: a randomised study comparing analgesia, antinociception and gastrointestinal effects. *Pain.* **91**: 23–31.
26 Rodriguez RF *et al.* (2007) Incidence of weak opioids adverse events in the management of cancer pain: a double-blind comparative trial. *Journal of Palliative Medicine.* **10**: 56–60.
27 Wu SD *et al.* (2004) Effects of narcotic analgesic drugs on human Oddi's sphincter motility. *World Journal of Gastroenterology.* **10**: 2901–2904.
28 Preston K *et al.* (1991) Abuse potential and pharmacological comparison of tramadol and morphine. *Drug and Alcohol Dependency.* **27**: 7–18.
29 Soyka M *et al.* (2004) Tramadol use and dependence in chronic noncancer pain patients. *Pharmacopsychiatry.* **37**: 191–192.
30 FDA (2010) Safety alerts for human medical products Ultram (tramadol hydrochloride), Ultracet (tramadol hydrochloride/acetaminophen). Available from: www.fda.gov/Safety/MedWatch/SafetyInformation/SafetyAlertsforHumanMedicalProducts/ucm213264.htm (accessed 10th Aug 2010)
31 Vickers M *et al.* (1992) Tramadol: pain relief by an opioid without depression of respiration. *Anaesthesia.* **47**: 291–296.
32 Naguib M *et al.* (1998) Perioperative antinociceptive effects of tramadol. A prospective, randomized, double-blind comparison with morphine. *Canadian Journal of Anaesthesia.* **45**: 1168–1175.
33 Pang WW *et al.* (1999) Comparison of patient-controlled analgesia (PCA) with tramadol or morphine. *Canadian Journal of Anaesthesia.* **46**: 1030–1035.
34 Leppert W (2001) Analgesic efficacy and side effects of oral tramadol and morphine administered orally in the treatment of cancer pain. *Nowotwory.* **51**: 257–266.
35 Wilder-Smith CH *et al.* (1994) Oral tramadol, a mu-opioid agonist and monoamine reuptake-blocker, and morphine for strong cancer-related pain. *Annals of Oncology.* **5**: 141–146.
36 Tawfik MO *et al.* (1990) Tramadol hydrochloride in the relief of cancer pain: a double blind comparison against sustained release morphine. *Pain.* **41 (Suppl 1)**: S377.
37 Leppert W and Luczak J (2005) The role of tramadol in cancer pain treatment--a review. *Supportive Care in Cancer.* **13**: 5–17.
38 Grond S *et al.* (1999) High-dose tramadol in comparison to low-dose morphine for cancer pain relief. *Journal of Pain and Symptom Management.* **18**: 174–179.
39 Palliativedrugs.com (2008) Tramadol - What is your experience? *March/April Survey.* www.palliativedrugs.com
40 Gibson T (1996) Pharmacokinetics, efficacy, and safety of analgesia with a focus on tramadol HCl. *American Journal of Medicine.* **101 (Suppl 1A)**: 47s–53s.
41 Mercadante S *et al.* (2005) Randomized double-blind, double-dummy crossover clinical trial of oral tramadol versus rectal tramadol administration in opioid-naive cancer patients with pain. *Supportive Care in Cancer.* **13**: 702–707.
42 Lintz W *et al.* (1998) Pharmacokinetics of tramadol and bioavailability of enteral tramadol formulations. 3rd Communication: suppositories. *Arzneimittelforschung.* **48**: 889–899.
43 FDA (2017) FDA restricts use of prescription codeine pain and cough medicines and tramadol pain medicines in children; recommend against use in breastfeeding women. *Drug Safety Communication.* www.fda.gov/drugs/drugsafety
44 Boyd IW (2005) Tramadol and seizures. *Medical Journal of Australia.* **182**: 595–596.
45 Spiller HA *et al.* (1997) Prospective multicenter evaluation of tramadol exposure. *Journal of Toxicology and Clinical Toxicology.* **35**: 361–364.
46 Close BR (2005) Tramadol: does it have a role in emergency medicine? *Emergency Medicine Australasia.* **17**: 73–83.
47 Park SH *et al.* (2014) Serotonin syndrome: is it a reason to avoid the use of tramadol with antidepressants? *Journal of Pharmacy Practice.* **27**: 71–78.
48 Fournier JP *et al.* (2015) Tramadol use and the risk of hospitalization for hypoglycemia in patients with noncancer pain. *JAMA Internal Medicine.* **175**: 186–193.
49 Pilgrim JL *et al.* (2011) Deaths involving contraindicated and inappropriate combinations of serotonergic drugs. *International Journal of Legal Medicine.* **125**: 803–815.
50 Saarikoski T *et al.* (2013) Rifampicin markedly decreases the exposure to oral and intravenous tramadol. *European Journal of Clinical Pharmacology.* **69**: 1293–1301.
51 Laugesen S *et al.* (2005) Paroxetine, a cytochrome P450 2D6 inhibitor, diminishes the stereoselective O-demethylation and reduces the hypoalgesic effect of tramadol. *Clin Pharmacol Ther.* **77**: 312–323.
52 Sabbe JR *et al.* (1998) Tramadol-warfarin interaction. *Pharmacotherapy.* **18**: 871–873.
53 Juel J *et al.* (2013) Administration of tramadol or ibuprofen increases the INR level in patients on warfarin. *European Journal of Clinical Pharmacology.* **69**: 291–292.
54 De Witte JL *et al.* (2001) The analgesic efficacy of tramadol is impaired by concurrent administration of ondansetron. *Anesthesia and Analgesia.* **92**: 1319–1321.
55 Arcioni R *et al.* (2002) Ondansetron inhibits the analgesic effects of tramadol: a possible 5-HT(3) spinal receptor involvement in acute pain in humans. *Anesthesia and Analgesia.* **94**: 1553–1557.
56 Rauers NI *et al.* (2010) Antagonistic effects of ondansetron and tramadol? A randomized placebo and active drug controlled study. *Journal of Pain.* **11**: 1274–1281.

57 Gautam SK *et al.* (2013) Urinary incontinence induced by tramadol. *Indian Journal of Palliative Care.* **19**: 76–77.
58 King S *et al.* (2011) A systematic review of the use of opioid medication for those with moderate to severe cancer pain and renal impairment: A European palliative care research collaborative opioid guidelines project. *Palliative Medicine.* **25**: 525–552.
59 Senay EC *et al.* (2003) Physical dependence on Ultram (tramadol hydrochloride): both opioid-like and atypical withdrawal symptoms occur. *Drug Alcohol Dependence.* **69**: 233–241.
60 Rajabizadeh G *et al.* (2009) Psychosis following Tramadol Withdrawal. *Addiction and Health.* **1**: 58–61.

Updated September 2017

STRONG OPIOIDS

Strong opioids are essential drugs in palliative care; their use should be dictated by therapeutic need and response, not by brevity of prognosis.[1,2]

Contra-indications: Provided the dose of an opioid is carefully titrated against the patient's pain, there are generally no absolute contra-indications to the use of strong opioids for cancer pain. However, there are circumstances, e.g. renal or hepatic impairment, when it may be better to avoid the use of certain opioids and/or positively choose certain other ones (also see Chapter 17, p.693 and Chapter 18, p.709).

Chemical classes

Opioids can be divided into four chemical classes (Table 1). Knowledge of the different chemical classes is of value when dealing with cases of intolerance to a particular opioid, e.g. cutaneous histamine release causing a rash and pruritus. However, in many situations switching from one phenanthrene to another phenanthrene is satisfactory, e.g. neurotoxicity (see p.368).

Table 1 Chemical classification of opioids

Phenanthrenes	*Benzomorphans*	*Phenylpiperidines*	*Diphenylheptanes*
Codeine	Diphenoxylate	Fentanils	Dextropropoxyphene
Dextromethorphan	Loperamide	Pethidine[a]	Methadone
Dihydrocodeine	Pentazocine[a]		
Hydrocodone			
Tramadol			
Morphine			
Diamorphine			
Buprenorphine			
Hydromorphone			
Oxycodone			
Oxymorphone			
Tapentadol			

a. *not* recommended for use in palliative care.

Opioid receptors

There are four main opioid receptors (μ, κ, δ and opioid receptor-like 1, OPRL-1) distributed in varying densities throughout the body, particularly in nervous tissue. Their naturally-occurring ligands are opioid peptides, and together they contribute to various physiological functions including the modulation of pain, hormones and the immune system (Table 2).[3,4]

In nervous tissue, opioid peptides function as neurotransmitters. Like other peptides, they are synthesized as large inactive precursors in the neuronal cell body, and are then cleaved while being transported to the nerve terminals. The active fragment is released into the synapse and binds to one or more receptors.

Opioid receptors are found both pre- and post-synaptically, with the former predominating, controlling the release of several neurotransmitters. Endogenous peptides are rapidly degraded, and have a relatively short duration of action. In contrast, exogenous opioids such as **morphine** have a prolonged effect. They produce analgesia primarily by interacting with μ-opioid receptors in the CNS, e.g. in the dorsal horn of the spinal cord and peri-aqueductal grey area of the midbrain.

Opioid receptors, synthesized in the dorsal root ganglion, are transported to peripheral as well as central nerve terminals. In the presence of tissue injury and inflammation, the number of peripheral opioid receptors increases, and exogenous and endogenous opioids (released by activated inflammatory cells in close proximity to nerve fibres) thereby exert a peripheral analgesic action. Conversely, in bone and neuropathic pain, opioid receptor expression is reduced, contributing towards a reduced response to opioids.[5,6]

All clinically important opioid analgesics act as agonists at the μ-opioid receptor (Table 2). 'Broad-spectrum' opioid agonists, active at all four receptor subtypes, are in development, e.g. **cebranopadol**.[7] Some opioids are mixed agonist-antagonists, e.g. **buprenorphine** is a *partial agonist* at the μ-opioid and OPRL-1 receptors, and an *antagonist* at the κ- and δ-opioid receptors.[8,9] (Note. At usual analgesic doses, **buprenorphine** acts as a *full* μ agonist, see p.397).

Undesirable effects generally relate to both central and peripheral μ-opioid receptor activation, mainly in the CNS and GI tract.

Some opioids also possess non-opioid activity. Thus, **methadone** blocks the pre-synaptic re-uptake of serotonin and the NMDA-receptor-channel (see p.437), **tapentadol** blocks re-uptake of noradrenaline (norepinephrine; see p.453), and **tramadol** blocks re-uptake of both serotonin and noradrenaline (see p.354).

Opioid receptors are classified as G-protein coupled receptors. In the absence of a ligand, the receptor constantly oscillates through a range of possible active and inactive states. Once an opioid agonist binds to the receptor, conformational changes occur allowing interaction with a G-protein which subsequently dissociates into its various subunits responsible for multiple 'downstream' effects. For example, in opioid-related analgesia, the G-protein is inhibitory (Gi/o) and its subunits close Ca^{2+} and other ion channels, open rectifying K+ channels, and reduce cyclic adenosine monophosphate production, thereby reducing neurotransmitter release and nerve impulse transmission. Several kinase cascades are also activated, e.g. signal regulated kinase (ERK1/2), c-Jun N-terminal kinases (JNKs) and AKT/protein kinase B, which have a wide impact on cell function, e.g. through changes in protein expression, receptor activation. Conversely, some G-proteins (Gs) have stimulatory (pronociceptive) effects, which may play a role in opioid-induced hyperalgesia (see p.368).

Following agonist binding and G-protein activation, the opioid receptor is phosphorylated, enhancing the binding of the protein β-arrestin2. This prevents G-protein coupling and facilitates receptor internalization (for recycling or destruction), desensitizing the receptor and contributing towards the development of tolerance. Further, β-arrestin2 also independently modulates cell signalling and this may also contribute towards tolerance and other undesirable effects of opioids, e.g. constipation, respiratory depression.[10] This has led to the development of μ-opioid 'biased agonists', which show functional selectivity, i.e. although activating the same receptor, they evoke different signalling cascades, probably through the induction of different receptor conformations.[11] Thus, **oliceridine** stimulates μ-opioid receptor coupling with G-proteins as usual, but subsequently less phosphorylation and recruitment of β-arrestin2. Phase III trials of **oliceridine** in postoperative pain are ongoing.[11]

Thus, the pharmacology of opioid receptors is complex. Further, opioid receptors have additional (allosteric) binding sites which can modulate their function, and they can exist as:

- homodimers, e.g. two μ-opioid receptors
- heterodimers, with another opioid receptor, e.g. μ–δ, δ–κ, or non-opioid receptor, e.g. μ–$5HT_{1A}$, μ–D_1, μ–D_1, δ–CB_1
- 'splice variants' of the μ-opioid receptor, with 1, 6 and 7 transmembrane proteins.

All are considered potential targets for novel analgesic approaches.[11]

Finally, genetic variation in the μ-opioid receptor gene may contribute to inter-individual response to opioids (see Chapter 19, p.717).

Table 2 Opioid receptors, ligands,[12] and effects[a]

Receptors	*Mu (μ)*	*Delta (δ)*	*Kappa (κ)*	*Opioid receptor-like 1 (OPRL-1)*
Endogenous opioid	β-Endorphin Endormorphins	Enkephalins	Dynorphins	Nociceptin
Exogenous agonist	Morphine Buprenorphine[b] Codeine Dextropropoxphene Diamorphine Dihydrocodeine Fentanils Hydromorphone Methadone[c] Oxycodone Pethidine Tapentadol[c] Tramadol[c]	DSTBULET	U50488H Pentazocine	Buprenorphine[b]
Antagonists	Naloxone Naltrexone Pentazocine	Buprenorphine Naloxone	Buprenorphine Naloxone	
Effector mechanism	G protein opens K^+ channel	G protein opens K^+ channel	G protein closes Ca^{++} channel	G protein opens K^+ channel
Effects[d]	*Hyperpolarization of neurons, inhibition of neurotransmitter release*			
	Analgesia Euphoria Nausea Constipation Cough suppression Dependence Respiratory depression Miosis	Similar to μ but less marked	Analgesia Aversion Diuresis Dysphoria	Mixed analgesia (spinal) and anti-analgesia (brain)

a. also see individual drug monographs

b. partial agonist. Note. At usual analgesic doses, buprenorphine behaves as a full μ agonist, see p.397

c. non-opioid effects also contribute towards analgesia (see text)

d. not an exhaustive list; other roles include hormone and immune system regulation.

Clinical use

The focus of this section of *PCF* is on the use of strong opioids for *cancer* pain. Because the use of strong opioids for chronic *non-cancer* pain is generally associated with lower benefits and higher risks,[13] specialist advice should be followed (e.g. Faculty of Pain Medicine)[14] and/or sought from chronic pain teams.

Based on familiarity, availability and cost, **morphine** (p.375) is the strong opioid of choice for moderate–severe cancer pain management.[15–18] Other strong opioids are used mostly when:

- **morphine** is not readily available
- the TD route is preferable (**buprenorphine, fentanyl**)
- the patient has unacceptable undesirable effects with **morphine**, e.g. **oxycodone**.[15]

Some patients report better pain relief after switching opioids (see p.370). Similarly, the pattern and severity of undesirable effects may be altered, e.g. when switching from **morphine** to **oxycodone** (p.447) or TD **fentanyl** (p.409). Explanations for these observations include differences between opioids in their pharmacology, intrinsic activity at different opioid receptor subtypes and the plasticity of the response of the opioid receptor to different ligands (see above).

Both **methadone** (p.437) and **tapentadol** (p.453) have opioid and non-opioid effects which, in the case of **tapentadol**, are analgesically synergistic.

Strong opioids are not the panacea for cancer pain; effective analgesia generally requires the use of both a strong opioid and a non-opioid. Further, even combined use does not guarantee success, particularly with neuropathic pain or if the psychosocial dimension of pain and suffering is ignored. Other reasons for poor relief include:

- underdosing (failure to titrate the dose upwards or dose at the correct interval)
- poor patient adherence (patient not taking medication)
- poor alimentary absorption (e.g. because of vomiting).

Pentazocine should *not* be used; it is a weak opioid by mouth,[19,20] and often causes undesirable psychotropic effects (dysphoria, depersonalization, frightening dreams, hallucinations).[21] **Pethidine** also should *not* be used (Box A).

The dose of strong opioid should be individualized by careful titration against the patient's pain. Once an effective dose is determined, the regular dose should be rationalized as far as possible, e.g. by conversion to m/r products. P.r.n. doses should also be prescribed for break-through pain (see p.295). Both the pain and use of p.r.n medications should be reviewed regularly.

Although branded and generic versions of the same PO opioid formulations are often bio-equivalent, names and appearances vary. In addition, for some opioids, there are a wide range of different formulations available, some of which are not interchangeable, or have different durations of action (see Cautions). Consequently, to reduce the risk of error and avoid confusing patients and carers, prescribing by brand for oral m/r products, transmucosal and transdermal products is recommended.[22,23]

Box A Pethidine

The use of pethidine is actively discouraged in palliative care.

Pethidine is a synthetic μ agonist. In typical doses PO it is little more than a weak opioid (see Table 4, p.371). It has a relatively short duration of action (2–3h) and is thus a bad choice for round-the-clock analgesia.

Pethidine has a toxic metabolite, norpethidine, which accumulates when pethidine is given regularly. Particularly in renal impairment, norpethidine causes tremors, multifocal myoclonus, agitation, and occasionally seizures.[24]

Pethidine:

- is not antitussive
- is less constipating than morphine but causes more vomiting
- causes less smooth muscle spasm (e.g. sphincter of Oddi)
- is antimuscarinic (anticholinergic)
- is associated with a higher risk of post-operative delirium compared with other opioids[25]
- does not cause constriction of the pupils.[26]

continued

Box A Continued

Drug-drug interaction with:
- phenobarbital
- chlorpromazine } increased production of norpethidine.
- MAOIs

Serotonin toxicity
Pethidine must not be given concurrently with an MAOI because of the risk of serotonin toxicity (see p.200).[27–29]

Overdose and effect of naloxone
Overdose is a mixed picture of CNS depression (pethidine) and excitation (norpethidine), with both stupor and seizures.

Naloxone will reverse the pethidine-induced stupor but not the stimulant effects of norpethidine. Seizures should be treated with a benzodiazepine (see p.149).

Cautions

Because of reports of serious incidents and the potential for toxicity with strong opioids, diligent prescribing, dispensing, administration, monitoring and counselling is required to reduce the risk of error and/or confusion, particularly between:
- immediate-release and m/r products
- products with different durations of action, e.g. 12-hourly vs 24-hourly m/r products, 7-day vs 3- or 4-day transdermal patches
- products with both low and high strength concentrates, e.g. oral solutions, injections
- products with different bio-availabilities that are not interchangeable, e.g. **fentanyl** transmucosal products.

Also see individual monographs.

Because of the wide number of different formulations and brands available, prescribing by brand for PO m/r, transmucosal and transdermal products is recommended to reduce the risk of error and/or avoid confusing patients and carers.

All opioids can impair driving ability and patients should be counselled accordingly. Further, **morphine**, **diamorphine** and **methadone** are included in a new law in England and Wales relating to driving with certain drugs above specified plasma concentrations (see p.743).

Renal or hepatic impairment
Opioids differ in their potential to cause toxicity when renal or hepatic function is impaired. For general information on the choice of opioids, and use in ESRF or severe hepatic impairment, see p.693 and p.709.

When there is an acute deterioration in renal or hepatic function, an opioid may rapidly accumulate because of reduced excretion or metabolism (see individual monographs, also p.681 and p.703); consider a dose reduction pre-emptively, and always when there is evidence of toxicity, e.g. sedation, myoclonus, delirium. When toxicity is moderate–severe, e.g. marked sedation, respiratory depression (see QCG: Reveral of opioid-induced respiratory depression, p.464), discontinue the regular opioid, and allow only a reduced p.r.n. dose. Subsequently, if the situation stabilizes/improves, a regular dose can be restarted, based on p.r.n. use. Alternatively, consider a switch to a 'renally/hepatically safer' opioid according to circumstances.

Drug interactions
Many opioids are metabolized by the CYP450 enzyme pathway (see Chapter 19, Table 1, p.719) and interactions may occur with drugs which induce or inhibit these enzymes, see the individual monographs and also Chapter 19, Table 8, p.725).

For opioids associated with serotonin toxicity, see below.

Undesirable effects

Strong opioids tend to cause the same undesirable effects (Box B), although to a varying degree. Strategies are necessary to deal with them, particularly nausea and vomiting (see QCG: Nausea and vomiting, p.240), and constipation (see QCG: Opioid-induced constipation, p.42).[30] For opioid-induced pruritus, see Chapter 26, p.757.

Box B Undesirable effects of opioids when used for analgesia

Common initial
Nausea and vomiting[a]
Drowsiness
Light-headedness/unsteadiness
Delirium (acute confusional state)

Common ongoing
Constipation
Nausea and vomiting[a]
Dry mouth

Possible ongoing
Suppression of hypothalamic-pituitary axis
Suppression of immune system

Less common
Neurotoxicity:
- hyperalgesia
- allodynia
- myoclonus
- cognitive failure/delirium
- hallucinations

Sweating
Urinary retention
Postural hypotension
Spasm of the sphincter of Oddi
Pruritus (see Chapter 26, p.757)

Rare
Respiratory depression
Psychological dependence

a. generally, opioid-related nausea and vomiting is transient and improves after 5–7 days; if persistent despite an anti-emetic (see QCG: Nausea and vomiting, p.240), consider other possible causes before switching to another opioid (see p.370).

Respiratory depression

When appropriately titrated against the patient's pain, strong opioids do not cause clinically important respiratory depression in patients in pain.[31–33] Strong opioids also relieve moderate–severe breathlessness at rest at doses which do not cause respiratory depression (see p.382).

Naloxone, a specific opioid antagonist, is rarely needed in palliative care (see p.457). In contrast to postoperative patients, cancer patients with pain:

- have generally been receiving a weak opioid for some time, i.e. are not opioid-naïve
- take medication PO (slower absorption, lower peak concentration)
- titrate the dose upwards step by step (less likelihood of an excessive dose being given).

The relationship of the therapeutic dose to the lethal dose of a strong opioid (the therapeutic ratio) is greater than commonly supposed. For example, patients who take a double dose of immediate-release **morphine** at bedtime are no more likely to die during the night than those who do not.[34]

Nonetheless, there is an association between the use of opioids and sleep-disordered breathing, e.g. nocturnal apnoeas resulting in hypoxaemia.[35] Opioids cause this by reducing the central respiratory drive and/or relaxing the upper airway. It appears to be common, with central apnoeas affecting half of patients in one study (all receiving a morphine equivalent dose >100mg/24h PO), which resolved completely when the opioid was stopped.[35] Although the full clinical relevance is unknown, it has been suggested as an explanation for the increased deaths and cardiovascular events reported in patients receiving opioids, and as another reason to avoid opioids when possible in chronic non-cancer pain.[35]

Tolerance and dependence

Generally, tolerance to strong opioids is not a practical problem.[36,37] Psychological dependence (addiction) to **morphine** is rare in patients with cancer pain.[33,38,39] Caution in this respect should be reserved for patients with a present or past history of substance abuse; even then strong opioids should be used when there is clinical need.[40,41] Nonetheless, sensible precautions include the provision of opioid by a single prescriber, close liaison with addiction medicine services and the use of an opioid contract (Box C). Physical dependence does not prevent a reduction in the dose if the patient's pain ameliorates, e.g. as a result of radiotherapy or a nerve block.[42]

Box C Example of a contract for controlled substance prescriptions with addicts[a]

Controlled substance medications (narcotics, tranquillizers and barbiturates) are very useful, but have high potential for misuse and are therefore closely controlled by the local, state, and federal government. They are intended to relieve pain, to improve function and/or ability to work, not simply to feel good. Because my physician is prescribing such medication for me to help manage my condition, I agree to the following conditions:

1 I am responsible for my controlled substance medications. If the prescription of medication is lost, misplaced, or stolen, or if I use it up sooner than prescribed, I understand that it will not be replaced.

2 I will not request or accept controlled substance medication from any other physicians or individual while I am receiving such medication from Dr.________________. Besides being illegal to do so, it may endanger my health. The only exception is if it is prescribed while I am admitted in a hospital.

3 Refills of controlled substance medication:
- Will be made only during Dr.__________________ regular office hours, in person, once each month during a scheduled office visit. Refills will not be made at night, on holidays, or weekends.
- Will not be made if I "run out early". I am responsible for taking the medication in the dose prescribed and for keeping track of the amount remaining.
- Will not be made as an "emergency", such as on Friday afternoon because I suddenly realize I will "run out tomorrow". I will call at least seventy-two hours ahead if I need assistance with a controlled substance medication prescription.

4 I will bring in the containers of all medications prescribed by Dr. ________________ each time I see him even if there is no medication remaining. These will be in the original containers from the pharmacy for each medication.

5 I understand that if I violate any of the above conditions, my controlled substances prescription and/or treatment with Dr.__________________ may be ended immediately. If the violation involves obtaining controlled substances from another individual, as described above, I may also be reported to my physician, medical facilities, and other authorities.

6 I understand that the main treatment goal is to improve my ability to function and/or work. In consideration of that goal and the fact that I am being given potent medication to help me reach that goal, I agree to help myself by the following better health habits: exercise, weight control, and the non-use of tobacco and alcohol. I understand that only through following a healthier life-style can I hope to have the most successful outcome to my treatment.

I have been fully informed by Dr.______________ and his staff regarding psychological dependence (addiction) of a controlled substance, which I understand is rare. I know that some persons may develop a tolerance, which is the need to increase the dose of the medication to achieve the same effect of pain control, and I do know that I will become physically dependent on the medication. This will occur if I am on the medication for several weeks, and, when I stop the medication, I must do so slowly and under medical supervision or I may have withdrawal symptoms.

I have read this contract and it has been explained to me by Dr.__________________ and/or his staff. In addition, I fully understand the consequences of violating said contract.

____________________	________	____________________	________
Patient's Signature	Date	Witness	Date

a. reproduced with permission from Hansen 1999.[43] © Southern Medical Association.

However, with the dramatic increase in the use of opioids for chronic non-cancer pain there have been corresponding increases in rates of misuse, abuse and addiction, along with fatal overdose, particularly with concurrent benzodiazepine use.[44,45] Further, deaths from causes other than overdose are also increased.[46] These concerns have led to a re-appraisal of the place of opioids in chronic non-cancer pain and to the introduction of opioid products which reduce abuse potential. For example, some m/r products form insoluble precipitates if an attempt is made to crush and dissolve them, preventing their injection.[47] Others contain a sequestered opioid antagonist which, if the tablet is crushed or dissolved, is released in sufficient amounts to antagonize the opioid and prevent a 'high' (see p.457).

For the use of strong opioids for chronic non-cancer pain, specialist advice should be followed (e.g. Faculty of Pain Medicine)[14] and/or sought from chronic pain teams.

Opioid-related serotonin toxicity

Serotonin toxicity results from the ingestion of drug(s) which increase brain serotonin above a critical level (see p.200).[48] Toxicity manifests as a triad of neuro-excitatory features:

- *autonomic hyperactivity*; sweating, fever, mydriasis, tachycardia, hypertension, tachypnea, sialorrhoea, diarrhoea
- *neuromuscular hyperactivity*; tremor, clonus, myoclonus, hyperreflexia, and pyramidal rigidity (advanced stage)
- *altered mental status*; agitation, hypomania, and delirium (advanced stage).

Clonus (inducible, spontaneous or ocular), agitation, sweating, tremor and hyperreflexia are essential features. Spontaneous clonus, in the presence of a serotoninergic drug, is the most reliable indicator of serotonin toxicity.[49]

Opioids are relatively weak serotonin re-uptake inhibitors and only cause symptoms in higher doses or susceptible individuals, or when used concurrently with a second drug with serotoninergic potency, notably an MAOI but also with many other antidepressants and some psychostimulants (see Antidepressants, Box A, p.200).

Fatalities from serotonin toxicity have occurred with **dextromethorphan**, **pethidine** (see Box A), **tramadol**, and possibly **fentanyl** when used in conjunction with an MAOI.[50] Non-fatal serotonin toxicity has also been observed with other fentanils, **dextropropoxyphene**, **methadone**, and **pentazocine**. Concurrent administration of these opioids with an MAOI (or within 2 weeks of cessation of an MAOI) is generally best avoided. It has *not* been observed with other opioids, and the 'blanket' warning against the concurrent use of an MAOI and other opioids is misplaced.

The onset of toxicity is generally rapid and progressive, typically as the second drug reaches effective blood levels (one or two doses). Occasionally, recurrent mild symptoms may occur for weeks before the development of severe toxicity. The patient is often alert or agitated, with tremor (sometimes severe), myoclonus and hyperreflexia. Ankle clonus is generally demonstrable or, in severe toxicity, occurs spontaneously. Neuromuscular signs are initially greater in the lower limbs, then become more generalized as toxicity increases. Other symptoms include shaking, shivering (often including chattering of the teeth), and sometimes trismus. Pyramidal rigidity is a late development in severe cases, and can impair respiration. Rigidity, a fever of >38.5°C or deteriorating blood gases indicate life-threatening toxicity.

Opioid-induced endocrinopathy

Opioids are associated with wide ranging endocrine effects, including interference with the production of various hypothalamic, pituitary, gonadal and adrenal hormones, e.g.:[51–55]

- inhibition of gonadotrophin-releasing hormone from the hypothalamus:
  - ▷ ↓ luteinizing hormone (LH) release from the pituitary → ↓ production of testosterone (testes) or oestrogen (ovaries)
  - ▷ ↓ follicle-stimulating hormone (FSH) release from the pituitary → ↓ production of sperm or ovarian follicles
  - ▷ associated with loss of libido, impotence, irregular menses or amenorrhoea, subfertility and other consequences of hypogonadism, e.g. reduced muscle mass, osteoporosis, fatigue
- inhibition of adrenocorticotrophic hormone (ACTH) from the pituitary:
  - ▷ ↓ cortisol production and release (adrenals)
  - ▷ ↓ androgen release (adrenals); an important source in women, also converted to oestrogens
  - ▷ associated with symptoms such as fatigue, weight loss, anorexia, vomiting, diarrhoea, abdominal pain, hypoglycaemia, hypotension and those caused by sex hormone deficiency (see above)

- inhibition of growth hormone from the pituitary:
  - ▷ associated with decreased cognitive function and possibly other effects.

In patients with chronic non-cancer pain, hormone suppression is evident after 1 week of opioid administration and appears dose-related. In one study, abnormally low levels of sex hormones were found in three quarters of men receiving opioids equivalent to <150mg **morphine**/24h PO, and in all receiving >150mg/24h PO.[56] The risk appears greater with m/r compared with immediate-release formulations; it is hypothesized that the greater fluctuation in plasma opioid level with the latter results in only intermittent inhibition of endocrine function.[57]

IT **morphine** (mean doses 5–12mg/24h) produced hypogonadism in most subjects, both men and women.[58–60] In one study, one third of patients also developed hypocortisolism ± growth hormone deficiency, leading to an Addisonian crisis in one patient.[58] Thus, in patients due to receive long-term IT opioids, it is recommended to measure sex hormone levels at baseline, and annually thereafter (see Spinal analgesia, Table 4, p.845).

The clinical implications of opioid-induced endocrinopathy in those with advanced life-limiting illnesses is unclear. However, when any patient receiving long-term opioids has symptoms suggestive of an endocrinopathy, it may be necessary to refer to an endocrinologist for investigation and possible replacement hormone therapy.[58] In men receiving opioids for chronic non-cancer pain, sexual function, mood, bone density and pain tolerance can benefit from testosterone replacement.[61]

Compared with **morphine** and other opioids, **buprenorphine** appears less likely to suppress the gonadal axis or testosterone levels (see p.397). If the opioid treatment is stopped, although testosterone levels generally increase within 24–72h, hypogonadism may persist for months–years.

Opioids and immune function

Opioids modulate immune cell function directly (by binding to opioid and Toll-like receptors on immune cells) and indirectly via activation of the hypothalamic-pituitary-adrenal (HPA) axis and the sympathetic nervous system.[62] Immune function is suppressed by the opioid-induced release of glucocorticoids and catecholamines (e.g. adrenaline (epinephrine), noradrenaline (norepinephrine)) from the adrenal medulla, and the release of catecholamines and neuropeptide Y from sympathetic nerve fibres which innervate lymphoid tissue (e.g. lymph nodes, spleen).[62] Thus, in some studies, **morphine** depresses natural killer cell activity, T-lymphocyte proliferation, monocyte/macrophage function and cytokine release function (e.g. interleukin (IL)-2, interferon (IFN)-γ), potentially reducing host resistance to bacterial, fungal and viral infections and impeding cancer immunosurveillance.[63–66] Further, partly through its effects on the immune system, **morphine** can influence cancer cell growth and metastasis. However, it is unclear if the overall effect is beneficial or deleterious.[62] Cancer cells also express opioid receptors, further complicating this area of research. In animal models of cancer, their overexpression is associated with cancer growth and metastasis, with contrasting reports of exogenous opioids either stimulating or inhibiting angiogenesis.[62,67]

Compared with **morphine** (and **diamorphine**), other opioids appear less immunosuppressive and **buprenorphine**, **hydromorphone**, **methadone**, **oxycodone**, **oxymorphone** and **tramadol** have little or no effect.[68–71] Neither **buprenorphine** nor **fentanyl** affected CD4+/CD8+ counts in patients with AIDS.[72] In patients with cancer pain, although one small retrospective study found the incidence of infections to be less in those receiving **oxycodone** compared to **morphine**, another found no difference between **fentanyl**, **morphine** and **oxycodone**.[73,74] Nonetheless, there was a dose relationship, with the risk of infection increasing by 2% per 10mg increase in daily oral **morphine** equivalent dose.[74]

However, overall, data are limited and inconsistent, and the clinical implications of these effects are uncertain.[62,71,75,76] Nonetheless, they may help to explain the increased susceptibility to infection seen in opioid abusers.[77] On the other hand, because pain is immunosuppressive, opioid analgesia may improve immune function in patients with pain.[62,78]

Opioid-induced hyperalgesia

Opioid-induced hyperalgesia (OIH) is an increased response to a painful stimulus associated with exposure to opioids. Although well demonstrated in animals, the findings in human studies are inconsistent and their relevance debated. For example, although in a recent large epidemiological study, OIH is suggested by the finding that the regular use of opioids was associated with greater pain sensitivity than non-opioids (which in turn, was greater than those taking no analgesic), the authors conceded that an increased pain sensitivity could also be both a cause and a consequence of chronic pain *per se*.[79]

OIH has been shown in both acute and chronic pain and appears to result from sustained sensitization of the nervous system in which excitatory neurotransmitters and the NMDA-receptor-channel complex play important roles.[80] The exact cause is unclear, but possibly includes the following opioid-related mechanisms:[80–83]

- activation of glial cells (via toll-like (TLR4) receptors), which play a role in inflammation, pain signal transmission, pain hypersensitivity and opioid tolerance
- activation of excitatory pathways, e.g.:
  - ▷ adenylyl cyclase and cyclic adenosine monophosphate levels increase, resulting in greater protein kinase activity, ultimately facilitating pain signal transmission, e.g. through activation of the NMDA-receptor-channel complex
  - ▷ μ-opioid receptors are G protein coupled receptors, generally containing 7-transmembrane domains (7TM) and binding with $G_{i/o}$ which leads to an inhibitory effect. Ongoing opioid exposure increases the expression of the splice variant 6TM μ-opioid receptor; this couples to G_s which leads to an excitatory effect
  - ▷ increased expression/sensitivity of transient receptor potential vanilloid 1 (TRPV1) receptors
- in the case of **morphine**, accumulation of M3G, which can activate glial cells via TLR4.

Susceptibility to OIH appears to vary widely and genetic make-up probably plays an important part in its development.[80,82]

Clinical features

In surgical pain, OIH may contribute to exaggerated levels of pain in the immediate postoperative period and the development of a chronic pain state. In patients with cancer, OIH may manifest in various ways:

- rapidly developing tolerance to opioids
- short-lived benefit from increased doses
- a change of pain pattern (Table 3).

OIH probably also contributes towards 'narcotic bowel syndrome' which presents with chronic or frequently recurring abdominal pain, unexplained by GI pathology; additional features include continuing/progressive pain despite increasing doses of opioids.[84]

Table 3 Opioid-induced hyperalgesia[85]

What the patient says	*What the doctor finds*
Increased sensitivity to pain stimulus (hyperalgesia)	Any dose of any opioid, but particularly with high-dose morphine or hydromorphone, and in renal failure
Worsening pain despite increasing doses of opioids	Pain elicited from ordinary non-painful stimuli, e.g. stroking skin with cotton (allodynia)
Pain which becomes more diffuse, extending beyond the distribution of the pre-existing pain	Presence of other manifestations of opioid-induced neural hyperexcitability: myoclonus, seizures, delirium

The extreme upper end of the spectrum may be those patients who manifest evidence of severe neural hyperexcitability (myoclonus, allodynia, and/or hyperalgesia), particularly when taking high doses of **morphine** or an alternative strong opioid. This may be accompanied by sedation and delirium (when it is often described as opioid neurotoxicity). However, OIH:

- is *not* limited to very high doses, or to any one opioid
- is probably under-diagnosed
- is more common than generally thought.

Severe pain which does not respond to increasing doses of opioids, or is complicated by severe undesirable effects, should raise the *possibility* of OIH.[85]

Evaluation

A diagnosis of OIH is generally made on the basis of a high level of clinical suspicion, probability, and pattern recognition. OIH must be differentiated from increased pain caused by disease progression or the development of opioid tolerance, both of which may be managed by increasing the opioid dose.

Management

Management is based largely on theoretical grounds and clinical observation.[80]

Prophylaxis

Use a multimodal approach to analgesia, e.g.:

- an NSAID may help to reduce inflammation and production of excitatory amino acid neurotransmitters which activate the pronociceptive and anti-opioid systems
- **gabapentin** may block calcium channels which may contribute to hyperalgesia in nerve pain.

Treatment

- progressively and rapidly reduce the dose of the causal opioid to about 25% of the peak dose
- switch conservatively (as a dose reduction will likely be needed) to an opioid with less risk of OIH, i.e. **fentanyl** (highest)® **morphine**® **methadone**® **buprenorphine** (lowest)[86], see opioid switching below
- (rarely) if occurring at very low doses (<10mg/24h), discontinue the opioid completely
- use a multimodal approach to analgesia, i.e. use non-opioids, e.g. **paracetamol** or an NSAID, and adjuvant analgesics, e.g. **gabapentin**
- consider **ketamine** (p.641) an NMDA-receptor-channel blocker.[87]

When switching from **morphine** because of severe neural hyperexcitability, a lower than expected dose of the alternative opioid is likely to be needed unless the dose of **morphine** has recently been much reduced (as suggested above).[88,89]

If these steps do not lead to a resolution of the OIH:

- consider spinal, regional or local analgesia (with local anaesthetics), and tail off systemic opioids completely
- check for hypomagnesaemia because this can aggravate OIH[90,91]
- consider treatment with ultralow doses of an opioid antagonist.[92,93]

Opioid switching ('rotation')

It is crucial to appreciate that conversion ratios are *never* more than an approximate guide. Thus, careful monitoring during conversion is necessary to avoid both underdosing and excessive dosing. For general considerations when switching opioids, see p.855.

Generally, switching from **morphine** (or other strong opioid) to an alternative is undertaken in an attempt to improve analgesia and/or reduce undesirable effects. It is reported necessary in about 10–44% of patients.[94–96] Before switching, it is worth considering if other options may be more appropriate, e.g. the use of adjuvant analgesics or modifying the management of the undesirable effects.

There is a lack of high quality RCT data to support switching. One open-label prospective study which randomized patients to either **morphine** or **oxycodone** first-line found that about one third required a switch to the alternative opioid, generally for undesirable effects (e.g. drowsiness, nausea/vomiting, confusion/hallucinations); these improved in similar proportions, such that using these two opioids, overall 95% of patients found an effective and tolerable dose. Apart from supporting the use of **morphine** over **oxycodone** first-line (i.e. similar efficacy and tolerability at a lower cost), these findings suggest that only a small proportion of patients (~5%) will require multiple switches in opioid.[97]

Examples of when more specific switches may be appropriate include:

- poor adherence or *intractable* constipation (→ TD **fentanyl**)
- significant decline in the patient's renal function (**morphine** → **alfentanil**, **buprenorphine**, **fentanyl**, **methadone**, see Chapter 17, p.693)
- opioid-induced hyperalgesia or other manifestations of neurotoxicity, e.g. cognitive failure/delirium, hallucinations, myoclonus, allodynia.

In cases of neurotoxicity, **fentanyl**, **hydromorphone**, **oxycodone** and **methadone** have all been substituted successfully for **morphine**.[98–101] Similarly, in the presence of inadequate pain relief and intolerable undesirable effects, TD **buprenorphine** has been substituted successfully for TD **fentanyl**, and vice versa.[102]

When converting from **morphine** to an alternative strong opioid, or vice versa, the initial dose depends on the relative potency of the two drugs (Table 4). (See also Opioid dose conversion ratios, p.855).

Table 4 Approximate potency of opioids relative to morphine; PO and immediate-release formulations unless stated otherwise[a]

Analgesic	*Potency relative to morphine*	*Duration of action (h)*[b]
Codeine Dihydrocodeine	1/10	3–6
Tramadol	1/10	4–6
Pethidine	1/8	2–4
Tapentadol	1/3	4–6
Hydrocodone (not UK)	2/3	4–8
Papaveretum	2/3[c]	3–5
Oxycodone	1.5 (2)[d]	3–4
Methadone	5–10[e]	8–12
Hydromorphone	4–5 (5–7.5)[d]	4–5
Buprenorphine (SL)	80	6–8
Buprenorphine (TD)	100 (75–115)[d]	Formulation dependent (72–168)
Fentanyl (TD)	100 (150)[d]	72

a. multiply dose of opioid in first column by relative potency in the second column to determine the equivalent dose of morphine sulfate/hydrochloride; conversely, divide morphine dose by the relative potency to determine the equivalent dose of another opioid

b. dependent in part on severity of pain and on dose; often longer lasting in very elderly and those with renal impairment

c. papaveretum (strong opium) is standardized to contain 50% morphine base; potency expressed in relation to morphine sulfate

d. the numbers in parenthesis are the manufacturers' preferred relative potencies; for explanation of divergence, see individual drug monographs

e. a single 5mg dose of methadone is equivalent to morphine 7.5mg, but a variable long plasma halflife and broad-spectrum receptor affinity result in a much higher than expected relative potency when administered regularly, sometimes much higher than the range given above; *it is essential to read the methadone monograph*, p.437.[88,103]

However, relative potencies and thus conversion ratios are *never* more than an approximate guide because of:[104–107]

- wide interindividual variation in opioid pharmacokinetics; influencing factors include age, ethnicity, renal or hepatic impairment
- other variables including dose and duration of opioid treatment, direction of switch in opioid, nutritional status and concurrent medications
- their method of derivation, e.g. single dose rather than chronic dose studies, using typical doses.

Thus, careful monitoring during conversion is necessary to avoid both underdosing and excessive dosing.

Providing explicit guidance on switching opioids is difficult because the reasons for switching are varied, as are the patient's circumstances. One guideline, based on expert consensus, recommends routinely reducing the calculated equivalent dose of the new opioid by 25–50%.[108] Various patient factors are then taken into account to modify the reduction, which potentially could see it removed (e.g. young patient, no undesirable effects, in severe pain, switching at low dose) or increased further (e.g. older patient, delirious, in moderate pain, switching at high dose).

Certainly, a dose reduction of at least 50% would seem prudent when switching at high doses (e.g. **morphine** or equivalent doses of ≥1g/24h PO), in elderly or frail patients, because of intolerable undesirable effects (e.g. delirium), or when there has been a recent rapid escalation of the first opioid (possibly due to opioid-induced hyperalgesia). In such circumstances, p.r.n. doses can be relied on to make up any deficit while re-titrating to a satisfactory dose of the new opioid.

A separate strategy is necessary for **methadone** (see p.437).

Combining opioids

It is generally considered to be bad practice to prescribe more than one strong opioid for simultaneous use. Thus, for example, regular **morphine** is best backed up by p.r.n **morphine** for break-through pain (see p.297). However, there are circumstances when this may be necessary, for example TD **fentanyl** backed up by p.r.n. **morphine** (see QCG: Use of transdermal fentanyl patches, p.417). Also, someone with good pain relief from a regular weak opioid may have a supply of **morphine** for back-up use in case of severe break-through pain.

However, there are reports of two strong opioids being used successfully in combination, i.e. providing better pain relief at relatively lower doses and reduced undesirable effects.[109–111] For example, in one, regular **oxycodone** plus p.r.n. **morphine** was more beneficial than regular **morphine** plus p.r.n. **morphine**.[109] In another, patients on regular **morphine** benefited from the addition of a second regular opioid in low dose (either **methadone** or TD **fentanyl**).[110] However, the quality of this evidence is low or very low.[112] Thus, despite such reports, because of the increased complexity and scope for error, patients should *not* normally have two opioids prescribed concurrently on a regular basis.[113,114]

1 Portenoy RK *et al.* (2006) Opioid use and survival at the end of life: a survey of a hospice population. *Journal of Pain and Symptom Management.* **32**: 532–540.
2 Ballantyne JC (2007) Regulation of opioid prescribing. *British Medical Journal.* **334**: 811–812.
3 Mika J (2008) The opioid systems and the role of glial cells in the effects of opioids. *Advances in Palliative Medicine.* **7**: 185–196.
4 Sauriyal DS *et al.* (2011) Extending pharmacological spectrum of opioids beyond analgesia: Multifunctional aspects in different pathophysiological states. *Neuropeptides.* **45**: 175–188.
5 Zhu C *et al.* (2017) Neuron-restrictive silencer factor-mediated downregulation of mu-opioid receptor contributes to the reduced morphine analgesia in bone cancer pain. *Pain.* **158**: 879–890.
6 Sun L *et al.* (2017) Nerve injury-induced epigenetic silencing of opioid receptors controlled by DNMT3a in primary afferent neurons. *Pain.* **158**: 1153–1165.
7 Raffa RB *et al.* (2017) Cebranopadol: novel dual opioid/NOP receptor agonist analgesic. *Journal of Clinical Pharmacy and Therapeutics.* **42**: 8–17.
8 Lutfy K *et al.* (2003) Buprenorphine-induced antinociception is mediated by mu-opioid receptors and compromised by concomitant activation of opioid receptor-like receptors. *Journal of Neuroscience.* **23**: 10331–10337.
9 Virk MS *et al.* (2009) Buprenorphine is a weak partial agonist that inhibits opioid receptor desensitization. *Journal of Neuroscience.* **29**: 7341–7348.
10 Siuda ER *et al.* (2017) Biased mu-opioid receptor ligands: a promising new generation of pain therapeutics. *Current Opinion in Pharmacology.* **32**: 77–84.
11 Olson KM *et al.* (2017) Novel molecular strategies and targets for opioid drug discovery for the treatment of chronic pain. *Yale Journal of Biology and Medicine.* **90**: 97–110.
12 McDonald J and Lambert DG (2005) Opioid receptors. Continuing education in anaesthesia. *Critical Care and Pain.* **5**: 22–25.
13 Manchikanti L *et al.* (2017) Responsible, safe, and effective prescription of opioids for chronic non-cancer pain: American Society of Interventional Pain Physicians (ASIPP) guidelines. *Pain Physician.* **20**: S3–S92.
14 Faculty of Pain Medicine (2017) Opioids aware: a resource for patients and healthcare professionals to support prescribing of opioid medicines for pain. Available from: www.rcoa.ac.uk/faculty-of-pain-medicine/opioids-aware
15 Caraceni A *et al.* (2012) Use of opioid analgesics in the treatment of cancer pain: evidence-based recommendations from the EAPC. *Lancet Oncology.* **13**: e58–68.
16 WHO (1986). *Cancer Pain Relief.* World Health Organization, Geneva.
17 Quigley C (2005) The role of opioids in cancer pain. *British Medical Journal.* **331**: 825–829.
18 NICE (2012) Opioids in palliative care: safe and effective prescribing of strong opioids for pain in palliative care adults. *Clinical Guideline.* CG140 www.nice.org.uk
19 Hoskin P and Hanks G (1991) Opioid agonist-antagonist drugs in acute and chronic pain states. *Drugs.* **41**: 326–344.
20 Twycross RG (1994) Pentazocine. In: *Pain Relief in Advanced Cancer.* Churchill Livingstone, Edinburgh, pp. 247–248.
21 Woods A *et al.* (1974) Medicines evaluation and monitoring group: central nervous system effects of pentazocine. *British Medical Journal.* **1**: 305–307.
22 Smith J (2004) Building a safer NHS for patients - Improving medication safety. A Report by the Chief Pharmacuetical Officer. Gateway ref 1459. 105–111 Department of Health, London
23 Care Quality Commission and NHS England (2013) Safer use of controlled drugs - preventing harms from fentanyl and buprenorphine transdermal patches. *Use of controlled drugs supporting information.* www.cqc.org.uk
24 Plummer JL *et al.* (2001) Norpethidine toxicity. *Pain Reviews.* **8**: 159–170.
25 Swart LM *et al.* (2017) The comparative risk of delirium with different opioids: a systematic review. *Drugs and Aging.* **34**: 437–443.

26 Sweetman SC (ed) (2005) Martindale: The Complete Drug Reference. (34e). Pharmaceutical Press, London, pp. 80–82.
27 Shee JC (1960) Dangerous potentiation of pethidine by iproniazid, and its treatment. *British Medical Journal*. **ii**: 507–509.
28 Taylor D (1962) Alarming reaction to pethidine in patients on phenelzine. *Lancet*. **2**: 401–402.
29 Rogers KJ and Thornton JA (1969) The interaction between monoamine oxidase inhibitors and narcotic analgesics in mice. *British Journal of Pharmacology*. **36**: 470–480.
30 Cherny N *et al.* (2001) Strategies to manage the adverse effects of oral morphine: an evidence-based report. *Journal of Clinical Oncology*. **19**: 2542–2554.
31 Borgbjerg FM *et al.* (1996) Experimental pain stimulates respiration and attenuates morphine-induced respiratory depression: a controlled study in human volunteers. *Pain*. **64**: 123–128.
32 Estfan B *et al.* (2007) Respiratory function during parenteral opioid titration for cancer pain. *Palliative Medicine*. **21**: 81–86.
33 Sykes NP (2007) Morphine kills the pain, not the patient. *Lancet*. **369**: 1325–1326.
34 Regnard CFB and Badger C (1987) Opioids, sleep and the time of death. *Palliative Medicine*. **1**: 107–110.
35 Schwarzer A *et al.* (2015) Sleep-disordered breathing decreases after opioid withdrawal: results of a prospective controlled trial. *Pain*. **156**: 2167–2174.
36 Collin E *et al.* (1993) Is disease progression the major factor in morphine 'tolerance' in cancer pain treatment? *Pain*. **55**: 319–326.
37 Portenoy RK (1994) Tolerance to opioid analgesics: clinical aspects. *Cancer Surveys*. **21**: 49–65.
38 Passik S and Portenoy R (1998) Substance abuse issues in palliative care. In: A Berger (ed) *Principles and Practice of Supportive Oncology*. Lippincott-Raven, Philadelphia, pp. 513–529.
39 Joranson D *et al.* (2000) Trends in medical use and abuse of opioid analgesics. *Journal of the American Medical Association*. **283**: 1710–1714.
40 Passik S *et al.* (1998) Substance abuse issues in cancer patients. Part 1: prevalence and diagnosis. *Oncology*. **12**: 517–521.
41 Passik S *et al.* (1998) Substance abuse issues in cancer patients. Part 2: evaluation and treatment. *Oncology*. **12**: 729–734.
42 Twycross RG and Wald SJ (1976) Longterm use of diamorphine in advanced cancer. In: JJ Bonica and D Albe-Fessard (eds) *Advances in Pain Research and Therapy* Vol 1. Raven Press, New York, pp. 653–661.
43 Hansen H (1999) Treatment of chronic pain with antiepileptic drugs. *Southern Medical Journal*. **92**: 642–649.
44 Babalonis S and Walsh SL (2015) Warnings unheeded: the risks of co-prescribing opioids and benzodiazepines. *Pain: Clinical Updates*. **23**: 6.
45 Ballantyne JC *et al.* (2016) WHO analgesic ladder: a good concept gone astray. *British Medical Journal*. **352**: i20.
46 Ray WA *et al.* (2016) Prescription of long-acting opioids and mortality in patients with chronic noncancer pain. *JAMA*. **315**: 2415–2423.
47 Cicero TJ *et al.* (2012) Effect of abuse-deterrent formulation of OxyContin. *New England Journal of Medicine*. **367**: 187–189.
48 Gillman K (2006) Serotonin toxicity, serotonin syndrome. *Psycho Tropical Research*. www.psychotropical.com (accessed April 2013).
49 Dunkley EJ *et al.* (2003) The Hunter Serotonin Toxicity Criteria: simple and accurate diagnostic decision rules for serotonin toxicity. *Quarterly Journal of Medicine*. **96**: 635–642.
50 Gillman PK (2005) Monoamine oxidase inhibitors, opioid analgesics and serotonin toxicity. *British Journal of Anaesthesia*. **95**: 434–441.
51 McWilliams K *et al.* (2014) A systematic review of opioid effects on the hypogonadal axis of cancer patients. *Supportive Care in Cancer*. **22**: 1699–1704.
52 Thosani S and Jimenez C (2011) Opioid-induced biochemical alterations of the neuroendocrine axis. *Expert Reviews of Endocrinology and Metabolism*. **6**: 705–713.
53 Debono M *et al.* (2011) Tramadol-induced adrenal insufficiency. *European Journal of Clinical Pharmacology*. **67**: 865–867.
54 Rhodin A *et al.* (2014) Recombinant human growth hormone improves cognitive capacity in a pain patient exposed to chronic opioids. *Acta Anaesthesiologica Scandinavica*. **58**: 759–765.
55 NICE (2003) Human Growth hormone (somatropin) in adults with growth hormone deficiency. *Technology appraisal guidance*. TA64. www.nice.org.uk
56 Daniell HW (2002) Hypogonadism in men consuming sustained-action oral opioids. *The Journal of Pain*. **3**: 377–384.
57 Rubinstein A and Carpenter DM (2014) Elucidating risk factors for androgen deficiency associated with daily opioid use. *American Journal of Medicine*. **127**: 1195–1201.
58 Abs R *et al.* (2000) Endocrine consequences of long-term intrathecal administration of opioids. *Journal of Clinical Endocrinology and Metabolism*. **85**: 2215–2222.
59 Finch PM *et al.* (2000) Hypogonadism in patients treated with intrathecal morphine. *Clinical Journal of Pain*. **16**: 251–254.
60 Roberts LJ *et al.* (2002) Sex hormone suppression by intrathecal opioids: a prospective study. *Clinical Journal of Pain*. **18**: 144–148.
61 O'Rourke TK, Jr. and Wosnitzer MS (2016) Opioid-induced androgen deficiency (OPIAD): diagnosis, management, and literature review. *Current Urology Reports*. **17**: 76.
62 Boland JW and Pockley AG (2017) Influence of opioids on immune function in patients with cancer pain: from bench to bedside. *British Journal of Pharmacology*. In press.
63 Sacerdote P *et al.* (1997) Antinociceptive and immunosuppressive effects of opiate drugs: a structure-related activity study. *British Journal of Pharmacology*. **121**: 834–840.
64 Risdahl JM *et al.* (1998) Opiates and infection. *Journal of Neuroimmunology*. **83**: 4–18.
65 McCarthy L *et al.* (2001) Opioids, opioid receptors, and the immune response. *Drug and Alcohol Dependence*. **62**: 111–123.
66 Boland JW *et al.* (2014) Effects of opioids on immunologic parameters that are relevant to anti-tumour immune potential in patients with cancer: a systematic literature review. *British Journal of Cancer*. **111**: 866–873.
67 Ondrovics M *et al.* (2017) Opioids: Modulators of angiogenesis in wound healing and cancer. *Oncotarget*. **8**: 25783–25796.
68 Sacerdote P *et al.* (2000) The effects of tramadol and morphine on immune responses and pain after surgery in cancer patients. *Anesthesia and Analgesia*. **90**: 1411–1414.
69 Budd K and Shipton E (2004) Acute pain and the immune system and opioimmunosuppression. *Acute Pain*. **6**: 123–135.
70 Budd K and Raffa R (eds) (2005) Buprenorphine - the unique opioid analgesic. Georg Thieme Verlag, Stuttgart, Germany, p. 134.
71 Sacerdote P *et al.* (2008) Buprenorphine and methadone maintenance treatment of heroin addicts preserves immune function. *Brain, Behavior, and Immunity*. **22**: 606–613.
72 Canneti A *et al.* (2013) Safety and efficacy of transdermal buprenorphine and transdermal fentanyl in the treatment of neuropathic pain in AIDS patients. *Minerva Anestesiologica*. **79**: 871–883.
73 Suzuki M *et al.* (2013) Correlation between the administration of morphine or oxycodone and the development of infections in patients with cancer pain. *American Journal of Hospice and Palliative Care*. **30**: 712–716.
74 Shao YJ *et al.* (2017) Contribution of opiate analgesics to the development of infections in advanced cancer patients. *Clinical Journal of Pain*. **33**: 295–299.

75 Rittner HL *et al.* (2010) The clinical (ir)relevance of opioid-induced immune suppression. *Current Opinion in Anaesthesiology.* **23**: 588–592.

76 Boland JW *et al.* (2014) A preliminary evaluation of the effects of opioids on innate and adaptive human in vitro immune function. *BMJ Supportive and Palliative Care.* **4**: 357–367.

77 Alonzo NC and Bayer BM (2002) Opioids, immunology, and host defenses of intravenous drug abusers. *Infectious Disease Clinics of North America.* **16**: 553–569.

78 Page GG (2005) Immunologic effects of opioids in the presence or absence of pain. *Journal of Pain and Symptom Management.* **29**: S25–31.

79 Samuelsen PJ *et al.* (2017) Pain sensitivity and analgesic use among 10,486 adults: the Tromso study. *BMC Pharmacology and Toxicology.* **18**: 45.

80 Edwards DA and Chen L (2014) The evidence for opioid-induced hyperalgesia today. *Austin Journal of Anesthesia and Analgesia.* **2**: 12.

81 Milligan ED and Watkins LR (2009) Pathological and protective roles of glia in chronic pain. *Nature Reviews Neurosciene.* **10**: 23–36.

82 Roeckel LA *et al.* (2016) Opioid-induced hyperalgesia: Cellular and molecular mechanisms. *Neuroscience.* **338**: 160–182.

83 Shah M and Choi S (2017) Toll-like receptor-dependent negative effects of opioids: a battle between analgesia and hyperalgesia. *Frontiers in Immunology.* **8**: 642.

84 Lee AA and Hasler WL (2016) Opioids and GI motility-friend or foe? *Current Treatment Options in Gastroenterology.* **14**: 478–494.

85 Zylicz Z and Twycross R (2008) Opioid-induced hyperalgesia may be more frequent than previously thought. *Journal of Clinical Oncology.* **26**: 1564.

86 Koppert W (2007) Opioid-induced hyperalgesia. Pathophysiology and clinical relevance. *Acute Pain.* **9**: 21–24.

87 Walker SM and Cousins MJ (1997) Reduction in hyperalgesia and intrathecal morphine requirements by low-dose ketamine infusion. *Journal of Pain and Symptom Management.* **14**: 129–133.

88 Bruera E *et al.* (1996) Opioid rotation in patients with cancer pain. *Cancer.* **78**: 852–857.

89 Lawlor P *et al.* (1998) Dose ratio between morphine and methadone in patients with cancer pain. *Cancer.* **82**: 1167–1173.

90 Dubray C *et al.* (1997) Magnesium deficiency induces an hyperalgesia reversed by the NMDA receptor antagonist MK801. *Neuroreport.* **8**: 1383–1386.

91 Begon S *et al.* (2002) Magnesium increases morphine analgesic effect in different experimental models of pain. *Anesthesiology.* **96**: 627–632.

92 Gan T *et al.* (1997) Opioid-sparing effects of a low-dose infusion of naloxone in patient-administered morphine sulfate. *Anesthesiology.* **87**: 1075–1081.

93 Chindalore VL *et al.* (2005) Adding ultralow-dose naltrexone to oxycodone enhances and prolongs analgesia: a randomized, controlled trial of Oxytrex. *Journal of Pain.* **6**: 392–399.

94 Wiffen PJ *et al.* (2017) Opioids for cancer pain - an overview of Cochrane reviews. *Cochrane Database of Systematic Reviews.* **7**: CD012592. www.thecochranelibrary.com

95 Corli O *et al.* (2016) Are strong opioids equally effective and safe in the treatment of chronic cancer pain? A multicenter randomized phase IV 'real life' trial on the variability of response to opioids. *Annals of Oncology.* **27**: 1107–1115.

96 Mercadante S and Bruera E (2016) Opioid switching in cancer pain: From the beginning to nowadays. *Critical Reviews in Oncology/Hematology.* **99**: 241–248.

97 Riley J *et al.* (2015) Morphine or oxycodone for cancer-related pain? A randomized, open-label, controlled trial. *Journal of Pain and Symptom Management.* **49**: 161–172.

98 Sjogren P *et al.* (1994) Disappearance of morphine-induced hyperalgesia after discontinuing or substituting morphine with other opioid agonists. *Pain.* **59**: 313–316.

99 Hagen N and Swanson R (1997) Strychnine-like multifocal myoclonus and seizures in extremely high-dose opioid administration: treatment strategies. *Journal of Pain and Symptom Management.* **14**: 51–58.

100 Ashby M *et al.* (1999) Opioid substitution to reduce adverse effects in cancer pain management. *Medical Journal of Australia.* **170**: 68–71.

101 Morita T *et al.* (2005) Opioid rotation from morphine to fentanyl in delirious cancer patients: an open-label trial. *Journal of Pain and Symptom Management.* **30**: 96–103.

102 Aurilio C *et al.* (2009) Opioids switching with transdermal systems in chronic cancer pain. *Journal of Experimental and Clinical Cancer Research.* **28**: 61.

103 Nixon AJ (2005) Methadone for cancer pain: a case report. *American Journal of Hospice and Palliative Care.* **22**: 337.

104 Anderson R *et al.* (2001) Accuracy in equianalgesic dosing: conversion dilemmas. *Journal of Pain and Symptom Management.* **21**: 397–406.

105 Pasternak G (2001) Incomplete cross tolerance and multiple mu opioid peptide receptors. *Trends in Pharmacological Sciences.* **22**: 67–70.

106 Pereira J *et al.* (2001) Equianalgesic dose ratios for opioids: a critical review and proposals for long-term dosing. *Journal of Pain and Symptom Management.* **22**: 672–687.

107 Knotkova H *et al.* (2009) Opioid rotation: the science and the limitations of the equianalgesic dose table. *Journal of Pain and Symptom Management.* **38**: 426–439.

108 Fine PG and Portenoy RK (2009) Establishing "best practices" for opioid rotation: conclusions of an expert panel. *Journal of Pain and Symptom Management.* **38**: 418–425.

109 Lauretti GR *et al.* (2003) Comparison of sustained-release morphine with sustained-release oxycodone in advanced cancer patients. *British Journal of Cancer.* **89**: 2027–2030.

110 Mercadante S *et al.* (2004) Addition of a second opioid may improve opioid response in cancer pain: preliminary data. *Supportive Care Cancer.* **12**: 762–766.

111 Kotlinska-Lemieszek A (2010) Rotation, partial rotation (semi-switch), combining opioids, and titration. Does "opioid plus opioid" strategy make a step forward on our way to improving the outcome of pain treatment? *Journal of Pain and Symptom Management.* **40**: e10–12.

112 Fallon MT and Laird BJA (2011) A systematic review of comination strong opioid therapy in cancer pain (in press). *Palliative Medicine.*

113 Davis MP *et al.* (2005) Look before leaping: combined opioids may not be the rave. *Supportive Care in Cancer.* **13**: 769–774.

114 Strasser F (2005) Promoting science in a pragmatic world: not (yet) time for partial opioid rotation. *Supportive Care in Cancer.* **13**: 765–768.

Updated September 2017

MORPHINE

Class: Strong opioid analgesic.

Indications: Severe or †moderate pain, †diarrhoea, †cough, †breathlessness.

Contra-indications: None absolute if titrated carefully against a patient's pain (also see Strong opioids, p.360).

5

Pharmacology

Morphine is the main pharmacologically active constituent of opium. Its effects are mediated by specific opioid receptors both within the CNS and peripherally. Under normal circumstances, its main peripheral action is on smooth muscle. However, in the presence of tissue injury and inflammation, the number of opioid receptors at the peripheral end of a nociceptive afferent nerve fibre increases, and exogenous and endogenous opioids (released by activated inflammatory cells in close proximity to the nerve fibre) thereby exert a peripheral analgesic action.[1] Thus, there is increasing interest in the role of topical morphine (see below). Conversely, in bone and neuropathic pain, opioid receptor expression is reduced, contributing towards a reduced response to opioids. Nonetheless, in pooled data from RCTs in pure neuropathic pain states, morphine provides a 25–33% improvement in pain in 2/3 of patients (NNT 3.7 (95% CI 2.6–6.5)). However, this is considered very low quality evidence, mostly because of the small number of participants (≤152).[2] In practice, a multimodal approach to pain relief is followed (see p.295).

Morphine, like all μ-opioid receptor agonists (μ agonists) increases intestinal transit time by decreasing propulsive activity and increasing non-propulsive activity via its effect on the myenteric plexus in the longitudinal muscle layer. This causes predictable opioid-induced constipation, which requires prophylactic regular laxatives when used regularly for pain (see Dose and use). Conversely, it can also be used for diarrhoea, although generally **loperamide**, a peripherally acting μ agonist, is preferred (see p.35). All opioids can be used for cough and act by suppressing the cough reflex centre in the brain stem (see p.144). Morphine is also used to relieve breathlessness (see Dose and use).

The liver is the principal site of morphine metabolism.[3] Metabolism also occurs in other organs,[4] including the CNS.[5] Glucuronidation, the main metabolic pathway, is rarely impaired except in severe hepatic impairment, and morphine is well tolerated in patients with mild–moderate hepatic impairment.[6] However, with impairment severe enough to prolong the prothrombin time, the plasma halflife of morphine may be increased (see p.703).[4]

The major metabolites of morphine are morphine-3-glucuronide (M3G; 55–80%) and morphine-6-glucuronide (M6G; 10–15%) which are excreted by the kidneys.[7] M6G binds to opioid receptors and contributes substantially to the effects of morphine, both desirable (e.g. analgesia) and undesirable (e.g. nausea and vomiting, sedation and respiratory depression).[8–10] In renal failure, the plasma halflife of M6G increases from 2.5h up to 7.5h, and is likely to lead to accumulation and enhanced toxicity (see p.681). Similarly, in the last week of life, M6G accumulates as renal function deteriorates, increasing the risk of opioid toxicity and thereby terminal delirium;[11] this may also explain why some RCTs of IV hydration at the end of life found a reduced incidence of sedation, myoclonus and delirium.[12] M3G will also accumulate, but the significance of this is unclear; it binds poorly to opioid receptors and is considered devoid of an analgesic effect. Although animal studies suggest a neuro-excitatory effect, this has not been clearly demonstrated in humans.[13]

Morphine is administered by a range of routes. Systemic absorption from topical application to ulcers or inflamed surfaces varies with the amount and concentration of the gel used; bio-availability ranges from negligible (with 0.06–0.125% gel) to almost the same as SC (0.125–0.5% gel applied to large ulcers).[14–17]

Because of the wide range in PO bio-availability, when switching from PO to SC/IM/IV morphine, the dose required is between 1/2–1/3 of the PO dose.[18,19] In practice, for morphine, most centres use a conversion ratio of PO:SC/IM/IV of 2:1. Conversely, when switching from SC/IM/IV to PO, the PO dose should be 2–3 times greater than the SC/IM/IV dose. In a recent observational study, about 80% of patients achieved a satisfactory 24h PO dose at 3 times the previous 24h IV dose, rounded down to convenient strength m/r tablets.[20]

Bio-availability 35% PO, ranging from 15–64%; 25% PR.
Peak effect ≤60min PO (immediate-release tablets); 20min IV; 30–60min IM; 50–90min SC.

Time to peak plasma concentration 15–60min PO (immediate-release tablets), 1–6h m/r (product dependent); 10–20min IM; 15min SC; 45–60min PR.
Plasma halflife 1.5–4.5h PO; 1.5h IV.
Duration of action 3–6h; 12–24h m/r (product dependent).

Cautions

Renal impairment and severe hepatic impairment (see Dose and use, Chapter 17, p.693 and Chapter 18, p.709).

Drug interactions

The following have been reported with PO morphine, although their clinical relevance is unknown:

- **rifampicin** may reduce plasma levels of morphine, possibly via the induction of p-glycoprotein in the GI tract
- **quinidine** may increase plasma levels of morphine via the inhibition of p-glycoprotein in the GI tract
- morphine may increase plasma levels of **gabapentin** by slowing GI transit time
- **metoclopramide** may increase the rate of absorption of morphine via increased gastric emptying. (Conversely, morphine can also reduce the pro-kinetic effects of **metoclopramide** on gastric emptying.)

Undesirable effects

See Table 1 and Strong opioids, Box B, p.365.

Dose and use

As with all opioids, patients must be monitored for undesirable effects, particularly nausea and vomiting, and constipation. Depending on individual circumstances, an anti-emetic should be prescribed for regular or p.r.n. use (see QCG Nausea and vomiting, p.240) and, routinely, a laxative prescribed (see QCG Opioid-induced constipation, p.42).

Opioids can impair driving ability and patients should be counselled accordingly. Morphine is included in a new law in England and Wales relating to driving with certain drugs above specified plasma concentrations (see p.743).

Based on familiarity, availability and cost, morphine is the strong opioid of choice for moderate–severe cancer pain.[22] However, in terms of efficacy and undesirable effects, morphine, **hydromorphone** and **oxycodone** are essentially similar.[23] Morphine is generally prescribed with a non-opioid when the non-opioid + a weak opioid does not provide adequate relief (see p.295).

There is no pharmacological need for weak opioids in cancer pain (see p.295). Moving directly from a non-opioid to a strong opioid is increasingly preferred in adults, and is the norm in children in whom weak opioids are no longer recommended.[24]

Oral

Morphine is available as immediate-release tablets and solutions, and m/r tablets, capsules and suspensions. Most m/r products are administered b.d., some once daily. Because the pharmacokinetic profiles of m/r products differ,[25–27] it is best to keep individual patients on the same brand. M/r tablets should be swallowed whole; crushing or chewing them will lead to a rapid release of an overdose of morphine. For administration of immediate-release and m/r morphine to patients with swallowing difficulties or enteral feeding tubes, see p.785.

Patients can be started on either an ordinary (immediate-release) or an m/r formulation (Box A).[28,29] An observational study supports a starting dose of 5mg q4h as generally safe for opioid-naïve patients, and 10mg q4h for those being switched from a regular weak opioid.[30] However, slight variation exists between guidelines, e.g. in the recommended starting dose.[31] It is important to recognize that guidelines are just guidelines; and for each patient, when deciding the starting dose, it is necessary to consider the individual circumstances, e.g. severity of the pain, current analgesia, presence of renal impairment, increasing age or frailty. In every case, the patient must be monitored closely, and the dose titrated as necessary.

Table 1 Potential intolerable effects of morphine

Type	*Effects*	*Initial action*	*Comment*
For general undesirable effects of opioid analgesics, see Strong opioids Box B, p.000.			
Gastric stasis	Epigastric fullness, flatulence, anorexia, hiccup, persistent nausea	Prescribe a prokinetic, e.g. metoclopramide 10mg PO/SC t.d.s. (see p.244)	If the problem persists, change to an alternative opioid, with less impact on the GI tract
Sedation	Intolerable persistent sedation	Reduce dose of morphine; consider a psychostimulant, e.g. methylphenidate 5mg PO b.d. (see p.225)	Sedation may be caused by other factors; stimulant rarely appropriate
Cognitive failure	Agitated delirium with hallucinations	Prescribe an antipsychotic, e.g. haloperidol 500microgram PO/SC stat & q2h p.r.n. (see p.180); reduce dose of morphine and, if no improvement, switch to an alternative opioid	Some patients develop intractable delirium with one opioid but not with an alternative opioid
Myoclonus	Multifocal twitching ± jerking of limbs	Prescribe a benzodiazepine, e.g. diazepam PO/ midazolam SC 5mg stat & q1h p.r.n.; reduce dose of morphine but increase again if pain recurs	Uncommon with typical oral doses; more common with high dose IV and spinal morphine
Neurotoxicity	Abdominal muscle spasms, symmetrical jerking of legs; whole-body allodynia, hyperalgesia (manifests as excruciating pain)	Prescribe a benzodiazepine, e.g. diazepam PO/ midazolam SC 5mg stat & q1h p.r.n.; reduce dose of morphine; consider changing to an alternative opioid	A rare syndrome in patients receiving intrathecal or high dose IV morphine; occasionally seen with typical oral and SC doses
Vestibular stimulation	Movement-induced nausea and vomiting	Prescribe an antihistaminic antimuscarinic anti-emetic, e.g. cyclizine 50mg PO/SC t.d.s. or promethazine 25mg PO t.d.s.–q.d.s. (see p.249)	If intractable, try levomepromazine or switch to an alternative opioid
Pruritus	Whole-body itch with systemic morphine; localized to upper body or face/nose with spinal morphine	With systemic opioids, prescribe PO H_1-antihistamine (e.g. chlorphenamine 4mg stat; if beneficial continue with 4mg t.d.s. or p.r.n. for 2–3 days). Possibly switch opioids, e.g. morphine → oxycodone. For spinal opioids, see p.839.	Pruritus after systemic opioids is uncommon. It can sometimes be caused by cutaneous histamine release and be self-limiting but the most distressing cases are chronic and antihistamine-resistant. Centrally-acting opioid antagonists also relieve the pruritus but will also antagonize analgesia[21]
Histamine release	Bronchoconstriction → breathlessness	Treat as for anaphylaxis (see p.000); change to a chemically distinct opioid immediately, e.g. methadone	Rare

5

Box A Starting a patient on PO morphine

The starting dose of morphine is calculated to give a greater analgesic effect than the medication already in use:

- if the patient was previously receiving a weak opioid regularly (e.g. codeine 240mg/24h or equivalent), give 10mg q4h or m/r 20–30mg q12h, but less if suspected to be a poor codeine metabolizer (see p.349)
- if changing from an alternative strong opioid (e.g. fentanyl, methadone) a much higher dose of morphine may be needed
- if the patient is frail and elderly, or opioid-naïve, a lower dose helps to reduce initial drowsiness, confusion and unsteadiness, e.g. 5mg q4h
- because of accumulation of an active metabolite, a lower and/or less frequent regular dose may suffice in mild–moderate renal impairment, e.g. 5–10mg q8h–q6h (but the use of a 'renally safer' opioid is generally advisable with moderate–severe renal impairment, see p.681 and p.703).

When adjusting the dose of morphine, p.r.n. use should be taken into account; increments should not exceed 33–50% every 24h.
As with all opioids, patients must be monitored for undesirable effects, particularly nausea and vomiting, and constipation (see Strong opioids, Box B, p.365). Depending on individual circumstances, an anti-emetic should be prescribed for regular or p.r.n. use (see QCG: Nausea and vomiting, p.240) and, routinely, a laxative prescribed (see QCG: Opioid-induced constipation, p.42).

Opioids can impair driving ability and patients should be counselled accordingly. Diamorphine is included in a new law in England and Wales relating to driving with certain drugs above specified plasma concentrations (see p.743).

Upward titration of the dose of morphine stops when either the pain is relieved or unacceptable undesirable effects occur. In the latter case, it is generally necessary to consider alternative measures. The aim is to have the patient free of pain and mentally alert after the initial drowsiness has cleared.

Because of poor absorption, m/r morphine may not be satisfactory in patients troubled by frequent vomiting or those with diarrhoea or an ileostomy.

Scheme 1: immediate-release morphine oral solution or tablets

- morphine given q4h 'by the clock' with p.r.n. doses 1/10–1/6 of the 24h dose
- after 1–2 days, recalculate q4h dose by dividing the total used in previous 24h (regular + p.r.n. use) by 6
- continue q4h and p.r.n. doses
- increase the regular dose until there is adequate relief throughout each 4h period, taking p.r.n. use into account
- a double dose at bedtime obviates the need to wake the patient for a dose during the night
- >90% of patients achieve satisfactory pain relief within 5 days.

Scheme 2: immediate-release morphine and modified-release (m/r) morphine

- begin as for Scheme 1
- when the q4h dose is stable, replace with m/r morphine q12h, or once daily if a 24h product is prescribed
- the q12h dose will be three times the previous q4h dose; a q24h dose will be six times the previous q4h dose, rounded to a convenient number of tablets or capsules
- continue to provide immediate-release morphine solution or tablets for p.r.n. use; give 1/10–1/6 of the 24h dose.

Scheme 3: m/r morphine and immediate-release morphine

- generally start with m/r morphine 20–30mg q12h, or 10mg q12h in frail elderly patients
- use immediate-release morphine solution or tablets for p.r.n. medication; give 1/10–1/6 of the 24h dose
- if necessary, increase the dose of m/r morphine every 2–3 days until there is adequate relief throughout each 12h period, guided by p.r.n. use.

Traditionally, to make things easier for patients, morphine q4h has been given on waking, 1000h, 1400h, 1800h with a double dose at bedtime. Despite contrary results in a non-blinded study,[32] RCT evidence has shown that this approach results in less pain through the night, better sleep, and no increase in early morning pain.[33]

When adjusting the dose of morphine, p.r.n. use should be taken into account; increments should not exceed 33–50% every 24h.[34] Two-thirds of patients never need >30mg q4h (or m/r morphine 100mg q12h); the rest need up to 200mg q4h (or m/r morphine 600mg q12h), and occasionally more.[35] Instructions must be clear: extra p.r.n. morphine does not mean that the next regular dose is omitted.

P.r.n. doses of morphine for break-through cancer pain are typically 1/10–1/6 of the regular 24h dose but, as with the regular dose, there is need to consider individual variation. In practice, satisfactory p.r.n. doses vary from 1/20 (5%) to 1/5 (20%) of the 24h dose.[36]

As a general rule, the p.r.n. dose should be increased when the regular dose is increased. A p.r.n. dose is generally permitted every q2–4h as required (up to q1h when pain severe, or in the last days of life). However, frequent use of p.r.n. doses, i.e. ≥2 a day, should prompt a review of pain management. The mean time to onset of effect is 15min with a solution of morphine compared with 30min after an immediate-release tablet, suggesting that morphine solution is the better option for p.r.n. use (see also p.419).

An anti-emetic, e.g. **haloperidol** 500microgram PO, should be supplied for p.r.n. use during the first week or prescribed regularly if the patient has had nausea with a weak opioid (see QCG: Nausea and vomiting, p.240). Warn patients about the possibility of initial drowsiness. A laxative should be prescribed routinely unless there is a definite reason for not doing so, e.g. the patient has an ileostomy (see QCG: Opioid-induced constipation, p.42). *Constipation may be more difficult to manage than the pain.* Laxative suppositories and enemas continue to be necessary in about one third of patients.[37]

SC/CSCI

In the UK, if the PO route becomes an unreliable means of administering regular morphine, e.g. because of difficulty swallowing or vomiting, generally the CSCI route is used (see Chapter 29, p.817). In strong opioid-naïve patients:

- start with 20mg/24h CSCI and 5mg SC p.r.n. (halve both doses in the frail elderly, or mild–moderate renal impairment)
- if necessary, titrate the dose upwards, guided by p.r.n. use.

For general considerations when switching routes, see p.855. When switching morphine PO to CSCI, most centres divide the total daily PO dose by 2 and re-titrate as necessary, e.g.:

- patient taking m/r morphine 30mg PO b.d. = 60mg/24h PO
- divide 60mg/24h by 2 = 30mg/24h CSCI
- the p.r.n. dose is 1/10–1/6 of the 24h dose, i.e. 3–5mg SC p.r.n.

For CSCI dilute with WFI, 0.9% saline or 5% glucose.

CSCI compatibility with other drugs: There are 2-drug compatibility data for morphine sulfate in WFI with **clonazepam**, **cyclizine**, **glycopyrronium**, **hyoscine *butylbromide***, **hyoscine *hydrobromide***, **ketamine**, **levomepromazine**, **metoclopramide**, and **octreotide**.

Morphine sulfate is *incompatible* with **ketorolac** and may be *incompatible* with higher concentrations of **haloperidol** or **midazolam**.

For more details and 3-drug compatibility data, see Appendix 3 Chart 1 (p.863) and Chart 5 (p.874).

Compatibility charts for mixing drugs in 0.9% saline can be found in the extended appendix section of the on-line *PCF* on *www.palliativedrugs.com*.

Renal or hepatic impairment

Because of the risk of impaired metabolism or elimination:

- lower than usual starting doses are advised in mild–moderate renal impairment, e.g. 5–10mg PO q8h–q6h and severe hepatic impairment (see p.709)
- the use of a 'renally safer' opioid is generally advisable with severe renal impairment or ESRF. If unavoidable, start with 1.25–2.5mg PO/SC p.r.n. and once the pain is controlled consider switching to an equivalent dose of **fentanyl** TD (see p.693).

For a general approach when renal or hepatic function deteriorates rapidly, see p.364.

IV/CIVI

IV morphine is widely used for the rapid relief of severe pain caused by acute trauma or medical emergencies.

In opioid-naïve patients:

- give a prophylactic anti-emetic IV, e.g. **metoclopramide** 10mg
- over 5–10min, give a total of morphine 5–10mg (2.5–5mg in the elderly) IV
- when insufficient, give additional morphine at a rate not exceeding 1–2mg/min until satisfactory relief obtained; monitor for undesirable effects, e.g. excessive sedation, respiratory depression
- the dose can be repeated q2–4h as required.

Although uncommon in UK, CIVI morphine and/or p.r.n. IV morphine are used in palliative care units in Europe and North America.[38,39] Generally, this is in the context of the first few days of an inpatient admission for pain control. Subsequently, patients can be switched from IV to PO (see Pharmacology).

Rapid IV/SC titration of morphine dose for severe cancer pain

Although rapid IV/SC titration of morphine is generally *not* necessary, it can be useful in patients with severe acute pain, whether already taking opioids ('opioid-tolerant') or 'opioid-naïve'.[40,41] Further, because of difficulties in relation to follow-up, rapid IV titration is the norm at some centres in India for new patients presenting with pain of ≥5/10.

Two IV methods are included here; the first with 10min and the second with 1min intervals between each IV bolus (Box B and Box C).[41–45] In India, a single cumulative IV dose is given, followed immediately by PO medication (Box B). About 80% of patients obtain relief with 10mg or less.[42,43] At the Cleveland Clinic (USA), patients are maintained on CIVI for several days before conversion to PO medication (Box C). Although these methods have been used safely in many patients, **naloxone** should be readily available (see QCG: Reversal of opioid-induced respiratory deression, p.464).

IV patient-controlled analgesia (PCA) can also be used but is more costly, requires inpatient admission and may take >10h to achieve relief.[46,47] Some centres use a more rapidly acting strong opioid, e.g. IV **fentanyl**, with subsequent doses given after pauses of only 5–10min.[48]

Note. Patients who have required a rapid escalation in opioid requirements must be monitored closely. The underlying cause may be transient, e.g. haemorrhage into a liver metastasis, and a subsequent reduction in dose will be necessary.

Buccal morphine

Morphine is only slowly absorbed through the buccal mucosa.[49] Thus, most of a morphine solution given sublingually or into the gingival gutter will be swallowed and absorbed from the GI tract. Nonetheless, in the past, this route was successfully used in moribund patients.

Rectal morphine

Morphine is absorbed from suppositories.[50] From the lower and middle rectum, it will enter the systemic circulation bypassing the liver. From the upper rectum, it will undergo hepatic first-pass metabolism after it enters the portal circulation. However, there are extensive anastomoses between the rectal veins which make it impossible to predict how much will enter the portal circulation.[51,52] Despite the uncertainty, in practice the same dose is given PR as PO and titrated as necessary.

Although not authorized for this route and not generally recommended, m/r morphine tablets have been used PR to provide analgesia in moribund patients, generally while organizing a more reliable delivery method.[53]

Spinal morphine

In the UK, <5% of cancer patients needing morphine receive it spinally, i.e. ED or IT. This route of administration (see p.839) is normally undertaken by an anaesthetist. Particularly with neuropathic pain, morphine is generally combined with a local anaesthetic (e.g. **bupivacaine**), and sometimes with **clonidine**.

Topical morphine

The number of peripheral opioid receptors increases in nociceptive afferent nerve fibres in the presence of local inflammation.[1,15,54] This property is exploited in joint surgery where morphine is given intra-articularly at the end of the operation.[55] Topical morphine has also been used

Box B Rapid titration of morphine dose in 'opioid-naïve' patients (Institute of Palliative Medicine, India)[42,43]

Prerequisites
Pain ≥5/10 on a numerical scale.
Probability of a partial or complete response to morphine.[a]

Method
Obtain venous access with a butterfly cannula.
Give metoclopramide 10mg IV routinely, if no contra-indications.
Dilute the contents of 15mg morphine ampoule in a 10mL syringe.[b]
Inject 1.5mg (1mL) every 10min until the patient is pain-free or complains of undue sedation.[c]
If patients experience nausea, give additional metoclopramide 5mg IV.

Results
Dose required (with approximate percentages):
- 1.5–4.5mg (40%)
- 6–9mg (40%)
- 10.5–15mg (15%)
- >15mg (5%).

Complete relief in 80%; none in 1%.
Drop outs 2%.
Undesirable effects: sedation 32%; other 3%.

Ongoing treatment
Prescribe a dose of oral morphine q4h similar to the IV dose, rounded to nearest 5mg, e.g. needed morphine 3–6mg IV → 5mg PO; the minimum dose is 5mg.
Advise about p.r.n. doses and, if >2/24h needed, to increase the dose the next day.
In practice, 20% of patients need a dose increase within 3 days.

a. most patients will already be taking an NSAID
b. ampoule strengths varies from country to country; use local standard
c. if ampoule = 10mg/mL (diluted to 10mg in 10mL), a bolus dose of 2mg would be reasonable.

Box C Rapid titration of morphine dose in both 'opioid-tolerant' and 'opioid-naïve' patients (based on practice at Cleveland Clinic, Ohio, USA)[40,44,45]

Sequence	*IV*	*SC*
Dose	1mg/min up to 10mg	2mg q5min up to 10mg
Pause	5min	10min
Dose	1mg/min up to 10mg	2mg q5min up to 10mg
Pause	5min	10min
Dose	1mg/min up to 10mg[a]	2mg q5min up to 10mg[a]

Maintenance IV/SC dose
Regard cumulative effective dose as the equivalent of a q4h dose, and prescribe accordingly.

Example
Cumulative effective IV dose = 9mg.
If giving intermittent injections, dose = 9mg q4h, rounded to 10mg.
If CIVI, total daily IV dose = 9mg x 6 = 54mg/24h.
Round this up or down to convenient number of ampoules, i.e. 50mg or 60mg.
P.r.n. dose = 5–10mg q1h.

a. review cause if relief inadequate after a total of 30mg.

successfully to relieve otherwise intractable pain associated with cutaneous ulceration, often decubitus ulcers.[56–59] It is often given as a 0.1% (1mg/mL) gel, using IntraSite®. If prepared under sterile conditions, morphine sulfate is stable for at least 28 days when mixed with IntraSite® gel at a concentration of 0.125% (1.25mg/mL). This preparation can be made by thoroughly mixing 1mL of morphine sulfate 10mg/mL injection with an 8g sachet of IntraSite® gel.[60] A fact sheet with further information can be obtained from the www.palliativedrugs.com Document library.

Higher concentrations, namely 0.3–0.5%, have been used when managing pain associated with:
- vaginal inflammation associated with a fistula
- rectal ulceration.[57]

The amount of gel applied varies according to the size and the site of the ulcer, but is typically 5–10mL applied b.d.–t.d.s. The topical morphine is kept in place with either a non-absorbable pad or dressing, e.g. Opsite® or Tegaderm®, or gauze coated with petroleum jelly. Other opioids, e.g. **diamorphine**, **methadone**, and other carriers, e.g. Stomahesive® paste, **medronidazole** gel have also been used.[61]

For cancer treatment related oral mucositis, an oral morphine solution *without alcohol* of 2mg/mL can be used. Use 15mL to rinse the mouth for 2min q2–3h (see p.619). It provides better pain relief than a placebo mouthwash, or one containing **co-magaldrox** + **lidocaine** + **diphenhydramine.**[62,63] Significant relief occurs after about 30min, and lasts about 3.5h.[64]

In vitro and animal studies suggest that topical morphine may also aid wound healing by stimulating angiogenesis.[65] However, no such benefit was seen in an RCT of patients with ulcerative oral lichen planus;[66] studies in other settings are ongoing.

Morphine for breathlessness

Opioids are used for breathlessness which persists despite optimal treatment of the underlying cause along with non-drug approaches relevant to the performance status and prognosis of the patient.[67] Most experience is with morphine.

Current evidence and clinical experience supports the use of regular opioids for patients who are breathless at rest but not for those breathless only on exertion.[68] For the latter group, a p.r.n. dose of an opioid also has limited utility because exertional breathlessness generally recovers within 5–20min, much quicker than the time it takes to locate, administer and obtain benefit from an opioid.[69] Thus, non-drug measures are of primary importance in this circumstance.[67]

Systematic reviews ± meta-analyses of RCTs mostly in COPD, CHF and cancer support the use of opioids by the oral and parenteral but *not* the nebulized route.[70–72] A specific review of nebulized (and nasal) opioids concluded the same, and these should not be used outside of a clinical trial.[67,73]

Morphine and other opioids reduce the ventilatory response to hypercapnia, hypoxia and exercise, decreasing respiratory effort and breathlessness.[67] Improvements are seen at doses which do *not* cause respiratory depression.[74]

Generally, small doses are sufficient, typically PO morphine 10–20mg/24h, but often less, and only rarely more.[75–80] For opioid-naïve patients, some advocate starting with a m/r product, others an immediate-release one (Box D). Both approaches have specific advantages, e.g. the m/r approach is simpler, provides relief more quickly for some patients and opioid plasma concentrations fluctuate less over a 24h period; the immediate-release approach identifies those patients who benefit from doses <10mg/24h and appears to be associated with fewer withdrawals because of undesirable effects.[79,80]

In patients already taking morphine for pain, there are limited data to guide practice. One study suggests a reasonable starting point to be:[81]
- divide the 24h dose by 6 (e.g. morphine 60mg/24h ÷ 6 = 10mg q4h)
- start with p.r.n. doses equivalent to 25% of what would be the q4h analgesic dose (e.g. 10mg ÷ 4 = 2.5mg); this may suffice in those with mild–moderate breathlessness at rest
- if necessary, increase to 50% of the q4h analgesic dose (e.g. 10mg ÷ 2 = 5mg)
- if frequent p.r.n. doses are needed, the regular background opioid dose should be increased accordingly.

As with pain, individual titration is required for optimal benefit, and p.r.n. doses equal to or higher than the q4h analgesic dose may be required. In some patients, morphine by CSCI is better tolerated

Box D Starting morphine for breathlessness in opioid-naïve patients[79,80]

Approaches using either m/r or immediate-release morphine products have been described for patients with moderate–severe breathlessness, mostly with COPD or lung cancer. Whichever is used, because of the risk of undesirable effects, it is important to provide appropriate explanation, laxatives, anti-emetics and monitoring. In studies of 3–6 months duration, benefit is generally maintained at the same dose after the initial titration.

M/r approach

- start with MST Continus® 5mg PO b.d. for 1 week
- if baseline breathlessness not reduced ≥10%, increase by 10mg/24h weekly
- usual maximum 30mg/24h.

In one study using this approach,[80] about 60% of patients benefited from morphine, most at 10mg/24h. However, undesirable effects, e.g. dowsiness, confusion, nausea and vomiting, constipation, were a common cause of discontinuation during initial titration (20%).

Immediate-release approach

Mostly in an attempt to minimize the risk of undesirable effects and maintain the confidence of patients who may be wary of taking an opioid, others advocate slower initial titration with immediate-release morphine solution, increased until breathlessness is tolerable, e.g.:

- in the first week, start with 500microgram PO b.d. and increase at 48h intervals → 500microgram q.d.s. → 1mg q4h
- then at weekly intervals, increase the q4h dose to 2mg → 3mg → 5mg
- if necessary, continue to adjust each week using 30–50% dose increments
- reduce dose if undesirable effects occur
- if persistent, consider a switch to an alternate opioid
- when the dose is unchanged for 2 weeks, consider switching to a m/r formulation.

In one study using this approach,[79] a similar overall response rate of 60% was obtained, with most of those switched to a m/r formulation requiring 10–15mg/24h (only 1 required 20mg/24h). However, 40% remained on an immediate-release formulation requiring doses ≤10mg/24h.

Undesirable effects were a less frequent cause of discontinuation during initial titration (7%). However, unlike the m/r study, a switch to an alternative opioid was permitted in cases of intolerance, and was necessary in about 10%.

and provides greater relief, possibly by avoiding the peaks (with undesirable effects) and troughs (with loss of effect) of oral medication. If using an alternative opioid to morphine, adopt the same approach.

Generally, the average reduction in breathlessness as assessed by NRS (0–10) or VAS (0–100mm) is relatively small, e.g. about 1 point/10mm respectively. Nonetheless, this represents a change that is clinically important.[82]

Several adverse effects (e.g. excess exacerbations, emergency room visits, hospitalizations, deaths) have been associated with the use of opioids and/or benzodiazepines in patients with COPD.[71,83] Although some found a relationship with any opioid dose, others reported no excess deaths or hospitalizations with lower opioid doses (± benzodiazepines) equivalent to morphine ≤30mg/24h PO.[71] This supports limiting the dose of morphine to within this dose range in this group of patients.

Breathlessness in the last days of life

The incidence of breathlessness increases as death approaches. For severe breathlessness in the last days of life:

- patients often fear suffocating to death and a positive approach to the patient, their family and colleagues about the relief of terminal breathlessness is important
- no patient should die with distressing breathlessness
- failure to relieve terminal breathlessness is a failure to utilize drug treatment correctly.

Because of the distress, inability to sleep and exhaustion, patients and their carers generally accept that drug-related drowsiness may need to be the price paid for greater comfort. However, unless there is overwhelming distress, sedation is not the primary aim of treatment and some patients become mentally brighter when their breathlessness is reduced.

Even so, because increasing drowsiness also generally reflects the deteriorating clinical condition, it is important to stress the gravity of the situation and the aim of treatment to the relatives. Drug treatment typically comprises:

- parenteral administration of an opioid and a sedative-anxiolytic, e.g. for opioid naïve patients, start with:
  - ▷ morphine 5–10mg/24h + **midazolam** 10mg/24h by CSCI *and*
  - ▷ morphine 2.5mg + **midazolam** 2.5mg SC p.r.n. q1h
  - ▷ for those already receiving PO morphine or another opioid, convert to the equivalent parenteral 24h and p.r.n. doses
  - ▷ titrate both p.r.n. and regular doses to obtain satisfactory relief.
- **haloperidol** or **levomepromazine** if the patient develops an agitated delirium, see p.156 (may be aggravated by a benzodiazepine).[84,85]

Supply

Unless indicated otherwise, all products are Schedule 2 **CD**.

Immediate-release oral products

Morphine solution is available in two strengths, 2mg/mL and a high potency concentrate of 20mg/mL supplied with a calibrated syringe. *Deaths have occurred from accidental overdose with the concentrated solution*, mostly when doses prescribed in *mg* were administered as *mL*. Prescribing should be in *mg* not mL to minimise the risk of *20 times* the prescribed dose being given.[86]

Sevredol® (Napp)
Tablets 10mg, 20mg, 50mg; 10mg and 100mg dose = £0.10 and £1 respectively.

Morphine sulfate (generic)
Oral solution 2mg/mL (**PoM**); 10mg dose = £0.10; *may contain alcohol.*
Oral solution 2mg/mL (**PoM**), 10mg dose = £1.50; *alcohol-free* (Unauthorized, available as a special order; see Chapter 24, p.751.)

Oramorph® (Boehringer Ingelheim)
Oral solution 2mg/mL (**PoM**); 10mg dose = £0.10; *contains alcohol.*
Concentrated oral solution 20mg/mL, 100mg dose = £1.

Modified-release products

Because the pharmacokinetic profiles of m/r products differ, and to minimize the risk of mistakes (e.g. mixing up immediate-release and m/r products), it is best to keep individual patients on the same m/r brand, and to label with both the generic and proprietary names.

Modified-release 12-hourly oral products
Morphgesic® SR (Concordia)
Tablets m/r 10mg, 30mg, 60mg, 100mg, 28 days @ 30mg q12h = £9.

MST Continus® (Napp)
Tablets m/r 5mg, 10mg, 15mg, 30mg, 60mg, 100mg, 200mg, 28 days @ 30mg q12h = £12.
Oral suspension (sachet of m/r granules) 20mg, 30mg, 60mg, 100mg, 200mg/sachet, 28 days @ 30mg q12h = £51. *May be mixed with 10mL water, or the granules sprinkled on cold soft food and swallowed whole.*

Zomorph® (Ethypharm)
Capsules containing m/r granules 10mg, 30mg, 60mg, 100mg, 200mg, 28 days @ 30mg q12h = £8. *May be swallowed whole or opened and the granules sprinkled on cold soft food and swallowed whole.*

Modified-release 24-hourly oral products
MXL® (Napp)

Capsules containing m/r granules 30mg, 60mg, 90mg, 120mg, 150mg, 200mg, 28 days @ 60mg *once daily = £15. May be swallowed whole or opened and the granules sprinkled on cold soft food and swallowed whole.*

Rectal products
Morphine *sulfate* (generic)
Suppositories 10mg, one suppository = £1.50; *the salt should be specified on the prescription.*

Parenteral products
Morphine *sulfate* (generic)
Injection 1mg/mL (1mL, 5mL and 10mL amp = £2.50, £3.50 and £1.50); 10mg/mL and 15mg/mL (1mL amps = £1); 20mg/mL (1mL amp = £5); 30mg/mL (1mL and 2mL amp = £1 and £2).
Infusion 1mg/mL 50mL vial = £5, 2mg/mL 50mL vial = £6.50.

Other injectable morphine formulations are available including morphine sulfate 1mg/mL (10mL disposable syringe, Minijet®), combination products with anti-emetics, e.g. cyclimorph®.

1 Smith HS (2008) Peripherally-acting opioids. *Pain Physician*. **11**: S121–132.
2 Cooper TE *et al.* (2017) Morphine for chronic neuropathic pain in adults. *Cochrane Database of Systematic Reviews*. **5**: CD011669. www.thecochranelibrary.com
3 Hasselstrom J *et al.* (1986) The metabolism and bioavailability of morphine in patients with severe liver cirrhosis. *British Journal of Clinical Pharmacology*. **29**: 289–297.
4 Mazoit J-X *et al.* (1987) Pharmacokinetics of unchanged morphine in normal and cirrhotic subjects. *Anesthesia and Analgesia*. **66**: 293–298.
5 Sandouk P *et al.* (1991) Presence of morphine metabolites in human cerebrospinal fluid after intracerebroventricular administration of morphine. *European Journal of Drug Metabolism and Pharmacology*. **16**: 166–171.
6 Regnard CFB and Twycross RG (1984) Metabolism of narcotics (letter). *British Medical Journal*. **288**: 860.
7 McQuay HJ *et al.* (1990) Oral morphine in cancer pain: influences on morphine and metabolite concentration. *Clinical Pharmacology and Therapeutics*. **48**: 236–244.
8 Osborne RJ *et al.* (1986) Morphine intoxication in renal failure: the role of morphine-6-glucuronide. *British Medical Journal*. **292**: 1548–1549.
9 Thompson P *et al.* (1992) Mophine-6-glucuronide: a metabolite of morphine with greater emetic potency than morphine in the ferret. *British Journal of Pharmacology*. **106**: 3–8.
10 Klimas R and Mikus G (2014) Morphine-6-glucuronide is responsible for the analgesic effect after morphine administration: a quantitative review of morphine, morphine-6-glucuronide, and morphine-3-glucuronide. *British Journal of Anaesthesia*. **113**: 935–944.
11 Franken LG *et al.* (2016) Pharmacokinetics of morphine,morphine-3-glucuronide and morphine-6-glucuronide in terminally ill adult patients. *Clinical Pharmacokinetics*. **55**: 697–709.
12 Good P *et al.* (2014) Medically assisted hydration for adult palliative care patients. *Cochrane Database of Systematic Reviews*. **4**: CD006273. www.thecochranelibrary.com
13 Gretton S and Riley J (2008) Morphine metabolites: a review of their clinical effects. *European Journal of Palliative Care*. **15**: 110–114.
14 Westerling D *et al.* (1994) Transdermal administration of morphine to healthy subjects. *British Journal of Clinical Pharmacology*. **37**: 571–576.
15 Ribeiro MD *et al.* (2004) The bioavailability of morphine applied topically to cutaneous ulcers. *Journal of Pain and Symptom Management*. **27**: 434–439.
16 Watterson G *et al.* (2004) Peripheral opioids in inflammatory pain. *Archives of Disease in Childhood*. **89**: 679–681.
17 Jansen M (2006) Morphine gel. Palliativedrugs.com bulletin board message. Available from: www.palliativedrugs.com/forum/read.php?f=1&i=9271&t=9189
18 Hanks G *et al.* (2001) Morphine and alternative opioids in cancer pain: the EAPC recommendations. *British Journal of Cancer*. **84**: 587–593.
19 Takahashi M *et al.* (2003) The oral-to-intravenous equianalgesic ratio of morphine based on plasma concentrations of morphine and metabolites in advanced cancer patients receiving chronic morphine treatment. *Palliative Medicine*. **17**: 673–678.
20 Lasheen W *et al.* (2010) The intravenous to oral relative milligram potency ratio of morphine during chronic dosing in cancer pain. *Palliative Medicine*. **24**: 9–16.
21 Twycross RG *et al.* (2003) Itch: scratching more than the surface. *Quarterly Journal of Medicine*. **96**: 7–26.
22 Caraceni A *et al.* (2012) Use of opioid analgesics in the treatment of cancer pain: evidence-based recommendations from the EAPC. *Lancet Oncology*. **13**: e58–68.
23 Caraceni A *et al.* (2011) Is oral morphine still the first choice opioid for moderate to severe cancer pain? A systematic review within the European Palliative Care Research Collaborative guidelines project. *Palliative Medicine*. **25**: 402–409.
24 WHO (2012) WHO guidelines on the pharmacological treatment of persistent pain in children with medical illness. Available from: http://www.palliativedrugs.com/news/march/who-guidelines-for-treating-persistent-pain-in-children.html
25 Bloomfield S *et al.* (1993) Analgesic efficacy and potency of two oral controlled-release morphine preparations. *Clinical Pharmacology and Therapeutics*. **53**: 469–478.
26 Gourlay G *et al.* (1993) A comparison of Kapanol (a new sustained-release morphine formulation), MST Continus and morphine solution in cancer patients: pharmacokinetic aspects. In: *The Seventh World Congress on Pain*; Seattle. IASP Press.
27 West R and Maccarrone C (1993) Single dose pharmacokinetics of a new oral sustained-release morphine formulation, Kapanol capsules. In: *The Seventh World Congress on Pain*; Seattle. IASP Press.
28 Mercadante S (2007) Opioid titration in cancer pain: a critical review. *European Journal of Pain*. **11**: 823–830.

29 De Conno F *et al.* (2008) The MERITO Study: a multicentre trial of the analgesic effect and tolerability of normal-release oral morphine during 'titration phase' in patients with cancer pain. *Palliative Medicine*. **22**: 214–221.
30 Ripamonti CI *et al.* (2009) Normal-release oral morphine starting dose in cancer patients with pain. *Clinical Journal of Pain*. **25**: 386–390.
31 Taubert M *et al.* (2010) Re: Update on cancer pain guidelines. *Journal of Pain and Symptom Management*. **24**: 1–5.
32 Todd J *et al.* (2002) An assessment of the efficacy and tolerability of a 'double dose' of normal-release morphine sulphate at bedtime. *Palliative Medicine*. **16**: 507–512.
33 Dale O *et al.* (2009) A double-blind, randomized, crossover comparison between single-dose and double-dose immediate-release oral morphine at bedtime in cancer patients. *Journal of Pain and Symptom Management*. **37**: 68–76.
34 Carver AC and Foley KM (2001) Symptom assessment and management. *Neurologic Clinics*. **19**: 921–947.
35 Schug SA *et al.* (1992) A long-term survey of morphine in cancer pain patients. *Journal of Pain and Symptom Management*. **7**: 259–266.
36 Donnelly S *et al.* (2002) Morphine in cancer pain management: a practical guide. *Supportive Care in Cancer*. **10**: 13–35.
37 Twycross RG and Harcourt JMV (1991) The use of laxatives at a palliative care centre. *Palliative Medicine*. **5**: 27–33.
38 Mercadante S *et al.* (2008) Intravenous morphine for breakthrough (episodic-) pain in an acute palliative care unit: a confirmatory study. *Journal of Pain and Symptom Management*. **35**: 307–313.
39 Mercadante S (2010) Intravenous morphine for management of cancer pain. *Lancet Oncology*. **11**: 484–489.
40 Hagen N *et al.* (1997) Cancer pain emergencies: a protocol for management. *Journal of Pain and Symptom Management*. **14**: 45–50.
41 Davis MP *et al.* (2004) Opioid dose titration for severe cancer pain: a systematic evidence-based review. *Journal of Palliative Medicine*. **7**: 462–468.
42 Kumar K *et al.* (2000) Intravenous morphine for emergency treatment of cancer pain. *Palliative Medicine*. **14**: 183–188.
43 Harris JT *et al.* (2003) Intravenous morphine for rapid control of severe cancer pain. *Palliative Medicine*. **17**: 248–256.
44 Davis MP (2004) Acute pain in advanced cancer: an opioid dosing strategy and illustration. *American Journal of Hospice and Palliative Care*. **21**: 47–50.
45 Davis MP (2005) Rapid opioid titration in severe cancer pain. *European Journal of Palliative Care*. **12**: 11–14.
46 Radbruch L *et al.* (1999) Intravenous titration with morphine for severe cancer pain: report of 28 cases. *Clinical Journal of Pain*. **15**: 173–178.
47 Schiessl C *et al.* (2010) Rhythmic pattern of PCA opioid demand in adults with cancer pain. *European Journal of Pain*. **14**: 372–379.
48 Soares LG *et al.* (2003) Intravenous fentanyl for cancer pain: a "fast titration" protocol for the emergency room. *Journal of Pain and Symptom Management*. **26**: 876–881.
49 Coluzzi P (1998) Sublingual morphine: efficacy reviewed. *Journal of Pain and Symptom Management*. **16**: 184–192.
50 deBoer AG *et al.* (1982) Rectal drug administration: clinical pharmacokinetic considerations. *Clinical Pharmacokinetics*. **7**: 285–311.
51 Johnson AG and Lux G (1988) *Progress in the Treatment of Gastrointestinal Motility Disorder. The role of cisapride*. Excerpta Medica, Amsterdam.
52 Ripamonti C and Bruera E (1991) Rectal, buccal and sublingual narcotics for the management of cancer pain. *Journal of Palliative Care*. **7** 30–35.
53 Wilkinson T *et al.* (1992) Pharmacokinetics and efficacy of rectal versus oral sustained-release morphine in cancer patients. *Cancer Chemotherapy and Pharmacology*. **31**: 251–254.
54 Krajnik M and Zylicz Z (1997) Topical opioids - fact or fiction? *Progress in Palliative Care*. **5**: 101–106.
55 Likar R *et al.* (1999) Dose-dependency of intra-articular morphine analgesia. *British Journal of Anaesthesia*. **83**: 241–244.
56 Back NI and Finlay I (1995) Analgesic effect of topical opioids on painful skin ulcers. *Journal of Pain and Symptom Management*. **10**: 493.
57 Krajnik M *et al.* (1999) Potential uses of topical opioids in palliative care - report of 6 cases. *Pain*. **80**: 121–125.
58 Twillman R *et al.* (1999) Treatment of painful skin ulcers with topical opioids. *Journal of Pain and Symptom Management*. **17**: 288–292.
59 Zeppetella G *et al.* (2003) Analgesic efficacy of morphine applied topically to painful ulcers. *Journal of Pain and Symptom Management*. **25**: 555–558.
60 Zeppetella G and Ribeiro MD (2005) Morphine in intrasite gel applied topically to painful ulcers. *Journal of Pain and Symptom Management*. **29**: 118–119.
61 Le Bon B *et al.* (2009) Effectiveness of topical administration of opiods inpalliative care a systematic review. *Journal of Pain and Symptom Management*. **37**: 913–917.
62 Cerchietti LC *et al.* (2002) Effect of topical morphine for mucositis-associated pain following concomitant chemoradiotherapy for head and neck carcinoma. *Cancer*. **95**: 2230–2236.
63 Vayne-Bossert P *et al.* (2010) Effect of topical morphine (mouthwash) on oral pain due to chemotherapy- and/or radiotherapy-induced mucositis: a randomized double-blinded study. *Journal of Palliative Medicine*. **13**: 125–128.
64 Cerchietti LC *et al.* (2003) Potential utility of the peripheral analgesic properties of morphine in stomatitis-related pain: a pilot study. *Pain*. **105**: 265–273.
65 Ondrovics M *et al.* (2017) Opioids: Modulators of angiogenesis in wound healing and cancer. *Oncotarget*. **8**: 25783–25796.
66 Zaslansky R *et al.* (2017) Topical application of morphine for wound healing and analgesia in patients with oral lichen planus: a randomized, double-blind, placebo-controlled study. *Clinical Oral Investigations*. (Epub ahead of print).
67 Twycross R and Wilcock A (eds) (2016) *Introducing Palliative Care* (5e). palliativedrugs.com, pp. 145–155.
68 Johnson MJ *et al.* (2016) Opioids, exertion, and dyspnea: a review of the evidence. *American Journal of Hospital Palliative Care*. **33**: 194–200.
69 Mercadante S *et al.* (2016) Epidemiology and characteristics of episodic breathlessness in advanced cancer patients: an observational study. *Journal of Pain and Symptom Management*. **51**: 17–24.
70 Barnes H *et al.* (2016) Opioids for the palliation of refractory breathlessness in adults with advanced disease and terminal illness. *Cochrane Database of Systematic Reviews*. **3**: CD011008. www.thecochranelibrary.com
71 Ekstrom M *et al.* (2017) One evidence base; three stories: do opioids relieve chronic breathlessness? *Thorax*. (Epub ahead of print).
72 Kohberg C *et al.* (2016) Opioids: an unexplored option for treatment of dyspnea in IPF. *European Clinical Respiratory Journal*. **3**: 30629.
73 Bausewein C and Simon ST (2014) Inhaled nebulized and intranasal opioids for the relief of breathlessness. *Current Opinion in Supportive and Palliative Care*. **8**: 208–212.
74 Lopez-Saca JM and Centeno C (2014) Opioids prescription for symptoms relief and the impact on respiratory function: updated evidence. *Current Opinion in Supportive and Palliative Care*. **8**: 383–390.
75 Cohen M *et al.* (1991) Continuous intravenous infusion of morphine for severe dyspnoea. *Southern Medical Journal*. **84**: 229–234.
76 Boyd K and Kelly M (1997) Oral morphine as symptomatic treatment of dyspnoea in patients with advanced cancer. *Palliative Medicine*. **11**: 277–281.
77 Abernethy AP *et al.* (2003) Randomised, double blind, placebo controlled crossover trial of sustained release morphine for the management of refractory dyspnoea. *British Medical Journal*. **327**: 523–528.
78 Allen S *et al.* (2005) Low dose diamorphine reduces breathlessness without causing a fall in oxygen saturation in elderly patients with end-stage idiopathic pulmonary fibrosis. *Palliative Medicine*. **19**: 128–130.

79 Rocker GM *et al.* (2013) Opioid therapy for refractory dyspnea in patients with advanced chronic obstructive pulmonary disease: patients' experiences and outcomes. *Canadian Medical Association Journal Open.* **1**: E27-36.
80 Currow DC *et al.* (2011) Once-daily opioids for chronic dyspnea: a dose increment and pharmacovigilance study. *Journal of Pain and Symptom Management.* **42**: 388–399.
81 Allard P *et al.* (1999) How effective are supplementary doses of opioids for dyspnea in terminally ill cancer patients? A randomized continuous sequential clinical trial. *Journal of Pain and Symptom Management.* **17**: 256–265.
82 Johnson MJ *et al.* (2013) Clinically important differences in the intensity of chronic refractory breathlessness. *Journal of Pain and Symptom Management.* **46**: 957–963.
83 Vozoris NT *et al.* (2016) Incident opioid drug use and adverse respiratory outcomes among older adults with COPD. *European Respiratory Journal.* **48**: 683–693.
84 Navigante AH *et al.* (2006) Midazolam as adjunct therapy to morphine in the alleviation of severe dyspnea perception in patients with advanced cancer. *Journal of Pain and Symptom Management.* **31**: 38–47.
85 Matsuda Y *et al.* (2017) Low-dose morphine for dyspnea in terminally ill patients with idiopathic interstitial pneumonias. *Journal of Palliative Medicine.* **20**: 879–883.
86 FDA (2011) Medwatch safety alert. Morphine sulfate oral solution 100mg per 5mL (20mg/mL): medication use error - reports of accidental overdose. Available from: www.fda.gov/Safety/MedWatch/SafetyInformation (archived).

Updated September 2017

5

DIAMORPHINE

Class: Strong opioid analgesic (available only in the UK).

Indications: As for **morphine**; used in the UK instead of parenteral **morphine** because of its greater solubility, particularly when large doses are necessary.

Contra-indications: None absolute if titrated carefully against a patient's pain (also see Strong opioids, p.360 and p.367).

Pharmacology

Diamorphine (di-acetylmorphine, heroin) is available for medicinal analgesic use only in the UK. It is generally considered to be a pro-drug without intrinsic activity.[1] *In vivo*, it is rapidly de-acetylated (plasma halflife 3min) to an active metabolite, 6-mono-acetylmorphine (6-MAM) (plasma halflife 20min), and then to **morphine** itself.[2] Thus, similar considerations as for **morphine** apply regarding the use of diamorphine in patients with renal or hepatic impairment/failure (see p.375).[3]

IM diamorphine is more than twice as potent as IM **morphine**.[4–6] The greater potency of parenteral diamorphine could be because 6-MAM is more potent than **morphine**[7] or because diamorphine and 6-MAM cross the blood-brain barrier more readily than **morphine**. However, by mouth the two opioids are almost equipotent.[8]

Diamorphine IM acts more quickly than **morphine**,[6,9] but **morphine** acts more quickly IV.[10] This paradox is not easily explained, but it could relate to differences in plasma protein-binding (diamorphine 40%, **morphine** 20%).

In terms of analgesic efficacy and effect on mood, diamorphine has no clinical advantage over **morphine** by oral or SC/IM routes.[4,5,8] Diamorphine hydrochloride is much more water-soluble than **morphine** sulfate/hydrochloride and, in the UK, is the strong opioid of choice when high-dose injections are needed (Table 1). In some countries, **hydromorphone** is used instead (see p.434).

Table 1 Solubility of selected opioids[11]

Preparation	*Amount of water needed to dissolve 1g at 25°C (mL)*
Morphine	5000
Morphine hydrochloride	24
Morphine sulfate	21
Diamorphine hydrochloride	1.6[a]
Hydromorphone	3

a. 1g of diamorphine hydrochloride dissolved in 1.6mL has a volume of 2.4mL.

Like **morphine**, diamorphine can be given by many different routes, including spinally. Diamorphine can also be given intranasally using a nasal dosing device, a route used mainly in children.[12] It can be used for the same range of indications as **morphine**, including bladder spasms (intravesical administration)[13,14] and painful decubitus ulcers (topically in Intrasite® gel).[15,16]
Bio-availability (as 6-MAM) no data.
Onset of action 5–10min SC.
Time to peak plasma concentration 1.5–2h PO as 6-MAM and **morphine**.
Plasma halflife 3min IV; metabolized to active metabolites.
Duration of action 4h.

Cautions

Renal impairment and severe hepatic impairment (see Dose and use, Chapter 17, p.693 and Chapter 18, p.709).

Stability

Diamorphine hydrochloride is stable indefinitely when stored as a powder[17] but de-acetylates when in solution, first to 6-mono-acetylmorphine (6-MAM) and then to **morphine**. The rate of de-acetylation is situation dependent. Thus, *in vivo*, diamorphine is converted to 6-MAM in minutes, whereas the stability of diamorphine hydrochloride in simple solution is much longer. Further, because 6-MAM is the primary active agent, there is no loss of potency until 6-MAM is degraded to **morphine**.[7]

In one study, after 3 months in simple solution, 30% of the diamorphine had degraded to 6-MAM, but it was only at 12 months that a trace of **morphine** became detectable.[18] A second study looked at the effect of ambient temperature.[19,20] The loss of 10% of diamorphine to 6-MAM took 8 weeks when kept at 22°C, but only 2 weeks at 37°C. Other studies have produced comparable results.[21,22]

Undesirable effects

See Strong opioids, p.360 and **morphine**, Table 1 p.377.

Dose and use

As with all opioids, patients must be monitored for undesirable effects, particularly nausea and vomiting, and constipation. Depending on individual circumstances, an anti-emetic should be prescribed for regular or p.r.n. use (see QCG: Nausea and vomiting, p.240) and, routinely, a laxative prescribed (see QCG: Opioid-induced constipation, p.42).

Opioids can impair driving ability and patients should be counselled accordingly. Diamorphine is included in a new law in England and Wales relating to driving with certain drugs above specified plasma concentrations (see p.743).

In the UK, diamorphine has been used for all the same indications as **morphine**, and by the same range of routes, including topically and spinally (see p.375). An intranasal spray is now commercially available, authorized for the relief of acute severe pain in children 2–15 years of age in a hospital setting, originating from off-label use in Emergency Departments in England and Wales.[12,23]

Although in the past it was widely used PO, diamorphine is now generally reserved for SC/CSCI use (see p.820).

SC/CSCI

In strong opioid-naïve patients:

- start with 15mg/24h CSCI and 2.5mg SC p.r.n. (halve doses in the frail elderly, mild–moderate renal impairment or severe hepatic impairment)
- if necessary, titrate the dose upwards, guided by p.r.n. use; conventionally, p.r.n. SC doses are 1/6–1/10 of the total 24h CSCI dose.

For general considerations when switching opioids, see p.855. The following are practical clinical conversion ratios:

- PO **morphine** to CSCI diamorphine, give one third of the 24h dose, e.g. **morphine** 60mg/24h PO = diamorphine 20mg/24h CSCI
- CSCI **morphine** to CSCI diamorphine, divide the 24h dose by 1.5 (i.e. decrease by one third), e.g. **morphine** 30mg/24h = diamorphine 20mg/24h
- if necessary, titrate the dose upwards, guided by p.r.n. use; conventionally, p.r.n. SC doses are 1/6–1/10 of the total 24h CSCI dose.

For CSCI dilute with WFI, concentration-dependent *incompatibility* occurs with 0.9% saline at higher doses (see p.819).

CSCI compatibility with other drugs: There are 2-drug compatibility data for diamorphine in WFI with **clonazepam, dexamethasone, glycopyrronium, hyoscine *butylbromide*, hyoscine *hydrobromide*, ketorolac, levomepromazine, metoclopramide, midazolam, octreotide,** and **ondansetron.**

Concentration-dependent *incompatibility* occurs with **cyclizine** or **haloperidol** at higher concentrations. For more details and 3-drug compatibility data, see Appendix 3 charts 1 (p.866) and 3 (p.870).

Compatibility charts for mixing drugs in 0.9% saline can be found in the extended appendix section of the on-line *PCF* on *www.palliativedrugs.com.*

Renal or hepatic impairment

Because of the risk of impaired metabolism or elimination:

- halve the usual starting doses in mild–moderate renal impairment or severe hepatic impairment (also see p.709)
- the use of a 'renally safer' opioid is generally advisable with severe renal impairment or ESRF. If unavoidable, see p.693.

For a general approach when renal of hepatic function deteriorates rapidly, see p.364.

Supply

Because diamorphine ampoules cost about 3 times more than **morphine** ampoules, many palliative care units in the UK now use **morphine** as their standard parenteral strong opioid, unless the need for high doses makes diamorphine more convenient because of its greater solubility.[24] All preparations are Schedule 2 **CD**.

Diamorphine (generic)
Tablets 10mg, 10mg dose = £0.25.
Injection (powder for reconstitution) 5mg amp = £2.25; 10mg amp = £3.75; 30mg amp = £3.75; 100mg amp = £8.50; 500mg amp = £38.

Ayendi (Wockhardt)
Nasal Spray (powder for reconstitution with 0.5% saline and 9 disposable nasal tips provided for multiple patient use) 720microgram/metered dose spray, 1600microgram/metered dose spray, 160 metered dose spray bottle = £113 and £124 respectively; *stable for 14 days after reconstitution.*

1 Inturrisi CE *et al.* (1984) The pharmacokinetics of heroin in patients with chronic pain. *New England Journal of Medicine.* **310**: 1213–1217.
2 Barrett DA *et al.* (1992) The effect of temperature and pH on the deacetylation of diamorphine in aqueous solution and in human plasma. *Journal of Pharmacy and Pharmacology.* **44**: 606–608.
3 King S *et al.* (2011) A systematic review of the use of opioid medication for those with moderate to severe cancer pain and renal impairment: A European palliative care research collaborative opioid guidelines project. *Palliative Medicine.* **25**: 525–552.
4 Kaiko RF *et al.* (1981) Analgesic and mood effects of heroin and morphine in cancer patients with postoperative pain. *New England Journal of Medicine.* **304**: 1501–1505.
5 Beaver WT *et al.* (1981) Comparison of the analgesic effect of intramuscular heroin and morphine in patients with cancer pain. *Clinical Pharmacology and Therapeutics.* **29**: 232.
6 Reichle CW *et al.* (1962) Comparative analgesic potency of heroin and morphine in postoperative patients. *Journal of Pharmacology and Experimental Therapeutics.* **136**: 43–46.
7 Wright CI and Barbour FA (1935) The respiratory effects of morphine, codeine and related substances. *Journal of Pharmacology and Experimental Therapeutics.* **54**: 25–33.
8 Twycross RG (1977) Choice of strong analgesic in terminal cancer: diamorphine or morphine? *Pain* **3**: 93–104.
9 Dundee JW *et al.* (1966) Studies of drugs given before anaesthesia XI: diamorphine (heroin) and morphine. *British Journal of Anaesthesia.* **38**: 610–619.
10 Morrison L *et al.* (1991) Comparison of speed of onset of analgesic effect of diamorphine and morphine. *British Journal of Anaesthesia.* **66**: 656–659.
11 Hanks GW and Hoskin PJ (1987) Opioid analgesics in the management of pain in patients with cancer: a review. *Palliative Medicine.* **1**: 1–25.
12 Kendall J *et al.* (2015) A novel multipatient intranasal diamorphine spray for use in acute pain in children: pharmacovigilance data from an observational study. *Emergency Medical Journal.* **32**: 269–273.
13 McCoubrie R and Jeffrey D (2003) Intravesical diamorphine for bladder spasm. *Journal of Pain and Symptom Management.* **25**: 1–3.
14 Duckett J (1997) Intravesical morphine analgesia after bladder surgery. *Journal of Urology.* **157**: 1407–1409.

15 Abbas SQ (2004) Diamorphine-Intrasite dressings for painful pressure ulcers. *Journal of Pain and Symptom Management.* **28**: 532–534.
16 Flock P (2003) Pilot study to determine the effectiveness of diamorphine gel to control pressure ulcer pain. *Journal of Pain and Symptom Management.* **25**: 547–554.
17 Lerner M and Mills A (1963) Some modern aspects of heroin analysis. *Bulletin on Narcotics.* **15**: 37–42.
18 Rizzotti G (1935) Contributo allo studio delle alterazioni delle soluzioni acquose di eroina. *Archives Internationales de Pharmacodynamie et de Therapie.* **52**: 87–96.
19 Twycross RG and Gilhooley RA (1973) Euporiant elixirs. *British Medical Journal.* **4**: 552.
20 Twycross RG (1974) Diamorphine and cocaine elixir BPC. *Pharmaceutical Journal.* **212**: 153 & 159.
21 Kleinberg ML *et al.* (1990) Stability of heroin hydrochloride in infusion devices and containers for intravenous administration. *American Journal of Hospital Pharmacy.* **47**: 377–381.
22 Omar OA *et al.* (1989) Diamorphine stability in aqueous solution for subcutaneous infusion. *Journal of Pharmacy and Pharmacology.* **41**: 275–277.
23 Hadley G *et al.* (2010) A survey of intranasal medication use in the paediatric emergency setting in England and Wales. *Emergency Medical Journal.* **27**: 553–554.
24 Palliativedrugs.com (2010) Diamorphine essential opioid or time to say goodbye? Available from: www.palliativedrugs.com/download/100223_diamorphine_essential_opioid.pdf

Updated September 2017

*ALFENTANIL

Class: Strong opioid analgesic.

Indications: Intra-operative analgesia, analgesia and procedure-related pain in mechanically ventilated patients on intensive care units, †an alternative in cases of intolerance to other strong opioids, particularly in renal failure,[1] †procedure-related pain in non-ventilated patients,[2–4] †break-through pain.[5]

Contra-indications: Do not administer concurrently with MAOIs or within two weeks of their discontinuation. Generally, none absolute if titrated carefully against a patient's pain (see also Strong opioids, p.360).

Pharmacology

Alfentanil is a synthetic lipophilic μ-opioid receptor agonist in the same class as **fentanyl** and **sufentanil**. Compared with these, it has a more rapid onset of action and time to peak effect, and a shorter duration of action (Table 1). Its potency is approximately one quarter that of **fentanyl**[6] (and 10–20 times more than parenteral **morphine**).

Alfentanil is less lipophilic than **fentanyl** and is 90% bound to mainly α_1-acid glycoprotein.[7] However, because most of the unbound alfentanil is unionized, it rapidly enters the CNS. It is metabolized in the liver by CYP3A4 to inactive metabolites that are excreted in the urine. Alfentanil can accumulate with chronic administration, particularly in the elderly and the obese, and even with only mild hepatic impairment.[8,9] Renal impairment does not significantly alter the clearance of alfentanil and consequently, alfentanil is used at some centres when a parenteral opioid is required in severely reduced renal function or ESRF. Lower doses may be sufficient because of changes in protein binding (see p.693).[1] However, unless the volume is prohibitive, **fentanyl** is generally recommended as the first-line parenteral opioid in ESRF at the end of life (see p.693).[1]

It has been suggested that analgesic tolerance occurs rapidly with alfentanil,[10] but this has been refuted.[11] However, tolerance does not seem to be a problem in palliative care.[1]

Because alfentanil is available in a more concentrated form (500microgram/mL) than **fentanyl** (50microgram/mL), a smaller equivalent dose volume is needed, and this facilitates administration by CSCI or SL. For similar reasons, in countries where alfentanil is not available, **sufentanil** is used instead (Table 1 and Box A).[12]

Alfentanil has been used successfully by short-term PCA, CSCI or SL for procedure-related pain, e.g. dressing changes in burns or trauma patients.[2,4,13] It has also been used SL and nasally for break-through pain, including severe intractable angina in inoperable coronary artery disease.[5,14,15] In the UK, an unauthorized spray for buccal or nasal use containing alfentanil 5mg/5mL, can be obtained via special order. It is expensive compared to using the injection formulation (see Supply). A dose of 140microgram/0.14mL spray is delivered. Details and instructions for use can be downloaded from the Document library of palliativedrugs.com. In an audit of patients already on regular strong opioids, about three quarters benefited from SL alfentanil in doses of 560–1,680microgram (4–12 sprays; titrated as necessary). Pain relief was seen within 10min. However, such use has diminished since transmucosal **fentanyl** products have become available (see p.419) which cost about the same as the special order alfentanil spray.

Spinal administration of lipophilic opioids remains controversial because of the rapid clearance into the systemic circulation (see Chapter 32).[16]

Opioid withdrawal symptoms can occur when switching from **morphine** (or other less lipophilic/less potent opioid) to CSCI alfentanil.[17] These manifest with symptoms like gastric flu and last for a few days; p.r.n. doses of the original opioid will relieve troublesome symptoms.

Table 1 Pharmacokinetics of single IV doses of fentanils[18–20]

	Alfentanil	*Sufentanil*	*Fentanyl*
Onset of action (min)	0.75[a]	1	1.5[b]
Time to peak effect (min)	1.5	2.5	4.5
Plasma halflife (min)	95	165	220
Duration of action (min)	30[a]	60	60

a. onset slower if given IM (<5min), and duration of action longer (60min)
b. onset slower if given IM (7–15min), and duration of action longer (1–2h).

Box A Sufentanil injection (not UK)

A lipophilic opioid with a strong affinity for the μ-opioid receptor. Time to onset of action and to peak effect is mid-way between that of alfentanil and fentanyl (see Table 1).[19]

Sufentanil is about 7.5–10 times more potent than fentanyl,[21,22] and this allows a smaller volume to be given by injection. Divide the parenteral dose of fentanyl by 10 to obtain an easy-to-calculate starting dose.

Example
Fentanyl 1,000microgram/24h CSCI (i.e. 20mL of 50microgram/mL)
→ sufentanil 100microgram/24h CSCI (i.e. 2mL of 50microgram/mL).

Sufentanil can be administered SC, IV, or spinally.[23] By CSCI, it is compatible with other commonly prescribed drugs.[24]

Also given by intranasal or SL routes as pre-operative sedation, analgesia for moderate–severe acute trauma pain[25] and for rescue analgesia for break-through cancer pain.[26]

Accumulates in fat tissue when given continuously;[27] monitor carefully when switching to another opioid.

Is not dependent on renal function for elimination, and is thus useful in renal impairment.

Cautions

Hepatic or renal impairment (also see p.681 and p.703).

Drug interactions

Alfentanil is metabolized by CYP3A4. Caution is required with concurrent use of drugs which inhibit or induce these enzymes, (see p.721). Reports of interactions where closer monitoring ± dose adjustment are required are listed in Box B.[28]

Box B Interactions between alfentanil and other drugs involving CYP450

Plasma concentrations of alfentanil

Increased by	**Decreased by**
Aprepitant[a]	Aprepitant[a]
Azoles, e.g. fluconazole, voriconazole	Efavirenz
Cimetidine	Rifampicin
Diltiazem	
Macrolide antibiotics, e.g. clarithromycin, erythromycin	
Protease inhibitors, e.g. indinavir, nelfinavir, ritonavir	

a. aprepitant can increase the exposure to CYP3A4 substrates in the short-term, then reduce their exposure within 2 weeks.

Undesirable effects

See Strong opioids, p.360.

Dose and use

As with all opioids, patients must be monitored for undesirable effects, particularly nausea and vomiting, and constipation (see p.000). Depending on individual circumstances, an anti-emetic should be prescribed for regular or p.r.n. use (see QCG: Nausea and vomiting, p.240) and, routinely, a laxative prescribed (see QCG: Opioid-induced constipation, p.42).

Opioids can impair driving ability and patients should be counselled accordingly (see p.743).

Procedure-related pain (see Quick Clinical Guide, p.395)

- give 250–500microgram alfentanil SL (using the 500microgram/mL injection formulation) or SC/IV.

CSCI as an alternative to morphine

Used mostly for patients with severe renal impairment/ESRF in whom there is evidence of **morphine** neurotoxicity (see p.368), or when volume restrictions prevent the use of **fentanyl**.

For general considerations when switching opioids, see p.855. Given the shorter duration of action of alfentanil, it is difficult to give a single precise dose conversion ratio. However, the following are safe practical conversion ratios:

- PO **morphine** to CSCI alfentanil, give one thirtieth of the 24h dose, e.g. **morphine** 60mg/24h PO = alfentanil 2mg/24h CSCI
- CSCI **morphine** to CSCI alfentanil, give one fifteenth of the 24h dose, e.g. **morphine** 30mg/24h = alfentanil 2mg/24h
- CSCI **diamorphine** to CSCI alfentanil, give one tenth of the 24h dose, e.g. **diamorphine** 30mg/24h = alfentanil 3mg/24h.

Conventionally, p.r.n. SC doses of alfentanil are 1/6–1/10 of the total 24h CSCI dose. Because of the short duration of action of alfentanil (≤30min), even with an optimally titrated p.r.n. dose, frequent dosing may be required; this is one reason why **fentanyl** is recommended first-line in these circumstances (see Pharmacology).

The CSCI dose of alfentanil should be reviewed at least daily, and titrated accordingly. For CSCI dilute with WFI, 0.9% saline or 5% glucose.

CSCI compatibility with other drugs: There are 2-drug compatibility data for alfentanil in WFI with **clonazepam**, **dexamethasone**, **glycopyrronium**, **haloperidol**, **hyoscine** ***butylbromide***, **levomepromazine**, **metoclopramide**, **midazolam**, **octreotide**, and **ondansetron**.

Concentration-dependent *incompatibility* occurs with **cyclizine**. For more details, and 3-drug compatibility data, see Appendix 3 Chart 1 (p.866) and Chart 2 (p.868).

Compatibility charts for mixing drugs in 0.9% saline can be found in the extended appendix section of the on-line *PCF* on *www.palliativedrugs.com*.

An alternative CSCI dosing schedule

The recommendations above may well be too conservative for some patients. It is important to review sooner rather than later, and increase the dose if necessary. At one centre, a conversion ratio for **diamorphine** to alfentanil of one sixth has been used for many years without clinical evidence of respiratory depression, e.g.[29,30]

- CSCI **diamorphine** to CSCI alfentanil, give one sixth of the 24h dose, e.g. **diamorphine** 30mg/24h = alfentanil 5mg/24h.

At this centre, p.r.n. SC **diamorphine/morphine** is given to supplement CSCI alfentanil, giving the same p.r.n. dose as used before the switch to alfentanil. When the switch has been prompted by opioid neurotoxicity, a recurrence has not been observed with 1–2 p.r.n. doses/24h of **diamorphine/morphine**.

Break-through cancer pain, SL administration

Given the variability in the intensity of break-through pains, p.r.n. recommendations are best expressed as a range of doses rather than a single fixed dose. There is a poor relationship between the effective SL p.r.n. dose and regular CSCI dose. Individual dose titration is necessary, e.g. starting with 1/10–1/6 of the daily alfentanil CSCI dose, and titrating upwards if necessary. The alfentanil 500microgram/mL injection formulation can be used SL. However, retaining even 2mL in the mouth (sublingually or buccally) for 5–10min is difficult (Table 2). Generally, authorized **fentanyl** transmucosal products would now be used (p.419).

Table 2 Equivalent volumes of parenteral formulations of alfentanil, fentanyl and sufentanil for SL use[a]

Alfentanil 500microgram/mL		*Fentanyl 50microgram/mL*		*Sufentanil 50microgram/mL (not UK)*	
Dose (microgram)	*Volume (mL)*	*Dose (microgram)*	*Volume (mL)*	*Dose (microgram)*	*Volume (mL)*
100	0.2	25	0.5	2.5	N/A
200	0.4	50	1	5	0.1
300	0.6	75	1.5	7.5	0.15
400	0.8	100[b]	2	10	0.2
500	1	125	N/O[c]	12.5	0.25
600	1.2	150	N/O	15	0.3
800	1.6	200[b]	N/O	20	0.4
1,000	2	250	N/O	25	0.5

a. this is *not* a true dose conversion chart. Alfentanil, fentanyl and sufentanil have differing properties (see Table 1). As always with analgesics, individual patient dose titration is required

b. fentanyl SL product commercially available (see p.419); generally use in preference

c. N/O = not optimal, because ≥2mL.

Supply

All preparations are Schedule 2 **CD**.

Alfentanil (generic)

Nasal spray (with attachment for buccal/SL use) 140microgram/spray, 5mg/5mL bottle = £55–£99. (Unauthorized, available as a special order from the pharmacy manufacturing unit, Torbay hospital, see Chapter 24, p.751). *Telephone number for enquiries: 01803 664707; orders must be faxed to the manufacturing unit on 01803 664354. The solution is stable for 1 year unopened and for 28 days after opening.*

Injection 500microgram/mL, 2mL amp = £0.75, 10mL amp = £2.75.

Injection (for dilution and use as a continuous infusion) 5mg/mL, 1mL amp = £2.50.

The high-strength 5mg/mL injection is used at some centres when the CSCI/CIVI dose is >5mg/24h. However, to avoid the risk of the high-strength injection being administered by mistake, in many hospitals its availability is restricted to the Intensive Care Unit.

1 King S *et al.* (2011) A systematic review of the use of opioid medication for those with moderate to severe cancer pain and renal impairment: A European palliative care research collaborative opioid guidelines project. *Palliative Medicine.* **25**: 525–552.

2 Gallagher G *et al.* (2001) Target-controlled alfentanil analgesia for dressing change following extensive reconstructive surgery for trauma. *Journal of Pain and Symptom Management.* **21**: 1–2.

3 Miner JR *et al.* (2011) Alfentanil for procedural sedation in the emergency department. *Annals of Emergency Medicine.* **57**: 117–121.

4 Fontaine M *et al.* (2016) Feasibility of monomodal analgesia with IV alfentanil during burn dressing changes at bedside (in spontaneously breathing non-intubated patients). *Burns.* Epud ahead of print.

5 Duncan A (2002) The use of fentanyl and alfentanil sprays for episodic pain. *Palliative Medicine.* **16**: 550.

6 Larijani G and Goldberg M (1987) Alfentanil hydrochloride: a new short acting narcotic analgesic for surgical procedures. *Clinical Pharmacy.* **6**: 275–282.

7 Bernards C (1999) Clinical implications of physicochemical properties of opioids. In: C Stein (ed) *Opioids in Pain Control: basic and clinical aspects*. Cambridge University Press, Cambridge, pp. 166–187.
8 Bodenham A and Park GR (1988) Alfentanil infusions in patients requiring intensive care. *Clinical Pharmacokinetics*. **15**: 216–226.
9 Bosilkovska M *et al.* (2012) Analgesics in patients with hepatic impairment: pharmacology and clinical implications. *Drugs*. **72**: 1645–1669.
10 Kissin I *et al.* (2000) Acute tolerance to continuously infused alfentanil: the role of cholecystokinin and N-methyl-D-aspartate-nitric oxide systems. *Anesthesia and Analgesia*. **91**: 110–116.
11 Schraag S *et al.* (1999) Lack of rapid development of opioid tolerance during alfentanil and remifentanil infusions for postoperative pain. *Anesthesia and Analgesia*. **89**: 753–757.
12 Gardner-Nix J (2001) Oral transmucosal fentanyl and sufentanil for incident pain. *Journal of Pain and Symptom Management*. **22**: 627–630.
13 Kwon YS *et al.* (2016) A comparison of oxycodone and alfentanil in intravenous patient-controlled analgesia with a time-scheduled decremental infusion after laparoscopic cholecystectomy. *Pain Research and Management*. Epub ahead of print.
14 Osborn H and Jefferson M (2010) Intranasal alfentanil for severe intractable angina in inoperable coronary artery disease. *Palliative Medicine*. **24**: 94–95.
15 Brenchley J and Ramlakhan S (2006) Intranasal alfentanil for acute pain in children. *Emergency Medical Journal*. **23**: 488.
16 Bujedo BM (2014) Spinal opioid bioavailability in postoperative pain. *Pain Practice*. **14**: 350–364.
17 Carmichael JP and Lee MA (2010) Symptoms of opioid withdrawal syndrome after switch from oxycodone to alfentanil. *Journal of Pain and Symptom Management*. **40**: e4–6.
18 Willens JS and Myslinski NR (1993) Pharmacodynamics, pharmacokinetics, and clinical uses of fentanyl, sufentanil, and alfentanil. *Heart Lung*. **22**: 239–251.
19 Scholz J *et al.* (1996) Clinical pharmacokinetics of alfentanil, fentanyl and sufentanil. An update. *Clinical Pharmacokinetics*. **31**: 275–292.
20 Hall T and Hardy J (2005) The lipophilic opioids: fentanyl, alfentanil, sufentanil and remifentanil. In: M Davis *et al.* (eds) *Opioids in Cancer Pain*. Oxford University Press, Oxford.
21 Reynolds L *et al.* (2004) Relative analgesic potency of fentanyl and sufentanil during intermediate-term infusions in patients after long-term opioid treatment for chronic pain. *Pain*. **110**: 182–188.
22 Scott JC *et al.* (1991) Electroencephalographic quantitation of opioid effect: comparative pharmacodynamics of fentanyl and sufentanil. *Anesthesiology*. **74**: 34–42.
23 Waara-Wolleat KL *et al.* (2006) A review of intrathecal fentanyl and sufentanil for the treatment of chronic pain. *Pain Medicine*. **7**: 251–259.
24 White C *et al.* (2008) Subcutaneous sufentanil for palliative care patients in a hospital setting. *Palliative Medicine*. **22**: 89–90.
25 Steenblik J *et al.* (2012) Intranasal sufentanil for the treatment of acute pain in a winter resort clinic. *American Journal of Emergency Medicine*. **30**: 1817–1821.
26 Good P *et al.* (2009) Intranasal sufentanil for cancer-associated breakthrough pain. *Palliative Medicine*. **23**: 54–58.
27 Alazia M *et al.* (1992) Pharmacokinetics of long term sufentanil infusion (72 hours) used for sedation in ICU patients. *Anesthesiology*. **77**: A364 (abstract).
28 Baxter K and Preston CL. *Stockley's Drug Interactions*. London: Pharmaceutical Press www.medicinescomplete.com (accessed May 2017).
29 Cran A *et al.* (2017) Opioid rotation to alfentanil: comparative evaluation of conversion ratios. *BMJ Supportive and Palliative Care*. **7**: 265–266.
30 Dorman S (2017). *Personal communication*.

Updated September 2017

Quick Clinical Guide: Procedure-related pain

1 Palliative care patients may experience pain while undergoing procedures, e.g.:
- position change
- investigation, e.g. MRI
- wound dressing change
- venous cannulation
- urethral catheterization
- removing impacted faeces
- insertion of nasogastric tube
- insertion/removal of central line
- insertion/removal of spinal line
- drainage of chest/abdomen
- treatment, e.g. radiation therapy.

2 The goal is adequate pain relief without undesirable effects. What is appropriate depends on the anticipated pain severity, procedure duration, current opioid use, and the patient's past personal experience. Thus, severe procedure-related pain may necessitate parenteral analgesia and sedation as first-line therapy.

3 Always include non-drug approaches:
- discuss past experiences of procedure-related pain, identify what was helpful or unhelpful, and clarify present concerns
- explain the procedure thoroughly before starting
- assure that you will stop immediately if requested
- as far as possible, choose the most comfortable position for the patient
- distract and relax, e.g. through talking, music, hypnosis and other relaxation techniques.

4 Use a local anaesthetic for:
- venous cannulation; if needle phobic or if requested, e.g. EMLA® cream (wait 60min)
- urethral catheterization; use lidocaine 2% gel, e.g. Instillagel® (wait 5min)
- chest aspiration; infiltrate tissue with lidocaine injection, e.g. 5mL of 1% (wait 5min).

5 If available, consider nitrous oxide-oxygen (Entonox®) inhalation if only mild–moderate pain anticipated, the procedure is short and the patient is able to use the mask or mouthpiece effectively.

6 Give analgesia from the appropriate step of the ladder (also see Box). Note. General anaesthetic approaches are beyond the scope of these guidelines.

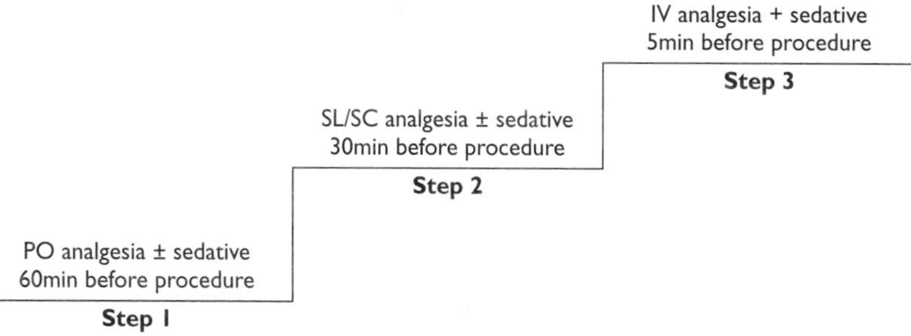

7 If pain relief inadequate, give a repeat dose and wait again; if still inadequate, move to the next step.

8 When a sedative or sedative analgesic is used, practitioners must be competent in airway management. Monitor the patient to ensure that the airway remains patent, and intervene if the patient becomes cyanosed because of severely depressed respiration.

Examples of analgesia for procedure-related pain in adults

Use lower doses in older or frail patients and those with renal or hepatic impairment.

Step 1: If anticipating mild–moderate pain
Give 60min before the procedure:
PO morphine, give the patient's usual rescue dose for break-through pain.
If necessary, combine with:
- PO diazepam 5mg *or*
- SL lorazepam 500microgram–1mg *or*
- an alternative sedative.

Step 2: If anticipating moderate–severe pain
Give 30min before procedure:
SC morphine, give 50% of the patient's usual PO morphine rescue dose.
If necessary, combine with:
- SC midazolam 2.5–5mg *or*
- SL lorazepam 500microgram–1mg *or*
- an alternative sedative.

Step 3: If anticipating severe–excruciating pain
Give 5min before procedure:
IV morphine, give 50% of the patient's usual PO morphine rescue dose *or*
IV ketamine 0.5–1mg/kg (typically 25–50mg).
Combine with:
- IV midazolam 2mg over 1–2min, followed by 1mg every 2min until adequate sedation *or*
- an alternative sedative.

There is a risk of marked sedation when ketamine and a sedative such as midazolam are combined in this way; use only if competent in airway management.

Alternatives to SC/IV morphine
- fentanyl 50–100microgram or more transmucosally using an authorized product (see p.419) or SC/IV
- alfentanil 250–500microgram SL (*from ampoule for injection or spray*) or SC/IV
- sufentanil 12.5–25microgram SL (*from ampoule for injection, not UK*) or SC/IV.

9 An opioid antagonist (naloxone) and a benzodiazepine antagonist (flumazenil) should be available in case of need. To prevent the complete reversal of any background regular opioid analgesic therapy, use naloxone 100microgram IV, repeated every 2min until the respiratory rate and cyanosis have improved. The initial dose of flumazenil is 200microgram IV over 15 seconds; if the desired level of consciousness is not obtained after 1 minute, further 100microgram doses can be given at 1 minute intervals p.r.n. up to a maximum total dose of 1mg.

10 If the procedure is to be repeated, give analgesia based on previous experience, e.g. drugs used and the patient's comments.

Updated September 2017

BUPRENORPHINE

Buprenorphine is experiencing a renaissance in the management of chronic cancer and non-cancer pain, and opioid dependence (high-dose SL formulation ± **naloxone**).[1–7] Preliminary data suggests that compared to **morphine** and other opioids, buprenorphine appears to cause less hyperalgesia (see p.361) and tolerance, and has less effect on the immune and endocrine systems. However, clinical trials are needed to find out whether such differences represent real clinical advantages.

5

Class: Strong opioid analgesic.

Indications: ***SL tablet (200 and 400microgram) and injection*** moderate–severe pain, premedication and peri-operative analgesia, †intolerance to other strong opioids.
SL higher-dose tablet (400microgram, 2mg, 8mg) withthdrawal and maintenance therapy for opioid addicts (also available as a combined formulation with naloxone, to prevent parenteral misuse).
TD patches (5–20microgram/h) moderate non-cancer pain; †intolerance to other strong opioids.
TD higher-dose patches (35–70microgram/h) severe non-cancer pain; moderate–severe cancer pain, †intolerance to other strong opioids.

Contra-indications: None absolute if titrated carefully against a patient's pain (also see Strong opioids, p.360). TD buprenorphine should not be used for acute (transient, intermittent or short-term) pain, e.g. postoperative, or when there is need for rapid dose titration for severe uncontrolled pain.

Pharmacology

Buprenorphine is a partial μ-opioid receptor and opioid-receptor-like (ORL-1) *agonist* and a κ- and δ-opioid receptor *antagonist*.[8–10] It has high affinity at the μ-, κ- and δ-opioid receptors, but affinity at the ORL-1 receptor is 500-fold less. It associates and dissociates slowly from receptors.[11] Analgesia is via the μ-opioid receptor and subjective and physiological effects are generally similar to **morphine**. A common polymorphism of the μ-opioid receptor (N40D), present in ≤50% of people, reduces the efficacy of buprenorphine at the receptor (but not **fentanyl** (p.409), **methadone** (p.437), **morphine** (p.375) or **oxycodone** (p.447)) and may contribute towards a reduced clinical effect.[12]

Buprenorphine is effective in cancer pain, but because of very low quality evidence, particularly for the TD patch, the authors of a systematic review positioned its use after **morphine** and the common alternatives, **oxycodone** and **fentanyl**.[13]

Studies in volunteers suggest that compared with **morphine** and other opioids, buprenorphine exerts a more prominent antihyperalgesic than analgesic effect;[14,15] however, this is not a consistent finding.[16] Animal studies, case reports and one RCT (in diabetic neuropathy) suggest that buprenorphine may be of particular benefit in neuropathic pain.[2,6,17–21] However, high quality RCTs are needed to confirm this. The co-administration of an ultra-low dose of an opioid antagonist potentiated the analgesic effect of buprenorphine (as with other opioids) in healthy volunteers but not patients (also see p.457).[22,23]

Antagonist effects at the κ-opioid receptor may limit spinal analgesia, sedation and psychotomimetic effects.[24] It is also thought to explain the antidepressant effect of buprenorphine reported in patients refractory to usual approaches.[25,26]

In animal studies, buprenorphine shows a ceiling effect or a bell-shaped dose-response curve for analgesic (>1mg/kg) and respiratory effects (0.1mg/kg). This is thought to be due to its partial agonist effect at the μ-opioid receptor. An agonist effect at the pronociceptive supraspinal ORL-1 receptor may also contribute.[27] In humans, a ceiling effect has been shown for respiratory depression (~200microgram/70kg IV)[28,29] and other effects, e.g. euphoria (4–8mg SL),[30,31] but *not* for analgesia.[29] Total daily doses up to 32mg SL are reported to provide effective analgesia.[32] Thus, the ceiling dose for analgesia in humans is much higher than the 'maximum' TD dose recommended by the UK manufacturers, namely 3.36mg/day (70microgram/h patches x 2).

Studies of buprenorphine TD or SL up to 1.6mg/day have confirmed that it is possible to use **morphine** (or other μ agonist) for break-through pain,[33,34] and to switch either way between buprenorphine and **morphine** (or other μ agonist) without loss of analgesia.[35,36]

However, greater difficulties are experienced when switching patients on higher doses of opioids, using larger doses of buprenorphine.[37] When patients on various opioids (oral **morphine** equivalent 15–450mg/24h) were switched using doses of buprenorphine 2mg SL (resulting in maximum post-switch doses of 6–24mg/24h), over half experienced intolerable undesirable effects and abandoned the switch. Generally, undesirable effects related to opioid excess in patients receiving low doses of oral **morphine** equivalent (≤20mg/24h) and opioid withdrawal in those receiving high doses (>300mg/24h). This experience guided the development of a clinical protocol, although the dosing algorithm has not yet been tested formally.[37]

The use of other μ agonists for break-through pain in patients on higher doses of buprenorphine may also be less straightforward (see SL opioid-maintenance therapy in addicts). Nonetheless, various μ agonists have been used in patients on SL buprenorphine 2–32mg/24h, although higher doses than usual may be required.[38,39]

Buprenorphine has either no effect or a smaller effect than **morphine** on pressure within the biliary and pancreatic ducts.[40,41] Buprenorphine does slow intestinal transit, but possibly less so than **morphine**.[42,43] Constipation may be less severe.[44]

Compared with **morphine** and other opioids, buprenorphine appears less likely to suppress the gonadal axis or testosterone levels (see p.367).[45] This may relate to its κ *antagonist* effect.[46] Because hypogonadism is associated with reduced sexual desire and function, mood disturbance, fatigue and other physiological effects, e.g. muscle wasting, osteoporosis, this may become an important consideration in patients requiring long-term opioid therapy.[47–49]

Compared with **morphine** and other opioids, buprenorphine has little or no immunosuppressive effect (see p.368).[2,50–53]

Compared with **methadone**, buprenorphine has little or no effect on the QT interval, even at high doses used for opioid maintenance treatment (see p.731).[54–56]

In an anecdotal report, 2 out of 5 patients with cholestatic pruritus responded to treatment with buprenorphine.[57,58] However, there are insufficient data at present to recommend its use in this circumstance.

TD buprenorphine

Buprenorphine is highly lipid-soluble making it suitable for TD delivery. It is available in the UK in formulations delivering lower and higher doses, i.e. 5, 10 15, or 20microgram/h as 7-day patches[59–61] and 35, 52.5 or 70microgram/h as 3- or 4-day patches (see Dose and use).[62] Like other strong opioids, buprenorphine is an alternative to both weak opioids and **morphine**.[63] Buprenorphine is evenly distributed in a drug-in-adhesive matrix. Its release is controlled by the physical characteristics of the matrix and is proportional to the surface area of the patch. Absorption of the buprenorphine through the skin and into the systemic circulation is influenced by the stratum corneum and blood flow. Thus, if the skin is warm and vasodilated, the rate of absorption increases.

There are few practical differences in the use of the buprenorphine or **fentanyl** matrix patches, and similar safety considerations apply (see Cautions). Compared with **fentanyl**, TD buprenorphine (as Transtec®) adheres better. However, after patch removal, it is associated with more persistent erythema (± localized pruritus), and sometimes a more definite dermatitis.[64] This is generally caused by the adhesive, but occasionally buprenorphine itself causes a contact dermatitis ± more widespread skin rash.[65]

Retrospective analysis suggests that, compared with TD **fentanyl**, patients receiving TD buprenorphine (as Transtec®) have a slower rate of dose increase and longer periods of dose stability.[66] This requires confirmation in an RCT. Indeed, systematic reviews have highlighted a lack of high quality studies of TD buprenorphine.[67,68]

SL opioid-maintenance therapy in addicts

Buprenorphine binds to the μ-opioid receptor with a higher affinity than other μ-opioid agonists. Studies in addicts indicate that buprenorphine ≥16mg SL is required to suppress illicit opioid use;[69] at this dose level, ≥80% of the μ-opioid receptors in the brain are occupied by buprenorphine which is sufficient to antagonize the subjective and respiratory depressant effects of **hydromorphone**, a μ agonist.[11,70] This has implications for the management of acute pain in these patients, e.g. postoperative or traumatic pain (see Chapter 25, p.753) and potentially for patients on higher-dose buprenorphine for chronic pain (see above).

Respiratory depression

Buprenorphine demonstrates a ceiling effect for respiratory depression. Thus, unlike other opioids where progressive doses reduce ventilation to the point of apnoea, with buprenorphine, the level of respiratory depression plateaus once a certain dose is reached. In a healthy volunteer study, this equated to a maximum reduction of 50% in minute ventilation at doses >3microgram/kg IV.[28] Although significant respiratory depression is rarely seen with clinically recommended doses, *it can still occur, particularly in opioid naïve patients in the acute pain setting.*[71]

A lower risk of respiratory depression may explain why buprenorphine (mainly SL ± **naloxone**) appears to have a better safety profile than **methadone**.[72] However, serious or fatal respiratory depression has occurred in addicts misusing buprenorphine, generally in high-dose IV and in combination with benzodiazepines or other CNS depressants, e.g. alcohol.[73,74] Because buprenorphine has both high receptor affinity and prolonged receptor binding, **naloxone** in standard doses does not reverse the effects of buprenorphine and higher doses must be used (Box A).[2,75] The non-specific respiratory stimulant **doxapram** can also be used, 1–1.5mg/kg IV over 30sec, repeated if necessary at hourly intervals or *1.5–4mg/min* CIVI.[75–77]

Box A Reversal of buprenorphine-induced respiratory depression

1. Discontinue buprenorphine (stop CSCI/CIVI, remove TD patch).
2. Give oxygen by mask.
3. Give IV naloxone *2mg* stat over 90sec.
4. Commence naloxone *4mg/h* by CIVI.
5. Continue CIVI until the patient's condition is satisfactory (probably <90min).
6. Monitor the patient frequently for the next 24h, and restart CIVI if respiratory depression recurs.
7. If the patient's condition remains satisfactory, restart buprenorphine at a reduced dose, e.g. half the previous dose.

Potency

Buprenorphine has a longer duration of action than **morphine**. In postoperative single-dose studies, buprenorphine provided analgesia for 6–7h compared with 4–5h with **morphine**.[78] This is reflected in the recommended dose frequency (q8h–q6h vs. q4h for **morphine**). However, the longer duration of action of buprenorphine almost certainly means *single-dose* studies will *underestimate* the relative potency of buprenorphine. Thus, the following should be *not* be regarded as 'cast iron'. They merely provide a rough guide for use when switching route or opioids (also see Appendix 2, p.855):

- SL buprenorphine is about half as potent as IV/IM/SC buprenorphine; thus, in round figures, 200microgram SL is equivalent to 100microgram by injection[79,80]
- SL buprenorphine is about 80 times more potent than PO **morphine**;[35] thus, in round figures, 200microgram SL buprenorphine is equivalent to 15mg PO **morphine**
- IV/IM/SC buprenorphine is 30–40 times more potent than IV/IM/SC **morphine**;[81] thus, in round figures, 300microgram IV buprenorphine is equivalent to 10mg IV **morphine**
- TD buprenorphine is 70–115 times more potent than PO **morphine**; the lower limit is based on a small prospective study and the upper limit a large retrospective chart review.[82–84]

Thus, *PCF* considers TD buprenorphine being 100 times more potent than PO **morphine** a convenient compromise. A PO **morphine**:TD buprenorphine conversion ratio of 100:1 makes a 5microgram/h TD buprenorphine patch equivalent to about 12mg/24h PO **morphine**. (Note. A lack of definitive data explains the wide variation seen in recommendations and clinical practice).[85–87]

A conversion ratio of PO **morphine**:TD buprenorphine of 100:1 also means that TD buprenorphine and TD **fentanyl** can be considered essentially equipotent (see Appendix 2, Table 2, p.858). However, others suggest that TD **fentanyl** is 1.4 times more potent than TD buprenorphine,[36,84] making TD **fentanyl** 25 and 50microgram/h patches equivalent to buprenorphine 35 and 70microgram/h patches respectively. Even so, when switching opioids because of possible opioid-induced hyperalgesia, it is prudent to reduce the calculated equivalent dose of the new opioid by 25–50% (see Opioid switching, p.370).

Switching opioids

As with any opioid switch, patients changing from another opioid to buprenorphine may experience worsening pain and/or opioid-withdrawal symptoms. Careful monitoring and titration of buprenorphine is required to ensure any worsening pain is dealt with promptly.

Opioid-withdrawal manifests with GI and flu-like symptoms, e.g. abdominal pain, diarrhoea, arthralgia, myalgia, and last for a few days. With TD and lower doses of SL buprenorphine, p.r.n. doses of the previous opioid will relieve troublesome symptoms.

However, in addiction medicine, when switching generally involves high-dose SL buprenorphine, the practice is to discontinue the first opioid, await the development of withdrawal symptoms and only then commence buprenorphine. In this way, opioid withdrawal will not be precipitated by buprenorphine (because of its greater affinity for the μ-opioid receptor) but, rather, once withdrawal symptoms are present, they should be relieved by it.

Pharmacokinetics

The bio-availability of PO buprenorphine is low (15%); it undergoes extensive first-pass metabolism in the GI mucosa and liver, where it is almost completely converted by CYP3A4 to norbuprenorphine. Norbuprenorphine has similar opioid receptor-binding affinities to buprenorphine but does not readily cross the blood-brain barrier and has little, if any, central effect.[88] Both buprenorphine and norbuprenorphine undergo glucuronidation to what have traditionally been considered inactive metabolites, although animal work has questioned this.[89,90]

The bio-availability of SL buprenorphine is about 50%; it is rapidly absorbed into the oral mucosa (2–3min), followed by a slower absorption into the systemic circulation (t_{max} 30min–3.5h after a single dose; 1–2h with repeat dosing).[88] This, together with a duration of action of 6–8h, suggests that SL buprenorphine is *not* ideal for the treatment of break-through pain. Nonetheless, onset of analgesia in 10–20min is reported for SL buprenorphine,[42] and it has been successfully used as a rescue analgesic in patients receiving higher dose TD buprenorphine (i.e. Transtec®).[91] After parenteral and SL administration, 70% of buprenorphine is excreted unchanged in the faeces and some enterohepatic recirculation is likely; whereas norbuprenorphine is mainly excreted in the urine.[92] Vomiting is more common with SL administration than IM or TD.

Buprenorphine has a large volume of distribution and is highly protein-bound (96%; α- and β-globulins).[88] It does not accumulate in renal impairment nor is it generally removed by haemodialysis, and thus analgesia is unaffected.[93,94] Although accumulation of norbuprenorphine can occur, this is of uncertain clinical relevance given its lack of central effect.[88,93] Thus, buprenorphine is potentially a reasonable option for patients with renal impairment (see p.693). However, clinical experience is more limited compared to other opioids, e.g. **fentanyl** (p.409).[95]

Data are limited,[96] but smaller starting doses and careful titration are advisable in patients with severe (but not mild–moderate) hepatic impairment (see p.709). Buprenorphine crosses the placenta and enters breast milk. The incidence, severity and duration of the neonatal abstinence syndrome appears to be less than with **methadone**.[97,98]

Table 1 Pharmacokinetic details for buprenorphine

	IV	*TD (Hapoctasin®)*	*TD (Transtec®)*	*TD (BuTrans®)*	*SL*
Onset of action	5–15min[78]	4–12h	21h for 35microgram/h patch; 11h for 70microgram/h patch	18–24h	10–20min[42]
Time to peak plasma concentration	5min	34h for 35microgram/h patch; 29h for 70microgram/h patch	60h	3 days	30min–3.5h single dose; 1–2h multiple doses[24,88]
Plasma halflife	3–16h[88]	24–27h[a]	25–36h[a]	13–35h[a]	24–69h[88]
Duration of action	6–8h	3 days	4 days	7 days	6–8h

a. the halflife after a patch has been removed and not replaced.

The bio-availability of IV buprenorphine is by definition 100%, and that of SC essentially the same. Bio-availability is irrelevant in relation to TD patches; the stated delivery rates reflect the mean amount of drug delivered to patients throughout the patch's recommended duration of use. Inevitably, there will be interindividual variation in the amount delivered. Extrapolating from data relating to TD fentanyl, the absorption of TD buprenorphine could also be impaired in patients with cachexia, possibly because of a loss of skin hydration.[99] Pharmacokinetic data are summarized in Table 1.

Cautions

Although most of the safety warnings and cautions from the regulatory authorities regarding the use of TD patches have been issued for **fentanyl** (p.411), adverse events have also occurred with the use of buprenorphine TD patches.[100] Thus, the same cautions are applicable, i.e. health professionals and patients/carers must be made aware:[101]

- buprenorphine is a strong opioid analgesic
- buprenorphine TD patches are inappropriate for short-term, intermittent or postoperative pain in patients who had not previously been receiving a strong opioid
- of directions for safe use, storage and disposal
- of the signs of an overdose and when to seek attention
- that the rate of absorption of buprenorphine may be increased if the skin under the patch becomes vasodilated, e.g. in febrile patients, high ambient temperatures, or by an external heat source, e.g. electric blanket, heat lamps, saunas, hot tubs or MRI scans
- of drug interactions which can increase buprenorphine levels.

Additional errors reported for TD patches include the failure to remove old patches, the dispensing and application of higher strength patches than prescribed and incorrect disposal. The latter is associated with accidental exposure and deaths in others, particularly children.

Severe renal or hepatic impairment (also see p.681 and p.703).

The combination of high-dose buprenorphine SL with antiretrovirals, particularly **delavirdine** and **ritonavir** increases the QT interval, but the clinical significance of this is uncertain.[102] Although the SPC contra-indicates the use of buprenorphine within 14 days of MAOI use, this appears a blanket precaution, see Strong opioids, p.367.

Drug interactions

A single case report describes respiratory depression when IM **ketorolac** was added to ED buprenorphine.[103]

Buprenorphine is mainly a substrate of CYP3A4, and the manufacturers and others advise caution if prescribed concurrently with CYP3A4 inhibitors (e.g. **clarithromycin**, **erythromycin**, **itraconazole**, protease inhibitors), or avoiding concurrent use, because of the potential to increase buprenorphine levels. Although for most CYP3A4 inhibitors this is a theoretical concern, **atazanavir**, **ritonavir** and **delavirdine** (not UK) have been shown to significantly increase buprenorphine levels in patients receiving high-doses SL (8–16mg/day).[104] Accordingly, it is recommended that the dose of buprenorphine is halved in patients receiving high-dose buprenorphine SL if used concurrently with a CYP3A4 inhibitor (see Chapter 19, Table 8, p.725).[104]

Conversely, CYP3A4 inducers (e.g. **carbamazepine**, **phenobarbital**, **phenytoin**, **rifampicin**) could reduce buprenorphine levels. For **rifampicin**, reduced levels are seen following SL but not IV buprenorphine.[105]

Undesirable effects

Also see Strong opioids, Box B, p.365.

Very common (>10%): nausea; erythema and pruritus at the patch application site.

Common (<10%, >1%): asthenia, drowsiness, dizziness, headache, oedema, vomiting, constipation, sweating.

Dose and use

As with all opioids, patients must be monitored for undesirable effects, particularly nausea and vomiting, and constipation. Depending on individual circumstances, an anti-emetic should be prescribed for regular or p.r.n. use, (see QCG: Nausea and vomiting, p.240) and, routinely, a laxative prescribed (see QCG Opioid-induced constipation, p.42).

Opioids can impair driving ability and patients should be counselled accordingly (see p.743).

TD

The use of TD buprenorphine patches is summarized in the Quick Clinical Guide (see QCG: Use of transdermal buprenorphine patches, p.407). This is based on a dose conversion ratio of PO **morphine** to TD buprenorphine of 100:1. Prescribers using the manufacturer's ratio of 75−115:1 should follow the dose conversion guidelines in the SPC (Appendix 2, Box A, p.859).

In 2013, in response to large numbers of safety incident reports about buprenorphine and **fentanyl** TD patches, the Care Quality Commission highlighted the need to ensure that:
- use is appropriate, e.g. chronic *not* acute pain
- dose is appropriate, i.e. in line with published conversion charts
- dose is titrated appropriately, i.e. no more than 50% of the previous daily dose
- date and site of application are recorded to avoid inadvertent dose omission or duplication.

Further, to avoid confusing patients and carers, prescribing by brand was recommended.[100]

TD patches and MRI scans: Buprenorphine patches should be removed before the patient enters the scan room due to the risks from heating. Patients should be advised to bring a replacement patch with them to facilitate this (also see p.831).

In Europe, the TD patches are the commonest formulation of buprenorphine used in chronic cancer and non-cancer pain. Particularly for patients unable to swallow or take PO/SL products reliably, TD buprenorphine provide an alternative non-invasive route for opioid administration.[85]

Compared to the SL and parenteral routes, the TD patches permit smaller initial doses of buprenorphine to be delivered more consistently (without large peaks and troughs) and are thus better tolerated.[106] In the UK, TD buprenorphine patches are available:
- as 5, 10, 15 and 20microgram/h 7-day patches
- as 35, 52.5 and 70microgram/h 3-day or 4-day patches; the 4-day patches can be replaced on fixed days in the week, i.e. after 3 and 4 days alternatively.

Because of the wide number of different formulations and brands available (see supply), prescribing by brand is recommended to avoid confusing patients and carers.[100]

For patients who have not already been taking an opioid, a low patch strength should be prescribed, i.e. 5–10microgram/h (equivalent to **morphine** 12–24mg/24h PO). For patients switching from another strong opioid, see QCG: Use of transdermal buprenorphine patches, p.407. General advice and recommended starting doses are also detailed in the manufacturer's SPC.

Absorption of buprenorphine through the skin and into the systemic circulation is influenced by both the condition of the skin and cutaneous blood flow. Thus, if the skin is warm and vasodilated, the rate of absorption will be increased.

It is important to give adequate rescue doses of **morphine** (see QCG: Use of transdermal buprenorphine patches, p.407) or other strong opioid. Adjusting the patch strength on a daily basis is not recommended. With inpatients, the use of a monitoring chart is recommended (see Document Library, www.palliativedrugs.com).[107]

SL

The tablet should not be chewed or swallowed as this will reduce efficacy:
- manufacturer's recommended starting dose 200microgram SL (equivalent to approximately **morphine** 15mg PO) q8h; this may be too much for some patients
- moisten the mouth with a sip of water beforehand, if the mouth is dry
- use an appropriate dose of a strong opioid as a rescue analgesic. Note. SL buprenorphine is *not* an ideal rescue analgesic but, if used, allow one tenth of the total daily dose, rounded to a convenient tablet size, q3h p.r.n.; some limit this to a maximum of four doses per 24h
- titrate the dose every 4–5 days, based on p.r.n. use
- typical dose 800–1,200microgram/day, given as 200–400microgram q8h–q6h
- doses of 2–24mg/day have been reported in chronic pain patients switched from other opioids.[37,108]

SC/IM/IV

- manufacturer's recommended starting dose 300microgram (equivalent to approximately **morphine** 10mg SC/IM/IV) q8h; this may be too much for some patients
- give IV over ≥2min
- if necessary, titrate to 600microgram q8h–q6h (the recommended maximum in acute pain; in chronic pain higher doses may be required).

CSCI/CIVI

- buprenorphine has been given CIVI diluted in 0.9% saline or 5% glucose at a concentration of 15microgram/mL; there are no compatibility data for mixing with other drugs used in palliative care
- for patients receiving CSCI/CIVI buprenorphine, p.r.n. injections about one tenth of the total daily dose can be used for break-through pain.

Supply

All preparations are Schedule 3 **CD**.

Buprenorphine (generic)
Tablets SL 200microgram, 400microgram, 28 days @ 200microgram t.d.s. = £8.50.
Injection 300microgram/mL, 1mL amp = £0.50.

Note. SL buprenorphine tablets 400microgram, 2mg and 8mg for substitution treatment for opioid dependence are available in 7 tablet packs. A combined formulation with **naloxone** is also available (Suboxone®, Reckitt Benckiser).

Transdermal products
Buprenorphine (generic)
Matrix patches (for 7 days) 5microgram/h, 10microgram/h, 15microgram/h, 20microgram/h, 1 = £4.50, £8, £12.50 and £14 respectively.
Brands include Butec®, Butrans®, Panitaz®, Reletrans® and Sevodyne®.
Matrix patches (for 3 or 4 days) 35microgram/h, 52.5microgram/h, 70microgram/h, 1 = £4, £6 and £8 respectively.
Brands include Hapoctasin® (3 days only), Prenotrix® (3 days only), Bupeaze®, Buplast®, Relevtec®, Transtec®.

1 Resnick RB (2003) Food and Drug Administration approval of buprenorphine-naloxone for office treatment of addiction. *Annals of Internal Medicine.* **138**: 360.

2 Budd K and Raffa R (eds) (2005) Buprenorphine - the unique opioid analgesic. Georg Thieme Verlag, Stuttgart, Germany, p. 134.

3 Griessinger N *et al.* (2005) Transdermal buprenorphine in clinical practice–a post-marketing surveillance study in 13,179 patients. *Current Medical Research and Opinion.* **21**: 1147–1156.

4 Gowing L *et al.* (2006) Buprenorphine for the management of opioid withdrawal. *Cochrane Database Systematic Reviews.* **2**: CD002025. www.thecochranelibrary.com

5 Landau CJ *et al.* (2007) Buprenorphine transdermal delivery system in adults with persistent noncancer-related pain syndromes who require opioid therapy: a multicenter, 5-week run-in and randomized, double-blind maintenance-of-analgesia study. *Clinical Therapeutics.* **29**: 2179–2193.

6 Kress HG (2009) Clinical update on the pharmacology, efficacy and safety of transdermal buprenorphine. *European Journal of Pain.* **13**: 219–230.

7 Przeklasa-Muszynska A and Dobrogowski J (2011) Transdermal buprenorphine for the treatment of moderate to severe chronic pain: results from a large multicenter, non-interventional post-marketing study in Poland. *Current Medical Research Opinion.* **27**: 1109–1117.

8 Rothman R (1995) Buprenorphine: a review of the binding literature. In: A Cowan and J Lewis (eds) *Buprenorphine: combatting drug abuse with a unique opioid.* Wiley-Liss, New York, pp. 19–29.

9 Zaki P *et al.* (2000) Ligand-induced changes in surface mu-opioid receptor number: relationship to G protein activation? *Journal of Pharmacology and Experimental Therapeutics.* **292**: 1127–1134.

10 Lewis JW and Husbands SM (2004) The orvinols and related opioids--high affinity ligands with diverse efficacy profiles. *Current Pharmaceutical Design.* **10**: 717–732.

11 Greenwald M *et al.* (2007) Buprenorphine duration of action: mu-opioid receptor availability and pharmacokinetic and behavioral indices. *Biological Psychiatry.* **61**: 101–110.

12 Knapman A *et al.* (2014) Buprenorphine signalling is compromised at the N40D polymorphism of the human mu opioid receptor in vitro. *British Journal of Pharmacology.* **171**: 4273–4288.

13 Schmidt-Hansen M *et al.* (2015) Buprenorphine for treating cancer pain. *Cochrane Database of Systematic Reviews.* **3**: CD009596. www.thecochranelibrary.com

14 Koppert W *et al.* (2005) Different profiles of buprenorphine-induced analgesia and antihyperalgesia in a human pain model. *Pain.* **118**: 15–22.

15 Simonnet G (2005) Opioids: from analgesia to anti-hyperalgesia? *Pain.* **118**: 8–9.

16 Ravn P *et al.* (2013) Morphine- and buprenorphine-induced analgesia and antihyperalgesia in a human inflammatory pain model: a double-blind, randomized, placebo-controlled, five-arm crossover study. *Journal of Pain Research.* **6**: 23–38.

17 Hans G (2007) Buprenorphine--a review of its role in neuropathic pain. *Journal of Opioid Management.* **3**: 195–206.

18 Sanchez-Blazquez P and Garzon J (1988) Pertussis toxin differentially reduces the efficacy of opioids to produce supraspinal analgesia in the mouse. *European Journal of Pharmacology.* **152**: 357–361.

19 Likar R and Sittl R (2005) Transdermal buprenorphine for treating nociceptive and neuropathic pain: four case studies. *Anesthesia and Analgesia.* **100**: 781–785.

20 Penza P *et al.* (2008) Short- and intermediate-term efficacy of buprenorphine TDS in chronic painful neuropathies. *Journal of the Peripheral Nervous System*. **13**: 283–288.
21 Simpson RW and Wlodarczyk JH (2016) Transdermal buprenorphine relieves neuropathic pain: a randomized, double-blind, parallel-group, placebo-controlled trial in diabetic peripheral neuropathic pain. *Diabetes Care*. **39**: 1493–1500.
22 Hay JL *et al.* (2011) Potentiation of buprenorphine antinociception with ultra-low dose naltrexone in healthy subjects. *European Journal of Pain*. **15**: 293–298.
23 Ling W *et al.* (2012) Comparisons of analgesic potency and side effects of buprenorphine and buprenorphine with ultra-low-dose naloxone. *Journal of Addiction Medicine*. **6**: 118–123.
24 Johnson RE *et al.* (2005) Buprenorphine: considerations for pain management. *Journal of Pain and Symptom Management*. **29**: 297–326.
25 Falcon E *et al.* (2016) Antidepressant-like effects of buprenorphine are mediated by kappa opioid receptors. *Neuropsychopharmacology*. **41**: 2344-2351.
26 Stanciu CN *et al.* (2017) Use of Buprenorphine in treatment of refractory depression-A review of current literature. *Asian Journal of Psychiatry*. **26**: 94–98.
27 Lutfy K *et al.* (2003) Buprenorphine-induced antinociception is mediated by mu-opioid receptors and compromised by concomitant activation of opioid receptor-like receptors. *Journal of Neuroscience*. **23**: 10331–10337.
28 Dahan A *et al.* (2005) Comparison of the respiratory effects of intravenous buprenorphine and fentanyl in humans and rats. *British Journal Anaesthesia*. **94**: 825–834.
29 Dahan A *et al.* (2006) Buprenorphine induces ceiling in respiratory depression but not in analgesia. *British Journal of Anaesthesia*. **96**: 627–632.
30 Budd K (2002) *Buprenorphine: a review. Evidence Based Medicine in Practice*. Hayward Medical Communications, Newmarket.
31 Walsh S *et al.* (1994) Clinical pharmacology of buprenorphine: ceiling effects at high doses. *Clinical Pharmacology and Therapeutics*. **55**: 569–580.
32 Cote J and Montgomery L (2014) Sublingual buprenorphine as an analgesic in chronic pain: a systematic review. *Pain Medicine*. **15**: 1171–1178.
33 Mercadante S *et al.* (2006) Safety and effectiveness of intravenous morphine for episodic breakthrough pain in patients receiving transdermal buprenorphine. *Journal of Pain and Symptom Management*. **32**: 175–179.
34 van Niel JC *et al.* (2016) Efficacy of full micro-opioid receptor agonists is not impaired by concomitant buprenorphine or mixed opioid agonists/antagonists - preclinical and clinical evidence. *Drug Research*. **66**: 562–570.
35 Atkinson R *et al.* (1990) The efficacy in sequential use of buprenorphine and morphine in advanced cancer pain. In: D Doyle (ed) *Opioids in the treatment of cancer pain*. Royal Society of Medicine Services, London, pp. 81–87.
36 Mercadante S *et al.* (2007) Switching from transdermal drugs: an observational "N of 1" study of fentanyl and buprenorphine. *Journal of Pain and Symptom Management*. **34**: 532–538.
37 Rosenblum A *et al.* (2012) Sublingual buprenorphine/naloxone for chronic pain in at-risk patients: development and pilot test of a clinical protocol. *Journal of Opioid Management*. **8**: 369–382.
38 Kornfeld H and Manfredi L (2010) Effectiveness of full agonist opioids in patients stabilized on buprenorphine undergoing major surgery: a case series. *American Journal of Therapeutics*. **17**: 523–528.
39 Heit HA and Gourlay DL (2008) Buprenorphine: new tricks with an old molecule for pain management. *Clinical Journal of Pain*. **24**: 93–97.
40 Pausawasdi S *et al.* (1984) The effect of buprenorphine and morphine on intraluminal pressure of the common bile duct. *Journal of the Medical Association of Thailand*. **67**: 329–333.
41 Staritz M *et al.* (1986) Effect of modern analgesic drugs (tramadol, pentazocine, and buprenorphine) on the bile duct sphincter in man. *Gut*. **27**: 567–569.
42 Robbie DS (1979) A trial of sublingual buprenorphine in cancer pain. *British Journal of Clinical Pharmacology*. **7 (Suppl 3)**: S315–S317.
43 Bach V *et al.* (1991) Buprenorphine and sustained release morphine - effect and side-effects in chronic use. *The Pain Clinic*. **4**: 87–93.
44 Pace MC *et al.* (2007) Buprenorphine in long-term control of chronic pain in cancer patients. *Frontiers in Bioscience*. **12**: 1291–1299.
45 Hallinan R *et al.* (2009) Hypogonadism in men receiving methadone and buprenorphine maintenance treatment. *International Journal of Andrology*. **32**: 131–139.
46 Bliesener N *et al.* (2005) Plasma testosterone and sexual function in men receiving buprenorphine maintenance for opioid dependence. *Journal of Clinical Endocrinology and Metabolism*. **90**: 203–206.
47 Daniell HW (2002) Hypogonadism in men consuming sustained-action oral opioids. *The Journal of Pain*. **3**: 377–384.
48 Rajagopal A *et al.* (2004) Symptomatic hypogonadism in male survivors of cancer with chronic exposure to opioids. *Cancer*. **100**: 851–858.
49 Hallinan R *et al.* (2008) Erectile dysfunction in men receiving methadone and buprenorphine maintenance treatment. *Journal of Sexual Medicine*. **5**: 684–692.
50 Sacerdote P *et al.* (2000) The effects of tramadol and morphine on immune responses and pain after surgery in cancer patients. *Anesthesia and Analgesia*. **90**: 1411–1414.
51 Budd K and Shipton E (2004) Acute pain and the immune system and opioimmunosuppression. *Acute Pain*. **6**: 123–135.
52 Sacerdote P *et al.* (2008) Buprenorphine and methadone maintenance treatment of heroin addicts preserves immune function. *Brain, Behavior, and Immunity*. **22**: 606–613.
53 Canneti A *et al.* (2013) Safety and efficacy of transdermal buprenorphine and transdermal fentanyl in the treatment of neuropathic pain in AIDS patients. *Minerva Anestesiologica*. **79**: 871–883.
54 Wedam EF *et al.* (2007) QT-interval effects of methadone, levomethadyl, and buprenorphine in a randomized trial. *Archives of Internal Medicine*. **167**: 2469–2475.
55 Esses JL *et al.* (2008) Successful transition to buprenorphine in a patient with methadone-induced torsades de pointes. *Journal of Interventional Cardiac Electrophysiology*. **23**: 117–119.
56 Isbister GK *et al.* (2017) QT interval prolongation in opioid agonist treatment: analysis of continuous 12-lead electrocardiogram recordings. *British Journal of Clinical Pharmacology*. **83**: 2274–2282.
57 Juby L *et al.* (1994) Buprenorphine and hepatic pruritus. *British Journal of Clinical Practice*. **48**: 331.
58 Reddy L *et al.* (2007) Transdermal buprenorphine may be effective in the treatment of pruritus in primary biliary cirrhosis. *Journal of Pain and Symptom Management*. **34**: 455–456.
59 Steiner DJ *et al.* (2011) Efficacy and safety of the seven-day buprenorphine transdermal system in opioid-naive patients with moderate to severe chronic low back pain: an enriched, randomized, double-blind, placebo-controlled study. *Journal of Pain and Symptom Management*. **42**: 903–917.
60 Conaghan PG *et al.* (2011) Transdermal buprenorphine plus oral paracetamol vs an oral codeine-paracetamol combination for osteoarthritis of hip and/or knee: a randomised trial. *Osteoarthritis and Cartilage*. **19**: 930–938.

61 Steiner D *et al.* (2011) Efficacy and safety of buprenorphine transdermal system (BTDS) for chronic moderate to severe low back pain: a randomized, double-blind study. *Journal of Pain and Symptom Management.* **12**: 1163–1173.
62 Likar R *et al.* (2007) Transdermal buprenorphine patches applied in a 4-day regimen versus a 3-day regimen: a single-site, Phase III, randomized, open-label, crossover comparison. *Clinical Therapeutics.* **29**: 1591–1606.
63 Davis MP (2005) Buprenorphine in cancer pain. *Supportive Care in Cancer.* **13**: 878–887.
64 Schmid-Grendelmeier P *et al.* (2006) A comparison of the skin irritation potential of transdermal fentanyl versus transdermal buprenorphine in middle-aged to elderly healthy volunteers. *Current Medical Research Opinion.* **22**: 501–509.
65 Vander Hulst K *et al.* (2008) Allergic contact dermatitis from transdermal buprenorphine. *Contact Dermatitis.* **59**: 366–369.
66 Sittl R *et al.* (2006) Patterns of dosage changes with transdermal buprenorphine and transdermal fentanyl for the treatment of noncancer and cancer pain: a retrospective data analysis in Germany. *Clinical Therapeutics.* **28**: 1144–1154.
67 Deandrea S *et al.* (2009) Managing severe cancer pain: the role of transdermal buprenorphine: a systematic review. *Therapeutics and Clinical Risk Management.* **5**: 707–718.
68 Tassinari D *et al.* (2011) Transdermal opioids as front line treatment of moderate to severe cancer pain: a systemic review. *Palliative Medicine.* **25**: 478–487.
69 Mattick RP *et al.* (2014) Buprenorphine maintenance versus placebo or methadone maintenance for opioid dependence. *Cochrane Database of Systematic Reviews.* **2**: CD002207. www.thecochranelibrary.com
70 Greenwald MK *et al.* (2003) Effects of buprenorphine maintenance dose on mu-opioid receptor availability, plasma concentrations, and antagonist blockade in heroin-dependent volunteers. *Neuropsychopharmacology.* **28**: 2000–2009.
71 Richards S *et al.* (2017) Buprenorphine-related complications in elderly hospitalised patients: a case series. *Anaesthesia and Intensive Care.* **45**: 256–261.
72 Dasgupta N *et al.* (2010) Post-marketing surveillance of methadone and buprenorphine in the United States. *Pain Medicine.* **11**: 1078–1091.
73 Kintz P (2001) Deaths involving buprenorphine: a compendium of French cases. *Forensic Science International.* **121**: 65–69.
74 Hakkinen M *et al.* (2012) Benzodiazepines and alcohol are associated with cases of fatal buprenorphine poisoning. *European Journal of Clinical Pharmacology.* **68**: 301–309.
75 Dahan A *et al.* (2010) Incidence, reversal, and prevention of opioid-induced respiratory depression. *Anesthesiology.* **112**: 226–238.
76 British National Formulary Section 3.5.1 Respiratory stimulants London: BMJ Group and Pharmaceutical Press www.bnf.org (accessed December 2012).
77 Orwin JM (1977) The effect of doxapram on buprenorphine induced respiratory depression. *Acta anaesthesiologica Belgica.* **28**: 93–106.
78 Heel RC *et al.* (1979) Buprenorphine: a review of its pharmacological properties and therapeutic efficiency. *Drugs.* **17**: 81–110.
79 Ellis R *et al.* (1982) Pain relief after abdominal surgery-a comparison of i.m. morphine, sublingual buprenorphine and self-administered i.v. pethidine. *British Journal of Anaesthesia.* **54**: 421–428.
80 Bullingham RE *et al.* (1984) Mandatory sublingual buprenorphine for postoperative pain. *Anaesthesia.* **39**: 329–334.
81 Cuschieri RJ *et al.* (1984) Comparison of morphine and sublingual buprenorphine following abdominal surgery. *British Journal of Anaesthesia.* **56**: 855–859.
82 Sittl R *et al.* (2005) Equipotent doses of transdermal fentanyl and transdermal buprenorphine in patients with cancer and noncancer pain: results of a retrospective cohort study. *Clinical Therapeutics.* **27**: 225–237.
83 Likar R *et al.* (2008) Challenging the equipotency calculation for transdermal buprenorphine: four case studies. *International Journal of Clinical Practice.* **62**: 152–156.
84 Mercadante S *et al.* (2009) Equipotent doses to switch from high doses of opioids to transdermal buprenorphine. *Supportive Care in Cancer.* **17**: 715–718.
85 Caraceni A *et al.* (2012) Use of opioid analgesics in the treatment of cancer pain: evidence-based recommendations from the EAPC. *Lancet Oncology.* **13**: e58–68.
86 NICE (2012) Opioids in palliative care: safe and effective prescribing of strong opioids for pain in palliative care adults. *Clinical Guideline.* CG104. www.nice.org.uk
87 Palliativedrugs.com (2013) The oral morphine equivalent of buprenorphine TD patches - What conversion do you use? Survey Results. *Additions Archive.* **March**: www.palliativedrugs.com
88 Elkader A and Sproule B (2005) Buprenorphine: clinical pharmacokinetics in the treatment of opioid dependence. *Clinical Pharmacokinetics.* **44**: 661–680.
89 McQuay H and Moore R (1995) Buprenorphine kinetics in humans. In: A Cowan and J Lewis (eds) *Buprenorphine: combatting drug abuse with a unique opioid.* Wiley-Liss, New York, pp. 137–147.
90 Brown SM *et al.* (2011) Buprenorphine metabolites, buprenorphine-3-glucuronide and norbuprenorphine-3-glucuronide, are biologically active. *Anesthesiology.* **115**: 1251–1260.
91 Poulain P *et al.* (2008) Efficacy and safety of transdermal buprenorphine: a randomized, placebo-controlled trial in 289 patients with severe cancer pain. *Journal of Pain and Symptom Management.* **36**: 117–125.
92 Cone EJ *et al.* (1984) The metabolism and excretion of buprenorphine in humans. *Drug Metabolism and Disposition.* **12**: 577–581.
93 Hand CW *et al.* (1990) Buprenorphine disposition in patients with renal impairment: single and continuous dosing, with special reference to metabolites. *British Journal of Anaesthesia.* **64**: 276–282.
94 Filitz J *et al.* (2006) Effect of intermittent hemodialysis on buprenorphine and norbuprenorphine plasma concentrations in chronic pain patients treated with transdermal buprenorphine. *European Journal of Pain.* **10**: 743–748.
95 King S *et al.* (2011) A systematic review of the use of opioid medication for those with moderate to severe cancer pain and renal impairment: A European palliative care research collaborative opioid guidelines project. *Palliative Medicine.* **25**: 525–552.
96 Bosilkovska M *et al.* (2012) Analgesics in patients with hepatic impairment: pharmacology and clinical implications. *Drugs.* **72**: 1645–1669.
97 Fischer G (2000) Treatment of opioid dependence in pregnant women. *Addiction.* **95**: 1141–1144.
98 Lacroix I *et al.* (2004) Buprenorphine in pregnant opioid-dependent women: first results of a prospective study. *Addiction.* **99**: 209–214.
99 Heiskanen T *et al.* (2009) Transdermal fentanyl in cachectic cancer patients. *Pain.* **144**: 218–222.
100 Care Quality Commission and NHS England (2013) Safer use of controlled drugs - preventing harms from fentanyl and buprenorphine transdermal patches. *Use of controlled drugs supporting information.* www.cqc.org.uk
101 All Wales Medicine Strategy Group (2016) Safeguarding users of opioid patches by standardising patient/caregiver counselling. www.awmsg.org
102 Baker JR *et al.* (2006) Effect of buprenorphine and antiretroviral agents on the QT interval in opioid-dependent patients. *Annals of Pharmacotherpy.* **40**: 392–396.

103 Jain PN and Shah SC (1993) Respiratory depression following combination of epidural buprenorphine and intramuscular ketorolac. *Anaesthesia*. **48**: 898–899.

104 Baxter K and Preston CL (2012). *Stockley's Drug Interactions*. London: Pharmaceutical Press www.medicinescomplete.com (accessed December 2012).

105 Hagelberg NM *et al.* (2016) Rifampicin decreases exposure to sublingual buprenorphine in healthy subjects. *Pharmacology Research and Perspectives*. **4**: e00271.

106 James IG *et al.* (2010) A randomized, double-blind, double-dummy comparison of the efficacy and tolerability of low-dose transdermal buprenorphine (BuTrans seven-day patches) with buprenorphine sublingual tablets (Temgesic) in patients with osteoarthritis pain. *Journal of Pain and Symptom Management*. **40**: 266–278.

107 Palliativedrugs.com (2017) Strong opioid transdermal patch monitoring chart. *Document Library*. Pain (strong opioids): www.palliativedrugs.com

108 Malinoff HL *et al.* (2005) Sublingual buprenorphine is effective in the treatment of chronic pain syndrome. *American Journal of Therapeutics*. **12**: 379–384.

Updated September 2017

Quick Clinical Guide: Use of transdermal buprenorphine patches

1 Indications for using transdermal (TD) buprenorphine instead of morphine include:
- intolerable undesirable effects with morphine, e.g. nausea and vomiting, constipation, hallucinations, dysphagia
- renal failure (no centrally active metabolites)
- 'tablet phobia' or poor compliance with oral medication
- high risk of tablet misuse/diversion (although the patch can still be abused).

2 TD buprenorphine is contra-indicated in patients with acute (short-term) pain and in those who need rapid dose titration for severe uncontrolled pain.

3 TD buprenorphine patches are available:
- as 5, 10, 15 and 20microgram/h 7-day patches
- as 35, 52.5, and 70microgram/h 3-day or 4-day patches.

The patch brand, dose and duration should be stated on the prescription to avoid confusion. The maximum authorized dose is two 70microgram/h patches.

Use the Table below to decide a safe starting dose for TD buprenorphine and an appropriate rescue dose of morphine. These recommendations are based on a PO morphine:TD buprenorphine dose conversion ratio of 100:1 derived from published data, which is in keeping with the manufacturer's dose ratio range of 75–115:1 (see SPC). It is an approximation, and inevitably there will be individual variation. If switching to buprenorphine because of possible opioid-induced hyperalgesia, reduce the calculated equivalent dose by 25–50%.

4 Patients not previously receiving opioids should start on 5 or 10microgram/h patches; patients with unrelieved pain despite maximum dose of a weak opioid should commence on 20 or 35microgram/h patches, according to circumstances.

5 For patients taking a dose of morphine that is not the exact equivalent of a buprenorphine patch, it will be necessary to opt for a patch which is either slightly more or slightly less than the morphine dose. Thus, if the patient still has pain, round up to a higher patch strength; if pain-free and frail, round down.

Comparative doses based on dose conversion ratio 100:1

PO Morphine[a]		*SC/IV Morphine*[a]		*TD Buprenorphine*	
mg/24h	*p.r.n. mg*[b]	*mg/24h*[c]	*p.r.n. mg*[b]	*microgram/h*	*microgram/24h*
				7-day patch	
12	2[d]	6	1	5	120
24	5[d]	12	2.5	10	240
36	6[d]	18	3	15	360
48	10	24	5	20	480
				3- or 4-day patches	
84	15	42	7.5	35	840
126	20	63	10	52.5	1,260
168	30	84	15	70[e]	1,680

a. an alternative strong opioid can be used, calculated using the appropriate conversion factor.
Note. SL buprenorphine is *not* an ideal rescue medication but some centres use an initial dose of 200microgram SL q3h, up to 4 doses per 24h, for patients receiving any strength of the 3- or 4-day patches

b. using traditional one sixth of total daily dose as p.r.n. dose and rounded to a convenient dose; give up to q1h; some centres opt for one tenth of total daily dose

c. assuming conversion ratio of PO morphine to SC/IV morphine of 2:1

d. at these doses, p.r.n. codeine/dihydrocodeine (30–60mg) or tramadol (50mg) may suffice

e. for combinations of patches, add the p.r.n. doses together, e.g. 70 + 52.5microgram/h patches = 15 + 10mg morphine SC/IV = 25mg morphine SC/IV, but can round up to 30mg or down to 20mg for convenience.

6 The date of application and/or the date for renewal should be written in a consistent manner on the patch. Apply to dry, non-inflamed, non-irradiated, hairless skin on the upper trunk or arm. Body hair may be clipped with scissors but not shaved. If the skin is washed beforehand, use only water; do not use soap and do not apply oils, cream or ointment to the area. Press patch firmly in place for at least 30 seconds. Micropore® or Tegaderm® can be used to ensure adherence. Careful removal of the patch helps to minimize local skin irritation.

7 Systemic analgesic concentrations are generally reached within 12–24h but levels continue to rise for 32–54h. If converting from:
- 4-hourly PO morphine, give regular doses for the first 12h after applying the patch
- 12-hourly m/r morphine, apply the patch and the final m/r dose at the same time
- 24-hourly m/r morphine, apply the patch 12h after the final m/r dose
- CSCI/CIVI opioids, continue the infusion for about 12h after applying the patch.

8 Steady-state plasma concentrations of buprenorphine are reached after 9 days (1–2 days with patch strength of ≤20microgram/h); the patient should use p.r.n. doses liberally, particularly during the first 24h, either the previously used weak opioid, or morphine/other strong opioid, or buprenorphine (see Table above).

9 After 72h, if a patient continues to need 2 or more rescue doses of analgesic/day, the next strength patch should be used.

10 Patients could experience opioid-withdrawal symptoms when changed from another opioid (particularly large doses) to TD buprenorphine. These manifest with symptoms like gastric flu and last for a few days; p.r.n. doses of the previous opioid will relieve troublesome symptoms.

11 Buprenorphine is less constipating than morphine; halve the dose of laxatives when starting buprenorphine and re-titrate.

12 Buprenorphine may cause nausea and vomiting; if necessary, prescribe an anti-emetic, e.g. haloperidol 500microgram–1.5mg PO stat & at bedtime.

13 In febrile patients, the rate of absorption of buprenorphine increases, and may cause toxicity, e.g. drowsiness. Absorption is also enhanced by an external heat source over the patch, e.g. electric blanket or hot-water bottle; patients should be warned about this. Patients may swim or shower with a patch but should not soak in a hot bath. Remove patches before MRI scans.

14 Remove and replace patches once (7-day patch) or twice (3- and 4-day patches) a week. The 4-day patch can be replaced on fixed days in the week, i.e. after 3 and 4 days alternatively. Change the position of the new patches so as to rest the underlying skin for at least 9 days. The use of a monitoring chart is recommended for inpatients.

15 A reservoir of buprenorphine cumulates in the body, particularly in adipose tissue, and significant plasma levels persist for at least 24h after discontinuing TD buprenorphine.

16 TD buprenorphine is unsatisfactory in <5% of patients.

17 In moribund patients, continue TD buprenorphine and give additional SC morphine p.r.n. (see Table above). If >2 p.r.n. doses are required/24h, give morphine by CSCI, starting with a dose equal to the sum of the p.r.n. doses over the preceding 24h. If necessary, adjust the p.r.n. dose taking into account the total opioid dose (i.e. TD buprenorphine + CSCI morphine).

18 Used patches still contain buprenorphine; after removal, fold the patch with the adhesive side inwards, and then discard in a sharps container (hospital) or dustbin (home), and wash hands. Ultimately, any unused patches should be returned to a pharmacy.

Updated September 2017

FENTANYL

For transmucosal fentanyl for cancer-related break-through pain or procedure-related pain, see p.419.

Class: Strong opioid analgesic.

Indications: ***TD*** severe, chronic (persistent, long-term) pain, including cancer, †AIDS,[1,2] †intolerance to other strong opioids.[3] An iontophoretic fentanyl TD system is authorized for postoperative pain but is beyond the remit of this monograph.[4]
Injection severe pain, premedication and peri-operative analgesia, analgesic/respiratory depressant in patients requiring assisted ventilation, neuroleptanalgesia (i.e. in combination with an antipsychotic/neuroleptic), †an alternative in cases of intolerance to other strong opioids, particularly in renal failure.[5]

Contra-indications: TD fentanyl should not be used for acute (transient, intermittent or short-term) pain, e.g. postoperative, or when there is need for rapid dose titration for severe uncontrolled pain.

In the UK, most manufacturers and the Care Quality Commission/NHS England recommend against its use in opioid-naïve patients (see Dose and use).[6]

In the USA and Canada, TD fentanyl is contra-indicated in opioid-naïve patients because of reports of unintentional overdoses, with serious (sometimes fatal) consequences.[7]

Pharmacology

Fentanyl (*like* **morphine**) is a strong μ-opioid receptor agonist. It has a relatively low molecular weight and (*unlike* **morphine**) is lipophilic. This makes it suitable for TD and transmucosal administration (see p.419). Generally, TD fentanyl is used only when PO opioids, e.g. **morphine**, **oxycodone**, are not tolerated.[3] In some patients, it may be the preferred strong opioid, e.g. those unable to swallow.[8]

Fentanyl is sequestrated in body fats, including epidural fat and the white matter of the CNS.[9,10] Thus, by any route (including spinally), after systemic redistribution, fentanyl acts supraspinally mainly in the thalamus (white matter). Any effect in the dorsal horn (grey matter) is probably minimal.[9]

The lipophilic nature of fentanyl also provides one explanation for the difference in undesirable effects compared with **morphine** (Figure 1).[11] Thus, when converting from PO or parenteral **morphine** to TD or parenteral fentanyl, there is a massive decrease in opioid molecules outside the CNS with, in consequence, less constipation. This also explains why peripherally-mediated withdrawal symptoms are also sometimes seen.

Elimination of fentanyl mainly involves biotransformation in the liver by CYP3A4 to inactive norfentanyl which is excreted in the urine. Less than 7% is excreted unchanged. The SPCs generally advise caution in patients with moderate–severe liver or renal impairment, but this is based on limited data which suggest reduced clearance of fentanyl because of, for example, alterations in metabolic clearance and plasma protein-binding. Given the risk of accumulation, close monitoring is indicated. Nonetheless, fentanyl is a reasonable option for patients with renal impairment or failure and is generally recommended as the first-line parenteral opioid in ESRF at the end of life (see Dose and use and also p.693).[5] It is also generally the opioid of choice in moderate–severe hepatic impairment (see p.709).[12]

TD fentanyl is used in the management of chronic severe pain,[13–15] particularly in cancer.[16–21] Like **morphine** (p.375), there is limited very low quality evidence of benefit in pure neuropathic pain states.[22] Steady-state plasma concentrations of fentanyl are generally achieved after 36–48h[1] but, according to manufacturer data[23] this is sometimes achieved only after 9–12 days.

For some patients, pain relief does not last for 3 days. As long as poor adhesion of the patch is not to blame, this is an end-of-dose phenomenon; as fentanyl in the patch is used up, the concentration gradient driving fentanyl absorption reduces thereby resulting in lower plasma concentrations. The correct response is to increase the patch strength. Even so, a minority of patients (<10%) do best if the patch is changed every 2 days.[20,24,25] Where available (not UK), an alternative is to use a fentanyl patch designed to be changed daily, e.g. Fentos® Tape.[26]

Matrix and reservoir patches are now available from several manufacturers. All the SPCs contain dose conversion recommendations from PO **morphine** which, although broadly similar, do vary. The original manufacturer in the UK initially recommended a dose conversion ratio for **morphine** and fentanyl of 150:1. However, several RCTs support a smaller ratio, ranging 70–125:1. Indeed, at the same time in Germany, the original manufacturer promoted 100:1. Consequently, *PCF* has opted for a ratio of 100:1, as have others.[8,27–29]

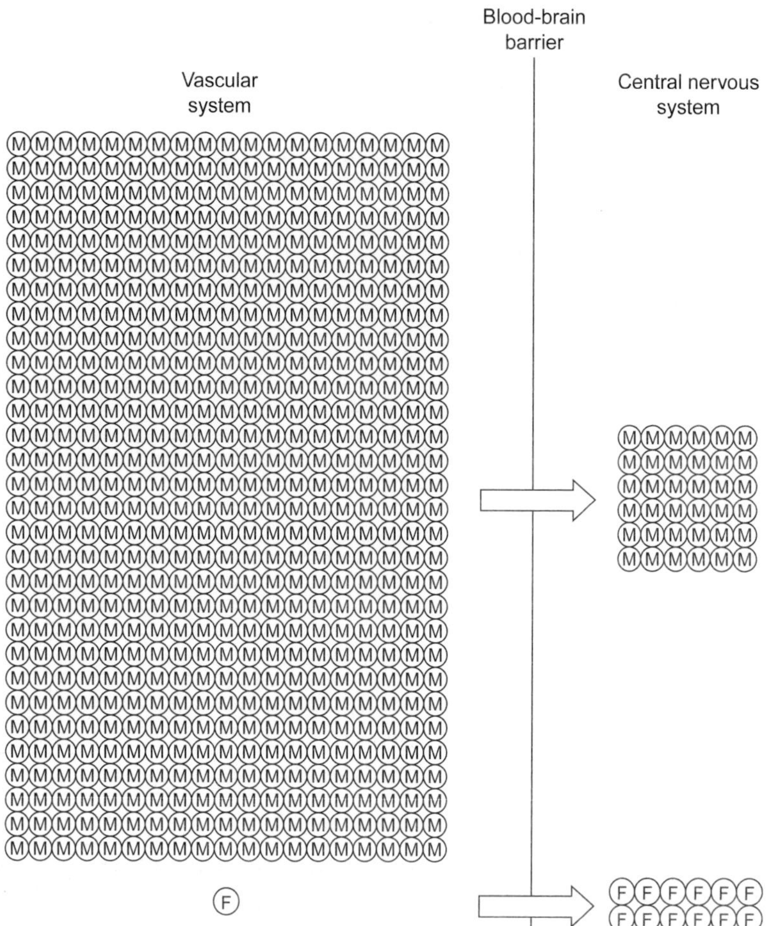

Figure 1 Distribution of equipotent doses of morphine and fentanyl in the vascular and central nervous systems based on animal data.[11]

The original manufacturer's SPC now contains conversion tables based on both 150:1 and 100:1, with the former recommended for patients who have a need for opioid rotation (e.g. because of undesirable effects) or who are less clinically stable, and the latter for patients on a stable and well-tolerated opioid regimen (see Appendix 2, Box B, p.860). It is unclear on what evidence this distinction is made. Studies exploring patient factors that may influence conversion ratios, e.g. reason for switching, prior dose of opioid, show inconsistent findings.[30,31]

PCF also favours a PO **morphine**:TD **buprenorphine** conversion ratio of 100:1 and this means that TD **buprenorphine** and TD fentanyl can be considered essentially equipotent (see Appendix 2, Table 2, p.858). However, others suggest that fentanyl is 1.4 times more potent than TD **buprenorphine**,[32,33] which would make TD fentanyl 25 and 50microgram/h patches equivalent to **buprenorphine** 35 and 70microgram/h patches respectively. Even so, when switching opioids because of possible opioid-induced hyperalgesia, it is prudent to reduce the calculated equivalent dose of the new opioid by 25–50% (see p.370).

Because fentanyl is less constipating than **morphine**,[21,24,34,35] when converting from **morphine** to fentanyl, the dose of laxative should be halved and subsequently adjusted according to need. Some patients experience withdrawal symptoms (e.g. diarrhoea, colic, nausea, sweating, restlessness) when changed from PO **morphine** to TD fentanyl despite satisfactory pain relief. This is probably related to differences between the two opioids in relation to their relative impact on peripheral and central μ-opioid receptors (see Figure 1). Such symptoms are easily treatable by using rescue doses of **morphine** until they resolve after a few days. Like **buprenorphine**, fentanyl appears to have little effect on the sphincter of Oddi.[36]

At one PCU, it was noted that patients admitted on fentanyl TD were receiving relatively higher equivalent opioid doses than other patients.[37] The reasons for this are not clear but may include a failure to appreciate the potency of fentanyl, and the induction of opioid-induced hyperalgesia by inappropriately high doses.[38] It is noteworthy that fentanyl TD was successfully reduced or discontinued in 60% of patients.[37]

5

Pharmacokinetic data are summarized in Table 1. Bio-availability is irrelevant in relation to TD patches; the stated delivery rates reflect the mean amount of drug delivered to patients throughout the patch's recommended duration of use. Inevitably, there will be interindividual variation in the amount delivered, e.g. for the 100microgram/h patch, the mean (±SD) delivery is 97 (±15) microgram/h,[39] and the amount of unused fentanyl in the patch after 3 days can vary from 30–85% of the original contents.[40]

In cachectic patients, plasma concentrations of fentanyl are reduced by 1/3–1/2.[41] The reason for this is unclear; it appears not to relate to loss of subcutaneous adipose tissue,[42] but loss of skin hydration is a possibility.[41]

Table 1 Pharmacokinetic data for fentanyl

	TD	*SC/IM*	*IV*
Onset of action	3–23h[43]	7–15min IM	1.5min
Time to peak plasma concentration	24–72h	Median 15min, range 10–30min [44]	<5min
Plasma halflife	13–22h[a,45]	Median 10h, range 6–16h[44]	4h
Duration of action	72h; for some patients, 48h[46]	1–2h IM	60min

a. the halflife after a patch has been removed and not replaced.

Cautions

The reservoir patches should not be cut because damage to the rate-controlling membrane can lead to a rapid release of fentanyl and overdose. Although cutting matrix patches is theoretically safer, some strongly discourage it because of similar concerns.[47] However, cutting has become unnecessary with the introduction of a 12microgram/h patch.

After reports of serious adverse events (overdoses and deaths), regulatory authorities in the UK, USA and Canada have issued safety warnings about the use of TD fentanyl.[6,7,48,49] Factors contributing to adverse drug events include:

- lack of appreciation that fentanyl is a strong opioid analgesic
- inappropriate use for short-term, intermittent or postoperative pain in patients who had not previously been receiving a strong opioid
- lack of patient education regarding directions for safe use, storage and disposal
- lack of awareness of the signs of an overdose and when to seek attention
- lack of awareness that the rate of absorption of fentanyl may be increased if the skin under the patch becomes vasodilated, e.g. in febrile patients, high ambient temperatures,[50] or by an external heat source, e.g. electric blanket, heat lamps, saunas, hot tubs or MRI scans
- lack of awareness of drug interactions which can increase fentanyl levels.

Deaths continue to occur from incorrect use.[51] Additional errors include the failure to remove old patches, the dispensing and application of higher strength patches than prescribed and incorrect disposal. The latter is associated with accidental exposure and deaths in others, particularly children.

Patients with COPD or other medical conditions which predispose to respiratory depression (e.g. myasthenia gravis) or who are susceptible to the intracranial effects of hypercapnia (e.g.

those with raised intracranial pressure). Caution is also needed if bradyarrhythmic (symptomatic bradycardia can occur),[52] elderly, cachectic, debilitated, moderate–severe renal or hepatic impairment (also see p.681 and p.703), hypovolaemic, hypotensive, and if a history or high risk of abuse or diversion. Muscle rigidity can occur (generally transiently following IV injection).

Addicts misuse TD fentanyl in various ways, e.g. heating the patch, applying buccally, chewing, ingesting, inhaling, IV injection of patch contents, sometimes with fatal consequences.[53,54] In the USA, tighter controls on the prescription of opioids has seen increasing abuse (and deaths) from illicit fentanyl.[55]

Drug interactions

Fentanyl is metabolized by CYP3A4. Caution is required with concurrent use of drugs which inhibit or induce these enzymes (see Chapter 19, table 8, p.725). Reports of interactions where closer monitoring ± dose adjustment are required are listed in Box B.[56–60]

Box B Interactions between fentanyl and other drugs involving CYP450

Plasma concentrations of fentanyl	
Increased by	**Decreased by**
Aprepitant[a]	Aprepitant[a]
Azoles, e.g. fluconazole[b], voriconazole	Carbamazepine
Cimetidine	Phenytoin
Macrolide antibiotics, e.g. clarithromycin, erythromycin	Phenobarbital
Protease inhibitors, e.g. indinavir, nelfinavir, ritonavir	Rifampicin

a. aprepitant can increase the exposure to CYP3A4 substrates in the short-term, then reduce their exposure within 2 weeks

b. a case report of a fatality with oral fluconazole and TD fentanyl has been attributed to this interaction.

Fentanyl has been reported to reduce the metabolism of **midazolam**, reducing the clearance by 30% and extending the half-life by 50%.[56]

Fentanyl is best avoided in patients who have used a MAOI within the past 2 weeks. Although they have been used safely together, serotonin toxicity (sometimes fatal) has occurred (also see p.200), manufacturers' SPCs warn of a risk of serotonin toxicity when fentanyl is *used in combination* with other serotoninergic drugs.[56]

Undesirable effects

Also see Strong opioids, Box B, p.365.

Very common (>10%): drowsiness, dizziness, headache, insomnia, nausea, vomiting, constipation; muscle rigidity (including thoracic muscles) when given IV.

Common (<10%, >1%): anxiety, visual disturbance, palpitations, dry mouth, anorexia, dyspepsia, abdominal pain, diarrhoea, sweating, vasodilation.

Topical effects: Occasional skin irritation, hypersensitivity.

Dose and use

As with all opioids, patients must be monitored for undesirable effects, particularly nausea and vomiting, and constipation. Depending on individual circumstances, an anti-emetic should be prescribed for regular or p.r.n. use, (see QCG: Nausea and vomiting, p.240) and, routinely, a laxative prescribed (see QCG: Opioid-induced constipation, p.42).

Opioids can impair driving ability and patients should be counselled accordingly (see p.743).

TD

The use of TD fentanyl patches is summarized in the Quick Clinical Guide (see p.417). These and the comments in this section are based on a dose conversion ratio of PO **morphine** to TD fentanyl of 100:1. Prescribers using the manufacturer's ratio of 150:1 should follow the dose conversion guidelines in the SPC (Appendix 2, Box B, p.860).

Prescribers considering the use of TD fentanyl as a first-line strong opioid, particularly in opioid-naïve patients, should be sufficiently experienced and able to closely monitor the patient; otherwise seek specialist advice.

In 2013, in response to large numbers of safety incident reports about **buprenorphine** and fentanyl TD patches, the Care Quality Commission highlighted the need to ensure that:

- use is appropriate, e.g. chronic *not* acute pain
- dose is appropriate, i.e. in line with published conversion charts
- dose is titrated appropriately, i.e. no more than 50% of the previous daily dose
- date and site of application are recorded to avoid inadvertent dose omission or duplication.

Further, to avoid confusing patients and carers, prescribing by brand was recommended.[6]

Under no circumstances should a *reservoir* patch be cut in an attempt to reduce the dose (see Cautions).

TD patches and MRI scans: Fentanyl patches should be removed before the patient enters the scan room due to the risks from heating. Patients should be advised to bring a replacement patch with them to facilitate this (also see p.831).

Two different TD formulations are currently available:

- *matrix* patch (e.g. Durogesic DTrans®, Matrifen Matrix®) the fentanyl is evenly distributed throughout a drug-in-adhesive matrix, and the release of fentanyl is controlled by the physical characteristics of the matrix
- *reservoir* patch (e.g. Fentalis Reservoir®, Tilofyl®) the fentanyl is contained within a reservoir, and the release of fentanyl is controlled by a rate-limiting membrane.

Absorption of the fentanyl through the skin and into the systemic circulation is influenced by both the condition of the skin and cutaneous blood flow. Thus, if the skin is warm and vasodilated, the rate of absorption will be increased.

Bio-equivalence has been demonstrated between two different makes of *matrix* patches, and between the *matrix* and *reservoir* patches.[23,61–63] However, the matrix patch is thinner (because there is no reservoir) and, for equal strengths, more than one-third smaller. Consequently, to avoid confusing patients and carers, prescribing by brand is recommended.[6]

In North America, the manufacturer stresses that TD fentanyl should be commenced *only* in patients who have been receiving strong opioids in a dose at least equivalent to a 25microgram/h patch for ≥1 week, such as:

- **morphine** 60mg/day PO
- **oxycodone** 30mg/day PO
- **hydromorphone** 8mg/day PO.

In the UK, most manufacturers and the Care Quality Commission/NHS England recommend against use in opioid-naïve patients, advising initial titration with immediate-release **morphine**.[6] Nonetheless, there are reports where TD fentanyl has been used satisfactorily as a first-line strong opioid in, for example, patients with severe dysphagia, renal failure or who are living in social circumstances where there is a high risk of diversion and tablet misuse. (Note. Misuse of TD fentanyl can also occur; see Cautions). TD fentanyl is also used in totally opioid-naïve patients at centres which do not use weak opioids.[64–67] However, prescribers considering the use of TD fentanyl as a first-line strong opioid, particularly in opioid-naïve patients, should be sufficiently experienced and able to closely monitor the patient; otherwise specialist advice should be sought. Authorized starting doses for TD fentanyl as a first-line strong opioid in the UK are 12–25microgram/h, depending on the individual product, equivalent to **morphine** 30–60mg/24h PO. Thus, the 12microgram/h dose will be a safer starting dose for *totally opioid-naïve* patients and for some *strong* (but not weak) *opioid-naïve* patients, e.g. frail patients using low doses of weak opioid with moderate pain. Undesirable effects, e.g. nausea and vomiting, are more frequent in strong opioid-naïve patients and, in separate studies, resulted in one-sixth and one-third of patients discontinuing TD fentanyl 12microgram/h and 25microgram/h respectively.[68,69]

It is important to give adequate rescue doses of **morphine** (see QCG: Use of transdermal fentanyl patches, p.417) or other strong opioid. Adjusting the patch strength on a daily basis is not recommended.[70] With inpatients, the use of a monitoring chart is recommended (for an example, see www.palliativedrugs.com).[71]

SC/IM/IV

- start with a stat dose of 50–200microgram, and subsequently 50microgram p.r.n.
- reduce the dose in the elderly and debilitated, e.g. 12.5–25microgram SC p.r.n.
- traditionally p.r.n. dosing intervals are q1h, but more frequent dosing with close monitoring may be required in severe acute pain
- give IV by slow injection; this reduces the risk of muscular rigidity.

CSCI

In the UK, this route is recommended mostly in the setting of severe and end-stage renal impairment (eGFR<30mL/min) when pain is uncontrolled:[5]

- *opioid-naïve*
  - ▷ initial dose 100–300microgram/24h CSCI
  - ▷ allow 12.5–25microgram SC p.r.n q1h
- *converting from another opioid*
  - ▷ calculate equivalent dose (see Appendix 2, p.855)
  - ▷ reduce by 20% and use as initial dose
  - ▷ allow a suitable p.r.n. SC dose (conventionally, 1/6–1/10 of the total 24h CSCI dose).

If the patient is not in the last days of life, a switch to TD fentanyl may be possible once stable pain control is achieved. Select a patch which delivers a similar rate of fentanyl in microgram/h as the CSCI, discontinuing the CSCI at the same time as the first patch is applied.

For CSCI, dilute with WFI, 0.9% saline or 5% glucose. Volume constraints for a syringe driver can limit the use of higher doses of fentanyl and/or the ability to combine it with other drugs.

CSCI compatibility with other drugs: limited clinical experience suggests that fentanyl in doses <500microgram is compatible with **haloperidol**, **levomepromazine**, or **midazolam**, using WFI as diluent (also see Chapter 29, p.817). For further information, see www.palliativedrugs.com Syringe Driver Survey Database (SDSD).

Health professionals are encouraged to add details of any successful or unsuccessful combinations to the existing list of fentanyl combinations on the www.palliativedrugs.com SDSD.

If the required dose of CSCI fentanyl causes volume issues, consider using **alfentanil** instead (see p.390). However, because **alfentanil** has a shorter half-life, continue to use fentanyl SC p.r.n. for break-through pain.

Transmucosal fentanyl formulations could be used as an alternative p.r.n. analgesic, but only when the patient has sufficient time and ability to co-operate with the necessary titration (see p.419). Because bio-availability of transmucosal fentanyl is less than SC and varies widely, apply an appropriate reduction when adjusting the background CSCI dose based on the p.r.n. dose and frequency of use. Monitor the patient closely for signs of toxicity.

CIVI

Fentanyl CIVI is used in some centres (generally *not* UK) for initial control of cancer pain. When an effective stable dose is found, the route is switched to TD; continue the infusion unchanged for 6h after applying the patch, then discontinue.[72] This appears satisfactory for most patients; other methods exist, but are more complex.[72]

Supply

All preparations are Schedule 2 **CD**.

Transdermal products
Fentanyl (generic)
Matrix patches (for 3 days) 12microgram/h, 25microgram/h, 37.5microgram/h (Mezolar Matrix® only), 50microgram/h, 75microgram/h, 100microgram/h, 1 = £2.50, £3.50, £3, £6.50, £9.50 and £12 respectively.
Brands include Durogesic Dtrans®, Fencino®, Matrifen®, Mezolar Matrix®, Mylafent®, Opiodur®, Osmanil®, Victanyl®, Yemex®.
Reservoir patches (for 3 days) 25microgram/h, 50microgram/h, 75microgram/h, 100microgram/h, 1 = £3.50, £7, £10 and £12 respectively.
Brands include Fentalis Reservoir®, Tilofyl®.

Parenteral products
Fentanyl citrate (generic)
Injection 50microgram/mL, 2mL amp = £1, 10mL amp = £1.50.

1 Newshan G and Lefkowitz M (2001) Transdermal fentanyl for chronic pain in AIDS: a pilot study. *Journal of Pain and Symptom Management*. **21**: 69–77.
2 Canneti A *et al.* (2013) Safety and efficacy of transdermal buprenorphine and transdermal fentanyl in the treatment of neuropathic pain in AIDS patients. *Minerva Anestesiologica*. **79**: 871–883.
3 Tassinari D *et al.* (2011) Transdermal opioids as front line treatment of moderate to severe cancer pain: a systemic review. *Palliative Medicine*. **25**: 478–487.
4 NICE (2016) Moderate to severe acute post-operative pain: fentanyl transdermal system. *Evidence summary* ESNM77. www.nice.org.uk
5 King S *et al.* (2011) A systematic review of the use of opioid medication for those with moderate to severe cancer pain and renal impairment: A European palliative care research collaborative opioid guidelines project. *Palliative Medicine*. **25**: 525–552.
6 Care Quality Commission and NHS England (2013) Safer use of controlled drugs - preventing harms from fentanyl and buprenorphine transdermal patches. *Use of controlled drugs supporting information*. www.cqc.org.uk
7 Health Canada (2008) Fentanyl transdermal patch and fatal adverse reactions. *Canadian Adverse Reaction Newsletter*. **18**: 1–2.
8 Caraceni A *et al.* (2012) Use of opioid analgesics in the treatment of cancer pain: evidence-based recommendations from the EAPC. *Lancet Oncology*. **13**: e58–68.
9 Bernards C (1999) Clinical implications of physicochemical properties of opioids. In: C Stein (ed) *Opioids in Pain Control: basic and clinical aspects*. Cambridge University Press, Cambridge, pp. 166–187.
10 Ummenhofer W *et al.* (2000) Comparative spinal distribution and clearance kinetics of intrathecally administered morphine, fentanyl, alfentanil, and sufentanil. *Anesthesiology*. **92**: 739–953.
11 Herz A and Teschemacher H-J (1971) Activities and sites of antinociceptive action of morphine-like analgesics and kinetics of distribution following intravenous, intracerebral and intraventricular application. *Advances in Drug Research*. **6**: 79–119.
12 Bosilkovska M *et al.* (2012) Analgesics in patients with hepatic impairment: pharmacology and clinical implications. *Drugs*. **72**: 1645–1669.
13 Simpson R *et al.* (1997) Transdermal fentanyl as treatment for chronic low back pain. *Journal of Pain and Symptom Management*. **14**: 218–224.
14 Milligan K and Campbell C (1999) Transdermal fentanyl in patients with chronic, nonmalignant pain: a case study series. *Advances in Therapy*. **16**: 73–77.
15 Allan L *et al.* (2001) Randomised crossover trial of transdermal fentanyl and sustained release oral morphine for treating chronic non-cancer pain. *British Medical Journal*. **322**: 1154–1158.
16 Yeo W *et al.* (1997) Transdermal fentanyl for severe cancer-related pain. *Palliative Medicine*. **11**: 233–239.
17 Payne R *et al.* (1998) Quality of life and cancer pain: satisfaction and side effects with transdermal fentanyl versus oral morphine. *Journal of Clinical Oncology*. **16**: 1588–1593.
18 Sloan P *et al.* (1998) A clinical evaluation of transdermal therapeutic system fentanyl for the treatment of cancer pain. *Journal of Pain and Symptom Management*. **16**: 102–111.
19 Nugent M *et al.* (2001) Long-term observations of patients receiving transdermal fentanyl after a randomized trial. *Journal of Pain and Symptom Management*. **21**: 385–391.
20 Radbruch L *et al.* (2001) Transdermal fentanyl for the management of cancer pain: a survey of 1005 patients. *Palliative Medicine*. **15**: 309–321.
21 Hadley G *et al.* (2013) Transdermal fentanyl for cancer pain. *Cochrane Database of Systematic Reviews*. **10**: CD010270. www.thecochranelibrary.com
22 Derry S *et al.* (2016) Fentanyl for neuropathic pain in adults. *Cochrane Database of Systemtic Reviews*. **10**: CD011605. www.thecochranelibrary.com
23 Janssen-Cilag Ltd *Data on file*.
24 Donner B *et al.* (1998) Long-term treatment of cancer pain with transdermal fentanyl. *Journal of Pain and Symptom Management*. **15**: 168–175.
25 Arnet I *et al.* (2016) Poor adhesion of fentanyl transdermal patches may mimic end-of-dosage failure after 48 hours and prompt early patch replacement in hospitalized cancer pain patients. *Journal of Pain Research*. **9**: 993–999.
26 Koike K *et al.* (2016) A new once-a-day fentanyl citrate patch (Fentos Tape) could be a new treatment option in patients with end-of-dose failure using a 72-h transdermal fentanyl matrix patch. *Supportive Care in Cancer*. **24**: 1053–1059.
27 Donner B *et al.* (1996) Direct conversion from oral morphine to transdermal fentanyl: a multicenter study in patients with cancer pain. *Pain*. **64**: 527–534.
28 Mercadante S and Caraceni A (2011) Conversion ratios for opioid switching in the treatment of cancer pain: a systematic review. *Palliative Medicine*. **25**: 504–515.
29 Reddy A *et al.* (2016) The opioid rotation ratio of strong opioids to transdermal fentanyl in cancer patients. *Cancer*. **122**: 149–156.
30 Jia SS *et al.* (2015) Modified Glasgow prognostic score predicting high conversion ratio in opioid switching from oral oxycodone to transdermal fentanyl in patients with cancer pain. *International Journal of Clinical Experimental Medicine*. **8**: 7606–7612.
31 Matsumura C *et al.* (2016) Indication of adequate transdermal fentanyl dose in opioid switching from oral cxycodone in patients with cancer. *American Journal of Hospice and Palliative Care*. **33**: 109–114.
32 Mercadante S *et al.* (2007) Switching from transdermal drugs: an observational "N of 1" study of fentanyl and buprenorphine. *Journal of Pain and Symptom Management*. **34**: 532–538.
33 Mercadante S *et al.* (2009) Equipotent doses to switch from high doses of opioids to transdermal buprenorphine. *Supportive Care in Cancer*. **17**: 715–718.
34 Tassinari D *et al.* (2008) Adverse effects of transdermal opiates treating moderate-severe cancer pain in comparison to long-acting morphine: a meta-analysis and systematic review of the literature. *Journal of Palliative Medicine*. **11**: 492–501.
35 Hannon B *et al.* (2013) The role of fentanyl in refractory opioid-related acute colonic pseudo-obstruction. *Journal of Pain and Symptom Management*. **45**: e1–3.
36 Koo HC *et al.* (2010) Effect of transdermal fentanyl patches on the motility of the sphincter of oddi. *Gut and Liver*. **4**: 368–372.

37 Botterman J and Criel N (2011) Inappropriate use of high doses of transdermal fentanyl at admission to a palliative care unit. *Palliative Medicine*. **25**: 111–116.
38 Mauermann E *et al.* (2016) Does fentanyl lead to opioid-induced hyperalgesia in healthy volunteers? a double-blind, randomized, crossover trial. *Anesthesiology*. **124**: 453–463.
39 Van Nimmen NF *et al.* (2010) Fentanyl transdermal absorption linked to pharmacokinetic characteristics in patients undergoing palliative care. *Journal of Clinical Pharmacology*. **50**: 667–678.
40 Marquardt KA *et al.* (1995) Fentanyl remaining in a transdermal system following three days of continuous use. *Annals of Pharmacotherpy*. **29**: 969–971.
41 Heiskanen T *et al.* (2009) Transdermal fentanyl in cachectic cancer patients. *Pain*. **144**: 218–222.
42 Hadgraft J and Lane ME (2005) Skin permeation: the years of enlightenment. *International Journal of Pharmaceutics*. **305**: 2–12.
43 Gourlay GK *et al.* (1989) The transdermal administration of fentanyl in the treatment of post-operative pain: pharmacokinetics and pharmacodynamic effects. *Pain*. **37**: 193–202.
44 Capper SJ *et al.* (2010) Pharmacokinetics of fentanyl after subcutaneous administration in volunteers. *European Journal of Anaesthesiology*. **27**: 241–246.
45 Portenoy RK *et al.* (1993) Transdermal fentanyl for cancer pain. *Anesthesiology*. **78**: 36–43.
46 Smith J and Ellershaw J (1999) Improvement in pain control by change of fentanyl patch after 48 hours compared with 72 hours. *Poster EAPC Congress, Geneva*. PO1/1376.
47 Anonymous (2007) Safe use of fentanyl (Duragesic) patches. *Pharmacist's Letter/Prescriber's Letter*. **23**: 1–5.
48 FDA (2007) Fentanyl transdermal system (marketed as Duragesic) information. *Post Market Drug Safety Information for Patients and Providers*. www.fda.gov/Drugs/DrugsSafety/default.htm
49 MHRA (2008) Fentanyl patches: serious and fatal overdose from dosing errors, accidental exposure, and inappropriate use. *Drug Safety Update*. **2** www.mhra.gov.uk/safetyinformation
50 Sindali K *et al.* (2012) Life-threatening coma and full-thickness sunburn in a patient treated with transdermal fentanyl patches: a case report. *Journal of Medical Case Reports*. **6**: 220.
51 Jumbelic MI (2010) Deaths with transdermal fentanyl patches. *American Journal of Forensic Medicine and Pathology*. **31**: 18–21.
52 Hawley P (2013) Case report of severe bradycardia due to transdermal fentanyl. *Palliative Medicine*. **27**: 793–795.
53 Prosser JM *et al.* (2010) Complications of oral exposure to fentanyl transdermal delivery system patches. *Journal of Medical Toxicology*. **6**: 443–447.
54 Carson HJ *et al.* (2010) A fatality involving an unusual route of fentanyl delivery: Chewing and aspirating the transdermal patch. *Legal Medicine (Tokyo)*. **12**: 157–159.
55 Beletsky L and Davis CS (2017) Today's fentanyl crisis: Prohibition's Iron Law, revisited. *International Journal of Drug Policy*. **46**: 156–159.
56 Baxter K and Preston CL. *Stockley's Drug Interactions*. London: Pharmaceutical Press www.medicinescomplete.com (accessed May 2017).
57 Kharasch ED *et al.* (2004) Influence of hepatic and intestinal cytochrome P4503A activity on the acute disposition and effects of oral transmucosal fentanyl citrate. *Anesthesiology*. **101**: 729–737.
58 Takane H *et al.* (2005) Rifampin reduces the analgesic effect of transdermal fentanyl. *Annals of Pharmacotherpy*. **39**: 2139–2140.
59 Sasson M and Shvartzman P (2006) Fentanyl patch sufficient analgesia for only one day. *Journal of Pain and Symptom Management*. **31**: 389–391.
60 Morii H *et al.* (2007) Failure of pain control using transdermal fentanyl during rifampicin treatment. *Journal of Pain and Symptom Management*. **33**: 5–6.
61 Freynhagen R *et al.* (2005) Switching from reservoir to matrix systems for the transdermal delivery of fentanyl: a prospective, multicenter pilot study in outpatients with chronic pain. *Journal of Pain and Symptom Management*. **30**: 289–297.
62 Marier JF *et al.* (2006) Pharmacokinetics, tolerability, and performance of a novel matrix transdermal delivery system of fentanyl relative to the commercially available reservoir formulation in healthy subjects. *Journal of Clinical Pharmacology*. **46**: 642–653.
63 Kress HG *et al.* (2010) Transdermal fentanyl matrix patches Matrifen and Durogesic DTrans are bioequivalent. *European Journal of Pharmceutics and Biopharmaceutics*. **75**: 225–231.
64 Vielvoye-Kerkmeer A *et al.* (2000) Transdermal fentanyl in opioid-naive cancer pain patients: an open trial using transdermal fentanyl for the treatment of chronic cancer pain in opioid-naive patients and a group using codeine. *Journal of Pain and Symptom Management*. **19**: 185–192.
65 van Seventer R *et al.* (2003) Comparison of TTS-fentanyl with sustained-release oral morphine in the treatment of patients not using opioids for mild-to-moderate pain. *Current Medical Research Opinion*. **19**: 457–469.
66 Tawfik MO *et al.* (2004) Use of transdermal fentanyl without prior opioid stabilization in patients with cancer pain. *Current Medical Research Opinion*. **20**: 259–267.
67 Othman AH *et al.* (2016) Transdermal fentanyl for cancer pain management in opioid-naive pediatric cancer patients. *Pain Medicine*. (Epub ahead of print).
68 Mercadante S *et al.* (2010) Low doses of transdermal fentanyl in opioid-naive patients with cancer pain. *Current Medical Research Opinion*. **26**: 2765–2768.
69 Chang JT *et al.* (2010) Transdermal fentanyl for pain caused by radiotherapy in head and neck cancer patients treated in an outpatient setting: a multicenter trial in Taiwan. *Japanese Journal of Clinical Oncology*. **40**: 307–312.
70 Korte W *et al.* (1996) Day-to-day titration to initiate transdermal fentanyl in patients with cancer pain: short and long term experiences in a prospective study of 39 patients. *Journal of Pain and Symptom Management*. **11**: 139–146.
71 Palliativedrugs.com (2017) Strong opioid transdermal patch monitoring chart. *Document Library*. Pain (strong opioids): www.palliativedrugs.com
72 Samala RV *et al.* (2014) Efficacy and safety of a six-hour continuous overlap method for converting intravenous to transdermal fentanyl in cancer pain. *Journal of Pain and Symptom Management*. **48**: 132–136.

Updated September 2017

Quick Clinical Guide: Use of transdermal fentanyl patches

These recommendations use only a dose conversion ratio for PO morphine to TD fentanyl of 100:1 and, as such, differ from those in UK SPCs. It is an approximation, and inevitably there will be individual variation.

Pain not relieved by morphine will generally not be relieved by fentanyl. If in doubt, seek specialist advice before prescribing TD fentanyl.

1 Indications for using TD fentanyl instead of morphine include:
- intolerable undesirable effects with morphine, e.g. nausea and vomiting, constipation, hallucinations, dysphagia
- renal failure (fentanyl has no active metabolite)
- 'tablet phobia' or poor compliance with oral medication
- high risk of tablet misuse/diversion.

2 TD fentanyl is contra-indicated in patients with acute (short-term) pain and in those who need rapid dose titration for severe uncontrolled pain. Generally, it is *not* recommended as a first-line strong opioid (seek specialist advice). Thus, TD fentanyl is most appropriate for patients already on a stable dose of morphine (or other strong opioid) for ≥1 week.

3 TD fentanyl patches are available in six strengths: 12, 25, 37.5, 50, 75 and 100microgram/h for 3 days. The patch brand, dose and duration should be stated on the prescription to avoid confusion.

4 Use the table below to decide a safe starting dose for TD fentanyl, and an appropriate rescue dose. The starting dose for patients taking a weak opioid should be 12microgram/h.

5 For patients taking a dose of morphine that is not the exact equivalent of a fentanyl patch, it will be necessary to opt for a patch which is either slightly more or slightly less than the morphine dose. Thus, if the patient still has pain, round up to a higher patch strength; if pain-free and frail, round down. However, if switching because of possible opioid-induced hyperalgesia, reduce the calculated equivalent dose by 25–50%.

Comparative doses of PO morphine and TD fentanyl (based on dose conversion ratio 100:1)

PO Morphine		*SC/IV Morphine*		*TD Fentanl*	
mg/24h	*p.r.n. mg*[a]	*mg/24h*[b]	*p.r.n. mg*[a]	*microgram/h*	*microgram/24h*
30	5	15	2.5	12	0.3
60	10	30	5	25	0.6
90	15	45	7.5	37.5	0.9
120	20	60	10	50	1.2
180	30	90	15	75	1.8
240	40	120	20	100[c]	2.4

a. using traditional 1/6 of total daily dose as p.r.n. dose

b. assuming morphine SC/IV is twice as potent as PO

c. for combinations of patches, add the p.r.n. doses together, e.g. 100 + 75microgram/h patches = 20 + 15mg morphine SC/IV = 35mg morphine SC/IV, but can round up to 40mg or down to 30mg for convenience.

6 The date of application and/or the date for renewal should be written on the patch. Apply to dry, non-inflamed, non-irradiated, hairless skin on the upper trunk or arm. Body hair may be clipped with scissors but not shaved. If the skin is washed beforehand, use only water; do not use soap and do not apply oils, cream or ointment to the area. Press patch firmly in place for at least 30 seconds. Micropore® or Tegaderm® can be used to ensure adherence. Careful removal of the patch helps to minimize local skin irritation.

7 Effective systemic analgesic concentrations are generally reached in <12h. When converting from:
   - 4-hourly PO morphine, give regular doses for the first 12h after applying the patch
   - 12-hourly m/r morphine, apply the patch and the final m/r dose at the same time
   - 24-hourly m/r morphine, apply the patch 12h after the final m/r dose
   - CSCI/CIVI morphine, continue the infusion unchanged for 8–12h after applying the patch, then discontinue
   - CSCI/CIVI fentanyl, continue the infusion unchanged for 6h after applying the patch, then discontinue.

8 Steady-state plasma concentrations of fentanyl are generally achieved in 36–48h; the patient should use p.r.n. doses liberally during the first 3 days, particularly the first 24h. Safe rescue doses of PO morphine are given in the table above.

9 After 48h, if a patient still needs 2 or more rescue doses of morphine/day, the strength of the next patch to be applied should be increased by 12–25microgram/h. (Note. With the manufacturer's recommended starting doses, about 50% of patients need to increase the patch strength after the first 3 days).

10 About 10% of patients experience opioid withdrawal symptoms when changed from morphine to TD fentanyl. These manifest with symptoms like gastric flu and last for a few days; p.r.n. doses of morphine will relieve troublesome symptoms.

11 Fentanyl is less constipating than morphine; halve the dose of laxatives when starting fentanyl and re-titrate.

12 Fentanyl may cause nausea and vomiting; if necessary, prescribe an anti-emetic, e.g. haloperidol 500microgram–1.5mg stat & at bedtime.

13 In febrile patients, the rate of absorption of fentanyl increases, and may cause toxicity, e.g. drowsiness. Absorption is also enhanced by high ambient temperatures or external heat sources over the patch, e.g. electric blanket or hot-water bottle; patients should be warned about this. Patients may shower with a patch but should not soak in a hot bath. Remove patches before MRI scans.

14 Remove patches after 72h; change the position of the new patches so as to rest the underlying skin for 3–6 days. The use of a monitoring chart is recommended for inpatients.

15 A reservoir of fentanyl accumulates in the body, and significant blood concentrations persist for at least 24h after discontinuing TD fentanyl.

16 TD fentanyl is unsatisfactory in <5% of patients. However, discontinuation is more common when TD fentanyl is used in strong opioid-naïve patients.

17 Additional or alternative analgesic approaches should be considered when the dose exceeds 300microgram/h.

18 In moribund patients, continue TD fentanyl and give additional SC morphine p.r.n. (see Table). If >2 p.r.n. doses are required/24h, give morphine by CSCI, starting with a dose equal to the sum of the p.r.n. doses over the preceding 24h. If necessary, adjust the p.r.n. dose taking into account the total opioid dose (i.e. TD fentanyl + CSCI morphine).

19 Used patches still contain fentanyl; after removal, fold the patch with the adhesive side inwards and discard in a sharps container (hospital) or dustbin (home), and wash hands. Ultimately, any unused patches should be returned to a pharmacy.

Updated September 2017

FENTANYL (TRANSMUCOSAL)

For information on transdermal and parenteral use of fentanyl, see p.409.

Relative to PO opioids, transmucosal fentanyl products are expensive (about £5–12/episode). They are more effective than placebo, but direct comparison with PO **morphine**, or each other, is limited. Careful patient selection, training, titration and monitoring are required to ensure optimum use. They are *not* interchangeable.

Medicine advisory boards (Scottish Medicines Consortium, All Wales Medicines Strategy Group) have recommended restricting their use to patients unsuitable for other short-acting opioids, e.g. PO **morphine**.

5

Class: Strong opioid analgesic.

Indications: Break-through cancer pain in patients on regular strong opioids. The use of fentanyl injection SL or nasally is off-label.

Contra-indications: Use in strong opioid-naïve patients, acute non-cancer pain (e.g. postoperative pain, migraine), severe obstructive airways disease. *Instanyl®*: previous facial radiotherapy, recurrent epistaxis.

Pharmacology

Fentanyl (*like* **morphine**) is a strong μ-opioid receptor agonist. It has a relatively low molecular weight and (*unlike* **morphine**) is lipophilic, which makes it suitable for TD (see p.409) and transmucosal administration. Multiple formulations are now authorized for the treatment of break-through cancer pain. In the UK, these include SL tablets (Abstral®), a lozenge (Actiq®), a buccal/SL tablet (Effentora®) and nasal sprays (Instanyl®, Pecfent®). Elsewhere, other formulations available may include a SL tablet (Recivit®), a SL spray (Subsys®) and a buccal film (Breakyl®).

Break-through cancer pain generally has a relatively rapid onset (median 5–10min) and short duration (45–60min), but ranges from <1min to 4–6h (see p.295).[1] By comparison, PO opioids such as **morphine**, on average, take about 30–40min to achieve meaningful pain relief and have a longer duration of effect (3–6h).[2] Thus, transmucosal fentanyl products aim to provide rapid onset pain relief which better matches the time course of a typical break-through pain.

Pharmacokinetics

The transmucosal formulations range from an aqueous solution of fentanyl (Instanyl®) to combinations which include bio-adhesive substances, e.g. croscarmellose (Abstral®), pectin (Pecfent®). The pharmacokinetic characteristics of the products vary and they are *not* interchangeable (Tables 1 and 2). Fentanyl is readily absorbed transmucosally and the bio-adhesive substances tend to *slow* its rate of absorption. Various justifications are given (e.g. to aid mucosal adherence, to attenuate the peak plasma concentration) but the fact that a novel delivery system can be patented (although not fentanyl itself) is also relevant.

With the buccal/SL products, the amount of fentanyl absorbed directly across the mucosa or swallowed varies with formulation and route of administration. A lack of saliva will impede dissolution of tablet formulations and patients with a dry mouth should moisten it with water beforehand. About two thirds of any swallowed fentanyl will be eliminated by intestinal or hepatic first-pass metabolism. Nonetheless, significant amounts of swallowed fentanyl are absorbed, e.g. about 25% and 15% of the systemically available Actiq® and Effentora® respectively is via GI absorption.[11,6,12] The effects of the GI absorption on the plasma concentration of fentanyl include producing a 'double peak', maintaining high levels for longer (e.g. >2h) and contributing to the wide range in T_{max}.[5]

The rate and degree of absorption of fentanyl from the nasal cavity is dependent on mucosal perfusion. Vasoconstrictive nasal decongestants, e.g. **oxymetazoline**, double the time to maximum plasma concentration and halve the maximum plasma concentration of a dose of nasal fentanyl. Thus, the concurrent use of vasoconstrictive nasal decongestants with Instanyl® or Pecfent® should be avoided.

Once absorbed, fentanyl is rapidly distributed to the best perfused tissues, i.e. brain, heart, lungs, and then to fat, muscle and other tissues. Subsequently, fentanyl is redistributed between the deep tissue compartment and plasma. This pattern of rapid distribution, followed by a slower

Table 1 Selected characteristics and pharmacokinetic data for *oromucosal* fentanyl products available in the UK[a,b]

	Abstral®	*Actiq*®	*Effentora*® [c]
Formulation	SL tablet	Buccal lozenge	Buccal/SL tablet
Dose range and presentation	100, 200, 300, 400, 600, 800microgram Different shapes; packs of 10 or 30	200, 400, 600, 800, 1,200, 1,600microgram On a stick, marked with dose and different colours; packs of 3 or 30	100, 200, 400, 600, 800microgram 100 smaller in size; embossed 1, 2, etc.; packs of 4 or 28
Maximum dose/episode	800microgram	1,600microgram	800microgram
Maximum frequency of use	Maximum 4 episodes/24h, ideally ≥4h apart (see Dose and use)	Maximum 4 episodes/24h, ideally ≥4h apart (see Dose and use)	Maximum 4 episodes/24h, ≥4h apart
Approximate cost per dose (also see Supply)	£5	£7	£5
Time to dissolution	<2min	Applied over 15min	Buccal 14–25min; SL quicker
Onset of action[d]	10min	15min	10min
Time to peak plasma concentration, median (range)	30–60min (15–240) Longer with highest dose	Across dose range 90min (30–480)[3,4] Longer with highest dose	Pooled data 53min (20–240)[5] Longer with highest dose
Plasma halflife	Mean 5–14h	Median 18h (7–49) 800microgram[3]	Median 12h (2–44), pooled data[5]
Duration of action	≥1h	≥1h (≤3.5h reported with higher doses)[6]	≥2h
Bio-availability	55%	50% (25% transmucosal, 25% PO)[6]	65% (50% transmucosal, 15% PO)
Comments		Requires continual movement around the mouth; less effective if finished <15min as more is swallowed	Absorption not affected by mild (grade 1) mucositis[7]

a. the source (i.e. healthy volunteers vs. patients) and quality (e.g. small number of subjects, whole dose range not studied, use of massage over buccal tablet) of the data varies widely

b. data based on venous blood sampling; with arterial sampling, a higher maximum concentration is achieved about 15min quicker[8]

c. pharmacokinetics are similar for either buccal or SL placement

d. earliest *statistically significant* difference between fentanyl product and placebo in mean pain intensity difference; a *clinically meaningful* difference has been variably defined and generally takes longer (see text).

Table 2 Selected characteristics and pharmacokinetic data for *intranasal* fentanyl products[a]

	Instanyl®	*Pecfent®*
Formulation	Nasal spray	Nasal spray
Dose range and presentation	50, 100, 200microgram/spray (100microL) 1 dose repeated once after 10min p.r.n.; colour coded and in single, 10 and 20 dose bottles	100, 200, 400 and 800microgram; given as 1 or 2 doses of 100 or 400microgram/spray (100microL); colour coded and in 8 and 32 dose bottles
Maximum dose/episode	400microgram	800microgram
Maximum frequency of use	Maximum 4 episodes/24h, ≥4h apart	Maximum 4 episodes/24h, ≥4h apart
Approximate cost per spray (also see Supply)	£6; up to 1/2 require 2 doses, thus average cost up to £9	£4.50; about 1/2 require 200 or 800microgram dose, thus average cost = £7
Time to dissolution	N/A	N/A
Onset of action[b]	5min	10min
Time to peak plasma concentration, median (range)	Across dose range 12–15min (6–90min)[9]	Across dose range 15–21min (5–180min)[4]
Plasma halflife	Median 19h (8–30); 200microgram, 2 doses 10min apart[10]	Mean 15–25h
Duration of action	≥1h	≥1h
Bio-availability	90%	No data
Comments	Non-preserved solution, pH 6.6, osmolality ~0.9% saline	Preserved solution containing pectin, adjusted for pH and osmolality. Cmax is about 1/3 of that of Instanyl. Audible click denotes dose administered; visual priming guide and dose counter, end-of-use lock

a. the source (i.e. healthy volunteers vs. patients) and quality (e.g. small number of subjects, whole dose range not studied) of the data varies widely

b. earliest *statistically significant* difference between fentanyl product and placebo in mean pain intensity difference; a *clinically meaningful* difference has been variably defined and can take longer (see text).

redistribution explains why fentanyl has a relatively short duration of action despite a long halflife (Tables 1 and 2). However, with repeat administration, saturation of the deep tissue compartment can occur, resulting in higher peak plasma concentrations of fentanyl and a more prolonged effect.

Up to 85% of fentanyl is protein bound, mainly to α_1-acid glycoprotein, but also to albumin and lipoproteins. Elimination mainly involves biotransformation in the liver by CYP3A4 to inactive norfentanyl, which is excreted in the urine. Less than 7% is excreted unchanged. The SPCs of all of the transmucosal fentanyl products advise caution in their use in patients with moderate–severe hepatic or renal impairment, but this is based on limited data which suggests a reduced clearance of fentanyl, e.g. via alterations in metabolic clearance and plasma protein binding. Nonetheless, fentanyl is a reasonable option for patients with renal impairment or failure (also see p.409 and p.693),[13] including those with hepatorenal syndrome (see p.709).[14]

Pharmacokinetic studies of repeat/chronic dosing of the transmucosal products are limited. Repeating a dose of Pecfent® after an interval of 1 or 2h significantly increases the maximum plasma concentration, but not when given 4h apart.[4] Accumulation of fentanyl can occur with regular use; when Abstral® (whole of dose range) or Effentora® (400microgram) are given q6h, steady state is reached after about 3–5 days, and the maximum plasma concentration becomes double that of the initial dose.[15,16] Thus, even when an effective and tolerable dose is identified through titration, with subsequent regular use, accumulation, and undesirable effects could occur.

Pharmacodynamics

Generally, patients recruited to the development studies for the fentanyl transmucosal products were relatively young (mean age 50–60 years), had a good performance status (ECOG PS 0–2), no clinically relevant renal or hepatic impairment and were taking regular scheduled doses of an opioid equivalent to 160–280mg morphine PO/24h. Thus, additional caution is required when giving these products to patients with characteristics which differ from this group, particularly those who are elderly. A sober critique of the published papers is also required for various reasons, including:

- many studies are sponsored by the manufacturer and thus lack impartiality
- although similar methods of evaluation are used across studies, the criteria used to define a response vary, making direct comparison difficult (see below)
- some approaches undertaken in the studies do not reflect recommended clinical practice, e.g.:
  - ▷ only single doses of Abstral® were used for titration and maintenance in the study on which its safety data is based, with the effective dose confirmed over several consecutive episodes; by comparison, in the SPC, a second dose is permitted during titration, with no mention of confirmation of the effective dose[17]
  - ▷ Effentora® tablet remnants were 'massaged' after 10–15min in the pharmacokinetic and some efficacy studies, potentially artificially enhancing absorption and efficacy data[18]
  - ▷ patients who had already used Instanyl® were enrolled into an efficacy study, artificially enhancing the proportion achieving successful titration (>90% vs. more usual 60–70%)[10]
  - ▷ in some instances the regulatory authorities expressed concerns about the amount and/or the quality of the data, e.g. Abstral® pharmacokinetic data, Instanyl® safety reporting.[10,19]

For speed of onset of analgesia, generally what is promoted is the earliest *statistically significant* difference in pain intensity between the fentanyl product and placebo (generally 5–15min). Although some patients report a reduction in pain intensity which is considered *clinically meaningful* by this time, this generally takes longer for most products. Reliable comparison of the different products is difficult because the definition and calculation of a clinically meaningful change varies, e.g. reduction in pain intensity score from baseline of ≥2/10 or 30–33%, by episode (at least one or all) or by patient. Further, applying different criteria to the same data can produce different times, e.g. for Pecfent®, half of the patients experience a reduction in pain intensity score of ≥2 by 15min, but a ≥33% reduction takes 30min.[4,20] (Note. It has been suggested that a ≥50% improvement in pain intensity is required to be of *substantial* clinical importance.[21]) However, data suggest that for half of the episodes, an improvement in pain intensity of at least moderate clinical importance appears by about 10min (Instanyl®[22]), 15min (Pecfent®[20]) or 30min (Abstral®—[23] Actiq®[24] Effentora®[25]). Even so, in up to a quarter of episodes, an alternative rescue analgesic is needed because of an inadequate response to the fentanyl product. Clinicians must provide careful explanation to ensure the patient uses both rescue analgesics correctly.

High-quality comparative data, either between products or with PO analgesics, are limited.[26] Generally, the transmucosal products perform statistically significantly better than the immediate-release PO formulations tested, but the absolute differences in outcomes are relatively small, making their clinical relevance uncertain (Box A).

Box A Higher quality active comparator studies of transmucosal fentanyl products

Actiq® vs. PO morphine tablets[24]

Actiq®, titrated to an effective dose, has been compared with morphine *tablets* (previously identified effective dose, encapsulated to maintain blinding) in a double-blind, double-dummy, multiple cross-over study. For the primary and secondary outcomes, Actiq® was statistically superior to PO morphine tablets. However, the differences were small and their clinical relevance uncertain.

For example, for Actiq® vs. PO morphine tablets, the proportion of episodes after 15min with clinical meaningful pain relief (defined as a ≥33% reduction in pain intensity) was 42 vs. 32%. Nonetheless, >90% of patients chose to continue with Actiq®.

continued

Box A Continued

Effentora® vs. PO oxycodone tablets[27,28]

Effentora® titrated to an effective dose, has been compared with oxycodone *tablets* (titrated to an effective dose and encapsulated to maintain blinding) in double-blind, double-dummy, cross-over studies in opioid-tolerant patients mostly with non-cancer break-through pain (only two had cancer pain). Findings were similar in both studies; for primary and most secondary outcomes, Effentora® was statistically superior to PO oxycodone tablets. However, the differences were small and their clinical relevance uncertain.

For example, in the larger of the two studies,[27] for Effentora® vs. PO oxycodone tablets:

- mean (SD) pain intensity difference at 15min (primary outcome) was 0.8 (1.1) vs. 0.6 (0.9)
- % of episodes with a reduction in pain intensity of ≥33% was 13 vs. 9% (15min) and 41 vs. 32% (30min); for a reduction ≥50%, it was 6 vs. 4% (15min) and 21 vs. 16% (30min)
- patients rated the overall medication performance as 'good' to 'excellent' in 41 vs. 26% of episodes at 30min and 79 vs. 71% at 60min.

Pecfent® vs. PO morphine tablets[29,30]

Pecfent®, titrated to an effective dose, has been compared with encapsulated morphine *tablets* (one sixth of the total daily dose, or previously identified effective dose) in a double-blind, double-dummy, multiple cross-over study. For the primary and most secondary outcomes, Pecfent® was statistically superior to PO morphine tablets. However, the differences were small and their clinical relevance uncertain.

For example, for Pecfent® vs. PO morphine tablets:

- mean (SD) pain intensity difference at 15min (primary outcome) was 3.0 (0.2) vs. 2.7 (0.2)
- % of episodes with clinical meaningful pain relief (defined as a ≥2 reduction in pain intensity) was 25 vs. 23% (5min); 52 vs. 45% (10min) and 76 vs. 69% (15min).

Instanyl® vs. Actiq® [10,31]

Instanyl® and Actiq® (both titrated to an effective dose) have been compared in an open label RCT. The primary outcome was time to meaningful pain relief, measured by stop-watch. The fastest time to meaningful pain relief was significantly more likely with Instanyl® than Actiq®, with a median difference of 5min (11 vs. 16min respectively). A second dose of Instanyl® or Actiq® was required in about 60% and 30% of episodes respectively. For Instanyl® this was permitted 10min after the first dose, and for Actiq® 15min after fully consuming the first dose, i.e. at least 30min after starting the first dose. Usual rescue analgesia was required in 5–8% of episodes. Patients found the administration of Instanyl® easier and overall preferred Instanyl® (75%) to Actiq® (25%).

Given the mismatch between the time-action relationship of PO **morphine** and the typical time course of a break-through pain, it is interesting how well PO **morphine** performs in these studies. Unlike the fentanyl product, the PO **morphine** was not optimized in a titration phase and was given as *tablets* rather than as a *solution*, which is absorbed and acts more quickly. Studies have reported a median (range) T_{max} of 60min (20–90) vs. 125min (40–240) and mean time to meaningful pain relief of about 15min vs. 30min for morphine solution vs. tablets respectively.[32,33] Only an inadequate comparison of Abstral® with PO **morphine** *solution* is currently available.[34]

Abstral® 100microgram has been compared with SC **morphine** 5mg in a single dose, double-blind, double-dummy, RCT.[35] The SL route was preferred by >90% of patients. Although pain relief over 30–60min was similar, the results favoured **morphine**, with fewer patients requiring a second dose compared to Abstral® (35% vs. 50%). Notably, for 70% of patients their regular opioid dose was equivalent to PO **morphine** 20–60mg/24h, i.e. lower than the minimum recommended by the manufacturer (see Dose and use).

The lack of high quality comparative data among the transmucosal products prevents conclusions about the best to use. However, the practical aspects of using some of the products have been compared in a patient satisfaction survey.[36] Following instruction, 30 patients were asked to use a single *placebo* version of Abstral®, Effentora® and Instanyl® and to rate factors such as ease of access from packaging, ease of administration and palatability; they also rated their current rescue analgesic (generally PO **morphine** or **oxycodone**) similarly. They were asked to indicate if they would be prepared to use the transmucosal product and, if so, which they felt was the best and why. Several themes emerged:

- *ease of access:* the fentanyl products were generally more difficult to access than usual rescue analgesia, particularly the child-proof container for Instanyl®
- *ease of use:* Abstral® and the usual rescue analgesia were equal best
- *palatability:* Abstral® was rated best
- *patients willing to use:* Abstral® (90%) vs. Effentora® and Instanyl® (about 60% each); three patients would not use any (did not like the product or could not open the packaging)
- *which is best and why?:*
  - ▷ Abstral® (~70%); easy to access and use, dissolved quickly
  - ▷ Instanyl® (~20%); quick to use (once you get into package), route familiar
  - ▷ Effentora® (~10%); liked sensation in the mouth
  - ▷ one could not choose between Abstral® and Effentora®.

The use of placebos means that overall satisfaction with the products could not be compared. Nonetheless, taking these practical issues and other factors into account, the *PCF* suggests the following in patients with cancer taking regular strong opioids and experiencing break-through cancer pain:

- use immediate-release PO strong opioids first-line and titrate accordingly (include a trial of a PO solution if tablets not adequate); only when inadequate with regards to speed of onset of action or prolonged undesirable effects should the transmucosal products be considered (echoed in recent NICE guidance)[37]
- a patient's circumstances should be considered carefully to ensure they fulfil the necessary requirements for use of a transmucosal product, e.g. current opioid dose, ability to access, use, store and dispose of the product reliably etc. (see Dose and use)
- decide which route and product is the most appropriate, i.e.:
  - ▷ *nasal:* generally works quicker and shorter lasting (less PO absorption) than the SL/buccal route; Pecfent® works slightly slower than Instanyl®, but has a safer, accountable delivery system, and is cheaper
  - ▷ *SL/buccal:* there is little to choose from in terms of efficacy; Abstral® dissolves the quickest, making it the most convenient to use.

There may be other more specific reasons which guide choice of route, e.g. patient preference, presence of severe dry mouth or mucositis (use nasal), or frequent nose bleeds (use SL/buccal).

In contrast to *PCF* and NICE guidance,[37] European guidelines recommend that either PO or transmucosal fentanyl products can be used for break-through cancer pain without clearly distinguishing a first-line preference.[38]

There are limited data on the wider impact of the transmucosal fentanyl products, e.g. on quality of life, mood, physical function and health care utilization.[39–41]

Unauthorized alternatives

Some palliative care services use the parenteral formulation of various fentanils for SL administration, e.g. fentanyl (50microgram/mL), **sufentanil** (50microgram/mL, not UK) and **alfentanil** (500microgram/mL and 5mg/mL).[42,43] Onset of analgesic effect may be broadly similar (5–10min) but duration of effect is likely to differ (fentanyl>**sufentanil**>**alfentanil**) (see **Alfentanil**, p.390). Although the availability of authorized transmucosal fentanyl products has largely rendered this practice unnecessary, it may still have a role when either the authorized products are unavailable or only small doses are required.

Using a 1mL graduated oral syringe:

- start with fentanyl 25–50microgram SL (0.5–1mL of 50microgram/mL injection formulation)
- if necessary, increase to 50–100microgram SL; many patients do not need more than this
- doses >100microgram are impractical because 2mL is the maximum volume that can be reliably kept in the mouth for transmucosal absorption (see p.393).[43]

The 50microgram/mL fentanyl injection solution has also been administered as a nasal spray. In adults this approach is limited by the large dose volume. However, it has provided effective analgesia in children 1–18 years old presenting pre-hospital or to the emergency department with acute moderate–severe pain.[44–46] A 1mL syringe attached to a mucosal atomizer device permits the appropriate amount of fentanyl to be converted into a spray. The initial dose is generally 1–2microgram/kg, administered in divided doses to a maximum of 1mL in each nostril, with some centres permitting a second dose of 0.5microgram/kg after 10min if required.[47]

To overcome the dose/volume issues, higher concentration fentanyl solutions up to 300microgram/mL have also been used. However, compared with the standard solution, they are less readily available, more expensive and, at least in children <50kg, no more effective.[44,48] Obviously, the authorized products avoid the dose/volume issue, and the use of Instanyl® 50–100microgram by paramedics for acute severe pain has been reported.[49]

Further dilution of the 50microgram/mL fentanyl injection solution to produce 10 and 25microgram/mL solutions, has permitted 1 and 2.5microgram/0.1mL doses to be administered intranasally to dying neonates and infants with respiratory distress.[50] However, evidence supporting the use of transmucosal fentanyl to relieve breathlessness in other circumstances is limited.[51–54]

5

Cautions

All companies provide additional information for prescribers, pharmacists and patients; these include check-lists to ensure proper patient selection and education around use, signs of opioid overdose, safe storage and disposal. Store out of reach of children (accidental deaths have occurred).

In 2007, after reports of serious overdoses and deaths in the USA, the FDA issued a safety warning about the use of Fentora® (Effentora®). Factors which contributed to the adverse drug events included improper:

- patient selection, e.g. non-opioid tolerant, acute (non-cancer) pain
- dosing, e.g. wrong dose prescribed, exceeding recommended maximum use
- product substitution, e.g. like for like swap from Actiq® to Fentora®.

Thus, these products need to be used correctly, specifically:

- do *not* use in opioid naïve (non-tolerant) patients, including those who only take strong opioids p.r.n.
- they are contra-indicated in the management of acute or postoperative pain, including headache/migraine
- they are not interchangeable; do *not* convert patients on a microgram per microgram basis from one to another; it is necessary to titrate the new formulation
- when dispensing, do *not* substitute one product for another.

Use with caution in patients with COPD or other medical conditions predisposing them to respiratory depression (e.g. myasthenia gravis) or susceptible to the intracranial effects of hypercapnia (e.g. those with raised intracranial pressure). Also if bradyarrhythmia, elderly, cachectic, debilitated, moderate–severe hepatic or renal impairment (also see p.681 and p.703), hypovolaemia, hypotension; and if a history or high risk of abuse or diversion.

Mouth wounds, mucositis (may enhance absorption); nasal vasoconstrictive decongestants (reduce the effect), other nasal medications (the SPC for Instanyl® recommends avoiding because of lack of data, whereas that for Pecfent® advises avoiding within 15min of a dose), epistaxis.

Actiq® contains 2g of sugars; inform diabetic patients, also risk of tooth decay (uncommon).

Drug interactions

Fentanyl is metabolized by CYP3A4. Caution is required with concurrent use of drugs which inhibit or induce these enzymes, (see Chapter 19, Table 8, p.725). Reports of interactions where closer monitoring ± dose adjustment are required are listed in Box B.[55–59]

Box B Interactions between fentanyl and other drugs involving CYP450

Plasma concentrations of fentanyl	
Increased by	**Decreased by**
Aprepitant[a]	Aprepitant[a]
Azoles, e.g. fluconazole[b], voriconazole	Carbamazepine
Cimetidine	Phenytoin
Macrolide antibiotics, e.g. clarithromycin, erythromycin	Phenobarbital
Protease inhibitors, e.g. indinavir, nelfinavir, ritonavir	Rifampicin

a. aprepitant can increase the exposure to CYP3A4 substrates in the short-term, then reduce their exposure within 2 weeks

b. a case report of a fatality with oral fluconazole and TD fentanyl has been attributed to this interaction.

Fentanyl has been reported to reduce the metabolism of **midazolam**, reducing the clearance by 30% and extending the halflife by 50%.[59]

Fentanyl is best avoided in patients who have used a MAOI within the past 2 weeks. Although they have been used safely together, serotonin toxicity (sometimes fatal) has occurred (also see p.200), manufacturers' SPCs warn of a risk of serotonin toxicity when fentanyl is *used in combination* with other serotoninergic drugs.[59]

Undesirable effects

Also see Strong opioids, p.360.

Very common (>1/10): drowsiness, dizziness, headache, confusion, nausea, vomiting, sweating.

Topical effects: less common and formulation-dependent, but include: oral and nasal discomfort, inflammation or ulceration, rhinorrhoea, epistaxis, sore throat, dysguesia, dental caries with Actiq® (uncommon).

Dose and use

As with all opioids, patients must be monitored for undesirable effects, particularly nausea and vomiting, and constipation. Depending on individual circumstances, an anti-emetic should be prescribed for regular or p.r.n. use, (see QCG: Nausea and vomiting, p.240) and, routinely, a laxative prescribed (see QCG: Opioid-induced constipation, p.42).

Opioids can impair driving ability and patients should be counselled accordingly (see p.743).

Prescribers of transmucosal fentanyl products should:

- be experienced in the management of opioid-therapy in cancer patients
- limit use to opioid-tolerant patients who can adhere to the instructions regarding indication, administration, storage and returns
- provide ongoing supervision
- keep in mind the potential for fentanyl to be misused[60–63]
- understand that the formulations are *not* bio-equivalent and *not* directly interchangeable, and thus:
  - ▷ prescribe by brand[64]
  - ▷ when switching transmucosal products, de novo titration from the lowest available dose is required; the only exception is Effentora®, when a starting dose higher than 100microgram may be considered (see Box E).

Transmucosal fentanyl products should be used only in adults on a regular strong opioid for chronic cancer pain for ≥1 week:

- **morphine** 60mg/24h PO
- fentanyl 25microgram/h TD (50microgram/h required in some studies)
- **hydromorphone** 8mg/24h PO
- **oxycodone** 30mg/24h PO
- an equivalent dose of another opioid.

Individual titration is required because the effective dose cannot be reliably predicted from the maintenance dose of opioid.[18,27,31,65–67] Despite this, the use of doses proportional to the maintenance dose has been suggested.[68–71]

Careful monitoring is required during initial or subsequent titration; the complexity of the titration schedules varies between products (Box C–G). Even so, transmucosal fentanyl products are unsatisfactory in about 1/4–1/3 of patients, either because they fail to provide relief at the highest practical dose or cause unacceptable undesirable effects.

The optimal dose found during successful titration (Box C–G) can be used to treat up to a maximum of 4 episodes/24h. The recommended minimum interval between treatments is generally ≥4h apart. This varies between products (e.g. Abstral® specifies ≥2h, Instanyl® allows a minimum interval of 2h in 'exceptional circumstances', and Actiq® does not specify a minimum) and even for the same product between countries (e.g. Pecfent® in the UK and USA). However, applying the ≥4h apart rule across all products would be reasonable because it was used by most studies and more frequent dosing than q4h appears to increase the maximum plasma concentration achieved with the subsequent dose of fentanyl.[4] Thus, an alternative p.r.n. analgesic, e.g. **morphine** PO, will be required to treat any additional, more frequent episodes. Further, in about 5–25% of episodes, the transmucosal products fail to provide adequate relief and an alternate analgesic is required.[67,72]

Box C Abstral® dose and use

Follow the manufacturer's guidance on administration, titration, storage and disposal in the SPC, Prescribers guide, Dose titration guide, and Patient Information Leaflet. A hospital/ hospice referral pad for GPs is also available.

Abstral® is a SL tablet, placed in the deepest part under the tongue. The tablets must not be chewed or sucked and patients should not eat or drink until they have dissolved. Those with a dry mouth should moisten it with water beforehand.[73] The tablet generally dissolves quickly (<5min), with the particles produced adhering to the oral mucosa from which the fentanyl is subsequently absorbed.

Evaluate each dose after 15–30min and if effective, i.e. a *single* dose provides adequate analgesia with little or no undesirable effects, this is the maintenance dose. If unsuccessful, during titration, a further dose can be given and subsequently a higher dose used for the next episode:

- start with 100microgram, if unsuccessful, give an additional 100microgram dose
- for the next episode give 200microgram, if unsuccessful, give an additional 100microgram tablet
- for the next episode give 300microgram, if unsuccessful, give an additional 100microgram tablet
- for the next episode give 400microgram, if unsuccessful, give an additional 200microgram tablet
- for the next episode give 600microgram, if unsuccessful, give an additional 200microgram tablet
- for the next episode give 800microgram, the maximum dose.

The SPC suggests that intermediate doses of 500 and 700microgram can be considered if there is adequate analgesia but undesirable effects at either the 600 or 800microgam doses. However, in practice, such doses are rarely used. It requires the use of a 100microgram tablet plus a 400 or 600microgram tablet, and doubles the cost of treating an episode (~£10).

Note. In the study on which its safety data is based, only single doses of Abstral® were used for titration and maintenance, with the effective dose confirmed over several consecutive episodes.[17]

More than two thirds of patients find an effective and tolerable dose; about one quarter require 800microgram.[74] However, because of inadequate relief after 30min, an alternative rescue analgesic is needed in about 10% of episodes.[17]

The maximum frequency of use is 4 episodes/24h. In studies, this had to be ≥2h apart (each pain episode was limited to treatment with a single dose)[17,75] and is the recommended interval in the SPC; nonetheless, ≥4h apart is the ideal (see text). Regular daily use of medication for break-through pain (traditionally ≥2/24h) should prompt a review and possible increase in the dose of the regular strong opioid. Subsequently, if a single dose of Abstral® fails to provide consistent relief, the dose should be further titrated as above.

Abstral® is generally well tolerated and remains effective. Use of a median dose of 600microgram treating a mean of 3 episodes/day for 5–6 months showed that:

- opioid-related undesirable effects (e.g. nausea) are common but not a major cause of discontinuation
- application site irritation rarely occurred
- about 75% of patients were satisfied or very satisfied with its use.[17,75]

Although only authorized for break-through cancer pain, some data exists for the use of Abstral® in non-cancer pain.[76]

Box D Actiq® dose and use

Follow the manufacturer's guidance on administration, titration, storage and disposal in the SPC, Patients and caregivers guide, Patient Information Leaflet and Health professionals guide.

Actiq® is a 'lozenge on a stick' containing fentanyl in a hard sweet matrix. In order to achieve maximum mucosal exposure to the fentanyl, the lozenge should be placed between the cheek and the gum and moved constantly up and down, and changed at intervals from one cheek to the other. It should not be chewed. The lozenge should be consumed completely over 15min; quicker than this and more fentanyl is swallowed. Patients with xerostomia (dry mouth) may find it hard to consume it in this time period.[77] If necessary, moisten the mouth with water beforehand. Initially, prescribe 6 doses of one strength at a time:

- start with fentanyl 200microgram and consume over 15min; drinking or eating is not permitted during administration
- wait 15min; if there is inadequate analgesia, use a second 200microgram lozenge
- not more than two lozenges should be used for any one episode of pain
- continue with 200microgram for a further 2 episodes of pain, allowing a second lozenge when necessary
- if on review, the break-through pain is not controlled satisfactorily with a single 200microgram dose, increase to 400microgram
- wait 15min; use a second 400microgram lozenge if necessary
- continue this upwards titration through the available dose strengths until a *single* dose provides adequate analgesia with little or no undesirable effects; this is the maintenance dose
- the maximum dose is 1,600microgram.

The lozenge should be removed from the mouth once the pain is relieved; partly consumed lozenges should be dissolved under hot running water and the handle discarded in a waste container out of reach of children.

About three quarters of patients find an effective and tolerable dose. An alternative rescue analgesic is required in 5–15% of episodes (permitted if inadequate response 15min after Actiq® dose fully completed).

The maximum frequency of use is 4 episodes/24h. In studies, this generally had to be ≥2h apart (each pain episode was limited to treatment with a single dose);[24] ≥4h apart is the ideal (see text). Regular daily use of medication for break-through pain (traditionally ≥2/24h) should prompt a review and possible increase in the dose of the regular strong opioid. Subsequently, if a single dose of Actiq® fails to provide consistent relief, the dose should be further titrated as detailed above.

Actiq® is generally well tolerated and remains effective. Follow up over a mean of about 3 months showed that:

- opioid-related undesirable effects are common (e.g. nausea) but not a major cause of discontinuation
- a single dose is effective in 85–90% of episodes
- about 1/2–3/4 of patients require a dose adjustment; mostly upwards, but sometimes downwards
- patient ratings of global medication performance remain the same (generally 'very good').[78,79]

5

Box E Effentora® dose and use

Follow the manufacturer's guidance on administration, titration, storage and disposal in the SPC, Patients and caregivers guide and Patient Information Leaflet.

Effentora ® is a tablet which can be placed either buccally (between the cheek and gum near a molar tooth) or SL. Absorption is similar from both sites, but it dissolves quicker SL.[80] A dry mouth should be moistened with water beforehand. Mild mucositis (grade 1) does not affect absorption,[7] but avoid use in more severe grades because the impact on absorption has not been examined.

The tablets must not be chewed or sucked and patients should not eat or drink until they have dissolved. The time to dissolution is generally 15–25min but can be longer. However, any tablet remnants should be swallowed after 30min with a glass of water.

Evaluate each dose after 30min and, if effective, this is the maintenance dose. If unsuccessful, during the titration phase, a further dose can be given and subsequently a higher dose used for the next episode. Titration packs, each containing 4 tablets, are available; prescribing 1 pack of 100microgram and 3 packs of 200microgram is sufficient to escalate through the dose range over 5 episodes:

- start with 100microgram, if unsuccessful, give an additional 100microgram dose
- for the next episode give 200microgram (2 x 100microgram tablets), if unsuccessful, give an additional 200microgram tablet
- for the next episode give 400microgram (2 x 200microgram tablets), if unsuccessful, give an additional 200microgram tablet
- for the next episode give 600microgram (3 x 200microgram tablets), if unsuccessful, give an additional 200microgram tablet
- for the next episode give the maximum dose of 800microgram (4 x 200microgram tablets).

If switching from another transmucosal fentanyl product, although titration is still necessary, a starting dose higher than 100microgram may be considered.

About two thirds of patients find an effective and tolerable dose. Subsequently only a *single* dose of the appropriate strength tablet is used per episode, which can be prescribed in 28 tablet packs. An alternative rescue analgesic is required in about 10–25% of episodes.

The maximum frequency of use is 4 episodes/24h, with at least 4h between doses (including any other rescue analgesic used). Regular daily use of medication for break-through pain (traditionally ≥2/24h) should prompt a review and possible increase in the dose of the regular strong opioid. Subsequently, if a single dose of Effentora® fails to provide consistent relief, the dose may require further titration as above.

Effentora® is generally well tolerated and remains effective. Follow up over a mean of 6 months showed that:

- opioid-related undesirable effects are common (e.g. nausea) but not a major cause of discontinuation
- application site problems (e.g. pain, irritation, ulceration) are seen in 6% and lead to discontinuation in <2%
- 70% of patients continue on the same dose
- patient ratings of global medication performance remain the same (generally 'good').[81]

Although only authorized for ≤800microgram in break-through cancer pain in patients receiving oral morphine equivalent of ≥60mg/24h, data exist for the use of Effentora® in:

- highly opioid-tolerant cancer patients (>700mg oral morphine equivalent/24h) in doses of 1,200–3,200microgram[82]
- opioid-tolerant Japanese cancer patients receiving an oral morphine equivalent of 30–59mg/24h using a 50microgram tablet (not UK) as the starting dose[83]
- opioid-tolerant patients with non-cancer break-through pain, e.g. degenerative back pain, complex regional pain syndrome[27,60,84–86]
- opioid-naïve patients with severe pain attending emergency departments with possible or definite fractures or dislocations (single dose of 100microgram), or undergoing invasive procedures.[87,88]

The use of Effentora® in non-cancer patients is controversial, and concerns exist around safety and the potential for misuse.[60–62]

Box F Instanyl® dose and use

Follow the guidance on priming, administration, storage and disposal in the manufacturer's SPC, Physician's guides, Patient Brochure/Information Leaflet.

Instanyl® is a nasal spray. Not all patients feel the spray and they should be warned not to repeat the dose because of this. There is no dose counter.

Evaluate each dose after 10min and if effective, this is the maintenance dose; if unsuccessful, a maximum of one further dose can be given.

Evaluate each dose strength over 3–4 episodes; increase to the next higher strength if there is frequent need for a second dose:

- start with 50microgram in one nostril, if unsuccessful give an additional 50microgram in the other nostril
- if unsuccessful over several episodes, give 100microgram in one nostril, if necessary give an additional 100microgram in the other nostril
- if unsuccessful over several episodes, give 200microgram in one nostril, if necessary give an additional 200microgram in the other nostril; this is the *maximum* dose.

About 2/3–3/4 of patients find an effective and tolerable dose. Although the aim is to use only one dose per episode, 30–50% require a second dose. An alternative rescue analgesic is required in about 15% of episodes; this is given after waiting ≥10min after a dose of Instanyl®.

The maximum frequency of use is 4 episodes/24h, with at least 4h between doses (including any other rescue analgesic used). Although, the SPC states that Instanyl® can be used after 2h 'in exceptional circumstances', ≥4h apart is the ideal (see text). Regular daily use of medication for break-through pain (traditionally ≥2/24h) should prompt a review and possible increase in the dose of the regular strong opioid. The dose of Instanyl® may subsequently need to be re-titrated.

Instanyl® is generally well tolerated and remains effective; opioid-related undesirable effects are common (e.g. nausea) but not a major cause of discontinuation. Follow up for ≤3 months showed that:

- 65% of patients continue on the same dose
- <3% of patients dropped out because of drug-related undesirable effects
- 15% of patients dropped out because of a lack of efficacy.[89]

The multi-dose bottles should be stored upright in the child-resistant container for safety; if not used for >1 week, they need to be primed again by spraying a single dose in the air.

Supply

All formulations are fentanyl citrate and schedule 2 **CD**. All costs per dose for each transmucosal product are independent of strength or pack size and are NHS list price. Not all pack sizes are available for every strength.

Oromucosal formulations
Abstral® (Kyowa Kirin)
Tablets sublingual 100microgram, 200microgram, 300microgram, 400microgram, 600microgram, 800microgram, pack sizes 10 and 30, 1 tablet = £4.99.

Actiq® (Teva UK)
Lozenge buccal with oromucosal applicator 200microgram, 400microgram, 600microgram, 800microgram, 1,200microgram and 1,600microgram, pack sizes 3 and 30, 1 lozenge = £7.01.

Effentora® (Teva UK)
Tablets buccal 100microgram, 200microgram, 400microgram, 600microgram, 800microgram, pack sizes 4 and 28, 1 tablet = £4.99.

Box G Pecfent® dose and use

Follow the guidance on priming, administration, storage and disposal in the manufacturer's SPC, Physician and Pharmacist guides, Patient Brochure/Information Leaflet.

Pecfent ® is a nasal spray. Not all patients feel the spray, but there is an audible click when the dose is administered, and the dose counter advances by one. Advise patients not to blow their nose for 1h after administration:

- start with 100microgram in one nostril
- if unsuccessful, for the next episode, give 200microgram (100microgram in each nostril)
- if unsuccessful, for the next episode, prescribe higher concentration formulation and give 400microgram in one nostril
- if unsuccessful, for the next episode, increase to the maximum dose of 800microgram (400microgram in each nostril).

Evaluate each dose after 30min and, if ineffective, an alternative rescue analgesic can be given.

If any of the above doses are effective, this should be confirmed in the next episode. About three quarters of patients find an effective and tolerable dose; an alternative rescue analgesic is needed in about 5–10% of episodes. Subsequently, if a previously effective dose fails to provide relief over several episodes, consider titration to a higher dose.

The maximum frequency of use is 4 episodes/24h, with at least 4h between doses (including any other rescue analgesic used). Regular daily use of medication for break-through pain (traditionally ≥2/24h) should prompt a review and a possible increase in the dose of the regular strong opioid. The dose of Pecfent® may subsequently need to be re-titrated.

Pecfent® is generally well tolerated and remains effective.[20,72] Follow up over a mean of about 10 months showed that:

- 70% continued on the same dose
- <7% of patients dropped out because of drug-related undesirable effects
- <3% of patients dropped out because of a lack of efficacy.[90]

Preliminary data exists on the pre-emptive use of Pecfent® in opioid-tolerant patients to relieve predictable break-through pain related to cancer treatment, e.g. positioning/immobilization required for radiotherapy, odynophagia or painful defecation due to mucositis;[91,92] the dose is administered 20–30min prior to the activity.

The bottles should be kept in the child-resistant container for safety; if not used for >5 days, they need to be primed again by spraying a single dose in the air. Discard 60 days after first opening.

Intranasal formulations
Instanyl® (Takeda)
Nasal spray 50micrograms/metered dose spray, 100microgram/metered dose spray and 200microgram/metered dose spray, single-dose, 10 and 20 dose, 1 spray = £5.95.

Pecfent® (Kyowa Kirin)
Nasal spray 100microgram/metered dose spray, 400microgram/metered dose spray, 8 or 32 dose, 1 spray = £4.56; the dose required may consist of 1 or 2 sprays.

Parenteral formulations
Fentanyl (generic)
Injection 50microgram/mL, 2mL amp = £1, 10mL amp = £1.50.

---

1 Davies A *et al.* (2013) Breakthrough cancer pain: an observational study of 1000 European oncology patients. *Journal of Pain and Symptom Management.* **46**: 619–628.

2 Zeppetella G (2008) Opioids for cancer breakthrough pain: a pilot study reporting patient assessment of time to meaningful pain relief. *Journal of Pain and Symptom Management.* **35**: 563–567.

3 Darwish M *et al.* (2007) Absolute and relative bioavailability of fentanyl buccal tablet and oral transmucosal fentanyl citrate. *Journal of Clinical Pharmacology*. **47**: 343–350.
4 European Medicines Agency (2010) Assessment report for Pecfent. Procedure No. EMA/H/C/001164.
5 European Medicines Agency (2008) Effentora: EPAR - Scientific discussion.
6 Lichtor J *et al.* (1999) The relative potency of oral transmucosal fentanyl citrate compared with intravenous morphine in the treatment of moderate to severe postoperative pain. *Anesthesia and Analgesia*. **89**: 732–738.
7 Darwish M *et al.* (2007) Absorption of fentanyl from fentanyl buccal tablet in cancer patients with or without oral mucositis: a pilot study. *Clinical Drug Investigation*. **27**: 605–611.
8 Darwish M *et al.* (2006) Comparison of equivalent doses of fentanyl buccal tablets and arteriovenous differences in fentanyl pharmacokinetics. *Clinical Pharmacokinetics*. **45**: 843–850.
9 Kaasa S et *al.* (2010) Pharmacokinetics of intranasal fentanyl spray in patients with cancer and breakthrough pain. *Journal of Opioid Management*. **6**: 17–26.
10 European Medicines Agency (2009) Assessment report for Instanyl. Procedure No. EMEA/H/C/959. London.
11 Vasisht N *et al.* (2010) Single-dose pharmacokinetics of fentanyl buccal soluble film. *Pain Medicine*. **11**: 1017–1023.
12 Darwish M *et al.* (2006) Pharmacokinetic properties of fentanyl effervescent buccal tablets: a phase I, open-label, crossover study of single-dose 100, 200, 400, and 800 microgram in healthy adult volunteers. *Clinical Therapeutics*. **28**: 707–714.
13 King S *et al.* (2011) A systematic review of the use of opioid medication for those with moderate to severe cancer pain and renal impairment: A European palliative care research collaborative opioid guidelines project. *Palliative Medicine*. **25**: 525–552.
14 Bosilkovska M *et al.* (2012) Analgesics in patients with hepatic impairment: pharmacology and clinical implications. *Drugs*. **72**: 1645–1669.
15 Darwish M *et al.* (2007) Single-dose and steady-state pharmacokinetics of fentanyl buccal tablet in healthy volunteers. *Journal of Clinical Pharmacology*. **47**: 56–63.
16 Lister N *et al.* (2011) Pharmacokinetics, safety, and tolerability of ascending doses of sublingual fentanyl, with and without naltrexone, in Japanese subjects. *Journal of Clinical Pharmacology*. **51**: 1195–1204.
17 Rauck RL *et al.* (2009) Efficacy and long-term tolerability of sublingual fentanyl orally disintegrating tablet in the treatment of breakthrough cancer pain. *Current Medical Research Opinion*. **25**: 2877–2885.
18 Slatkin NE *et al.* (2007) Fentanyl buccal tablet for relief of breakthrough pain in opioid-tolerant patients with cancer-related chronic pain. *Journal of Supportive Oncology*. **5**: 327–334.
19 European Medicines Agency (2008) Committee for medicinal products for human use (CHMP). Opinion following article 29(4) referral for Rapinyl.
20 Portenoy RK *et al.* (2010) A multicenter, placebo-controlled, double-blind, multiple-crossover study of Fentanyl Pectin Nasal Spray (FPNS) in the treatment of breakthrough cancer pain. *Pain*. **151**: 617–624.
21 Dworkin RH *et al.* (2008) Interpreting the clinical importance of treatment outcomes in chronic pain clinical trials: IMMPACT recommendations. *Journal of Pain*. **9**: 105–121.
22 Kress HG *et al.* (2009) Efficacy and tolerability of intranasal fentanyl spray 50 to 200 microg for breakthrough pain in patients with cancer: a phase III, multinational, randomized, double-blind, placebo-controlled, crossover trial with a 10-month, open-label extension treatment period. *Clinical Therapeutics*. **31**: 1177–1191.
23 Prostraken (2010) *Personal communication.*
24 Coluzzi P *et al.* (2001) Breakthrough cancer pain: a randomized trial comparing oral transmucosal fentanyl citrate (OTFC) and morphine sulfate immediate release (MSIR). *Pain*. **91**: 123–130.
25 Zeppetella G *et al.* (2010) Consistent and clinically relevant effects with fentanyl buccal tablet in the treatment of patients receiving maintenance opioid therapy and experiencing cancer-related breakthrough pain. *Pain Practice*. **10**: 287–293.
26 Zeppetella G and Davies AN (2013) Opioids for the management of breakthrough pain in cancer patients. *Cochrane Database of Systematic Reviews*. **10**: CD004311. www.thecochranelibrary.com
27 Ashburn MA *et al.* (2011) The efficacy and safety of fentanyl buccal tablet compared with immediate-release oxycodone for the management of breakthrough pain in opioid-tolerant patients with chronic pain. *Anesthesia and Analgesia*. **112**: 693–702.
28 Webster LR *et al.* (2013) Fentanyl buccal tablet compared with immediate-release oxycodone for the management of breakthrough pain in opioid-tolerant patients with chronic cancer and noncancer pain: a randomized, double-blind, crossover study followed by a 12-week open-label phase to evaluate patient outcomes. *Pain Medicine*. **14**: 1332–1345.
29 Fallon M *et al.* (2011) Efficacy and safety of fentanyl pectin nasal spray compared with immediate-release morphine sulfate tablets in the treatment of breakthrough cancer pain: a multicenter, randomized, controlled, double-blind, double-dummy multiple-crossover study. *Journal of Supportive Oncology*. **9**: 224–231.
30 Davies A *et al.* (2011) Consistency of efficacy, patient acceptability, and nasal tolerability of fentanyl pectin nasal spray compared with immediate-release morphine sulfate in breakthrough cancer pain. *Journal of Pain and Symptom Management*. **41**: 358–366.
31 Mercadante S *et al.* (2009) A comparison of intranasal fentanyl spray with oral transmucosal fentanyl citrate for the treatment of breakthrough cancer pain: an open label, randomised, crossover trial. *Current Medical Research Opinion*. **25**: 2805–2815.
32 Sawe J *et al.* (1983) Steady-state kinetics and analgesic effect of oral morphine in cancer patients. *European Journal of Clinical Pharmacology*. **24**: 537–542.
33 Freye E *et al.* (2007) Effervescent morphine results in faster relief of breakthrough pain in patients compared to immediate release morphine sulfate tablet. *Pain Practice*. **7**: 324–331.
34 Velazquez Rivera I *et al.* (2014) Efficacy of sublingual fentanyl vs. oral morphine for cancer-related breakthrough pain. *Advances in Therapy*. **31**: 107–117.
35 Zecca E *et al.* (2017) Fentanyl sublingual tablets versus subcutaneous morphine for the management of severe cancer pain episodes in patients receiving opioid treatment: a double-blind, randomized, noninferiority trial. *Journal of Clinical Oncology*. **35**: 759–765.
36 England R *et al.* (2011) How practical are transmuscosal fentanyl products for breakthrough cancer pain? Novel use of placebo formulations to survey user opinion. *BMJ Supportive and Palliative Care*. **1**: 349–351.
37 NICE (2012) Opioids in palliative care: safe and effective prescribing of strong opioids for pain in palliative care adults. *Clinical Guideline*. CG104. www.nice.org.uk
38 Caraceni A *et al.* (2012) Use of opioid analgesics in the treatment of cancer pain: evidence-based recommendations from the EAPC. *Lancet Oncology*. **13**: e58–68.
39 Guitart J *et al.* (2015) Sublingual fentanyl tablets for relief of breakthrough pain in cancer patients and association with quality-of-life outcomes. *Clinical Drug Investigation*. **35**: 815–822.
40 Davies A *et al.* (2015) Improved patient functioning after treatment of breakthrough cancer pain: an open-label study of fentanyl buccal tablet in patients with cancer pain. *Supportive Care in Cancer*. **23**: 2135–2143.
41 Ueberall MA *et al.* (2016) Efficacy, safety, and tolerability of fentanyl pectin nasal spray in patients with breakthrough cancer pain. *Journal of Pain Research*. **9**: 571–585.

42 Gardner-Nix J (2001) Oral transmucosal fentanyl and sufentanil for incident pain. *Journal of Pain and Symptom Management*. **22**: 627–630.
43 Zeppetella G (2001) Sublingual fentanyl citrate for cancer-related breakthrough pain: a pilot study. *Palliative Medicine*. **15**: 323–328.
44 Murphy A et al. (2014) Intranasal fentanyl for the management of acute pain in children. *Cochrane Database Systematic Reviews*. **10**: CD009942. www.thecochranelibrary.com
45 Fein DM et al. (2017) Intranasal fentanyl for initial treatment of vaso-occlusive crisis in sickle cell disease. *Pediatric Blood Cancer*. **64**.
46 Hansen MS and Dahl JB (2013) Limited evidence for intranasal fentanyl in the emergency department and the prehospital setting--a systematic review. *Danish Medical Journal*. **60**:A4563.
47 Cole J et al. (2009) Intranasal fentanyl in 1-3-year-olds: a prospective study of the effectiveness of intranasal fentanyl as acute analgesia. *Emergency Medicine Australasia*. **21**: 395–400.
48 Borland M et al. (2011) Equivalency of two concentrations of fentanyl administered by the intranasal route for acute analgesia in children in a paediatric emergency department: a randomized controlled trial. *Emergency Medicine Australasia*. **23**: 202–208.
49 Karlsen AP et al. (2014) Safety of intranasal fentanyl in the out-of-hospital setting: a prospective observational study. *Annals of Emergency Medicine*. **63**: 699–703.
50 Harlos MS et al. (2013) Intranasal fentanyl in the palliative care of newborns and infants. *Journal of Pain and Symptom Management*. **46**: 265–274.
51 Simon ST et al. (2013) Fentanyl for the relief of refractory breathlessness: a systematic review. *Journal of Pain and Symptom Management*. **46**: 874–886.
52 Pinna MA et al. (2013) A Randomized Crossover Clinical Trial to Evaluate the Efficacy of Oral Transmucosal Fentanyl Citrate in the Treatment of Dyspnea on Exertion in Patients With Advanced Cancer. *American Journal of Hospice and Palliative Care*.
53 Simon ST et al. (2016) EffenDys-Fentanyl buccal tablet for the relief of episodic breathlessness in patients with advanced cancer: a multicenter, open-label, randomized, morphine-controlled, crossover, phase II trial. *Journal of Pain and Symptom Management*. **52**: 617–625.
54 Hui D et al. (2016) Impact of prophylactic fentanyl pectin nasal spray on exercise-induced episodic dyspnea in cancer patients: a double-blind, randomized controlled trial. *Journal of Pain and Symptom Management*. **52**: 459–468.
55 Kharasch ED et al. (2004) Influence of hepatic and intestinal cytochrome P4503A activity on the acute disposition and effects of oral transmucosal fentanyl citrate. *Anesthesiology*. **101**: 729–737.
56 Takane H et al. (2005) Rifampin reduces the analgesic effect of transdermal fentanyl. *Annals of Pharmacotherpy*. **39**: 2139–2140.
57 Sasson M and Shvartzman P (2006) Fentanyl patch sufficient analgesia for only one day. *Journal of Pain and Symptom Management*. **31**: 389–391.
58 Morii H et al. (2007) Failure of pain control using transdermal fentanyl during rifampicin treatment. *Journal of Pain and Symptom Management*. **33**: 5–6.
59 Baxter K and Preston CL. *Stockley's Drug Interactions*. London: Pharmaceutical Press www.medicinescomplete.com (accessed May 2017).
60 Fine PG et al. (2010) Long-term safety and tolerability of fentanyl buccal tablet for the treatment of breakthrough pain in opioid-tolerant patients with chronic pain: an 18-month study. *Journal of Pain and Symptom Management*. **40**: 747–760.
61 Markman JD (2008) Not so fast: the reformulation of fentanyl and breakthrough chronic non-cancer pain. *Pain*. **136**: 227–229.
62 Passik SD et al. (2011) Aberrant Drug-Related Behavior Observed During Clinical Studies Involving Patients Taking Chronic Opioid Therapy for Persistent Pain and Fentanyl Buccal Tablet for Breakthrough Pain. *Journal of Pain and Symptom Management*. **41**: 116–125.
63 Nunez-Olarte JM and Alvarez-Jimenez P (2011) Emerging opioid abuse in terminal cancer patients taking oral transmucosal fentanyl citrate for breakthrough pain. *Journal of Pain and Symptom Management*. **42**: e6–8.
64 NHS PrescQuipp (2016) Immediate release fentanyl (DROP-List). *Bulletin*. **132**: www.prescquipp.info
65 Christie J et al. (1998) Dose-titration, multicenter study of oral transmucosal fentanyl citrate for the treatment of breakthrough pain in cancer patients using transdermal fentanyl for persistent pain. *Journal of Clinical Oncology*. **16**: 3238–3248.
66 Portenoy R et al. (1999) Oral transmucosal fentanyl citrate (OTFC) for the treatment of breakthrough pain in cancer patients: a controlled use titration study. *Pain*. **79**: 303–312.
67 Portenoy RK et al. (2006) A randomized, placebo-controlled study of fentanyl buccal tablet for breakthrough pain in opioid-treated patients with cancer. *Clinical Journal of Pain*. **22**: 805–811.
68 Mercadante S et al. (2014) Intranasal fentanyl versus fentanyl pectin nasal spray for the management of breakthrough cancer pain in doses proportional to basal opioid regimen. *Journal of Pain*. **15**: 602–607.
69 Shimoyama N et al. (2015) Efficacy and safety of sublingual fentanyl orally disintegrating tablet at doses determined from oral morphine rescue doses in the treatment of breakthrough cancer pain. *Japanese Journal of Clinical Oncology*. **45**: 189–196.
70 Mercadante S et al. (2016) Fentanyl pectin nasal spray versus oral morphine in doses proportional to the basal opioid regimen for the management of breakthrough cancer pain: a comparative study. *Journal of Pain and Symptom Management*. **52**: 27–34.
71 Mercadante S et al. (2015) Fentanyl buccal tablet vs. oral morphine in doses proportional to the basal opioid regimen for the management of breakthrough cancer pain: a randomized, crossover, comparison study. *Journal of Pain and Symptom Management*. **50**: 579–586.
72 Portenoy RK et al. (2010) Long-term safety, tolerability, and consistency of effect of fentanyl pectin nasal spray for breakthrough cancer pain in opioid-tolerant patients. *Journal of Opioid Management*. **6**: 319–328.
73 Davies A et al. (2016) The influence of low salivary flow rates on the absorption of a sublingual fentanyl citrate formulation for breakthrough cancer pain. *Journal of Pain and Symptom Management*. **51**: 538–545.
74 Nalamachu SR et al. (2012) Successful dose finding with sublingual fentanyl tablet: Combined results from 2 0pen-label titration studies. *Pain Practice*. **12**: 449–456.
75 Nalamachu S et al. (2011) Long-term effectiveness and tolerability of sublingual fentanyl orally disintegrating tablet for the treatment of breakthrough cancer pain. *Current Medical Research Opinion*. **27**: 519–530.
76 Guitart J et al. (2013) Efficacy and safety of sublingual fentanyl orally disintegrating tablets in patients with breakthrough pain: multicentre prospective study. *Clinical Drug Investigation*. **33**: 675–683.
77 Davies AN and Vriens J (2005) Oral transmucosal fentanyl citrate and xerostomia. *Journal of Pain and Symptom Management*. **30**: 496–497.
78 Payne R et al. (2001) Long-term safety of oral transmucosal fentanyl citrate for breakthrough cancer pain. *Journal of Pain and Symptom Management*. **22**: 575–583.
79 Hanks GW et al. (2004) Oral transmucosal fentanyl citrate in the management of breakthrough pain in cancer: an open, multicentre, dose-titration and long-term use study. *Palliative Medicine*. **18**: 698–704.
80 Darwish M et al. (2008) Bioequivalence following buccal and sublingual placement of fentanyl buccal tablet 400 microg in healthy subjects. *Clinical Drug Investigation*. **28**: 1–7.

81 Weinstein SM *et al.* (2009) Fentanyl buccal tablet for the treatment of breakthrough pain in opioid-tolerant patients with chronic cancer pain:A long-term, open-label safety study. *Cancer.* **115**: 2571–2579.
82 Mercadante S *et al.* (2011) Fentanyl buccal tablets for breakthrough pain in highly tolerant cancer patients: preliminary data on the proportionality between breakthrough pain dose and background dose. *Journal of Pain and Symptom Management.* **42**: 464–469.
83 Kosugi T *et al.* (2014) A randomized, double-blind, placebo-controlled study of fentanyl buccal tablets for breakthrough pain: efficacy and safety in Japanese cancer patients. *Journal of Pain and Symptom Management.* **47**: 990–1000.
84 Simpson DM *et al.* (2007) Fentanyl buccal tablet for the relief of breakthrough pain in opioid-tolerant adult patients with chronic neuropathic pain: a multicenter, randomized, double-blind, placebo-controlled study. *Clinical Therapy.* **29**: 588–601.
85 Portenoy RK *et al.* (2007) Fentanyl buccal tablet (FBT) for relief of breakthrough pain in opioid-treated patients with chronic low back pain: a randomized, placebo-controlled study. *Current Medical Research Opinion.* **23**: 223–233.
86 Farrar JT *et al.* (2010) A novel 12-week study, with three randomized, double-blind placebo-controlled periods to evaluate fentanyl buccal tablets for the relief of breakthrough pain in opioid-tolerant patients with noncancer-related chronic pain. *Pain Medicine.* **11**: 1313–1327.
87 Shear ML *et al.* (2010) Transbuccal fentanyl for rapid relief of orthopedic pain in the ED. *American Journal of Emergency Medicine.* **28**: 847–852.
88 Bortolussi R *et al.* (2016) A phase II study on the efficacy and safety of procedural analgesia with fentanyl buccal tablet in cancer patients for the placement of indwelling central venous access systems. *Supportive Care in Cancer.* **24**: 1537–1543.
89 Kongsgaard UE *et al.* (2014) The use of Instanyl(R) in the treatment of breakthrough pain in cancer patients: a 3-month observational, prospective, cohort study. *Support Care Cancer.* **22**: 1655–1662.
90 Taylor D *et al.* (2014) A report on the long-term use of fentanyl pectin nasal spray in patients with recurrent breakthrough pain. *Journal of Pain and Symptom Management.* **47**: 1001–1007.
91 Mazzola R *et al.* (2017) Fentanyl pectin nasal spray for painful mucositis in head and neck cancers during intensity-modulated radiation therapy with or without chemotherapy. *Clinical and Translational Oncology.* **19**: 593–598.
92 Bell BC and Butler EB (2013) Management of predictable pain using fentanyl pectin nasal spray in patients undergoing radiotherapy. *Journal of Pain Research.* **6**: 843–848.

Updated September 2017

HYDROMORPHONE

Class: Strong opioid analgesic.

Indications: Severe pain in cancer; †an alternative in cases of intolerance to other strong opioids.[1,2]

Contra-indications: None absolute if titrated carefully against a patient's pain. (Also see Cautions below, and Strong opioids, p.360).

Pharmacology

Hydromorphone is an analogue of **morphine** with similar pharmacokinetic and pharmacodynamic properties.[3] Thus, it is both analgesic and antitussive. Hydromorphone, **morphine** and **oxycodone** are comparable in terms of analgesic efficacy, although differ in potency.[1,2] Undesirable effects are similar but, as with all opioids, these can vary in severity between individuals. Hydromorphone can be used as an alternative in cases of intolerance to **morphine** or another opioid.[1]

PO hydromorphone is absorbed mainly in the small intestine. As with **morphine**, bio-availability is subject to wide inter-individual variation.[4] Hydromorphone is metabolized in the liver by 6-ketoreduction with subsequent glucuronidation. The main metabolite is hydromorphone-3-glucuronide (H3G). All the metabolites are renally excreted and can accumulate in renal impairment.[5]

H3G has no analgesic activity but is estimated to be about 2.5 times more potent than morphine-3-glucuronide as a neuro-excitant.[6] In animal studies, dose-dependent allodynia, myoclonus, and seizures are seen.[7] Neurotoxicity (e.g. tremor, myoclonus, delirium) has been reported with hydromorphone, generally with higher doses and/or renal impairment.[8]

Hydromorphone is available in PO (immediate-release, modified-release) and injectable formulations. Compared with **morphine**, hydromorphone costs more. However, hydromorphone is more soluble than **morphine**, and is available as a high concentration injection (50mg/mL). Because hydromorphone is more potent (see below), this permits a high dose to be delivered in a small volume. Thus, in countries where **diamorphine** (p.387) is not available, hydromorphone is used CSCI, particularly when higher doses are required.

An osmotic-release oral delivery system (OROS®) for once daily administration has been developed, but as yet is unauthorized in the UK and Ireland. This 'extended-release' hydromorphone displays dose-dependent linear pharmacokinetics which are not significantly affected by food or alcohol.[9,10]

According to the UK manufacturer, hydromorphone PO is about 7.5 times more potent than **morphine** PO,[11,12] and this accounts for the choice of capsule content (1.3mg and 2.6mg; stated to be equivalent to **morphine** 10mg and 20mg PO respectively). However, independent reviews and guidelines recommend that when switching from PO **morphine** to PO hydromorphone, a conversion ratio of 5:1 is used, i.e. the hydromorphone dose should be one fifth of the **morphine** dose.[2,13] A conversion ratio of 5:1 is also appropriate for switching from **morphine** CSCI to hydromorphone CSCI. (Also see Opioid switching p.370 and Appendix 2, Table 1, p.857 and Table 4, p.862).

When switching from PO hydromorphone to SC/IV hydromorphone, the UK manufacturer recommends a conversion ratio of 3:1. However, this may be too conservative for some patients and clinical experience is that a conversion ratio of 2:1 can be used, i.e. the hydromorphone SC/IV 24h dose should be half of the hydromorphone PO 24h dose. (Also see Opioid switching p.370 and Appendix 2, Table 3, p.861). For switching from other oral opioids to CSCI-hydromorphone, see Dose and use.

Bio-availability 37–62% PO.[4]
Onset of action <5min IV;[14] 15min SC/IM; 30min PO.[15]
Time to peak plasma concentration 45min PO.[16]
Plasma halflife 2.5h early phase, with a prolonged late phase.
Duration of action 4–5h immediate-release; 12–24h m/r (product-dependent).[17–19]

Cautions

In 2005, the FDA warned that the concurrent ingestion of alcohol could hasten the release of hydromorphone from one m/r product resulting in 'dose dumping', i.e. a rapid rise in plasma concentrations. In 2011, the EMEA reported the results of a review of the interaction between alcohol and opioid m/r mechanisms, and concluded that the risk is minor for most m/r products except those using polymethylmethacrylate-triethylcitrate (none in the UK).[20]

Moderate–severe renal or hepatic impairment (see Dose and use, Chapter 17, p.693 and Chapter 18, p.709).

Undesirable effects

Also see Strong opioids, p.360.

Dose and use

As with all opioids, patients must be monitored for undesirable effects, particularly nausea and vomiting, and constipation (see p.365). Depending on individual circumstances, an anti-emetic should be prescribed for regular or p.r.n. use (see QCG: Nausea and vomiting, p.240) and, routinely, a laxative prescribed (see QCG: Opioid-induced constipation, p.42).

Opioids can impair driving ability and patients should be counselled accordingly (see p.743).

Oral

PO hydromorphone is used in the same way as PO **morphine**, generally q4h as immediate-release capsules or q12h as m/r capsules; both formulations can be swallowed whole or, if necessary, opened and the contents sprinkled on a small amount of soft food, e.g. yoghurt. The m/r granules should not be crushed or chewed because this could lead to a rapid release of an overdose (see Chapter 28, Box B, p.788).

In the UK, hydromorphone is unlikely to be used primarily as an antitussive but theoretically could be (see Antitussives, p.144).

CSCI

For general considerations when switching routes ± converting opioids, see p.855. A large case series suggests the following calculations are suitable across a range of doses:

- PO hydromorphone to CSCI hydromorphone, give half of the 24h dose, e.g. hydromorphone 32mg/24h PO = hydromorphone 16mg/24h CSCI

- PO **morphine** to CSCI hydromorphone, give a tenth of the 24h dose, e.g. **morphine** 60mg/24h PO = hydromorphone 6mg/24h CSCI
- PO **oxycodone** to CSCI hydromorphone, give an eighth of the 24h dose, e.g. **oxycodone** 40mg/24h PO = hydromorphone 5mg/24h CSCI.[21]

When switching from **morphine** CSCI to hydromorphone CSCI, *PCF* recommends a conversion ratio of 5:1 (see Pharmacology):

- CSCI **morphine** to CSCI hydromorphone, give a fifth of the 24h dose, e.g. **morphine** 30mg/24h CSCI = hydromorphone 6mg/24h CSCI.

Conventionally, p.r.n. SC doses of hydromorphone are 1/6–1/10 of the total 24h CSCI dose. For CSCI dilute with WFI, 0.9% saline or 5% glucose.

CSCI compatibility with other drugs: Although most data are for dilution in 0.9% saline, there are 2-drug compatibility data for hydromorphone in WFI with **glycopyrronium**, **hyoscine *butylbromide***, **hyoscine *hydrobromide***, **ketamine**, **levomepromazine metoclopramide** and **midazolam**.

Concentration-dependent *incompatibility* may occur with **cyclizine**, **dexamethasone**, **haloperidol** and **ketorolac**. For more details and 3-drug compatibility data, see Appendix 3 charts 1 (p.866) and 4 (p.872).

Compatibility charts for mixing drugs in 0.9% saline can be found in the extended appendix section of the on-line *PCF* on *www.palliativedrugs.com*.

Renal or hepatic impairment

Because of the risk of impaired metabolism or elimination:[22–24]

- lower than usual starting doses are advised in moderate–severe renal, or moderate hepatic impairment
- avoid if possible in severe hepatic impairment; if unavoidable lower the usual starting dose *and* increase the dosing interval of immediate-release products to q8h (see p.709)
- hydromorphone is advised against in hepatorenal syndrome.

Despite the risk of accumulation of H3G and other glucuronide metabolites, hydromorphone is successfully used in some centres in severe renal impairment and ESRF (see p.693).

For a general approach when renal of hepatic function deteriorates rapidly, see p.364.

Supply

All products are Schedule 2 **CD**.

Palladone® (Napp)
Capsules 1.3mg, 2.6mg, 1.3mg dose = £0.16.
Injection 2mg/mL, 10mg/mL; 20mg/mL and 50mg/mL, 1mL amp = £1.50, £13, £26 and £34 respectively.

Modified-release oral formulation

As for all m/r opioids, brand prescribing is recommended to reduce the risk of confusion and error in dispensing and administration (see p.xvii).

Palladone® SR (Napp)
Capsules enclosing m/r granules 2mg, 4mg, 8mg, 16mg, 24mg, 28 days @ 2mg, 8mg or 24mg every 12h = £21, £56 and £160 respectively.

1 Bao YJ *et al.* (2016) Hydromorphone for cancer pain. *Cochrane Database of Systematic Reviews.* **10**: CD011108. www.thecochranelibrary.com

2 Caraceni A *et al.* (2012) Use of opioid analgesics in the treatment of cancer pain: evidence-based recommendations from the EAPC. *Lancet Oncology.* **13**: e58–68.

3 Quigley C and Glare P (2009) Hydromorphone. In: M Davis *et al.* (eds) *Opioids in Cancer Pain* (2e). Oxford University Press, Oxford, pp. 245–252.

4 Vallner J *et al.* (1981) Pharmacokinetics and bioavailability of hydromorphone following intravenous and oral administration to human subjects. *Journal of Clinical Pharmacology.* **21**: 152–156.

5 King S *et al.* (2011) A systematic review of the use of opioid medication for those with moderate to severe cancer pain and renal impairment: A European palliative care research collaborative opioid guidelines project. *Palliative Medicine.* **25**: 525–552.

6 Wright AW *et al.* (2001) Hydromorphone-3-glucuronide: a more potent neuro-excitant than its structural analogue, morphine-3-glucuronide. *Life Sciences*. **69**: 409–420.
7 Babul N and Darke AC (1992) Putative role of hydromorphone metabolites in myoclonus. *Pain*. **51**: 260–261.
8 Lee KA *et al.* (2016) Evidence for neurotoxicity due to morphine or hydromorphone use in renal impairment: a systematic review. *Journal of Palliative Medicine*. **19**: 1179–1187.
9 Hale ME *et al.* (2012) Safety and tolerability of OROS(R) hydromorphone ER in adults with chronic noncancer and cancer pain: pooled analysis of 13 studies. *Journal of Opioid Management*. **8**: 299–314.
10 Vandenbossche J *et al.* (2012) Repeat-dose steady-state pharmacokinetic evaluation of once-daily hydromorphone extended-release (OROS((R)) hydromorphone ER) in patients with chronic pain. *Journal of Pain Research*. **5**: 523–533.
11 McDonald C and Miller A (1997) A comparative potency study of a controlled release tablet formulation of hydromorphone with controlled release morphine in patients with cancer pain. *European Journal of Palliative Care Abstracts of the Fifth Congress*.
12 Moriarty M *et al.* (1999) A randomised crossover comparison of controlled release hydromorphone tablets with controlled release morphine tablets in patients with cancer pain. *Journal of Clinical Research*. **2**: 1–8.
13 Mercadante S and Caraceni A (2011) Conversion ratios for opioid switching in the treatment of cancer pain: a systematic review. *Palliative Medicine*. **25**: 504–515.
14 Coda B *et al.* (1997) Hydromorphone analgesia after intravenous bolus administration. *Pain*. **71**: 41–48.
15 Benedetti CB and Butler SH (1990) Systemic analgesics. In: Bonica J.J (ed) *The Management of Pain*. Lea and Febiger, Philedelphia.
16 Durnin C *et al.* (2001) Pharmacokinetics of oral immediate-release hydromorphone (Dilaudid IR) in young and elderly subjects. *Proceedings of the Western Pharmacology Society*. **44**: 79–80.
17 Hagen N *et al.* (1995) Steady-state pharmacokinetics of hydromorphone and hydromorphone-3-glucuronide in cancer patients after immediate and controlled-release hydromorphone. *Journal of Clinical Pharmacology*. **35**: 37–44.
18 Bruera E *et al.* (1996) A randomized, double-blind, double-dummy, crossover trial comparing the safety and efficacy of oral sustained-release hydromorphone with immediate-release hydromorphone in patients with cancer pain. Canadian Palliative Care Clinical Trials Group. *Journal of Clinical Oncology*. **14**: 1713–1717.
19 Hays H *et al.* (1994) Comparative clinical efficacy and safety of immediate release and controlled release hydromorphone for chronic severe cancer pain. *Cancer*. **74**: 1808–1816.
20 European Medicines Agency (2010) EMA concludes review of modified-release oral opioids of the WHO level III scale management of pain. *Press release* 23 July 2010: www.ema.europa.eu
21 Reddy A *et al.* (2017) The conversion ratio from intravenous hydromorphone to oral opioids in cancer patients. *Journal of Pain and Symptom Management*. **54**: 280–288.
22 Durnin C *et al.* (2001) Pharmacokinetics of oral immediate-release hydromorphone (Dilaudid IR) in subjects with moderate hepatic impairment. *Proceedings of the Western Pharmacology Society*. **44**: 83–84.
23 Bosilkovska M *et al.* (2012) Analgesics in patients with hepatic impairment: pharmacology and clinical implications. *Drugs*. **72**: 1645–1669.
24 Durnin C *et al.* (2001) Pharmacokinetics of oral immediate-release hydromorphone (Dilaudid IR) in subjects with renal impairment. *Proceedings of the Western Pharmacology Society*. **44**: 81–82.

Updated September 2017

*METHADONE

Class: Strong opioid analgesic.

Methadone should be used as a strong opioid analgesic only by those fully conversant with its pharmacology.[1] It is generally best reserved for patients who fail to respond well to **morphine** or another μ-opioid receptor agonist. Important facts about methadone include:

- a widely variable plasma halflife
- dosing which is more complicated than for other strong opioids
- metabolism which is modified to a clinically important extent by other drugs which may be used in palliative care
- an association with a potentially fatal cardiac arrhythmia (see Cautions below and Prolongation of the QT interval in palliative care, p.731).

In addition, because methadone is used to treat opioid addiction, there is a social stigma attached to its use.

Indications: Moderate–severe pain, †cough, †an alternative in cases of intolerance to other strong opioids, †**morphine** poorly-responsive pain, †pain relief in severe renal impairment.[2,3] Also treatment of opioid addiction.

Contra-indications: None absolute if titrated carefully against a patient's pain (also see Strong opioids, p.360).

Pharmacology

Methadone is a synthetic strong opioid with mixed properties.[4,5] Thus, it is a μ-opioid receptor agonist, an NMDA-receptor-channel blocker,[6,7] and a pre-synaptic blocker of serotonin and noradrenaline (norepinephrine) re-uptake.[8] However, the analgesic relevance of the non-opioid effects is debated.[9] Differential effects at the μ-opioid receptor may alone explain the reported benefit from switching one opioid to another. Thus, compared to **morphine**, methadone (like **fentanyl**) is associated with higher levels of receptor internalisation, β-arrestin recruitment and little or no stimulation of Na^+,K^+-ATPase activity (also see p.361).[9,10] Although some suggest that the non-opioid effects make methadone of particular benefit in neuropathic pain,[11,12] RCT evidence is limited, of very low quality and insufficient to make any reliable conclusion.[13]

Methadone is a racemic mixture (*R*− and *S*−enantiomers); *R*−methadone is responsible for most of the analgesic and undesirable effects, whereas *S*−methadone is antitussive and has a more potent effect on cardiac conduction. Methadone is a non-acidic and lipophilic drug which is generally well absorbed from all routes of administration. However, PO bio-availability shows wide variation, in part explained by methadone being a substrate for p-glycoprotein (see Chapter 19, p.717).

Partly because of its lipid-solubility, methadone has a high volume of distribution with only about 1% of the drug in the blood.[14] Methadone accumulates in tissues when given repeatedly, creating an extensive reservoir.[15] Protein-binding (principally to a glycoprotein) is 60–90%;[16] this is double that of **morphine**. Both volume of distribution and protein-binding contribute to the long plasma halflife (it takes 4–7 days to achieve steady state), and accumulation is a potential problem. Methadone is metabolized mainly in the liver by cytochrome P450 to several inactive metabolites.[17] About half of the drug and its metabolites are excreted by the intestines and half by the kidneys, most of the latter unchanged.[18] Renal and hepatic impairment do not affect methadone clearance.[19,20] Even so, in renal and hepatic failure (see Chapter 17, p.681 and Chapter 18, p.703), it is generally best to reduce the starting dose, e.g. by at least 50%, and titrate according to response.

IM methadone is equivalent to half the PO methadone dose (i.e. a PO:IM conversion ratio of 2:1).[21] In single doses, IM methadone is marginally more potent than IM **morphine**. However, with repeated doses, methadone is several times more potent and longer-acting; analgesia lasts 8–12h and sometimes more.[22,23] There is no single conversion ratio between methadone and **morphine**. When patients with inadequate pain relief or undesirable effects with **morphine** are switched, the eventual 24h dose of methadone *is typically 5–10 times smaller than the previous dose of* ***morphine****, but sometimes 20–30 times smaller, and occasionally even smaller.*[24–27] The relative potency of methadone tends to increase as the dose of **morphine** increases, i.e. proportionately less methadone is required as the **morphine** dose increases.[25–27]

When considering the use of methadone, the difficulty of a subsequent switch from methadone to another opioid should also be borne in mind. For such switches, typically the PO **morphine** equivalent dose will be 5–10 times greater than the PO methadone dose with a wide range again reported, e.g. from 1−75 times.[28] Thus, it is prudent to use conservative dose calculations and monitor the patient closely.

Methadone is used in several different settings. Because it is relatively inexpensive, it is a popular first-line opioid in resource poor countries. RCT evidence is limited for both cancer and non-cancer pain, and insufficient for meta-analysis.[29–31] Nonetheless, when used first-line in cancer pain, methadone appears to provide similar analgesia to **morphine** but, in some studies, more undesirable effects.[1] For example, in one RCT, 20% of patients allocated to PO methadone 7.5mg b.d. discontinued treatment compared with 5% of those who received **morphine** 15mg b.d. Half of the withdrawals occurred in the first week, and most were because of sedation or nausea. For patients remaining in the study, there was no difference in efficacy or undesirable effects.[23] This suggests that a smaller starting dose of PO methadone (e.g. 2.5–5mg b.d., or even 1–2mg b.d.) would have been more appropriate.[32,33] Indeed, in one large case series of patients with cancer and non-cancer pain receiving methadone first-line, the median effective PO dose was 2.5mg b.d., with only 20% requiring ≥10mg/24h.[34]

Second-line, patients who experience inadequate analgesia with **morphine** (or another opioid), with or without unacceptable undesirable effects such as nausea, vomiting, hallucinations or sedation, when switched to relatively low-dose methadone can obtain good relief with few undesirable effects.[35–38] Patients who experience more specific neurotoxicity with **morphine**, e.g. hyperalgesia, allodynia and/or myoclonus ± sedation and delirium, generally also benefit by switching to methadone. However, switching to other opioids also helps.[39–42] Thus, when switching from **morphine**, it would seem sensible to choose an opioid which is easier and safer to use than methadone, e.g. **oxycodone**, **hydromorphone**, **fentanyl**.

Methadone is an alternative strong opioid for patients with severe renal impairment at risk of excessive drowsiness ± delirium with **morphine** because of accumulation of morphine-6-glucuronide.[3] Methadone is poorly removed by haemodialysis.[43] However, for moribund patients, **alfentanil** or **fentanyl** are probably better choices (see p.681). Methadone can also be used as a strong opioid analgesic in former opioid addicts who are being maintained on methadone.[44,45] The once daily maintenance dose (typically 60–120mg) is halved and given q12h and subsequently titrated as necessary. An alternate strategy is to add another strong opioid and titrate this to achieve analgesia, leaving the methadone maintenance dose unchanged.[46] Successful use of a locally prepared TD gel has been described in patients unable to tolerate administration by other routes.[47]

5

Methadone has been successfully used for cancer break-through pain, either PO or SL (1mL of extemporaneously produced solutions ranging 1–40mg/mL held for 2min); the average time to meaningful pain relief is 30min and 10min respectively.[48,49] However, given that the time to peak plasma concentration takes ≤4h, together with a long halflife and duration of action, this approach is unsuitable for patients with frequent short-lasting occurrences of break-through pain (see p.297).

Bio-availability 80% (range 40–100%) PO.

Onset of action <30min PO, 15min IM.

Time to peak plasma concentration 4h PO; 1h IM.

Plasma halflife highly variable, mean 20–35h (range 5–130h);[50] longer in older patients; acidifying the urine results in a shorter halflife (20h) and raising the pH with sodium bicarbonate a longer halflife (>40h).[51]

Duration of action 4–5h PO and 3–5h IM single dose; 8–12h repeated doses.

Cautions

In 2006, after a review of deaths and life-threatening adverse events (e.g. respiratory depression, cardiac arrhythmia) associated with unintentional overdose, drug interactions, and prolongation of the QT interval, the FDA in the USA issued a safety warning about the use of methadone. This highlighted the need for:

- physicians to be fully aware of the pharmacology of methadone
- close monitoring of the patient when starting methadone, particularly when switching from a high dose of another opioid
- slow dose titration, and close monitoring of the patient when changing the dose of methadone
- warning the patient not to exceed the prescribed dose.

Because methadone generally has a long plasma halflife, accumulation to a variable extent should be anticipated, particularly in the frail elderly, or severe renal or hepatic impairment (see Chapter 17, p.693 and Chapter 18, p.709). Drowsiness and respiratory depression may develop after several days/weeks on a steady dose. *PCF* recommends p.r.n. dose titration to minimize the risk of this occurring (see below).[52]

QT interval prolongation and, rarely, a serious ventricular arrhythmia (*torsade de pointes*) have been observed during treatment with methadone. Generally, the latter is associated with, but not limited to, higher dose treatment (>120mg/24h), see Chapter 20, p.731.[53] The SPC recommends that methadone is administered with caution to patients at risk of developing QT prolongation, e.g. those with:

- a history of cardiac conduction abnormalities
- a family history of sudden death
- advanced heart disease or ischaemic heart disease
- liver disease
- electrolyte abnormalities
- concurrent treatment with drugs which:
  - ▷ may cause electrolyte abnormalities
  - ▷ have a potential to prolong QT
  - ▷ inhibit CYP3A4.

Note. The IV formulation of methadone in the USA (but *not* the UK), contains a preservative chlorobutanol, which has an additive QT prolonging effect.[54]

The risk this rare but potentially fatal cardiac complication poses must be considered in the context of the patient's circumstances. A commonsense approach should prevail, and ECG monitoring will be largely irrelevant in the last days of life. On the other hand, for a patient with a prognosis of several months or longer, it may be appropriate to identify any risk factors for QT prolongation and consider ECG ± electrolyte monitoring (see Chapter 20, p.731).

Even so, research is needed to establish the magnitude of the risk of *torsade de pointes* with methadone, and the overall value of monitoring in the palliative care setting.[53]

Plasma levels of methadone are increased in CYP2D6 poor metabolizers resulting in a greater risk of undesirable effects, including fatal overdose.[55] Similarly, plasma levels of *S*−methadone are increased in CYP2B6 poor metabolizers which, because it is a more potent blocker of the potassium channels in the cardiac myocytes than *R*−methadone, may increase their risk of prolonged QTc and arrhythmia (also see Chapter 19, p.717).[56]

Drug interactions

Methadone is metabolized by several cytochrome P450 iso-enzymes, mainly CYP3A4 and CYP2B6, with CYP2D6, CYP2C9, CYP2C19, and CYP1A2 also involved to varying degrees; this differs between the enantiomers with CYP3A4 and CYP2B6 preferentially metabolizing *R*−methadone and *S*−methadone respectively. Clinically relevant and well-established CYP-related drug-drug interactions are listed in Table 1. Note particularly that **carbamazepine**, **phenobarbital**, **phenytoin**, **rifampicin** and **St John's wort** increase the metabolism of methadone, and may reverse previously satisfactory pain relief, or even precipitate withdrawal symptoms.[57,58] Conversely, methadone overdose has occurred when such inducers have been stopped, including after cessation of smoking (polycyclic aromatic hydrocarbons in tobacco smoke are CYP1A2 inducers).[59]

Symptomatic bradycardia has been reported in a patient on **thalidomide** given methadone.[60]

Table 1 Cytochrome P450 interactions with methadone resulting in changed drug plasma concentrations[57]

Methadone increased by	*Methadone decreased by*	*Increased by methadone*	*Decreased by methadone*
SSRIs Cimetidine Ciprofloxacin Diazepam (high-dose) Itraconazole Fluconazole Voriconazole	Carbamazepine Phenobarbital Phenytoin Rifampicin St John's wort Antiretroviral, e.g. abacavir, amprenavir, efavirenz, lopinavir, nelfinavir, nevirapine, ritonavir, saquinavir, telaprevir, tipranavir Tobacco smoking	Desipramine Zidovudine (AZT)	Amprenavir

Avoid concurrent use with other drugs that prolong the QT interval.

Risk of serotonin toxicity when used in combination with other serotoninergic drugs, e.g. **selegiline**, SSRIs, see Antidepressants Box A, p.200.

The concurrent use of MAOIs and methadone is contra-indicated in the SPC, however see Strong opioids, p.367.

Undesirable effects

Also see Strong opioids, Box B, p.365. Methadone may occasionally cause neurotoxicity, e.g. myoclonus,[61] or more florid opioid-induced hyperalgesia.[62–64] Local erythema and induration when given by CSCI.[65]

Rarely, hypoglycaemia (particularly with IV methadone and PO doses >40mg/24h)[66] and sensorineural hearing loss (generally following overdose; can be permanent).[67,68]

Dose and use

As with all opioids, patients must be monitored for undesirable effects, particularly nausea and vomiting, and constipation. Depending on individual circumstances, an anti-emetic should be prescribed for regular or p.r.n. use (see QCG: Nausea and vomiting, p.240) and a laxative prescribed routinely (see QCG: Opioid-induced constipation, p.42).

Opioids can impair driving ability and patients should be counselled accordingly. Methadone is included in a new law in England and Wales relating to driving with certain drugs above specified plasma concentrations (see p.743).

Because of the wide interindividual variation in the pharmacokinetics of methadone, dose titration is different from **morphine**. The implication of its large volume of distribution must be considered. During the first few days, while the body tissues become saturated, a greater daily dose of methadone will be required for satisfactory analgesia than subsequently; once saturation is complete, a smaller daily dose of methadone will then be sufficient. Continuing on the initial daily dose is likely to result in sedation after a few days, and possibly respiratory depression and even death.[69,70]

Several methods exist for switching from **morphine** to methadone, e.g.:[71–78]

- *three-day switch*: **morphine** is tailed off and the methadone progressively introduced over three days; methadone dose based on conversion ratios which differ according to **morphine** dose
- *stop and go, regular dose*: **morphine** is abruptly stopped and switched to a regular dose of methadone, based on conversion ratios which differ according to **morphine** dose
- *stop and go, p.r.n. dose*: **morphine** is abruptly stopped and for the first week p.r.n. doses of methadone are used to establish the regular dose required thereafter.

Direct comparisons are limited, but a systematic review considered the last approach likely to be the safest and most effective,[78] and is the one favoured by the *PCF* (see QCG: Use of methadone for cancer pain, p.445). These guidelines are an evolution from earlier ones, incorporating feedback to www.palliativedrugs.com from clinicians.[3,24,79] A single loading dose aids tissue saturation and helps to reduce the number of p.r.n. doses required in the first 48h.[24] The recommendations may be overcautious but are safer, particularly in the elderly and for those switching from large doses of **morphine**.

Regardless of the method used, all require practitioners to be experienced in the use of methadone and the importance of close supervision cannot be overemphasized, generally as an inpatient. [78] There are reports of carefully controlled outpatient regimens, but in some, pain relief can take weeks rather than days to achieve.[38,80,81] Caution is also required when there has been rapid dose escalation of the pre-switch opioid; in these circumstances it is probably safer to calculate the initial dose of methadone using the pre-escalation dose.[82] Maintenance doses vary considerably, but most are <80mg/24h PO.[83] *Subsequent switching from methadone to other opioids can be difficult. In one series 12/13 patients experienced increased pain ± dysphoria.*

Because of the difficulties associated with a complete swap from **morphine** to methadone, some clinicians add a small dose of methadone (as per first-line use) alongside **morphine** (or other strong opioid).[84] The dose of **morphine** is progressively reduced if opioid toxicity occurs. Although simpler, this approach does *not* avoid the need for close supervision. Only low-level evidence (grade D) exists to support this approach.[85]

Methadone SC (generally doses >25mg) or CSCI can cause marked local inflammation necessitating site rotation, and possibly other measures (see QCG: Use of methadone for cancer pain, p.445).[86,87] When switching from methadone PO to SC, a safe conversion is to halve the methadone PO dose. However, for some patients, particularly those receiving a small dose of PO methadone (<80mg/24h), a 1:1 conversion ratio may be more appropriate and subsequent upwards dose titration may be required.[87] For switching from other CSCI opioids to CSCI methadone, see QCG: Use of methadone for cancer pain, p.445. Methadone can also be given buccally, SL, PR, IV, CIVI ± PCA.[71,88–91] It has also been used as a topical analgesic for mouth ulcers (as a mouthwash),[92] and for open wounds and ulcers (in powder form mixed with Stomahesive®).[93]

For CSCI, dilute with WFI, 0.9% saline or 5% glucose. There are limited compatibility data for mixing methadone with other drugs for CSCI. Health professionals are encouraged to add details of any successful or unsuccessful combinations to the existing list of methadone combinations on the www.palliativedrugs.com Syringe Driver Survey Database (SDSD).

Supply

All preparations are Schedule 2 **CD**.

Ensure the correct concentration is prescribed; incidents have occurred because of confusion between methadone oral solution 1mg/mL with methadone oral concentrates 10mg/mL and 20mg/mL (authorized for opioid dependence) which require further dilution with Methadose® diluent to the required strength.[94]

Methadone (generic)
Tablets 5mg, 28 days @ 5mg b.d. = £3.
Oral solution 1mg/mL, 28 days @ 5mg b.d. = £3; *sugar-free available.*
Injection 10mg/mL, (1mL, 2mL, 3.5mL and 5mL amp = £1.25); 25mg/mL, (2mL amp = £1.50; 50mg/mL, (1mL amp = £1.50).

1 Caraceni A *et al.* (2012) Use of opioid analgesics in the treatment of cancer pain: evidence-based recommendations from the EAPC. *Lancet Oncology.* **13**: e58–68.
2 Gannon C (1997) The use of methadone in the care of the dying. *European Journal of Palliative Care.* **4**: 152–158.
3 Morley J and Makin M (1998) The use of methadone in cancer pain poorly responsive to other opioids. *Pain Reviews.* **5**: 51–58.
4 Watanabe S (2001) Methadone the renaissance. *Journal of Palliative Care.* **17 (2)**: 117–120.
5 Davis MP and Walsh D (2001) Methadone for relief of cancer pain: a review of pharmacokinetics, pharmacodynamics, drug interactions and protocols of administration. *Supportive Care in Cancer.* **9**: 73–83.
6 Ebert B *et al.* (1995) Ketobemidone, methadone and pethidine are non-competitive N-methyl-D-aspartate (NMDA) antagonists in the rat cortex and spinal cord. *Neuroscience Letter.* **187**: 165–168.
7 Gorman A *et al.* (1997) The d- and l- isomers of methadone bind to the non-competitive site on the N-methyl-D-aspartate (NMDA) receptor in rat forebrain and spinal cord. *Neuroscience Letters.* **223**: 5–8.
8 Codd E *et al.* (1995) Serotonin and norepinephrine uptake inhibiting activity of centrally acting analgesics: structural determinants and role in antinociception. *Journal of Pharmacology and Experimental Therapeutics.* **274**: 1263–1270.
9 Doi S *et al.* (2016) Characterization of methadone as a beta-arrestin-biased mu-opioid receptor agonist. *Molecular Pain.* **12**: 1–9.
10 Masocha W *et al.* (2016) Distinguishing subgroups among mu-opioid receptor agonists using Na(+),K(+)-ATPase as an effector mechanism. *European Journal of Pharmacology.* **774**: 43–49.
11 Takase N *et al.* (2015) Methadone for patients with malignant psoas syndrome: case series of three patients. *Journal of Palliative Medicine.* **18**: 645–652.
12 Sugiyama Y *et al.* (2016) A retrospective study on the effectiveness of switching to oral methadone for relieving severe cancer-related neuropathic pain and limiting adjuvant analgesic use in Japan. *Journal of Palliative Medicine.* **19**: 1051–1059.
13 McNicol ED *et al.* (2017) Methadone for neuropathic pain in adults. *Cochrane Database of Systematic Reviews.* **5**: CD012499. www.thecochranelibrary.com
14 Ferrari A *et al.* (2004) Methadone-metabolism, pharmacokinetics and interactions. *Pharmacological Research.* **50**: 551–559.
15 Robinson AE and Williams FM (1971) The distribution of methadone in man. *Journal of Pharmacy and Pharmacology.* **23**: 353–358.
16 Eap CB *et al.* (1990) Binding of D-methadone, L-methadone and DL-methadone to proteins in plasma of healthy volunteers: role of variants of X1-acid glycoprotein. *Clinical Pharmacology and Therapeutics.* **47**: 338–346.
17 Fainsinger R *et al.* (1993) Methadone in the management of cancer pain: clinical review. *Pain.* **52**: 137–147.
18 Inturrisi CE and Verebely K (1972) The levels of methadone in the plasma in methadone maintenance. *Clinical Pharmacology and Therapeutics.* **13**: 633–637.
19 King S *et al.* (2011) A systematic review of the use of opioid medication for those with moderate to severe cancer pain and renal impairment: A European palliative care research collaborative opioid guidelines project. *Palliative Medicine.* **25**: 525–552.
20 Bosilkovska M *et al.* (2012) Analgesics in patients with hepatic impairment: pharmacology and clinical implications. *Drugs.* **72**: 1645–1669.
21 Beaver WT *et al.* (1967) A clinical comparison of the analgesic effects of methadone and morphine administered intramuscularly, and of orally and parenterally administered methadone. *Clinical Pharmacology and Therapeutics.* **8**: 415–426.
22 Sawe J *et al.* (1981) Patient-controlled dose regimen of methadone for chronic cancer pain. *British Medical Journal.* **282**: 771–773.
23 Bruera E *et al.* (2004) Methadone versus morphine as a first-line strong opioid for cancer pain: a randomized, double-blind study. *Journal of Clinical Oncology.* **22**: 185–192.
24 Cornish CJ and Keen JC (2003) An alternative low-dose ad libitum schedule for conversion of other opioids to methadone. *Palliative Medicine.* **17**: 643–644.
25 Benitez-Rosario MA *et al.* (2009) Morphine-methadone opioid rotation in cancer patients: analysis of dose ratio predicting factors. *Journal of Pain and Symptom Management.* **37**: 1061–1068.
26 Mercadante S and Caraceni A (2011) Conversion ratios for opioid switching in the treatment of cancer pain: a systematic review. *Palliative Medicine.* **25**: 504–515.
27 Chatham MS *et al.* (2013) Dose ratios between high dose oral morphine or equivalents and oral methadone. *Journal of Palliative Medicine.* **16**: 947–950.
28 Walker PW *et al.* (2008) Switching from methadone to a different opioid: what is the equianalgesic dose ratio? *Journal of Palliative Medicine.* **11**: 1103–1108.
29 Nicholson AB *et al.* (2017) Methadone for cancer pain. *Cochrane Database of Systematic Reviews.* **2**: CD003971. www.thecochranelibrary.com
30 Cherny N (2011) Is oral methadone better than placebo or other oral/transdermal opioids in the management of pain? *Palliative Medicine.* **25**: 488–493.
31 Haroutiunian S *et al.* (2012) Methadone for chronic non-cancer pain in adults. *Cochrane Database of Systematic Reviews.* **11**: CD008025. www.thecochranelibrary.com
32 Mercadante S *et al.* (2008) Sustained-release oral morphine versus transdermal fentanyl and oral methadone in cancer pain management. *European Journal of Pain.* **12**: 1040–1046.

33 Gallagher R (2009) Methadone: an effective, safe drug of first choice for pain management in frail older adults. *Pain Medicine*. **10**: 319–326.
34 Salpeter SR *et al.* (2013) The use of very-low-dose methadone for palliative pain control and the prevention of opioid hyperalgesia. *Journal of Palliative Medicine*. **16**: 616–622.
35 Tse DM *et al.* (2003) An ad libitum schedule for conversion of morphine to methadone in advanced cancer patients: an open uncontrolled prospective study in a Chinese population. *Palliative Medicine*. **17**: 206–211.
36 Mercadante S *et al.* (2001) Switching from morphine to methadone to improve analgesia and tolerability in cancer patients: a prospective study. *Journal of Clinical Oncology*. **19**: 2898–2904.
37 Mercadante S *et al.* (1999) Rapid switching from morphine to methadone in cancer patients with poor response to morphine. *Journal of Clinical Oncology*. **17**: 3307–3312.
38 Porta-Sales J *et al.* (2016) Efficacy and safety of methadone as a second-line opioid for cancer pain in an outpatient clinic: a prospective open-label study. *Oncologist*. **21**: 981–987.
39 Sjogren P *et al.* (1994) Disappearance of morphine-induced hyperalgesia after discontinuing or substituting morphine with other opioid agonists. *Pain*. **59**: 313–316.
40 Hagen N and Swanson R (1997) Strychnine-like multifocal myoclonus and seizures in extremely high-dose opioid administration: treatment strategies. *Journal of Pain and Symptom Management*. **14**: 51–58.
41 Ashby M *et al.* (1999) Opioid substitution to reduce adverse effects in cancer pain management. *Medical Journal of Australia*. **170**: 68–71.
42 Morita T *et al.* (2005) Opioid rotation from morphine to fentanyl in delirious cancer patients: an open-label trial. *Journal of Pain and Symptom Management*. **30**: 96–103.
43 Furlan V *et al.* (1999) Methadone is poorly removed by haemodialysis. *Nephrology, Dialysis, Transplantation*. **14**: 254–255.
44 Manfredi P *et al.* (2001) Methadone analgesia in cancer pain patients on chronic methadone maintenance therapy. *Journal of Pain and Symptom Management*. **21**: 169–174.
45 Rowley D *et al.* (2011) Review of cancer pain management in patients receiving maintenance methadone therapy. *American Journal of Hospice and Palliative Care*. **28**: 183–187.
46 Taveros MC and Chuang EJ (2016) Pain management strategies for patients on methadone maintenance therapy: a systematic review of the literature. *BMJ Supportive and Palliative Care*. 1–7.
47 Love R and Bourgeois K (2014) Topical methadone: an alternative for pain control in end-of-life management. *Journal of Palliative Medicine*. **17**: 128.
48 Fisher K *et al.* (2004) Characterization of the early pharmacodynamic profile of oral methadone for cancer-related breakthrough pain: a pilot study. *Journal of Pain and Symptom Management*. **28**: 619–625.
49 Hagen NA *et al.* (2010) A formal feasibility study of sublingual methadone for breakthrough cancer pain. *Palliative Medicine*. **24**: 696–706.
50 Lugo RA *et al.* (2005) Pharmacokinetics of methadone. *Journal of Pain and Palliative Care Pharmacotherapy*. **19**: 13–24.
51 Nilsson MI *et al.* (1982) Pharmacokinetics of methadone during maintenance treatment: adaptive changes during the induction phase. *European Journal of Clinical Pharmarcology*. **22**: 343–349.
52 Hendra T *et al.* (1996) Fatal methadone overdose. *British Medical Journal*. **313**: 481–482.
53 Wilcock A and Beattie JM (2009) Prolonged QT interval and methadone: implications for palliative care. *Current Opinion in Supportive and Palliative Care*. **3**: 252–257.
54 Kornick CA *et al.* (2003) QTc interval prolongation associated with intravenous methadone. *Pain*. **105**: 499–506.
55 Bunten H *et al.* (2011) CYP2B6 and OPRM1 gene variations predict methadone-related deaths. *Addiction Biology*. **16**: 142–144.
56 Eap CB *et al.* (2007) Stereoselective block of hERG channel by (S)-methadone and QT interval prolongation in CYP2B6 slow metabolizers. *Clinical Pharmacology and Therapeutics*. **81**: 719–728.
57 Baxter K and Preston CL. *Stockley's Drug Interactions*. London: Pharmaceutical Press www.medicinescomplete.com (accessed May 2017).
58 Kreek MJ *et al.* (1976) Rifampin-induced methadone withdrawal. *New England Journal of Medicine*. **294**: 1104–1106.
59 Wahawisan J *et al.* (2011) Methadone toxicity due to smoking cessation--a case report on the drug-drug interaction involving cytochrome P450 isoenzyme 1A2. *Annals of Pharmacotherapy*. **45**: e34.
60 Buchanan D (2010) Sinus bradycardia related to methadone in a patient with myeloma receiving thalidomide therapy. *Palliative Medicine*. **24**: 742–743.
61 Sarhill N *et al.* (2001) Methadone-induced myoclonus in advanced cancer. *American Journal of Hospice and Palliative Care*. **18 (1)**: 51–53.
62 Davis MP *et al.* (2007) When opioids cause pain. *Journal of Clinical Oncology*. **25**: 4497–4498.
63 El Osta B *et al.* (2007) Intractable pain: intoxication or undermedication? *Journal of Palliative Medicine*. **10**: 811–814.
64 Hoff AM *et al.* (2017) Methadone-induced neurotoxicity in advanced cancer: a case report. *Journal of Palliative Medicine*. **20**: 1042–1044.
65 Bruera E *et al.* (1991) Local toxicity with subcutaneous methadone. Experience of two centers. *Pain*. **45**: 141–143.
66 Flory JH *et al.* (2016) Methadone use and the risk of hypoglycemia for inpatients with cancer pain. *Journal of Pain and Symptom Management*. **51**: 79–87.
67 Saifan C *et al.* (2013) Methadone induced sensorineural hearing loss. *Case Reports in Medicine*. **2013**: Article ID 242730.
68 Vorasubin N *et al.* (2013) Methadone-induced bilateral severe sensorineural hearing loss. *American Journal of Otolaryngology*. **34**: 735–738.
69 Twycross RG (1977) A comparison of diamorphine with cocaine and methadone. *British Journal of Clinical Pharmacology* **4**: 691–692.
70 Lipman AG (2005) Methadone: effective analgesia, confusion, and risk. *Journal of Pain and Palliative Care Pharmacotherapy*. **19** 3–5.
71 Santiago-Palma J *et al.* (2001) Intravenous methadone in the management of chronic cancer pain: safe and effective starting doses when substituting methadone for fentanyl. *Cancer*. **92**: 1919–1925.
72 Blackburn D *et al.* (2002) Methadone: an alternative conversion regime. *European Journal of Palliative Care*. **9**: 93–96.
73 Blackburn D (2005) Methadone: the analgesic. *European Journal of Palliative Care*. **12**: 188–191.
74 Bruera E *et al.* (1996) Opioid rotation in patients with cancer pain. *Cancer*. **78**: 852–857.
75 Auret K *et al.* (2006) Pharmacokinetics and pharmacodynamics of methadone enantiomers in hospice patients with cancer pain. *Therapeutic Drug Monitoring*. **28**: 359–366.
76 Moksnes K *et al.* (2011) How to switch from morphine or oxycodone to methadone in cancer patients? a randomised clinical phase II trial. *European Journal of Cancer*. **47**: 2463–2470.
77 Moksnes K *et al.* (2012) Serum concentrations of opioids when comparing two switching strategies to methadone for cancer pain. *European Journal of Clinical Pharmacology*. **68**: 1147–1156.
78 McLean S and Twomey F (2015) Methods of rotation from another strong opioid to methadone for the management of cancer pain: a systematic review of the available evidence. *Journal of Pain and Symptom Management*. **50**: 248–259.e241.

79 Palliativedrugs.com (2005) Hot Topics: new draft methadone monograph. In: *September Newsletter*. Available from: www.palliativedrugs.com
80 Soares LG (2005) Methadone for cancer pain: what have we learned from clinical studies? *American Journal of Hospice and Palliative Care*. **22**: 223–227.
81 Hagen N and Wasylenko E (1999) Methadone: outpatient titration and monitoring strategies in cancer patients. *Journal of Pain and Symptom Management*. **18**: 369–375.
82 Zimmermann C *et al.* (2005) Rotation to methadone after opioid dose escalation: How should individualization of dosing occur? *Journal of Pain and Palliative Care Pharmacotherapy*. **19**: 25–31.
83 Scholes C *et al.* (1999) Methadone titration in opioid-resistant cancer pain. *European Journal of Cancer Care*. **8**: 26–29.
84 Courtemanche F *et al.* (2016) Methadone as a coanalgesic for palliative care cancer patients. *Journal of Palliative Medicine*. **19**: 972–978.
85 Fallon MT and Laird BJ (2011) A systematic review of combination step III opioid therapy in cancer pain: an EPCRC opioid guideline project. *Palliative Medicine*. **25**: 597–603.
86 Mathew P and Storey P (1999) Subcutaneous methadone in terminally ill patients: manageable local toxicity. *Journal of Pain and Symptom Management*. **18**: 49–52.
87 Centeno C and Vara F (2005) Intermittent subcutaneous methadone administration in the management of cancer pain. *Journal of Pain and Palliative Care Pharmacotherapy*. **19**: 7–12.
88 Fitzgibbon D and Ready L (1997) Intravenous high-dose methadone administered by patient controlled analgesia and continuous infusion for the treatment of cancer pain refractory to high-dose morphine. *Pain*. **73**: 259–261.
89 Davis M and Walsh D (2001) Methadone for relief of cancer pain: a review of pharmacokinetics, pharmacodynamics, drug interactions and protocols of administration. *Supportive Care in Cancer*. **9**: 73–83.
90 Manfredi PL and Houde RW (2003) Prescribing methadone, a unique analgesic. *Journal of Supportive Oncology*. **1**: 216–220.
91 Spaner D (2014) Effectiveness of the buccal mucosa route for methadone administration at the end of life. *Journal of Palliative Medicine*. **17**: 1262–1265.
92 Gallagher R (2004) Methadone mouthwash for the management of oral ulcer pain. *Journal of Pain and Symptom Management*. **27**: 390–391.
93 Gallagher RE *et al.* (2005) Analgesic effects of topical methadone: a report of four cases. *Clinical Journal of Pain*. **21**: 190–192.
94 Care Quality Commission (2014) Safer use of controlled drugs - preventing harms from methadone. *Use of controlled drugs supporting information*. www.cqc.org.uk

Updated September 2017

Quick Clinical Guide: Use of methadone for cancer pain

Methadone has both opioid and non-opioid properties, and a long variable halflife (range 5–130h vs. 2.5h for morphine). Thus, there is no single conversion ratio for methadone and other opioids. When switching from morphine, the eventual 24h dose of methadone is typically 5–10 times smaller than the dose of morphine, sometimes 20–30 times smaller, and occasionally even smaller. Inevitable accumulation is the reason for the week-long intervals between dose adjustments. *Switching must be closely supervised by specialists*, generally as an inpatient.

Indications for use

- any of the following, when switching to another easier-to-use opioid (e.g. fentanyl, hydromorphone, oxycodone) is not possible:
  - ▷ neurotoxicity with morphine (e.g. myoclonus, allodynia, hyperalgesia) which does not respond to a reduction in dose
  - ▷ morphine poorly-responsive pain, e.g. mixed nociceptive–neuropathic pain despite additional use of NSAID + adjuvant analgesics
  - ▷ end-stage renal failure
- the strong opioid of choice, instead of morphine.

Dose titration

1. When prescribing PO methadone as first-line strong opioid:
   - start with methadone 2.5mg (1–2mg in the elderly) q12h regularly and q3h p.r.n.
   - if necessary, titrate the regular dose upwards once a week, guided by p.r.n. use
   - continue with 2.5mg p.r.n., or 1–2mg in the elderly
   - with doses ≥30mg q12h, increase the p.r.n. dose to 1/6–1/10 of the q24h dose, rounded to a convenient tablet size or volume.
2. If the patient is already receiving morphine, use the following method.

PO morphine to PO methadone

Morphine is stopped abruptly when methadone is started.
If switching from:

- immediate-release morphine, give the first dose of methadone ≥2h (pain present) or 4h (pain-free) after last dose of morphine
- m/r morphine, give the first dose of methadone ≥6h (pain present) or 12h (pain-free) after the last dose of a 12h preparation, or ≥12h (pain present) or 24h (pain-free) after the last dose of a 24h preparation.

Give a single loading dose of PO methadone 1/10 of the previous total 24h PO morphine dose, up to a maximum of 30mg.

Give q3h p.r.n. doses of PO methadone 1/30 of the previous total 24h PO morphine dose, rounded to a convenient tablet size or volume, up to a maximum of 30mg per dose.

Example 1: Morphine 300mg/24h PO = loading dose of methadone 30mg PO, and 10mg q3h p.r.n.

Example 2: Morphine 1,200mg/24h PO = loading dose of methadone 120mg PO, and 40mg q3h p.r.n.; however, both are limited to the maximum of 30mg.

For patients in severe pain who need more analgesia in <3h, see point 6 below.

On Day 6, the amount of methadone taken *in total* over the previous 2 days is noted and divided by 4 to give a regular q12h dose, with 1/6–1/10 of the 24h dose q3h p.r.n., e.g. *methadone 80mg PO in previous 48h → 20mg q12h and 5mg PO q3h p.r.n.*

If ≥2 doses/day of p.r.n. methadone continue to be needed, the dose of regular methadone should be increased once a week, guided by p.r.n. use.

3 If using another strong opioid, calculate the morphine equivalent daily dose and then follow the guidelines for morphine.

4 If converting from PO methadone to SC/IV methadone, or from another CSCI/CIVI opioid, see the respective boxes below.

5 If there has been recent rapid escalation of the pre-switch opioid dose, calculate the initial dose of methadone using the pre-escalation dose of the opioid.

6 For patients in severe pain and who need more analgesia in <3h, options include:
   - taking the previously used opioid q1h p.r.n. (50–100% of the p.r.n. dose used before switching)
   - if neurotoxicity with the pre-switch opioid, use an appropriate dose of an alternative strong opioid.

7 The switch to methadone is successful (i.e. improved pain relief and/or reduced toxicity) in about 75% of patients.

8 If a patient:
   - becomes oversedated, reduce the dose generally by 33–50% (some centres monitor the level of consciousness and respirations q4h for 24h)
   - develops opioid abstinence symptoms, give p.r.n. doses of the previous opioid to control these.

PO methadone to SC/IV or CSCI/CIVI methadone

To convert PO methadone to SC/IV methadone, halve the PO dose, e.g. methadone 80mg/24h PO = 40mg/24h SC/IV, this is a safe conversion ratio. For some patients, particularly those receiving <80mg/24h, the SC/IV dose = PO dose.

Because of its long halflife, methadone (10mg/mL injection) can be given SC q12h–q8h. If SC injection is painful or causes local inflammation, give by CSCI/CIVI instead.

If CSCI methadone causes a skin reaction:
- administer as a more dilute solution in a 20–30mL syringe
- change the site daily
- consider applying hydrocortisone cream 1% topically around the needle entry site (under an occlusive dressing)
- consider adding dexamethasone 1mg to the diluted combination of drugs (compatibility data permitting).

For additional rescue doses of methadone SC/IV, give 1/6–1/10 of the 24h SC/IV dose q3h p.r.n., e.g. methadone 20mg CIVI/24h = 2mg q3h p.r.n. SC/IV.

If ≥2 p.r.n doses/day continue to be needed, the 24h SC/IV dose should be increased once a week, guided by p.r.n. use.

For patients in severe pain who need more analgesia in <3h, see point 6 above.

Other CSCI/CIVI opioids to CSCI/CIVI methadone

The safest approach is to follow the method for PO switching, using bolus injections of SC/IV methadone instead of PO doses.

Convert the opioid 24h CSCI/CIVI dose to its PO equivalent and determine the PO methadone dose (Dose titration, point 2).

The SC/IV dose of methadone is half the PO dose; the maximum initial dose of SC/IV methadone will be 15mg. This is a safe conversion ratio; for some patients the SC/IV dose = PO dose.

Updated September 2017

OXYCODONE

Class: Strong opioid analgesic.

Indications: Moderate–severe cancer and non-cancer pain, †an alternative in cases of intolerance to other strong opioids.[1,2] Restless legs syndrome (Targinact®, see Box A).

Contra-indications: Moderate–severe hepatic impairment. Otherwise none absolute if titrated carefully against a patient's pain (also see Strong opioids, p.360).

Pharmacology

Oxycodone is a strong opioid with similar properties to **morphine** (p.375).[3–5] Its main effects are the result of activity at the μ-opioid receptor, although this may involve different G-protein subunits and thereby different downstream effects to **morphine** (also see p.361).[6–9] Studies in rodents suggest oxycodone may also possess activity at δ- and κ-opioid receptors.[10,11]

Like **morphine**, oxycodone shows efficacy in pure neuropathic pain states (diabetic and postherpetic neuropathy), with a NNT of 5.7 (95% CI 4.0–9.9) for moderate benefit. However, as with **morphine**, the evidence is considered very low quality.[12]

Oxycodone appears to be less immunosuppressive than **morphine**. In patients with cancer pain, although one small retrospective study found the incidence of infections to be less in those receiving **oxycodone** compared to **morphine**, another found no difference between **fentanyl**, **morphine** and **oxycodone**, with the risk of infection increasing with dose (see p.360).

Most of the analgesic effect arises from oxycodone itself.[13] The main metabolite, noroxycodone (via CYP3A4), is active at the μ-opioid receptor but to a much lesser degree. Another metabolite, **oxymorphone** (via CYP2D6), is produced in relatively small amounts but has ≥10 times the affinity and activity of oxycodone.[13] However, studies in postoperative and cancer pain found no differences between CYP2D6 ultra-rapid, extensive or poor metabolizers in the dose requirements or analgesic efficacy of oxycodone, suggesting **oxymorphone** contributes little overall.[14,15] Nonetheless, case reports suggest that opioid-naïve CYP2D6 ultra-rapid metabolizers may be at greater risk of undesirable CNS effects when starting oxycodone because of an enhanced production of **oxymorphone** (also see Chapter 19, p.717).[16] (Note. **Oxymorphone** is commercially available in some countries (not UK) and is 3 times and 10 times more potent than PO and parenteral **morphine** respectively.[17])

By mouth, oxycodone has a mean bio-availability of 75%, whereas **morphine**'s is about half this (see p.375). This partly explains why PO oxycodone is more potent than PO **morphine** (i.e. *fewer* mg of oxycodone are needed than **morphine** to have a comparable analgesic effect).[18–23]

According to the UK manufacturer, oxycodone PO is twice as potent as **morphine** PO. Although reasonable in terms of caution and safety, this almost certainly exaggerates the actual potency of oxycodone, and a conversion ratio of **morphine** to oxycodone of 1.5:1 is generally used in clinical practice, i.e. the dose of oxycodone PO should be two thirds of the **morphine** PO dose (e.g. oxycodone 10mg PO is equivalent to **morphine** 15mg PO).

Parenterally, when the bio-availability of **morphine** and oxycodone is comparable, the situation is different. Despite a short-term (2h) postoperative PCA study which suggested that **morphine** is less potent parenterally than oxycodone (i.e. *more* mg of **morphine** will be needed, as with PO administration),[24] earlier single-dose studies and two more recent longer PCA studies (1–2 days) suggest that by injection **morphine** is more potent than oxycodone, in the region of 4:3. Thus, *fewer* mg of **morphine** will be needed (**morphine** 10mg being approximately equivalent to oxycodone 13mg).[17,18,25] However, given the modest difference in potency, together with the constraints of ampoule size, it is reasonable in clinical practice to use a conversion ratio of 1:1, i.e. when converting from **morphine** injection to oxycodone injections (or vice versa) regard SC/IV **morphine** 10mg as equivalent to SC/IV oxycodone 10mg.

When switching from PO oxycodone to SC/IV oxycodone, although the UK manufacturer recommends a conversion ratio of 2:1, because mean PO bio-availability is 75%, this may be too conservative for some patients. Thus, some centres use a conversion ratio of 1.5:1, i.e. the oxycodone SC/IV 24h dose should be two thirds of the oxycodone PO 24h dose. (Also see Opioid switching p.370 and Appendix 2, Table 3, p.861). For switching from PO **morphine** to CSCI oxycodone, see Dose and use.

About 20% of oxycodone is excreted unchanged in the urine. In mild–moderate hepatic impairment, oxycodone and noroxycodone concentrations increase by 50% and 20% respectively (but the **oxymorphone** concentration decreases) and the elimination halflife increases by about 2h. In renal impairment the clearance of oxycodone, noroxycodone and conjugated **oxymorphone** are reduced. Oxycodone plasma concentration increases by 50% and the halflife lengthens by 1h.[19,26] Nonetheless, oxycodone is used as an alternative to **morphine** in mild–moderate renal impairment and is used cautiously in some centres in severe renal impairment for initial pain management (see Dose and use and p.693).

Although reports are not consistent, most suggest that the clearance of oxycodone is unaffected by increasing age *per se*; any reduction most likely relating to associated renal impairment.[27,28] However, in the presence of systemic inflammation sufficient to increase C-RP and IL-6 levels, there is inhibition of CYP3A, resulting in higher plasma levels of oxycodone.[29]

Bio-availability 75% PO, ranging from 60–87%.[30,31]
Onset of action 20–30min PO.
Time to peak plasma concentration 1–1.5h; 3h m/r.
Plasma halflife 3.5h; 4.5h in renal failure.
Duration of action 4–6h; 12h m/r.

Cautions

Renal and mild hepatic impairment (see Dose and use, Chapter 17, p.693 and Chapter 18, p.709).

Drug interactions

Inhibitors of CYP3A4 (e.g. **voriconazole**, **erythromycin**, **fluconazole**, **telithromycin** and **ritonavir**) can inhibit oxycodone metabolism, and may enhance its effects.[32–36] However, inhibition of CYP2D6 (e.g. with **quinidine**) appears to have no detectable clinical impact.[37]

The enzyme inducers **rifampicin** and **St John's Wort** decrease plasma concentrations of oxycodone.[32,38,39]

Undesirable effects

See Strong opioids, Box B, p.365. Various studies have suggested possible differences in the undesirable effect profiles of oxycodone and **morphine**.[40] However, systematic reviews comparing efficacy and tolerability of oxycodone versus other opioids found no overall difference in the undesirable effect profile between oxycodone and either **morphine** or **hydromorphone**.[4,5]

Dose and use

As with all opioids, patients must be monitored for undesirable effects, particularly nausea and vomiting, and constipation. Depending on individual circumstances, an anti-emetic should be prescribed for regular or p.r.n. use, (see QCG, Nausea and vomiting, p.240) and, routinely, a laxative prescribed (see QCG Opioid-induced constipation, p.42).

Opioids can impair driving ability and patients should be counselled accordingly (see p.743).

Although oxycodone is similar to **morphine** (and **hydromorphone**) in terms of efficacy and undesirable effects,[2] because it is more expensive it should generally be reserved for patients who cannot tolerate **morphine**. In Scotland, oxycodone injections are restricted to cancer patients who cannot tolerate **diamorphine** or **morphine** injections.

A combination product of oxycodone with **naloxone** is available (Targinact® Box A).

Remains of m/r tablets (e.g. Oxycontin®, Longtec® and Targinact®) may appear in the patient's faeces ('ghost tablets'), but these are inert residues, and do not affect the efficacy of the products.

Oral

Immediate-release oxycodone is generally given q4h but, in some patients, q6h is satisfactory.[41] Oxycodone m/r tablets are biphasic in their release of oxycodone, i.e. there is an initial fast release which leads to the early onset of analgesia and a slow release which provides a prolonged duration of action. M/r tablets should be swallowed whole; crushing or chewing them will lead to a rapid release of an overdose of oxycodone.

Box A Oxycodone combined with naloxone (Targinact®)

Targinact® is marketed as a range of tablets containing m/r formulations of oxycodone and naloxone in a fixed-dose ratio of 2:1, i.e. oxycodone 5mg/naloxone 2.5mg; 10mg/5mg; 20mg/10mg and 40mg/20mg. The addition of naloxone is to antagonize the constipating effect of oxycodone. The desire to develop a formulation which deters misuse (e.g. by crushing and injecting IV) is also relevant.

Targinact® is authorized for severe pain. Evidence to support claims of improved pain control, better GI tolerability, and improved quality of life are based mainly on uncontrolled, observational studies.[42–47]

RCTs have mostly involved relatively young non-cancer (mid–late 50s) and cancer patients (early 60s) with either moderate or severe pain, and with no significant hepatic or renal impairment. Reported use in older non-cancer (early 80s) and cancer patients (mean age 70) is limited to open-label studies.[44,48,49]

In the non-cancer studies, those unwilling or unable to tolerate a 'restricted laxative regimen' were excluded, i.e. the most severely constipated. Although Targinact® improved bowel function and reduced the number of patients requiring laxatives, the absolute differences were small (e.g. on average, one extra bowel action/week and a reduction of 0.6mg/24h in bisacodyl dose). However, laxatives were taken only p.r.n.[50–52]

In RCTs including cancer patients, Targinact® improved bowel function and there was a trend towards a reduction in laxative use. However, absolute differences were of similar magnitudes as above, and laxatives were taken only p.r.n.[52,53]

Targinact® is 40% more expensive than the equivalent dose of m/r oxycodone alone, and 2–3 times more expensive than an equivalent dose of morphine + regular laxatives. Because the benefit of Targinact® in patients taking laxatives *regularly* is uncertain, the Scottish Medicines Consortium, the Drugs and Therapeutics Bulletin and *PCF* do *not* recommend its use.[54]

Although Targinact® is also authorized as a second-line treatment for restless legs syndrome refractory to dopaminergic therapy, the available evidence is limited.[55,56]

If clinicians choose to prescribe Targinact®, its use should be restricted to occasions when the upward titration of regularly administered laxatives is ineffective (see p.46). Because constipation is generally multifactorial in origin,[57] Targinact® is likely to augment rather than replace laxatives.[50,51]

The m/r formulation of naloxone avoids a 'bolus dose', and >97% is removed by first-pass metabolism in the liver. Thus, the main effect of naloxone is on the GI tract, with insufficient amounts reaching the systemic circulation to adversely affect analgesia.[58,59] However, plasma concentrations of naloxone can increase significantly in:

- *hepatic impairment:* use of Targinact® requires caution in mild impairment and is contra-indicated in moderate–severe impairment
- *renal impairment:* use Targinact® with caution.

The increase in naloxone can antagonize the analgesic effect of oxycodone, resulting in either frank opioid withdrawal or the need to increase to an 'artifically' higher dose.[60] Thus, in a patient with progressive hepatic impairment, a switch from Targinact® to the same dose of oxycodone m/r, resulted in opioid-induced respiratory depression within 12h.[60]

Dose recommendations:

- in opioid-naïve patients, generally start with oxycodone/naloxone 10mg/5mg b.d.
- in elderly/frail patients, start with 5mg/2.5mg b.d.
- in those already taking strong opioids, switch to the equivalent dose of oxycodone
- maximum dose 80mg/40mg b.d.

When higher analgesic doses are required, the manufacturer recommends supplemental oxycodone m/r tablets, taken at the same time as the m/r combination tablets. However, this reduces the impact of the naloxone, and oxycodone:naloxone ratios >4:1 have no significant effect on bowel function.[51,61] However, a recent study used doses ≤90mg/45mg b.d.[62]

Common undesirable effects include nausea, vomiting, abdominal pain and diarrhoea. The manufacturer warns that patients on long-term opioids may develop opioid withdrawal symptoms when switched to Targinact®.

For strong opioid-naïve patients:

- start with 5mg q6h–q4h for immediate-release capsules and oral solutions
- start with 10mg b.d. for m/r tablets
- halve the above doses in elderly/frail patients or those with mild–moderate renal impairment or mild hepatic impairment (also see below)
- if necessary, titrate the dose upwards, guided by p.r.n. use; conventionally, p.r.n. PO doses are 1/6–1/10 of the total 24h PO dose.

For patients switching from PO **morphine** to PO oxycodone, *PCF* recommends a conversion ratio of 1.5:1 (see Pharmacology):

- PO **morphine** to PO oxycodone, decrease the dose by one third, e.g. **morphine** 15mg PO → oxycodone 10mg PO.

For general considerations when converting opioids, see p.855.

SC/CSCI

Oxycodone injection may be given SC as a bolus or by CSCI (and also IV by bolus and by CIVI). For CSCI, dilute with WFI, 0.9% saline or 5% glucose.

For strong opioid-naïve patients:

start with 7.5mg/24h CSCI

if necessary, titrate the dose upwards, guided by p.r.n. use; conventionally, p.r.n. SC doses are 1/6–1/10 of the total 24h CSCI dose.

For general considerations when switching routes ± converting opioids, see p.855. The following are practical clinical conversion ratios:

- PO oxycodone to CSCI oxycodone, decrease the dose by one third, e.g. oxycodone 30mg/24h PO → oxycodone 20mg/24h CSCI (see Pharmacology)
- PO **morphine** to CSCI oxycodone, decrease the dose by half, e.g. **morphine** 60mg/24h PO → oxycodone 30mg/24h CSCI.

When switching from **morphine** CSCI to oxycodone CSCI, *PCF* recommends a dose conversion ratio of 1:1 (see Pharmacology):

- CSCI **morphine** to CSCI oxycodone, give the same dose, e.g. **morphine** 30mg/24h CSCI → oxycodone 30mg/24h CSCI
- if necessary, titrate the dose upwards, guided by p.r.n. use.

Two strengths of injection are available, 10mg/mL and high-strength 50mg/mL. The latter may be useful in situations where high doses cause volume difficulties for CSCI. However, there is an increased risk of serious mistakes being made when more than one strength is readily available.[63,64] There are also differences in compatibility with other drugs (see below) and, on a mg for mg basis, the high-strength injection costs about twice as much.

CSCI with oxycodone 10mg/mL

There are 2-drug compatibility data for mixtures in WFI with **clonazepam, dexamethasone, glycopyrronium, haloperidol, hyoscine *butylbromide*, hyoscine *hydrobromide*, levomepromazine, metoclopramide, midazolam,** and **octreotide**.

Concentration-dependent incompatibility may occur when oxycodone (hydrochloride) is mixed with **cyclizine** (lactate); for more details see Appendix 3, Chart 1, p866.

CSCI with oxycodone 50mg/mL

Differences in compatibility with other drugs for the 10mg/mL and 50mg/mL formulations of oxycodone have been reported.[65,66] This may be due to the different ratios of excipients in each formulation (see Appendix 3, Table 1, p.880). It is important *not* to extrapolate compatibility information from one formulation to the other.

More details

For 2-drug and 3-drug compatibility data for oxycodone 10mg/mL in WFI, and for currently available data for oxycodone 50mg/mL, see Appendix 3, Charts 1 (p.866), 6 (p.000) and Table 1 (p.880).

Information on compatibility in 0.9% saline can be found in the extended appendix section of the on-line *PCF* on *www.palliativedrugs.com*.

5

Renal or hepatic impairment

Because of the risk of impaired metabolism or elimination:

- lower than usual starting doses are advised in mild–moderate renal impairment or mild hepatic impairment, i.e. start with a maximum of 10mg/24h PO as for frail/elderly patients
- in severe *renal impairment* or ESRF start with 1–2mg PO q6–8h and p.r.n; once pain is controlled consider switching to an equivalent dose of TD fentanyl (see p.693)
- oxycodone is contra-indicated in moderate–severe hepatic impairment. If unavoidable, lower the usual starting dose *and* increase the dosing interval of immediate release products to q8h (see p.709).

For a general approach when renal of hepatic function deteriorates rapidly, see p.364.

Supply

All preparations are Schedule 2 **CD**.

Immediate-release oral products

> Oxycodone oral solution is available in two strengths, 1mg/mL and a high potency concentrate of 10mg/mL.; incidents have occurred from confusion between the two formulations.[67,68] Prescribing should be in *mg* not mL to minimise the risk of 10 times the intended dose being given.

Oxycodone (generic)
Capsules 5mg, 10mg, 20mg, 5mg dose = £0.13.
Oral solution 5mg/5mL, 5mg dose = £0.20.
Concentrated oral solution 10mg/mL, 5mg dose = £0.20.
Injection 10mg/mL, 1mL and 2mL amp = £1.50 and £3 respectively.
Injection 50mg/mL, 1mL amp = £14.

Modified-release 12-hourly oral products

> As for all m/r opioids, brand prescribing is recommended to reduce the risk of confusion and error in dispensing and administration (see p.xvii).[68]

Oxycodone (generic)
Tablets m/r 5mg, 10mg, 15mg, 20mg, 30mg, 40mg, 60mg, 80mg, 120mg 28 days @ 5mg or 120mg b.d. = £13 and £153 respectively. *Note. The 15mg, 30mg, 60mg and 120mg are not available for all brands; only Longtec® and Oxycontin® have the full range of strengths available.*
Brands include Abtard®, Carexil®, Leveraxo®, Longtec®, Onexila® XL, Oxeltra®, Oxycontin®, Oxylan®, Reltebon®, Zomestine®.

Oxycodone/naloxone combined
Targinact® (Napp)
Tablets m/r containing oxycodone/naloxone in a fixed ratio of 2:1, 5mg/2.5mg, 10mg/5mg, 20mg/10mg, 40mg/20mg, 28 days @10mg/5mg b.d. = £42.

1 King S *et al.* (2011) A systematic review of the use of opioid medication for those with moderate to severe cancer pain and renal impairment: A European palliative care research collaborative opioid guidelines project. *Palliative Medicine*. **25**: 525–552.
2 Caraceni A *et al.* (2012) Use of opioid analgesics in the treatment of cancer pain: evidence-based recommendations from the EAPC. *Lancet Oncology*. **13**: e58–68.
3 Kalso E (2005) Oxycodone. *Journal of Pain and Symptom Management*. **29 (Suppl 5)**: S47–S56.
4 Schmidt-Hansen M *et al.* (2015) Oxycodone for cancer-related pain. *Cochrane Database of Systematic Reviews*. **2**: CD003870. www.thecochranelibrary.com
5 Ma H (2016) The adverse events of oxycodone in cancer-related pain. *Medicine*. **95**: 1–9.
6 Gaspari S *et al.* (2017) RGS9-2 Modulates responses to oxycodone in pain-free and chronic pain states. *Neuropsychopharmacology*. **42**: 1548–1556.
7 Lemberg KK *et al.* (2006) Antinociception by spinal and systemic oxycodone: why does the route make a difference? In vitro and in vivo studies in rats. *Anesthesiology*. **105**: 801–812.
8 Kalso E *et al.* (1990) Morphine and oxycodone in the management of cancer pain: plasma levels determined by chemical and radioreceptor assays. *Pharmacology and Toxicology*. **67**: 322–328.
9 Nakamura A *et al.* (2013) Differential activation of the mu-opioid receptor by oxycodone and morphine in pain-related brain regions in a bone cancer pain model. *British Journal of Pharmacology*. **168**: 375–388.

10 Yang PP *et al.* (2016) Activation of delta-opioid receptor contributes to the antinociceptive effect of oxycodone in mice. *Pharmacological Research.* **111**: 867–876.
11 Ross F and Smith M (1997) The intrinsic antinociceptive effects of oxycodone appear to be kappa-opioid receptor mediated. *Pain.* **73**: 151–157.
12 Gaskell H *et al.* (2016) Oxycodone for neuropathic pain in adults. *Cochrane Database of Systematic Reviews.* **7**: CD010692. www.thecochranelibrary.com
13 Ruan X *et al.* (2017) Revisiting oxycodone analgesia: a review and hypothesis. *Anesthesiology Clinics.* **35**: e163–e174.
14 Zwisler ST *et al.* (2010) Impact of the CYP2D6 genotype on post-operative intravenous oxycodone analgesia. *Acta Anaesthesiologica Scandinavica.* **54**: 232–240.
15 Andreassen TN *et al.* (2012) Do CYP2D6 genotypes reflect oxycodone requirements for cancer patients treated for cancer pain? A cross-sectional multicentre study. *European Journal of Clinical Pharmacology.* **68**: 55–64.
16 de Leon J *et al.* (2003) Adverse drug reactions to oxycodone and hydrocodone in CYP2D6 ultrarapid metabolizers. *Journal of Clinical Psychopharmacology.* **23**: 420–421.
17 Beaver WT *et al.* (1978) Analgesic studies of codeine and oxycodone in patients with cancer. II. Comparisons of intramuscular oxycodone with intramuscular morphine and codeine. *Journal Pharmacology and Experiemental Therapeutics.* **207**: 101–108.
18 Kalso E and Vainio A (1990) Morphine and oxycodone in the management of cancer pain. *Clinical Pharmacology and Therapeutics.* **47**: 639–646.
19 Heiskanen T and Kalso E (1997) Controlled-release oxycodone and morphine in cancer related pain. *Pain.* **73**: 37–45.
20 Bruera E *et al.* (1998) Randomized, double-blind, cross-over trial comparing safety and efficacy of oral controlled-release oxycodone with controlled-release morphine in patients with cancer pain. *Journal of Clinical Oncology.* **16**: 3222–3229.
21 Mucci-LoRusso P *et al.* (1998) Controlled-release oxycodone compared with controlled-release morphine in the treatment of cancer pain: a randomized, double-blind, parallel-group study. *European Journal of Pain.* **2**: 239–249.
22 Curtis GB *et al.* (1999) Relative potency of controlled-release oxycodone and controlled-release morphine in a postoperative pain model. *European Journal of Clinical Pharmacology.* **55**: 425–429.
23 Lauretti GR *et al.* (2003) Comparison of sustained-release morphine with sustained-release oxycodone in advanced cancer patients. *British Journal of Cancer.* **89**: 2027–2030.
24 Kalso E et *al.* (1991) Intravenous morphine and oxycodone for pain after abdominal surgery. *Acta anaesthesiologica Scandinavica.* **35**: 642–646.
25 Silvasti M et *al.* (1998) Comparison of analgesic efficacy of oxycodone and morphine in postoperative intravenous patient-controlled analgesia. *Acta anaesthesiologica Scandinavica.* **42**: 576–580.
26 Glare P and Davis MP (2009) Oxycodone. In: MP Davis *et al.* (eds) *Opioids in Cancer Pain* (2e). Oxford University Press, Oxford, pp. 155–173.
27 Liukas A *et al.* (2011) Elimination of intravenous oxycodone in the elderly: a pharmacokinetic study in postoperative orthopaedic patients of different age groups. *Drugs Aging.* **28**: 41–50.
28 Charles B *et al.* (2014) Should the dosage of controlled-release oxycodone in advanced cancer be modified on the basis of patient characteristics? *Supportive Care in Cancer.* **22**: 325–330.
29 Sato H and Naito T (2016) Relationships between oxycodone pharmacokinetics, central symptoms, and serum interleukin-6 in cachectic cancer patients. *European Journal of Clinical Pharmacology.* **72**: 1463–1470.
30 Leow K *et al.* (1992) Single-dose and steady-state pharmacokinetics and pharmacodynamics of oxycodone in patients with cancer. *Clinical Pharmacology and Therapeutics.* **52**: 487–495.
31 Poyhia R *et al.* (1992) The pharmacokinetics and metabolism of oxycodone after intramuscular and oral administration to healthy subjects. *British Journal of Clinical Pharmacology.* **33**: 617–621.
32 Baxter K, Preston CL *Stockley's Drug Interactions.* London: Pharmaceutical Press www.medicinescomplete.com (accessed January 2017).
33 Hagelberg NM *et al.* (2009) Voriconazole drastically increases exposure to oral oxycodone. *European Journal of Clinical Pharmacology.* **65**: 263–271.
34 Nieminen TH *et al.* (2010) Oxycodone concentrations are greatly increased by the concomitant use of ritonavir or lopinavir/ritonavir. *European Journal of Clinical Pharmacology.* **66**: 977–985.
35 Hagelberg NM *et al.* (2011) Interaction of oxycodone and voriconazole-a case series of patients with cancer pain supports the findings of randomised controlled studies with healthy subjects. *European Journal of Clinical Pharmacology.* **67**: 863–864.
36 Charpiat B *et al.* (2017) Respiratory depression related to multiple drug-drug interactions precipitated by a fluconazole loading dose in a patient treated with oxycodone. *European Journal of Clinical Pharmacology.* **73**: 787–788.
37 Kleine-Bruggeney (2010) Pharmacogenetics in palliative care. *Forensic Science International.* **203**: 63–70.
38 Nieminen TH *et al.* (2009) Rifampin greatly reduces the plasma concentrations of intravenous and oral oxycodone. *Anesthesiology.* **110**: 1371–1378.
39 Nieminen TH *et al.* (2010) St John's wort greatly reduces the concentrations of oral oxycodone. *European Journal of Pain.* **14**: 854–859.
40 Leppert W (2010) Role of oxycodone and oxycodone/naloxone in cancer pain management. *Pharmacological Reports.* **62**: 578–591.
41 Lugo RA and Kern SE (2004) The pharmacokinetics of oxycodone. *Journal of Pain and Palliative Care Pharmacotherapy.* **18**: 17–30.
42 Amato F *et al.* (2017) High dosage of a fixed combination oxycodone/naloxone prolonged release: efficacy and tolerability in patients with chronic cancer pain. *Supportive Care in Cancer.* **25**: 3051–3058.
43 Schutter U *et al.* (2010) Innovative pain therapy with a fixed combination of prolonged-release oxycodone/naloxone: a large observational study under conditions of daily practice. *Current Medical Research Opinion.* **26**: 1377–1387.
44 Clemens KE *et al.* (2011) Bowel function during pain therapy with oxycodone/naloxone prolonged-release tablets in patients with advanced cancer. *International Journal of Clinical Practice.* **65**: 472–478.
45 Hermanns K *et al.* (2012) Prolonged-release oxycodone/naloxone in the treatment of neuropathic pain - results from a large observational study. *Expert Opinion on Pharmacotherapy.* **13**: 299–311.
46 Gatti A *et al.* (2013) Prolonged-release oxycodone/naloxone in nonmalignant pain: single-center study in patients with constipation. *Advances in Therapy.* **30**: 41–59.
47 Poelaert J *et al.* (2015) Treatment with prolonged-release oxycodone/naloxone improves pain relief and opioid-induced constipation compared with prolonged-release oxycodone in patients with chronic severe pain and laxative-refractory constipation. *Clinical Therapeutics.* **37**: 784–792.
48 Lazzari M *et al.* (2016) Switching to low-dose oral prolonged-release oxycodone/naloxone from WHO-Step I drugs in elderly patients with chronic pain at high risk of early opioid discontinuation. *Clinical Interventions in Aging.* **11**: 641–649.
49 Petro E *et al.* (2016) Low-dose oral prolonged-release oxycodone/naloxone for chronic pain in elderly patients with cognitive impairment: an efficacy-tolerability pilot study. *Neuropsychiatric Disease and Treatment.* **12**: 559–569.

50 Simpson K *et al.* (2008) Fixed-ratio combination oxycodone/naloxone compared with oxycodone alone for the relief of opioid-induced constipation in moderate-to-severe noncancer pain. *Current Medical Research Opinion.* **24**: 3503–3512.
51 Lowenstein O *et al.* (2009) Combined prolonged-release oxycodone and naloxone improves bowel function in patients receiving opioids for moderate-to-severe non-malignant chronic pain: a randomised controlled trial. *Expert Opinion in Pharmacotherapy.* **10**: 531–543.
52 Dupoiron D *et al.* (2017) A phase III randomized controlled study on the efficacy and improved bowel function of prolonged-release (PR) oxycodone-naloxone (up to 160/80 mg daily) vs oxycodone PR. *European Journal of Pain.*
53 Ahmedzai SH *et al.* (2012) A randomized, double-blind, active-controlled, double-dummy, parallel-group study to determine the safety and efficacy of oxycodone/naloxone prolonged-release tablets in patients with moderate/severe, chronic cancer pain. *Palliative Medicine.* **26**: 50–60.
54 Anonymous (2010) Targinact - opioid relief without constipation? *Drugs and Therapeutics Bulletin.* **48**: 138–141.
55 de Oliveira CO *et al.* (2016) Opioids for restless legs syndrome. *Cochrane Database of Systematic Reviews.* **6**: CD006941. www.thecochranelibrary.com
56 Anonymous (2016) Targinact for restless legs syndrome. *Drugs and Therapeutics Bulletin.* **54**: 42.
57 Larkin PJ *et al.* (2008) The management of constipation in palliative care: clinical practice recommendations. *Palliative Medicine.* **22**: 796–807.
58 Vondrackova D *et al.* (2008) Analgesic efficacy and safety of oxycodone in combination with naloxone as prolonged release tablets in patients with moderate to severe chronic pain. *Journal of Pain.* **9**: 1144–1154.
59 Sandner-Kiesling A *et al.* (2010) Long-term efficacy and safety of combined prolonged-release oxycodone and naloxone in the management of non-cancer chronic pain. *International Journal of Clinical Practice.* **64**: 763–774.
60 Franklin AE *et al.* (2017) A case of opioid toxicity on conversion from extended-release oxycodone and naloxone to extended-release oxycodone in a patient with liver dysfunction. *Journal of Pain and Symptom Management.* **53**: e1–e2.
61 Meissner W *et al.* (2009) A randomised controlled trial with prolonged-release oral oxycodone and naloxone to prevent and reverse opioid-induced constipation. *European Journal of Pain.* **13**: 56–64.
62 Dupoiron D *et al.* (2017) Long-term efficacy and safety of oxycodone-naloxone prolonged-release formulation (up to 180/90 mg daily) - results of the open-label extension phase of a phase III multicenter, multiple-dose, randomized, controlled study. *European Journal of Pain.* **21**: 1485–1494.
63 National Patient Safety Agency (2008) Reducing risk of overdose with midazolam injection in adults. *Rapid response report.* NPSA/2008/RRR2011. http://www.nrls.npsa.uk
64 National Patient Safety Agency (2006) Ensuring safer practice with high dose ampoules of diamorphine and morphine. *Safer Practice Notice.* NPSA/2006/2012. http://www.nrls.npsa.nhs.uk
65 Gardiner P (2003) Compatibility of an injectable oxycodone formulation with typical diluents, syringes, tubings, infusion bags and drugs for potential co-administration. *Hospital Pharmacist* **10**: 354–361.
66 Hines S and Pleasance S (2009) Compatibility of an injectable high strength oxycodone formulation with typical diluents, syrings, tubings and infusion bags and drugs for potential co-administration. *European Journal of Hospital Pharmacy Practice.* **15**: 32–38.
67 National Pharmacy Association (2015) Potential risk of error in selecting incorrect oxycodone strength. www.npa.co.uk
68 Care Quality Commission and NHS England (2013) Safer use of controlled drugs - preventing harms from oral oxycodone medicines. *Use of controlled drugs supporting information.* www.cqc.org.uk

Updated September 2017

TAPENTADOL

Class: Strong opioid analgesic (but see below).

Indications: Moderate–severe acute pain (immediate-release products); severe chronic pain (m/r products).

Contra-indications: None absolute if titrated carefully against a patient's pain. (Also see Cautions below, and Strong opioids, p.360).

Pharmacology

Tapentadol is a centrally-acting analgesic which is both a μ agonist and an inhibitor of synaptic re-uptake of noradrenaline (norepinephrine); the latter enhances the action of the descending pain inhibitory pathway, contributing to a synergistic analgesic effect.[1–3] This possibly explains why tapentadol is only about ≤3 times less potent than **morphine**, despite an affinity for the μ-opioid receptor some ≥18 times lower (see **Tramadol**, Table 1, p.355).[1–3] Tapentadol also has some serotoninergic activity, but this is not considered relevant to its analgesic effect.

Tramadol, like tapentadol, is also a synthetic centrally-acting analgesic with both non-opioid and opioid properties. However, at recommended maximum doses, tapentadol is equivalent to a much higher dose of PO **morphine** than **tramadol**, namely 150mg/24h vs. 40mg/24h (see p.354). Thus, for practical purposes, **tramadol** is best considered a weak opioid (alongside **codeine**) and tapentadol a strong opioid (alongside **morphine**; see p.295).

RCTs of tapentadol, using mainly **oxycodone** as the comparator, have been conducted in both acute (e.g. postoperative orthopaedic, low back pain)[4–6] and chronic pain (e.g. osteo-arthritis, low back pain, diabetic neuropathy, cancer-related).[7,8] These have shown tapentadol to be superior to placebo and/or non-inferior to **oxycodone** *at the lower end of its dose range*, i.e. in the RCTs used to obtain regulatory approval for tapentadol m/r, the maximum comparative dose was **oxycodone** m/r ≤50mg b.d. Further, median doses in the cancer pain study were only tapentadol m/r 25mg b.d. and **oxycodone** m/r 5mg b.d.[8]

Tapentadol is comparable in cost to **oxycodone**. However, a lack of comparative studies with other cheaper strong opioid products resulted in recommendations *against* its use in acute pain,[9] and its restriction in chronic pain to patients who fail to get satisfactory analgesia from **morphine**.[10,11] Subsequent studies have found the analgesic effect of tapentadol m/r non-inferior to **oxycodone** + **naloxone** m/r (Targinact®, see p.449) in chronic pain, and to **morphine** m/r in cancer pain.[7]

Undesirable effects include those typical of an opioid agonist. However, during initial titration, GI effects are generally less than with **oxycodone** (e.g. less nausea, vomiting, constipation).[7] In non-cancer chronic pain studies, drug-related treatment withdrawals were about 20% for tapentadol vs. 30–40% for **oxycodone**.[7] In cancer pain studies, compared with **oxycodone** (median dose 5mg m/r b.d.) rates of constipation and nausea were about 7% lower with tapentadol,[8] compared with **morphine** (median dose 60mg m/r b.d.) rates of nausea and vomiting were 10% lower with tapentadol, but only during intital titration.[12] There were similar rates of treatment withdrawal for all three drugs (≤9%). Data are mixed over whether tapentadol m/r is associated with similar or greater degrees of constipation compared with **oxycodone** + **naloxone** m/r.[7]

A Cochrane review of tapentadol in chronic musculoskeletal pain concluded it was associated with better pain relief than placebo or **oxycodone** (although the difference with the latter is of uncertain clinical significance) and fewer undesirable effects.[13] A similar review in cancer pain was unable to pool RCT data and concluded that analgesic efficacy and undesirable effects were similar between tapentadol, **oxycodone** and **morphine**.[14] A systematic review of treatments for neuropathic pain considered the evidence insufficient to make a conclusive recommendation for tapentadol but noted a NNT of 10.2, much higher than, e.g. tricyclic antidepressants (3.6), other strong opioids (4.3) or **tramadol** (4.7).[15,16]

Food does not alter absorption to a clinically relevant degree. Tapentadol is extensively metabolized in the liver to inactive metabolites by glucuronidation, with ≤15% of a dose metabolized via CYP450 (mostly 2C9 and 2C19), thus reducing the likelihood of pharmacokinetic drug–drug interactions; only 3% is excreted unchanged in the urine. Systemic exposure to tapentadol is increased by hepatic but not renal impairment, although in the latter, levels of tapentadol-O-glucuronide (considered inactive) are increased. It has no effect on the QT interval (see Chapter 20, p.731).

By mouth, it is about 5 times *less* potent than **oxycodone** (i.e. tapentadol 50mg is approximately equivalent to **oxycodone** 10mg). By extrapolation, this suggests that it is about 3 times *less* potent than PO **morphine** (i.e. tapentadol 50mg is approximately equivalent to **morphine** 15mg) and study data supports this.[12,17] Thus, the maximum recommended m/r dose of tapentadol 250mg b.d. is approximately equivalent to **oxycodone** 50mg b.d. or **morphine** 75mg b.d.

Bio-availability 32% PO.

Onset of action <1h immediate-release.

Time to peak plasma concentration 75min immediate-release; 3–6h m/r.

Plasma halflife 4h immediate-release; 5–6h m/r.

Duration of action 4–6h immediate-release; 12h m/r.

Cautions

Renal or hepatic impairment (see Dose and use). Epilepsy or risk of seizures (lack of clinical trial data). Switching from another μ agonist (e.g. **morphine**, **oxycodone**) to tapentadol may cause low-grade opioid withdrawal (see Dose and use).

Abrupt discontinuation of tapentadol may result in symptoms of opioid withdrawal and the SPC advises tapering gradually. On the other hand, the SPC also notes that even with ≤12 months of use, withdrawal symptoms were either absent or mild.

Tapentadol has the potential for abuse and addiction.[18]

Drug interactions

Avoid concurrent administration with an MAOI, or within 2 weeks of the cessation of one, due to potential additive effects on synaptic noradrenaline concentrations.

Tapentadol is not completely devoid of serotoninergic activity.[2] There have been isolated reports of serotonin toxicity involving the use of tapentadol in conjunction with serotoninergic drugs (e.g. SSRIs); also see p.200.

Undesirable effects

See Strong opioids, Box B, p.365.

Dose and use

As with all opioids, patients must be monitored for undesirable effects, particularly nausea and vomiting, and constipation. Depending on individual circumstances, an anti-emetic should be prescribed for regular or p.r.n. use, (see QCG Nausea and vomiting, p.240) and, routinely, a laxative prescribed (see QCG Opioid-induced constipation, p.42).

Opioids can impair driving ability and patients should be counselled accordingly (see p.743).

Moderate–severe acute pain

Use immediate-release products:

- start with 50mg PO q4–6h if moderate pain/strong opioid naïve
- a higher starting dose may be necessary for severe pain/previous strong opioid use
- if the first dose is inadequate, a second dose can be taken after 1h (once only)
- if required, increase progressively to 100mg q4h or 150mg q6h
- maximum dose 600mg/24h (700mg in first 24h of use).

Severe chronic pain

Use m/r products:

- start with 50mg PO q12h if strong opioid-naïve
- a higher starting dose may be necessary when switching from another strong opioid; recommendations vary widely,[19] but the following is adapted from a cancer pain trial based on existing oral **morphine** equivalent (OME) use:[20]
  - ▷ OME ≤30mg/24h → tapentadol 50mg b.d.
  - ▷ 31–60mg/24h → 100mg b.d.
  - ▷ 61–90mg/24h → 150mg b.d.
  - ▷ 91–120mg/24h → 200mg b.d.
  - ▷ 121–150mg/24h → 250mg b.d.
  - ▷ within the first week, 30% required a dose increase and 8% a decrease
- if necessary, increase by 50mg b.d. every 3 days
- maximum dose 250mg b.d.

In the cancer pain studies, break-through pain was treated with appropriate doses of immediate-release **morphine** or **oxycodone** p.r.n.; conventionally, p.r.n. PO doses are 1/6–1/10 of the total 24h PO dose (see Pharmacology for dose equivalents).[19]

Switching from another μ agonist (e.g. **morphine**, **oxycodone**) to tapentadol may cause low-grade opioid withdrawal, and p.r.n. doses of the *original* opioid should be used to counter this (e.g. give an immediate-release product at 1/4–1/2 of the original dose).

M/r tablets should be swallowed whole; crushing or chewing them will lead to a rapid release of an overdose of tapentadol (see Chapter 28, Box B, p.788).

Renal or hepatic impairment

Dose reduction is not required in mild–moderate renal impairment.

In moderate hepatic impairment, systemic exposure to tapentadol is increased >4 times, and the maximum recommended starting dose is 50mg q8h (immediate-release) or once daily (m/r).

Because of a lack of clinical trial data, the SPC recommends against the use of tapentadol in patients with severe hepatic or renal impairment.

For a general approach when renal of hepatic function deteriorates rapidly, see p.364.

Supply

All products are Schedule 2 **CD**.

Immediate-release oral products

Palexia® (Grünenthal)

Tablets 50mg, 75mg, 50mg dose =£0.45

Oral solution 20mg/mL, 50mg dose = £0.45; *can be diluted in water or a non-alcoholic cold drink and is suitable for administration via EFT.*

Modified-release oral products

As for all m/r opioids, brand prescribing is recommended to reduce the risk of confusion and error in dispensing and administration (see p.xvii).

Palexia® SR (Grünenthal)

Tablets m/r 50mg, 100mg, 150mg, 200mg, 250mg 28 days @ 100mg q12h = £50.

1 Tzschentke TM *et al.* (2014) The mu-opioid receptor agonist/noradrenaline reuptake inhibition (MOR-NRI) concept in analgesia: the case of tapentadol. *CNS Drugs*. **28**: 319–329.

2 Hoy SM (2012) Tapentadol extended release: in adults with chronic pain. *Drugs*. **72**: 375–393.

3 Schroder W *et al.* (2011) Synergistic interaction between the two mechanisms of action of tapentadol in analgesia. *Journal of Pharmacology and Experimental Therapeutics*. **337**: 312–320.

4 Frampton JE (2010) Tapentadol immediate release: a review of its use in the treatment of moderate to severe acute pain. *Drugs*. **70**: 1719–1743.

5 Biondi D *et al.* (2013) Tapentadol immediate release versus oxycodone immediate release for treatment of acute low back pain. *Pain Physician*. **16**: E237–246.

6 Vorsanger GJ *et al.* (2013) Immediate-release tapentadol or oxycodone for treatment of acute postoperative pain after elective arthroscopic shoulder surgery: a randomized, phase IIIb study. *Journal of Opioid Management*. **9**: 281–290.

7 Baron R *et al.* (2017) Tapentadol prolonged release for chronic pain: a review of clinical trials and 5 years of routine clinical practice data. *Pain Practice*. **17**: 678–700.

8 Imanaka K *et al.* (2013) Efficacy and safety of oral tapentadol extended release in Japanese and Korean patients with moderate to severe, chronic malignant tumor-related pain. *Current Medical Research and Opinion*. **29**: 1399-1409.

9 Anonymous (2012) Tapentadol (Palexia) for moderate to severe acute pain. *Drug and Therapeutics Bulletin*. **50**: 30–33.

10 Scottish Medicines Consortium (2011) Tapentadol prolonged-release tablets (Palexia SR). www.scottishmedicines.org

11 All Wales Medicine Strategy Group (2011) Tapentadol prolonged-release tablets (Palexia SR). www.awmsg.org

12 Kress HG *et al.* (2014) Tapentadol prolonged release for managing moderate to severe, chronic malignant tumor-related pain. *Pain Physician*. **17**: 329–343.

13 Santos J *et al.* (2015) Tapentadol for chronic musculoskeletal pain in adults. *Cochrane Database of Systematic Reviews*. **5**: CD009923. www.thecochranelibrary.com

14 Wiffen PJ *et al.* (2015) Oral tapentadol for cancer pain. *Cochrane Database of Systematic Reviews*. **9**: CD011460. www.thecochranelibrary.com

15 Finnerup NB *et al.* (2016) Pharmacotherapy for neuropathic pain in adults: a systematic review and meta-analysis. *Lancet Neurology*. **14**: 162–173.

16 Finnerup NB and Attal N (2015) Tapentadol prolonged release in the treatment of neuropathic pain related to diabetic polyneuropathy-authors' reply. *Lancet Neurology*. **14**: 685–686.

17 Galvez R *et al.* (2013) Tapentadol prolonged release versus strong opioids for severe, chronic low back pain: results of an open-label, phase 3b study. *Advances in Therapy*. **30**: 229–259.

18 Cepeda MS *et al.* (2013) Comparison of opioid doctor shopping for tapentadol and oxycodone: a cohort study. *Journal of Pain*. **14**: 158–164.

19 Sanchez Del Aguila MJ *et al.* (2015) Practical considerations for the use of tapentadol prolonged release for the management of severe chronic pain. *Clinical Therapeutics*. **37**: 94–113.

20 Imanaka K *et al.* (2014) Ready conversion of patients with well-controlled, moderate to severe, chronic malignant tumor-related pain on other opioids to tapentadol extended release. *Clinical Drug Investigation*. **34**: 501–511.

Updated September 2017

OPIOID ANTAGONISTS (THERAPEUTIC TARGET WITHIN THE CNS)

For *Opioid antagonists (therapeutic target outside the CNS)*, see p.466; these are authorized for opioid-induced constipation, with effects limited to the periphery and leaving CNS opioid analgesic effects unaltered. Generally, this is because of an inability to penetrate the blood-brain barrier. The exception is **naloxone** in Targinact®, where use of a m/r formulation limits systemic absorption (see p.449), and thereby limits central antagonism.

5

Indications: Reversal of opioid-induced respiratory depression (**naloxone**), acute opioid overdose (**naloxone**), prevention of relapse in opioid and †alcohol addiction (**naloxone, naltrexone**), †pruritus caused by cholestasis[1] or spinal opioids (**naloxone, naltrexone**) and possibly chronic renal failure (**naltrexone**).[1,2]

Contra-indications: Naloxone: none when used to reverse life-threatening opioid-induced respiratory depression or acute opioid overdose.
Naltrexone: patients physically dependent on opioids (i.e. after 2 weeks of regular PO use), acute hepatitis, hepatic failure, severe renal impairment (creatinine clearance <30mL/min).

Pharmacology

For **naloxone, naltrexone** and **nalmefene** the main therapeutic target is within the CNS. They reversibly block access to opioid receptors and, if given after an opioid agonist, they displace the latter because of their higher receptor affinity.

Although generally thought of as pure antagonists (i.e. having a high affinity for opioid receptors but no intrinsic activity), the reality is more complex. High doses of opioid antagonists reverse opioid-analgesia (as expected), but *ultra-low* doses potentiate the opioid analgesic effect and/or reduce opioid undesirable effects (e.g. nausea and vomiting, and pruritus). This has mostly been explored using *ultra-low* dose **naloxone** (e.g. 0.25microgram/kg/h IVI) in postoperative pain.[3–11] In other settings, *ultra-low* dose **naltrexone** (e.g. ≤1mg/24h PO) has shown similar effects.[12–15]

These phenomena are best explained by opioid antagonists having other effects in addition to classical opioid receptor antagonism. These may include interfering with G protein coupling and/or acting as antagonists at toll-like receptor 4 (TLR4).

Interfering with G protein coupling: A ligand binding to an opioid receptor can trigger either an inhibitory or excitatory response, dependent on the type of G protein coupled to the receptor, either G_I/G_O (inhibitory) or G_s (excitatory). Typically, with an opioid agonist, the G_I/G_O (inhibitory) activity predominates resulting in analgesia and other opioid effects. In such circumstances, a typical clinical dose of an opioid antagonist like **naloxone** will displace the opioid agonist from the receptor and thereby reverse its effects. However, the G_s excitatory response can increase in various circumstances, e.g. chronic opioid use, nerve damage.[16] This may contribute to opioid tolerance and, when predominant, to opioid-induced hyperalgesia (p.368).[17] Ultra-low levels of **naloxone** interfere with the scaffolding protein (filamin A), which couples G_s to the opioid receptor and thereby inhibits the excitatory response.[18]

TLR4 antagonism: **naloxone** and **naltrexone** are TLR4 antagonists.[19] The TLR4 receptor is expressed in dorsal root ganglion neurones and widely in the CNS, particularly glial cells. Its activation promotes inflammation and other changes, and it is an important mediator of CNS sensitization and thereby inflammatory and neuropathic pain (and also drug reward and reinforcement). Apart from products released in nerve damage, opioids also activate TLR4 which may counteract their analgesic effect, contribute towards tolerance and, when predominant, opioid-induced hyperalgesia (p.368).[20] Thus, in animal models of nerve injury, ultra-low dose **naloxone** enhanced the analgesic effect of **morphine** and ultra-low dose (+)-**naltrexone** prevented mechanical allodynia and its potentiation by **morphine**.[20–22]

Note. **Naloxone** and **naltrexone** products are the (-)-isomers which bind to opioid receptors, filamin A, and TLR4. In contrast, their (+)-isomers bind to filamin A and TLR4 but *not* to opioid receptors. However, the (+)-isomers are not commercially available despite the fact that their use would avoid the risk of reversal of analgesia.

Specific TLR4 antagonists are likely to be developed for clinical use. However, currently, despite the potential benefits of *ultra-low* dose **naloxone** or **naltrexone**, the inherent risk of reversal of opioid analgesia limits the clinical application of this approach which should be undertaken only by specialists in pain or palliative medicine. In practice, if opioid-induced hyperalgesia is suspected, the first and most important step is to reduce the dose of the offending opioid (also see p.368).

Compared with **naloxone**, **naltrexone** has a higher PO bio-availability and a longer duration of action; it undergoes extensive first-pass metabolism.[23,24] The major metabolite, 6-β-naltrexol, is a *neutral* antagonist, i.e. it inhibits activation of opioid receptors but, unlike **naloxone** and **naltrexone**, it does not suppress basal receptor signalling, thereby reducing the risk of severe withdrawal.

Pharmacokinetic details are summarized in Table 1.

Table 1 Pharmacokinetic details for naloxone and naltrexone

	Naloxone	*Naltrexone*
Bio-availability (%)	6 PO	5–40 PO
Onset of action	1–2min IV; 2–5min SC/IM	may precipitate withdrawal symptoms in <5min in opioid-dependent patients
Time to peak plasma concentration		1–2h PO
Plasma halflife	about 1h	4h; 13h for 6-β-naltrexol[25]

Reversal of opioid-induced respiratory depression

The most important clinical property of **naloxone** is reversal of opioid-induced respiratory depression (and other opioid effects). In addition to a deliberate overdose, accidental overdose can occur in those misusing opioids and, less commonly, in patients requiring opioids for analgesia.

Increasingly, 'traditional doses' of **naloxone** (e.g. 400microgram IV stat) are recommended only for use in *immediately life-threatening situations*, i.e. unconscious patient with minimal/no respiratory effort. In other circumstances, careful titration using lower doses of **naloxone** (e.g. 20–100microgram) is recommended to avoid precipitating a severe acute withdrawal syndrome and, in those receiving opioids for analgesia, severe pain and hyperalgesia (see QCG: Reversal of opioid-induced respiratory depression, p.464).[26,27] Acute opioid withdrawal causes the release of catecholamines which can result in vomiting, shivering, sweating, tremor, agitation, anxiety, aggression, tachycardia, hypertension and, rarely, life-threatening pulmonary oedema (also see below) and cardiac arrhythmia.

However, compared with other opioids, antagonism of **buprenorphine** requires higher doses of **naloxone** because **buprenorphine** has both high receptor affinity and prolonged receptor binding (see QCG: Reversal of opioid-induced respiratory depression, p.464 and also p.397). **Naloxone** has been reported to be only partially effective in reversing the effects of **tramadol**.[28,29] However, in a series of 11 patients with a **tramadol** overdose, seven had a good response to **naloxone**, and only one had no response.[30]

Patients with opioid overdose may develop pulmonary oedema. Because pulmonary oedema has been seen both in older patients with typical doses of **naloxone**, e.g. 200–400microgram, and in healthy teenagers with doses as low as 40–80microgram, it has been suggested that **naloxone** can trigger a central neurogenic response which leads to vasoconstriction of the pulmonary vasculature followed by pulmonary oedema.[31] Alternatively, because pulmonary oedema is almost universal in fatal opioid overdose,[32,33] **naloxone** by increasing respiratory rate and tidal volume may simply unmask pulmonary oedema which has developed secondary to severe hypoxaemia and acidaemia.[34]

Delayed-onset pulmonary oedema (48h after overdose treated with **naloxone**) due to acute cardiomyopathy has also been reported, possibly the result of cardiac muscle damage caused by hypoxaemia.[35]

Prevention of relapse in opioid addiction

Naltrexone 100mg PO blocks the effect of a challenge of IV **diamorphine** 25mg by 96% at 24h, and 46% at 72h.[36] Thus, **naltrexone** is primarily used to prevent relapse in opioid addiction by blocking opioid 'highs'. It is also used PO off-label to reduce the relapse rate in alcohol addiction. **Naltrexone** is given PO either once daily or three times per week. It is also available as a long-acting depot IM injection (duration of action >1 month; authorized for use in alcohol and opioid addiction) and a SC pellet implant (duration of action weeks–months).[37] Both injectable products are unauthorized in the UK, but are available through private addiction clinics.

Opioid combination products to deter opioid abuse

In an attempt to reduce the risk of opioid abuse, PO/SL formulations containing both a strong opioid and an opioid antagonist have been developed, e.g.:

- Suboxone® (**buprenorphine** + **naloxone**) given SL for opioid dependency
- Targinact® (**oxycodone** + **naloxone**) for PO use (see p.447)
- Embeda® (**morphine** + **naltrexone**) for PO use (not UK)
- Troxyca® ER (**oxycodone** + **naltrexone**) for PO use (not UK).

When administered as indicated, the opioid antagonist either remains sequestered (Embeda®, Troxyca® ER) or the amount absorbed is insufficient to antagonize the analgesic effect of the opioid (Suboxone®, Targinact®). However, if abused (e.g. the tablets crushed and administered by insufflation or IV), the opioid antagonist is then released and available in sufficient amounts to antagonize the opioid.

Pruritus

In cholestasis, pruritus is partly a consequence of increased opioidergic tone caused by a raised plasma enkephalin concentration.[38–41] Centrally-acting opioid antagonists are thought to counteract the increased tone within the CNS, and thus improve the pruritus (also see Chapter 26, p.757).

Naloxone by CIVI/CSCI decreases scratching activity by patients with cholestatic pruritus[42–44] and has a place in the emergency treatment of acute exacerbations of cholestatic pruritus. PO **naltrexone**[1,45] (or **nalmefene**;[46] not UK) can then be used long-term.

However, opioid antagonists can precipitate an opioid withdrawal-like reaction in patients with cholestasis, including hallucinations and dysphoria.[40,47] To avoid or minimize such a reaction, treatment must be started cautiously with a low dose (see Dose and use).

The use of **naltrexone** to relieve cholestatic jaundice may sometimes unmask or exacerbate underlying pain, necessitating discontinuation of **naltrexone**.[48] Thus, patients with cholestatic jaundice and pruritus and severe pain should *not* be treated with a centrally acting opioid antagonist.[49] However, case reports suggest benefit from **methylnaltrexone**, a peripherally acting opioid antagonist (see p.466). In two jaundiced patients with cancer, pruritus resolved completely 30min–12h after a dose of **methylnaltrexone**, with a duration of benefit ranging between 24h and 3 weeks.[50] This approach avoids the risk of opioid-withdrawal and/or reversal of opioid analgesia, making it a reasonable option to trial in patients receiving opioids. For other treatments for cholestatic pruritus, see Chapter 26, Table 1, p.761.

There are reports of patients with cholestatic pruritus who have responded to **buprenorphine** alone or in combination with ultra-low doses of **naloxone**.[51–54] Sometimes ultra-low doses of **naloxone** or **naltrexone** improved both the pruritus and the pain.[55] However, there are insufficient data at present to recommend this approach.

In uraemic pruritus, the situation is more complex because there are several causal mechanisms, both peripheral (cutaneous) and central (neural).[56] The opioid system is involved, but in uraemia there is no increase in opioidergic tone (and thus no danger of a withdrawal syndrome if an opioid antagonist is given). Instead, the ratio between μ-opioid (pruritus-inducible) and κ-opioid (pruritus-suppressive) receptors alters in favour of the former.[57,58] This predisposes to the onset or exacerbation of pruritus. It also suggests that both κ *agonists* and μ *antagonists* could bring relief. Thus, RCTs have found **nalfurafine** (not UK), a novel κ agonist, to be more effective than placebo in relieving uraemic itch in haemodialysis patients.[1]

Naltrexone has also been tried in this setting. However, RCTs have given conflicting results, e.g. benefit was seen in uraemic patients with very severe pruritus but not in those with moderately severe pruritus.[1] One explanation is that, in uraemia, an opioid mechanism is important only in severe pruritus. The fact that **naltrexone** is non-selective and antagonizes both μ- and κ-opioid receptors may also be relevant.

In a RCT of patients with atopic eczema, **naltrexone** provided greater relief than placebo.[1] Open studies report benefit from **naltrexone** in various other skin and systemic disorders associated with pruritus.[39,59] However, further studies are required. Pruritus associated with chronic disease generally requires alternative specific measures (see p.757).

Ultra-low dose **naloxone** is also used to relieve pruritus caused by spinal opioids, when other treatments have failed (see p.839).

Miscellaneous

Naloxone is reported to benefit patients with septic shock,[60] **morphine**-induced peripheral vasodilation,[61] ischaemic central neurological deficits[62,63] and post-stroke central pain.[64]

Endogenous opioids inhibit cell proliferation, an effect which intermittent low-dose **naltrexone** appears to augment by provoking a compensatory elevation in opioid growth factor (OGF, an enkephalin) and OGF receptor (a non-classical opioid receptor). This interaction impacts upon the cell cycle, inhibiting proliferation. The potential roles of low-dose **naltrexone** and OGF in cancer and auto-immune diseases (e.g. multiple sclerosis, Crohn's disease) are being explored.[65]

In the past, PO **naloxone** and **naltrexone** have been used to correct delayed gastric emptying and constipation.[66] However, because both act centrally as well as peripherally, there is a risk of analgesic reversal and systemic withdrawal. Consequently, opioid antagonists which do not readily cross the blood-brain-barrier are preferable (p.466).

Cautions

In patients receiving opioids for pain relief, **naloxone** should *not* be used for drowsiness and/or delirium which is not life-threatening because of the danger of reversing the opioid analgesia and precipitating a major physical withdrawal syndrome. Instead, omit or reduce the next regular dose, and subsequently continue at a reduced dose.

The use of **naltrexone** will also impede opioid analgesia (see below),[67] and can precipitate an opioid withdrawal-like syndrome in patients with cholestatic pruritus. **Naltrexone** may cause occasional hepatotoxicity.[68] The manufacturer advises checking LFTs before and at intervals during treatment.

Undesirable effects

Naloxone: nausea and vomiting; occasionally severe hypertension, pulmonary oedema (see above), rarely tachycardia, arrhythmias, and even cardiac arrest.[69]

Naltrexone: *very common (>10% in detoxifying opioid addicts)* insomnia, headaches, anxiety, nausea and vomiting, intestinal colic, lack of energy, joint and muscle pain.

The long-term use of **naltrexone** increases the concentration of opioid receptors in the CNS and results in a temporary enhanced response to the subsequent administration of opioid analgesics.[70] The management of severe acute and postoperative pain in patients receiving long-term **naltrexone** requires careful consideration (Box A).[67,71]

Box A Management of acute pain in patients receiving naltrexone

Elective surgery

The use of naltrexone must be identified well before the operation.

Ensure effective liaison between the substance misuse and acute pain teams.

Consider switching patients on IM depot injections to PO tablets before surgery.

For minor surgery, when non-opioids are considered sufficient to manage the postoperative pain, leave SC pellet *in situ*; if severe postoperative pain anticipated, remove SC pellet.

Discontinue PO naltrexone 72h before the operation.

Maximize the use of non-opioid analgesics, e.g. IV paracetamol, NSAID.

Note. If an opioid analgesic is required, a bigger than usual dose may be needed but, conversely, there may be an increased response to opioids (see Pharmacology above).

To avoid precipitating opioid withdrawal, do not restart naltrexone until 3–7 days after the last dose of opioid, depending on the duration of use and halflife of the opioid.

continued

Box A Continued

Unexpected severe acute pain, e.g. trauma, emergency surgery
If possible use non-opioid analgesics, e.g.:
- IV paracetamol and/or NSAID
- ketamine 100microgram/kg IV every 5min until satisfactory analgesia obtained, plus a single dose of midazolam 20–40microgram/kg IV to minimize dysphoria; may be repeated after 30min; give further midazolam only if dysphoria present.

There is a risk of marked sedation when ketamine and midazolam are combined in this way; to be used only by those competent in airway management.

If venous access is difficult, ketamine can be given SC; use the same doses as for IV but allow 15min between doses.

The above are generally used to achieve rapid pain relief until other measures can be instituted, e.g.:
- local anaesthetic blocks
- epidural analgesia (local anaesthetic ± clonidine).

Dose and use

Reversal of opioid-induced respiratory depression (naloxone)

Naloxone is best given IV but, if not practical, may be given IM or SC. The intranasal route has also been used, with specific nasal-spray products becoming available.[72,73]

Dose recommendations vary.[26,27] For *PCF* recommendations, see QCG: Reversal of opioid-induced respiratory depression (p.464).

Cholestatic pruritus (naloxone, naltrexone, nalmefene)

To try and avoid or minimize an opioid withdrawal-like syndrome, start with a low dose. Although some recommend the initial use of **naloxone** CIVI, others have successfully used **naltrexone** *de novo* 12.5–25mg PO b.d. and subsequently titrated as below:
- start with a low dose of **naloxone** by CIVI, e.g. 0.002microgram/kg/min (about 160–200microgram/24h)[40]; long-term administration by CSCI has also been reported[44]
- if no withdrawal-like symptoms occur, the rate can be doubled every 3–4h; but if symptoms occur, continue with the current dose until resolved
- after 18–24h, when a rate known to be associated with opioid antagonistic effects is reached (0.2microgram/kg/min), the infusion is stopped and **naltrexone** 12.5–25mg PO b.d. is started)[40,45,47]
- the dose is increased every few days until a satisfactory clinical response is obtained; at this stage the effective dose should be consolidated into a single daily maintenance dose
- the effective dose range for PO **naltrexone** is 25–250mg once daily[40]
- for **nalmefene** (not UK) start with 2mg PO b.d.; double the dose every 2 days until pruritus is relieved or no further improvement; individual maximum doses 30–120mg b.d.[74]

Uraemic pruritus (naltrexone)

- start with **naltrexone** 50mg PO once daily
- if necessary, after 1 week, increase dose to 100mg once daily.

Supply

Naloxone

Naloxone hydrochloride (generic)
Injection 20microgram/mL, 2mL amp = £5.50; 400microgram/mL, 1mL amp = £4; 1mg/mL, 2mL prefilled syringe = £17.

Minijet® Naloxone (UCB Pharma)
Injection (prefilled syringe) 400microgram/mL, 1mL = £20, 2mL= £13, 5mL = £21.

Naltrexone

Naltrexone hydrochloride (generic)

Tablets *(scored)* 50mg, 28 days @ 50mg once daily = £22.

Capsules 0.5mg, 1mg, 1.5mg, 3mg, 4mg, 4.5mg; 100 x all strengths = £180 (unauthorized, available as a special order from Martindale, see p.751).

Oral solution 5mg/5mL, 28 days @ 50mg once daily = £674 (unauthorized, available as a special order, see p.751); *price based on specials tariff in community.*

1 Pongcharoen P and Fleischer AB, Jr. (2016) An evidence-based review of systemic treatments for itch. *European Jourrnal of Pain.* **20**: 24–31.

2 Legroux-Crespel E *et al.* (2004) A comparative study on the effects of naltrexone and loratadine on uremic pruritus. *Dermatology.* **208**: 326–330.

3 Firouzian A *et al.* (2016) Ultra-low-dose naloxone as an adjuvant to patient controlled analgesia (PCA) with morphine for postoperative pain relief following lumber discectomy: a double-blind, randomized, placebo-controlled trial. *Journal of Neurosurgocal Anesthesiology (Epub ahead of print).*

4 Xiao Y *et al.* (2015) A randomized clinical trial of the effects of ultra-low-dose naloxone infusion on postoperative opioid requirements and recovery. *Acta Anaesthesiologica Scandinavica.* **59**: 1194–1203.

5 He F *et al.* (2016) The effect of naloxone treatment on opioid-induced side effects: A meta-analysis of randomized and controlled trails. *Medicine (Baltimore).* **95**: e4729.

6 Largent-Milnes TM *et al.* (2008) Oxycodone plus ultra-low-dose naltrexone attenuates neuropathic pain and associated mu-opioid receptor-Gs coupling. *Journal of Pain.* **9**: 700–713.

7 Hay JL *et al.* (2011) Potentiation of buprenorphine antinociception with ultra-low dose naltrexone in healthy subjects. *European Journal of Pain.* **15**: 293–298.

8 Cepeda MS *et al.* (2004) Addition of ultralow dose naloxone to postoperative morphine PCA: unchanged analgesia and opioid requirement but decreased incidence of opioid side effects. *Pain.* **107**: 41–46.

9Maxwell LG *et al.* (2005) The effects of a small-dose naloxone infusion on opioid-induced side effects and analgesia in children and adolescents treated with intravenous patient-controlled analgesia: a double-blind, prospective, randomized, controlled study. *Anesthesia and Analgesia.* **100**: 953–958.

10 Murphy JD *et al.* (2011) Analgesic efficacy of intravenous naloxone for the treatment of postoperative pruritus: a meta-analysis. *Journal of Opioid Management.* **7**: 321–327.

11 Joshi G *et al.* (1999) Effects of prophylactic nalmefene on the incidence of morphine-related side effects in patients receiving intravenous patient-controlled analgesia. *Anesthesiology.* **90**: 1007–1011.

12 Cruciani RA *et al.* (2003) Ultra-low dose oral naltrexone decreases side effects and potentiates the effect of methadone. *Journal of Pain and Symptom Management.* **25**: 491–494.

13 Hamann S and Sloan P (2007) Oral naltrexone to enhance analgesia in patients receiving continuous intrathecal morphine for chronic pain: a randomized, double-blind, prospective pilot study. *Journal of Opioid Management.* **3**: 137–144.

14 Chindalore VL *et al.* (2005) Adding ultralow-dose naltrexone to oxycodone enhances and prolongs analgesia: a randomized, controlled trial of Oxytrex. *Journal of Pain.* **6**: 392–399.

15 Raffaeli W and Indovina P (2015) Low-dose naltrexone to prevent intolerable morphine adverse events: a forgotten remedy for a neglected, global clinical need. *Pain Medicine.* **16**: 1239–1242.

16 Crain S and Shen K (2000) Antagonists of excitatory opioid receptor functions enhance morphine's analgesic potency and attenuate opioid tolerance/dependence liability. *Pain.* **84**: 121–131.

17 Sjogren P *et al.* (1994) Disappearance of morphine-induced hyperalgesia after discontinuing or substituting morphine with other opioid antagonists. *Pain.* **59**: 313–316.

18 Wang HY and Burns LH (2009) Naloxone's pentapeptide binding site on filamin A blocks Mu opioid receptor-Gs coupling and CREB activation of acute morphine. *PLoS One.* **4**: e4282.

19 Wang X *et al.* (2016) Pharmacological characterization of the opioid inactive isomers (+)-naltrexone and (+)-naloxone as antagonists of toll-like receptor 4. *British Journal of Pharmacology.* **173**: 856–869.

20 Ellis A *et al.* (2016) Morphine amplifies mechanical allodynia via TLR4 in a rat model of spinal cord injury. *Brain Behaviour and Immunity.* **58**: 348–356.

21 Yang CP *et al.* (2013) Intrathecal ultra-low dose naloxone enhances the antihyperalgesic effects of morphine and attenuates tumour necrosis factor-α and tumour necrosis factor-α receptor 1 expression in the dorsal horn of rats with partial sciatic nerve transection. *Anesthesia and Analgesia.* **117**: 1493–1502.

22 Ellis A *et al.* (2014) Systemic administration of propentofylline, ibudilast, and (+)-naltrexone each reverses mechanical allodynia in a novel rat model of central neuropathic pain. *Journal of Pain.* **15**: 407–421.

23 Gonzalez J and Brogden R (1988) Naltrexone: a review of its pharmacodynamic and pharmacokinetic properties and therapeutic efficacy in the management of opioid dependence. *Drugs.* **35**: 192–213.

24 Crabtree B (1984) Review of naltrexone: a long-acting opiate antagonist. *Clinical Pharmacy.* **3**: 273–280.

25 Gutstein H and Akil H (2001) Opioid analgesics. In: J Hardman *et al.* (eds) *Goodman & Gilman's The Pharmacological Basis of Therapeutics* (10e). McGraw-Hill, New York ; London.

26 Connors NJ and Nelson LS (2016) The evolution of recommended naloxone dosing for opioid overdose by medical specialty. *Journal of Medical Toxicology.* **12**: 276–281.

27 UK Medicines Information (2015) What naloxone doses should be used in adults to reverse urgently the effects of opioids or opiates? *Medicines Q&A.* 227.221. www.evidence.nhs.uk

28 Raffa RB *et al.* (1992) Opioid and nonopioid components independently contribute to the mechanism of action of tramadol, an 'atypical' opioid analgesic. *Journal of Pharmacology and Therapeutics.* **260**: 275–285.

29 Shipton EA (2000) Tramadol - present and future. *Anaesthesia and Intensive Care.* **28**: 363–374.

30 Marquardt KA *et al.* (2005) Tramadol exposures reported to statewide poison control system. *Annals of Pharmacotherapy.* **39**: 1039–1044.

31 Horng HC *et al.* (2010) Negative pressure pulmonary edema following naloxone administration in a patient with fentanyl-induced respiratory depression. *Acta Anaesthesiology Taiwan.* **48**: 155–157.

32 Ridgway ZA and Pountney AJ (2007) Acute respiratory distress syndrome induced by oral methadone managed with non-invasive ventilation. *Emergency Medicine Journal.* **24**: 681.

33 Feeney C *et al.* (2011) Morphine-induced cardiogenic shock. *Annals of Pharmacotherpy.* **45**: e30.

34 Clarke SF *et al.* (2005) Naloxone in opioid poisoning: walking the tightrope. *Emergency Medicine Journal.* **22**: 612–616.

35 Paranthaman SK and Khan F (1976) Acute cardiomyopathy with recurrent pulmonary edema and hypotension following heroin overdosage. *Chest.* **69**: 117–119.

36 Verebey K (1981) The clinical pharmacology of naltrexone: pharmacology and pharmacodynamics. *NIDA Research Monograph.* **28**: 147–158.

37 Sudakin D (2016) Naltrexone: Not just for opioids anymore. *Journal of Medical Toxicology.* **12**: 71–75.

38 Davis M (2007) Cholestasis and endogenous opioids: liver disease and exogenous opioid pharmacokinetics. *Clinical Pharmacokinetics.* **46**: 825–850.

39 Metze D *et al.* (1999) Efficacy and safety of naltrexone, an oral opiate receptor antagonist, in the treatment of pruritus in internal and dermatological diseases. *Journal of the American Academy of Dermatology.* **41**: 533–539.

40 Jones E *et al.* (2002) Opiate antagonist therapy for the pruritus of cholestasis: the avoidance of opioid withdrawal-like reactions. *Quarterly Journal of Medicine.* **95**: 547–552.

41 Tandon P *et al.* (2007) The efficacy and safety of bile acid binding agents, opioid antagonists, or rifampin in the treatment of cholestasis-associated pruritus. *American Journal of Gastroenterology.* **102**: 1528–1536.

42 Bergasa N *et al.* (1992) A controlled trial of naloxone infusions for the pruritus of chronic cholestasis. *Gastroenterology.* **102**: 544–549.

43 Bergasa N *et al.* (1995) Effects of naloxone infusions in patients with the pruritus of cholestasis. *Annals of Internal Medicine.* **123**: 161–167.

44 Kumar N *et al.* (2013) Opiate receptor antagonists for treatment of severe pruritus associated with advanced cholestatic liver disease. *Journal of Palliative Medicine.* **16**: 122–123.

45 Terg R *et al.* (2002) Efficacy and safety of oral naltrexone treatment for pruritus of cholestasis, a crossover, double blind, placebo-controlled study. *Journal of Hepatology.* **37**: 717–722.

46 Bergasa N *et al.* (1999) Oral nalmefene therapy reduces scratching activity due to the pruritus of cholestasis: a controlled study. *Journal of the American Academy of Dermatology.* **41**: 431–434.

47 Jones E and Dekker L (2000) Florid opioid withdrawal-like reaction precipitated by naltrexone in a patient with chronic cholestasis. *Gastroenterology.* **118**: 431–432.

48 McRae CA *et al.* (2003) Pain as a complication of use of opiate antagonists for symptom control in cholestasis. *Gastroenterology.* **125**: 591–596.

49 Lonsdale-Eccles AA and Carmichael AJ (2009) Opioid antagonist for pruritus of cholestasis unmasking bony metastases. *Acta Dermato Venereologica.* **89**: 90.

50 Hohl CM *et al.* (2015) Methylnaltrexone to palliate pruritus in terminal hepatic disease. *Journal of Palliative Care.* **31**: 124–126.

51 Juby L *et al.* (1994) Buprenorphine and hepatic pruritus. *British Journal of Clinical Practice.* **48**: 331.

52 Reddy L *et al.* (2007) Transdermal buprenorphine may be effective in the treatment of pruritus in primary biliary cirrhosis. *Journal of Pain and Symptom Management.* **34**: 455–456.

53 Marinangeli F *et al.* (2009) Intravenous naloxone plus transdermal buprenorphine in cancer pain associated with intractable cholestatic pruritus. *Journal of Pain and Symptom Management.* **38**: e5–8.

54 Zylicz Z *et al.* (2005) Severe pruritus of cholestasis in disseminated cancer: developing a rational treatment strategy. A case report. *Journal of Pain and Symptom Management.* **29**: 100–103.

55 Jones EA and Zylicz Z (2005) Treatment of pruritus caused by cholestasis with opioid antagonists. *Journal of Palliative Medicine.* **8**: 1290–1294.

56 Manenti L *et al.* (2009) Uraemic pruritus: clinical characteristics, pathophysiology and treatment. *Drugs.* **69**: 251–263.

57 Kumagai H *et al.* (2000) Endogenous opioid system in uraemic patients. In: *Joint Meeting of the Seventh World Conference on Clinical Pharmacology and IUPHAR - Division of Clinical Pharmacology and the Fourth Congress of the European Association for Clinical Pharmacology and Therapeutics.*

58 Odou P *et al.* (2001) A hypothesis for endogenous opioid peptides in uraemic pruritus: role of enkephalin. *Nephrology, Dialysis, Transplantation.* **16**: 1953–1954.

59 Bottcher B and Wildt L (2014) Treatment of refractory vulvovaginal pruritus with naltrexone, a specific opiate antagonist. *European Journal of Obstetrics and Gynecology Reproductive Biology.* **174**: 115–116.

60 Peters WP *et al.* (1981) Pressor effect of naloxone in septic shock. *Lancet.* **i**: 529–532.

61 Cohen RA and Coffman JD (1980) Naloxone reversal of morphine-induced peripheral vasodilatation. *Clinical Pharmacology and Therapeutics.* **28**: 541–544.

62 Baskin DS and Hosobuchi Y (1981) Naloxone reversal of ischaemic neurological deficits in man. *Lancet.* **ii**: 272–275.

63 Bousigue J-Y *et al.* (1982) Naloxone reversal of neurological deficit. *Lancet.* **ii**: 618–619.

64 Ray D and Tai Y (1988) Infusions of naloxone in thalamic pain. *British Medical Journal.* **296**: 969–970.

65 McLaughlin PJ and Zagon IS (2015) Duration of opioid receptor blockade determines biotherapeutic response. *Biochemical Pharmacology.* **97**: 236–246.

66 McNicol ED (2008) Mu-opioid antagonists for opioid-induced bowel dysfunction. *Cochrane Database of Systematic Reviews.* **2**: CD006332.

67 Vickers AP and Jolly A (2006) Naltrexone and problems in pain management. *British Medical Journal.* **332 (7534)**: 132–133.

68 Mitchell J (1986) Naltrexone and hepatotoxicity. *Lancet.* **1**: 1215.

69 Partridge BL and Ward CF (1986) Pulmonary oedema following low-dose naloxone administration. *Anesthesiology.* **65**: 709–710.

70 Yoburn BC *et al.* (1988) Upregulation of opioid receptor subtypes correlates with potency changes of morphine and DADLE. *Life Sciences.* **43**: 1319–1324.

71 WHO (2009) Guidelines for the psychosocially assisted pharmacological treatment of opioid dependence. www.who.int

72 Sabzghabaee AM *et al.* (2014) Naloxone therapy in opioid overdose patients: intranasal or intravenous? A randomized clinical trial. *Archives of Medical Science.* **10**: 309–314.

73 Dietze P and Cantwell K (2016) Intranasal naloxone soon to become part of evolving clinical practice around opioid overdose prevention. *Addiction.* **111**: 584–586.

74 Bergasa N *et al.* (1998) Open-label trial of oral nalmefene therapy for the pruritus of cholestasis. *Hepatology.* **27**: 679–684.

Added February 2017

Quick Clinical Guide: Reversal of opioid-induced respiratory depression

Traditional IV doses of naloxone (e.g. 400microgram stat) should be used only in immediately life-threatening situations (i.e. unconscious patient with minimal/no respiratory effort).

In other circumstances, careful titration using lower doses of naloxone (e.g. 20–100microgram IV) should be used to avoid a severe acute withdrawal syndrome and, in those receiving opioids for analgesia, severe pain and hyperalgesia.

The dose should be titrated against respiratory function (i.e. to achieve a respiratory rate ≥8 breaths/min and no cyanosis) and level of consciousness (i.e. patient easily rousable; they do not have to be fully alert).

Because buprenorphine has both high receptor affinity and prolonged receptor binding, naloxone in standard doses does not reverse the effects of buprenorphine and higher doses must be used (see Box below).

Diagnosis

Most episodes are preceded by a progressive reduction in consciousness. Significant respiratory depression can be present despite a respiratory rate ≥8 breaths/min, thus:

- patients with a reduced level of consciousness and respiratory rate <8 breaths/min require naloxone
- if respiratory rate ≥8 breaths/min, and the patient difficult to rouse and cyanosed, give naloxone
- If respiratory rate ≥8 breaths/min, and the patient easily rousable and not cyanosed, adopt a policy of 'watchful waiting'; consider omitting or reducing the next regular dose of opioid, and then continuing at the lower dose.

Initial treatment

General approaches include:

- maintain airway
- administer oxygen to maintain SaO_2 >95%
- discontinue opioid (e.g. stop CSCI/CIVI, remove TD patch)
- obtain IV access
- administer naloxone IV (if not practical can be given IM or SC).

Immediately life-threatening respiratory depression

In this situation, i.e. unconscious patient with minimal/no respiratory effort, 'traditional doses' of naloxone are used. Administer each dose over 30 seconds. Assess after 1min and, if no response, move to the next dose:

- start with 400microgram IV → 800microgram → 800microgram → 2–4mg
- if no response to 2–4mg, consider an alternate diagnosis.

Severe but not immediately life-threatening respiratory depression

This is written from the perspective of an iatrogenic overdose in a patient receiving opioid analgesia, but it can also be applied to overdose from drug misuse.

When naloxone is indicated (see Diagnosis):

- dilute a 1mL ampoule containing naloxone 400microgram to 4mL with 0.9% saline for injection
- administer 1mL (100microgram) IV every 2min until respirations are satisfactory.

Even lower doses may be used:

- dilute a 1mL ampoule containing naloxone 400microgram to 10mL with 0.9% saline for injection
- administer 0.5mL (20microgram) IV every 2min until respirations are satisfactory.

Ongoing treatment

After the last dose of naloxone, monitor level of consciousness and respiratory rate every 15min for 2h, then hourly for 6h after immediate-release opioid, 12h after modified-release opioid, or 24h after methadone.

Further boluses are likely to be necessary because naloxone is shorter-acting than morphine and other opioids. If more than three repeat bolus doses are required, consider IVI naloxone for up to 24h, sometimes longer:

- dilute 10 ampoules containing naloxone 400microgram in 1mL to 20mL with 0.9% saline or 5% glucose to produce a 200microgram/mL solution
- administer via a large peripheral vein or central venous catheter
- use an IVI device (e.g. syringe pump) to deliver an hourly dose which is 60% of the stat dose which had previously maintained satisfactory ventilation for ≥15min
- titrate the IVI as necessary.

Naloxone IVI requires close monitoring; some centres recommend use only within a Critical Care Unit.

Rarely, an opioid overdose is complicated by pulmonary oedema, but the signs may be absent until naloxone improves the respiratory rate and tidal volume. Consider if there is unexpected breathlessness and persistent hypoxaemia despite oxygen. Treat with oxygen, IV furosemide, IVI nitrates, and ventilation as necessary. Generally the pulmonary oedema responds to these approaches in 24–48h.

Review opioid regimen

Consider:

- possible causes for the opioid overdose, e.g.:
  - ▷ excessive dosing (e.g. opioid poorly responsive pain)
  - ▷ drug–drug interaction (e.g. fentanyl and clarithromycin)
  - ▷ drug accumulation because of an opioid with a long halflife (e.g. methadone)
  - ▷ reduced elimination because of renal impairment (e.g. morphine)
- only when there is sustained respiratory improvement, restarting on a lower dose of opioid
- switching to another opioid; seek specialist advice.

Reversal of buprenorphine-induced respiratory depression

1 Discontinue buprenorphine (stop CSCI/CIVI, remove TD patch).

2 Give oxygen by mask.

3 Give IV naloxone *2mg* stat over 90sec.

4 Commence naloxone *4mg/h* by CIVI.

5 Continue CIVI until the patient's condition is satisfactory (probably <90min).

6 Monitor the patient frequently for the next 24h, and restart CIVI if respiratory depression recurs.

7 If the patient's condition remains satisfactory, restart buprenorphine at a reduced dose, e.g. half the previous dose.

The non-specific respiratory stimulant doxapram can also be used, 1–1.5mg/kg IV over 30sec, repeated if necessary at hourly intervals or 1.5–*4mg/min* CIVI.

Added March 2017

OPIOID ANTAGONISTS (THERAPEUTIC TARGET OUTSIDE THE CNS)

For *Opioid antagonists (therapeutic target within the CNS)*, see p.457; these are authorized for reversal of opioid-induced respiratory depression and acute opioid overdose. Because they reverse opioid-induced analgesia, their use for reversing the peripheral effects of opioids (e.g. constipation) is restricted. The exception is **naloxone** in Targinact®, where use of a m/r formulation limits systemic absorption (see p.449), and thereby limits central antagonism.

Indications: Opioid-induced constipation in adults whose *response to laxatives is insufficient* (**methylnaltrexone** SC) *or inadequate* (**naloxegol** PO); post-operative ileus (**methylnaltrexone** SC, **alvimopan** (not UK) PO).[1,2]

Contra-indications: Methylnaltrexone: known or suspected bowel obstruction; acute surgical abdomen.
Naloxegol: known or suspected bowel obstruction; increased risk of GI perforation (i.e. those at risk of recurrent bowel obstruction, recurrent or advanced ovarian cancer, other cancers of the GI tract or peritoneum, concurrent use of a VEGF inhibitor); concurrent use of a *strong CYP3A4 inhibitor* (see Drug interactions).

Pharmacology

Alvimopan (not UK), **methylnaltrexone** and **naloxegol** do not readily cross the blood-brain barrier, and thus act as peripheral opioid antagonists. Although referred to as PAMORA (*p*eripherally-*a*cting *m*u-*o*pioid *r*eceptor *a*ntagonists), they also bind to other types of opioid receptor, albeit with lower and differing levels of affinity.

Methylnaltrexone

Authorized for SC use in adults to treat opioid-induced constipation when there has been an insufficient response to laxatives. A PO product is likely to become available. RCTs have been undertaken in those with advanced illness (palliative care patients) using doses based on body weight, and in those with chronic pain (mostly back pain) using a fixed dose of 12mg SC.[3,4]

In patients with advanced illness, **methylnaltrexone** was used alongside existing laxative therapy, whereas in patients with chronic pain, only p.r.n. rescue laxatives were permitted. One systematic review based on these RCTs reported an overall NNT of 3 (95% CI 2–10) and a NNH (for diarrhoea) of 30 (95% CI 18–111);[3] another found only the risk of abdominal pain to be significantly higher than placebo, and a serious adverse event rate of 0.2%.[4]

Off-label uses of **methylnaltrexone** include opioid-induced constipation in children,[5–7] post-operative[8–10] or non-surgical critical care patients[11,12] and opioid-related acute colonic pseudo-obstruction.[13] **Methylnaltrexone** may also improve other peripheral effects of opioids, e.g. delayed gastric emptying, urinary retention.[8] Case reports also suggest benefit in cholestatic pruritus (see p.459).[14]

After SC **methylnaltrexone**, peak plasma concentration is reached in about 30min. Elimination is mostly as unchanged drug (85%), via the urine (50%) and faeces. The main metabolites (methylnaltrexone sulfate, methyl-6-naltrexol) are inactive. Mild–moderate hepatic impairment does not affect the metabolism of **methylnaltrexone** to a clinically relevant degree; the effect of severe hepatic impairment has not been evaluated.

The clearance of **methylnaltrexone** reduces with increasing renal impairment. When severe, overall exposure (AUC) is doubled and dose reduction is required (see Dose and use). For pharmacokinetic data see Table 1.

Naloxegol

In RCTs, **naloxegol** 25mg PO consistently improved bowel function and symptoms, but *only* in the subset of patients defined as having an inadequate response to laxatives, i.e. those with moderate symptoms of opioid-induced constipation (≥1 of: hard or lumpy stools, straining, or a sensation of incomplete bowel movement or anorectal obstruction) despite taking ≥1 type of laxative for ≥4 days during the previous 2 weeks. In this group, about half respond to **naloxegol** (compared with one third to placebo), with a NNT of 5–7.[15]

However, laxatives were only taken p.r.n. and in small amounts, i.e. on average **bisacodyl** ≤10mg *weekly*.[15,16] This suggests a very different population to that typically seen in palliative care. Further, severely constipated patients were excluded from the RCTs, i.e. those with faecal impaction or no bowel movement for 2 weeks.

RCTs involved relatively young patients (early 50s; only 10% ≥65, 2% ≥75) with non-cancer pain (mostly back pain) and, at most, mild hepatic/renal impairment with a mean oral **morphine** equivalent dose of 140mg/day.[15] *Thus, data to support the use of **naloxegol** in patients with cancer-related pain is currently lacking.* Consequently, in the USA, authorization is limited to patients with chronic non-cancer pain.

5

PO absorption of **naloxegol** is rapid and enhanced by food (a high-fat meal increases C_{max} and AUC by about 30% and 45% respectively). A secondary plasma concentration peak occurs 0.5–3h after the first, probably reflecting enterohepatic recirculation. Metabolism is mostly via CYP3A and elimination via the faeces (70%). Mild–moderate hepatic impairment does not affect the metabolism of **naloxegol** to a clinically relevant degree; the effect of severe hepatic impairment has not been evaluated.

Generally, because renal excretion is a minor route of elimination (≤5% unchanged **naloxegol**), pharmacokinetics are not significantly altered by renal impairment. Nonetheless, unpredictable increases in exposure to **naloxegol** can occur, possibly because of the effect of renal impairment on other clearance pathways (e.g. liver, GI wall). Consequently, a lower initial dose is recommended in patients with moderate–severe renal impairment. Haemodialysis has no effect on the pharmacokinetics of **naloxegol**. For pharmacokinetic data see Table 1.

Table 1 Pharmacokinetic details for methylnaltrexone and naloxegol

	Methylnaltrexone	*Naloxegol*
Bio-availability (%)	80% (SC)	60% (PO, estimate)
Onset of action	can be rapid (within 30min); median time to bowel movement ranges 1–6h	median time to bowel movement ranges 5–21h
Time to peak plasma concentration	0.5h (SC)	≤2h
Plasma halflife	8h	6–11h
Duration of action	<24h	<24h

Cautions

Methylnaltrexone: known or suspected lesions of the GI tract; patients with colostomy, active diverticular disease, faecal impaction, peritoneal catheter (excluded from studies); increased risk of perforation (e.g. GI cancer, peptic ulcer, pseudo-obstruction).

Naloxegol: increased risk of GI perforation from other causes not constituting a contra-indication, e.g. Crohn's disease, active/recurrent diverticulitis, infiltrative GI cancers or peritoneal metastases, severe peptic ulcer disease; potential disruption of the blood-brain barrier (trials excluded patients with Alzheimer's disease, brain tumours or multiple sclerosis); use of **methadone** or high doses of opioid (i.e. ≥200mg/day oral **morphine** equivalent) increases risk of GI symptoms, e.g. abdominal pain and diarrhoea; cardiovascular disease (trials excluded patients with recent myocardial infarction, symptomatic CHF, overt cardiovascular disease, or QT interval >500ms, although QT was unaffected in a healthy volunteer study).

Drug interactions

Concurrent use of a *strong CYP3A4 inhibitor* increases exposure to **naloxegol** ≥10 times, e.g. **clarithromycin**, grapefruit juice (specifically large quantities), **itraconazole**, protease inhibitors, **telithromycin** and is contra-indicated.

Naloxegol is rendered ineffective by *strong CYP3A4 inducers*, which reduce exposure to **naloxegol** by ≥75%, e.g. **carbamazepine, rifampicin, St. John's Wort**.

Undesirable effects

Methylnaltrexone

Very common (≥10%): abdominal pain (generally mild–moderate),[17] diarrhoea, flatulence, nausea (these generally resolve after a bowel movement).
Common (<10%, >1%): vomiting, dizziness, mild peripheral opioid-withdrawal symptoms (see **naloxegol** below), injection site reactions.
Not known: GI perforation (stomach, small and large bowel).[18]

Naloxegol

Very common (≥10%): abdominal pain and diarrhoea. GI symptoms are most likely in the first ≤4 weeks of treatment.
Common (<10%, >1%): headache, nasopharyngitis, flatulence, nausea, vomiting, hyperhidrosis.
Uncommon (<1%, >0.1%): opioid-withdrawal syndrome (defined as ≥3 of the following: diarrhoea, dysphoria, fever, insomnia, lacrimation or rhinorrhoea, muscle aches, nausea or vomiting, pupillary dilation or piloerection or sweating, yawning). Generally, occurs in the first few days of treatment and is mild–moderate in intensity.

Dose and use

Naloxegol has been approved by NICE[19] and the Scottish Medicines Consortium,[20] but both the *Drugs and Therapeutics Bulletin* and *PCF* consider **naloxegol** to be of very limited value clinically.[21] Its benefit compared with an optimized laxative regimen is unknown, and there is a lack of experience in patients with cancer. It is much more expensive than even high doses of stimulant laxatives.

By comparison, **methylnaltrexone**, although a SC injection and more expensive, has the advantages of a higher response rate (≤70% vs. ≤50%), a lower NNT (3 vs. 5–7) and has been widely used in palliative care.

Thus, if a clinician chooses to prescribe **naloxegol**, its use should be restricted (as with **methylnaltrexone**) to occasions when upward titration of regularly administered laxatives is ineffective, poorly tolerated or not adhered to (see p.38).

Because constipation in advanced disease is generally multifactorial in origin,[22] **methylnaltrexone** and **naloxegol** will augment rather than replace laxatives.

Methylnaltrexone

Injection sites should be rotated, using soft, non-bruised areas of the abdomen or upper legs/arms.

Between 1/3–2/3 of patients given **methylnaltrexone** defaecate within 30min–4h.[23–28] Patients should be warned of the possibility of a rapid effect; those with reduced mobility should have immediate access to a commode.

Patients should discontinue **methylnaltrexone** and seek advice if they develop severe, persistent or worsening symptoms, e.g. abdominal pain, diarrhoea.

Patients with advanced illness (palliative care patients)

- continue all other laxative treatment
- the dose is based on the patient's weight:
  - ▷ 38–61kg, start with 8mg SC on alternate days
  - ▷ 62–114kg, start with 12mg SC on alternate days
  - ▷ outside this range, give *0.15mg/kg (150microgram/kg)* on alternate days
- for dose adjustment in renal and hepatic impairment, see below
- the interval between administrations can be varied, either extended or reduced, but not more than once daily; in open-label extension studies, the median (range) interval between doses was 3 (1–39) days.

Trial data does not extend beyond 4 months in patients with advanced illness.

Patients with chronic pain but not advanced illness

- stop all other laxative treatment until the response to **methylnaltrexone** is known
- start with 12mg SC on alternate days, irrespective of the patients weight
- if after 3 days there is an insufficient response, resume laxatives
- otherwise, follow guidance as above.

Trial data does not extend beyond 12 months in patients with chronic pain.

In severe renal impairment (creatinine clearance <30mL/min) reduce the dose:
- for patients weighing 62–114kg, reduce to 8mg
- outside this range, reduce to *0.075mg/kg (75microgram/kg)*, rounding up the dose volume to the nearest 0.1mL.

Methylnaltrexone has not been studied in patients requiring dialysis and is not recommended in this setting.

No dose adjustment is required in mild–moderate hepatic impairment but use in severe hepatic impairment has not been studied, and is not recommended.

Naloxegol

Half of subjects experience a bowel action after 6–12h, and about 2/3 within 24h.[15,29] Patients should discontinue **naloxegol** and seek advice if they develop severe, persistent or worsening symptoms, e.g. abdominal pain, diarrhoea:
- stop all other laxative treatment until the response to **naloxegol** is known
- start with **naloxegol** 25mg PO once daily, taken in the morning on an empty stomach, i.e. 30min before or 2h after breakfast
- ideally, the tablet should be swallowed whole; if necessary, it can be crushed to a powder, mixed in half a glass of water (120mL) and drunk immediately
- if there is unacceptable abdominal pain/diarrhoea, reduce the dose to 12.5mg once daily
- if after 3 days there is an insufficient response, resume laxatives (necessary in about half of trial participants)
- also use a starting dose of 12.5mg PO once daily if:
  - ▷ moderate–severe renal impairment (Cr Cl <60mL/min)
  - ▷ concurrent use of a *moderate* CYP3A4 *inhibitor* (e.g. **diltiazem, erythromycin, verapamil**; also see p.721).

If tolerated and if necessary, increase after 2 days to 25mg once daily.

No dose adjustment is required in mild–moderate hepatic impairment but use in severe hepatic impairment has not been studied, and cannot be recommended.

Supply

Methylnaltrexone

Relistor® (Wyeth)

Injection methylnaltrexone bromide 12mg/0.6mL, 1mL vial = £21.

Naloxegol

Moventig® (Astra Zeneca)

Tablets naloxegol 12.5mg, 25mg, 28 days @ 12.5mg or 25mg each morning = £55.

1 McNicol ED (2008) Mu-opioid antagonists for opioid-induced bowel dysfunction. *Cochrane Database of Systematic Reviews*. **2**: CD006332. www.thecochranelibrary.com

2 Becker G and Blum HE (2009) Novel opioid antagonists for opioid-induced bowel dysfunction and postoperative ileus. *Lancet*. **373**: 1198–1206.

3 Ford AC *et al.* (2013) Efficacy of pharmacological therapies for the treatment of opioid-induced constipation: systematic review and meta-analysis. *American Journal of Gastroenterology*. **108**: 1566–1574.

4 Siemens W and Becker G (2016) Methylnaltrexone for opioid-induced constipation: review and meta-analyses for objective plus subjective efficacy and safety outcomes. *Therapeutics and Clinical Risk Management*. **12**: 401–412.

5 Lopez J *et al.* (2016) Methylnaltrexone for the treatment of constipation in critically ill children. *Journal of Clinical Gastroenterology*. **50**: 351–352.

6 Flerlage JE and Baker JN (2015) Methylnaltrexone for opioid-induced constipation in children and adolescents and young adults with progressive incurable cancer at the end of life. *Journal of Palliative Medicine*. **18**: 631–633.

7 Rodrigues A *et al.* (2013) Methylnaltrexone for opioid-induced constipation in pediatric oncology patients. *Pediatric Blood and Cancer*. **60**: 1667–1670.

8 Deibert P *et al.* (2010) Methylnaltrexone: the evidence for its use in the management of opioid-induced constipation. *Core Evidence*. **4**: 247–258.

9 Anissian L *et al.* (2012) Subcutaneous methylnaltrexone for treatment of acute opioid-induced constipation: phase 2 study in rehabilitation after orthopedic surgery. *Journal of Hospital Medicine*. **7**: 67–72.

10 Zand F *et al.* (2015) The effect of methylnaltrexone on the side effects of intrathecal morphine after orthopedic surgery under spinal anesthesia. *Pain Practice*. **15**: 348–354.

11 Sawh SB *et al.* (2012) Use of methylnaltrexone for the treatment of opioid-induced constipation in critical care patients. *Mayo Clinic Proceedings*. **87**: 255–259.

12 Hewitt K *et al.* (2014) Use of methylnaltrexone to induce laxation in acutely injured patients with burns and necrotizing soft-tissue infections. *Journal of Burn Care and Research*. **35**: e106–111.

13 Weinstock LB and Chang AC (2011) Methylnaltrexone for treatment of acute colonic pseudo-obstruction. *Journal of Clinical Gastroenterology*. **45**: 883–884.

14 Hohl CM *et al.* (2015) Methylnaltrexone to palliate pruritus in terminal hepatic disease. *Journal of Palliative Care*. **31**: 124–126.

15 Chey WD *et al.* (2014) Naloxegol for opioid-induced constipation in patients with noncancer pain. *New England Journal of Medicine*. **370**: 2387–2396.

16 Astra Zeneca (2016) Personal communication.

17 Slatkin NE *et al.* (2011) Characterization of abdominal pain during methylnaltrexone treatment of opioid-induced constipation in advanced illness: a post hoc analysis of two clinical trials. *Journal of Pain and Symptom Management*. **42**: 754–760.

18 Mackey AC *et al.* (2010) Methylnaltrexone and gastrointestinal perforation. *Journal of Pain and Symptom Management*. **40**: e1–3.

19 NICE (2015) Naloxegol for opioid-induced constipation. *Drugs and Therapeutics Bulletin*. **53**: 138–140.

20 Scottish Medicines Consortium (2015) Naloxegol (1106/15).

21 Anonymous (2015) Naloxegol for opioid-induced constitpation. *Drugs and Therapeutics Bulletin*. **53**: 138–140.

22 Larkin PJ *et al.* (2008) The management of constipation in palliative care: clinical practice recommendations. *Palliative Medicine*. **22**: 796–807.

23 Portenoy RK *et al.* (2008) Subcutaneous methylnaltrexone for the treatment of opioid-induced constipation in patients with advanced illness: a double-blind, randomized, parallel group, dose-ranging study. *Journal of Pain and Symptom Management*. **35**: 458–468.

24 Thomas J *et al.* (2008) Methylnaltrexone for opioid-induced constipation in advanced illness. *New England Journal of Medicine*. **358**: 2332–2343.

25 Slatkin N *et al.* (2009) Methylnaltrexone for treatment of opioid-induced constipation in advanced illness patients. *Journal of Supportive Oncology*. **7**: 39–46.

26 Michna E *et al.* (2011) Subcutaneous methylnaltrexone for treatment of opioid-induced constipation in patients with chronic, nonmalignant pain: A randomized controlled study. *Journal of Pain*. **12**: 554–562.

27 Candy B *et al.* (2011) Laxatives or methylnaltrexone for the management of constipation in palliative care patients. *Cochrane Database of Systematic Reviews*. **19**: CD003448. www.thecochranelibrary.com

28 Bull J *et al.* (2015) Fixed-dose subcutaneous methylnaltrexone in patients with advanced illness and opioid-induced constipation: results of a randomized, placebo-controlled study and open-label extension. *Journal of Palliative Medicine*. **18**: 593–600.

29 Webster L *et al.* (2014) Randomised clinical trial: the long-term safety and tolerability of naloxegol in patients with pain and opioid-induced constipation. *Alimentary Pharmacology and Therapeutics*. **40**: 771–779.

Added February 2017

6: INFECTIONS

6

ANTIBACTERIALS IN PALLIATIVE CARE

Remember: always ask about drug allergies before prescribing an antibacterial.

The dose and frequency of many antibacterials are reduced in renal impairment.

The BNF contains a comprehensive account of antibacterial use,[1] and many hospitals have antibacterial policies which govern local infection control and treatment, e.g. the prevention of methicillin-resistant *Staphylococcus aureus* (MRSA) infection and the prevention of *Clostridium difficile* infection. Thus, any specific recommendations about antibacterials in *PCF* should be considered in conjunction with local policy. When in doubt, seek advice from a local medical microbiologist.

Be aware that rigorously applied screening and infection control protocols will impose significant burdens at the end of life.[2]

Penicillin allergy

Allergic reactions to penicillins occur in 1–10% of exposed individuals, and anaphylaxis in <0.05%. Those with a history of urticaria, rash or anaphylaxis immediately after starting a course of a penicillin should not be prescribed a penicillin, a cephalosporin, or other beta-lactam antibacterial.

Those with a history of a minor rash (e.g. non-confluent, non-pruritic rash restricted to a small area of the body) or a rash which occurs >72h after a penicillin is started are probably *not* allergic to penicillin, and a penicillin need not be withheld if indicated. However, the possibility of an allergic reaction should be kept in mind. Other beta-lactam antibacterials (including cephalosporins) can be used in these patients.[1]

Stop and think!

In a moribund patient with progressive incurable disease, are you justified in giving antibacterials for an intercurrent infection which may be the natural endpoint of the dying process?

Antibacterials in end-stage disease should have the primary purpose of ameliorating distressing symptoms (including fever and malaise), and not simply delaying inevitable death. It is important to *stop and think:* if antibacterials are automatically prescribed when infection is diagnosed, they may simply serve to prolong suffering.[3–5]

The potential for antibacterials to impact on the survival of patients with advanced cancer varies with the type of infection and setting of the patient. For example, in hospital inpatients referred to a palliative care service, a prolonged survival was associated with the recent use of antibacterials for septicaemia but not focal infection.[6] Overall, compared to patients with infections who did not receive antibacterials, this amounted to a difference in median survival of about 2–3 weeks. However, median survival differed by about 5 months (septicaemia) and 2 months (focal infection) between patients deemed to have had a good vs. a poor initial response to the antibacterials, with the latter only surviving about 1 and 3 weeks respectively.[6] On the other hand, in a community-based hospice programme, the presence of infection or the use of antibacterials made no difference to the median survival of patients of about 30 days.[7]

Nonetheless, whatever the setting, in addition to symptom relief, clinicians should balance the potential for any benefit from extra time gained by the use of antibacterials with the burden of irreversible progressive physical deterioration. Thus, antibacterials are generally appropriate for a patient with advanced cancer who develops a chest infection while still relatively active and independent. However, in someone who has become bedbound as a result of general progressive deterioration and who seems close to death, pneumonia should still be allowed to be 'the old person's friend'. In such circumstances it is generally appropriate *not* to prescribe antibacterials and to 'give death a chance'.

Although some terminally ill patients recover from a chest infection without an antibacterial, others progress to a 'grumbling pneumonia'. A continuing wet cough may cause much distress, and possibly loss of sleep. If this is the case, an antibacterial may well be indicated for symptom relief.

When it is difficult to make a decision, a '2-day rule' could be invoked: if after 2 days of general symptom management the patient is clinically stable, prescribe an antibacterial but, if the patient is clearly much worse, do not. Conversely, given the poor survival of those who fail to have a good initial response to antibacterials,[6] there is need also for a reverse '2-day rule', namely discontinue antibacterials after a few days if there is no apparent response, particularly if the patient is now moribund.

General considerations

Evidence for symptom improvement with antibacterials at the end of life remains patchy. Only 8 of 11 studies in a recent systematic review of antibacterial use in hospice patients considered symptom response as an outcome following antibacterial therapy.[8]

Several surveys give similar prevalence rates for *symptomatic* infection in palliative care patients, namely about 40%,[7] and show that the response to antibacterials varies according to the site of infection (Table 1). Provided a patient does not have an indwelling urinary catheter, UTIs should generally be treated routinely unless there is an overriding reason for not doing so (see p.485 = UTI m/g).[6,9] Cough caused by infection is also significantly reduced by antibacterials.[9] On the other hand, in patients with end-stage progressive disease being cared for at home, the use of antibacterials to treat septicaemia in a patient is generally futile (Table 1).

Table 1 Response to antimicrobials[a] in >600 home care patients[7]

Type of infection	*Number*	*Response (%)*[b]
UTI	265	79
RTI	221	43
Oral cavity[a]	63	46
Skin or SC	59	41
Septicaemia	25	0

a. includes the use of antibacterials for infections at all sites, and of antifungals for oral candidosis
b. reduction of fever ± amelioration of site-specific symptoms within 3 days.

Specific recommendations

The specific information given in this chapter is limited to selected situations which may occur in palliative care:

- local infection causing severe pain
- ascending cholangitis associated with a biliary stent
- infection associated with an airway stent
- respiratory tract infection in the dying patient
- cellulitis in patients with lymphoedema (see p.490).

Note. Generally, to ensure adequate plasma concentrations, it is recommended that antibacterials are prescribed at consistent regular intervals, e.g. q6h, q8h or q12h, and this should be adhered to in patients with severe infection, particularly requiring IV antibacterials. However, in patients approaching last days of life, particularly taking PO antibacterials, a more pragmatic and less rigorous administration, e.g. q.d.s, t.d.s, b.d. can be considered.

Antibacterials to relieve infection-related pain

Antibacterials are essential in some patients for the relief of severe pain associated with infection around a malignant tumour in, for example, the neck, the gluteal muscles underlying an ulcerated cancer, or the perineum.[10] Sometimes there is a history of a rapid increase in pain intensity over several days which is poorly responsive to escalating doses of a strong opioid. The pain is often associated with fever and malaise, and may be complicated by delirium. Commonly, there will be a mixture of more superficial aerobic infection with deeper anaerobic infection. Treatment is similar to that recommended for ascending cholangitis (see below).

Ascending cholangitis

Ascending cholangitis may occur in patients with a partially obstructed or stented common bile duct. It often causes severe systemic disturbance and should be treated promptly:

- **piperacillin/tazobactam** 4.5g IV t.d.s.
- if a minor rash with a penicillin in the past (see p.471), **cefuroxime** 1.5g IV t.d.s. plus **metronidazole** 500mg IV t.d.s.
- if the patient is in septic shock, also give a single dose of **gentamicin** 5mg/kg (maximum dose 500mg) IV over 20–30min
- if a risk of multiresistant Gram-negative bacilli, serious penicillin allergy or in any doubt, consult a medical microbiologist.

When IV administration is difficult, alternatives include:

- **ceftazidime** 1g IM t.d.s., reconstituted with 3mL of WFI or 0.5–1% **lidocaine hydrochloride** solution (total injection volume ~3.8mL)
- in countries where it is available (not UK) **cefepime** 1g SC t.d.s. reconstituted with 2.4mL of either 0.9% saline, 5% glucose (dextrose), WFI or 0.5–1% **lidocaine hydrochloride** solution (total injection volume ~3.6mL).

The doses and/or frequency of **cefuroxime**, **ceftazidime**, **cefepime**, **piperacillin/ tazobactam** and **gentamicin** should be reduced in renal impairment.

Infection associated with an airway stent

The presence of an airway stent, whether for cancer or other obstruction, increases the risk of serious respiratory tract infection.[11] In a systematic review of 500 patients, mortality rate was almost 70%.[12] Commonest pathogens are *Staphylococcus aureus* and *Pseudomonas aeruginosa*. Treatment should be commenced promptly and guided by the advice of a medical microbiologist.

Respiratory tract infection in the imminently dying patient

Occasionally, death rattle (noisy respiratory secretions) is caused by profuse purulent sputum from a chest infection, and an antibacterial is prescribed in the hope that it will reduce the copious purulent malodorous discharge from the mouth.[13] In this circumstance, the IV route is generally the best. However, if not practical, the IM or SC routes can be used instead.[14–17]

Some centres use single doses of **ceftriaxone**; either 1–2g IV, or 1g IM reconstituted with 3.5mL **lidocaine** 1% (total injection volume ~4.1mL).[13] **Ceftriaxone** is a broad-spectrum antibacterial and has a long duration of action. Patients who responded did so within hours (marked reduction in purulent sputum and resolution of associated halitosis). Non-responders appeared not to benefit from a second dose after 24h.

Other centres give **ceftriaxone** by SC injection[16–19] and administer multiple doses if a patient survives >1 day, e.g. **ceftriaxone** 1g vial reconstituted with 2.2mL **lidocaine** 1% (total injection volume ~2.8mL) 250mg–1g SC once daily. If a larger volume of **lidocaine** is added, e.g. 3.3mL (total injection volume ~3.9mL), the mixture can be administered as a divided dose, given at the same time but using two or more separate SC/IM sites[20] (see manufacturer's SPC for additional information and guidance).

The result of surveys suggest that the above is reasonably well tolerated, and has been used for ≤10 days when patients have not been imminently dying.[14,16]

The bio-availability (in volunteers) of **cefepime** SC is comparable with IM.[21] Further, when 1g is infused over 30min, pain at the injection site is absent or minimal. Thus, **cefepime** (not UK) could be a better option. Concern about the safety of **cefepime**[22] has been shown to be groundless.[23]

Although other antimicrobials have also been given SC, apart from **ertapenem**,[24] supporting data are generally lacking.[17]

Supply

Cefuroxime (generic)
Injection (powder for reconstitution) 250mg, 750mg, 1.5g (IV only), 2 days @ 1.5g t.d.s. = £30.

Ceftazidime (generic)
Injection (powder for reconstitution) 1g, 2g, 2 days @ 1g t.d.s. = £51.

Ceftriaxone (generic)
Injection (powder for reconstitution) 1g vial = £10, 2g vial = £20.

Gentamicin sulfate (generic)
Injection 40mg/mL, 1mL amp, 2mL vial = £1.50; 2mL amp = £1.

Piperacillin/tazobactam (generic)
Injection (powder for reconstitution) piperacillin 2g / tazobactam 250mg, piperacillin 4g / tazobactam 500mg, 2 days @ 4.5g t.d.s = £90.

Also see **metronidazole**, p.478.

1 British National Formulary Chapter 5 Infections: Antibacterials, principles of therapy. London: BMJ Groupo and Pharmaceutical Press. www.medicinescomplete.com (accessed April 2016).
2 Bukki J *et al.* (2013) Methicillin-resistant Staphylococcus aureus (MRSA) management in palliative care units and hospices in Germany: a nationwide survey on patient isolation policies and quality of life. *Palliative Medicine.* **27**: 84–90.
3 Lam PT *et al.* (2005) Retrospective analysis of antibiotic use and survival in advanced cancer patients with infections. *Journal of Pain and Symptom Management.* **30**: 536–543.
4 Thompson AJ *et al.* (2012) Antimicrobial use at the end of life among hospitalized patients with advanced cancer. *American Journal of Hospice and Palliative Care.* **29**: 599–603.
5 Albrecht JS *et al.* (2013) A nationwide analysis of antibiotic use in hospice care in the final week of life. *Journal of Pain and Symptom Management.* **46**: 483–490.
6 Thai V *et al.* (2012) Impact of infections on the survival of hospitalized advanced cancer patients. *Journal of Pain and Symptom Management.* **43**: 549–557.
7 Reinbolt RE *et al.* (2005) Symptomatic treatment of infections in patients with advanced cancer receiving hospice care. *Journal of Pain and Symptom Management.* **30**: 175–182.
8 Rosenberg JH *et al.* (2013) Antimicrobial use for symptom management in patients receiving hospice and palliative care: a systematic review. *Journal of Palliative Medicine.* **16**: 1568–1574.
9 Mirhosseini M *et al.* (2006) The role of antibiotics in the management of infection-related symptoms in advanced cancer patients. *Journal of Palliative Care.* **22**: 69–74.
10 Bruera E and MacDonald N (1986) Intractable pain in patients with advanced head and neck tumors: a possible role of local infection. *Cancer Treatment Reports.* **70**: 691–692.
11 Grosu HB *et al.* (2013) Stents are associated with increased risk of respiratory infections in patients undergoing airway interventions for malignant airways disease. *Chest.* **144**: 441–449.
12 Agrafiotis M *et al.* (2009) Infections related to airway stenting: a systematic review. *Respiration.* **78**: 69–74.
13 Spruyt O and Kausae A (1998) Antibiotic use for infective terminal respiratory secretions. *Journal of Pain and Symptom Management.* **15**: 263–264.
14 palliativedrugs.com (2010) Survey: SC/IM antibiotics - Do you use this route? Available from: www.palliativedrugs.com
15 Azevedo EF (2012) Administration of antibiotics subcutaneously: an integrative literature review. *Acta Paulista de Enfermagem.* **25**: 817–822.
16 Gauthier D *et al.* (2014) Subcutaneous and intravenous ceftriaxone administration in patients more than 75 years of age. *Medicine et Mal Infectieuses.* **44**: 275–280.
17 Forestier E *et al.* (2015) Subcutaneously administered antibiotics: a national survey of current practice from the French Infectious Diseases (SPILF) and Geriatric Medicine (SFGG) society networks. *Clinical Microbiology and Infection.* **21**: 370.e371–373.
18 Borner K *et al.* (1985) Comparative pharmacokinetics of ceftriaxone after subcutaneous and intravenous administration. *Chemotherapy.* **31**: 237–245.
19 Bricaire F *et al.* (1988) Pharmacokinetics and tolerance of ceftriaxone after subcutaneous administration. *Pathologie Biologie (Paris).* **36**: 702–705.
20 Tahmasebi M S/C injection of antibiotics. *Bulletin board (August 2005).* http://www.palliativedrugs.com

21 Walker P *et al.* (2005) Subcutaneous administration of cefepime. *Journal of Pain and Symptom Management*. **30**: 170–174.
22 Yahav D *et al.* (2007) Efficacy and safety of cefepime: a systematic review and meta-analysis. *The Lancet Infectious Diseases*. **7**: 338–348.
23 FDA (2009) Cefepime (marketed as Maxipime) update of ongoing safety review. www.fda.gov/drugs/drugsafety (Archived).
24 Ferry T *et al.* (2012) Prolonged subcutaneous high dose (1 g bid) of Ertapenem as salvage therapy in patients with difficult-to-treat bone and joint infection. *Journal of Infection*. **65**: 579–582.

Updated February 2017

ORAL CANDIDOSIS

Oral yeast carriage is present in about one third of the general population. The prevalence in patients with advanced cancer is significantly higher (about 50–90%).[1] Thus, it is not surprising that oral candidosis is a common fungal infection in the palliative care population of patients (13–30%).[2,3]

Many patients with oral candidosis have concurrent oesophageal infection,[4] and some patients develop systemic fungal infections. Oral candidosis is associated with:
- poor performance status
- dry mouth
- dentures
- topical antibacterials and/or corticosteroids
- in AIDS with CD4 cell count <200cells/mm^3.[1–3]

Oral candidosis is *not* associated with the use of oral/parenteral antibacterials, and most data suggest that it is *not* associated with the use of oral/parenteral corticosteroids.[5]

Non-*Candida albicans* species are increasingly being isolated from patients with oral candidosis.[2,3] The reason for this is thought to be related to increased use of antifungal drugs; the consequence of this change is an increased incidence of azole drug resistance (many non-*Candida albicans* species exhibit inherent azole drug resistance).[6]

Management strategy

Correct the correctable

Underlying causal factors must be considered and corrected if possible, particularly dry mouth and poor denture hygiene.

Dentures must be thoroughly cleaned at least once daily, brushing the denture with a nailbrush or denture brush, and using soap and water or an appropriate commercial product.[7] Dentures should also be soaked overnight in an appropriate antiseptic, e.g. **chlorhexidine** or dilute **sodium hypochlorite**. The latter should not be used for dentures with metal parts. Failure to sterilize the denture will lead to failure of antifungal treatment. The dentures should be thoroughly rinsed before re-insertion.

Drug treatment

A systematic review concluded that there was limited evidence about the efficacy of antifungal drugs in patients with cancer, but that there was some evidence that drugs absorbed from the GI tract are more effective than drugs not absorbed from the GI tract.[8]

Nystatin is a good choice for mild oral candidosis in non-immunocompromised patients. **Miconazole** oral gel is a more expensive topical alternative.

Fluconazole is the preferred choice for moderate–severe infections, and in patients who cannot use **nystatin**.[9] **Itraconazole** is generally second-line; it is more expensive, drug interactions are more likely (see below), and PO bio-availability is variable.

The non-fasting PO bio-availability of **itraconazole** is around 55%. Because an acidic environment is needed to obtain maximal absorption from *capsules*, administration with food is recommended. Hypochlorhydria and acid-reducing drugs decrease absorption (also see Drug interactions). In contrast, the *oral solution* is not dependent on an acidic environment for absorption, and the PO bio-availability is >80% when administered on an empty stomach. Because of the difference in bio-availability, the formulations are *not* interchangeable. (Note. The capsules are authorized for oral candidosis generally but the higher bio-available oral solution only for use in oral/oesophageal candidosis in immunocompromised patients.)

Cross-resistance and cross-infection do occur and, if there is a high prevalence of azole resistance within the local patient population, then even azole-naïve patients may be infected with azole-resistant organisms.[10] Local treatment protocols must take this into account.

Potential topical treatments in resistant cases (or other special circumstances) include **chlorhexidine**,[1] **gentian violet** (e.g. 0.5–1%, 1.5mL applied twice daily),[11] and tea tree oil.[12]

Cautions

Because of a teratogenic risk with **fluconazole** and **itraconazole**, the manufacturers advise that women of child-bearing potential should use contraceptive precautions until the next menstrual period after completing treatment. Because of similar toxicological findings in animal studies with other azoles, it would be wise to extend this precaution to **miconazole**.

Itraconazole may cause or worsen left ventricular dysfunction or CHF, and is contra-indicated unless its use is necessitated by life-threatening infection.
Renal impairment: reduce dose of **fluconazole** by 50% if creatinine clearance is <50mL/min; the bio-availability of oral **itraconazole** may be reduced in renal impairment (also see Chapter 17, p.681).
Hepatic impairment: serious or fatal hepatotoxicity may occur with **fluconazole** and **itraconazole**. The manufacturers advise monitoring liver function in patients receiving large doses and/or prolonged courses, and in patients with known liver dysfunction. With both drugs, treatment should be discontinued if symptoms suggestive of hepatotoxicity develop, e.g. jaundice, dark urine.

MHRA has issued an alert for products or medical devices containing **chlorhexidine** following reports of anaphylaxis.[13]

Drug interactions

Azole antifungals have a strong inhibitory effect on human cytochrome P450 enzymes, particularly CYP3A4 (see Chapter 19, p.717). This results in inhibition of adrenal steroid synthesis (cortisol, testosterone, oestrogens and progesterone) and the metabolism of many drugs.

Drug interactions are most likely with **itraconazole**. They are generally less likely and less pronounced with **fluconazole** (a weaker CYP inhibitor), although several clinically important interactions have been reported.[14] With maximum doses of **miconazole** oromucosal gel, systemic absorption can be suffficient to cause interactions.[15]

Avoid concurrent administration of **fluconazole**, **itraconazole** or **miconazole** with:

- drugs metabolized by CYP3A4 which are known to prolong the QT-interval, e.g. **amiodarone**, **astemizole** (not UK), **domperidone**, **erythromycin**, **methadone**, **pimozide** or **quinidine** because of a risk of fatal cardiac arrhythmias (also see Chapter 20, p.731)
- statins metabolized by CYP3A4, e.g. **atorvastatin**, **lovastatin** and **simvastatin**
- ergot alkaloids, e.g. **ergotamine**
- **eletriptan**, **naloxegol**, **triazolam** (not UK) and PO **midazolam** (not UK).

Fluconazole, **itraconazole** or **miconazole** may increase the plasma concentration of all drugs metabolized by CYP3A4 (see Chapter 19, Table 8, p.725), and thus increase undesirable effects or toxicity. Box A list drugs used in palliative care where increased plasma concentrations have been reported.

Box A Drugs which may require dose reduction if used concurrently with an azole[a,14]

Alfentanil	Haloperidol
Alprazolam	Loperamide
Aprepitant	Methylprednisolone
Budesonide (inhaled)	Midazolam
Carbamazepine	Nifedipine
Dexamethasone	Phenytoin
Digoxin	Risperidone
Fentanyl	Theopylline
Fluticasone (inhaled)	TCAs
Glibenclamide	Warfarin
Glipizide	

a. generally, drug interactions are more likely with itraconazole>fluconazole>miconazole.

Table 1 Antifungal treatment[17]

Class	*Drug*	*Recommended regimen*	*Comments*	*Cost for specified duration*
Polyene group	Nystatin	***Oral suspension*** 100,000 units/mL; 5mL q.d.s for 7 days (continue for 48h after lesions disappear); hold against lesions for at least 1min, and then swallow	Smaller volumes make it more difficult to hold against lesions	£8.50
	Amphotericin (not UK)	***Lozenges*** 10mg; 1 lozenge q.d.s for 10–14 days (continue for 48h after lesions disappear); place in the mouth and allow to dissolve	Up to 2 lozenges q.d.s. in severe infections	Not available in the UK
Azole group (imidazoles)	Miconazole	***Oral gel*** 20mg/g; 5–10mL oral gel q.d.s for 5–7 days (continue for ≥7 days after lesions disappear); hold against lesions for as long as possible, and then swallow	Useful in management of angular cheilitis (has anti-staphylococcal action)	£13
Azole group (triazoles)	Fluconazole	***Capsules*** 50mg, 150mg, 200mg or ***Oral suspension*** 50mg/5mL and 200mg/5mL; 50–100mg once daily for 7 days	May need higher doses/longer courses if immunosuppressed, and for severe infection	£1 (capsules) £17 (oral suspension)
	Itraconazole	***Capsules*** 100mg; 100mg once daily for 2 weeks	Generally *not* used as first-line treatment. May need higher doses/longer courses if immunosuppressed, and for severe infection	£4 (capsules)
		Oral solution[a] 10mg/mL; 100mg (10mL) b.d. or 200mg (20mL) once daily for 2 weeks; use as a mouthwash and swallow	Authorized only for immunosuppressed patients (see text); for fluconazole-resistant infection can increase to 200mg (20mL) b.d. (see SPC)	£116 (oral solution)

a. because of the difference in bio-availability, the oral solution is *not* interchangeable with the capsules on a mg for mg basis (see Management strategy: Drug treatment above).

6

Strong CYP3A4 inducers, e.g. **carbamazepine**, **phenytoin**, **phenobarbital**, **rifampicin**, **rifabutin** and possibly *Hypericum perforatum* (St. John's wort), reduce **fluconazole** and **itraconazole** plasma concentrations, which may result in antifungal treatment failure.

The absorption of **itraconazole** (but not **fluconazole**) is affected by antacids, **sucralfate**, H_2-receptor antagonists, PPIs or food (see above).

Undesirable effects

Common (<10%, >1%): headache (azole antifungals), dizziness (**fluconazole** and **itraconazole**), GI symptoms, i.e. dyspepsia, nausea and vomiting, abdominal pain, diarrhoea (**fluconazole** and **itraconazole**), rashes, pruritus, hypokalaemia (**fluconazole** and **itraconazole**).

Uncommon, rare or very rare (<1%): anaphylaxis, hepatitis, cholestasis, hepatic failure, adrenal suppression (**itraconazole**), reduced libido, gynaecomastia, impotence, menstrual disturbances.

Dose, use and supply

See Table 1. With topical treatment, dentures should be removed temporarily before each dose is given. With topical treatment and **itraconazole** *oral solution*, food and drink should be avoided for 1h after each dose. Note:

- because **chlorhexidine** binds to **nystatin** and leads to inactivation of both drugs, **chlorhexidine** mouthwash should *not* be used at the same time as **nystatin** oral suspension.[16] The problem can be avoided if **chlorhexidine** is used ≥30min before **nystatin**
- the absorption of **itraconazole** capsules is improved if taken with an acidic drink, e.g. cola.

1 Finlay I and Davies A (2005) Fungal Infections. In: A Davies and I Finlay (eds) *Oral Care in Advanced Disease*. Oxford University Press, Oxford, pp. 55–71.

2 Davies AN *et al.* (2006) Oral candidosis in patients with advanced cancer. *Oral Oncology*. **42**: 698–702.

3 Davies AN *et al.* (2008) Oral candidosis in community-based patients with advanced cancer. *Journal of Pain and Symptom Management*. **35**: 508–514.

4 Samonis G *et al.* (1998) Oropharyngeal candidiasis as a marker for esophageal candidiasis in patients with cancer. *Clinical Infectious Diseases*. **27**: 283–286.

5 Samaranayake L (1990) Host factors and oral candidosis. In: L Samaranayake and T MacFarlane (eds) *Oral Candidosis*. Wright, London, pp. 66–103.

6 Bagg J *et al.* (2003) High prevalence of non-albicans yeasts and detection of anti-fungal resistance in the oral flora of patients with advanced cancer. *Palliative Medicine*. **17**: 477–481.

7 Sweeney P and Davies A (2010) Oral hygiene. In: A Davies and J Epstein (eds) *Oral Complications of Cancer and its Management*. Oxford University Press, Oxford, pp. 43–51.

8 Worthington HV *et al.* (2010) Interventions for treating oral candidiasis for patients with cancer receiving treatment. *Cochrane Database of Systematic Reviews*. **7**: CD001972. www.thecochranelibrary.com

9 Pappas PG *et al.* (2009) Clinical practice guidelines for the management of candidiasis: 2009 update by the Infectious Diseases Society of America. *Clinical Infectious Diseases*. **48**: 503–535.

10 Davies A *et al.* (2006) Antifungal drug resistance amongst yeasts isolated from patients with advanced cancer. *Supportive Care in Cancer*. **14**: 645.

11 Nyst MJ *et al.* (1992) Gentian violet, ketoconazole and nystatin in oropharyngeal and esophageal candidiasis in Zairian AIDS patients. *Annales de la Societe Belge de Medecine Tropicale*. **72**: 45–52.

12 Vazquez J (1999) Options for the management of mucosal candidiasis in patients with AIDS and HIV infection. *Pharmacotherapy*. **19**: 76–87.

13 MHRA (2012) All medical devices and medicinal products containing chlorhexidine. Risk of anaphylactic reaction due to chlorhexidine allery. *Medical Devices Alert*. MDA/2012/2075 www.gov.uk/drug-device-alerts

14 Baxter K and Preston CL. *Stockley's Drug Interactions*. London: Pharmaceutical Press www.medicinescomplete.com (accessed April 2017).

15 MHRA (2016) Topical miconazole, including oral gel: reminder of potential for serious interactions with warfarin. *drug Safety Update*. www.gov.uk/drug-safety-update

16 Barkvoll P and Attramadal A (1989) Effect of nystatin and chlorhexidine digluconate on Candida albicans. *Oral Surgery Oral Medicine and Oral Pathology*. **67**: 279–281.

17 Samaranayake K and Sitheeque M (2010) Oral fungal infections. In: A Davies and J Epstein (eds) *Oral Complications of Cancer and its Management*. Oxford University Press, Oxford, pp. 171–183.

Updated July 2017

METRONIDAZOLE

Class: Antibacterial and antiprotozoal.

Indications: Anaerobic and protozoal infections, *Helicobacter pylori* eradication, malodour caused by fungating cancers (topical gel), †pseudomembranous colitis (see *Clostridium difficile* infection, p.496) bacterial vaginosis.

Pharmacology

Metronidazole is highly active against anaerobic bacteria and protozoa. Although it has no activity against aerobic organisms *in vitro*, in mixed infections *in vivo* both aerobes and anaerobes appear susceptible. Unlike most other antibacterials, resistance to metronidazole among anaerobes is uncommon.

Metronidazole, either systemically (PO or IV) or topically, is used to reduce malodour from fungating cancers and decubitus ulcers.[1] The malodour is caused by dimethyl trisulfide and volatile fatty acids produced by bacteria colonizing moist necrotic tissue.[2]

Metronidazole is metabolized in the liver; the main hydroxy metabolite has antibacterial activity. Accumulation may occur in severe hepatic impairment, and can exacerbate hepatic encephalopathy (see Chapter 18, p.703). In renal failure, there is no accumulation of metronidazole and no dose adjustment is necessary. The hydroxy metabolite does accumulate; this is of uncertain clinical significance.

6

Tinidazole is similar to metronidazole with a longer duration of action (is given either b.d. or once daily).[3] It causes less GI disturbance than metronidazole.

Bio-availability 80–100% PO; 60–80% PR; 60% gel PV, 25% pessary PV.
Onset of action 20–60min PO; 5–12h PR.
Time to peak plasma concentration 1–2h PO; 3h PR.
Plasma halflife 6–11h.
Duration of action 8–12h.

Cautions

Hepatic impairment (see Dose and use). Monitoring of FBC and LFTs advised with systemic use >10 days (see Undesirable effects). Concurrent use of alcohol (see Drug interactions). May exacerbate existing neurological disease. Photosensitivity (topical gel).

Drug interactions

Metronidazole may impair the metabolism or excretion of several drugs, e.g. **ciclosporin**, **fluorouracil**, **lithium**, **phenytoin**, **warfarin** and coumarins thus potentially increasing their toxicity. On the other hand, plasma concentrations of metronidazole are decreased by **phenobarbital** and **phenytoin**; consider a 2–3 fold increase in dose of metronidazole if not achieving the desired clinical effect.[4]

Metronidazole has been linked to **disulfiram**-like reaction with alcohol.[5] Like **disulfiram**, metabolites of metronidazole can inhibit alcohol dehydrogenase, xanthine oxidase and aldehyde dehydrogenase. This could lead to acidosis, noradrenaline (norepinephrine) excess, and accumulation of acetaldehyde,[6] the latter being responsible for symptoms such as flushing, headaches, epigastric discomfort, nausea and vomiting. However, there is *no* hard evidence of a clinically important reaction between alcohol and metronidazole, rather the reverse.[4,5]

Even so, because of warnings in the PIL and SPC, patients should be advised that they may experience mild anorexia, and sometimes vomiting, if they drink alcohol when taking metronidazole. Any risk with topical or PV metronidazole is presumably lower because of smaller doses and lower systemic absorption.[7] In the USA (but not the UK), patients are advised to avoid liquid medicines containing alcohol during metronidazole treatment.

Undesirable effects

Very common (>10%): abdominal pain, nausea and vomiting, diarrhoea.
Common (<10%, >1%): skin irritation (topical use).
Very rare (<0.01%): epilepsy, encephalopathy, aseptic meningitis, optic and peripheral neuropathy (sometimes irreversible), blood dyscrasias (neutropenia, thrombocytopenia, pancytopenia), cholestatic hepatitis, pancreatitis (generally reversible on discontinuation), darkening of urine (due to metabolite).

Dose and use

Limit dose to a maximum of 400mg PO b.d. in elderly debilitated patients and 400mg PO once daily if significant hepatic impairment, i.e. patients with incipient or actual hepatic encephalopathy.

Anaerobic infections

- metronidazole 400mg PO t.d.s. for 7 days; administration with food may reduce the risk of nausea and vomiting.

Oral suspensions are available for those with swallowing difficulties, but are significantly more expensive and best taken on an empty stomach (also see Chapter 28, Table 2, p.793).

If PO is not possible, metronidazole can be given IV or PR. Standard practice is 500mg IV q8h for 7 days or 1g PR t.d.s for 3 days, then 1g b.d. for a further 4 days.

Clostridium difficile infection (see p.496)

Malodour caused by a fungating cancer

Topical

High quality evidence of topical use is limited,[8,9] but most patients are said to benefit.[10,11] About half report complete resolution of the odour. Improvement generally occurs within 2 days but can take up to one month.[9]

Topical application to a fungating cancer can be considered when:

- the cancer is relatively small (and thus easily accessible for topical application)
- the cancer is very sloughy and poorly vascularized (which will reduce systemic access by metronidazole)
- systemic therapy is impractical, e.g. because of dysphagia
- systemic therapy causes unacceptable effects.

The metronidazole is applied as a 0.75% gel:[1,12]

- after cleansing the wound, apply the gel liberally, about 1g/cm^2
- pack large cavities with paraffin gauze smeared in the gel
- cover with a non-adherent and then an absorbent dressing
- repeat once daily–b.d. as long as beneficial.

Traditionally, some centres have used a crushed 200mg tablet in lubricating gel (off-label, but cheaper, see Supply).

Systemic

Supporting data for topical use relate mostly to patients in richer countries. The situation in poorer countries is generally different, with typically late referrals and deeper inaccessible infection. In these circumstances, PO treatment is better. After the initial treatment, a maintenance dose of metronidazole is continued indefinitely (Box A).[13]

Box A Metronidazole for malodourous fungating cancer[13]

Odour classification

SNIFFF: Smell *Nil* (absent), *Faint* (not offensive), *Foul* (offensive but tolerable) or *Forbidding* (offensive and intolerable).

Malodour regimen

Regardless of severity, start with metronidazole 400mg PO t.d.s.

Review after 1 week and continue treatment based on *SNIFFF* test:

- *Nil or Faint*: 200mg once daily indefinitely
- *Foul*: continue 400mg t.d.s. for 1 more week; then 200mg once daily indefinitely
- *Forbidding*: continue 400mg t.d.s. for 2 more weeks; then 200mg once daily indefinitely.

If there is concern that the patient may not attend for review, information about continuing treatment is given at the initial appointment.

General care

Teach low-cost home-based wound care, and environmental hygiene.

Supply

Metronidazole (generic)

Tablets 200mg, 400mg, 7 days @ 400mg t.d.s. = £8.

Tablets 500mg, 7 days @ 500mg t.d.s. = £38.

Oral suspension (as benzoate) 200mg/5mL, 7 days @ 400mg t.d.s. = £69.

IV infusion 5mg/mL, 100mL = £3.

Flagyl® (Winthrop)
Tablets 200mg, 400mg, 7 days @ 400mg t.d.s. = £9.50.
Suppositories 500mg, 1g, 3 days @ 1g t.d.s. and 4 days @ 1g b.d. = £40.

Topical products
Anabact® (CHS)
Gel 0.75%, 15g = £4.50, 30g = £8.

Metrogel® (Galderma)
Gel 0.75%, 40g = £23.

Other topical metronidazole creams and gels are available; they are authorized for exacerbation of rosacea and are generally more expensive.
Crushed tablets in lubricating gel cost about £0.70 per topical application compared with £4.50 for proprietary gel.

Metronidazole (generic)
Vaginal gel 0.75%, 40g pack with 5 applicators = £4.50. *One applicator delivers a 5g dose of metronidazole 0.75%.*

Tinidazole
Fasigyn® (Pfizer)
Tablets 500mg, 2g stat and then 1g daily for 6 days = £11.

1 Finlay IG *et al.* (1996) The effect of topical 0.75% metronidazole gel on malodorous cutaneous ulcers. *Journal of Pain and Symptom Management.* **11**: 158–162.
2 Shirasu M *et al.* (2009) Dimethyl trisulfide as a characteristic odor associated with fungating cancer wounds. *Bioscience, Biotechnology and Biochemistry.* **73**: 2117–2120.
3 Carmine AA *et al.* (1982) Tinidazole in anaerobic infections: a review of its antibacterial activity, pharmacological properties and therapeutic efficacy. *Drugs.* **24**: 85–117.
4 Baxter K and Preston CL. *Stockley's Drug Interactions.* London: Pharmaceutical Press www.medicinescomplete.com (accessed May 2017).
5 Williams CS and Woodcock KR (2000) Do ethanol and metronidazole interact to produce a disulfiram-like reaction? *Annals of Pharmacotherapy.* **34**: 255–257.
6 Harries D *et al.* (1990) Metronidazole and alcohol: potential problems. *Scottish Medical Journal.* **35**: 179–180.
7 Plosker G (1987) Possible interaction between ethanol and vaginally administered metronidazole. *Clinical Pharmacy.* **6**: 189–193.
8 Adderley U and Holt IG (2014) Topical agents and dressings for fungating wounds. *Cochrane Database of Systematic Reviews.* CD003948. www.thecochranelibrary.com
9 Kalinski C *et al.* (2005) Effectiveness of a topical formulation containing metronidazole for wound odor and exudate control. *Wounds.* **17**: 84–90.
10 da Costa Santos CM *et al.* (2010) A systematic review of topical treatments to control the odor of malignant fungating wounds. *Journal of Pain and Symptom Management.* **39**: 1065–1076.
11 Gethin G *et al.* (2014) Current practice in the management of wound odour: an international survey. *International Journal of Nursing Studies.* **51**: 865–874.
12 Thomas S and Hay N (1991) The antimicrobial properties of two metronidazole medicated dressings used to treat malodorous wounds. *Pharmaceutical Journal.* **246**: 264–266.
13 George R *et al.* (2017) Improving malodour management in advanced cancer: a 10-year retrospective study of topical, oral and maintenance metronidazole. *BMJ Supportive and Palliative Care.* **7**: 286–291.

Updated August 2017

RIFAMPICIN

Class: Rifamycin antibacterial.

Indications: Infection (notably tuberculosis and leprosy; meningococcal prophylaxis), †cholestatic pruritus.[1–3]

Pharmacology

The bactericidal activity of rifampicin is due to inhibition of bacterial RNA polymerase. Rifampicin is also a pregnane X receptor (PXR) agonist, one of several receptors involved in upregulating enzymes and transporters required for the removal of xenobiotics, e.g. drugs, and endogenous metabolites, e.g. bile acids.[4,5]

Pooled RCT data (n=61) support the efficacy of rifampicin in cholestatic pruritus with an NNT of 1.75.[6] Participants had various non-cancer causes of cholestasis, mostly (80%) primary biliary cirrhosis (PBC). The RCTs were short-term (≤2 weeks), but longer-term benefit (≤2 years) has been reported.[7]

It has been suggested that the benefit of rifampicin in cholestatic pruritus is via an effect on bile acid metabolism. However, plasma concentrations of bile acids do not correlate with the severity of pruritus, nor with the response to antipruritic treatments.[8,9] Further, other drugs with similar enzyme and transporter-inducing properties, e.g. **phenobarbital**, have little or no antipruritic effect.[5,10]

However, activation of the PXR receptor by rifampicin also inhibits the synthesis of the enzyme autotaxin, the plasma concentration of which correlates with the antipruritic effect of rifampicin. Autotaxin catalyzes the conversion of cell membrane phospholipids into the lipid signalling molecule lysophosphatidic acid (LPA), the plasma concentration of which also correlates with the severity of pruritus and falls when there is benefit from rifampicin, bile acid sequestrants or biliary drainage.[11]

How LPA causes pruritus in cholestasis is uncertain, but may include immune and/or neuromodulation; LPA is known to affect histamine release from mast cells, eosinophil and lymphocyte trafficking, and neuronal synaptic plasticity.[12–14] However, because levels of LPA can be increased in diseases which are not associated with pruritus, additional cofactors may be involved.[15]

The absorption of rifampicin is halved by food. Metabolites also have antibacterial effects and are excreted in bile (70%). Up to 30% of a dose is excreted in the urine, about half as unchanged drug. Halflife doubles in cirrhosis, and acute or chronic hepatitis.[16,17]

Bio-availability ≥95%.[17]
Onset of action ≥2 days (for pruritus).[18]
Peak plasma concentration 2–4h.
Plasma halflife 3–5h initially; 2–3h after repeat dosing (due to auto-induction).
Duration of action no data for pruritus.

Cautions

Jaundice is listed as a contra-indication by the UK manufacturer and a warning by the US manufacturer, but rifampicin was well tolerated in eight patients with jaundice and pruritus associated with hepatic metastases.[18] The risk of hepatotoxicity is increased with pre-existing hepatic impairment; monitor carefully when used for cholestatic pruritus.

Drug interactions

Concurrent use with **isoniazid** and some antiretrovirals increases the risk of serious hepatotoxicity; concurrent use of **saquinavir/ritonavir** is contra-indicated.

Concurrent use of **atazanavir**, **darunavir**, **fosamprenavir**, **saquinavir** and **tipranavir** is contra-indicated, due to substantially decreased plasma concentrations which may lead to loss of antiviral efficacy and/or development of viral resistance.

Rifampicin induces various enzymes involved in drug metabolism, including oxidation (a potent inducer of CYP2B6, CYP2C19, and CYP3A4), glucuronidation (UGT1A1) and glutathione conjugation (GSTA1). Thus, caution is required with concurrent use of drugs which are metabolised by these enzymes, as rifampicin may reduce their effect. Reports of interactions where close monitoring ± dose adjustment are required are listed in Table 1. Onset and offset of enzyme induction is gradual (see Chapter 19, p.721) thus, clinical effects may not become fully evident for 2–3 weeks after rifampicin is started or discontinued.

Conversely, some drugs may reduce the effect of rifampicin:

- antacids (reduced absorption); generally avoided by separating the administration time by ≥2h
- **phenobarbital** (may increase clearance).

Undesirable effects

Nausea and anorexia (3% of patients with cholestatic pruritus[6]), diarrhoea (check for *Clostridium difficile* toxin; pseudomembranous colitis reported), orange discolouration of sweat, saliva, urine,

Table 1 Clinically important cytochrome P450 interactions with rifampicin[a,19]

Drug effect ↓ by rifampicin	*Specific drugs within a class*
Anticoagulants	Dabigatran[b], rivaroxaban[b], warfarin (and other coumarins)[c]
Antidiabetics	Canagliflozin, glibenclamide, gliclazide, repaglinide, linagliptin, pioglitazone, rosiglitazone (not UK), tolbutamide
Antipsychotics	Aripiprazole, haloperidol, lurasidone[b], risperidone
Aprepitant	
Azole antifungals	Fluconazole[d], itraconazole[b], ketoconazole[b], voriconazole[b]
Benzodiazepines	Diazepam, lorazepam, (IV only), midazolam[e], nitrazepam, triazolam[b] (not UK)
Bronchodilators	Aminophylline, theophylline
Calcium channel blockers	Diltiazem, nifedipine (PO only, not IV), verapamil
Cannabinoids	Cannabis extract (Sativex®)
Corticosteroids	Dexamethasone, prednisolone
Digoxin	
Doxycycline	
Fesoterodine[b]	
Fexofenadine	
Hormonal contraceptives[b]	All, including emergency hormonal contraceptives
Lamotrigine	
Macrolides	Clarithromycin, telithromycin[b]
NSAIDs	Celecoxib, diclofenac, etoricoxib
Opioids	Alfentanil, codeine, fentanyl (all routes), methadone, morphine, oxycodone
Phenytoin	
Ramelteon (not UK)	
Statins[f]	All
Terbinafine	
Tolvaptan	
Z-drug hypnotics	Zaleplon, zolpidem, zopiclone

a. *not* an exhaustive list; limited to drugs most likely to be encountered in palliative care and *excludes* anticancer, antiviral, HIV and immunosuppressive drugs (seek specialist advice)
b. likely to be ineffective PO (and IV, where available); avoid concurrent use
c. onset within one week of starting rifampicin and persists for about ≤5 weeks after its withdrawal
d. generally with IV but not PO fluconazole; however, reports of therapeutic failure with PO fluconazole in patients with severe fungal infection
e. likely to be ineffective PO, avoid concurrent use; up to 60% reduction in the area under the plasma concentration-time curve for IV
f. effect may increase or decrease depending on timing of administration and duration of concurrent use.

faeces and tears (may stain contact lenses), flushing or rash (generally mild and transient, discontinue if purpuric or urticaric).

Adrenal insufficiency (increased catabolism of adrenal steroids).

Hepatotoxicity occurs in ~10% of patients with PBC, 1–14 months after starting rifampicin.[7,20]

Hypersensitivity reactions (flu-like symptoms, urticarial, thrombocytopenia, haemolysis, renal failure) are more common with intermittent therapy used for some infections, but occurred in <2% of patients using rifampicin continuously for cholestatic pruritus.[6] Generally resolve if rifampicin is stopped.

Dose and use

Monitoring

Check LFTs, U+E and FBC before starting treatment and if symptoms suggestive of hepatotoxicity occur (e.g. nausea, vomiting, abdominal pain, worsening LFTs, pruritus). Repeat at intervals; there is no consensus as to frequency.[1,2,21]

With tuberculosis, it is recommended that rifampicin is stopped if ALT increases three times the upper limit of normal (when jaundice and/or symptoms of hepatitis present) or five times (when asymptomatic).[21] In cancer patients with complete biliary obstruction, worsening LFTs are inevitable, and rifampicin-induced hepatotoxicity cannot be diagnosed with certainty.

Cholestatic pruritus

Although experience with **sertraline** is limited, its tolerability, familiarity and limited interactions compared with rifampicin generally means that it is tried first (see Chapter 26, Table 1, p.761).

- start with rifampicin 150mg PO at bedtime
- if necessary, increase to 150mg twice daily after 1 week (sooner if pruritus is severe and prognosis short)
- some patients need 600mg/24h.

Although generally advised to take rifampicin on an empty stomach to optimise absorption, when used for pruritus, strict adherence to this is probably unnecessary.

When PO administration is not possible, the same dose of rifampicin may be given by intravenous infusion (see Supply for further details).

Supply

Rifampicin (generic)
Capsules 150mg, 300mg, 28 days @ 150mg b.d. = £8.50.

Rimactane (Sandoz)
Capsules 150mg, 300mg, 28 days @ 150mg b.d. = £15.

Rifadin (Sanofi-Aventis)
Capsules 150mg, 300mg, 28 days @ 150mg b.d. = £10.
Oral syrup 100mg/5mL, 28 days @ 150mg b.d. = £15.
Intravenous infusion (powder for reconstitution) 600mg vial, supplied with 10mL solvent = £9.
Reconstitute with solvent provided; the displacement value of the powder may be significant, e.g. 0.48mL consult local reconstitution guidelines. Further dilute the required dose with glucose 5% or sodium chloride 0.9% to a final concentration of 1.2mg/mL and infuse over 2–3h.

1 EASL (2009) Clinical Practice Guidelines: management of cholestatic liver diseases. *Journal of Hepatology*. **51**: 237–267.
2 Lindor KD (2009) AASLD Practice Guidelines: Primary biliary cirrhosis. *Hepatology*. **50**: 291–308.
3 Hegade VS *et al.* (2015) Drug treatment of pruritus in liver diseases. *Clinical Medicine*. **4**: 351–357.
4 Tolson AH and Wang H (2010) Regulation of drug-metabolizing enzymes by xenobiotic receptors: PXR and CAR. *Advanced Drug Delivery Reviews*. **62**: 1238–1249.
5 Halilbasic E *et al.* (2013) Bile acid transporters and regulatory nuclear receptors in the liver and beyond. *Journal of Hepatology*. **58**: 155–168.
6 Khurana S and Singh P (2006) Rifampin is safe for treatment of pruritus due to chronic cholestasis: a meta-analysis of prospective randomized-controlled trials. *Liver International*. **26**: 943–948.
7 Bachs L *et al.* (1992) Effects of long-term rifampicin administration in primary biliary cirrhosis. *Gastroenterology*. **102**: 2077–2080.
8 Kremer AE *et al.* (2012) Serum autotaxin is increased in pruritus of cholestasis, but not of other origin, and responds to therapeutic interventions. *Hepatology*. **56**: 1391–1400.
9 Kuiper EM *et al.* (2010) The potent bile acid sequestrant colesevelam is not effective in cholestatic pruritus: results of a double-blind, randomized, placebo-controlled trial. *Hepatology*. **52**: 1334–1340.
10 Bachs L *et al.* (1989) Comparison of rifampicin with phenobarbitone for treatment of pruritus in biliary cirrhosis. *Lancet*. **1**: 574–576.
11 Kremer AE *et al.* (2014) Advances in pathogenesis and management of pruritus in cholestasis. *Digestive Diseases*. **32**: 637–645.
12 Garcia-Morales V *et al.* (2015) Membrane-derived phospholipids control synaptic neurotransmission and plasticity. *PLoS Biol.* **13**: e1002153.
13 Yung YC *et al.* (2014) LPA receptor signaling: pharmacology, physiology, and pathophysiology. *Journal of Lipid Research*. **55**: 1192–1214.
14 Knowlden S and Georas SN (2014) The autotaxin-LPA axis emerges as a novel regulator of lymphocyte homing and inflammation. *Journal of Immunology*. **192**: 851–857.
15 Jones DE (2012) Pathogenesis of cholestatic itch: old questions, new answers, and future opportunities. *Hepatology*. **56**: 1194–1196.

16 Acocella G (1978) Clinical pharmacokinetics of rifampicin. *Clinical Pharmacokinetics*. **3**: 108–127.
17 Riess W (1969) Pharmacokinetic studies in the field of rifamycins. Proceedings of the 6th International Congress of Chemotherapy. *University of Tokyo Press*. **2**: 905–913.
18 Price TJ *et al.* (1998) Rifampicin as treatment for pruritus in malignant cholestasis. *Supportive Care in Cancer*. **6**: 533–535.
19 Baxter K and Preston CL. *Stockley's Drug Interactions*. London: Pharmaceutical Press www.medicinescomplete.com (accessed March 2015).
20 Prince MI *et al.* (2002) Hepatitis and liver dysfunction with rifampicin therapy for pruritus in primary biliary cirrhosis. *Gut*. **50**: 436–439.
21 ATS (2006) An Official ATS Statement: Hepatotoxicity of antituberculosis therapy. *American Journal of Respiratory and Critical Care Medicine*. **174**.

Added November 2015

6

URINARY TRACT INFECTIONS

Infections with strains of *Escherichia coli* and other Gram-negative bacilli which are resistant to several antibacterials, i.e. ESBL (Extended Spectrum Beta-Lactamase) positive enterobacteria, are increasing. Some are resistant to **gentamicin**, quinolones and cephalosporins as well as other antibacterials.[1]

This possibility should be considered in patients with recurrent urinary infection. Appropriate specimens (including blood cultures) should be taken and any previous microbiology reviewed.

If a multiresistant isolate has been identified previously, e.g. a **gentamicin**-resistant coliform in urine, treatment should be discussed with a medical microbiologist because the usual first-line treatment may not be appropriate.

Cystitis is the commonest form of urinary tract infection (UTI) in terminally ill patients and, as in general medicine, is often caused by *E. coli*.[2,3] UTIs are more common in women and, in the community, 60% of women with suggestive symptoms have a UTI confirmed by microscopy and culture.[4]

UTIs are generally classified as 'uncomplicated' if they occur in otherwise healthy, premenopausal women with normal urinary tracts. 'Complicated' UTIs occur in men, children, pregnant women, women with abnormal urinary tracts and the elderly particularly if they have co-morbidities, e.g. dementia, that make diagnosis challenging. Complicated UTIs are caused by a broader range of bacteria that are more likely to be resistant to antibacterials.[5]

Pyelonephritis should be suspected if the patient has a fever >38°C, loin pain and/or costovertebral angle tenderness, whether or not there are associated symptoms of cystitis. Pyelonephritis *without* evidence of urosepsis (i.e. septicaemia secondary to UTI) in a woman with a normal urinary tract may be classed as 'uncomplicated'. Pyelonephritis occurring in any other patient group or with evidence of urosepsis is classed as 'complicated'.[6]

Diagnosis

Uncomplicated UTI

If a woman has typical or severe symptoms and signs of a UTI, without vaginal irritation or discharge suggestive of an alternative diagnosis, prompt empirical antibacterial treatment is indicated; *dipstick testing (see below) and urine culture are irrelevant.*

In the community in non-catheterized women, three symptoms independently predict UTI: cloudy urine, dysuria and recent-onset nocturia:

- presence of all three symptoms has a positive predictive value of 82%
- absence of all three symptoms had a negative predictive value of 67%.[4,7]

Thus, using a symptom score alone will lead to a missed diagnosis in about one third of UTIs.

With dipsticks, nitrites are most predictive, followed by leucocytes (leucocyte esterase+ or greater) and blood (haemolysed trace or greater). For dipstick tests in combination:

- nitrite+ and *either* blood+ *or* leucocyte esterase+; positive predictive value 92%
- nitrite+ or leucocyte esterase and blood *both*+; positive predictive value about 80%
- nitrite, leucocyte esterase and blood *all* –; negative predictive value 76% (Box A).[4,7]

Thus, the use of a dipstick alone will lead to a missed diagnosis in about one quarter of UTIs.

Box A Urine dipsticks and the diagnosis of UTIs in non-catheterized women with few or mild symptoms

Use a urine dipstick which measures urinary pH and specific gravity, and the presence and amount of:

- glucose
- ketone
- blood
- protein
- nitrite, a bacterial metabolite
- leucocyte esterase (produced by inflammation/infection).

When to do the test

- if patient has few or mild symptoms of UTI
- if typical or severe symptoms of UTI, prescribe an antibacterial in accord with local policy without using a dipstick.

How to do the test

- clean external genitalia with sterile 0.9% sodium chloride
- take a mid-stream specimen of urine (or in-and-out catheter sample under aseptic conditions)
- dip the whole strip into the urine container and remove immediately
- drag the edge of the strip against the container rim to remove excess urine and start timing
- compare each test pad on the strip to the corresponding row of colour blocks on the bottle label
- read each test pad at the time shown on the bottle, starting with the shortest time first.

Late readings are of no value.

Significance of the results

Nitrite positive or leucocyte and blood positive or all three positive: make a working diagnosis of UTI; prescribe an antibacterial in accord with local policy. Urine specimen for culture *not* required unless risk factors present, e.g. recent hospital admission, recurrent UTIs.

Nitrite, leucocyte and blood all negative: tentatively exclude UTI; do *not* send urine specimen for culture unless definite urinary tract symptoms.

A negative culture may suggest an alternative diagnosis, e.g. urethritis caused by sexually transmitted infections (STIs, e.g. *Chlamydia, Neisseria, Trichomonas*) or interstitial cystitis. Although the traditional criterion for a positive urine culture is 10^5 colony-forming units (cfu)/mL, some studies have demonstrated that this is insensitive in 30–50% of women who have lower UTI confirmed by bladder aspirate but have only 10^2–10^4 cfu/mL in voided urine. Thus, in a woman with symptoms of uncomplicated UTI, a culture report of 'no growth' should be treated with caution and a colony count of $\geq 10^3$ cfu/mL is microbiologically diagnostic.[3,5,8]

Complicated UTI

To confirm the presence of bacteria and identify antibacterial sensitivity, mid-stream urine should be collected before starting antibacterial therapy in patients at risk of a complicated UTI, i.e. those associated with:

- recurrent UTI
- suspected pyelonephritis
- impaired immunity, e.g. from immunosuppressive treatment or poorly controlled diabetes mellitus
- moderate–severe renal impairment
- an abnormal urinary tract
- a recent hospital admission
- men.

In frail, elderly and hospitalized patients, diagnosis of a UTI is harder because a complicated UTI may present with atypical clinical symptoms (e.g. features of systemic infection but no localizing features such as dysuria, frequency, urgency or loin pain, or just suspected because of the onset of delirium). When there are *no* urinary symptoms and *no* signs of systemic infection, delay starting an antibacterial until the results of urine culture is available, even if urinalysis is positive.[9,10,11] *Dipsticks are less reliable in these circumstances.*

Management

Remember: always ask about drug allergies before prescribing an antibacterial.
The dose and frequency of many antibacterials are reduced in renal impairment.

Uncomplicated UTIs

If symptoms are moderate–severe, or urine dipstick test is positive (unless elderly, see above), start antibacterial treatment according to local guidelines. Alternatively, consider:

- **nitrofurantoin** 50mg PO q.d.s. or 100mg m/r PO b.d.; generally avoid when eGFR <45mL/min/1.73m^2 (unless no alternatives and eGFR >30mL/min/1.73m^2, see SPC) *or*
- **co-amoxiclav** 375mg PO t.d.s. and **amoxicillin** 250mg PO t.d.s. (or **co-amoxiclav** 625mg PO t.d.s. whichever is cheaper locally)
- **trimethoprim** 200mg PO b.d. (*now third-line because of increasing resistance*[5,12] unless history of penicillin allergy and/or renal impairment)[10]
- **ciprofloxacin** 500mg PO b.d. is sometimes recommended for uncomplicated pyelonephritis in the outpatient setting.[4,12]

Recommendations vary in relation to duration of antibacterial treatment:

- for an uncomplicated UTI in a woman, 3 days is generally sufficient[13,14]
- for complicated UTI, e.g. in diabetic patients, those who have undergone recent urinary surgery, children, men, and women with fever and/or loin pain (i.e. possible pyelonephritis), 7–14 days is recommended.

Note:

- fully sensitive bacteria respond to two 3g doses of **amoxicillin** given 12h apart[15]
- in some European countries **fosfomycin trometamol** (not UK) 3g single dose is recommended as first-line treatment for premenopausal women with uncomplicated UTI.[5,12]

Single dose treatment may be useful for frail patients. However, when compared in elderly patients, the *bacteriological* cure rate is higher in short (3–6 days) and long courses (7–14 days). On the other hand, *clinical* cure rates are similar and the acceptability of single-dose treatment is greater. The longer halflives of fluoroquinolones, **co-trimoxazole** and **fosfomycin trometamol** (not UK) may make them more efficacious for single-dose therapy, compared with the short halflives of several penicillins and cephalosporins.[16]

MRSA UTI

In confirmed MRSA UTI, treat according to local guidelines. Alternatively, consider:

- *lower UTI without systemic sepsis:* **nitrofurantoin** 50mg PO q.d.s. or 100mg m/r PO b.d. for 7 days; *generally avoid* when eGFR <45mL/min/1.73m^2 (unless no alternatives and eGFR >30mL/min/1.73m^2, see SPC)
- *if pyelonephritis or with systemic sepsis:* **vancomycin** 1–1.5g IVI q12h at a maximum rate of 10mg/min; reduce to 500mg IVI q12h in patients ≥65 years and in renal impairment (see SPC); each 500mg must be diluted in 100mL 0.9% saline or 5% glucose and given via a large peripheral vein; *plasma concentration monitoring is required.*

Systemically unwell patients

If the patient is systemically unwell, or has pyelonephritis, consider:

- IV **co-amoxiclav** 1.2g t.d.s.
- if history of penicillin allergy, give **ciprofloxacin** 500mg PO b.d. or 400mg IVI q12h over 60min via a large peripheral vein, according to local guidelines.

A single dose of IV **gentamicin** 5mg/kg should be given if there is severe sepsis or septic shock. Second-line antibacterials vary from region to region; if necessary, consult a medical microbiologist.[10]

Catheter-Associated UTI (CA-UTI)

In catheterized patients, bacterial colonization is common, occurring in up to 30% of patients catheterized for >7 days and almost universally in those catheterized for >28 days. It should not be investigated or treated unless symptomatic because generally bacteriuria does not progress to UTI.

Unfortunately, patients who develop CA-UTI are unlikely to present with fever or symptoms referable to the urinary tract. Non-specific symptoms such as rigors and new-onset delirium are more commonly associated with CA-UTI, so thorough evaluation for alternative sources of infection should also be conducted.[17]

If UTI is clinically suspected, do *not* perform a urine dipstick test because it is unreliable but send urine for culture, and then start empirical treatment with either **nitrofurantoin** or **co-amoxiclav** (as above) for 7 days.[10,18] Changing the catheter before starting antibacterials for UTI improves clinical and bacteriological cure rates,[19] and should be considered particularly if the catheter has been in place for >7 days.[4,200]

Prophylactic antibacterials for routine catheter changes are *not* recommended unless the patient has a history of UTI associated with catheter changes, is significantly immunosuppressed (e.g. neutropenic from recent chemotherapy) or experiences trauma during catheter change, i.e. frank haematuria following two or more attempts at catheterization. In such cases, single dose treatment according to local guidelines is sufficient.[4,21]

Because of the risk of increasing antibacterial resistance, continuous prophylaxis against UTI in catheterized patients is not recommended, even though there is some evidence to suggest it reduces the risk of symptomatic UTI.[22–24]

Elderly female patients may require treatment of persistent bacteriuria following catheter removal to reduce the risk of symptomatic UTI. Antibacterial treatment for 2 days before or at the time of catheter removal significantly reduces the risk of a subsequent UTI.[25–27] In patients with symptoms of a UTI after catheter removal, the cure rate for a single dose of **trimethoprim** was 79%, compared with a 10-day treatment cure rate of 81%, i.e. statistically identical.[25]

Alternative approaches

In catheterized patients, consider a urinary antiseptic to help prevent recurrent UTIs (but *not* for treatment), e.g. **methenamine hippurate** (see p.570).

For women with recurrent uncomplicated UTI, prophylaxis with PO/intravaginal probiotics containing *Lactobacillus rhamnosus GR-1* and *L. reuteri RC-14* may be considered.[5]

Although **cranberry** supplementation has generated much interest, it should no longer be encouraged as a means of preventing recurrent UTI (Box B).

Supply

Amoxicillin (generic)
Capsules 250mg, 500mg, 7 days @ 250mg t.d.s. = £1; two doses of 3g = £2.50.
Oral suspension 125mg/5mL, 250mg/5mL, 7 days @ 250mg t.d.s. = £1.50.
Oral suspension (sachet of powder to mix with water) 3g, two doses = £9.

Co-amoxiclav (generic)
Tablets 250/125 (amoxicillin 250mg, clavulanic acid 125mg), 7 days @ 375mg t.d.s. = £2.50.
Tablets 500/125 (amoxicillin 500mg, clavulanic acid 125mg), 7 days @ 625mg t.d.s. = £3.50.
Oral suspension 250/62 (amoxicillin 250mg as trihydrate, clavulanic acid 62.5mg as potassium salt)/5mL 7 days @ 10mL t.d.s = £14.
Injection (powder for reconstitution) 1000/200 (amoxicillin 1,000mg as sodium salt, clavulanic acid 200mg as potassium salt) 1.2g = £2.50.

Ciprofloxacin (generic)
Tablets 100mg, 250mg, 500mg, 750mg, 7 days @ 500mg b.d. = £1.
Infusion 2mg/mL, 400mg (200mL) bottle = £22.

Gentamicin sulfate (generic)
Injection 40mg/mL, 1mL amp and 2mL vial = £1.50, 2mL amp = £1.

Nitrofurantoin (generic)
Tablets 50mg, 100mg, 7 days @ 50mg q.d.s. = £2.
Oral suspension 25mg/5mL, 7 days @ 50mg q.d.s. = £99.

Box B Cranberry supplementation for recurrent UTI

Cranberry juice inhibits bacterial adherence to the urinary tract mucosa by disrupting the binding of bacterial macromolecules to receptors on mucosal epithelial cells.[28] This effect has been shown *in vitro* with *Escherichia coli*, and is produced by pro-anthocyanidins (PAC) present in cranberries (and blueberries).[28]

Cranberry juice does not cure established infection but its use has generated popular and scientific interest as a means of preventing UTIs.[29,30] The evidence is mixed and interpretation made difficult by the use of different formulations (with widely differing PAC content, e.g. juice or powder), doses, outcomes and patient populations.

However, almost all of the recent large RCTs have been negative, and the overwhelming evidence is for little or no effect.[31–36] Thus, the use of cranberry supplementation should *not* be encouraged as a means of preventing recurrent UTI.[37] Prophylactic antibiotics are more effective and cheaper, and should be considered with advice from a microbiologist.[38,39]

Patients who do take cranberry juice should be made aware of the potential for this to inhibit cytochrome P450 activity (see Chapter 19, p.717).[40] Regular use of cranberry juice has been linked to an increase in or fluctuation of INR values in patients taking **warfarin** (predominantly metabolized by CYP2C9).[41] This prompted the recommendation in the UK that the concurrent use of cranberry products and **warfarin** should be avoided.[42,43] If a patient taking **warfarin** consumes variable amounts of cranberry juice or other cranberry supplements, the INR should be monitored more closely.

A possible interaction between cranberry juice extracts and **tacrolimus**, resulting in sub-therapeutic levels of the latter, has also been reported.[44]

6

Macrobid® (Goldshield)
Capsules m/r 100mg, 7 days @ 100mg b.d. = £5.

Trimethoprim (generic)
Tablets 100mg, 200mg, 7 days @ 200mg b.d. = £1.
Oral suspension 50mg/5mL, 7 days @ 200mg b.d. = £6.

Vancomycin (generic)
Injection (powder for reconstitution) for IVI 500mg = £7.50, 1g = £15.

1 Nicolle LE (2011) Update in adult urinary tract infection. *Current Infectious Disease Reports.* **13**: 552–560.
2 Vitetta L *et al.* (2000) Bacterial infections in terminally ill hospice patients. *Journal of Pain and Symptom Management.* **20**: 326–334.
3 Hooton TM (2012) Clinical practice. Uncomplicated urinary tract infection. *New England Journal of Medicine.* **366**: 1028–1037.
4 NICE (2009) Urinary tract infection (lower) - women. *Clinical Knowledsge Summaries.* http://cks.nice.org.uk
5 Grabe M *et al.* (2012) Guidelines on Urological Infections. *European Association of Urology.* 1–110.
6 Johansen TE *et al.* (2011) Critical review of current definitions of urinary tract infections and proposal of an EAU/ESIU classification system. *International Journal of Antimicrobial Agents.* **38 Suppl**: 64–70.
7 Little P *et al.* (2009) Dipsticks and diagnostic algorithms in urinary tract infection: development and validation, randomised trial, economic analysis, observational cohort and qualitative study. *Health Technology Assessment.* **13**: iii–iv, ix–xi, 1–73.
8 Stamm WE *et al.* (1982) Diagnosis of coliform infection in acutely dysuric women. *New England Journal of Medicine.* **307**: 463–468.
9 Singh S *et al.* (2007) *Treatment of urinary tract infections in the older person. Medicines information leaflet.* Vol 4 No.10. Oxford Radcliffe Hospital, Oxford.
10 Oxford Hospitals Adult Inpatient Pocket Antimicrobial Guide (2011) *Urinary tract infection.*
11 NICE (2010) Urinary tract infection (lower) - men. *Clinical Knowledge Summaries.* http://cks/nice.org.uk
12 Gupta K *et al.* (2011) International clinical practice guidelines for the treatment of acute uncomplicated cystitis and pyelonephritis in women: A 2010 update by the Infectious Diseases Society of America and the European Society for Microbiology and Infectious Diseases. *Clinical Infectious Diseases.* **52**: e103–120.
13 Guay DR (2008) Contemporary management of uncomplicated urinary tract infections. *Drugs.* **68**: 1169–1205.
14 Milo G *et al.* (2005) Duration of antibacterial treatment for uncomplicated urinary tract infection in women. *Cochrane Database of Systematic Reviews.* CD004682. www.thecochranelibrary.com
15 British National Formulary Section 5.1. 13 Urinary-tract infections. London: BMJ Group and Pharmaceutical Press. www.medicinescomplete.com (accessed November 2014).
16 Lutters. M and Vogt-Ferrier. MB (2008) Antibiotic duration for treating uncomplicated, symptomatic lower urinary tract infections in elderly women. *Cochrane Database of Systematic Reviews.* **3**: CD001535. www.thecochranelibrary.com

17 Hooton TM *et al.* (2010) Diagnosis, prevention, and treatment of catheter-associated urinary tract infection in adults: 2009 International Clinical Practice Guidelines from the Infectious Diseases Society of America. *Clinical Infectious Diseases*. **50**: 625–663.
18 Schwartz DS and Barone JE (2006) Correlation of urinalysis and dipstick results with catheter-associated urinary tract infections in surgical ICU patients. *Intensive Care Medicine*. **32**: 1797–1801.
19 Raz R *et al.* (2000) Chronic indwelling catheter replacement before antimicrobial therapy for symptomatic urinary tract infection. *Journal of Urology*. **164**: 1254–1258.
20 Tenke P *et al.* (2008) European and Asian gudelines on management and prevention of catheter-associated urinary tract infections. *International Journal of Antimicrobial Agents*. **31 (Suppl 1)**: 68–78.
21 NICE (2012) Infection: prevention and control of healthcare-associated infections in primary and community care. *Clinical Guideline*. CG139. www.nice.org.uk
22 Niel-Weise BS and van den Broek PJ (2005) Antibiotic policies for short-term catheter bladder drainage in adults. *Cochrane Database of Systematic Reviews*. CD005428 (archived).
23 Rutschmann O and Zwahlen. A (1995) Use of norfloxacin for prevention of symptomatic urinary tract infection in chronically catheterized patients. *Journal of Clinical Microbiology and Infectious Diseases*. **14**: 441–444.
24 Niel-Weise BS and van den Broek PJ (2005) Urinary catheter policies for long-term bladder drainage. *Cochrane Database of Systematic Reviews*. **2**: CD004201. www.thecochranelibrary.com
25 Harding GK *et al.* (1991) How long should catheter-acquired urinary tract infection in women be treated? A randomized controlled study. *Annals of Internal Medicine*. **114**: 713–719.
26 Hustinx W *et al.* (1991) Impact of concurrent antimicrobial therapy on catheter-associated urinary tract infection. *Journal of Hospital Infection*. **18**: 45–56.
27 Pfefferkorn U *et al.* (2009) Antibiotic prophylaxis at urinary catheter removal prevents urinary tract infections: a prospective randomized trial. *Annals of Surgery*. **249**: 573–575.
28 Micali S *et al.* (2014) Cranberry and recurrent cystitis: more than marketing? *Critical Reviews in Food Science and Nutrition*. **54**: 1063–1075.
29 Natural Medicines Comprehensive Database (2008) Cranberry. www.naturaldatabase.com (accessed 2008).
30 Tong H *et al.* (2006) Effect of ingesting cranberry juice on bacterial growth in urine. *American Journal of Health-System Pharmacy*. **63**: 1417–1419.
31 Jepson RG *et al.* (2012) Cranberries for preventing urinary tract infections. *Cochrane Database of Systematic Reviews*. **10**: CD001321 www.thecochranelibrary.com
32 Caljouw MA *et al.* (2014) Effectiveness of cranberry capsules to prevent urinary tract infections in vulnerable older persons: a double-blind randomized placebo-controlled trial in long-term care facilities. *Journal of the American Geriatrics Society*. **62**: 103–110.
33 Gallien P *et al.* (2014) Cranberry versus placebo in the prevention of urinary infections in multiple sclerosis: a multicenter, randomized, placebo-controlled, double-blind trial. *Multiple Sclerosis Journal*. **20**: 1252–1259.
34 Juthani-Mehta M *et al.* (2016) Effect of cranberry capsules on bacteriuria plus pyuria among older women in nursing homes: a randomized clinical trial. *Journal of the American Medical Association*. **316**: 1879–1887.
35 Letouzey V *et al.* (2017) Cranberry capsules to prevent nosocomial urinary tract bacteriuria after pelvic surgery: a randomised controlled trial. *British Journal of Obstetrics and Gynaecology*. **124**: 912–917.
36 Wang CH *et al.* (2012) Cranberry-containing products for prevention of urinary tract infections in susceptible populations: a systematic review and meta-analysis of randomized controlled trials. *Archives of Internal Medicine*. **172**: 988–996.
37 Nicolle LE (2016) Cranberry for prevention of urinary tract infection?: time to move on. *Journal of the American Medical Association*. **316**: 1873–1874.
38 Bosmans JE *et al.* (2014) Cost-effectiveness of cranberries vs antibiotics to prevent urinary tract infections in premenopausal women: a randomized clinical trial. *PLoS One*. **9**: e91939.
39 van den Hout WB *et al.* (2014) Cost-effectiveness of cranberry capsules to prevent urinary tract infection in long-term care facilities: economic evaluation with a randomized controlled trial. *Journal of the American Geriatrics Society*. **62**: 111–116.
40 Hodek P *et al.* (2002) Flavonoids-potent and versatile biologically active compounds interacting with cytochromes P450. *Chemico-Biological Interactions*. **139**: 1–21.
41 Rettie AE *et al.* (1992) Hydroxylation of warfarin by human cDNA-expressed cytochrome P-450: a role for P-4502C9 in the etiology of (S)-warfarin-drug interactions. *Chemical Research in Toxicology*. **5**: 54–59.
42 CSM (Committee on Safety of Medicines) (2004) Interaction between warfarin and cranberry juice: new advice. *Current Problems in Pharmacovigilance*. **30**: 10.
43 MHRA (2009) Warfarin: changes to product safety information *Public assessment report*. December.
44 Dave AA and Samuel J (2016) Suspected interaction of cranberry juice extracts and tacrolimus serum levels: a case report. *Cureus*. **8**: e610.

Updated August 2017

CELLULITIS IN A LYMPHOEDEMATOUS LIMB

The following should be read in conjunction with *Consensus Document on the Management of Cellulitis in Lymphoedema* produced by the British Lymphology Society.[1]

Cellulitis, also called an acute inflammatory episode (AIE), is common in lymphoedema:
- mild: pain, increased swelling, erythema (well-defined or blotchy)
- severe: pain, increased swelling, extensive erythema with well-defined margins, blistering and weeping skin; there may be fever, nausea and vomiting and other features of septicaemia, and when the leg is affected, difficulty in walking.[2]

Management strategy

Preventive measures

Patients should be educated about:

- why they are susceptible to cellulitis, i.e. skin crevices harbour bacteria, reduced local immunity[3]
- the consequences of cellulitis, i.e. increased swelling, more fibrosis, decreased response to compression treatment
- the importance of daily skin care to improve and maintain skin integrity. Risk factors for cellulitis include cracked or macerated interdigital skin, dermatitis, limb wounds (including leg ulcers), and weeping lymphangiectasia (leaking lymph blisters on the skin surface)
- reducing risk by, for example, reducing the swelling, protecting hands when gardening, cleaning cuts, treating fungal infections (e.g. **terbinafine** 1% cream once daily for 2 weeks) and ingrowing toenails[4]
- the importance of seeking prompt medical attention and treatment if they suspect they may be developing cellulitis.

Patients who have had cellulitis in the past and who are travelling away from home should be supplied with an emergency 2-week supply of antibacterials (see QCG: Cellulitis in lymphoedema, p.495, point 14).

Non-drug treatment

- compression garments should not be worn until the limb is comfortable
- daily skin hygiene should be continued; washing and gentle drying
- emollients should not be used where the skin is broken
- *if severe, bed rest is essential* with the affected limb elevated in a comfortable position and supported on pillows.[4,5]

Drug treatment

The dose and frequency of many antibacterials are reduced in renal impairment.

Cellulitis should be treated promptly with antibacterials to prevent increased morbidity from increased swelling and accelerated fibrosis (Table 1 and QCG: Cellulitis in lymphoedema, p.494). In a lymphoedematous limb, beta-haemolytic *Streptococci* are the most common causal pathogens,[2,6,7] not *Staphylococcus aureus* as is typically the case in the absence of lymphoedema.[8] However, because it is effective against both *Streptococci* and *Staph. aureus*, **flucloxacillin** is often used as first choice PO antibacterial in lymphoedematous limbs, rather than **amoxicillin** (effective against *Streptococci* but not against *Staph. Aureus*).[1,9,10]

Folliculitis, pus formation, and crusting are indicative of *Staph. aureus* infection, and flucloxacillin should definitely be used.

The advice of a medical microbiologist should be obtained in unusual circumstances, e.g.:

- in anogenital cellulitis
- cellulitis developing shortly after an animal lick or bite
- failure to respond to the recommended antibacterials.

Remember: cellulitis is painful, and analgesics should be prescribed regularly and p.r.n. Because of a possible relationship between skin infections, NSAIDs and necrotizing fasciitis,[11] **paracetamol** and opioids are the preferred analgesics.[12]

Supply

Amoxicillin (generic)
Capsules 250mg, 500mg, 14 days @ 500mg t.d.s. = £3.25.
Oral suspension 125mg/5mL, 250mg/5mL, 14 days @ 500mg t.d.s. = £5.50.
Injection (powder for reconstitution) 250mg, 500mg, 1g vial, 2g dose = £2.25.

Clarithromycin (generic)
Tablets 250mg, 500mg, 14 days @ 500mg b.d. = £6.
Oral suspension 125mg/5mL, 250mg/5mL, 14 days @ 500mg b.d. = £25.

Table 1 Antibacterials for cellulitis: PO unless stated otherwise[a]

Situation	*First-line antibacterials*	*If allergic to penicillin*	*Second-line antibacterials*	*Comments*
Acute cellulitis (home care) or emergency back-up supply of antibacterials	Flucloxacillin 500mg q.d.s. *or* amoxicillin 500mg t.d.s.	Erythromycin[b] 500mg q.d.s. *or* clarithromycin[b] 500mg b.d.	Clindamycin 300mg q.d.s. If fails to resolve, convert to first-line IV regimen below	Continue antibacterials until the inflammation has been completely resolved for two weeks; this may take 1–2 months. Note. Residual 'staining' may persist beyond this.
Acute cellulitis + septicaemia (inpatient admission)	Flucloxacillin 2g IV q6h[c,7]	Clindamycin 600mg IV q6h[13]	Clindamycin 600mg IV q6h (if poor or no response by 48h)	Switch to PO flucloxacillin 500mg q.d.s. *or* clindamycin 300mg q.d.s. when: • no fever for 48h *and* • inflammation much resolved *and* • falling CRP. Then continue as above.
Prophylaxis if 2+ episodes of cellulitis per year	Phenoxymethylpenicillin 250mg b.d. (500mg b.d. if BMI $\geq$33)[d,14,15]	Erythromycin[b] 250mg b.d. *or* clarithromycin[b] 250mg once daily	Clindamycin 150mg once daily *or* cefalexin 125mg once daily *or* doxycycline 50mg once daily[e]	Continue for 2 years, after 1 year, halve the dose of phenoxymethylpenicillin; if an AIE develops after dose reduction/ discontinuation, treat the acute episode and then commence *life-long* prophylaxis.

a. but take note of local guidelines, particularly for IV antibacterials
b. if use contra-indicated (see SPC and QCG: Cellulitis in lymphoedema, p.494), use cefalexin (but not in patients with a history of serious penicillin allergy, i.e. anaphylaxis) or doxycycline as an alternative
c. add gentamicin 5mg/kg IV daily for 1 week if anogenital region involved, adjust dose according to renal function and gentamicin plasma concentration
d. trimethoprim 100mg at night for prophylaxis of anogenital cellulitis
e. in these circumstances, review by local specialist lymphoedema service and advice from a microbiologist are recommended. There is a need to balance the use of certain antibiotics (e.g. clindamycin, cefalexin) as prophylaxis against the risk of predisposing to *C. difficile* infection.

Clindamycin (generic)
Capsules 150mg, 14 days @ 300mg q.d.s. £16.
Injection 150mg/mL, 2mL, 4mL amp, 600mg dose = £12.

Erythromycin (generic)
Capsules (enclosing e/c granules) 250mg, 14 days @ 500mg q.d.s. = £22.
Tablets e/c 250mg, 14 days @ 500mg q.d.s. = £7.50.
Oral suspension (as ethyl succinate) 125mg/5mL, 250mg/5mL, 500mg/5mL, 14 days @ 500mg q.d.s. = £29.

Flucloxacillin (generic)
Capsules 250mg, 500mg, 14 days @ 500mg q.d.s. = £5.
Oral solution 125mg/5mL, 250mg/5mL, 14 days @ 500mg q.d.s. = £146.
Injection (powder for reconstitution) 250mg, 500mg, 1g vial, 2g dose = £10.

Gentamicin sulphate (generic)
Injection 40mg/mL, 1mL amp = £1.50, 2mL amp = £1, 2mL vial = £4.

Phenoxymethylpenicillin (generic)
Tablets 250mg, 14 days @ 250mg b.d. = £1.50.
Oral solution 125mg/5mL, 250mg/5mL, 14 days @ 250mg b.d. = £21.

1 British Lymphology Society (2015) Consensus document on the management of cellulitis in lymphoedema. Available from: www.thebls.com
2 Mortimer P (2000) Acute inflammatory episodes. In: RG Twycross *et al.* (eds) *Lymphoedema*. Radcliffe Medical Press, Oxford, pp. 130–139.
3 Mallon E *et al.* (1997) Evidence for altered cell-mediated immunity in postmastectomy lymphoedema. *British Journal of Dermatology*. **137**: 928–933.
4 Twycross R *et al.* (2000) *Lymphoedema*. Radcliffe Medical Press, Oxford.
5 Twycross R and Wilcock A (eds) (2016) *Introducting Palliative Care* (5e). palliativedrugs.com Ltd, Nottingham.
6 Cox NH (2008) Streptococcal cellulitis/erysipelas of the lower leg. In: William H et al (ed) *Evidence-Based Dermatology 2nd edition*. Blackwell Publishing, Oxford, pp. 406–417.
7 Leman P and Mukherjee D (2005) Flucloxacillin alone or combined with benzylpenicillin to treat lower limb cellulitis: a randomised controlled trial. *Emergency Medical Journal*. **22**: 342–346.
8 Chira S and Miller LG (2010) Staphylococcus aureus is the most common identified cause of cellulitis: a systematic review. *Epidemiology Infection*. **138**: 313–317.
9 British Lymphology Society (2010) Consensus document on the management of cellulitis in lymphoedema: flucloxacillin versus amoxicillin. Available from: www.thebls.com
10 CREST (2005) Guidelines on the management of cellulitis in adults. Available from: http://www.gain-ni.org/images/Uploads/Guidelines/cellulitis-guide.pdf
11 Sultan HY *et al.* (2012) Necrotising fasciitis. *British Medical Journal* **345**: e4274.
12 Anonymous (2007) Necrotising fasciitis, dermal infections and NSAIDs: caution. *Prescrire International*. **16**: 17.
13 Bisno AL and Stevens DL (1996) Streptococcal infections of skin and soft tissues. *New England Journal of Medicine*. **334**: 240–245.
14 Team UKDCTNs PT *et al.* (2012) Prophylastic antibiotics for the prevention of cellulitis (erysipelas) of the leg: results of the UK Dermatology Clinical Trials Network's PATCH II trial. *British Journal of Dermatology*. **166**: 169–178.
15 Thomas KS *et al.* (2013) Dermatology Clinical Trials Network's PATCH I Trial Team. Penicillin to prevent recurrent leg cellulitis. *New England Journal of Medicine*. **368**: 1695–1703.

Updated January 2016

Quick Clinical Guide: Cellulitis in lymphoedema

Cellulitis is often associated with septicaemia (e.g. fever, flu-like symptoms, hypotension, tachycardia, delirium, nausea and vomiting). It may be difficult to identify the pathogen but, in lymphoedema, *group A Streptococcus* is the most common.

Evaluation

1 Clinical features
- mild: pain, increased swelling, erythema (well-defined or blotchy)
- severe: pain, increased swelling, extensive erythema with well-defined margins, blistering and weeping skin; there may be features of septicaemia, and when the leg is affected, difficulty in walking.

2 Diagnosis is based on pattern recognition and clinical judgement. Elicit:
- present history: date of onset, precipitating factor (e.g. insect bite or trauma), treatment received to date
- past history: details of past cellulitis, precipitating factors, antibacterials taken
- examination: include sites of lymphatic drainage to and from inflamed area.

3 Establish a baseline
- extent and severity of rash: if well demarcated outline with pen and date
- level of systemic upset: temperature, pulse, BP, CRP, WBC
- swab cuts or breaks in skin for microbiology before starting antibacterials.

4 Arrange admission to hospital for patients:
- with septicaemia (e.g. low BP, tachycardia, high temperature, vomiting)
- failing to respond to antibacterials (see ladder below).

Antibacterials

5 To prevent increased swelling and accelerated fibrosis, cellulitis should be treated promptly with antibacterials. Continue antibacterials until the inflammation has been completely resolved for 2 weeks; this may take 1–2 months.

6 The advice of a microbiologist should be obtained in unusual circumstances, e.g. cellulitis developing shortly after an animal bite, and when the inflammation fails to respond to the recommended antibacterials.

7 Standard treatment at home (PO)

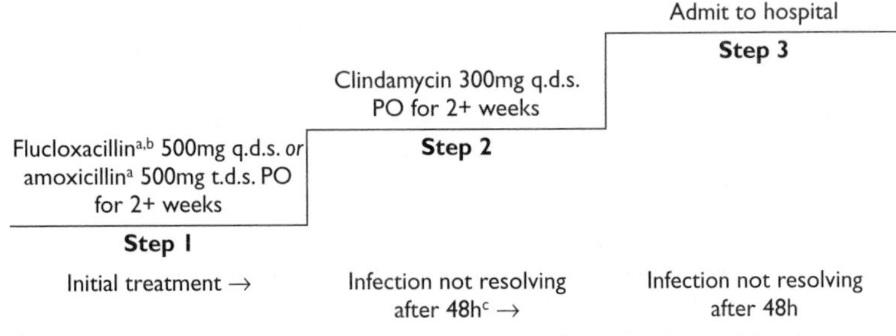

a. if a history of penicillin allergy, erythromycin 500mg q.d.s. or clarithromycin 500mg b.d. (but also see point 11 below)

b. if features suggest *Staph. aureus* infection (e.g. folliculitis, pus, crusted dermatitis), flucloxacillin should definitely be used

c. if despite 48h of a Step 1 antibacterial there are continuing or deteriorating systemic signs (± deteriorating local signs), admit to hospital; otherwise change to Step 2 antibacterial.

8 Standard treatment in hospital (IV): follow local guidelines. The following reflect the recommendations of the British Lymphology Society and Lymphoedema Support Network. Switch to PO flucloxacillin, amoxicillin or clindamycin when no fever for 48h, inflammation settling and CRP falling (see 7 above).

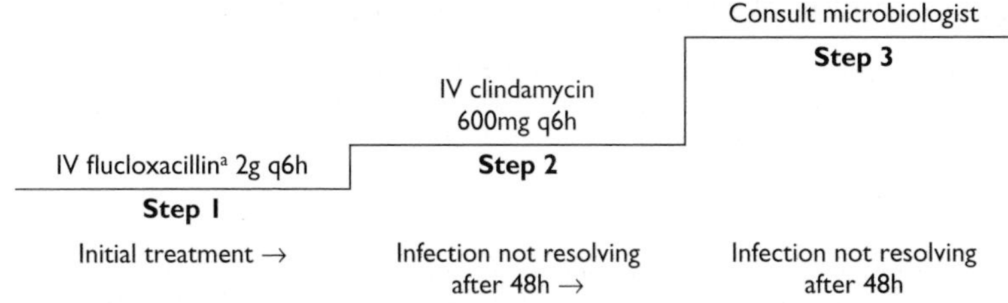

a. if a history of penicillin allergy, start on Step 2.

6

9 For anogenital cellulitis, first line treatment is amoxicillin 2g IV q8h plus gentamicin 5mg/kg IV once daily; the dose of the latter to be adjusted according to renal function and gentamicin plasma concentration.

10 If ≥2 episodes of cellulitis/year, review skin condition and skin care regimen, and consider further steps to reduce limb swelling. Start PO antibacterial prophylaxis with:
- phenoxymethylpenicillin 250mg b.d. (500mg b.d. if BMI ≥33) for 2 years; halve the dose after one year if no recurrence
- if allergic to penicillins, prescribe erythromycin 250mg b.d.; if not tolerated use clarithromycin 250mg once daily (but see 11 below)
- if cellulitis develops despite the above antibacterials, consider other once daily alternatives, e.g. clindamycin 150mg, cefalexin 125mg or doxycycline 50mg; seek advice from a microbiologist and local specialist lymphoedema service
- if cellulitis develops after discontinuation of antibacterials after 2 years, treat the acute episode, and then commence life-long prophylaxis
- if recurrent anogenital cellulitis, prescribe trimethoprim 100mg at bedtime.

11 Check for important drug interactions with macrolides (clarithromycin, erythromycin); certain combinations are contra-indicated (e.g. domperidone, statins) or require close monitoring ± dose adjustment. Alternative PO antibacterials: cefalexin 500mg t.d.s. (but not if a history of severe penicillin allergy) or doxycycline 200mg once daily stat, then 100mg once daily. For prophylaxis, prescribe cefalexin 125mg or doxycycline 50mg once daily. Some antibacterials also interact with coumarins, e.g. warfarin.

General

12 Remember:
- if severe, bed rest and elevation of the affected limb on pillows are essential
- cellulitis is painful; analgesics should be prescribed regularly and p.r.n. Avoid NSAIDs because there is an increased risk of necrotizing fasciitis
- compression garments should not be worn until limb is comfortable
- daily skin hygiene should be continued; washing and gentle drying
- emollients should not be used in the affected area if the skin is broken.

13 Patients should be educated about cellulitis:
- why susceptible (skin crevices harbour bacteria, reduced immunity)
- causes increased swelling, more fibrosis, decreased response to compression
- daily skin care to improve and maintain skin integrity
- reduce risk, e.g. protect hands when gardening, clean cuts, treat fungal infections (terbinafine cream once daily for 2 weeks) and ingrowing toenails
- obtain prompt medical attention if cellulitis occurs.

14 When away from home, take a 2-week supply of PO flucloxacillin 500mg q.d.s. (or amoxicillin 500mg t.d.s.) for emergency use. If allergic to penicillins, erythromycin 500mg q.d.s. or clarithromycin 500mg b.d. (also see point 11 above).

Updated (minor change) August 2016

CLOSTRIDIUM DIFFICILE INFECTION

Clostridium difficile is a bacterium that frequently inhabits the human bowel. It is spread indirectly by spores left on surfaces which are transmitted by the faecal–oral route.

C. difficile infection (CDI) is associated with hospital admission, the use of antibacterials, and the presence of other risk factors (Box A). However, community-acquired infection accounts for about 20–30% of cases, many of which lack 'traditional' risk factors, including antibacterial use.[1–3] CDI can range from mild and self-limiting to severe and life-threatening (Box A).

Box A Clinical features and risk factors for *Clostridium difficile* infection

Clinical features

Watery diarrhoea + mucus ± blood
Abdominal pain and tenderness ± tenesmus
Fever and malaise
± Nausea, vomiting, and anorexia
± Dehydration and delirium
± Leukocytosis
Symptoms generally begin within 1 week of starting antibacterial treatment or shortly after stopping, but may occur up to 2 months later.

Clinical grading of severity

Mild: <3 loose/liquid stools/day and normal WBC
Moderate: 3–5 loose/liquid stools/day and WBC $<15 \times 10^9$/L
Severe: if any of the following are present:
- WBC $>15 \times 10^9$/L
- Temperature >38.5°C
- Acutely rising plasma creatinine (>50% above baseline)
- Clinical or radiographic evidence of severe colitis, e.g. abdominal signs, hypotension, ileus.

Life-threatening: hypotension, partial or complete ileus or toxic megacolon, or CT evidence of severe disease.[4]

Risk factors

Patient-related

Age >65 years
Previous infection with *C. difficile*
Exposure to others with *C.difficile* (infections can occur in outbreaks)
Co-morbidity: cancer, chronic kidney disease, inflammatory bowel disease, immunosuppression

Treatment-related

Hospital admission
GI procedures (non-surgical or surgical)
Nasogastric feeding
Acid-suppressing drugs (H_2-receptor antagonists and particularly PPIs)

Antibacterial use

Prolonged antibacterial treatment, multiple courses, concurrent use of multiple antibacterials.[5]

Highest risk:
Cephalosporins (second/third generation)
Clindamycin
Fluoroquinolones

Medium risk:
Amoxicillin/ampicillin
Co-amoxiclav
Macrolides

Low risk:
Aminoglycosides
Benzylpenicillin
Piptazobactam
Tetracyclines
Trimethoprim
Vancomycin

Toxins are produced which damage the intestinal mucosa. In severe cases a pseudomembranous colitis develops, with sloughing of the inflamed colonic epithelium. This manifests as foul-smelling diarrhoea mingled with mucus and blood. Toxic megacolon and death can follow. CDI has an overall mortality of about 10%, higher (≤40%) in the frail elderly.[6]

In England, NHS Trusts are obliged to report all cases of CDI in anyone over 2 years old, and regular updates on infection rates and outcomes are published by the Public Health England (available from: https://www.gov.uk/government/collections/clostridium-difficile-guidance-data-and-analysis). Improved adherence to infection control measures has led to a dramatic fall in the number of cases of CDI.

Diagnosis

Based on the most recent Department of Health advice.[7]

When to test for C. difficile

- a faecal sample should be sent as soon as possible for testing in patients with diarrhoea (ranging from soft 'blobs' to watery faeces) not clearly attributable to another cause, e.g. laxatives; this includes any hospital patient ≥2 years and all community patients ≥65 years (or those <65 years when clinically indicated)
- if *C. difficile* infection is suspected in the absence of diarrhoea, e.g. with ileus or toxic megacolon, alternative investigations may be required, e.g. colonoscopy, CT abdomen; *seek specialist advice.*

How to test for C. difficile

C. difficile is difficult to culture. A two stage testing approach is recommended:

- initial screening test using either:
  - ▷ a glutamate dehydrogenase test which detects an antigen produced by all *C. difficile* strains, including those which are not toxigenic *or*
  - ▷ a toxin gene test, which detects the presence of toxin gene(s)
- when the screening test is positive, a second test is undertaken, either:
  - ▷ a sensitive toxin test, which detects toxin(s) specific for *C. difficile* colitis *or*
  - ▷ a cytotoxin assay, which detects toxins, but takes longer.

The screening test confirms the likely presence of *C. difficile* and, the second test, the presence or absence of toxins, which indicates if the patient has *C. difficile* infection or is merely colonized by *C. difficile*. For the latter, a toxin gene test (if not already done) can be used as an optional third test to identify toxigenic strains of *C. difficile*, which would make the patient a cross-infection risk to others. The presence of non-toxigenic strains of *C. difficile* can be regarded as normal bowel flora and are of no clinical or infection control relevance.

For those patients with a negative screening test, or who are toxin negative *C. difficile* excretors, other causes for their diarrhoea should be considered.

Management strategy

Based on the most recent Public Health England advice[4]

When there is high clinical suspicion of CDI, particularly when severe, consider starting treatment before test results are available. Stop the precipitating antibacterial if possible. When there is an underlying infection which requires treatment, use an antibacterial associated with a low risk of CDI (Box A). Discontinue PPIs if possible.

Seek specialist advice (e.g. surgical/gastro-enterological/microbiological) when there is life-threatening CDI, or severe CDI not responding to first-line treatment.

Spread of *C. difficile* is by the ingestion of spores from the environment around symptomatic patients or asymptomatic carriers of toxigenic strains of *C. difficile*. Environmental controls ('universal precautions') will generally prevent the spread of outbreaks:

- patients should be isolated while they have diarrhoea, and have their own commode or separate *en suite* toilet
- carers should use gloves, gowns and disposable aprons when caring for infected patients and handling body fluids

- carers should thoroughly wash their hands before and after patient contact using antibacterial soap and water; *alcohol-based hand rubs are ineffective against C. difficile spores*[1]
  - ▷ the WHO produces a downloadable chart illustrating correct hand-washing technique (available from: www.who.int/gpsc/tools/Pocket-Leaflet.pdf)
- areas where there are patients with *C. difficile* should be thoroughly cleaned using chlorine disinfectants.

Antibacterial prescribing policies should aim to minimize the use of broad-spectrum antibacterials, and to regulate treatment duration.

Acid-suppressing drugs, particularly PPIs, may be a risk factor for infection with *C. difficile*, see PPIs, p.31. Thus, it is important to review the need for PPIs in patients with or at high risk of CDI.

General measures

Attention should be given to hydration, electrolytes and nutrition. Antiperistaltic drugs should be avoided because of the theoretical risk of precipitating toxic megacolon by slowing the clearance of *C. difficile* toxin from the intestine.

Drug treatment

Grades of severity are defined in Box A.

Patients with mild CDI may not require specific antibacterial treatment. If treatment is required, **metronidazole** (p.478) is the treatment of choice for mild and moderate CDI; it is as effective as **vancomycin** and much cheaper.

PO **vancomycin** is recommended for severe CDI. ***Vancomycin** must be given PO (or PR), because it is not secreted into the GI tract after IV administration.*

Fidaxomicin 200mg b.d. PO for 10–14 days should be considered for patients with severe CDI who are considered at high risk for recurrence. These include elderly patients with multiple comorbidities who are receiving antibacterials.

In severe CDI not responding to **vancomycin**, PO **fidaxomicin** is an alternative or high-dose PO **vancomycin** + IV **metronidazole**. For other options, e.g. PO **rifampicin**, IV immunoglobulin, seek specialist microbiological advice.

In life-threatening CDI, high-dose **vancomycin** (administered via nasogastric tube or PR) + IV **metronidazole** is used.

Most patients show some symptom improvement in <2 days, e.g. reduction of fever. However, resolution of diarrhoea may take 1–2 weeks.

Symptoms failing to improve or worsening should generally not be considered a treatment failure until after 7 days of treatment. However, at any time, treatment should be escalated if mild–moderate CDI becomes severe, or when severe CDI continues or worsens.

If diarrhoea persists after 20 days of treatment and the patient is otherwise improved and stable, they may have a post-infective irritable bowel syndrome. Treat with **loperamide** 2mg PO p.r.n.

Recurrence

About 15–30% of patients treated with **metronidazole** or **vancomycin** will have a recurrence of CDI, most in ≤3 weeks. This may be caused by germination of residual spores within the colon (more likely if recurrence within 2 weeks)[8] or re-infection with *C. difficile*. Relapse because of antibacterial resistance in *C. difficile* is rare.

PO **fidaxomicin** is the recommended treatment for recurrent CDI, of all severities, except life-threatening. PO **vancomycin** can be used as an alternative if necessary, in a decreasing dose regimen, e.g. over 6 weeks:

- week 1, 125mg q.d.s.
- week 2, 125mg b.d.
- week 3, 125mg once daily
- week 4, 125mg every other day
- week 5 and 6, 125mg every 3 days.

Intermittent therapy in week 4 and 5 allows spores to germinate on 'no antibacterial' days with subsequent destruction on 'antibacterial' days. However, the use of such a regimen must be balanced against the risk of colonization with **vancomycin** resistant organisms such as enterococcus. Seek microbiological advice when there are multiple recurrences.

Probiotics may reduce the incidence of relapse,[9–11] but are not used routinely, and are not recommended by UK guidelines.[4] Various other approaches, including faecal transplant, and vaccines/monoclonal antibodies against *C. difficile* toxins are under investigation.

Dose and use

Grades of severity are defined in Box A.

Metronidazole

- give 400–500mg PO t.d.s. for 10–14 days for treatment of mild–moderate CDI.

Vancomycin

6

- give 125mg PO q.d.s. for 10–14 days for treatment of severe CDI
- an oral solution can be prepared using the injection powder and is significantly cheaper than the capsules (see Supply)
- if not responding, consider:
  - ▷ switching to **fidaxomicin** (see below), *or*
  - ▷ increasing **vancomycin** to 500mg PO (or by nasogastric tube) q.d.s. and combining with **metronidazole** 500mg IV t.d.s.
- for life-threatening CDI, use IV **metronidazole** as above + **vancomycin** 500mg administered via:
  - ▷ nasogastric tube q.d.s. *or*
  - ▷ intracolonic (rectal) route q4h–q12h (see supply).

Fidaxomicin

- give 200mg PO b.d. for 10–14 days for treatment of severe CDI. Generally used second-line when a failure to respond to **vancomycin**; can be used first-line when there is a high risk of recurrence
- give 200mg PO b.d. for 10–14 days for treatment of recurrent disease.

Supply

See **metronidazole**, p.478.

Vancomycin (generic)
Capsules 125mg, 250mg, 10 days @ 125mg q.d.s. = £190.
Injection (powder for reconstitution) 500mg, 1g vial = £7 and £13 respectively.

Vancocin® (Flynn)
Matrigel capsules 125mg, 10 days @ 125mg q.d.s. = £126.
Injection (powder for reconstitution) 500mg, 1g vial = £7 and £13 respectively.

Vancomycin *injection powder is authorized for the preparation of an oral solution; add 10mL WFI to a 500mg vial of powder and give 2.5mL (125mg) PO q.d.s. further diluted with 30mL water or fruit juice (other than grapefruit) prior to administration, 10-day course = £70 (based on using 1 vial/day; store reconstituted vials intended for oral administration in a refrigerator). When diluted with 30mL water it can also be administered by a nasogastric tube.*

Intracolonic vancomycin is prepared as 500mg in 100–500mL 0.9% saline and administered as a retention enema. Insert a 18G Foley catheter PR and inflate balloon with 30mL of water. Instill the vancomycin and clamp the catheter for 1h, after which deflate the balloon and remove.

Fidaxomicin
Dificlir® (Astellas)
Tablets 200mg, 10 days @ 200mg b.d. = £1350.

1 Shannon-Lowe J *et al.* (2010) Prevention and medical management of Clostridium difficile infection. *British Medical Journal.* **340**: c1296.
2 Leffler DA and Lamont JT (2012) Editorial: not so nosocomial anymore: the growing threat of community-acquired Clostridium difficile. *American Journal of Gastroenterology.* **107**: 96–98.
3 Fawley WN *et al.* (2016) Enhanced surveillance of Clostridium difficile infection occurring outside hospital, England, 2011 to 2013. *Euro Surveillance.* **21**.

4 Department of Health (2013) Updated guidance on the management and treatment of Clostridium Difficile infection. Available from: www.gov.uk/government/organisations/public-health-england
5 Monaghan T *et al.* (2008) Recent advances in Clostridium difficile-associated disease. *Gut.* **57**: 850–860.
6 Mitchell BG and Gardner A (2012) Mortality and Clostridium difficile infection: a review. *Antimicrobial Resistance and Infecton Control.* **1**: 20.
7 Department of Health (2012) Updated guidance on diagnosis and reporting of Clostridum Difficle. Available from: www.gov.uk/government/organisations/public-health-england
8 Figueroa I *et al.* (2012) Relapse versus reinfection: recurrent Clostridium difficile infection following treatment with fidaxomicin or vancomycin. *Clinical and Infectious Diseases.* **55 (Suppl 2)**: S104–109.
9 Surawicz CM *et al.* (2000) The search for a better treatment for recurrent Clostridium difficile disease: use of high-dose vancomycin combined with Saccharomyces boulardii. *Clinical Infectious Diseases.* **31**: 1012–1017.
10 Dendukuri N *et al.* (2005) Probiotic therapy for the prevention and treatment of Clostridium difficile-associated diarrhea: a systematic review. *Canadian Medical Association Journal.* **173**: 167–170.
11 Venuto C *et al.* (2010) Alternative therapies for Clostridium difficile infections. *Pharmacotherapy.* **30**: 1266–1278.

Updated April 2017

7: ENDOCRINE SYSTEM AND IMMUNOMODULATION

7

BISPHOSPHONATES

Indications: Authorized indications vary between products; consult SPC for details. They include hypercalcaemia; prophylaxis to reduce skeletal-related events (SRE) and pain associated with osteolytic bone metastases; osteoporosis; Paget's disease; †adjuvant analgesic in moderate–severe bone pain.

Contra-indications: *PO ibandronic acid*: Oesophageal abnormality (e.g. stricture or achalasia), inability to sit upright for 60min.

Pharmacology

The bisphosphonates are stable analogues of pyrophosphate, a naturally occurring regulator of bone metabolism. They have a high affinity for calcium ions, and bind rapidly to hydroxyapatite crystals in mineralized bone. Bisphosphonates are subsequently released and taken up by osteoclasts, interfering with their function and/or inducing their apoptosis (programmed cell death). Nitrogen-containing bisphosphonates (e.g. **alendronate**, **ibandronic acid**, **pamidronate disodium**, **zoledronic acid**) inhibit the mevalonate pathway vital for normal cellular function (e.g. vesicular trafficking, cell signalling, cytoskeleton function) and non-nitrogen-containing bisphosphonates (**sodium clodronate**, **disodium etidronate**) form cytotoxic adenosine triphosphate (ATP) analogues.[1,2] Nitrogen-containing bisphosphonates are more potent.

These cellular effects also extend to macrophages, reducing the production of cytokines. This anti-inflammatory effect may contribute to the analgesic effect of bisphosphonates. Bisphosphonates interfere with the cancer-related increase in the number and activity of osteoclasts which cause bone pain by:

- producing an increasingly acidic environment (stimulating acid-sensing receptors on sensory nerves)
- destroying sensory nerves (producing neuropathic pain)
- causing mechanical instability as a result of the loss of bone mineral (stimulating mechanoreceptors on sensory nerves in the periosteum).

In vitro and in animals, bisphosphonates also have a direct anticancer effect via inhibition of matrix metalloproteinase, altered cell adhesion, anti-angiogenic activity, reduction in release of local growth factors from bone and induction of apoptosis.[3] However, a cancer-promoting effect has been seen in some animal studies.[4] Bisphosphonates have no impact on the effect of parathyroid hormone-related protein (PTHrP) or on renal tubular resorption of calcium.

Bisphosphonates are poorly absorbed PO, and this is reduced further by food. They are rapidly taken up by the skeleton, particularly at sites of bone resorption and where the mineral is more exposed, and they remain there for weeks–months.[5] Most of the remainder is bound to plasma proteins. Bisphosphonates are not metabolized and are excreted unchanged via the kidneys. The plasma proportion of the drug is eliminated generally within 24h. Thereafter, elimination is much slower as the remainder gradually seeps out of bone.[6] Comparison of the halflives of different bisphosphonates is complicated by this multiphasic elimination.

Tumour-induced hypercalcaemia

Bisphosphonates given IV are the treatment of choice for hypercalcaemia of malignancy (Table 1).[7] With **zoledronic acid**, normocalcaemia is achieved after a median of 4 days (ranging up to 10), and pain relief ≤14 days.

Table 1 Bisphosphonates and the initial treatment of hypercalcaemia[8,9]

	Zoledronic acid	*Pamidronate disodium*	*Ibandronic acid*
IV dose	4mg	30–90mg	2–6mg
Onset of effect	<4 days	<3 days	<4 days
Maximum effect	4–7 days	5–7 days	7 days
Duration of effect	4 weeks	2.5 weeks	2.5 weeks (4mg) 4 weeks (6mg)
Restores normocalcaemia	90%	70–75%	75%

Zoledronic acid 8mg has been given to patients who do not respond to 4mg or to **pamidronate disodium**, and those who relapse within a few days of treatment. With the higher dose, normocalcaemia is achieved in 50% of the non-responders.[8] However, the median duration of response is only 2 weeks. Further, the incidence of renal impairment doubles with 8mg, so its use was abandoned in clinical trials and it is unauthorized.[10]

Prevention of skeletal-related events (SRE) in patients with myeloma or bone metastases

IV **pamidronate disodium**, IV **zoledronic acid** and PO/IV **ibandronic acid** are given long-term to patients with bone metastases to decrease the incidence of SRE (definition varies but includes pathological fracture, radiotherapy to bone, spinal cord compression, surgery to bone, and sometimes pain; see separate section below). Various national guidelines recommend with provisos the routine use of bisphosphonates for the treatment and prevention of SRE in patients with:

- symptomatic myeloma whether or not bone lesions are evident[11]
- breast cancer with bone metastases.[12,13]

There is no consensus on the use of bisphosphonates in other cancers, although it has been suggested that in any patient with a prognosis of ≥4–6 months and multiple bone metastases, it is reasonable to consider their use.[14,15]

Only studies ≥6 months in duration have shown a reduction in fractures, hypercalcaemia, and the need for radiotherapy. Studies ≥1 year in duration have also shown a reduced need for orthopaedic surgery. There is no impact on the occurrence of spinal cord compression.[16–18]

The optimal dosing schedule is not clearly established. Although **zoledronic acid** is generally given every 4 weeks, treatment every 12 weeks over 2 years in patients with bone metastases from breast or prostate cancer or myeloma appears to be equally effective.[19] The optimal duration of treatment is unclear, but bisphosphonates are generally continued for as long as they are tolerated or there is a substantial decline in the patient's performance status.

Myeloma

In patients with myeloma, bisphosphonates reduce SRE, including vertebral fracture, and are recommended for all patients with symptomatic myeloma. They may also reduce pain, both through prevention of painful SRE and through a possible direct anti-tumour effect. Meta-analyses are not wholly consistent but **zoledronic acid** is probably the most effective and prolongs overall and progression-free survival. Both **zoledronic acid** and **pamidronate disodium** are more effective than **disodium clodronate**.[11,20–22]

There is no consensus on duration of treatment, but treatment may be stopped when there is a complete response to therapy or no evidence of active bone disease.[11,20]

Breast cancer

In patients with breast cancer and bone metastases, bisphosphonates delay time to developing SRE and reduce the risk and rate of developing SRE. **Zoledronic acid** 4mg IV given every month for 1 year reduces the risk of an SRE by about 40%.[23] Treatment every 2 weeks provides no greater benefit.[24] After 1 year, a 12-weekly regimen has been shown to maintain benefit, and may be satisfactory from the start of treatment.[19,25]

Zoledronic acid is more effective than PO **ibandronic acid**; it may also be more effective than **pamidronate disodium** and IV **ibandronic acid**.[16,22,26] **Denosumab** is an alternative and is more effective than **zoledronic acid** at preventing SRE in breast cancer (see Box B). Current guidelines suggest that either IV **zoledronic acid** or SC **denosumab** should be started in all patients with breast cancer and bone metastases, whether or not they are symptomatic.[27]

7

In *post-menopausal* women with early or advanced breast cancer *without* bone metastases, bisphosphonates may reduce the incidence of bone metastases and lead to a small improvement in survival.[16,28,29] **Denosumab** given to post-menopausal women receiving an aromatase inhibitor (which leads to accelerated bone loss) prevents primary bone loss and increases time to first fracture. However, there are insufficient data to show if it increases survival. Consequently, bisphosphonates remain the treatment of choice in post-menopausal women with early (non-metastatic) breast cancer.[30,31]

Prostate cancer

In early and metastatic prostate cancer controlled by castration, there is little or no benefit from bisphosphonates in relation to SRE, quality of life, or survival.[32–36]

In patients with metastatic hormone-relapsed prostate cancer, **zoledronic acid** (but not **pamidronate**) given for >15 months may reduce the risk and rate of developing SRE.[37,38] Compared with **zoledronic acid**, **denosumab** reduces the risk of SRE (time to first SRE 21 vs. 17 months respectively). The rate of development of SRE was not reported.[39] However, the question of cost-effectiveness remains.[40] Neither **zoledronic acid** nor **denosumab** improve survival.

Further, the pivotal trials of both **zoledronic acid** and **denosumab** predate approval of newer treatment options for hormone-relapsed prostate cancer, e.g. **abiraterone**, **enzalutamide**, all of which reduce SRE. Thus, the place of **denosumab** and **zoledronic acid** in conjunction with these treatments is still to be determined.[22,41,42] As a result, bisphosphonates and **denosumab** are used more frequently in some regions (e.g. USA) than others (e.g. Europe).[40]

Bisphosphonates as adjuvant analgesics

The role of bisphosphonates as adjuvant analgesics for bone pain is unclear. Bisphosphonates are used in two ways:

- prophylactic use over months–years to reduce the risk and rate of developing potentially painful SRE
- as adjuvant analgesics for moderate–severe bone pain.

Prophylactic use

IV/PO bisphosphonates given over months–years are recommended in breast cancer, myeloma and, by some, in metastatic hormone-relapsed prostate cancer to reduce the risk and rate of developing potentially painful SRE (see above). This could lead to a delay in the development and/or worsening of bone pain. However, evidence in support of this is mixed. For example, in a systematic review, *no* analgesic benefit of bisphosphonates was seen in 22 of 28 RCTs, mostly involving patients with breast cancer, prostate cancer or myeloma.[43] Generally, bone pain was not the focus of these studies; few used it as a primary end-point and others did not require it as an inclusion criteria. Further, even when assessed, the use of differing and often non-validated measures of pain and analgesic use make comparisons difficult.

Of the studies showing benefit, most were in patients with breast cancer or myeloma and mild–moderate pain, with moderate relief obtained from an IV bisphosphonate given over several months.[16,21] A direct anti-cancer effect of bisphosphonates, seen particularly in breast cancer and myeloma, may be relevant. In this setting, the 'analgesic effect' is limited to preventing the development of more painful SRE.

Adjuvant analgesics for moderate–severe bone pain

IV bisphosphonates are given as adjuvant analgesics for moderate–severe bone pain, not responding to usual measures, with the expectation of a more rapid analgesic effect, potentially from their anti-inflammatory effect (see Pharmacology).[44] Onset of pain relief is about 2 weeks, and is most likely in patients with moderate pain receiving IV bisphosphonates.[23,45–48] However, supporting data are limited/low quality. Thus, for patients with painful bone metastases despite optimized analgesia, *PCF* advises:

- if localized, consider palliative radiotherapy[12,33]
- if more widespread, consider:
  - ▷ a radionuclide, e.g. radium-223, in patients with prostate cancer[41,49]
  - ▷ IV **zoledronic acid** or, if unavailable, IV **pamidronate** (see Dose and use) in patients with a prognosis of >2 weeks and not already receiving prophylactic bisphosphonates or **denosumab**.

Primary prevention of bone loss in patients treated for breast or prostate cancer

Oestrogen deficiency is induced in breast cancer by chemotherapy ± aromatase inhibitors. This increases the rate of bone loss and risk of fracture. All patients should be offered an axial bone density scan, and those with low bone mineral density offered treatment with **calcium** and **vitamin D** supplements and a bisphosphonate, e.g. **risedronate** 35mg once a week or **zoledronic acid** 4mg IV every 6 months.[13,50,51] **Denosumab** may be an alternative.[31]

Androgen deprivation treatment in men with prostate cancer is associated with increased risk of osteoporosis and fracture. In patients at high risk of osteoporosis, offer a bone density scan. **Calcium** and **vitamin D** supplements should be given and, if osteoporosis is found, **zoledronic acid** every 3–12 months.[41,52,53] **Denosumab** is an alternative if bisphosphonates are contra-indicated or poorly tolerated.[33,41,54]

Cautions

Renal impairment (see Dose and use, and p.695). Vitamin D deficiency (increased risk of hypocalcaemia).[55] Invasive dental procedures (risk of jaw osteonecrosis).

Drug interactions

Concurrent use increases the risk of:

- prolonged hypocalcaemia and hypomagnesaemia with an aminoglycoside[56]
- hypocalcaemia and dehydration with loop diuretics
- renal impairment with other nephrotoxic drugs
- renal impairment with **thalidomide** in multiple myeloma.

Undesirable effects

Very common (>10%): transient pyrexia and flu-like symptoms, more common with IV nitrogen-containing bisphosphonates (see below), fatigue, headache, anxiety, hypertension, anaemia, thrombocytopenia, cough, arthralgia, myalgia, bone pain, *asymptomatic* hypocalcaemia, hypomagnesaemia, hypophosphataemia.

Oral products in particular may cause anorexia, dyspepsia, nausea, vomiting, abdominal pain, diarrhoea or constipation.

Common (<10%, >1%): sleep disturbance, psychosis, tachycardia, atrial fibrillation or flutter, syncope, breathlessness, leucopenia, infusion site reactions, renal impairment (see below), hypokalaemia, jaw osteonecrosis (see below).

Rare (<0.1%, >0.01%): ocular inflammation (see below), angioedema, acute renal failure, nephrotic syndrome (**pamidronate disodium**), *symptomatic* hypocalcaemia (e.g. tetany), atypical femoral fractures, usually in patients treated for >5 years for osteoporosis.[57]

Very rare (<0.01%): osteonecrosis of the external auditory canal, generally in patients treated for >2 years.[58]

Acute systemic inflammatory reactions after IV bisphosphonates

Bone pain sometimes occurs <12h after IV bisphosphonates. Systemic reactions manifest as mild fever (occasionally rigors), myalgia, arthralgia, nausea and vomiting in 25–50% of patients, generally <2 days after IV infusion and lasting 1–2 days. Can be treated with **paracetamol** or NSAIDs. Generally lessen with repeat doses or with prophylactic **paracetamol** or NSAID.[59]

Renal toxicity

Bisphosphonates can affect renal function. Rarely, **pamidronate disodium** causes acute renal failure, particularly at high doses, e.g. 180mg every 2–4 weeks, probably as a direct toxic effect.

The more potent third-generation bisphosphonates are given in much smaller doses and reach lower concentrations in the renal tubules. Renal impairment has occurred with **zoledronic acid** but is uncommon with **ibandronic acid**.[10,60–62] In direct comparisons, the incidence of decreased renal function with **zoledronic acid** 4mg (about 10%) is similar to **pamidronate disodium** 90mg over 2h.[8]

With **zoledronic acid** 4mg, increases in plasma creatinine lead to treatment delay or discontinuation in about 1% and 3% of patients respectively.[63] Increases in creatinine levels >3 times the upper limit of normal were seen in 0.4% of patients.[64] There have been reports of life-threatening renal failure caused by toxic acute tubular necrosis in patients treated with **zoledronic acid**, e.g. 72 cases among >430,000 patients (<0.02%).[18,65,66] Other risk factors were often present, including dehydration, pre-existing renal impairment, and concurrent use of other nephrotoxic drugs.

Renal impairment often manifests <2 months after starting treatment. Mild impairment tends to recover a few days–several months after discontinuing **zoledronic acid** but, in those with renal failure, the damage is generally permanent.[16]

The risk of renal toxicity is reduced by adhering to the recommended dose and infusion rate, ensuring adequate hydration, monitoring renal function and adjusting the dose of bisphosphonate as appropriate or discontinuing treatment if there is deterioration, and avoiding the concurrent use of other nephrotoxic drugs.

Jaw osteonecrosis

All bisphosphonates (and **denosumab**) have been implicated as a risk factor for jaw osteonecrosis.[67,68] Most reports involve the long-term use of **zoledronic acid** or **pamidronate disodium** for metastatic bone disease.[69] Although osteonecrosis has been reported after 4 months, generally, patients have been receiving bisphosphonates for years (median duration 2–3 years). The true incidence of osteonecrosis is difficult to identify, but some studies put it as high as 10% of patients receiving long-term **zoledronic acid** and 4% of those receiving **pamidronate disodium**.[69] Other risk factors for jaw osteonecrosis include dental procedures (reported in about 60% of patients), poor dental health, blood clotting disorders, anaemia, and possibly chemotherapy and corticosteroids.

The jaw bones may be particularly susceptible to osteonecrosis because of the combination of repeated low-level local trauma (e.g. from chewing, dentures) and ease of infection from microbes. Trauma and infection increase the demand for bone repair which the bisphosphonate-inhibited bone cannot meet, resulting in localized bone necrosis; the anti-angiogenic effect of bisphosphonates may also contribute.[69]

Osteonecrosis can present as an asymptomatic bony exposure in one or more sites in the mandible or maxilla, or with orofacial pain, trismus, offensive discharge from a cutaneous fistula, chronic sinusitis because of an oro-antral fistula and numbness in the mandible or maxilla.[59] If probed, the necrotic bone is usually non-tender and may not bleed. There may be osteomyelitis with oral-cavity flora or *Actinomyces* species. Osteonecrosis may show as mottled bone on a plain radiograph and be confused with bone metastases on a bone scan. Pathological fracture can occur.

Management is based on clinical experience. Long-term outcomes are generally poor with relatively few patients experiencing improvement or resolution. Thus, prevention is an important part of the recommended approach:[59]

- explain the risk of osteonecrosis and give the patient a reminder card (supplied by manufacturers)
- undertake preventive dental treatment before commencing long-term bisphosphonates, e.g. treat infection, teeth extractions
- encourage good dental hygiene including regular dental cleaning by a dental hygienist
- avoid invasive dental procedures during treatment and advise patients to inform their dentist of bisphosphonate treatment
- minimize trauma, e.g. patients with dentures should wear soft liners
- advise patients to inform their doctor or dentist immediately if oral symptoms develop, e.g. loose teeth, pain, swelling, discharge or non-healing sores.[70]

If osteonecrosis occurs:

- discontinue the bisphosphonate but new lesions may continue to appear
- treat infection, e.g. antimicrobials, **chlorhexidine** mouthwash, periodic minor debridement and wound irrigation

- major debridement is avoided because it may exacerbate the situation
- avoid major surgery unless there is no alternative, e.g. due to sequestered bone, pathological fracture, or oro-antral fistula.

If urgent treatment precludes dental examination before starting a bisphosphonate, a dental referral and any treatment should be undertaken within 1–2 months for patients expected to receive long-term bisphosphonates.[69]

Ocular toxicity

A rare undesirable effect is ocular inflammation, causing eye pain, redness, swelling, abnormal vision or impaired eye movement (due to rectus muscle oedema).[71] Typically, the onset is <2 days after the first or second infusion and affects both eyes. There may be other symptoms of an acute systemic reaction (see above). An urgent ophthalmology assessment is required, followed by appropriate treatment.

Patients with mild reactions, e.g. those which settle quickly without treatment, can generally continue to receive the same bisphosphonate. Those with more severe reactions, e.g. uveitis or scleritis, should not receive the same bisphosphonate again. Some tolerate a switch to a non-nitrogen-containing bisphosphonate, but specialist advice should be sought from the ophthalmologist ± endocrinologist.[59]

Other emerging toxicities

Severe (sometimes incapacitating) musculoskeletal pain has been reported after days, months or years of bisphosphonate treatment. It is particularly associated with PO bisphosphonates used for osteoporosis and Paget's disease. The pain is distinct from the arthralgia/myalgia associated with an acute systemic reaction (see above), and may respond to temporary or permanent discontinuation of the bisphosphonate.[72]

Dose and use

Unless being treated for tumour-related hypercalcaemia, daily oral supplements of elemental **calcium** 500mg and **vitamin D** 400 units are recommended, e.g. Calcichew® D3 Forte.

Because **zoledronic acid** is more effective, it is replacing **pamidronate disodium** as the bisphosphonate of first choice.

Tumour-induced hypercalcaemia

Stop and think! Are you justified in correcting a potentially fatal complication in a moribund patient?

For **zoledronic acid** the SPC recommends treatment for an albumin-corrected plasma calcium ≥3mmol/L (see Box A):

- patients should be well hydrated, using 0.9% saline IV if necessary
- give 4mg IVI in 100mL 0.9% saline or 5% glucose over 15min
- if plasma calcium does not normalize, repeat after 1 week[7]
- in refractory hypercalcaemia 8mg has been used, but is unauthorized because of concerns about renal impairment (see Pharmacology)
- no dose adjustment is needed in mild–moderate renal impairment for patients being treated for tumour-induced hypercalcaemia; if possible, avoid use in severe renal impairment (see below).

For **pamidronate disodium** the SPC recommends a dose dependent on the initial albumin-corrected plasma calcium concentration (Box A and Table 2). However, it has been suggested that 90mg should be given irrespective of the initial calcium level to increase the probability of a response and to prolong its duration:[7]

- patients should be well hydrated, using 0.9% saline IV if necessary
- standard and maximum recommended dose is 90mg IVI in 500mL 0.9% saline over 4h
- repeat after 1 week if initial response inadequate
- repeat every 3–4 weeks according to plasma calcium concentration
- no dose adjustment is needed in mild–moderate renal impairment for patients being treated for tumour-induced hypercalcaemia; if possible, avoid use in severe renal impairment (see below).

Box A Correcting plasma calcium concentrations[a]

If the mean normal albumin for the local laboratory is 40g/L
Corrected calcium (mmol/L) = measured calcium + (0.022 x (40 – albumin g/L))
e.g. measured calcium = 2.45; albumin = 32
corrected calcium = 2.45 + (0.022 x 8) = 2.63mmol/L
(normal range = 2.12–2.65mmol/L)

a. most UK pathology laboratories automatically report an albumin-corrected plasma calcium concentration based on locally validated data.

Table 2 IV pamidronate disodium for tumour-induced hypercalcaemia[a]

Corrected plasma calcium concentration (mmol/L)	*Dose (mg)*
<3	15 or 30
3–3.5	30 or 60
3.5–4	60 or 90
>4	90

a. manufacturer's recommendations. Irrespective of the initial calcium level, many centres use 90mg to increase the probability of a response and to prolong its duration.[7]

7

Prophylactic use to reduce the incidence of skeletal-related events (SRE)

For **zoledronic acid**:

- patients should be well hydrated, using 0.9% saline IV if necessary
- give 4mg IVI in 100mL 0.9% saline or 5% glucose over 15min every 3–4 weeks; with appropriate support, this can be given at home[13]
- for dose in patients with mild–moderate renal impairment, see Table 3; avoid use in severe renal impairment (see below).

Table 3 Dose reduction for zoledronic acid in cancer patients and mild–moderate renal impairment[a,b,c]

Baseline creatinine clearance (mL/min)	*Recommended dose (mg)*
>60	4 (no reduction)
50–60	3.5
40–49	3.3
30–39	3

a. manufacturer's recommendations for patients with multiple myeloma or bone metastases
b. no data exist for severe renal impairment (creatinine clearance <30mL/min) because these patients were excluded from the studies
c. reduced doses are diluted in 100mL 0.9% saline or 5% glucose and given IVI over 15min; see SPC for preparation details.

For **pamidronate disodium**:

- patients should be well hydrated, using 0.9% saline IV if necessary
- in *breast cancer with bone metastases*, give 90mg IVI in 250mL 0.9% saline over 1.5−2h every 3–4 weeks
- in *multiple myeloma*, give 90mg IVI in 500mL 0.9% saline *over 4h* every 4 weeks because of greater risk of renal toxicity
- no dose adjustment is needed in mild–moderate renal impairment for prophylactic use to reduce the incidence of SRE, but the infusion rate should not exceed 90mg/4h; avoid use in severe renal impairment (see below).

Monitoring

For **zoledronic acid** and **pamidronate disodium**:

- measure plasma creatinine before each dose; withhold treatment if creatinine increases by:
  - ▷ ≥44micromol/L in patients with a normal baseline creatinine concentration (i.e. <124micromol/L), *or*
  - ▷ ≥88micromol/L in patients with a raised baseline creatinine concentration (i.e. >124micromol/L)
- treatment may be resumed at the same dose as before when plasma creatinine returns to within 10% of the baseline value
- discontinue treatment permanently if plasma creatinine fails to improve after 4–8 weeks.

Adjuvant analgesics for moderate–severe bone pain

High quality data are lacking and such use is unauthorized (see Pharmacology). Consider when analgesics and radiotherapy are unsatisfactory and the patient is not already receiving prophylactic bisphosphonates or **denusomab**. **Zoledronic acid** is the drug of choice (see Prophylactic use for SRE). If not available:

- give **pamidronate disodium** 90mg IVI (50% of patients respond, generally within 1–2 weeks); if helpful repeat 60–90mg every 3–4 weeks for as long as benefit is maintained.

Use in severe renal impairment or ESRF

The use of bisphosphonates in severe renal impairment or ESRF can be complex and specialist renal/endocrinology advice should be sought (also see p.695). Reasons include the need for caution with fluid administration, the presence of other potentially contributing factors, e.g. tertiary hyperparathyroidism, use of vitamin D analogues, calcium-based phosphate binders, and the risk of further renal toxicity (see Undesirable effects). 'Renally safer' options include **denosumab** (Box B) or reduced doses of **ibandronic acid** (Box C). Both are authorized for the prevention of SRE in patients with bone metastases from breast cancer/solid tumours in patients with severe renal impairment.

Subcutaneous administration

If the IV route is inaccessible, the following bisphosphonates can be administered by CSCI, together with SC hydration.[73,74]

- **pamidronate disodium** 90mg in 1L 0.9% saline over 12–24h
- **sodium clodronate** (not UK) 1,500mg in 50–250mL 0.9% saline or 5% glucose over 2–3h.

Denosumab is an alternative (Box B).

Box B Denosumab

Indications: recommended by NICE for:

- prevention of SRE in adults with bone metastases from breast cancer and other solid cancers (except prostate)[41,75]
- patients in whom bisphosphonates are contra-indicated or poorly tolerated in the following settings:
  - ▷ prevention of osteoporotic fragility fractures in postmenopausal women[76]
  - ▷ treatment of bone loss in men with prostate cancer receiving androgen deprivation.[33,41]

Denosumab is also an option for treating refractory hypercalcaemia of malignancy (unauthorized indication).[77]

Contra-indication: untreated severe hypocalcaemia; unhealed lesions from dental or oral surgery.

Pharmacology

Denosumab is a human monoclonal antibody that binds with receptor activator of nuclear factor kappa β ligand (RANKL), preventing the RANKL-RANK interaction and resulting in reduced osteoclast number and function, thus decreasing bone resorption and cancer-induced bone destruction.

continued

Box B Continued

Denosumab appears to be superior to zoledronic acid in reducing the risk and rate of SRE in patients with bone metastases from advanced cancer, particularly breast cancer.[27] Denosumab may reduce the risk of SRE in patients with metastatic hormone-relapsed prostate cancer (rate of SRE not reported). Thus, denosumab delays the development of painful SRE and the onset of moderate–severe pain in these patients.[43,78,79] However, this benefit does *not* translate into improved survival.[80–87]

The cost-effectiveness of denosumab has been questioned, particularly in prostate cancer and when symptomatic SRE are evaluated (see Prostate cancer above).[40,67,88,89] The role of denosumab has yet to be established in patients with symptomatic myeloma.

Denosumab can be used in patients with renal impairment without dose adjustment, and can be given SC. However, its long-term efficacy and safety are unknown.

Undesirable effects
Very common (>10%): breathlessness, diarrhoea.
Common (<10%, >1%): hypocalcaemia, hypophosphataemia, hyperhidrosis, osteonecrosis of jaw, tooth extraction.
Uncommon (<1%, >0.1%): cellulitis, drug hypersensitivity, atypical femoral fracture.[90]
The incidence of jaw osteonecrosis is comparable with zoledronic acid and similar precautions should be taken before and during treatment (see above); similarly, osteonecrosis of the external auditory canal has also been reported.[70,91] Hypocalcaemia is more common with denosumab and plasma calcium should be monitored.[92]

Dose and use
- *for prevention of SRE in patients with bone metastases from solid cancers*: 120mg administered as a single SC injection once every 4 weeks into the thigh, abdomen or upper arm (XGEVA®)
- *for treatment of postmenopausal osteoporosis in women at increased risk of fracture, and bone loss in men with prostate cancer receiving androgen deprivation therapy*: 60mg SC into thigh or upper arm once every 6 months (Prolia®).

The manufacturer recommends daily supplements of ≥500mg calcium and 400 IU Vitamin D unless the patient is hypercalcaemic.

Box C Ibandronic acid

Ibandronic acid is a third-generation bisphosphonate which can be taken PO. The tablet is smaller and more easily swallowed than sodium clodronate (not UK).

The incidence of undesirable events is low (see main text).[7,46] Renal impairment is no more frequent than with placebo, and it is the only bisphosphonate authorized for use in severe renal impairment (creatinine clearance <30mL/min).

Can be used PO in patients wanting to avoid IV treatment or at risk of renal impairment but is less effective than IV.[65,66,93] IV ibandronate may be as effective as zoledronic acid in reducing SRE in patients with myeloma or metastatic bone disease.[26,94]

Dose and use
For full details, see SPC.

Tumour-induced hypercalcaemia
- patients should be well hydrated, using 0.9% saline IV if necessary
- if the albumin-corrected plasma calcium:
  - ▷ is ≥3mmol/L give 4mg IVI
  - ▷ is <3mmol/L give 2mg IVI
- for both, the dose is given in 500mL 0.9% saline *or* 5% glucose over 2h.

continued

Box C Continued

Prevention of skeletal events in patients with bone metastases from breast cancer (PO/IV) or †moderate-severe bone pain (IV)

For oral use:

- give 50mg PO once daily
  - ▷ in moderate renal impairment, give 50mg PO *alternate days*
  - ▷ in severe renal impairment, give 50mg PO *once a week.*

To maximize absorption and to minimize undesirable gastro-oesophageal effects, patients should take ibandronic acid tablets whole after an overnight fast with a glass of *plain tap water*, followed by no food for ≥30min and remaining upright for 60min.

For parenteral use:

- give 6mg IVI in 100mL 0.9% saline *or* 5% glucose over 15min every 3–4 weeks
  - ▷ in moderate renal impairment, give 4mg in 500mL *over 1h* every 3–4 weeks
  - ▷ in severe renal impairment, give 2mg in 500mL *over 1h* every 3–4 weeks.

Supply

Pamidronate disodium (generic)

Injection (concentrate for dilution and use as an infusion) 3mg/mL, 5mL, 10mL, 20mL and 30mL vial = £30, £60, £110 and £165 respectively; 9mg/mL, 10mL vial = £170; 15mg/mL, 1mL, 2mL, 4mL and 6mL amp = £30, £60, £119 and £170 respectively.

Zoledronic acid (generic)

Injection (concentrate for dilution and use as an infusion) 4mg/5mL, 5mL vial = £10−£175.

Infusion 4mg/100mL, 100mL bag, vial, or bottle = £150−£175.

Note. Zoledronic acid 5mg/100mL is available but authorized for the treatment of Paget's disease and as an annual dose for osteoporosis in women (postmenopausal) or men.

Ibandronic acid (generic)

Tablets 50mg, 28 days @ 50mg once daily = £6.

Injection (concentrate for dilution) 1mg/mL, 2mL vial = £89; 6mL vial = £184.

Note. Ibandronic acid 150mg tablets and 1mg/mL, 3mL pre-filled syringe are available but authorized for the treatment of postmenopausal osteoporosis.

Denosumab

XGEVA® (Amgen)

Injection 70mg/mL, 120mg vial = £310.

Note. Denosumab 60mg/mL, 1mL pre-filled syringe (Prolia®) *is available but authorized for the treatment of postmenopausal osteoporosis in women and treatment of bone loss in men with prostate cancer receiving androgen deprivation therapy.*

1 Fleisch H (1998) Bisphosphonates: mechanisms of action. *Endocrine Reviews*. **19**: 80–100.

2 Russell R *et al.* (1999) Bisphosphonates: pharmacology, mechanisms of action and clinical uses. *Osteoporosis International*. **9 (Suppl 2)**: s66–s80.

3 Neville-Webbe H *et al.* (2002) The anti-tumour activity of bisphosphonates. *Cancer Treatment Reviews*. **28**: 305–319.

4 Sevcik MA *et al.* (2004) Bone cancer pain: the effects of the bisphosphonate alendronate on pain, skeletal remodeling, tumor growth and tumor necrosis. *Pain*. **111**: 169–180.

5 Rogers MJ *et al.* (2000) Cellular and molecular mechanisms of action of bisphosphonates. *Cancer*. **88 (Suppl 12)**: 2961–2978.

6 Barrett J *et al.* (2004) Ibandronate: a clinical pharmacological and pharmacokinetic update. *Journal of Clinical Pharmacology*. **44**: 951–965.

7 Saunders Y *et al.* (2004) Systematic review of bisphosphonates for hypercalcaemia of malignancy. *Palliative Medicine*. **18**: 418–431.

8 Major P *et al.* (2001) Zoledronic acid is superior to pamidronate in the treatment of hypercalcaemia of malignancy: a pooled analysis of two randomized, controlled clinical trials. *Journal of Clinical Oncology*. **19**: 558–567.

9 Ralston SH *et al.* (1997) Dose-response study of ibandronate in the treatment of cancer-associated hypercalcaemia. *British Journal of Cancer*. **75**: 295–300.

10 Rosen LS *et al.* (2001) Zoledronic acid versus pamidronate in the treatment of skeletal metastases in patients with breast cancer or osteolytic lesions of multiple myeloma: a phase III, double-blind, comparative trial. *Cancer Journal*. **7**: 377–387.

11 Snowden JA *et al.* (2017) Guidelines for screening and management of late and long-term consequences of myeloma and its treatment. *British Journal of Haematology*.
12 NICE (2014) Advanced breast cancer: diagnosis and treatment. *Clinical Guideline*. **CG81**: www.nice.org.uk
13 SIGN (2013) Treatment of primary breast cancer. *Clinical Guideline* 134. www.sign.ac.uk
14 Lopez-Olivo MA *et al.* (2012) Bisphosphonates in the treatment of patients with lung cancer and metastatic bone disease: a systematic review and meta-analysis. *Supportive Care in Cancer*. **20**: 2985–2998.
15 Aapro M *et al.* (2008) Guidance on the use of bisphosphonates in solid tumours: recommendations of an international expert panel. *Annals of Oncology*. **19**: 420–432.
16 Wong MH *et al.* (2012) Bisphosphonates and other bone agents for breast cancer. *Cochrane Database of Systematic Reviews*. **2**: CD003474. www.thecochranelibrary.com
17 Henk H *et al.* (2012) Evaluation of the clinical benefit of long-term (beyond 2 years) treatment of skeletal-related events in advanced cancers with zoledronic acid. *Current Medical Research and Opinion*. **28**: 1119–1127.
18 Ross JR *et al.* (2003) Systematic review of role of bisphosphonates on skeletal morbidity in metastatic cancer. *British Medical Journal*. **327**: 469.
19 Himelstein AL *et al.* (2017) Effect of longer-interval vs standard dosing of zoledronic acid on skeletal events in patients with bone metastases: a randomized clinical trial. *JAMA*. **317**: 48–58.
20 Morgan GJ *et al.* (2013) Long-term follow-up of MRC myeloma IX trial: survival outcomes with bisphosphonate and thalidomide treatment. *Clinical Cancer Research*. **19**: 6030–6038.
21 Mhaskar R *et al.* (2012) Bisphosphonates in multiple myeloma: a network meta-analysis. *Cochrane Database of Systematic Reviews*. **5**: CD003188. www.thecochranelibrary.com
22 Palmieri C *et al.* (2013) Comparative efficacy of bisphosphonates in metastatic breast and prostate cancer and multiple myeloma: a mixed-treatment meta-analysis. *Clinical Cancer Research*. **19**: 6863–6872.
23 Kohno N *et al.* (2005) Zoledronic acid significantly reduces skeletal complications compared with placebo in Japanese women with bone metastases from breast cancer: a randomized, placebo-controlled trial. *Journal of Clinical Oncology*. **23**: 3314–3321.
24 Mystakidou K *et al.* (2006) A prospective randomized controlled clinical trial of zoledronic acid for bone metastases. *American Journal of Hospice and Palliative Medicine*. **23**: 41–50.
25 Amadori D *et al.* (2013) Efficacy and safety of 12-weekly versus 4-weekly zoledronic acid for prolonged treatment of patients with bone metastases from breast cancer (ZOOM): a phase 3, open-label, randomised, non-inferiority trial. *Lancet Oncology*. **14**: 663–670.
26 Barrett-Lee P *et al.* (2014) Oral ibandronic acid versus intravenous zoledronic acid in treatment of bone metastases from breast cancer: a randomised, open label, non-inferiority phase 3 trial. *Lancet Oncology*. **15**: 114–122.
27 Coleman R *et al.* (2014) Bone health in cancer patients: ESMO Clinical Practice Guidelines. *Annals of Oncology*. **25 (Suppl 3)**: 124–137.
28 Early Breat Cancer Trialists' Collaborative Group (2015) Adjuvant biphosphonate treatment in early breast cancer: meta-analyses of individual patient data from randomised trials. *Lancet*. **386**: 1353–1361.
29 Coleman R *et al.* (2014) Adjuvant zoledronic acid in patients with early breast cancer: final efficacy analysis of the AZURE (BIG 01/04) randomised open-label phase 3 trial. *Lancet Oncology*. **15**: 997–1006.
30 Coleman R and Hadji P (2015) Denosumab and fracture risk in women with breast cancer. *Lancet*. **386**: 409–410.
31 Gnant M *et al.* (2015) Adjuvant denosumab in breast cancer (ABCSG-18): a multicentre, randomised, double-blind, placebo-controlled trial. *Lancet*. **386**: 433–443.
32 Yuen KK *et al.* (2006) Bisphosphonates for advanced prostate cancer. *Cochrane Database Systematic Reviews*. **4**: CD006250. www.thecochranelibrary.com
33 NICE (2014) Prostate cancer: diagnosis and management. *Clinical Guideline*. **CG175**: www.nice.org.uk
34 Denham JW *et al.* (2014) Short-term androgen suppression and radiotherapy versus intermediate-term androgen suppression and radiotherapy, with or without zoledronic acid, in men with locally advanced prostate cancer (TROG 03.04 RADAR): an open-label, randomised, phase 3 factorial trial. *Lancet Oncology*. **15**: 1076–1089.
35 Smith MR *et al.* (2014) Randomized controlled trial of early zoledronic acid in men with castration-sensitive prostate cancer and bone metastases: results of CALGB 90202 (alliance). *Journal of Clinical Oncology*. **32**: 1143–1150.
36 James ND *et al.* (2016) Addition of docetaxel, zoledronic acid, or both to first-line long-term hormone therapy in prostate cancer (STAMPEDE): survival results from an adaptive, multiarm, multistage, platform randomised controlled trial. *Lancet*. **387**: 1163–1177.
37 Saad F *et al.* (2002) A randomized, placebo-controlled trial of zoledronic acid in patients with hormone-refractory metastatic prostate carcinoma. *Journal of the National Cancer Institute*. **94**: 1458–1468.
38 James ND *et al.* (2016) Clinical outcomes and survival following treatment of metastatic castrate-refractory prostate cancer with docetaxel alone or with strontium-89, zoledronic acid, or both: the TRAPEZE randomized clinical trial. *JAMA Oncology*. **2**: 493–499.
39 Fizazi K *et al.* (2011) Denosumab versus zoledronic acid for treatment of bone metastases in men with castration-resistant prostate cancer: a randomised, double-blind study. *Lancet*. **377**: 813–822.
40 Tombal B (2015) Assessing the benefit of bone-targeted therapies in prostate cancer, is the devil in the end point's definition? *Annals of Oncology*. **26**: 257–258.
41 Mottet N and et al (2016). *European Association of Urology Prostate Cancer Guidelines*. www.uroweb.org (accessed February 2017).
42 Attard G *et al.* (2016) Prostate cancer. *Lancet*. **387**: 70–82.
43 Porta-Sales J *et al.* (2017) Evidence on the analgesic role of bisphosphonates and denosumab in the treatment of pain due to bone metastases: A systematic review within the European Association for Palliative Care guidelines project. *Palliative Medicine*. **31**: 5–25.
44 Mannix K *et al.* (2000) Using bisphosphonates to control the pain of bone metastases: evidence-based guidelines for palliative care. *Palliative Medicine*. **14**: 455–461.
45 Glover D *et al.* (1994) Intravenous pamidronate disodium treatment of bone metastases in patients with breast cancer. A dose-seeking study. *Cancer*. **74**: 2949–2955.
46 Wong R and Wiffen PJ (2002) Bisphosphonates for the relief of pain secondary to bone metastases. *Cochrane Database Systematic Reviews*. **2**: CD002068. www.thecochranelibrary.com
47 Groff L *et al.* (2001) The role of disodium pamidronate in the management of bone pain due to malignancy. *Palliative Medicine*. **15**: 297–307.
48 Kretzschmar A *et al.* (2007) Rapid and sustained influence of intravenous zoledronic Acid on course of pain and analgesics consumption in patients with cancer with bone metastases: a multicenter open-label study over 1 year. *Supportive Cancer Therapy*. **4**: 203–210.
49 Parker C *et al.* (2013) Alpha emitter radium-223 and survival in metastatic prostate cancer. *New England Journal of Medicine*. **369**: 213–223.
50 Reid DM *et al.* (2008) Guidance for the management of breast cancer treatment-induced bone loss: a consensus position statement from a UK Expert Group. *Cancer Treatment Reviews*. **34 (Suppl 1)**: S3–18.

51 Coleman RE *et al.* (2013) Management of cancer treatment-induced bone loss. *Nature Reviews Rheumatology*. **9**: 365–374.
52 Droz JP *et al.* (2014) Management of prostate cancer in older patients: updated recommendations of a working group of the International Society of Geriatric Oncology. *Lancet Oncology*. **15**: e404–414.
53 Wadhwa VK *et al.* (2010) Frequency of zoledronic acid to prevent further bone loss in osteoporotic patients undergoing androgen deprivation therapy for prostate cancer. *BJU International*. **105**: 1082–1088.
54 Smith MR *et al.* (2009) Denosumab in men receiving androgen-deprivation therapy for prostate cancer. *New England Journal of Medicine*. **361**: 745–755.
55 Broadbent A *et al.* (2005) Bisphosphonate-induced hypocalcemia associated with vitamin D deficiency in a patient with advanced cancer. *American Journal of Hospice and Palliative Care*. **22**: 382–384.
56 Johnson M and Fallon M (1998) Symptomatic hypocalcaemia with oral clodronate. *Journal of Pain and Symptom Management*. **15**: 140–142.
57 MHRA (2011) Biphosphonates: atypical femoral fractures. *Drug Safety Update*. **4**: www.gov.uk/drug-safety-update
58 MHRA (2015) Bisphosphonates: very rare reports of osteonecrosis of the external auditory canal. *Drug Safety Update*. **9:** www.gov.uk/drug-safety-update
59 Tanvetyanon T and Stiff PJ (2006) Management of the adverse effects associated with intravenous bisphosphonates. *Annals of Oncology*. **17**: 897–907.
60 Chang JT *et al.* (2003) Renal failure with the use of zoledronic acid. *New England Journal of Medicine*. **349**: 1676–1679.
61 Diel I *et al.* (2003) Renal safety of oral and intravenous ibandronate in metastatic bone disease: phase III clinical trial results. In: *15th Annual MASCC Meeting*; Berlin, 18–21 June.
62 Markowitz GS *et al.* (2003) Toxic acute tubular necrosis following treatment with zoledronate (Zometa). *Kidney International*. **64**: 281–289.
63 Vogel CL *et al.* (2004) Safety and pain palliation of zoledronic acid in patients with breast cancer, prostate cancer, or multiple myeloma who previously received bisphosphonate therapy. *Oncologist*. **9**: 687–695.
64 Rosen LS *et al.* (2003) Long-term efficacy and safety of zoledronic acid compared with pamidronate disodium in the treatment of skeletal complications in patients with advanced multiple myeloma or breast carcinoma: a randomized, double-blind, multicenter, comparative trial. *Cancer*. **98**: 1735–1744.
65 Body JJ *et al.* (2004) Oral ibandronate improves bone pain and preserves quality of life in patients with skeletal metastases due to breast cancer. *Pain*. **111**: 306–312.
66 Body JJ *et al.* (2004) Oral ibandronate reduces the risk of skeletal complications in breast cancer patients with metastatic bone disease: results from two randomised, placebo-controlled phase III studies. *British Journal of Cancer*. **90**: 1133–1137.
67 West H (2011) Denosumab for prevention of skeletal-related events in patients with bone metastases from solid tumors: incremental benefit, debatable value. *Journal of Clinical Oncology*. **29**: 1095–1098.
68 Ruggiero SL *et al.* (2004) Osteonecrosis of the jaws associated with the use of bisphosphonates: a review of 63 cases. *Journal of Oral and Maxillofacial Surgery*. **62**: 527–534.
69 Woo SB *et al.* (2006) Narrative review: bisphosphonates and osteonecrosis of the jaws. *Annals of Internal Medicine*. **144**: 753–761.
70 MHRA (2015) Denosumab (Xgeva, Prolia); intravenous biphosphonates: osteonecrosis of the jaw - further measures to minimise risk. *Drug Safety Update*. **8**: www.gov.uk/drug-safety-update
71 Fraunfelder FW and Fraunfelder FT (2003) Bisphosphonates and ocular inflammation. *New England Journal of Medicine*. **348**: 1187–1188.
72 FDA (2008) Information for healthcare professionals. Bisphosphonates (marketed as Actonel, Actonel+Ca, Aredia, Boniva, Didronel, Fosamax, Fosamax+D, Reclast, Skelid, and Zometa). Food and Drugs Administration. Available from: www.fda.gov/Drugs/DrugSafety/PostmarketDrugSafetyInformationforPatientsandProviders/ucm101551.htm
73 Roemer-Becuwe C *et al.* (2003) Safety of subcutaneous clodronate and efficacy in hypercalcemia of malignancy: a novel route of administration. *Journal of Pain and Symptom Management*. **26**: 843–848.
74 Duncan AR (2003) The use of subcutaneous pamidronate. *Journal of Pain and Symptom Management*. **26**: 592–593.
75 NICE (2012) Denosumab for the prevention of skeletal-related events adults with bone metasases from solid tumours. *Technology Appraisal Guidance* 265. www.nice.org.uk
76 NICE (2010) Denosumab for the prevention of osteoporotic fractures in postmenopausal women. *Technology Appraisal Guidance* 204. www.nice.org.uk
77 Hu MI (2016) Denosumab for treatment of hypercalcemia of malignancy. *Journal of Endocrinology and Metabolism*. **99**: 3144–3152.
78 von Moos R *et al.* (2013) Pain and health-related quality of life in patients with advanced solid tumours and bone metastases: integrated results from three randomized, double-blind studies of denosumab and zoledronic acid. *Supportive Care in Cancer*. **21**: 3497–3507.
79 Cleeland CS *et al.* (2013) Pain outcomes in patients with advanced breast cancer and bone metastases: results from a randomized, double-blind study of denosumab and zoledronic acid. *Cancer*. **119**: 832–838.
80 Stopeck AT *et al.* (2010) Denosumab compared with zoledronic acid for the treatment of bone metastases in patients with advanced breast cancer: a randomized, double-blind study. *Journal of Clinical Oncology*. **28**: 5132–5139.
81 Henry DH *et al.* (2011) Randomized, double-blind study of denosumab versus zoledronic acid in the treatment of bone metastases in patients with advanced cancer (excluding breast and prostate cancer) or multiple myeloma. *Journal of Clinical Oncology*. **29**: 1125–1132.
82 Lipton A *et al.* (2012) Superiority of denosumab to zoledronic acid for prevention of skeletal-related events: a combined analysis of 3 pivotal, randomised, phase 3 trials. *European Journal of Cancer*. **48**: 3082–3092.
83 Sun L and Yu S (2013) Efficacy and safety of denosumab versus zoledronic acid in patients with bone metastases: a systematic review and meta-analysis. *American Journal of Clinical Oncology*. **36**: 399–403.
84 Peddi P *et al.* (2013) Denosumab in patients with cancer and skeletal metastases: a systematic review and meta-analysis. *Cancer Treatment Reviews*. **39**: 97–104.
85 Martin M *et al.* (2012) Bone-related complications and quality of life in advanced breast cancer: results from a randomized phase III trial of denosumab versus zoledronic acid. *Clin Cancer Res*. **18**: 4841–4849.
86 Henry D *et al.* (2014) Delaying skeletal-related events in a randomized phase 3 study of denosumab versus zoledronic acid in patients with advanced cancer: an analysis of data from patients with solid tumors. *Supportive Care in Cancer*. **22**: 679–687.
87 Vadhan-Raj S *et al.* (2012) Clinical benefit in patients with metastatic bone disease: results of a phase 3 study of denosumab versus zoledronic acid. *Annals of Oncology*. **23**: 3045–3051.
88 Snedecor SJ *et al.* (2013) Denosumab versus zoledronic acid for treatment of bone metastases in men with castration-resistant prostate cancer: a cost-effectiveness analysis. *Journal of Medical Economics*. **16**: 19–29.
89 Smith MR *et al.* (2015) Denosumab for the prevention of skeletal complications in metastatic castration-resistant prostate cancer: comparison of skeletal-related events and symptomatic skeletal events. *Annals of Oncology*. **26**: 368–374.

90 MHRA (2013) Denosumab 60mg (Prolia). Rare cases if atypical femoral fracture with long-term use. *Drug Safety Update*. **6**: www.gov.uk/drug-safety-update
91 MHRA (2017) Denosumab (Prolia, Xgeva): reports of osteonecrosis of the external auditory canal. *Drug Safety Update* **10**: www.gov.uk/drug-safety-update
92 MHRA (2014) Denosumab: updated recommendations. *Drug Safety Update*. **8**: www.gov.uk/drug-safety-update
93 Costa L (2014) Which bisphosphonate to treat bone metastases? *Lancet Oncology*. **15**: 15–16.
94 Geng CJ *et al.* (2015) Ibandronate to treat skeletal-related events and bone pain in metastatic bone disease or multiple myeloma: a meta-analysis of randomised clinical trials. *British Medical Journal Open*. **5**: 1–10.

Updated September 2017

SYSTEMIC CORTICOSTEROIDS

7

Indications: Suppression of inflammatory and allergic disorders, cerebral oedema, nausea and vomiting with chemotherapy; †see Box A.

Box A Off-label indications for systemic corticosteroids in advanced cancer[1]

This list of off-label uses does not claim to be totally comprehensive. Inclusion does not mean that a systemic corticosteroid is necessarily the treatment of choice. Further, the evidence-base for some indications is only 'expert opinion'.

Specific
Spinal cord compression[2]
Nerve compression
Breathlessness
- pneumonitis (after radiation therapy)
- lymphangitic carcinomatosis
- tracheal compression/stridor

Superior vena caval obstruction[3]
Obstruction of hollow viscus
- bronchus[4]
- ureter
- GI[5,6]

Discharge from rectal tumour (can give either PO or PR)
Paraneoplastic fever
Nausea and vomiting in cancer resistant to standard measures (see p.238)

Pain relief[a]
Pain associated with spinal cord or nerve compression
Pain caused by a tumour in a confined organ or body cavity, e.g. raised intracranial pressure
Radiation-induced inflammation[7]

Anticancer hormone therapy
Prostate cancer[8]
Haematological malignancies
Lymphoproliferative disorders

General ('tonic')
To improve appetite
To enhance sense of wellbeing

a. RCT evidence is mixed, but overall suggests that the use of corticosteroids for cancer pain *per se* outside of the above indications has little benefit.[9,10] In an adequately powered study of cancer patients with moderate pain of various causes, 1 week of methylprednisolone 32mg/24h PO significantly improved anorexia and fatigue but not average daily pain or opioid use.[10]

Contra-indications: Systemic infection, unless considered to be life-saving and specific anti-infective therapy is employed.

Pharmacology

The adrenal cortex secretes **hydrocortisone** (cortisol) which has glucocorticoid activity and weak mineralocorticoid activity.[11] It also secretes aldosterone which has mineralocorticoid activity. Thus, in deficiency states, physiological replacement is best achieved with a combination of **hydrocortisone** and **fludrocortisone**, a mineralocorticoid.

In many disease states, corticosteroids are used primarily as potent anti-inflammatory agents. The anti-inflammatory action is mediated via several interacting mechanisms,[11] in contrast to the more specific impact of NSAIDs on prostaglandin synthesis (see p.296). Thus, as anti-inflammatory agents, corticosteroids are potentially more effective than NSAIDs. However, certainly when used long-term, corticosteroids are likely to cause more numerous and more serious undesirable effects (see below).

When comparing the relative anti-inflammatory (glucocorticoid) potencies of corticosteroids, their water-retaining properties (mineralocorticoid effect) should also be borne in mind (Table 1). Thus, **hydrocortisone** is not used for long-term disease suppression because large doses would be required and these would cause troublesome fluid retention. On the other hand, the moderate anti-inflammatory effect of **hydrocortisone** makes it a useful corticosteroid for topical use in inflammatory skin conditions; both topical and systemic undesirable effects are minimal.

Prednisolone is the most frequently used corticosteroid for disease suppression. **Dexamethasone**, with high glucocorticoid activity but insignificant mineralocorticoid effect, is particularly suitable for high-dose anti-inflammatory therapy. It is 7 times more potent than **prednisolone**, i.e. 2mg of **dexamethasone** is approximately equivalent to 15mg of **prednisolone** (Box B) and it has a long duration of action (Table 1). Some corticosteroid esters, e.g. of **betamethasone** and of **beclometasone**, exert a marked topical effect; use is made of this property with skin applications and bronchial inhalations (see p.627 and p.126).

General 'tonic' use

The non-specific 'tonic' use of corticosteroids is based on the known general effects of this group of drugs. In patients with advanced cancer, treatment with corticosteroids may result in increased appetite, reduced nausea and improved well-being. In one qualitative study, patients initially reported distressing symptoms, physical deterioration, decreased autonomy, and a feeling of apprehension and foreboding. After treatment for one week with **betamethasone** 4mg PO once daily, most patients had improved symptom relief, and reported enhanced physical abilities, increased autonomy, and renewed hope.[12]

RCTs of corticosteroids specifically as appetite stimulants have used daily doses of **prednisolone** 15–40mg (or equivalent).[11,12] All showed benefit compared with placebo. In one, benefit was comparable for daily doses of **dexamethasone** of either 3mg or 6mg (equivalent to **prednisolone** 20mg or 40mg). Overall, over 50% of the patients reported benefit, which was still apparent after 4 weeks.[11,12] A recent systematic review confirmed benefit, but there was insufficient evidence to recommend a particular regimen.[13]

However, both corticosteroids and progestogens (see p.552) should *not* be regarded as 'anticachexia' agents. Any weight gain relates to fluid retention ± increased fat, rather than to increased skeletal muscle mass. This could make mobilizing more difficult in an already debilitated patient. In addition, the catabolic effect of corticosteroids on skeletal muscle, exacerbated by reduced levels of physical activity, may well further weaken the patient, rendering corticosteroids suitable for short-term use only.

Nausea and vomiting

Dexamethasone is an integral part of standard management of severe chemotherapeutic vomiting.[14] Its anti-emetic effect may be mediated through a direct central action at the solitary tract nucleus, a direct anti-inflammatory effect on damaged tissue, or through reduced expression of serotonin receptors.[15]

In palliative care, **dexamethasone** is often used when all else fails as an 'add-on' anti-emetic (see QCG: Nausea and vomiting, p.240). However, there is some evidence that **dexamethasone** does not add to the anti-emetic efficacy of **metoclopramide** or phenothiazines in patients with advanced cancer.[16–18]

Obstructive syndromes

In obstructive syndromes (Box A), corticosteroids may help by reducing inflammation at the site of the obstruction, thereby increasing the lumen of the obstructed hollow viscus. Corticosteroids (e.g. **dexamethasone** 8mg/24h SC) may improve bowel obstruction but do not affect survival. The incidence of undesirable events is low.[5] High dose corticosteroids (**dexamethasone** equivalent 20–40mg/24h PO) relieved stridor within 12h in 3 patients with upper airway obstruction from infiltrating tumour.[4]

Brain metastases

Dexamethasone is recommended for treatment of adults with symptomatic brain metastases; no benefit is seen in patients with asymptomatic brain metastases. **Dexamethasone** 4–8mg/24h PO provides temporary symptomatic relief for patients with mild symptoms related to raised intracranial pressure from cerebral oedema. If patients have severe symptoms or are at risk of herniation, doses of ≥16mg/24h PO are recommended. Symptom relief from **dexamethasone** reduces over time and undesirable effects increase. Thus, ideally, the dose of **dexamethasone** should be reduced after one week and discontinued after 2–4 weeks.[19] However, unless patients receive additional treatment (e.g. palliative radiotherapy), they will experience a recurrence of their symptoms at some point as the dose of **dexamethasone** is decreased. Thus, it may be necessary to taper more slowly or continue 'maintenance' **dexamethasone** indefinitely in some patients.

Whole brain radiotherapy may cause nausea, vomiting, headache, fever and a transient worsening of neurological symptoms. **Dexamethasone** should be continued for one week after treatment and then tapered over 2–4 weeks.[20,21]

Spinal cord compression

Spinal cord compression must be treated as an emergency; patients with paraparesis do better than those who are totally paraplegic.[2,22,23] Because corticosteroids inhibit inflammation, stabilize vascular membranes, and reduce spinal cord oedema, their use in spinal cord compression often results in a dramatic reduction in pain, and an early improvement in the patient's physical status.

Traditionally, **dexamethasone** has been used as the corticosteroid of choice, sometimes initially given IV. However, given its high PO bio-availability (see Table 1), IV administration seems unnecessary. A typical PO regimen would be:[2]

- a stat dose of **dexamethasone** 16mg PO
- continue with 16mg PO each morning until surgery completed or radiotherapy started
- maintain on 8mg PO each morning until the completion of radiotherapy
- taper (and discontinue) over 1–2 weeks after the completion of radiotherapy or surgery.

If there is neurological deterioration during the dose reduction, the dose should be increased again to the previous satisfactory dose, and maintained at that level for a further 2 weeks before attempting to taper the dose again. About 1/4 require maintenance **dexamethasone** in order to preserve neural function.

Very high initial doses of **dexamethasone** (96–100mg stat and once daily for 3 days, then tapering to zero over 2 weeks) are not justified. They provide little or no more benefit than 16mg, but are associated with a definite risk of a major adverse event (>10%), particularly acute GI perforation (3%, at any level from the stomach to the sigmoid colon), GI haemorrhage, and sepsis, and possibly even death.[24]

For pharmacokinetic details, see Table 1.

Box B Approximate equivalent anti-inflammatory doses of corticosteroids[a]

Cortisone acetate	25mg
Hydrocortisone	20mg
Prednisone	5mg
Prednisolone	5mg
Methylprednisolone	4mg
Triamcinolone	4mg
Betamethasone	750microgram
Dexamethasone	750microgram

a. this list takes no account of either mineralocorticoid effects or variations in duration of action.

Cautions

Diabetes mellitus, psychotic illness. There is a small overall increased risk of GI bleed or perforation from the use of corticosteroids alone compared with placebo (2.9% vs. 2%; OR 1.42, 95%CI 1.22–1.66).[27] This is mostly explained by their high occurrence in hospitalized patients (38 vs. 26 per 1,000 patients), probably because of the association between severe illness and stress ulceration. In ambulatory patients, their occurrence was low (1.8 vs. 0.7 per 1,000 patients) with no significant difference in risk. *However, there is a 15 times increase in risk when corticosteroids are given concurrently with NSAIDs* (see p.316).[28–30]

Prolonged courses of corticosteroids increase susceptibility to infections and their severity. Clinical presentation may be atypical; the signs of infection (including peritonitis) may be masked.

Table 1 Selected pharmacokinetic details of commonly used corticosteroids[25,26]

Drug	*Anti-inflammatory potency*	*Approximate equivalent dose (mg)*	*Sodium-retaining potency*	*Oral bio-availability (%)*	*Onset of action*	*Peak plasma concentration*	*Plasma halflife (h)*	*Duration of action (h)*	*Relative affinity for lung tissue*	*Daily dose (mg) above which adrenal suppression possible*	
										Male	*Female*
Hydrocortisone	1	20	1	96	No data	1h PO	1.5	8–12	1	20–30	15–25
Prednisone[a] and prednisolone	4	5	0.25	75–85	No data	1h PO	3.5	12–36	1.6	7.5–10	7.5
Dexamethasone Betamethasone	25–50[b]	0.5–1	<0.01	78 98	8–24h IM[c] No data	1–2h PO 10–36min IV	4.5 6.5	36–54 24–48	1	1–1.15	1

a. biologically inert prednisone is converted by the liver to prednisolone

b. thymic involution assay

c. acute allergic reactions.

Serious infections (e.g. septicaemia and tuberculosis, pneumocystis pneumonia) may reach an advanced stage before diagnosis. Live vaccines should not be given; the antibody response to other vaccines may be diminished.[31]

In patients who have taken >10mg **prednisolone** (or equivalent) daily for 3 weeks, the occurrence of any significant intercurrent illness, trauma or surgical procedure necessitates a temporary increase in corticosteroid dose (or, if stopped within the past 3 months, a temporary re-introduction) to compensate for a reduced adrenocortical response caused by the corticosteroid treatment.[32]

Drug interactions

Corticosteroids antagonize oral hypoglycaemics and **insulin** (glucocorticoid effect), antihypertensives and diuretics (mineralocorticoid effect). Increased risk of hypokalaemia if high doses of corticosteroids are prescribed with β_2 agonists (e.g. **salbutamol**, **terbutaline**).

CYP3A4 is important in the metabolism of most corticosteroids and caution is required with the concurrent use of drugs which inhibit or induce this enzyme (see Chapter 19, Table 8, p.725). Reports of interactions include:

- **itraconazole** (potent CYP3A4 inhibitor) decreases the metabolism of corticosteroids, e.g. for **dexamethasone** this increases the area under the plasma concentration-time curve and maximum plasma concentration by up to 3-fold
- **carbamazepine**, **phenobarbital**, **phenytoin**, **primidone, rifabutin**, **rifampicin** (potent CYP3A4 inducers) increase the metabolism of corticosteroids. This is more pronounced with long-acting glucocorticoids; thus **phenytoin** may reduce the bio-availability of **dexamethasone** to 25–50%, and larger doses (double or more) will be needed when prescribed concurrently.[33]

Dexamethasone itself can affect plasma **phenytoin** concentrations (may either rise or fall). Concurrent prescription of a corticosteroid increases the INR in patients already taking **warfarin**, necessitating a dose reduction in about 50% of patients.[34] Thus, the INR should be checked weekly for 2–3 weeks when a corticosteroid is started or dose altered.

Undesirable effects

See Box C–Box F.

Box C Undesirable effects of corticosteroids[29]

Glucocorticoid effects

Avascular bone necrosis
Cataract (prednisolone 15mg/24h or equivalent for several years = 75% risk; also seen with long-term inhaled steroids)[35]
Diabetes mellitus or deterioration of glycaemic control in known diabetics (see p.539)
Infection (increased susceptibility):
candidosis (debatable, see p.475)
septicaemia (may delay recognition)
tuberculosis (may delay recognition)
PCP pneumonia
chickenpox[a], measles (increased severity)
Mental disturbances (Box D)
Muscle wasting and weakness (Box E)
Osteoporosis
Peptic ulceration (particularly if given with an NSAID)
Suppression of growth (in child)

Mineralocorticoid effects

Sodium and water retention → oedema
Potassium loss
Hypertension

Cushingoid features

Lipodystrophy after ≥8 weeks of treatment in 30–70% of patients (reversible on stopping treatment):
moon face
buffalo hump
increased abdominal fat
reduced subcutaneous fat in limbs
Acne
Bruising
Hirsuitism
Striae

a. if exposed to infection, non-immune patients should be given varicella-zoster immunoglobulin.[32]

Box D Corticosteroid-induced psychiatric disturbances[36–38]

Incidence

Reports range from 13–62% of those prescribed a corticosteroid.
Prevalence is higher in women, and more likely with higher doses.

Clinical manifestations

Symptoms generally occur 4–6 days after starting a corticosteroid, but this is highly variable and can occur even after cessation of treatment.

Manifestations are mostly mild or moderate, but can be severe, and include:

- depression (40%)
- mania (25%)
- paranoid ('steroid') psychosis (15%)
- delirium (10%)
- bipolar disorder (5%).

Educating patients about the possible risk of undesirable psychiatric effects may improve the reporting of symptoms.

Management

Reduce or discontinue the causal corticosteroid if possible.[36]
Environmental conditions should be optimized to minimize agitation.[39] Symptoms may take 1–2 weeks to resolve.[37]
If the corticosteroid cannot be stopped, or symptoms are intolerable, atypical antipsychotics should be prescribed for patients with psychosis, aggression or agitation.
Although antidepressants may exacerbate agitation and psychosis, they are generally helpful in depressed patients who require long-term corticosteroids.
All patients with corticosteroid-induced psychiatric disturbance should be evaluated for suicidal ideation.

Prognosis

A history of:

- psychiatric disease does not make a corticosteroid-induced psychiatric disturbance more likely
- previous corticosteroid-induced disturbance does not necessarily mean that a second disturbance will occur if corticosteroids are represcribed.[38]

Box E Systemic corticosteroid myopathy[40,41]

Glucocorticoids cause atrophy of limb and respiratory muscles. It is a dose-related effect which generally manifests only after ≥2 months of treatment with dexamethasone >4mg/24h or prednisolone >40mg/24h. Can occur earlier and with lower doses.

If the chronological sequence fits with corticosteroid myopathy, a presumptive diagnosis should be made and the following steps taken:

- explanation to patient and family
- discuss need to compromise between maximizing therapeutic benefit and minimizing undesirable effects
- halve corticosteroid dose (generally possible as a single step)
- consider changing from dexamethasone to prednisolone (non-fluorinated corticosteroids cause less myopathy)
- attempt further reductions in dose at intervals of 1–2 weeks
- arrange for physiotherapy (disuse exacerbates myopathy)
- emphasize that weakness should improve after 3–4 weeks (provided cancer-induced weakness does not supervene).

Box F Pseudorheumatism

Patients receiving corticosteroids for rheumatoid arthritis occasionally develop myalgia, arthralgia, malaise, rhinitis, conjunctivitis, painful itchy skin nodules, weight loss and pyrexia; so-called steroid pseudorheumatism.[42]

It is sometimes also seen in cancer patients receiving large doses of corticosteroids or when a very high dose is reduced rapidly to a lower dose. Most likely to be affected are those:

- receiving 100mg of prednisolone/24h for several days in association with chemotherapy
- with spinal cord compression given dexamethasone 96mg IV/24h for 3 days[43] (followed by a rapidly reducing oral dose)[a]
- on high doses of dexamethasone to reduce raised intracranial pressure associated with brain metastases
- reducing to an ordinary maintenance dose after a prolonged course.

a. such a high dose is unnecessary; 10mg IV is as effective as 96mg.[24]

Dose and use

Given the many and significant undesirable effects of corticosteroids, and the potentially deleterious effect of rapid withdrawal, corticosteroids should be prescribed cautiously:

- for defined symptoms potentially responsive to corticosteroid therapy
- always bearing in mind potential benefit vs. risk
- at a low–moderate dose, titrated to clinical effect
- for a time-limited trial
- discontinued if no clinical/symptomatic benefit seen *or*
- weaned to the lowest effective dose.[44]

Further:

- monitor blood glucose before starting, and regularly during treatment (e.g. every 1–2 weeks), particularly in patients at risk of diabetes (also see Box B, Drugs for diabetes, p.539)
- prescribe a PPI if patient is at high risk of peptic ulceration or bleeding, e.g. past history of either, acutely unwell, concurrent NSAID use (also see p.316)
- if expected to take corticosteroids for ≥3 weeks, give patients a *Steroid Treatment* card (Box G).

Box G Example of a *Steroid Treatment* card

I am a patient on STEROID treatment which must not be stopped suddenly.

- If you have been taking this medicine for more than 3 weeks, the dose should be reduced gradually when you stop taking steroids unless your doctor says otherwise.
- Read the patient information leaflet given with the medicine.
- Always carry this card with you and show it to anyone who treats you (for example a doctor, nurse, pharmacist, or dentist).
- For 1 year after you stop the treatment, you must mention that you have taken steroids.
- If you become ill, or if you come into contact with anyone who has an infectious disease, consult your doctor promptly.
- If you have never had chickenpox, you should avoid close contact with people who have chickenpox or shingles. If you do come into contact with chickenpox, see your doctor urgently.
- Make sure that the information on the card about your current dose is kept up to date.

For corticosteroid replacement therapy (e.g. in hypo-adrenalism), a typical regimen is **hydrocortisone** 20mg each morning, 10mg each evening with **fludrocortisone** 100–300microgram each morning.

Except for **hydrocortisone**, corticosteroids can be given in a single daily dose each morning. However, when 'tablet burden' is an issue, higher doses of **dexamethasone** (i.e. >8mg) can be halved and administered as a morning and a lunchtime dose. Giving doses later in the day should be generally avoided, as this increases the risk of corticosteroid-induced adrenal suppression and insomnia. Nonetheless, even with morning doses, **temazepam** or **diazepam** at bedtime is sometimes needed to counter insomnia or agitation.

PO

In palliative care, **dexamethasone** is generally the systemic corticosteroid of choice for anti-emesis, anorexia, raised intracranial pressure, obstruction of a hollow viscus and spinal cord compression. The initial dose varies according to indication (Table 2). For more information about dose adjustment and duration of treatment, see the relevant sections in Pharmacology above.

Table 2 Typical PO and SC/IV starting doses for dexamethasone, expressed as dexamethasone base[a]

Indication	*PO dose*	*SC/IV dose (volume)*	
		3.3mg/mL formulation	*3.8mg/mL formulation*
Anorexia[b]	2–6mg[9,45]	1.7–5mg (0.5–1.5mL)	1.9–5.7mg (0.5–1.5mL)
Anti-emetic[c]	8–16mg[14,46,47]	6.6–13.2mg (2–4mL)	7.6–15.2mg (2–4mL)
Obstruction of hollow viscus	8–16mg[5]	6.6–13.2mg (2–4mL)	7.6–15.2mg (2–4mL)
Raised intracranial pressure	8–16mg[48]	6.6–13.2mg (2–4mL)	7.6–15.2mg (2–4mL)
Spinal cord compression	16mg	13.2mg (4mL)	15.2mg (4mL)

a. generally given once daily in the morning (see text)

b. prednisolone 15–40mg each morning is an alternative

c. also see QCG: nausea and vomiting, p.240.

SC/IV

In the UK, **dexamethasone** is available in injectable formulations as the *sodium phosphate* salt. However, all dosing advice, prescribing and labelling must now be expressed as **dexamethasone** *base*.[49,50]

There is further potential for confusion because different brands of injection vary in their strength, presentation, preservative/solvent content and storage requirement. For more details, see Supply, Table 3.[51]

All the injectable formulations are suitable for SC use.

In palliative care, **dexamethasone** is traditionally given SC rather than IM/IV with the initial dose varying according to indication and strength of the injectable formulation (see Table 2).

Traditionally, for ease of prescribing, conversion of PO to SC/IV **dexamethasone** was made on a 1:1 basis (e.g. 4mg PO = 4mg SC/IV). Following recent labelling and formulation changes, the injectable formulations contain either 3.3mg/mL or 3.8mg/mL **dexamethasone** *base* (see Tables 2 and 3). Thus, continuing with an exact 1:1 conversion will lead to an unnecessarily complex and wasteful use of the ampoules and vials. Because the conversion between PO and SC/IV **dexamethasone** only requires the selection of a reasonable starting dose, *PCF* recommends that:

- for pragmatic purposes, when converting between PO and SC/IV routes, both 3.3mg and 3.8mg **dexamethasone** *base* of the injectable formulations can be considered approximately equivalent to **dexamethasone** *base* 4mg PO
- the SC/IV dose prescribed should take into account which injectable formulation is being used so as to avoid wasteful use of the vials/ampoules (see Tables 2 and 3)
- the dose should be subsequently titrated according to response
- *for consistency and to avoid confusion between colleagues and departments, clinicians should observe local guidelines and use the locally available injection formulation.*

Betamethasone *base* 4mg/mL injection provides an alternative of similar potency to **dexamethasone**. However, there is no cost advantage and there is less experience of its use.

CSCI

CSCI compatibility of dexamethasone with other drugs: Because it is an alkaline drug, therapeutic doses of **dexamethasone** often cause compatibility problems. To minimize the risk of precipitation, it should always be the last drug added to an already dilute combination of drugs. In addition, different injectable formulations may react differently when mixed (see p.817).

Dexamethasone has a long duration of action; therapeutic doses can generally be given as a bolus SC injection once daily, which avoids the risk of precipitation (see p.817).

To reduce CSCI site reactions, **dexamethasone** 1mg is sometimes added to other drugs, when compatibility data permits (see p.825).

Rectal use

For discharge from rectal tumour or acute post-radiation proctitis, use a retention enema of **hydrocortisone acetate** 125mg PR or **prednisolone** 20mg PR every 1–2 days. If local application is impractical, PO corticosteroids can be used instead.

Other uses

For use in the management of anaphylaxis, see p.851.
For inhaled corticosteroids, see p.126.
For depot corticosteroid injections, see p.599.
For topical corticosteroids, see p.629.

Stopping corticosteroids

If after 7–10 days the corticosteroid fails to achieve the desired effect, it should be stopped. It is often possible to stop corticosteroids abruptly (Box H).

However, if there is uncertainty about disease or symptom resolution, withdrawal should be guided by monitoring disease activity or the symptom.

Particularly if it has been taken for >3 weeks, rapid withdrawal of a corticosteroid may result in a corticosteroid withdrawal syndrome. This may cause an array of symptoms and signs similar to those of pseudorheumatism (Box F) together with adrenal insufficiency. The syndrome is treated by restarting the corticosteroid or increasing the dose to that given before the onset of withdrawal symptoms.[52]

In patients who are moribund and no longer able to swallow tablets, it is generally acceptable to discontinue corticosteroids abruptly,[44] although sometimes a maintenance dose may be indicated to prevent distress from symptomatic hypo-adrenalism.

Box H Recommendations for withdrawing systemic corticosteroids[32]

Abrupt withdrawal

Systemic corticosteroids may be stopped abruptly in those whose disease is unlikely to relapse *and* have received treatment for <3 weeks *and* are not in the groups below.

Gradual withdrawal

Gradual withdrawal of systemic corticosteroids is advisable in patients who:

- have received >3 weeks treatment
- have received prednisolone >40mg/24h or equivalent, e.g. dexamethasone 4–6mg for > one week
- have had a second dose in the evening
- have received repeated treatments
- are taking a short course within 1 year of stopping long-term treatment
- have other possible causes of adrenal suppression.

During corticosteroid withdrawal the dose may initially be reduced rapidly (e.g. halving the dose daily) to physiological doses (prednisolone 7.5mg/24h or equivalent) and then more slowly (e.g. 1–2mg per week) to allow the adrenals to recover and to prevent a hypo-adrenal crisis (malaise, profound weakness, hypotension, etc.). The patient should be monitored during withdrawal in case of deterioration.

If physiological stress, e.g. from infection, trauma, surgery, occurs within 1 week of stopping the corticosteroid, additional corticosteroid cover should be prescribed to compensate for adrenal suppression.

Occasionally, a patient with a brain tumour or multiple brain metastases requests that **dexamethasone** is stopped because, despite its continued use, there is progressive physical deterioration and/or cognitive impairment. In this circumstance, it is often best to reduce the **dexamethasone** step by step on a daily basis. This gives the patient time to reconsider. *Ensure appropriate analgesia is prescribed in case headache develops as the intracranial pressure increases.* If the patient becomes drowsy or swallowing becomes difficult, switch PO anti-epileptics to one which can be given parenterally, e.g. **midazolam** (see p.158), **levetiracetam** (see p.287), **valproate** (see p.282) or **phenobarbital** (see p.289).

If the patient becomes semicomatose and cannot communicate clearly, the presence of headache may manifest as grimacing or general restlessness. However, as in all moribund patients, it is important to exclude other common reasons for agitation, e.g. a full bladder or rectum, and discomfort and stiffness secondary to immobility.

Supply

Dexamethasone formulations in the UK

PO tablets are formulated as **dexamethasone** *base*; the oral solution and injectable formulations are formulated as **dexamethasone** *sodium phosphate*. BNF, SPCs and product labels now all use **dexamethasone** *base* for labelling and dosing advice.

Dexamethasone (generic)
Tablets 500microgram, 2mg, 28 days @ 2mg once daily = £24.
Oral solution (sugar-free) 2mg/5mL, 10mg/5mL, 20mg/5mL, 28 days @ 2mg (5mL) once daily = £40.
(In countries where an oral solution of dexamethasone is not available, the contents of an ampoule for injection can be used PO.)
Injection see Table 3.

Table 3 Dexamethasone injectable formulations (UK)[50,53]

	Aspen	*Hameln*	*Hospira/Pfizer*
Dexamethasone base	3.8mg/mL[a]	3.3mg/mL[b]	3.3mg/mL[b]
Presentation (all glass)	1mL vial	1mL, 2mL amp	1mL amp, 2mL vial
Storage	Refrigerate at 2–8°C	<25°C	<25°C
Other[c]		Contains propylene glycol 20mg/mL	2mL vial contains sodium sulphite 0.07mg/mL
Cost	£2	1mL, £1.25 2mL, £2.25	1mL, £2.50 2mL, £5

a. dexamethasone base 3.8mg ≈ dexamethasone sodium phosphate 5mg
b. dexamethasone base 3.3mg ≈ dexamethasone sodium phosphate 4.3mg
c. all formulations except the 1mL Hospira ampoule contain disodium edetate.

Betamethasone (generic)
Tablets (soluble) 500microgram, 28 days @ 2mg once daily = £48.
Injection betamethasone 4mg/mL (base) 1mL = £3.

Hydrocortisone (generic)
Tablets 10mg, 20mg 28days @ 20mg each morning and 10mg each evening = £168.

Colifoam® (Meda)
Retention foam enema hydrocortisone acetate 10% (100mg/mL), 1 metered application = 125mg **hydrocortisone *acetate***, 14-application cannister with applicator = £9.

Fludrocortisone (generic)
Tablets 100microgram, 28 days @ 100microgram each morning = £28.

Prednisolone (generic)
Tablets 1mg, 2.5mg, 5mg, 10mg, 20mg, 25mg, 30mg, 28 days @ 15mg once daily = £3.
Tablets e/c 1mg, 2.5mg, 5mg, 28 days @ 15mg once daily = £3.50.
Tablets soluble 5mg, 28 days @ 15mg once daily = £160.
Retention foam enema **prednisolone** (as ***metasulfobenzoate sodium***) 20mg/metered application, 14-application canister with applicators = £187.
Suppositories **prednisolone** (as ***sodium phosphate***) 5mg, 10 = £39.

Predsol® (Focus)
Retention enema **prednisolone** (as ***sodium phosphate***) 20mg in 100mL, 7-single enemas = £7.50.

Note. ***Budesonide*** *rectal products are also available.*

1 Hardy J *et al.* (2001) A prospective survey of the use of dexamethasone on a palliative care unit. *Palliative Medicine*. **15**: 3–8.
2 NICE (2014) Metastatic spinal cord compression. *Clinical Guideline* CG75. www.nice.org.uk
3 Rowell NP and Gleeson FV (2002) Steroids, radiotherapy, chemotherapy and stents for superior vena caval obstruction in carcinoma of the bronchus: a systematic review. *Clinical Oncology (Royal College of Radiologists)*. **14**: 338–351.
4 Elsayem A and Bruera E (2007) High-dose corticosteroids for the management of dyspnea in patients with tumor obstruction of the upper airway. *Supportive Care in Cancer*. **15**: 1437–1439.
5 Feuer DJ and Broadley KE (2009) Corticosteroids for the resolution of malignant bowel obstruction in advanced gynaecological and gastrointestinal cancer. *Cochrane Database of Systematic Reviews*. CD001219. www.thecochranelibrary.com
6 Laval G *et al.* (2000) The use of steroids in the management of inoperable intestinal obstruction in terminal cancer patients: do they remove the obstruction? *Palliative Medicine*. **14**: 3–10.
7 Yousef AA and El-Mashad NM (2014) Pre-emptive value of methylprednisolone intravenous infusion in patients with vertebral metastases. A double-blind randomized study. *Journal of Pain and Symptom Management*. **48**: 762–769.
8 Ndibe C *et al.* (2015) Corticosteroids in the management of prostate cancer: a critical review. *Current Treatment Options in Oncology*. **16**: 6.
9 Haywood A *et al.* (2015) Corticosteroids for the management of cancer-related pain in adults. *Cochrane Database of Systematic Reviews*. **4**: CD010756. www.thecochranelibrary.com
10 Paulsen O *et al.* (2014) Efficacy of methylprednisolone on pain, fatigue, and appetite loss in patients with advanced cancer using opioids: a randomized, placebo-controlled, double-blind trial. *Journal of Clinical Oncology*. **32**: 3221–3228.
11 Rhen T and Cidlowski JA (2005) Antiinflammatory action of glucocorticoids--new mechanisms for old drugs. *New England Journal of Medicine*. **353**: 1711–1723.
12 Lundstrom S *et al.* (2009) The existential impact of starting corticosteroid treatment as symptom control in advanced metastatic cancer. *Palliative Medicine*. **23**: 165–170.
13 Miller S *et al.* (2014) Use of corticosteroids for anorexia in palliative medicine: a systematic review. *Journal of Palliative Medicine*. **17**: 4824–4825.
14 Navari RM and Aapro M (2016) Antiemetic prophylaxis for chemotherapy-induced nausea and vomiting. *New England Journal of Medicine*. **374**: 1356–1367.
15 Chu CC *et al.* (2014) The cellular mechanisms of the antiemetic action of dexamethasone and related glucocorticoids against vomiting. *European Journal of Pharmacology*. **722**: 48–54.
16 Glare PA *et al.* (2008) Treatment of nausea and vomiting in terminally ill cancer patients. *Drugs*. **68**: 2575–2590.
17 Davis MP *et al.* (2010) A systematic review of the treatment of nausea and/or vomiting in cancer unrelated to chemotherapy or radiation. *Journal of Pain and Symptom Management*. **39**: 756–767.
18 Bruera E *et al.* (2004) Dexamethasone in addition to metoclopramide for chronic nausea in patients with advanced cancer: a randomized controlled trial. *Journal of Pain and Symptom Management*. **28**: 381–388.
19 Vecht C *et al.* (1994) Dose-effect relationship of dexamethasone on Karnofsky performance in metastatic brain tumors. A randomized study of doses of 4, 8 and 16 mg per day. *Neurology*. **44**: 675–680.
20 Soffieri R *et al.* (2011) Brain Metastases. In: Gilhus NE *et al.* (eds). *European Handbook of Neurological Management*. Volume 1. (2e). Blackwell Publishing Ltd.
21 Tsao MN (2015) Brain metastases: advances over the decades. *Annals of Palliative Medicine*. **4**: 225–232.
22 Cowap J *et al.* (2000) Outcome of malignant spinal cord compression at a cancer center: implications for palliative care services. *Journal of Pain and Symptom Management*. **19**: 257–264.
23 da Silva GT *et al.* (2015) Prognostic factors in patients with metastatic spinal cord compression secondary to lung cancer: a systematic review of the literature. *European Spine Jourmal*. **24**: 2107-2113.
24 George R *et al.* (2015) Interventions for the treatment of metastatic extradural spinal cord compression in adults. *Cochrane Database of Systematic Reviews*. **9**: CD006716. www.thecochranelibrary.com
25 Swartz S and Dluhy R (1978) Corticosteroids: clinical pharmacology and therapeutic use. *Drugs*. **16**: 238–255.
26 Demoly P and Chung K (1998) Pharmacology of corticosteroids. *Respiratory Medicine*. **92**: 385–394.
27 Narum S *et al.* (2014) Corticosteroids and risk of gastrointestinal bleeding: a systematic review and meta-analysis. *BMJ Open*. **4**: e004587.
28 Ellershaw J and Kelly M (1994) Corticosteroids and peptic ulceration. *Palliative Medicine*. **8**: 313–319.
29 Fardet L *et al.* (2007) Corticosteroid-induced adverse events in adults: frequency, screening and prevention. *Drug Safety*. **30**: 861–881.
30 Piper JM *et al.* (1991) Corticosteroid use and peptic ulcer disease: role of nonsteroidal anti-inflammatory drugs. *Annals of Internal Medicine*. **114**: 735–740.
31 Yamaguchi T *et al.* (2014) Pneumocystis pneumonia in patients treated with long-term steroid therapy for symptom palliation: a neglected infection in palliative care. *American Journal of Hospice and Palliative Care*. **31**: 857–861.
32 British National Formulary Section 6 Corticosreroids. London: BMJ Group and Pharmaceutical Press www.medicinescomplete.com (accessed July 2017).

33 Chalk J *et al.* (1984) Phenytoin impairs the bioavailability of dexamethasone in neurological and neurosurgical patients. *Journal of Neurology, Neurosurgery, and Psychiatry*. **47**: 1087–1090.
34 Hazlewood KA *et al.* (2006) Effect of oral corticosteroids on chronic warfarin therapy. *Annals of Pharmacotherapy*. **40**: 2101–2106.
35 Jick S *et al.* (2001) The risk of cataract among users of inhaled steroids. *Epidemiology*. **12**: 229–234.
36 Warrington TP and Bostwick JM (2006) Psychiatric adverse effects of corticosteroids. *Mayo Clinic Proceedings*. **81**: 1361–1367.
37 Brown ES and Suppes T (1998) Mood symptoms during corticosteroid therapy: a review. *Harvard Review of Psychiatry*. **5**: 239–246.
38 Stiefel FC *et al.* (1989) Corticosteroids in cancer: neuropsychiatric complications. *Cancer Investigation*. **7**: 479–491.
39 Twycross R and Wilcock A (eds) (2016) *Introducing Palliative Care* (5e). palliativedrugs.com, Nottingham, pp. 199–200.
40 Eidelberg D (1991) Steroid myopathy. In: DA Rottenberg (ed) *Neurological Complications of Cancer Treatment*. Butterworth-Heineman, Boston, pp. 185–191.
41 Schakman O *et al.* (2008) Mechanisms of glucocorticoid-induced myopathy. *Journal of Endocrinology*. **197**: 1–10.
42 Rotstein J and Good R (1957) Steroid pseudorheumatism. *AMA Archives of Internal Medicine*. **99**: 545–555.
43 Greenberg H *et al.* (1979) Epidural spinal cord compression from metastatic tumour: results with a new treatment protocol. *Annals of Neurology*. **8**: 361–366.
44 Rousseau P (2004) Sudden withdrawal of corticosteroids: a commentary. *American Journal of Hospice and Palliative Care*. **21**: 169–171.
45 Willox JC *et al.* (1984) Prednisolone as an appetite stimulant in patients with cancer. *British Medical Journal*. **288**: 27.
46 Gralla R *et al.* (1999) Recommendations for the use of antiemetics: evidence-based, clinical practice guidelines. *Journal of Clinical Oncology*. **17**: 2971–2994.
47 Editorial (1991) Ondansetron versus dexamethasone for chemotherapy-induced emesis. *Lancet*. **338**: 478.
48 Kirkham S (1988) The palliation of cerebral tumours with high-dose dexamethasone: a review. *Palliative Medicine*. **2**: 27–33.
49 MHRA (2014) Dexamethasone 4mg/mL injection (Organon Laboratories Limited) reformulation with changes in name, concentration, storage conditions, and presentation. *Drug Safety Update*. **3**: www.mhra.gov.uk/Safetyinformation
50 UK Medicines Information (2014) Dexamethasone injection. *In use product safety assessment report*. www.ukmi.nhs.uk
51 Palliativedrugs.com (2014) Use of dexamethasone formulations in palliative care: a palliativedrugs.com reponse to recent changes. *News (December)*. www.palliativedrugs.com
52 Margolin L *et al.* (2007) The steroid withdrawal syndrome: a review of the implications, etiology, and treatments. *Journal of Pain and Symptom Management*. **33**: 224–228.
53 MHRA (2014) Dexamethasone 4mg/mL injection (organon Laboratories Limited: reformulation with changes in name, concentration storage conditions, and presentation. *Drug Safety Update*. **3**: www.mhra.gov.uk/Safetyinformation

Updated September 2017

DEMECLOCYCLINE

Class: Tetracycline antibacterial and vasopressin receptor antagonist.

Indications: Symptomatic hyponatraemia caused by paraneoplastic syndrome of inappropriate antidiuretic hormone secretion (SIADH).

Contra-indications: Patients with hypovolaemic hyponatraemia, e.g. caused by severe diarrhoea, vomiting, or adrenal insufficiency.

Pathogenesis and clinical features of SIADH

There are many causes of SIADH, including a range of drugs (Box A). In paraneoplastic SIADH, there is ectopic secretion of arginine vasopressin (antidiuretic hormone, ADH) or vasopressin-like peptides by the cancer.[1] In small cell lung cancer (SCLC), an elevated arginine vasopressin can be detected in about 40% of patients, although in most it is asymptomatic.

Hyponatraemia (with consequential intracellular cerebral oedema), possibly caused by SIADH, should be considered in all patients who develop drowsiness, confusion or seizures while taking a TCA or SSRI. Risk factors for the development of SIADH with SSRIs include older age, female gender, low body weight and concurrent use of diuretics.[2]

Clinical features of SIADH depend on both the level and the rate of decline of the plasma sodium concentration (Box B). Asymptomatic hyponatraemia indicates chronic rather than acute SIADH. Treatment is necessary only if the hyponatraemia is symptomatic.

If suspected, paired urine and serum samples should be obtained from the patient. The diagnosis of SIADH is based on the following criteria:

- hyponatraemia (<130mmol/L)
- low plasma osmolality (<270mosmol/L)
- urine osmolality >300mosmol/L (i.e. higher than plasma osmolality)
- urine sodium concentration always >20mmol/L, and generally >40mmol/L
- normal or moderately expanded plasma volume.

Box A Causes of SIADH

Cancer	Miscellaneous
Acute myeloid leukaemia	Central nervous system
Carcinoid	cerebral thrombosis
Head and neck	encephalitis
Lymphoma	head injury
Pancreas	meningitis
Prostate	subarachnoid haemorrhage
Small cell lung	Psychiatric
	psychosis
Treatment	schizophrenia
Chemotherapy, e.g.	Pulmonary
cyclophosphamide	lung abscess
vincristine	pneumonia
Drugs	positive pressure ventilation
barbiturates	tuberculosis
carbamazepine	Recreational drugs
lorazepam	ethanol
phenothiazines	nicotine
SSRIs	
TCAs	
Post-neurosurgery	

7

Box B Clinical features of SIADH

Plasma sodium 110–120mmol/L	Plasma sodium <110mmol/L
Anorexia	Multifocal myoclonus
Nausea and vomiting	Drowsiness
Lassitude	Seizures
Confusion	Coma

Urine osmolality <300mosm/L but >100mosm/L may be consistent with a diagnosis of SIADH if there is co-existent renal tubular dysfunction, diuretic use or reset osmostat syndrome. In such cases, a raised urine sodium concentration (>30mmol/L) is more diagnostically reliable.[3,4]

In practice, a plasma sodium concentration of ≤120mmol/L is sufficient to make a clinical diagnosis of SIADH in the absence of:

- severe vomiting
- diuretic therapy
- hypo-adrenalism
- hypothyroidism
- severe renal impairment.

Pharmacology

Demeclocycline is a tetracycline derivative. It induces nephrogenic diabetes insipidus, i.e. inhibits the action of ADH on renal tubules, probably by antagonism of arginine-vasopressin V_2-receptors.[5] There are at least three arginine-vasopressin receptor subtypes. V_2-receptors are concentrated in renal collecting tubules where antagonism leads to aquaresis, i.e. the excretion of water without significantly changing the total level of electrolyte excretion. V_2-receptors also occur in vascular endothelium where antagonism results in vasodilation.

The European Society of Endocrinology guideline states that, in paraneoplastic SIADH, demeclocycline should be used only if fluid restriction and other options are ineffective.[5] However, in palliative care, fluid restriction to 700–1,000mL/24h (or a daily urine output of <500mL) is burdensome, and treatment with demeclocycline is generally preferable. The effect of demeclocycline is often apparent after 2–5 days, and persists for several days after stopping

treatment. There is no need to restrict fluid during treatment. It is effective in about 60% of patients with SIADH.[6]
Bio-availability 60–80%.
Onset of action 2–5days.
Time to peak plasma concentration 3–4h.
Plasma halflife 12h.
Duration of action several days.

Tolvaptan is a recently introduced alternative arginine-vasopressin V_2-receptor antagonist (Box C).

Box C Tolvaptan (Samsca®)

Tolvaptan is an alternative arginine-vasopressin V_2-receptor antagonist (VRA).[7,8] It decreases expression of aquaporin channels in the renal collecting ducts, resulting in increased free water clearance. Authorization differs in Europe and the USA (see country-specific SPCs/ Package Inserts).

European guidelines do not recommend tolvaptan for treatment of SIADH.[5] This is in contrast to American guidelines which recommend a limited role for tolvaptan in SIADH.[9,10]

Tolvaptan is contra-indicated in anuria, in patients with hypovolaemic hyponatraemia, and should not be used for treatment of patients with severe cerebral symptoms of SIADH. Tolvaptan may attenuate the effects of vasopressin analogues, e.g. desmopressin, used to control bleeding.[11]

RCTs of tolvaptan for patients with SIADH have generally excluded patients with a plasma sodium of <120mmol/L. Plasma sodium concentration increased by 3–5mmol/L after 4 days. After 1 month, there was a mean increase of 7mmol/L, and over 60% of patients achieved a normal plasma sodium.[12]

The impact of tolvaptan on long-term morbidity or mortality in SIADH of any cause is not known, although one study demonstrated acceptable safety in patients with various causes of hyponatraemia after 4 years.[8,13] Tolvaptan has *not* been compared with fluid restriction and/ or demeclocyline.

Patients with paraneoplastic SIADH may be more sensitive to tolvaptan, necessitating a lower starting dose, e.g. 15mg on alternate days.[14] With doses >60mg/day, there is a risk of liver toxicity.[15] Patients receiving tolvaptan should *not* be fluid-restricted, and should *not* receive IV normal or hypertonic saline.[16]

Irreversible osmotic demyelination is a risk with any treatment which causes a too rapid rise in plasma sodium (increase ≥12mmol/L in 24h).[11] Risk factors for osmotic demyelination include a baseline plasma sodium <120mmol/L, malnutrition, hypokalaemia, hypoxia, advanced liver disease and excessive alcohol use. When starting tolvaptan, plasma sodium levels should be checked at least every 6h for the first 48h.

Tolvaptan is expensive (see supply), and the need to closely monitor plasma sodium will restrict the use of tolvaptan in palliative care. However, it may have a role in recurrent severe hyponatraemia unresponsive to fluid restriction and demeclocycline.[17]

Cautions

Renal and hepatic impairment; lower doses (e.g. maximum dose <1g/24h) advised to avoid excessive systemic accumulation.[6] Risk of photosensitivity; warn patients not to expose skin to direct sunlight or sunlamps.

Drug interactions

The absorption of demeclocycline is reduced by the concurrent administration of **iron**, **calcium**, **magnesium**, **aluminium** and **zinc**.

Demeclocycline depresses plasma prothrombin activity and, if used concurrently, the dose of **warfarin** may need to be reduced. Risk of oral contraceptive failure (as with all antibacterials). Avoid concurrent **penicillin** use (tetracyclines possibly antagonize the effect of penicillins).

Undesirable effects

Nausea, vomiting, diarrhoea, renal impairment, photosensitivity (see Cautions), oesophagitis, discolouration of teeth during tooth development.
Rare (<0.1%, >0.01%): acute renal failure or nephritis.

Dose and use

Treat the patient and not the biochemical results.
If feasible, stop the causal drug and/or treat the underlying cause.

If symptomatic and cause of SIADH irreversible:

- start with 300mg PO t.d.s. on an empty stomach, e.g. 1h before food; take with plenty of water in an upright position to reduce the risk of oesophagitis; avoid milk, antacids, **iron** and **zinc** preparations at the same time
- if necessary, increase to 300mg q.d.s. after 2 weeks
- recommended maintenance dose = 300mg b.d.–t.d.s., but 150mg b.d.–t.d.s. is adequate in some patients.

In patients unable to take drugs PO, demeclocycline can be given PR dispersed in 5mL of a methylcellulose carrier.[18] However, the powder may cause local irritation and inflammation.

7

Supply

Demeclocycline hydrochloride (generic)
Capsules 150mg, 28 days @ 300mg b.d. = £644.

Tolvaptan

Samsca® (Otsuka)
Tablets 15mg, 30mg, 28 days @ 15mg or 30mg daily = £2,100.

Jinarc® (Otsuka)
Tablets 15mg, 30mg, 45mg, 60mg, 90mg, 28 days @ 15mg or 30mg daily = £1,200.
Jinarc® is authorized for use in autosomal dominant polycystic kidney disease. Combination packs of different strength tablets also available.

1 Sorensen J *et al.* (1995) Syndrome of inappropriate secretion of antidiuretic hormone (SIADH) in malignant disease. *Journal of Internal Medicine.* **238**: 97–110.
2 Jacob S and Spinler SA (2006) Hyponatremia associated with selective serotonin-reuptake inhibitors in older adults. *Annals of Pharmacotherapy.* **40**: 1618–1622.
3 Smellie WS and Heald A (2007) Hyponatraemia and hypernatraemia: pitfalls in testing. *British Medical Journal.* **334**: 473–476.
4 Ellison DH and Berl T (2007) Clinical practice. The syndrome of inappropriate antidiuresis. *N Engl J Med.* **356**: 2064–2072.
5 Spasovski G *et al.* (2014) Clinical practice guideline on diagnosis and treatment of hyponatraemia. *European Journal of Endocrinology.* **170**: G1–47.
6 Miell J *et al.* (2015) Evidence for the use of demeclocycline in the treatment of hyponatraemia secondary to SIADH: a systematic review. *International Journal of Clinical Practice.* **69**: 1396–1417.
7 Schrier RW *et al.* (2006) Tolvaptan, a selective oral vasopressin V2-receptor antagonist, for hyponatremia. *New England Journal of Medicine.* **355**: 2099–2112.
8 Amin A and Meeran K (2010) New drugs for hyponatraemia. *British Medical Journal.* **341**: c6219.
9 Verbalis JG *et al.* (2013) Diagnosis, evaluation, and treatment of hyponatremia: expert panel recommendations. *American Journal of Medicine.* **126**: S1–42.
10 Berl T (2015) Vasopressin antagonists. *New England Journal Medicine.* **372**: 2207–2216.
11 MHRA (2012) Tolvaptan (Samsca): over-rapid increase in serum sodium risking serious neurological events. *Drug Safety Update.* https://www.gov.uk/drug-safety-update.
12 Verbalis JG *et al.* (2011) Efficacy and safety of oral tolvaptan therapy in patients with the syndrome of inappropriate antidiuretic hormone secretion. *European Journal of Endocrinology.* **164**: 725–732.
13 Berl T *et al.* (2010) Oral tolvaptan is safe and effective in chronic hyponatremia. *Journal of the American Society of Nephrology.* **21**: 705–712.
14 Kenz S *et al.* (2011) High sensitivity to tolvaptan in paraneoplastic syndrome of inappropriate ADH secretion (SIADH). *Annals of Oncology.* **22**: 2696.
15 MHRA (2013) Tolvaptan (Samsca): risk of liver injury. *Drug Safety Update.* https://www.gov.uk/drug-safety-update.
16 Peri A and Combe C (2012) Considerations regarding the management of hyponatraemia secondary to SIADH. *Best Practice and Research Clinical Endocrinology and Metabolism.* **26 Suppl 1**: S16–26.
17 Mumby C and Adam S (2012) Tolvaptan use in a patient with metastatic small cell lung cancer. *Lung Cancer.* **75**: S59–S60.
18 Hussain I *et al.* (1998) Rectal administration of demeclocycline in a patient with syndrome of inappropriate ADH secretion. *International Journal of Clinical Practice.* **52**: 59.

Updated (minor change) July 2017

DESMOPRESSIN

Class: Vasopressin analogue.

Indications: Authorized indications vary between formulations and products; consult SPCs for full details. Pituitary diabetes insipidus, nocturnal enuresis and nocturia, mild–moderate haemophilia and von Willebrand's disease, †'last resort' treatment for severe bleeding associated with platelet dysfunction.[1]

Contra-indications: Current or previous hyponatraemia (including SIADH), coronary insufficiency, unstable angina, hypertension, concurrent use with diuretics, psychogenic and alcohol abuse-related polydipsia, renal impairment (creatinine clearance <50mL/min), type 2B and platelet-type (pseudo) von Willebrand's disease. ***Intranasal***: multiple sclerosis age >65 years.

Pharmacology

Desmopressin is an analogue of the pituitary antidiuretic hormone, **vasopressin**. It stimulates arginine-vasopressin V_2-receptors in the medullary collecting tubules, increasing water resorption by the renal tubules, thereby reducing urine volume. The antidiuretic effect of desmopressin is 3–10 times greater than that of **vasopressin**, and it has a longer duration of action. Unlike **vasopressin**, it has no vasoconstrictor effect. Desmopressin is ineffective in nephrogenic diabetes insipidus.[2]

Desmopressin also stimulates V_2-receptors on endothelial cells, leading to the release of stored von Willebrand factor and factor VIII. This augments platelet function and enhances haemostasis; hence its use as a last resort in certain bleeding states, including those associated with severe renal or hepatic impairment.[1,3,4]

Bio-availability 3–4% intranasal; 0.1–0.2% PO.
Onset of action 1h intranasal; 2h PO.
Plasma halflife 0.4–4h intranasal; 2–3h PO.
Duration of action 5–24h intranasal; 6–8h PO.

Cautions

CHF, raised intracranial pressure, cystic fibrosis. Take care to avoid fluid overload because with excessive water intake there is an increased risk of hyponatraemia. The effect of desmopressin may be potentiated by drugs which cause fluid retention, e.g. NSAIDs and corticosteroids. In renal impairment, the antidiuretic effect is less. Avoid in moderate–severe renal impairment. Food may reduce the absorption of tablets.

Drug interactions

Loperamide triples the desmopressin plasma concentration after PO administration.[5] The concurrent use of drugs which increase the endogenous secretion of vasopressin increases the risk of symptomatic hyponatraemia, notably **carbamazepine**, **chlorpromazine**, **lamotrigine**, NSAIDs, opioids, SSRIs, TCAs.

Undesirable effects

Water retention and hyponatraemia is a risk particularly in patients treated with desmopressin for an indication other than pituitary diabetes insipidus. In extreme cases this may result in hyponatraemic seizures.

Common (<10%, >1%): tablets and high doses of nasal spray (≥40microgram/24h): headache, dizziness, dry mouth, abdominal pain, nausea. Nasal spray: nosebleeds, nasal congestion or rhinitis, sore throat. IV: facial flushing, tachycardia, mild transient systemic arterial hypotension.[1]

Rare or very rare (<0.1%): IV: increase in thrombo-embolic events, e.g. myocardial infarction,[1] aggression in children.

Dose and use

Desmopressin products for SL administration are known as oral lyophilisates. Although all desmopressin products contain desmopressin *acetate*, the SL products and oral solution are labelled with the dose expressed as desmopressin *base*.

Global post-marketing data indicate a higher incidence of hyponatraemia in patients treated intranasally compared with PO,[3] reflecting the more favourable intranasal pharmacokinetics.

To minimize the risk of symptomatic hyponatraemia, keep to the recommended starting doses and take precautions to avoid fluid overload:

- advise all patients to avoid drinking large amounts of fluid (including when swimming)
- restrict fluid to the minimum which satisfies thirst:
  - ▷ from 1h before until 8h after the dose given for enuresis/nocturia
  - ▷ continually with repeated doses for bleeding.

The monitoring required to detect fluid retention (weight, blood pressure) ± hyponatraemia (plasma sodium) varies between reason for use; *see SPC and obtain advice from an endocrinologist.*

Treatment should be stopped if plasma sodium concentration <135mmol/L. In addition, fluid should be restricted if any of the following develop:

- unusually severe or prolonged headache, nausea or vomiting, confusion (symptoms associated with hyponatraemia); *advise patient to seek immediate medical help*
- progressive increase in blood pressure and/or body weight
- plasma sodium concentration <130mmol/L
- plasma osmolality <270mosmol/kg.

When a patient has fully recovered from an episode of fluid overload, desmopressin can be restarted at an appropriate dose, with strict fluid restriction enforced.

When given for enuresis/nocturia, desmopressin should also be stopped during an acute intercurrent illness impacting on fluid/electrolyte balance, e.g. diarrhoea, vomiting.

Pituitary diabetes insipidus

Tablets (PO or SL) should be used first-line. The nasal spray should be used only when tablets are not suitable:

- start with 100microgram PO t.d.s., 60microgram SL t.d.s. (or 10–20microgram intranasally at bedtime)
- if necessary, increase dose progressively every few days
- effective dose is generally 100–400microgram PO t.d.s., 120–240microgram SL t.d.s. (or 10–20microgram intranasally at bedtime–b.d.).

A parenteral formulation for SC/IM/IV use (1–4microgram daily) is available if necessary.

Nocturnal enuresis and nocturia

Primary nocturnal enuresis (children >5years, adults <65years)[6]

Exclude other causes of nocturia, e.g. diabetes mellitus. Treat only with PO or SL tablets:

- start with 200microgram PO or 120microgram SL at bedtime
- if necessary, after 1–2 weeks, increase dose to 400microgram PO or 240microgram SL at bedtime.[2]

Note. Women are more sensitive to the effects of desmopressin and more likely to develop hyponatraemia. A lower starting dose of desmopressin may thus be advisable in women, particularly those with other risk factors for hyponatraemia.[7,8]

†Nocturia associated with overactive bladder or urinary incontinence in women

Elderly women may be more sensitive to desmopressin; avoid use in those >65 years with cardiovascular disease or hypertension. Give if insufficient response to an antimuscarinic alone:

- start with 50–100microgram PO at bedtime
- check plasma sodium pretreatment and after 3 days
- if necessary, after 1–2 weeks, increase dose to maximum 200microgram.[9–11]

†Nocturia or nocturnal polyuria in men with lower urinary tract symptoms (LUTS)

Give only if insufficient response to treatment with an α-blocker ± anti-muscarinic ± 5α-reductase inhibitor (see p.565):

- start with 50–100microgram PO at bedtime
- check plasma sodium pretreatment and after 3 days
- if necessary, after 1–2 weeks, increase dose to maximum 200microgram.

A late afternoon loop diuretic is an alternative.[10–13]

Idiopathic nocturnal polyuria in adults (including adults >65 years)

This is the only type of nocturia authorized for treatment with desmopressin in patients aged >65 years (Noqdirna® SL).

Exclude other causes of nocturia, e.g. diabetes mellitus, overactive bladder in women or LUTS in men:

- in women, 25microgram SL 1h before bedtime
- in men, 50microgram SL 1h before bedtime
- in those >65 years, check plasma sodium pretreatment, after 3 days and 4 weeks
- dose increase is *not* recommended in patients aged >65 years.

Compared with placebo, time to first void is increased by 40–50min and the mean number of voids is reduced by 0.2–0.4, suggesting little or no benefit in some patients.

Clinical response is dose-related. In men, doses ≥100microgram are generally necessary. If higher doses are considered for patients <65 years, switch to an alternative SL desmopressin product to aid adherence because the largest tablet size of Noqdirna is 50microgram.[8,14–16]

Nocturia associated with multiple sclerosis

Give only in adults aged <65 years when other treatments have failed:

- do *not* give >1 dose/24h.[2,17,18]
- start with 10–20microgram intranasally at bedtime to reduce nocturia or in the morning to reduce daytime frequency[19]
- a trial of 40microgram may occasionally be justified but higher doses (e.g. 60microgram) are associated with a higher risk of hyponatraemia and generally do not provide additional benefit.[18]

†Severe surface bleeding associated with platelet dysfunction

Although the benefit is small, desmopressin is used as a 'last resort' treatment (i.e. when other measures are insufficient) for severe surface bleeding associated with platelet dysfunction caused by, for example, hepatic impairment,[20,21] renal impairment, paraproteinaemia:

- give a single dose of desmopressin 0.3–0.4microgram/kg IVI in 50mL 0.9% saline over 20min, by SC injection (using Octim® to minimize injection volume),[4]
- if necessary, give repeat injections once daily up to a total of 4 days[22]
- if inadequate, consider giving cryoprecipitate, e.g. 2 pooled packs.[23]

Because of the mechanism of action of desmopressin (releasing stored von Willebrand factor and factor VIII from the vascular endothelium), the second and subsequent injections provide only about two thirds of the benefit of the first injection.[22]

Supply

Table 1 Desmopressin formulations and use in palliative care

Indications	*PO*	*SL*	*Nasal*	*Parenteral*
Pituitary diabetes insipidus	Yes (DDAVP® or generic)	Yes (DDAVP® Melt)	Yes[a] (Desmospray®, DDAVP®, or generic)	Yes (DDAVP)
Primary nocturnal enuresis	Yes[b] (Desmotabs® or generic)	Yes[b] (DesmoMelt® or generic)	No	
Idiopathic nocturnal polyuria		Yes (Noqdirna®)		
Nocturia associated with MS (where other treatments have failed)			Yes[b] (Desmospray® DDAVP®, or generic)	
†Nocturia (other causes)	†Yes			
†Severe surface bleeding with platelet dysfunction				†Yes

a. intranasal formulations should *not* be used first-line

b. contra-indicated in adults over >65.

Desmopressin *acetate* (generic)
Tablets 100microgram, 200microgram, 28 days @ 200microgram t.d.s. = £21.
Oral solution desmopressin *base* 360microgram/mL (equivalent to 400microgram/mL desmopressin *acetate*), 28 days @ 180microgram (equivalent to 200microgram) t.d.s. = £84.

Desmotabs (Ferring)
Tablets 100microgram, 200microgram, 28 days @ 200microgram t.d.s. = £82.

DDAVP® (Ferring)
Tablets 100microgram, 200microgram, 28 days @ 200microgram t.d.s. = £82.

Oral lyophilisate products
Desmopressin *base* (generic)
Tablets SL 120microgram, 240microgram, 28 days @ 120microgram t.d.s. = £85.

7

DDAVP® Melt (Ferring)
Tablets SL 60microgram, 120microgram, 240microgram, 28 days @ 120microgram t.d.s. = £85.

DesmoMelt (Ferring)
Tablets SL 120microgram, 240microgram, 28 days @ 120microgram t.d.s. = £85.

Noqdirna® (Ferring)
Tablets SL 25microgram, 50microgram, 28 days@ 25microgram (women) or 50microgram (men) once daily = £15.

Nasal products
Desmopressin *acetate* (generic)
Nasal spray 10microgram/metered spray, 60 dose bottle = £23.

Desmospray (Ferring)
Nasal spray 10microgram/metered spray, 60 dose bottle = £25.

DDAVP (Ferring)
Intranasal solution 100microgram/mL (0.01%), 2.5mL bottle and graduated catheter = £10; *store in refrigerator at 2–8°C and protect from light.*

Octim® (Ferring)
Nasal spray 150microgram/metered spray, 25 dose bottle = £577.

Parenteral products
Desmopressin *acetate*
DDAVP (Ferring)
Injection 4microgram/mL, 1mL amp = £1.25; for SC/IM/IV injection or IVI.

Octim® (Ferring)
Injection 15microgram/mL, 1mL amp = £20; for SC injection or IVI; *store at room temperature and protect from light.*

1 Ozier Y and Bellamy L (2010) Pharmacological agents: antifibrinolytics and desmopressin. *Best Practice and Research Clinical Anaesthesiology*. **24**: 107–119.
2 Cvetkovic RS and Plosker GL (2005) Desmopressin: in adults with nocturia. *Drugs*. **65**: 99-107; discussion 108–109.
3 Van de Walle *et al.* (2007) Desmopressin 30 years in clinical use: A safety review. *Current Drug Safety*. **2**: 232–238.
4 Hedges SJ *et al.* (2006) Evidence-based treatment recommendations for uremic bleeding. *Nature Clinical Practice Oncology*. **3**: 138–153.
5 Callreus T *et al.* (1999) Changes in gastrointestinal motility influence the absorption of desmopressin. *European Journal of Clinical Pharmacology*. **55**: 305–309.
6 NICE (2010) Bedwetting in under 19s. *Clinical Guideline* CG11. www.nice.org.uk
7 Juul KV *et al.* (2011) Gender difference in antidiuretic response to desmopressin. *American Journal of Renal Physiology*. **300**: F1116–1122.
8 Weiss JP *et al.* (2012) Desmopressin orally disintegrating tablet effectively reduces nocturia: results of a randomized, double-blind, placebo-controlled trial. *Neurourology Urodynamics*. **31**: 441–447.
9 NICE (2013) Urinary incontinence in women: management. *Clinical Guideline* CG171. www.nice.org.uk
10 Ebell MH *et al.* (2014) A systematic review of the efficacy and safety of desmopressin for nocturia in adults. *Journal of Urology*. **192**: 829–835.
11 Friedman FM and Weiss JP (2013) Desmopressin in the treatment of nocturia: clinical evidence and experience. *Therapeutic Advances in Urology*. **5**: 310–317.

12 NICE (2013) Nocturia and nocturnal polyuria in men with lower urinary tract symptoms: oral desmopressin. *Evidence summary: unlicensed or off-label medicine* ESOUM. www.nice.org.uk
13 NICE (2010) Lower urinary tract symptoms. the managment of lower urinary tract symptoms in men. *Clinical Guideline* **CG97**: www.nice.org.uk
14 Sand PK *et al.* (2013) Efficacy and safety of low dose desmopressin orally disintegrating tablet in women with nocturia: results of a multicenter, randomized, double-blind, placebo controlled, parallel group study. *Journal of Urology*. **190**: 958–964.
15 Weiss JP *et al.* (2013) Efficacy and safety of low dose desmopressin orally disintegrating tablet in men with nocturia: results of a multicenter, randomized, double-blind, placebo controlled, parallel group study. *Journal of Urology*. **190**: 965–972.
16 Drugs and Therapeutics Bulletin (2017) Desmopressin for nocturia in adults. **55**: 30–32.
17 Zahariou A *et al.* (2008) Maximal bladder capacity is a positive predictor of response to desmopressin treatment in patients with MS and nocturia. *International Urology and Nephrology*. **40**: 65–69.
18 Fowler CJ *et al.* (2009) A UK consensus on the management of the bladder in multiple sclerosis. *Postgraduate Medical Journal*. **85**: 552–559.
19 Bosma R *et al.* (2005) Efficacy of desmopressin in patients with multiple sclerosis suffering from bladder dysfunction: a meta-analysis. *Acta Neurologica Scandinavica*. **112**: 1–5.
20 Blonski W *et al.* (2007) Coagulopathy in liver disease. *Current Treatment Options in Gastroenterology*. **10**: 464–473.
21 Lisman T *et al.* (2010) Hemostasis and thrombosis in patients with liver disease: the ups and downs. *Journal of Hepatology*. **53**: 362–371.
22 Mannucci PM *et al.* (1992) Patterns of development of tachyphylaxis in patients with haemophilia and von Willebrand disease after repeated doses of desmopressin (DDAVP). *British Journal of Haematology*. **82**: 87–93.
23 Mannucci PM and Levi M (2007) Prevention and treatment of major blood loss. *New England Journal of Medicine*. **356**: 2301–2311.

Updated August 2017

DRUGS FOR DIABETES MELLITUS

Diabetes UK have commissioned and published recommendations on the management of patients with diabetes at the end of life.[1] These should be read in conjunction with this monograph.

Indications: Diabetes mellitus not controlled by diet.

Contra-indications: Oral hypoglycaemics should not be used during severe infection, after major trauma, or peri-operatively.

Glibenclamide, **glimepiride** and **chlorpropamide** (not UK) should not be used in the elderly and those with severe renal (eGFR <30mL/min/1.73m², see Chapter 17, p.681) or hepatic impairment because their long plasma halflives increase the risk of hypoglycaemia. Avoid or use at reduced dose in mild–moderate renal impairment.

Metformin should not be used in patients with severe renal impairment (eGFR <30mL/min/1.73m²), and should be withheld during and for 48h after testing with IV iodinated contrast agents or until renal function is normal. Because of the risk of lactic acidosis, withhold in patients with acute conditions which could cause tissue hypoxia or sudden deterioration in renal function, e.g. dehydration, severe infection, sepsis, shock, acute heart failure, respiratory failure, hepatic impairment, excessive alcohol intake.

Glitazones, e.g. **pioglitazone**, should not be used in patients with CHF, severe hepatic impairment, at higher risk of fracture, with or at risk of bladder cancer.[2]

Background

Diabetes mellitus comprises a group of metabolic diseases characterized by hyperglycaemia resulting from defects in insulin secretion, insulin action or both. There are two main types of diabetes mellitus (Box A). Some patients can exhibit features of both type 1 and type 2 diabetes, making a definite classification difficult.

In the UK, 7% of the general population have diabetes mellitus,[3] and nearly 40% of cancer patients have impaired glucose tolerance demonstrated by an oral or IV glucose tolerance test.[4,5] In cancer, corticosteroids are the most common cause of drug-induced hyperglycaemia[6] (see Box B, p.539), but thiazides, **furosemide**, **levothyroxine**, **octreotide** and atypical antipsychotics (e.g. **olanzapine**, **risperidone**) are also potential precipitants.[7]

In patients with symptoms suggestive of diabetes mellitus (e.g. thirst, polydipsia and/or polyuria), a diagnosis can be made on the basis of the following criteria:

- fasting blood glucose concentrations of ≥7mmol/L (normal <5.6mmol/L) *or*
- random blood glucose concentrations of ≥11.1mmol/L *or*
- 2h post-load blood glucose ≥11.1mmol/L (normal = <7.8mmol/L) during oral glucose tolerance test *or*
- glycated haemoglobin (HbA_{1c}) ≥48mmol/mol (≥6.5%).

Box A Classification of diabetes mellitus

Type 1 (the minority, <10%)
Typically develops in children, young people, and adults <30 years old, but can occur at any age. There is a lack of insulin because of immune-mediated destruction of the β-cells in the pancreas. Symptoms develop rapidly and the diagnosis is based on the presence of characteristic symptoms plus a high blood glucose concentration.

Type 2 (the majority)
Typically develops in adults >40 years old, although it is increasingly manifesting in younger people because of obesity. The pancreas does not produce sufficient insulin for the body's needs and generally there is also marked insulin resistance, i.e. cells are not able to respond to the insulin that is produced. Symptoms tend to develop gradually, with a long delay (possibly years) before diagnosis. Treatment is based on modification of diet and weight loss, together with various glucose-lowering drugs. *Some patients with Type 2 diabetes need insulin.*

In *asymptomatic* patients, ≥2 of the above must be present. Measurement of HbA_{1c} is the recommended and most convenient diagnostic test for diabetes mellitus. However, HbA_{1c} reflects glycaemia in the preceding 2–3 months. Thus, it is *not* suitable as the sole test for patients with recent onset hyperglycaemia, e.g. in those:

- at high risk of diabetes and acutely ill
- taking medications which may cause a rapid rise in blood glucose, e.g. corticosteroids, atypical antipsychotics (see list above)
- with short duration of symptoms suggestive of diabetes mellitus
- with symptoms suggestive of type 1 diabetes at any age
- with acute pancreatitis or recent pancreatic surgery
- all symptomatic children and young people.[8]

Pharmacology

Drug treatment in type 1 diabetes mellitus

Insulin is an essential life-long treatment in type 1 diabetes and is sometimes needed in type 2 diabetes. Human sequence insulin can be produced by bacteria using recombinant DNA technology, or semi-synthetically by enzymatic modification of animal insulin (mainly porcine, sometimes beef). Care must be taken when prescribing animal insulin for patients of certain faith groups.

Insulin preparations can be classified according to duration of action (Table 1). Because the plasma halflife for insulin is a few minutes, the time-activity profile is determined by the absorption characteristics, e.g. dose, route, injection site, SC fat. Thus, there is significant intra- and inter-individual variation in the pharmacokinetics of any given dose. Further, sensitivity to insulin varies with body weight and renal function. Individual dose titration is required to identify the appropriate dose.

Table 1 Pharmacokinetics of different types of insulin given by SC administration

Duration of action	*Short*		*Intermediate*	*Long*
	Rapid	*Short*		
Example	Aspart	Soluble	Isophane	Glargine
Onset of action	10–20min	30min	2h	2h
Time to peak plasma concentration	40min	1.5–2.5h	5–8h	Plateau <4h[a]
Duration of action	3–5h	7–8h	13–22h	>30h

a. SC insulin glargine once daily takes 2–4 days to reach steady state.[9]

Most patients with type 1 diabetes will be on a multiple injection **insulin** regimen, e.g. short- or rapid-acting insulin before meals and intermediate or long-acting insulin once or twice daily. Some may be using mixtures of insulin preparations, e.g. **biphasic insulin aspart** or **biphasic insulin lispro**, or omitting pre-meal insulin, particularly if they have difficulty with or prefer not to use multiple injection therapy. The ability of the patient to use the necessary equipment for insulin delivery also influences the type of insulin used and the regimen, e.g. those with poor eyesight may not be able to safely use an insulin pen injector. Insulin pump therapy is used increasingly to manage patients with type 1 diabetes mellitus.[10]

Patients starting treatment with **insulin** must inform the Driver and Vehicle Licensing Agency (DVLA) if they intend to drive. Drivers need to be particularly careful to avoid hypoglycaemia (see below). Detailed guidance on eligibility to drive is available from the DVLA (www.gov.uk/diabetes-driving).

Drug treatment in type 2 diabetes mellitus

There are several different classes of antidiabetic drugs, with differing modes of action (Table 2). Guidelines recommend initial therapy with a single non-insulin hypoglycaemic agent (monotherapy). Treatment intensification to dual therapy (two non-insulin hypoglycaemic drugs), then to triple therapy (three non-insulin hypoglycaemic drugs or two non-insulin hypoglycaemic drugs with insulin) may be necessary.[11] However, choice of drugs in patients with advanced cancer requires additional consideration (see below). The risk of hypoglycaemia is greatest with **insulin** and sulfonylureas.

Metformin

Immediate-release **metformin** is generally recommended as first-line therapy for patients with type 2 diabetes.[11,21] However, it is unlikely to be appropriate in advanced cancer because it promotes weight loss, and initially causes nausea and diarrhoea or other undesirable effects in ≤20% of patients.

Metformin is best *not* used in elderly debilitated patients, particularly those with hepatic impairment or COPD.[1] The dose of **metformin** should be reduced in patients with an eGFR <60mL/min/1.73m^2 and avoided or withdrawn in those with an eGFR of <30mL/min/1.73m^2 (severe renal impairment) or creatinine >150micromol/L. It is contra-indicated in patients with acute heart failure, but not in those with CHF controlled on treatment.

Although **metformin** has been linked to lactic acidosis in patients with deteriorating renal function, CHF or tissue hypoxia, recent evidence suggests that the risk of this has been overestimated.[22,23] Hypoglycaemia is rare with **metformin**.

Sulfonylureas

In debilitated or elderly patients, consider intermediate-acting **gliclazide**. If episodes of hypoglycaemia occur, stop **gliclazide** and consider switching to a short-acting sulfonylurea, i.e. **tolbutamide** (Table 3). These are also good choices in mild–moderate renal impairment. Initially monitor blood glucose closely, e.g. by checking capillary (fingerstick) blood glucose twice daily before a meal.

Dose adjustment may be necessary if liver function deteriorates. After discontinuation, **glibenclamide** and **chlorpropamide** (not UK) can produce hypoglycaemia for 2–3 days, and up to 4 days if there is renal or hepatic impairment.

The plasma concentration of sulfonylureas may be increased (effect enhanced) by **fluconazole** and **miconazole**, and decreased (effect reduced) by **rifampicin** and **rifabutin**.

Meglitinides

Meglitinides, e.g. **repaglinide**, are insulin secretagogues. They provide similar glucose control to sulfonylureas but act more rapidly and for a shorter time (see Table 3). This permits flexible 'pulse dosing' before meals, which may be useful in patients with a variable appetite and oral intake. Meglitinides are significantly more expensive than sulfonylureas. If **metformin** is contra-indicated or not tolerated, **repaglinide** is clinically and cost-effective. **Nateglinide** is authorized only for use with **metformin**.[11]

Gemfibrozil (generally used as a second-line plasma lipid-lowering agent) increases plasma concentrations of **repaglinide**. Because this may result in severe hypoglycaemia, avoid concurrent use. However, in palliative care, the continued use of **gemfibrozil** is generally unnecessary.

Class	*Examples*	*Mechanism of action*	*Risk of hypoglycaemia*	*Comment*
Biguanides	Metformin	Decrease hepatic gluconeogenesis, increase uptake of glucose by muscle	–	Tend to cause weight loss; may cause nausea and diarrhoea; low risk of lactic acidosis. GI undesirable effects may be reduced with m/r metformin. Reduce dose if eGFR <60mL/min/1.73m^2; stop if eGFR of <30mL/min/1.73m^2 (severe renal impairment) or creatinine >150micromol/L
Sulfonylureas	Gliclazide, tolbutamide, glibenclamide, chlorpropamide (not UK)	Increase insulin secretion	++ with longer-acting glibenclamide, chlorpropamide	Original class of oral antidiabetic drugs; relatively inexpensive
Meglitinides	Repaglinide, nateglinide	Increase insulin secretion	±	Relatively fast onset and short duration of action; permits flexible regimen
Glitazones (thiazolidinediones)	Pioglitazone	Reduce peripheral insulin r esistance	±	1st line if metformin contra-indicated or not tolerated; or 2nd or 3rd line drug; causes fluid retention, exacerbates CHF. Contra-indicated in patients with macular oedema, hepatic impairment, bladder cancer; increases risk of myocardial infarction,[12] fracture[11] and bladder cancer[2]
Gliptins (DPP-4/dipeptidyl peptidase-4 inhibitors)	Linagliptin, saxagliptin, sitagliptin, vildagliptin	Incretin mimetics: increase insulin secretion and lower glucagon secretion	±	Linagliptin, sitagliptin and vildagliptin authorized as monotherapy if metformin inappropriate. 2nd or 3rd line drugs, for use particularly in patients at high risk of hypoglycaemia.[11] Some gliptins suitable for use in renal impairment/failure (seek advice). Can use with insulin. Stop if symptoms of pancreatitis develop.[a] May increase risk of developing heart failure[13]
GLP-1 (glucagon-like peptide-1) mimetic	Exenatide SC b.d., liraglutide SC once daily	Incretin mimetics: increase insulin secretion and lower glucagon secretion; slow gastric emptying and increase satiety	±	2nd or 3rd line drugs, for use particularly in patients with a BMI ≥35kg/m^2.[11] Only to be given with insulin after specialist advice. Stop if weight loss >1.5kg weekly or if symptoms of pancreatitis develop.[14,a] Initial nausea and vomiting common
SGLT-2 (sodium-glucose cotransporter) inhibitor	Canagliflozin, dapagliflozin, empagliflozin	Inhibits renal resorption of glucose, causing glycosuria		Newly introduced; authorized as monotherapy if metformin inappropriate. Can use as dual therapy with other hypoglycaemic drugs including insulin, or as triple therapy with metformin and a sulfonylurea. May promote weight loss. Stop if eGFR <60mL/min/1.73m^2. Consider stopping if patient develops foot complications, e.g. infection, skin ulcers[15–17]

a. the risk of pancreatitis is about one extra case per 10,000 patients.[18,19] Concern about pancreatic cancer is *not* supported by latest evidence.[20]

7

Table 3 Pharmacokinetics of selected oral hypoglycaemic drugs

	Repaglinide	*Tolbutamide*	*Gliclazide*
Bio-availability	56%	>95%	78%
Onset of action	15–60min	1–3h	3–4h
Time to peak plasma concentration	1h	3–5h	2–4h
Plasma halflife	1h	4.5–6.5h	10–12h
Duration of action	4–6h	≤12h	12–24h

Pioglitazone

Pioglitazone can be used as first-line treatment if **metformin** is contra-indicated or not tolerated, or as second- or third-line therapy with **metformin** and/or a sulfonylurea, or **insulin**. **Pioglitazone** is contra-indicated in patients with CHF or a history of CHF because it causes fluid retention. All patients taking **pioglitazone** should be monitored for symptoms and signs of CHF, e.g. excessive/rapid weight gain, cough, increasing breathlessness, and/or oedema.[11,24] It is also contra-indicated in patients with a high risk of fracture because it increases the risk of distal fracture, particularly in women.[25,26] Because of these concerns, it is unlikely to be appropriate for use in patients with advanced cancer.

Gemfibrozil (generally used as a second-line lipid-lowering agent) increases plasma concentrations of **pioglitazone**. Because this may result in severe hypoglycaemia, avoid concurrent use. However, in palliative care, the continued use of **gemfibrozil** is generally unnecessary.

Insulin in type 2 diabetes

Insulin is sometimes needed in patients with type 2 diabetes. When adding **insulin** to oral hypoglycaemics to improve blood glucose control, 6–12 units of **isophane insulin** or long-acting **insulin** at bedtime may suffice. However, it may be easier for patients with advanced cancer to switch to an insulin-only regimen rather than combining **insulin** with existing oral therapy.[1] All patients started on **insulin** should be provided with an Insulin Passport and information booklet.[27]

Management overview

The following sections provide advice about the management of common clinical scenarios in *the last few weeks of life*. Guidance from a diabetologist should be sought if in doubt. For corticosteroid-induced diabetes mellitus, see Box B (p.539).

Because the patient's prognosis is short (days, weeks, a few months), it is *not* necessary to maintain rigid dietary control or target theoretically ideal blood glucose levels to avoid long-term complications.[28,29] Measuring HbA_{1c} to determine the overall level of glycaemic control over 6–8 weeks is also irrelevant for most palliative care patients.

The goal is to preserve quality of life. Thus, the aim of treatment is the prevention of symptoms from hyper- or hypoglycaemia, keto-acidosis and hyperosmolar non-ketotic states. Set a realistic safe target, e.g. a pre-meal capillary (fingerstick) blood glucose of 6–15mmol/L. Because the threshold for symptomatic hyperglycaemia varies, the upper limit may need to be reduced in some patients.

Resetting blood glucose targets necessitates careful explanation to both patient and family.[1,30] When stable, monitor with a fasting fingerstick blood glucose test twice a week. Although not as accurate, urine tests for glucose may suffice: aim for <1+ glycosuria before evening meal.

> Patients with **insulin** pumps will generally be able to adjust pump settings to manage moderate variations in diet. However, advice from a diabetologist is essential when it is necessary to adjust pump settings in complex situations, e.g. marked reductions in oral intake, enteral feeding, starting corticosteroids.[31]

Management of existing type 1 diabetes mellitus

Injections of **insulin** are an essential life-long treatment, including the last days of life. However, for most patients, the **insulin** requirement decreases because of weight loss, anorexia, nausea and vomiting, and renal and/or hepatic impairment.

Generally, short-acting **insulins** (given to cover mealtimes) which produce a more rapid peak and have a greater risk of hypoglycaemia, are reduced or discontinued first. Intermediate- or long-acting **insulins** (given once daily or b.d. to provide background control) may subsequently need to be reduced as well.

Likewise, patients receiving mixed **insulins** may need to reduce or discontinue the short-acting **insulin** component. However, if a patient has months or weeks to live, it would be prudent to liaise with a diabetologist before making major changes to an established **insulin** regimen.

Sick day management in type 1 diabetes mellitus

To avoid serious metabolic complications, e.g. diabetic keto-acidosis, apply sick day rules when the patient is feeling particularly unwell and unable to manage normal oral intake or levels of activity:[1]

- do not stop the long-acting **insulin**
- encourage the patient to sip sugar-free fluids, aiming for 100mL/h
- offer frequent small meals, e.g. soup, ice cream, milky drinks
- if the patient has symptoms of hyperglycaemia and dehydration, check fingerstick blood glucose and test urine or blood for ketones
- if ketones are present, test blood glucose and ketones every 2h:
  - ▷ if ketones ++ in urine or >1.5mmol in blood, give additional 10% of current daily average insulin as short-acting **insulin**, e.g. Actrapid®, NovoRapid®
  - ▷ if ketone levels do not improve, and the patient is vomiting, seek urgent advice from a diabetologist; consider transfer to hospital for IV **insulin** and rehydration.

Note. Sick day rules are generally *not* relevant for patients entering the last days or hours of life.

Stopping insulin in type 1 diabetes mellitus

A decision to stop **insulin** completely should normally be taken only after discussion with the patient (if still has capacity) and the family. It is generally appropriate to stop **insulin** injections completely when the patient has become irreversibly unconscious as part of the dying process, and not because of hypoglycaemia or diabetic keto-acidosis, and when all other life-prolonging treatments have been stopped.[6]

If it is felt strongly that the **insulin** should be continued, a simple regimen can be used, e.g. once daily long-acting, or b.d. intermediate-acting **insulin**, with the minimum of routine monitoring, e.g. fingerstick blood glucose test once daily at teatime:

- if blood glucose is <8mmol/L, reduce **insulin** by 10–20%
- if blood glucose >20mmol/L, increase **insulin** dose by 10–20%.[1,32]

Management of type 2 diabetes

Newly diagnosed type 2 diabetes mellitus in advanced cancer

The relative advantages and disadvantages of **insulin** and oral hypoglycaemics need to be taken into account together with factors such as the patient's prognosis, food intake and the presence of other co-morbidities. **Insulin** provides rapid, effective and more predictable control, is easier to titrate, and has less risk of prolonged hypoglycaemia compared with some oral hypoglycaemics. It is a better choice in patients with:

- a short prognosis (<3 months)
- co-morbidity contributing to hyperglycaemia, e.g. infection
- poor or erratic food intake
- contra-indications to the use of oral hypoglycaemics
- severe symptoms from hyperglycaemia.

With oral hypoglycaemics, control may take several weeks, and be less effective, less predictable and harder to titrate than **insulin**. However, if oral hypoglycaemics are preferred, prescribe **tolbutamide** or **gliclazide**.

When deciding the starting dose of **insulin**, the patient's build, oral intake and the blood glucose levels must be considered. The dose is monitored to achieve a fasting blood glucose of 6–15mmol/L. Doses of 0.25 units/kg/day of a *long-acting* **insulin analogue**, e.g. **insulin glargine**, **insulin detemir** (both given once daily) or **isophane insulin** (given once daily or b.d.) will provide only a basal insulin supply, and thus it does not matter if a patient on this amount is not eating.

However, in patients who are still eating and require larger doses than this, **insulin glargine** or **insulin detemir** are a better choice than **isophane insulin** because there is less likelihood of interprandial hypoglycaemia. They still generally need to be given only once daily, and need not be given at the same time each day, thus easing the burden of injections on the patient/carer.[11,23,33] Given these advantages, it may be beneficial for patients on oral hypoglycaemics troubled by hypoglycaemic episodes or a burdensome tablet load to be switched to once daily injections of **insulin glargine** or **insulin detemir**. Blood glucose should be monitored before each dose until the **insulin** dose is stable. The frequency can then be reduced and the time of testing varied to monitor control during different parts of the day.

A variable dose SC scale (previously called 'sliding scale') of a *rapid-acting* **insulin analogue** (e.g. **insulin aspart, insulin lispro**, available as pen devices) is occasionally necessary. Treatment with a variable rate, continuous IV infusion of rapid-acting regular **soluble insulin** is generally reserved for patients with diabetic keto-acidosis or peri-operatively.

Isolated spikes of hyperglycaemia should *not* be treated with stat doses of short/rapid-acting **insulin**. Instead, monitor with regular fingerstick tests and adjust hypoglycaemic regimen if a particular pattern emerges.[34]

Rationalizing therapy in existing type 2 diabetes mellitus

If patients have a prognosis of weeks–months and are becoming increasingly dependent on carers to administer treatment, consider simplifying existing therapy:

- stop **pioglitazone**, gliptin inhibitors, GLP-1 agonists, and SGLT2 inhibitors if part of dual or triple therapy
- switch from combination of oral hypoglycaemic and **insulin** to **insulin** alone
- switch from b.d. to once daily **insulin** (start with 75% of total b.d. dose)
- if in doubt, consult a diabetologist.

Sick day management in type 2 diabetes mellitus

To avoid serious metabolic complications, apply sick day rules when the patient is feeling particularly unwell and unable to manage normal food intake or levels of activity:

- encourage the patient to sip sugar-free fluids, aiming for 100mL/h
- offer frequent small meals, e.g. soup, ice cream, milky drinks
- check blood glucose only if symptoms of hyperglycaemia and dehydration develop.

For patients on diet alone, **metformin, pioglitazone** or DPP4 inhibitor:

- aim to maintain blood glucose ≤15mmol/L
- stop **metformin** if the patient develops vomiting or diarrhoea.

For patients on a **sulfonylurea, meglitinide, insulin**, GLP1 agonist, SGLT-2 inhibitor:

- if blood glucose <6mmol/L, consider reducing dose of sulfonylurea or **insulin**
- if blood glucose >15mmol/L, consider increasing dose of sulfonylurea or **insulin**
- stop medicines for diabetes if the patient is not eating, has no symptoms of hyperglycaemia and blood glucose <15mmol/L.[1]

Note. Sick day rules are generally *not* relevant for patients entering the last days or hours of life.

Stopping treatment in patients with type 2 diabetes

In advanced cancer, patients with insulin-treated type 2 diabetes may be able to stop **insulin**, and those with tablet-treated type 2 diabetes may be able to stop tablets because of weight loss, anorexia, nausea and vomiting, renal and/or hepatic impairment.

As the patient approaches the last few days of life, they are unlikely to be able to swallow any remaining oral hypoglycaemics. These should be stopped, as should GLP-1 injections and blood glucose monitoring. Consider stopping low-dose **insulin** (e.g. intermediate or long-acting **insulin** <15units total daily dose).

In most cases it will be appropriate to stop blood glucose monitoring too. However, if it is felt necessary to continue monitoring, conduct daily urinalysis:

- if urine glucose >2+, check fingerstick glucose
- if fingerstick glucose >20mmol/L give 6 units SC rapid-acting **insulin**, e.g. Novorapid®
- recheck fingerstick glucose after 2h
- if rapid-acting **insulin** required more than b.d., consider starting daily **isophane insulin** or **insulin glargine**.

If a patient requires a total daily dose of >15 units of **insulin**, or a decision is made to continue **insulin** therapy, manage as for type 1 diabetes (see above).[1,35,36]

Corticosteroid-induced diabetes mellitus

Diabetes mellitus occurs in about 10% of patients treated with corticosteroids.[37] It can occur with any corticosteroid and any formulation (including inhaled and topical),[38] and is dose-related.[39] The greatest rise in blood glucose is likely to occur 2–3h after taking a corticosteroid, returning to normal 12–16h later with **prednisolone** and 24h with **dexamethasone**.[35] Thus, treatment with a longer acting product, either a sulfonylurea (see Table 3) or long-acting **insulin**, may cause nocturnal hypoglycaemia in patients with **prednisolone**-induced hyperglycaemia but is less likely when **dexamethasone**-induced.[40] This should be taken into account when planning treatment.

If corticosteroids are given b.d., consider switching to a once daily morning dose (Box B). If tablet load is a concern, soluble **prednisolone** tablets are available and **dexamethasone** can be given as an oral solution (see p.513).

If not possible to switch to a corticosteroid once daily, consider prescribing **gliclazide** or **isophane insulin** b.d. However, there is a risk of early morning hypoglycaemia. If early morning hypoglycaemia occurs on several occasions or the patient is struggling to manage **insulin** b.d., give **glargine** once daily in the morning. Obtain early advice from a diabetologist.

7

Box B Corticosteroids and diabetes: management of patients taking dexamethasone once daily in the morning[35,39]

Target glucose levels when antidiabetic treatment is indicated:
fingerstick blood glucose 6–15mmol/L or <1+ glycosuria before evening meal.

Before starting corticosteroids

Check random *fingerstick* blood glucose, if >8mmol/L take random *venous* blood glucose:

- if >7.8mmol/L, the patient is at risk of developing diabetes with corticosteroid therapy; check blood glucose every 1–2 weeks
- if ≥11.1mmol/L, check fasting venous blood glucose; ≥7mmol/L indicates pre-existing undiagnosed diabetes mellitus; manage accordingly (see text above).

Corticosteroid-induced diabetes

Start antidiabetic drugs only if the patient has symptomatic hyperglycaemia and a prolonged course of corticosteroid treatment is planned, e.g. >2 weeks.

If drug treatment is necessary, give corticosteroid + a once daily morning dose of:

- a sulfonylurea, e.g. gliclazide (see Dose and use below) *or*
- isophane insulin or glargine (e.g. 10 units). If blood glucose remains >15mmol/L before evening meal, increase insulin dose by 4 units.[1]

Corticosteroid-exacerbated pre-existing non-insulin dependent diabetes

If glycaemic control deteriorates when corticosteroids are started for a course of >3 days, antidiabetic treatment will need to be modified.

Diet-controlled diabetes or patient taking metformin alone or metformin and gliptin

Check fingerstick blood glucose or urine glucose before evening meal.
If two consecutive readings of blood glucose >15mmol/L or >2+ urine glucose:

- start gliclazide 40mg each morning
- if necessary, increase gliclazide 40mg each morning until blood glucose 6–15mmol/L or <1+ urine glucose before evening meal
- if no hypoglycaemia and blood glucose >15mmol/L or >2+ urine glucose despite gliclazide 240mg each morning, add in evening meal dose of gliclazide 40mg, increasing to 80mg if glucose remains above target levels
- if glucose remains above target levels, switch to a once daily morning dose of insulin, e.g. isophane insulin (see below).

continued

Box B Continued

Gliclazide-controlled diabetes

Check fingerstick blood glucose or urine glucose before evening meal.

If two consecutive readings of blood glucose >15mmol/L or >2+ urine glucose:

- in patients taking <320mg gliclazide daily, adjust dose up to a maximum of 240mg each morning and 80mg with evening meal
- in patients taking gliclazide 320mg daily, switch to morning isophane insulin 10 units SC
- if blood glucose remains >15mmol/L before evening meal, increase morning insulin dose by 4 units.

Corticosteroid-exacerbated pre-existing insulin-controlled diabetes mellitus

As above, target blood glucose is generally 6–15mmol/L. However, if a patient has episodes of hypoglycaemia despite between-meals ('mid-meal') snacks or has long gaps between meals, aim for blood glucose of 8–15mmol/L.

Twice daily insulin

Check fingerstick blood glucose before evening meal.

If blood glucose >15mmol/L *or* 10–15mmol/L and low risk of hypoglycaemia, consider increasing morning insulin:

- if insulin dose <20 units, increase dose by 2–5 units
- if insulin dose 20–50 units, increase insulin dose by 5–10 units
- if insulin dose 50–100 units, increase dose by 10–20 units.

Basal bolus insulin

Check fingerstick blood glucose before lunch and evening meals:

- if blood glucose >15mmol/L, increase breakfast or lunchtime rapid acting insulin doses (use same % increases as recommended for twice-daily insulin above)
- if blood glucose 10–15mmol/L, consider increasing breakfast or lunchtime rapid acting insulin doses if low risk of hypoglycaemia.

Reducing the corticosteroid dose

Insulin requirements decline in parallel.

Review hypoglycaemic therapy after each change in corticosteroid dose, and consider reverting to pre-corticosteroid regimen.

Hypoglycaemia

Hypoglycaemia is a lower than physiologically normal blood glucose concentration. It is the commonest undesirable effect of insulin and sulfonylureas. Elderly patients or those with renal failure are at particular risk.

Metformin, **pioglitazone**, gliptins, GLP-1 analogues and SLGT-2 inhibitors are unlikely to cause hypoglycaemia unless prescribed with either insulin or a sulfonylurea. Hypoglycaemia can be precipitated by several drugs including **warfarin**, **quinine**, fibrates, NSAIDs and SSRIs.

Hypoglycaemia can be described as 'mild' if self-treated and 'severe' if assistance by another person is needed.[41] Any blood glucose less than 4mmol/L should be treated (Box C). For patients at risk, it is helpful to have a 'hypo box' containing everything necessary for treating hypoglycaemia, and keep it in a prominent place.[34]

Malnourished patients with reduced hepatic glycogen stores have a reduced capacity to counteract hypoglycaemia, and glucagon treatment in these patients is likely to be less effective.

Driving and hypoglycaemia

Patients with diabetes should inform the DVLA if they:

- are taking **insulin**
- experience 2 episodes of severe hypoglycaemia in a year
- experience 1 episode of severe hypoglycaemia when driving
- develop impaired awareness of hypoglycaemia (and stop driving).

Box C Treatment of hypoglycaemia[34,42]

Conscious patient

1 Give *quick-acting* carbohydrate 15–20g PO:
- 200mL of pure fruit juice
- 200mL[a] of Lucozade® (*not* diet version); this is preferable in renal patients
- 150mL of Coca-Cola® (*not* diet version) *or* other non-diet fizzy drink
- 60mL GlucoJuice®
- 5–7 Dextrosol® glucose tablets (or 4 Glucotabs®)
- 3–4 heaped teaspoons *or* 4–5 lumps of sugar dissolved in water.

2 If the patient is not able to take tablets or drink but can still swallow, give 2 tubes of GlucoGel® or Dextrogel® squeezed into the mouth between the teeth and gums.

3 If the patient has a PEG, stop the feed and administer down the tube 30mL of undiluted Ribena® or 50mL Fortijuice® (*or* Lucozade® *or* Coca-Cola® as in point 1).

4 Repeat fingerstick test after 5min; if blood glucose <4mmol/L, *repeat above steps up to 3 times.*

5 Then, if blood glucose still remains <4mmol/L:
- *if well-nourished*, give glucagon 1mg IM (can be given SC but will act more slowly)
- *if malnourished or cachectic or PEG-fed*, give 10% glucose 150mL IV.

6 When the blood glucose is >4mmol/L and the patient has recovered, give a *long-acting* carbohydrate of the patient's choice, e.g.:
- two biscuits
- one slice of bread/toast
- 200–300mL glass of milk (not soya)
- normal meal if due (must contain carbohydrate)/restart PEG feed.

Note. Patients given glucagon require a larger portion of *long-acting* carbohydrate to replenish glycogen stores.

7 If the patient is aggressive, give IV glucose (as below).

Unconscious patient ± seizures
- treat patient using the **A**irway, **B**reathing, **C**irculation, **D**isability, **E**xposure (**ABCDE**) approach: ensure airway is clear and give high-flow oxygen via a mask, check breathing and circulation, obtain IV access. Stop insulin infusion if in situ.
- then give:
  - ▷ *if well-nourished*, glucagon 1mg IM (can be given SC but acts more slowly)
  - ▷ *if malnourished or cachectic or PEG-fed*, 10% glucose 150mL IV *or* 20% glucose 75mL IV
- repeat fingerstick test after 10min: repeat glucose infusion if blood glucose <4mmol/L
- when conscious, give *quick-acting* carbohydrate drink (see points 1–3), followed by a starchy snack (see point 6)
- consider 10% glucose 100mL/h IV until the hypoglycaemic drug has been metabolized and blood glucose levels are stable (or if patient 'nil by mouth' and unable to take carbohydrate drink or snack).

Further measures

Discuss with diabetes team and review diabetes management:
- consider reducing or stopping oral hypoglycaemics or insulin in patients with type 2 diabetes
- consider reducing but not stopping insulin in patients with type 1 diabetes.

a. the sugar content of Lucozade® was halved in 2017, thereby doubling the volume required to treat hypoglycaemia.

Drivers need to be particularly careful to avoid hypoglycaemia. Drivers treated with **insulin** should be advised to check their blood glucose before driving and, on long journeys, every 2h as specified by the DVLA (www.gov.uk/diabetes-driving).

These precautions may also be necessary for drivers taking oral antidiabetic drugs which carry a risk of hypoglycaemia (e.g. long-acting sulfonylureas, meglitinides). Drivers treated with **insulin** should ensure that a supply of sugar is always available in the vehicle, and they should avoid driving if a meal is delayed.

If warning signs hypoglycaemia develop, the driver should:

- stop the vehicle in a safe place
- switch off the ignition and move out of the driver's seat
- eat or drink a suitable source of sugar (see Box C)
- not drive again until 45min after the blood glucose has returned to normal.

Impaired awareness of hypoglycaemia (IAH)

This is an acquired syndrome associated with long-standing **insulin**-dependent diabetes. It is a consequence of autonomic neuropathy which removes both the warning symptoms (sweating, tremor, pounding heart beat) and the counter-regulatory mechanism of an adrenaline (epinephrine)-induced increase in blood glucose. Such patients tend to present with pallor, mental detachment ± drowsiness ± clumsiness. Some become irritable and aggressive, and others slip rapidly into hypoglycaemic coma.

Dose and use

To maximize safety, all regular and single **insulin** (bolus) doses must be measured and administered using an **insulin** syringe or commercial **insulin** pen device. IV syringes must never be used because they are calibrated in mL and not in **insulin** units. *'Units' must always be written in full.* Abbreviations, e.g. 'U' or 'IU', should not be used; e.g. 10U could be mistakenly read as 100.[43,44]

Gliclazide

- start with 40–80mg each morning with breakfast
- if necessary, increase every 3 days to a maximum of 160mg b.d.

Tolbutamide

- start with 500mg b.d. with meals
- if necessary, increase every 3 days to a maximum of 1g b.d.

Metformin

- start with 500mg each morning with breakfast
- if necessary, increase by 500mg at weekly intervals
- maximum dose = 1g t.d.s.

Repaglinide

- start with 500microgram within 30min of main meals (or 1mg in patients previously treated with an alternative oral hypoglycaemic agent)
- if necessary, increase the dose at 1–2 week intervals to a maximum of 4mg q.d.s.

Insulin

- if the patient is already taking the maximum dose of an oral hypoglycaemic, and the fasting blood glucose is >12mmol/L, prescribe **insulin glargine** 6–12 units once daily or **isophane insulin** 6–12 units once daily:
- adjust the dose according to the response
- a preprandial variable dose scale of SC short-acting **soluble insulin** is occasionally necessary (Table 4).

Table 4 Preprandial variable dose scale of SC soluble insulin[a]

Preprandial blood glucose (mmol/L)	*Insulin dose (units)*
10–15	6
15–18	8
18–22	10
>22[b]	12

a. responses to insulin vary widely and variable dose scales need to be individualized

b. patients with marked hyperglycaemia should have monitoring 2h after meals as well until the blood glucose is better controlled.

Supply

This is not a complete list; see BNF for additional details.

Gliclazide (generic)
Tablets 40mg, 80mg (scored), 28 days @ 80mg each morning = £1.
Oral suspension 40mg/5mL, 80mg/5mL, 28 days @ 80mg each morning = £67 (unauthorized; available as a special order, see Chapter 24, p.751). *Price based on specials tariff in the community.*

Tolbutamide (generic)
Tablets 500mg, 28 days @ 500mg b.d. = £14.

Metformin (generic)
Tablets 500mg, 850mg, 28 days @ 500mg each morning = £1.
Oral solution (sugar-free) 500mg/5mL, 28 days @ 500mg each morning = £15.

Repaglinide (generic)
Tablets 500microgram, 1mg, 2mg, 28 days @ 500microgram t.d.s. = £9.

Insulin

Most insulin products are also available as cartridges for use with dedicated re-usable injection pen devices or as prefilled disposable pen devices.

Note. All insulin products are 100 units/mL with the exception of insulin degludec which is available in strengths of 100 units/mL and 200 units/mL.

Short-acting insulin
Actrapid® (Novo Nordisk)
Injection human sequence insulin 100 units/mL, 10mL multidose vial = £7.50.

Rapid-acting insulin analogues (e.g. ***aspart, glulisine, lispro****) are double the price.*

Intermediate-acting insulin
Isophane insulin
Insulatard® (Novo Nordisk)
Injection human sequence insulin 100 units/mL, 10mL multidose vial = £7.50.

Mixed preparations of short-acting with intermediate-acting insulins are available (biphasic isophane insulin, biphasic insulin aspart, biphasic insulin lispro).

Long-acting insulin (e.g. detemir, degludec, glargine, zinc suspension)
Insulin glargine
Lantus® (Sanofi-Aventis)
Injection recombinant human insulin analogue 100 units/mL, 10mL multidose vial = £31; *once daily dosing.*

1. Diabetes UK (2013) End of Life Diabetes Care: Full Strategy Document Commissioned by Diabetes UK 2nd ed. Available from: www.diabetes.org.uk
2. MHRA (2011) Pioglitazone: risk of bladder cancer. *Drug Safety Update.* **5**: www.mhra.gov.uk/Safetyinformation
3. Holman N *et al.* (2011) The Association of Public Health Observatories (APHO) Diabetes Prevalence Model: estimates of total diabetes prevalence for England, 2010–2030. *Diabetic Medicine.* **28**: 575–582.
4. McCoubrie R *et al.* (2005) Managing diabetes mellitus in patients with advanced cancer: a case note audit and guidelines. *European Journal of Cancer Care (Engl).* **14**: 244–248.
5. Giovannucci E *et al.* (2010) Diabetes and cancer: a consensus report. *CA: A Cancer Journal for Clinicians.* **60**: 207–221.
6. Poulson J (1997) The management of diabetes in patients with advanced cancer. *Journal of Pain and Symptom Management.* **13**: 339–346.
7. Fathallah N *et al.* (2015) Drug-induced hyperglycaemia and diabetes. *Drug Safety.* **38**: 1153–1168.
8. WHO (2011) Use of glycated haemoglobin(HbA1c) in the diagnosis of diabetes mellitus. *World Healh Organization.*
9. Heinemann L *et al.* (2000) Time-action profile of the long-acting insulin analog insulin glargine (HOE901) in comparison with those of NPH insulin and placebo. *Diabetes Care.* **23**: 644–649.
10. NICE (2015) Type 1 diabetes in adults: diagnosis and management. NG17. www.nice.org.uk
11. NICE (2015) Type 2 diabetes in adults: management. NICE Guideline NG28. www.nice.org.uk
12. Loke YK *et al.* (2011) Comparative cardiovascular effects of thiazolidinediones: systematic review and meta-analysis of observational studies. *British Medical Journal.* **342**: d1309.
13. Li L *et al.* (2016) Dipeptidyl peptidase-4 inhibitors and risk of heart failure in type 2 diabetes: systematic review and meta-analysis of randomised and observational studies. *British Medical Journal.* **352**: i610.

14 NICE (2010) Liraglutide for the treatment of type 2 diabetes mellitus. *Technology Appraisal.* TA203. www.nice.org.uk
15 MHRA (2017) SGLT2 inhibitors: updated advice on increased risk of lower-limb amputation (mainly toes). *Drug Safety Update.* www.mhra.gov.uk/Safetyinformation
16 NICE (2016) Dapagliflozin in triple therapy for treating type 2 diabetes. *Technology Appraisal.* TA418. www.nice.org.uk
17 NICE (2016) Canaglifozin, dapaglifozin and empagliflozin as monotherapies for treating type 2 diabetes. *Technology Appraisal.* TA390. www.nice.org.uk
18 Li L *et al.* (2014) Incretin treatment and risk of pancreatitis in patients with type 2 diabetes mellitus: systematic review and meta-analysis of randomised and non-randomised studies. *British Medical Journal.* **348**: 2366.
19 Faillie JL *et al.* (2014) Incretin based drugs and risk of acute pancreatitis in patients with type 2 diabetes: cohort study. *British Medical Journal.* **348**: 2780.
20 Azoulay L *et al.* (2016) Incretin based drugs and the risk of pancreatic cancer: international multicentre cohort study. *British Medical Journal.* **352**: i581.
21 ADA (American Diabetes Association) (2008) Diagnosis and classification of diabetes mellitus. *Diabetes Care.* **31 (Suppl 1)**: S55–60.
22 Salpeter S *et al.* (2003) Risk of fatal and nonfatal lactic acidosis with metformin use in type 2 diabetes mellitus. *Cochrane Database of Systematic Reviews.* CD002967. www.thecochranelibrary.com
23 National Collaborating Centre for Chronic Conditions (2008) *Type 2 diabetes: national clinical guideline for management in primary and secondary care (update).* London: Royal College of Physicians and NICE 2009.
24 Yki-Jarvinen H *et al.* (1992) Comparison of insulin regimens in patients with non-insulin-dependent diabetes mellitus. *New England Journal of Medicine.* **327**: 1426–1433.
25 Loke YK *et al.* (2009) Long-term use of thiazolidinediones and fractures in type 2 diabetes: a meta-analysis. *Canadian Medical Association Journal.* **180**: 32–39.
26 Habib ZA *et al.* (2010) Thiazolidinedione use and the longitudinal risk of fractures in patients with type 2 diabetes mellitus. *Journal of Clinical Endocrinology and Metabolism.* **95**: 592–600.
27 National Patient Safety Agency (2011) The adult patient's passport for safer use of insulin. *Patient safety Alert.* NPSA/2011/PSA2003. www.nrls.npsa.nhs.uk
28 Angelo M *et al.* (2011) An approach to diabetes mellitus in hospice and palliative medicine. *Journal of Palliative Medicine.* **14**: 83–87.
29 Vandenhaute V (2010) Palliative care and type II diabetes: A need for new guidelines? *American Journal of Hospice and Palliative Care.* **27**: 444–445.
30 Dikkers MF *et al.* (2013) Information needs of family carers of people with diabetes at the end of life: a literature review. *Journal of Palliative Medicine.* **16**: 1617–1623.
31 Anonymous (2012) Insulin pump therapy. *Drug and Therapeutics Bulletin.* **50**: 105–108.
32 McCann M-A *et al.* (2006) Practical management of diabetes mellitus. *European Journal of Palliative Care.* **13**: 226–229.
33 Ciardullo AV *et al.* (2006) Effectiveness and safety of insulin glargine in the therapy of complicated or secondary diabetes: clinical audit. *Acta Diabetol.* **43**: 57–60.
34 Joint British Diabetes Societies Inpatient Care Group (2013) The hospital management of hypoglycaemia in adults with diabetes mellitus. Available from: www.diabetes.org.uk
35 Kilvert A *et al.* (2010) Diabetes and end of life care. Association of British Clinical Diabetologists. *ABCD Position Statement.* Available from: www.diabetologists-abcd.org.uk/
36 King EJ *et al.* (2012) The management of diabetes in terminal illness related to cancer. *Quarterly Journal of Medicine.* **105**: 3–9.
37 Pilkey J *et al.* (2012) Corticosteroid-induced diabetes in palliative care. *Journal of Palliative Medicine.* **15**: 681–689.
38 van der Linden MW *et al.* (2009) Topical corticosteroids and the risk of diabetes mellitus: a nested case-control study in the Netherlands. *Drug Safety.* **32**: 527–537.
39 Oyer DS *et al.* (2006) How to manage steroid diabetes in the patient with cancer. *Journal of Supportive Oncology.* **4**: 479–483.
40 Perez A *et al.* (2014) Glucocorticoid-induced hyperglycemia. *Journal of Diabetes.* **6**: 9–20.
41 DCCT (1993) The effect of intensive treatment of diabetes on the development and progression of long-term complications in insulin-dependent diabetes mellitus. The Diabetes Control and Complications Trial Research Group. *New England Journal of Medicine.* **329**: 977–986.
42 NHS Diabetes (2011) Recognition, treatment and prevention of hypoglycaemia in the community. Available from www.diabetesandprimarycare.co.uk
43 NICE (2017) Safer insulin prescribing. Key therapeutic topic ktt20. www.nice.org.uk
44 National Patient Safety Agency (2010) Safer administration of insulin. *Patient Safety Alert.* NPSA/2010/RRR2013. www.nrls.npsa.nhs.uk

Updated September 2017

*OCTREOTIDE

Class: Somatostatin analogue.

Indications: Symptoms associated with unresectable hormone-secreting tumours, e.g. carcinoid, VIPomas, glucagonomas and acromegaly; prevention of complications after elective pancreatic surgery;[1] bleeding oesophageal varices in cirrhosis; †salivary, buccal and enterocutaneous fistulas;[2–4] †intractable diarrhoea;[5–13] †inoperable bowel obstruction in patients with cancer;[14,15] †hypertrophic pulmonary osteo-arthropathy;[16] †ascites in cirrhosis and cancer;[17–19] †death rattle (noisy rattling breathing); †bronchorrhoea;[20,21] †reduction of tumour-related secretions.[19]

Pharmacology

Octreotide (and **lanreotide**) is a synthetic analogue of somatostatin with a longer duration of action.[22] Somatostatin is an inhibitory hormone found throughout the body. In the hypothalamus it inhibits the release of growth hormone, TSH, prolactin and ACTH. It inhibits the secretion of insulin, glucagon, gastrin and other peptides of the gastro-enteropancreatic system (i.e. peptide YY, neurotensin, VIP and substance P), reducing splanchnic blood flow, portal blood flow, GI motility, gastric, pancreatic and small bowel secretion, and increasing water and electrolyte absorption.[23]

In Type 1 diabetes mellitus, octreotide decreases insulin requirements. However, in Type 2 diabetes, octreotide suppresses both insulin and glucagon release, leaving blood glucose concentrations either unchanged or slightly elevated.[24,25] Thus, octreotide (with dextrose) has been suggested as treatment for refractory sulfonylurea-induced hypoglycaemia.[26]

Somatostatin acts as an inhibitory neurotransmitter in the CNS, has anti-inflammatory and analgesic effects and also inhibits cell proliferation.[27–30] Somatostatin analogues have a direct anticancer effect and improve time to progression ± prognosis in patients with neuroendocrine or solid tumours of the GI tract.[30–35] The combination of somatostatin analogues and targeted anticancer therapies (e.g. tyrosine kinase inhibitors) are now used in the treatment of some neuroendocrine tumours.

7

There are five somatostatin receptors (SST_{1-5}), each mediating a different biological action of somatostatin. Neuroendocrine tumours express various receptor profiles, but generally SST_2 or SST_5 predominate.[36] Octreotide and **lanreotide** bind with high affinity to SST_2 and with moderate affinity to SST_3 and SST_5. **Pasireotide**, developed more recently, has a broader receptor affinity profile ($SST_5 > SST_2 > SST_3 > SST_1$) and in acromegaly, provides higher rates of biochemical control than octreotide (30% vs. 20%). Further, of patients failing to respond to octreotide, ≤20% respond to **pasireotide**.[36] This suggests **pasireotide** has a potential role in patients who are or have become refractory to octreotide (tolerance can occur after 12–18 months).[34] However, compared with octreotide, the incidence of hyperglycaemia, diabetes mellitus, and potential for drug interactions are greater with **pasireotide**;[36] it is also more expensive (>£2,000 for the monthly depot injection).

Various radionuclides have been linked to somatostatin analogues for either diagnostic or therapeutic purposes. The latter are still in development and require the tumour to demonstrate high uptake on a somatostatin receptor radionuclide scan. Best results are seen in fitter patients without significant liver involvement.[34]

The inhibitory, antisecretory and absorptive effects of octreotide are utilized in a wide range of clinical settings:

Hormone-secreting tumours

Octreotide improves symptoms by inhibiting hormone secretion, e.g.:

- 5HT in carcinoid (improving flushing and diarrhoea)
- VIP in VIPomas (improving diarrhoea)
- glucagon in glucagonomas (improving rash and diarrhoea)
- TSH in pituitary adenomas.

Inoperable bowel obstruction in patients with cancer

For a suggested management approach, see QCG: Inoperable bowel obstruction (p.242).

Octreotide can provide rapid improvements in nausea and vomiting in this setting, although the evidence for benefit is generally low level and limited to short-term use.[37]

The optimal dose has not been formally identified, but reports suggest <50% of patients respond to the typical CSCI starting dose of 300microgram/24h,[38] and 75–90% respond to 600–800microgram/24h.[15,39] Although doses of up to 1,500microgram/24h have been used,[40] a dose of 600–800microgram/24h is generally sufficient to identify those likely to respond.[39,41] Benefit is less likely in obstruction of the gastric outlet or proximal small bowel.[38,42]

In a well-conducted RCT over 72h, there was no difference between octreotide 600microgram/24h CSCI and placebo in relation to the *complete* control of vomiting when given alongside a standardized regimen of bowel rest (IV hydration, PO clear fluids only ± NG tube) + SC/IV **dexamethasone** + SC/IV **ranitidine** (also chosen for its antisecretory effects, see p.253) and p.r.n. SC **hyoscine *butylbromide***.[43] No differences were seen in the number of patients free of vomiting for all 3 days (about 30%), mean number of days free of vomiting (about 2), nausea, or patient global impression of change. Although mean pain was the same in both groups, those receiving octreotide required more **hyoscine *butylbromide***. Nonetheless, octreotide about halved the overall number of vomiting episodes. These findings suggest that, in this setting, octreotide can be reserved for instances when such a regimen fails to reduce the frequency of vomiting to an acceptable level.

In comparisons with **hyoscine *butylbromide*** (60–80mg/24h CSCI; p.817), octreotide (300–800microgram/24h CSCI) provides more effective and rapid improvements in nausea and vomiting and reduction in NG tube output.[39,44] However, in those patients responding to either drug, after 3–6 days, overall symptom relief is similar, and NG tube removal possible with both.[39,44]

Depot (long-acting) preparations of octreotide and **lanreotide** have also been explored in RCTs in this setting.[45,46] Although there was suggestion of some benefit, both studies had methodological limitations.[37]

Ascites

Octreotide 300microgram SC b.d. can suppress diuretic-induced activation of the renin-aldosterone-angiotensin system. Its use has improved renal function and Na^+ and water excretion in patients with cirrhosis and ascites receiving **furosemide** and **spironolactone** (p.67).[18,47]

Octreotide is also reported to reduce the rate of formation of malignant ascites.[17,19] In a pilot RCT of depot octreotide 30mg IM monthly for malignant ascites, the median time to next paracentesis was doubled (28 vs. 14 days), although this did not reach statistical significance. Nonetheless, patients receiving octreotide had significantly less abdominal bloating, abdominal discomfort and shortness of breath.[48]

Octreotide may interfere with ascitic fluid formation in various ways, including a reduction in splanchnic blood flow, or by inhibiting vascular endothelial growth factor which increases vascular permeability and also promotes angiogenesis and tumour growth.

Octreotide could be considered in patients with rapidly accumulating ascites requiring frequent paracentesis despite diuretic therapy (if indicated; see **spironolactone** p.67) and/or when an indwelling catheter is inappropriate or declined. Octreotide may also help resolve chylous ascites and/or pleural effusion from various causes.[49–57]

Other antisecretory effects

Octreotide reduces salivary production and may be of use in salivary or buccal fistulas[2,4] Experience of its use in death rattle is limited.[58] The use of octreotide has led to rapid and sometimes complete control of bronchorrhoea (>1L/24h) in patients with diffuse adenocarcinoma of the lung.[20,21]

When given in conjunction with pancreatic surgery *for cancer* (but not for other conditions), octreotide reduces the risk of complications, e.g. fistula.[1] If enterocutaneous fistulas complicate abdominal surgery, somatostatin analogues reduce the time to closure and length of hospital stay.[3] However, in a review limited to pancreatic fistula, evidence of benefit was lacking.[59]

Octreotide has been used for intractable diarrhoea from various causes, e.g. high output ileostomies, AIDS, Crohn's disease, and following coeliac plexus block, radiation therapy, chemotherapy or bone marrow transplant.[6–13] It is recommended first-line for severe chemotherapy- or radiotherapy-induced diarrhoea (i.e. an increase of ≥7 stools/day over baseline, hospital admission and IV fluids >24h required), and second-line for less severe diarrhoea which does not respond to **loperamide** 16–24mg/24h PO (p.35).[8,9] For those who have experienced severe chemotherapy-induced diarrhoea, prophylactic depot octreotide is recommended for subsequent cycles. In an RCT, octreotide failed to improve diarrhoea in patients with ileal pouch anastomosis (± pouchitis) following total colectomy for ulcerative colitis.[60]

Octreotide has also been used for the treatment of enterovesical fistula,[61] to improve mucous discharge from rectal cancers[19] and, together with fasting ± TPN, for chylothorax of various aetiologies, including cancer.[62]

Pain

Octreotide is reported to have an analgesic effect in patients with cancer, e.g. in bone pain from metastatic carcinoid, in hypertrophic pulmonary osteo-arthropathy, pain arising from GI cancer, or when given IT.[16,63–65] However, a small RCT found octreotide to be no better than placebo.[66]

Although octreotide slows GI transit time, mostly via inhibitory effects on the small bowel,[67] there is no evidence of an antispasmodic effect. Indeed, patients receiving octreotide for bowel obstruction required 3 times more doses of **hyoscine *butylbromide*** than those receiving placebo.[43] This has implications for the management of patients with bowel obstruction associated with colic (see QCG inoperable bowel obstruction, p.242).

The development of somatostatin analogues with a greater affinity for the receptors predominantly responsible for an anti-inflammatory effect (SST_1, SST_4) may prove more effective.[27] Octreotide may also be of value in chronic pancreatitic pain caused by hypertension in scarred ducts.[68,69] Benefit may be secondary to its antisecretory action.[70] (Suppressing exocrine function by administering **pancreatin** supplements (p.58) can also reduce pain in patients with chronic pancreatitis).[71]

Miscellaneous

At doses far below those necessary for an antisecretory effect (e.g. 1 microgram SC t.d.s.), octreotide protects the stomach from NSAID-related injury, probably via its ability to reduce NSAID-induced neutrophil adhesion to the microvasculature.[72] Uncontrolled data suggest somatostatin analogues may reduce transfusion requirements in patients with angiodysplasia of the GI tract.[73] Benefit is also reported in the control of bleeding from peristomal varicies.[74] However, a systematic review casts doubt on the value of octreotide in the acute management of bleeding oesophageal varices.[75]

7

Octreotide improves tolerance to being upright, in part by reducing splanchnic blood flow. Potentially this could benefit patients with postural hypotension caused by the loss of the ability to vasoconstrict the splanchic blood vessels in response to standing.[76] Octreotide is used as an adjunct to IV dextrose in the treatment of hypoglycaemia caused by sulfonylurea overdose.[77]

Octreotide is generally given as a SC bolus or by CSCI[78] but can be given IV (after dilution) when a rapid effect is required. Octreotide has also been administered IT as an analgesic.[63] A long-acting IM depot formulation is also available but evaluation has been generally limited to hormone-secreting tumours.[79] Benefit from depot octreotide has been reported in an RCT for the prevention of chemotherapy-related diarrhoea[5] and in cancer patients with bowel obstruction.[80,81] **Lanreotide** is available in depot formulations only.

Onset of action 30min.

Time to peak plasma concentration 30min SC.

Plasma halflife 1.5h SC.

Duration of action 8h.

Cautions

In Type 1 diabetes mellitus, **insulin** requirements may be reduced by up to 50%; monitor blood glucose concentrations to guide dose reductions with both **insulin** and oral hypoglycaemic agents. Insulinoma: may exacerbate hypoglycaemia.

Cirrhosis, renal failure requiring dialysis (both lead to reduced elimination which may necessitate a dose reduction). May cause gallstones (although the manufacturer advises ultrasound examination of the gallbladder before treatment and then every 6–12 months, this is generally not necessary in palliative care). Avoid abrupt withdrawal of short-acting octreotide after long-term treatment (may precipitate biliary colic caused by gallstones/biliary sludge).

May cause bradycardia,[82] conduction defects or arrhythmias; use with caution in at-risk patients. Monitor thyroid function during long-term treatment (may cause hypothyroidism).

In patients with carcinoid, possibly by increasing catecholamine levels, anaesthesia and operations can provoke a sudden release of carcinoid hormones and cause a 'carcinoid crisis'. In addition to typical carcinoid symptoms (e.g. flushing, diarrhoea), life-threatening haemodynamic instability can occur. It is treated with IV octreotide and supportive measures, e.g. IV fluids. Traditionally, in an attempt to reduce the risk of a crisis, prophylactic octreotide is given peri-operatively, although the value of this has been questioned.[83]

Drug interactions

Octreotide increases the bio-availability of **bromocriptine** by about 40% (consider when using the combination in acromegaly).[84]

Octreotide markedly reduces plasma **ciclosporin** concentrations and inadequate immunosuppression may result. Increase the **ciclosporin** dose by 50% before starting octreotide, and monitor the plasma concentration daily to guide further adjustments.[84]

Undesirable effects

Dry mouth, flatulence (lowers oesophageal sphincter tone), nausea, abdominal pain, diarrhoea, steatorrhoea (GI undesirable effects may be reduced by administering octreotide between meals or at bedtime), impaired glucose tolerance, hypoglycaemia (shortly after starting treatment), persistent hyperglycaemia (during long-term treatment), gallstones (10–20% of patients on long-term treatment), pancreatitis (associated with gallstones).

Dose and use

Octreotide is painful if given as a SC bolus injection. Warming the ampoule or vial to body temperature before injection by holding it in the hand reduces the pain. With CSCI, to reduce the likelihood of inflammatory reactions at the skin injection site, dilute to the largest volume possible, preferably in 0.9% saline (see p.819).

The dose varies according to the indication (Table 1). To maximize the benefit (convenience and cost) of the multidose vials, the starting doses have been given in convenient fractions of 1mg (e.g. 250–500microgram rather than 300–600microgram). If necessary, the dose should be titrated upwards; higher doses are generally well tolerated.[85] However, after the desired response has been achieved, it may be possible to reduce to a lower maintenance dose.

Table 1 Dose recommendations for SC/CSCI octreotide

Indication	*Starting dose*[a]	*Maximum dose*[b]
Hormone-secreting tumours		
Acromegaly	100–200microgram t.d.s.	600microgram/24h[23]
Carcinoid, VIPomas, glucagonomas	50microgram once daily or b.d.	1,500microgram/24h; rarely 6,000microgram/24h[86]
Intractable diarrhoea (including that caused by chemotherapy and radiotherapy)	250–500microgram/24h	1,500microgram/24h,[8,9,87] occasionally higher
Inoperable bowel obstruction	250–500microgram/24h	750microgram/24h, occasionally higher
Tumour-antisecretory effect	50–100microgram b.d.	600microgram/24h[19]
Ascites	250–500microgram/24h	600microgram/24h[17]
Bronchorrhoea	250–500microgram/24h[20,21]	
Hypertrophic pulmonary osteo-arthropathy	100microgram b.d.[16]	

a. doses 'rounded' to maximize benefit from multidose vials

b. 'unrounded' doses from the literature.

CSCI compatibility with other drugs: There are 2-drug compatibility data for octreotide in 0.9% saline with **diamorphine**, **haloperidol**, **hyoscine *butylbromide***, **hyoscine *hydrobromide***, **midazolam**, **morphine sulfate**, **ondansetron**, and **oxycodone**.

Incompatibility may occur with **dexamethasone** or **levomepromazine**. More details and 3-drug compatibility data can be found on *www.palliativedrugs.com* Syringe Driver Survey Database.

For compatibility charts for mixing drugs in WFI, see Appendix 3, p.863.

Depot formulation

A depot formulation of octreotide 10–30mg, given IM every 4 weeks is available (Sandotatin LAR®). Higher (40–60mg) or more frequently administered (every 3 weeks) doses are sometimes required.[85] This has a relative bio-availability of about 60% compared with SC octreotide. Generally, the depot formulation is used only after symptoms have been controlled with SC octreotide.

Patients who have not previously received SC octreotide should have a test dose of 50–100microgram SC and, provided there are no unacceptable undesirable effects, then switch to the depot injection. The starting dose for those patients with acromegaly or gastro-enteropancreatic tumours who are adequately controlled is 20mg every 4 weeks. The depot formulation requires deep IM injection into the gluteal muscle; use alternate sides for subsequent injections.

In acromegaly, stop SC octreotide when the first depot injection is given; for other neuro-endocrine tumours, continue the SC dose for 2 weeks.

In a survey, 40% of respondents reported the use of depot formulations in cancer-related bowel obstruction.[88] There is limited published long-term experience of their use in this setting, although benefit in a small number of patients with ovarian cancer for up to 15 months has been reported.[80] A reduction in NG tube output and symptomatic benefit is evident within 24h.[81]

Lanreotide

Patients can be started directly on either of the long-acting formulations. However for palliative care, use of the Somatuline Autogel® may be preferable because it is given by deep SC injection into the superior external quadrant of the buttock:

- start with 60mg every 4 weeks for the first 3 months
- if necessary, increase to 120mg every 4 weeks.

If a switch between Sandotatin LAR® and Somatuline Autogel® is considered necessary, experience in patients with acromegaly suggests that Sandotatin LAR® 20mg is approximately equivalent to Somatuline Autogel® 90mg.[89]

Supply

For full details of storage and reconstitution details, see manufacturer's SPC.

For prolonged storage, keep all *unopened* ampoules, vials and pre-filled syringes in a refrigerator. Once opened, a multidose vial can be kept for up to 2 weeks at room temperature for day-to-day use.

Octreotide

Octreotide (generic)

Injection (as acetate) 50microgram/mL, 1mL amp = £3; 100microgram/mL, 1mL amp = £5.50; 500microgram/mL, 1mL amp = £27.

Injection (as acetate) 50microgram/mL, 1mL prefilled syringe = £4; 100microgram/mL, 1mL prefilled syringe = £6.50; 500microgram/mL, 1mL prefilled syringe = £34.

Injection (as acetate) 200microgram/mL multi-dose vial, 1mg in 5mL = £65.

Sandostatin LAR® (Novartis)

Depot injection (microsphere powder for aqueous suspension), octreotide (as acetate) 10mg vial = £550; 20mg vial = £800; 30mg vial = £998 (all supplied with diluent filled syringe) for deep IM injection every 28 days.

Lanreotide

Somatuline LA® (Ipsen)

Long acting injection (copolymer microparticles for aqueous suspension), lanreotide (as acetate) 30mg vial (with vehicle) = £323 for IM injection every 14 days.

Somatuline Autogel® (Ipsen)

Depot injection (prefilled syringe), lanreotide (as acetate) 60mg = £551; 90mg = £736; 120mg = £937 for deep SC injection into the superior, external quadrant of the buttock every 28 days.

1 Gurusamy KS *et al.* (2012) Somatostatin analogues for pancreatic surgery. *Cochrane Database of Systematic Reviews.* **6**: CD008370. www.thecochranelibrary.com

2 Spinell C *et al.* (1995) Postoperative salivary fistula: therapeutic action of octreotide. *Surgery.* **117**: 117–118.

3 Coughlin S *et al.* (2012) Somatostatin analogues for the treatment of enterocutaneous fistulas: a systematic review and meta-analysis. *World Journal of Surgery.* **36**: 1016–1029.

4 Lam C and Wong S (1996) Use of somatostatin analog in the management of traumatic parotid fistula. *Surgery.* **119**: 481–482.

5 Rosenoff SH *et al.* (2006) A multicenter, randomized trial of long-acting octreotide for the optimum prevention of chemotherapy-induced diarrhea: results of the STOP trial. *Journal of Supportive Oncology.* **4**: 289–294.

6 Crouch M *et al.* (1996) Octreotide acetate in refractory bone marrow transplant-associated diarrhea. *Annals of Pharmacotherapy.* **30**: 331–336.

7 Harris A (1992) Octreotide in the treatment of disorders of the gastrointestinal tract. *Drug Investigation.* **4**: 1–54.

8 Benson AB *et al.* (2004) Recommended guidelines for the treatment of cancer treatment-induced diarrhea *Journal of Clinical Oncology.* **22**: 2918–2926.

9 Maroun JA *et al.* (2007) Prevention and management of chemotherapy-induced diarrhea in patients with colorectal cancer: a consensus statement by the Canadian Working Group on Chemotherapy-Induced Diarrhea. *Current Oncology.* **14**: 13–20.
10 Dorta G (1999) Role of octreotide and somatostatin in the treatment of intestinal fistulae. *Digestion.* **60 (Suppl 2)**: 53–56.
11 Martelli L *et al.* (2017) Evaluation of the efficacy of octreotide LAR in the treatment of Crohn's disease associated refractory diarrhea. *Scandinavian Journal of Gastroenterology.* **52**: 564–569.
12 Yang A *et al.* (2016) Persistent diarrhea after celiac plexus block in a pancreatic cancer patient: case report and literature review. *Journal of Palliative Medicine.* **19**: 83–86.
13 Farthing MJ (1994) Octreotide in the treatment of refractory diarrhoea and intestinal fistulae. *Gut.* **35 (Suppl 3)**: s5–10.
14 Mercadante S and Porzio G (2012) Octreotide for malignant bowel obstruction: twenty years after. *Critical Reviews in Oncology/Hematology.* **83**: 388–392.
15 Ripamonti C and Mercadante S (2004) How to use octreotide for malignant bowel obstruction. *Journal of Supportive Oncology.* **2**: 357–364.
16 Birch E *et al.* (2011) Treatment of painful hypertrophic osteoarthropathy associated with non-small cell lung cancer with octreotide: a case report and review of the literature. *BMJ Supportive and Palliative Care.* **1**: 189–192.
17 Cairns W and Malone R (1999) Octreotide as an agent for the relief of malignant ascites in palliative care patients. *Palliative Medicine.* **13**: 429–430.
18 Kalambokis G *et al.* (2005) Renal effects of treatment with diuretics, octreotide or both, in non-azotemic cirrhotic patients with ascites. *Nephrology, Dialysis, Transplantation.* **20**: 1623–1629.
19 Harvey M and Dunlop R (1996) Octreotide and the secretory effects of advanced cancer. *Palliative Medicine.* **10**: 346–347.
20 Hudson E *et al.* (2006) Successful treatment of bronchorrhea with octreotide in a patient with adenocarcinoma of the lung. *Journal of Pain and Symptom Management.* **32**: 200–202.
21 Pahuja M *et al.* (2014) The use of octreotide to manage symptoms of bronchorrhea: a case report. *Journal of Pain and Symptom Management.* **47**: 814–818.
22 Lamberts SWJ *et al.* (1996) Octreotide. *New England Journal of Medicine.* **334**: 246–254.
23 Gyr K and Meier R (1993) Pharmacodynamic effects of sandostatin in the gastrointestinal tract. *Digestion.* **54**: 14–19.
24 Davies R *et al.* (1989) Somatostatin analogues in diabetes mellitus. *Diabetic Medicine.* **6**: 103–111.
25 Lunetta M *et al.* (1997) Effects of octreotide on glycaemic control, glucose disposal, hepatic glucose production and counterregulatory hormone secretion in type 1 and type 2 insulin treated diabetic patients. *Diabetes Research and Clinical Practice.* **38**: 81–89.
26 Dougherty PP and Klein-Schwartz W (2010) Octreotide's role in the management of sulfonylurea-induced hypoglycemia. *Journal of Medical Toxicology.* **6**: 199–206.
27 Heyles Z *et al.* (2006) Effects of the somatostatin receptor subtype 4 selective agonist j-2156 on sensory neuropeptide and inflammatory reactions in rodents. *British Journal of Pharmacology.* **149**: 405–415.
28 Pinter E *et al.* (2006) Inhibitory effect of somatostatin on inflammation and nociception. *Pharmacology and Therapeutics.* **112**: 440–456.
29 Gadelha MR *et al.* (2017) Somatostatin receptor ligands in the treatment of acromegaly. *Pituitary.* **20**: 100–108.
30 Rinke A *et al.* (2017) Placebo-controlled, double-blind, prospective, randomized study on the effect of octreotide LAR in the control of tumor growth in patients with metastatic neuroendocrine midgut tumors (PROMID): results of long-term survival. *Neuroendocrinology.* **104**: 26–32.
31 Deming DA *et al.* (2005) A dramatic response to long-acting octreotide in metastatic hepatocellular carcinoma. *Clinical Advances in Hematology and Oncology.* **3**: 468–472; discussion 472–464.
32 Kouroumalis E *et al.* (1998) Treatment of hepatocellular carcinoma with octreotide: a randomised controlled study. *Gut.* **42**: 442–447.
33 Cascinu S *et al.* (1995) A randomised trial of octreotide vs best supportive care only in advanced gastrointestinal cancer patients refractory to chemotherapy. *British Journal of Cancer.* **71**: 97–101.
34 Walter T *et al.* (2012) New treatment strategies in advanced neuroendocrine tumours. *Digestive and Liver Disease.* **44**: 95–105.
35 Miljkovic MD *et al.* (2012) Novel medical therapies of recurrent and metastatic gastroenteropancreatic neuroendocrine tumors. *Digestive Diseases and Sciences.* **57**: 9–18.
36 Cuevas-Ramos D and Fleseriu M (2016) Pasireotide: a novel treatment for patients with acromegaly. *Drug Design, Development and Therapy.* **10**: 227–239.
37 Obita GP *et al.* (2016) Somatostatin analogues compared with placebo and other pharmacologic agents in the management of symptoms of inoperable malignant bowel obstruction: a systematic review. *Journal of Pain and Symptom Management.* **52**: 901–919.
38 Shima Y *et al.* (2008) Clinical efficacy and safety of octreotide (SMS201-995) in terminally ill Japanese cancer patients with malignant bowel obstruction. *Japanese Journal of Clinical Oncology.* **38**: 354–359.
39 Mystakidou K *et al.* (2002) Comparison of octreotide administration vs conservative treatment in the management of inoperable bowel obstruction in patients with far advanced cancer: a randomized, double-blind, controlled clinical trial. *Anticancer Research.* **22**: 1187–1192.
40 Weber C and Zulian GB (2009) Malignant irreversible intestinal obstruction: the powerful association of octreotide to corticosteroids, antiemetics, and analgesics. *American Journal of Hospice and Palliative Care.* **26**: 84–88.
41 Riley J and Fallon M (1994) Octreotide in terminal malignant obstruction of the gastrointestinal tract. *European Journal of Palliative Care.* **1**: 23–25.
42 Hisanaga T *et al.* (2010) Multicenter prospective study on efficacy and safety of octreotide for inoperable malignant bowel obstruction. *Japanese Journal of Clinical Oncology.* **40**: 739–745.
43 Currow DC *et al.* (2015) Double-blind, placebo-controlled, randomized trial of octreotide in malignant bowel obstruction. *Journal of Pain and Symptom Management.* **49**: 814–821.
44 Peng X *et al.* (2015) Randomized clinical trial comparing octreotide and scopolamine butylbromide in symptom control of patients with inoperable bowel obstruction due to advanced ovarian cancer. *World Journal of Surgical Oncology.* **13**: 50.
45 Mariani P *et al.* (2012) Symptomatic treatment with lanreotide microparticles in inoperable bowel obstruction resulting from peritoneal carcinomatosis: a randomized, double-blind, placebo-controlled phase III study. *Journal of Clinical Oncology.* **30**: 4337–4343.
46 Laval G *et al.* (2012) SALTO: a randomized, multicenter study assessing octreotide LAR in inoperable bowel obstruction. *Bulletin Cancer.* **99**: E1–9.
47 Kalambokis G *et al.* (2006) The effects of treatment with octreotide, diuretics, or both on portal hemodynamics in nonazotemic cirrhotic patients with ascites. *Journal of Clinical Gastroenterology.* **40**: 342–346.
48 Jatoi A *et al.* (2012) A pilot study of long-acting octreotide for symptomatic malignant ascites. *Oncology.* **82**: 315–320.
49 Yildirim AE *et al.* (2011) Idiopathic chylous ascites treated with total parenteral nutrition and octreotide. A case report and review of the literature. *European Journal of Gastroenterology and Hepatology.* **23**: 961–963.
50 Widjaja A *et al.* (1999) Octreotide for therapy of chylous ascites in yellow nail syndrome. *Gastroenterology.* **116**: 1017–1018.

51 Ferrandiere M *et al.* (2000) Chylous ascites following radical nephrectomy: efficacy of octreotide as treatment of ruptured thoracic duct. *Intensive Care and Medicine*. **26**: 484–485.
52 Sharkey AJ and Rao JN (2012) The successful use of octreotide in the treatment of traumatic chylothorax. *Texas Heart Institute Journal*. **39**: 428–430.
53 Zhou DX *et al.* (2009) The effectiveness of the treatment of octreotide on chylous ascites after liver cirrhosis. *Digestive Diseases and Sciences*. **54**: 1783–1788.
54 Pfammatter R *et al.* (2001) Treatment of hepatic hydrothorax and reduction of chest tube output with octreotide. *European Journal of Gastroenterology and Hepatology*. **13**: 977–980.
55 Dumortier J *et al.* (2000) Successful treatment of hepatic hydrothorax with octreotide. *European Journal of Gastroenterology and Hepatology*. **12**: 817–820.
56 Lee PH *et al.* (2005) Octreotide therapy for chylous ascites in a chronic dialysis patient. *Nephrology (Carlton)*. **10**: 344–347.
57 Mincher L *et al.* (2005) The successful treatment of chylous effusions in malignant disease with octreotide. *Clinical Oncology*. **17**: 118–121.
58 Clark K *et al.* (2008) A pilot phase II randomized, cross-over, double-blinded, controlled efficacy study of octreotide versus hyoscine hydrobromide for control of noisy breathing at the end-of-life. *Journal of Pain and Palliative Care Pharmacotherapy*. **22**: 131–138.
59 Gans SL *et al.* (2012) Systematic review and meta-analysis of somatostatin analogues for the treatment of pancreatic fistula. *British Journal of Surgery*. **99**: 754–760.
60 Van Assche G *et al.* (2012) Octreotide for the treatment of diarrhoea in patients with ileal pouch anal anastomosis: a placebo-controlled crossover study. *Colorectal Disease*. **14**: e181–186.
61 Shinjo T *et al.* (2009) Treatment of malignant enterovesical fistula with octreotide. *Journal of Palliative Medicine*. **12**: 965–967.
62 Gupta A and Singh T (2016) Octreotide in malignant chylothorax: a case report. *BMJ Supportive and Palliative Care*. **6**: 122–124.
63 Penn RD *et al.* (1992) Octreotide: A potent new nonopiate analgesic for intrathecal infusion. *Pain*. **49**: 13–19.
64 Befon S *et al.* (2000) Continuous subcutaneous octreotide in gastrointestinal cancer patients: pain control and beta-endorphin levels. *Anticancer Research*. **20**: 4039–4046.
65 Katai M *et al.* (2005) Octreotide as a rapid and effective painkiller for metastatic carcinoid tumor. *Endocrine Journal*. **52**: 277–280.
66 De-Conno F *et al.* (1994) Subcutaneous octreotide in the treatment of pain in advanced cancer patients. *Journal of Pain and Symptom Management*. **9**: 34–38.
67 von der Ohe MR *et al.* (1995) Differential regional effects of octreotide on human gastrointestinal motor function. *Gut*. **36**: 743–748.
68 Donnelly PK *et al.* (1991) Somatostatin for chronic pancreatic pain. *Journal of Pain and Symptom Management*. **6**: 349–350.
69 Okazaki K *et al.* (1988) Pressure of papillary zone and pancreatic main duct in patients with chronic pancreatitis in the early state. *Scandinavian Journal of Gastroenterology*. **23**: 501–506.
70 Lembcke B *et al.* (1987) Effect of the somatostatin analogue sandostatin on gastrointestinal, pancreatic and biliary function and hormone release in man. *Digestion*. **36**: 108–124.
71 Draganov P and Toskes PP (2004) Chronic pancreatitis: controversies in etiology, diagnosis and treatment. *Revista Espanola de Enfermedades Digestivas*. **96**: 649–659.
72 Scheiman J *et al.* (1997) Reduction of NSAID induced gastric injury and leucocyte endothelial adhesion by octreotide. *Gut*. **40**: 720–725.
73 Sami SS *et al.* (2014) Review article: gastrointestinal angiodysplasia - pathogenesis, diagnosis and management. *Alimentary Pharmacology and Therapeutics*. **39**: 15–34.
74 Selby D and Jackson LD (2015) Octreotide for control of bleeding peristomal varices in palliative care. *Journal of Pain and Symptom Management*. **49**: e2–4.
75 Gotzsche PC and Hrobjartsson A (2008) Somatostatin analogues for acute bleeding oesophageal varices. *Cochrane Database of Systematic Reviews*. **3**: CD000193. www.thecochranelibrary.com
76 Jarvis SS *et al.* (2012) A somatostatin analog improves tilt table tolerance by decreasing splanchnic vascular conductance. *Journal of Applied Physiology*. **112**: 1504–1511.
77 Glatstein M *et al.* (2012) Octreotide for the treatment of sulfonylurea poisoning. *Clinical Toxicology*. **50**: 795–804.
78 Mercadante S (1995) Tolerability of continuous subcutaneous octreotide used in combination with other drugs. *Journal of Palliative Care*. **11**: 14–16.
79 Scherubl H *et al.* (1994) Treatment of the carcinoid syndrome with a depot formulation of the somatostatin analogue lanreotide. *European Journal of Cancer*. **30A**: 1590–1591.
80 Matulonis UA *et al.* (2005) Long-acting octreotide for the treatment and symptomatic relief of bowel obstruction in advanced ovarian cancer. *Journal of Pain and Symptom Management*. **30**: 563–569.
81 Massacesi C and Galeazzi G (2006) Sustained release octreotide may have a role in the treatment of malignant bowel obstruction. *Palliative Medicine*. **20**: 715–716.
82 Kubota K *et al.* (2013) Octreotide acetate administration for malignant bowel obstruction induces severe bradycardia in patients with terminal stage cancer: two case reports. *Journal of Palliative Medicine*. **16**: 596–597.
83 Condron ME *et al.* (2016) Continuous infusion of octreotide combined with perioperative octreotide bolus does not prevent intraoperative carcinoid crisis. *Surgery*. **159**: 358–365.
84 Baxter K (ed) (2008) Stockley's Drug Interactions. (8e). Pharmaceutical Press, London.
85 Ludlam WH and Anthony L (2011) Safety review: dose optimization of somatostatin analogs in patients with acromegaly and neuroendocrine tumors. *Advances in Therapy*. **28**: 825–841.
86 Harris A and Redfern J (1995) Octreotide treatment of carcinoid syndrome: analysis of published dose-titration data. *Alimentary Pharmacology and Therapeutics*. **9**: 387–394.
87 Cello J *et al.* (1991) Effect of octreotide on refractory AIDS-associated diarrhea. A prospective, multicenter clinical trial. *Annals of Internal Medicine*. **115**: 705–710.
88 Palliativedrugs.com (2010) Octreotide - What is your experience? Available from: www.palliativedrugs.com/download/100401_octreotide.pdf
89 Ashwell SG *et al.* (2004) The efficacy and safety of lanreotide Autogel in patients with acromegaly previously treated with octreotide LAR. *European Journal of Endocrinology*. **150**: 473–480.

Updated September 2017

PROGESTOGENS

Class: Sex hormones.

Indications: Authorized indications vary between products; consult SPC for details. Hormone therapy in endometrial cancer (use in breast, prostate and renal cancer has diminished);[1] anovulatory uterine bleeding; secondary amenorrhoea; mild–moderate endometriosis; †anorexia and cachexia in cancer and AIDS; †post-castration hot flushes in both women and men.

Contra-indications: Medroxyprogesterone acetate (MPA): oestrogen-progestogen-dependent cancer, hepatic impairment, history of (or high risk of developing) thrombo-embolism, active thrombophlebitis, undiagnosed abnormal vaginal bleeding, pregnancy (known or suspected).

Pharmacology

In addition to natural **progesterone**, there are several classes of synthetic progestogens, e.g. derivatives of retroprogesterone, progesterone, and 17α-hydroxyprogesterone (**cyproterone**, **MPA**, **megestrol acetate**).[2] Whereas all derivatives have a progestogenic effect on the uterus, there are differences in other biological effects (Table 1).

Table 1 Comparison of the biological effects of natural progesterone and selected synthetic progestogens[2]

Progestogen	*Effect*[a]		
	Androgenic	*Anti-androgenic*	*Anti-mineralocorticoid*
Progesterone	–	+	+
Cyproterone acetate	–	++	–
Megestrol acetate	+	+	–
MPA	+	–	–

++ = effect present; + = weak effect; – = no effect.

a. all the above possess similar progestogenic, anti-gonadotrophic, anti-oestrogenic and glucocorticoid effects.

In palliative care, progestogens are used mainly in selected patients with cachexia-anorexia, although their efficacy in cachexia is debatable (see next section). Progestogens may improve appetite by increasing levels of orexigenic neurotransmitters in the hypothalamus (e.g. neuropeptide Y), counteracting the anorexic effects of cytokines on the hypothalamus, or by interfering with the production of cytokines via their glucocorticoid anti-inflammatory effect.[3,4] *In vitro*, cytokine release from peripheral blood mononucleocytes are inhibited by both **MPA** and **megestrol acetate** in concentrations that would be achieved by daily doses of 1,500–2,000mg and 320–960mg respectively.[3] The release of serotonin was also inhibited and was considered one possible mechanism by which progestogens have an anti-emetic effect.[3]

Bio-availability of **MPA** and **megestrol acetate** is low (Table 2). Both **MPA** and **megestrol acetate** are highly protein-bound, mainly to albumin. **MPA** is metabolized extensively in the liver, and excreted mainly as glucuronides, whereas **megestrol acetate** is excreted mainly unchanged in the urine.

Table 2 Selected pharmacokinetic data[5,6]

	MPA	*Megestrol acetate*
Bio-availability	1–10%	No absolute data; reduced by 25% in fasting state
Time to peak plasma concentration	2–7h	1–3h
Plasma halflife	38–46h	24–42h

Cachexia and anorexia

Cachexia is common in cancer and other chronic diseases, impairing quality of life and increasing morbidity and mortality.[7] Cachexia is characterized by the loss of skeletal muscle ± body fat that cannot be fully reversed by conventional nutritional support. Loss of skeletal muscle is associated with impaired physical function and quality of life, whereas loss of fat (the body's main energy store) is associated with reduced survival. Recommended diagnostic criteria for cancer cachexia are:

- involuntary weight loss >5% in the past 6 months, *or*
- weight loss >2% in patients with either a BMI of <20kg/m^2 or skeletal muscle sarcopenia (absolute muscularity <5th centile of gender-specific norm).[8]

In cancer, a negative protein and energy balance is driven by the combination of reduced food intake (anorexia) and abnormal host metabolism resulting from factors produced by the cancer, e.g. proteolysis-inducing factor, or by the host in response to the cancer, e.g. cytokines.[9] One outcome of this is a chronic inflammatory state, as evidenced by a raised serum CRP, the level of which relates to the degree and rate of weight loss.[10] Cytokines such as interleukin-1 and tumour necrosis factor-α act on the hypothalamus and skeletal muscle leading to anorexia, inefficient energy expenditure, wasting of skeletal muscle and loss of body fat. Management needs to address both the reduced nutritional intake and the abnormal host metabolism; increasing nutritional intake alone is generally ineffective.[9,11–13]

Recent recommendations emphasize the importance of early identification and intervention, and recognize that once cancer cachexia is advanced (patient has severe muscle wasting, ongoing catabolism, WHO performance status 3–4, metastatic disease refractory to therapy and a prognosis of <3 months) a response to treatment is unlikely, and that the focus in these circumstances should be on symptom relief and psychosocial support.[8]

Megestrol acetate is used to stimulate appetite and weight gain. A recent systematic review included 35 RCTs, totalling about 4,000 patients, mostly with cancer, AIDS (n=475) or other conditions (n=270).[14] It concluded that the quality of the evidence was very low. Nonetheless, when compared with placebo, **megestrol acetate** increased appetite in about 1/4 and weight (≈2kg) in about 1/12, but not overall quality of life. There was little difference in efficacy when compared with other drugs, e.g. **prednisolone**, except in patients with cancer where **megestrol acetate** resulted in greater weight gain. For appetite stimulation, 160mg/day is probably the optimum dose; for weight gain higher doses (480mg) appear more effective.[14] However, the RCTs used body weight as a primary outcome measure; none accurately evaluated changes in body composition (see below). Data from individual RCTs indicates that impotence occurred in 10–25% of men.[4,15–22] Further, oedema, thrombo-embolism and deaths were more frequent in the patients treated with **megestrol acetate**.[14] Similar findings were reported in a study in frail elderly patients[23] and, in consequence, enthusiasm for its use in this setting has declined.

In studies which have evaluated body composition, both **megestrol acetate** and **MPA** appear to increase fat mass, but not fat-free mass, the part which includes skeletal muscle.[4,15,16,24] Thus it is likely that the gain in weight with progestogens (and corticosteroids), rather than representing the ideal increase in skeletal muscle *and* fat, is a less helpful retention of fluid or increase in fat only. This could make mobilizing more difficult in an already debilitated patient. In addition, the catabolic effect of progestogens on skeletal muscle could further weaken the patient. Catabolism may result from the glucocorticoid effect of progestogens but they also suppress the amount and function of testosterone, which is anabolic.

Progestogens generally cost more than the equivalent dose of **dexamethasone** or **prednisolone**. **Megestrol acetate** 800mg/day and **dexamethasone** 3mg/day are comparable with regard to appetite stimulation and non-fluid weight gain, although the latter was not accurately evaluated.[25] In this study, a high proportion of patients discontinued **dexamethasone** (36%) or **megestrol acetate** (25%) because of undesirable effects. **Dexamethasone** was more likely to cause cushingoid changes, myopathy, heartburn and peptic ulcers; **megestrol acetate** was associated with increased thrombo-embolism.[25] **Dexamethasone** is a fluorinated corticosteroid, a class which is more prone to cause muscle catabolism.[26] Thus, ideally, **dexamethasone** should be limited to short-term use only.

If long-term use of a corticosteroid is contemplated, a switch to the non-fluorinated **prednisolone** 10–20mg/day should be considered.[4] However, for patients expected to live months rather than weeks, progestogens may be more appropriate. Caution is still required as long-term progestogens can also cause cushingoid changes (25% of patients after 3 months in one study),[27] muscle catabolism and suppression of the hypothalamic-pituitary-adrenal axis. The latter may present with non-specific symptoms and a high level of clinical suspicion is required.[28] Additional corticosteroid replacement therapy would be a reasonable precaution in patients with serious infections or undergoing surgery.[4,29,30] Adrenal suppression is secondary to a central glucocorticoid effect on the hypothalamus and is dose-related; maximal suppression is seen with daily doses of **megestrol acetate** 200mg and **MPA** 1,000mg.[27]

In an attempt to improve outcomes, progestogens have been combined with other drugs, with the best evidence available for NSAIDs, e.g.:

- **megestrol acetate** 160mg t.d.s. + **ibuprofen** 400mg t.d.s.[31]
- **MPA** 500mg b.d. + **celecoxib** 200mg b.d.[32]
- **megestrol acetate** 160mg b.d. + **celecoxib** 300mg daily + l-carnitine + antioxidants. Note. In this study **celecoxib** was administered as 200mg once daily alternating with 400mg once daily, but this is unnecessary if both 100mg and 200mg tablets are available.[33]

NSAIDs provide benefit by reducing the chronic inflammatory response, and some have used **indometacin** or **celecoxib** alone.[34,35] Compared with progestogen alone, the combinations lead to greater improvements in fatigue, quality of life and lean body mass.[33] However, similar benefit is obtained with the combination of **celecoxib** + l-carnitine + antioxidants with or without **megestrol acetate**, suggesting the latter adds relatively little.[36]

In conclusion, progestogens and systemic corticosteroids (see p.513) are useful *appetite stimulants* which can increase calorie intake and as such may be indicated in selected patients for anorexia. Progestogens may be better for long-term use than corticosteroids, but significant undesirable effects can occur. Starting doses should be low and titrated to the lowest effective dose. Both progestogens and corticosteroids are best *not* regarded as 'anticachexia' agents; any weight gain is likely to be because of an increase in fat and fluid retention, and the catabolism of skeletal muscle *increased*, particularly in inactive people.

Cautions

Asthma, cardiac and renal impairment, diabetes (monitor), epilepsy; history of hypertension, depression, migraine.

MPA: hyperlipidaemia

Megestrol acetate: history of/susceptibility to thrombo-embolism (particular caution with high dose), severe hepatic impairment.

Undesirable effects

May suppress the hypothalamic-pituitary-adrenal axis.[37] Possibility of glucocorticoid effects. May cause or worsen diabetes mellitus. Thrombo-embolism (5%).

Frequency not stated: hyperglycaemia, depression, insomnia, fatigue, hypertension, oedema/fluid retention, nausea, vomiting, constipation, cushingoid changes, bone mineral density loss, reduced libido, impotence, altered menstruation, breast tenderness, urticaria, acne.

Rare (<0.1%): jaundice, alopecia, hirsutism.

MPA: discontinue if any of the following develop: jaundice, hepatic impairment, significant increase in blood pressure, thrombo-embolic event, new onset migraine, severe visual disturbances.

Dose and use

Appetite stimulation

Given the relatively poor benefit:risk ratio (see above), the use of progestogens requires careful consideration, particularly in patients with conditions other than cancer or AIDS:

- start with **megestrol acetate** 80–160mg PO each morning
- if initial response poor, consider doubling the dose after 2 weeks[38,39]
- maximum dose generally 800mg PO/24h.

MPA 400mg PO each morning–b.d. is an alternative in countries where higher strength tablets are available (e.g. 100mg, 200mg and 400mg).

Hot flushes after surgical or chemical castration

- **MPA** 5–20mg PO b.d.–q.d.s. *or*
- **megestrol acetate** 80mg PO each morning; 40mg is used in countries where the 40mg tablet or oral suspension is readily available. The effect manifests after 2–4 weeks.[40]

Supply

Megestrol acetate

Megace® (Bristol-Myers Squibb)
Tablets (scored) 160mg, 28 days @ 160mg each morning = £20.
Tablets 40mg, 28 days @ 40mg each morning = £10 (unauthorized in the UK, can import via IDIS, 100 tablets = £36 see Chapter 24, p.751).
Oral suspension 40mg/mL, 28 days @ 160mg each morning = £18 (unauthorized in the UK, can import via IDIS, 240mL bottle = £39 see Chapter 24, p.751).

Medroxyprogesterone acetate

Provera® (Pharmacia)
Tablets (scored) 2.5mg, 5mg, 10mg, 100mg, 200mg, 400mg (unscored), 28 days @ 5mg b.d. = £7; 28 days @ 400mg each morning = £55.

Climanor® (Resource Medical)
Tablets 5mg, 28 days @ 5mg b.d. = £6.50.

7

1 Decruze SB and Green JA (2007) Hormone therapy in advanced and recurrent endometrial cancer: a systematic review. *International Journal of Gynecology Cancer*. **17**: 964–978.
2 Schindler AE *et al.* (2003) Classification and pharmacology of progestins. *Maturitas*. **46 (Suppl 1)**: s7–s16.
3 Mantovani G *et al.* (1998) Cytokine involvement in cancer anorexia/cachexia: role of megestrol acetate and medroxyprogesterone acetate on cytokine downregulation and improvement of clinical symptoms. *Critical Reviews in Oncogenesis*. **9**: 99–106.
4 MacDonald N (2005) Anorexia-cachexia syndrome. *European Journal of Palliative Care*. **12 (Suppl)**: 8s–14s.
5 Par Pharmaceuticals *Data on file*.
6 Deschamps B *et al.* (2009) Food effect on the bioavailability of two distinct formulations of megestrol acetate oral suspension. *International Journal of Nanomedicine*. **4**: 185–192.
7 Laviano A *et al.* (2003) Cancer anorexia: clinical implications, pathogenesis, and therapeutic strategies. *Lancet Oncology*. **4**: 686–694.
8 Fearon K *et al.* (2010) Definition and classification of cancer cachexia: an international consensus framework. *Lancet Oncology*. **12**: 489–495.
9 Gordon JN *et al.* (2005) Cancer cachexia. *Quarterly Journal of Medicine*. **98**: 779–788.
10 Scott HR *et al.* (2002) The systemic inflammatory response, weight loss, performance status and survival in patients with inoperable non-small cell lung cancer. *British Journal of Cancer*. **87**: 264–267.
11 Davis MP *et al.* (2004) Appetite and cancer-associated anorexia: a review. *Journal of Clinical Oncology*. **22**: 1510–1517.
12 Ramos EJ *et al.* (2004) Cancer anorexia-cachexia syndrome: cytokines and neuropeptides. *Current Opinion in Clinical Nutrition and Metabolic Care*. **7**: 427–434.
13 Laviano A *et al.* (2005) Therapy insight: Cancer anorexia-cachexia syndrome--when all you can eat is yourself. *Nature Clinical Practice Oncology*. **2**: 158–165.
14 Ruiz Garcia V *et al.* (2013) Megestrol acetate for treatment of anorexia-cachexia syndrome. *Cochrane Database of Systemic Reviews*. **3**: CD004310. www.thecochranelibrary.com
15 Loprinzi CL *et al.* (1993) Phase III evaluation of four doses of megestrol acetate as therapy for patients with cancer anorexia and/or cachexia. *Journal of Clinical Oncology*. **11**: 762–767.
16 Simons JP *et al.* (1998) Effects of medroxyprogesterone acetate on food intake, body composition, and resting energy expenditure in patients with advanced, nonhormone-sensitive cancer: a randomized, placebo-controlled trial. *Cancer*. **82**: 553–560.
17 Jatoi A *et al.* (2002) Dronabinol versus megestrol acetate versus combination therapy for cancer-associated anorexia: a North Central Cancer Treatment Group study. *Journal of Clinical Oncology*. **20**: 567–573.
18 Jatoi A *et al.* (2003) On appetite and its loss. *Journal of Clinical Oncology*. **21 (Suppl 9)**: 79–81.
19 Jatoi A *et al.* (2004) An eicosapentaenoic acid supplement versus megestrol acetate versus both for patients with cancer-associated wasting: a North Central Cancer Treatment Group and National Cancer Institute of Canada collaborative effort. *Journal of Clinical Oncology*. **22**: 2469–2476.
20 Kropsky B *et al.* (2003) Incidence of deep-venous thrombosis in nursing home residents using megestrol acetate. *Journal of the American Medical Directors Association*. **4**: 255–256.
21 Garcia VR and Juan O (2005) Megestrol acetate-probably less effective than has been reported! *Journal of Pain and Symptom Management*. **30**: 4; author reply 5–6.
22 Payne C (2012) Interventions for fatigue and weight loss in adults with advanced progressive illness. *Cochrane Database of Systematic Reviews*. **1**: CD008427. www.thecochranelibrary.com
23 Bodenner D *et al.* (2007) A retrospective study of the association between megestrol acetate administration and mortality among nursing home residents with clinically significant weight loss. *American Journal Geriatric Pharmacotherapy*. **5**: 137–146.
24 Loprinzi C *et al.* (1993) Body-composition changes in patients who gain weight while receiving megestrol acetate. *Journal of Clinical Oncology*. **11**: 152–154.
25 Loprinzi CL *et al.* (1999) Randomized comparison of megestrol acetate versus dexamethasone versus fluoxymesterone for the treatment of cancer anorexia/cachexia. *Journal of Clinical Oncology*. **17**: 3299–3306.
26 Faludi G *et al.* (1966) Factors influencing the development of steroid-induced myopathies. *Annals of the New York Academy of Sciences*. **138**: 62–72.
27 Willemse PH *et al.* (1990) A randomized comparison of megestrol acetate (MA) and medroxyprogesterone acetate (MPA) in patients with advanced breast cancer. *European Journal of Cancer*. **26**: 337–343.
28 Dev R *et al.* (2007) Association between megestrol acetate treatment and symptomatic adrenal insufficiency with hypogonadism in male patients with cancer. *Cancer*. **110**: 1173–1177.

29 Naing KK *et al.* (1999) Megestrol acetate therapy and secondary adrenal suppression. *Cancer.* **86**: 1044–1049.
30 Lambert C *et al.* (2002) Effects of testosterone replacement and/or resistance exercise on the composition of megestrol acetate stimulated weight gain in elderly men: a randomized controlled trial. *Journal of Clinical Endocrinology and Metabolism.* **87**: 2100–2106.
31 McMillan DC *et al.* (1999) A prospective randomized study of megestrol acetate and ibuprofen in gastrointestinal cancer patients with weight loss. *British Journal of Cancer.* **79**: 495–500.
32 Cerchietti LC *et al.* (2004) Effects of celecoxib, medroxyprogesterone, and dietary intervention on systemic syndromes in patients with advanced lung adenocarcinoma: a pilot study. *Journal of Pain and Symptom Management.* **27**: 85–95.
33 Maccio A *et al.* (2012) A randomized phase III clinical trial of a combined treatment for cachexia in patients with gynecological cancers: evaluating the impact on metabolic and inflammatory profiles and quality of life. *Gynecologic Oncology.* **124**: 417–425.
34 Bosaeus I *et al.* (2002) Dietary intake, resting energy expenditure, weight loss and survival in cancer patients. *Journal of Nutrition.* **132 (Suppl 11)**: 3465s–3466s.
35 Lai V *et al.* (2008) Results of a pilot study of the effects of celecoxib on cancer cachexia in patients with cancer of the head, neck, and gastrointestinal tract. *Head & Neck.* **30**: 67–74.
36 Madeddu C *et al.* (2012) Randomized phase III clinical trial of a combined treatment with carnitine + celecoxib +/- megestrol acetate for patients with cancer-related anorexia/cachexia syndrome. *Clinical Nutrition.* **31**: 176–182.
37 Villarroel *et al.* (2008) Megestrol acetate-induced adrenal insufficiency. *Clinical Translational Oncology.* **10**: 235–237.
38 Donnelly S and Walsh TD (1995) Low-dose megestrol acetate for appetite stimulation in advanced cancer. *Journal of Pain and Symptom Management.* **10**: 182–183.
39 Vadell C *et al.* (1998) Anticachectic efficacy of megestrol acetate at different doses and versus placebo in patients with neoplastic cachexia. *American Journal of Clinical Oncology.* **21**: 347–351.
40 Loprinzi CL *et al.* (1996) Megestrol acetate for the prevention of hot flashes. *New England Journal of Medicine.* **331**: 347–352.

Updated April 2016

DANAZOL

Class: Anabolic steroid, 17α-alkyl androgen.

Indications: Endometriosis, severe pain in benign fibrocystic breast disease, †hereditary angioedema,[1,2] †cholestatic pruritus, †idiopathic immune thrombocytopenia, †gynaecomastia.

Contra-indications: Thrombo-embolic disorders; severe cardiac, hepatic or renal impairment (*except when indicated for cholestatic pruritus,* see Drugs for pruritus, Table 1, p.761); androgen-dependent tumour; undiagnosed genital bleeding; pregnancy; breast-feeding.

Pharmacology

Danazol is a chemically modified testosterone. It suppresses the pituitary-ovarian axis by inhibiting the pituitary output of gonadotrophins. The beneficial effect of 17α-alkyl androgens in cholestatic pruritus was discovered serendipitously some 60 years ago when the co-incidental use of **methyltestosterone** in a patient with primary biliary cirrhosis resulted in relief from the associated pruritus.[3] Cholestatic pruritus is central in origin and is associated with enhanced opioidergic tone, secondary to the increased production of endogenous opioids.[4–6] Thus, in some specialist liver units, an opioid antagonist (see p.459) such as **naloxone** or **naltrexone** is the treatment of choice for cholestatic pruritus.[7]

However, opioid antagonists are unsuitable for patients with cholestatic pruritus who need opioids for pain relief. In this setting, **sertraline**, **rifampicin** (see p.481) and 17α-alkyl androgens are alternatives (also see Drugs for pruritus, p.761).[8] The mechanism of action is uncertain, but 17α-alkyl androgens are directly toxic to hepatocytes.[9–11] Thus, it is possible that danazol causes focal cell damage which limits the ability of the cholestatic liver to produce enkephalins. Androgens themselves can cause cholestatic jaundice,[12,13] and have occasionally caused severe hepatic impairment.[14,15] By mouth, 17α-alkyl androgens (e.g. **methyltestosterone**) are more bio-available than other androgens (e.g. **testosterone**) because of the reduction in first-pass hepatic metabolism in androgens with a 17α-alkyl radical.[16] Danazol also has additional effects on the liver which are not shared by **testosterone**.[17] The antipruritic effect is maintained even if the cholestasis is exacerbated by the androgen itself.[16] Androgens and oestrogens sometimes relieve non-specific pruritus in the elderly.[18]

A meta-analysis suggests that anabolic steroids may increase body weight and lean body mass in HIV-infected individuals, though the change is small and may not be clinically significant.[19]

Bio-availability 11% (fasting), 44% (after lipid-rich meal);[20] doubling the dose increases the plasma concentration by only 35–40%.

Onset of action 5–10 days in cholestatic pruritus.

Time to peak plasma concentration <3h.
Plasma halflife 4.5h (single dose); >24h (multiple doses).
Duration of action >24h.

Cautions

Hepatic or renal disease, fluid retention, cardiovascular disease, hypertension, epilepsy, diabetes mellitus, lipoprotein disorder, polycythaemia, migraine. Discontinue if female virilization occurs (may become irreversible if treatment continued), or if symptoms of raised intracranial pressure or thrombo-embolism arise. Monitor LFTs and FBC every 6 months during long-term treatment. May cause false results with thyroid function tests. If contraception is required, a non-hormonal method will be necessary.

Drug interactions

Through an unknown mechanism, danazol inhibits the metabolism of several drugs, including **carbamazepine**, **ciclosporin**, **warfarin**, and possibly **tacrolimus**, and toxicity is sometimes seen. It can cause insulin resistance.

The concurrent use of danazol and a statin has been associated with acute renal impairment, pancreatitis and rhabdomyolysis.[21,22]

Undesirable effects

Related to inhibition of the pituitary-ovarian axis: amenorrhoea, hot flushes, sweating, reduction in breast size, reduced libido, vaginitis, emotional lability.
Related to androgenic activity: acne, oily skin or hair, mild hirsutism, deepening of the voice, androgenic alopecia, and rarely clitoral hypertrophy. Paradoxically, testicular atrophy may occur.
Other effects: include dizziness, seizures, benign intracranial hypertension (rare), thrombotic events, nausea, severe hepatotoxicity (occasional), muscle cramps, photosensitivity.

Dose and use

Cholestatic pruritus

Moisturizing the skin with an emollient is always the first step. In patients with an extrahepatic obstruction (e.g. because of pancreatic cancer, lymphadenopathy), the treatment of choice is generally stenting of the bile duct.

When this is not feasible or when associated with intrahepatic cholestasis, danazol is generally reserved for situations where **sertraline** or **rifampicin** (see p.481) are ineffective (see Chapter 26, Table 1, p.761):

- start with 200mg PO once daily–t.d.s. with food (to improve absorption).[20,23]

Benefit from danazol is generally seen after about 5–10 days.[24] Androgenic changes may be ameliorated by reducing the dose from once daily to 3 times weekly or even less.[16]

Alternative 17α-alkyl androgens in some countries (not UK) include:

- **norethandrolone** 10mg b.d.–t.d.s.
- **methyltestosterone** 25mg once daily SL.

Supply

All preparations are **CD** Schedule 4 part 2.

Danazol (generic)
Capsules 100mg, 200mg, 28 days @ 200mg once daily = £15–£33.

Danol® (Sanofi-Aventis)
Capsules 100mg, 200mg, 28 days @ 200mg once daily = £15.

1 Hosea SW and Frank MM (1980) Danazole in the treatment of hereditary angioedema. *Drugs*. **19**: 370–372.
2 MacFarlane JT and Davies D (1981) Management of hereditary angio-oedema with low-dose danazol. *British Medical Journal (Clin Res Ed)*. **282**: 1275.
3 Ahrens E *et al.* (1950) Primary biliary cirrhosis. *Medicine*. **29**: 299–364.
4 Jones E and Bergasa N (1990) The pruritus of cholestasis. From bile acids to opiate agonists. *Hepatology*. **11**: 884–887.

5 Jones E and Dekker L (2000) Florid opioid withdrawal-like reaction precipitated by naltrexone in a patient with chronic cholestasis. *Gastroenterology*. **118**: 431–432.
6 Jones EA and Bergasa N (2004) The pruritus of cholestasis and the opioid neurotransmitter system. In: Z Zylicz *et al.* (eds) *Pruritus in advanced desease*. Oxford University Press, Oxford, pp. 56–68.
7 Jones E and Bergasa N (1999) The pruritus of cholestasis. *Hepatology*. **29**: 1003–1006.
8 Twycross RG *et al.* (2003) Itch: scratching more than the surface. *Quarterly Journal of Medicine*. **96**: 7–26.
9 Welder A *et al.* (1995) Toxic effects of anabolic-androgen steroids in primary rat hepatic cell cultures. *Journal of Pharmacological and Toxicological Methods*. **33**: 187–195.
10 Ohsawa T and Iwashita S (1986) Hepatitis associated with danazol. *Drug Intelligence and Clinical Pharmacy*. **20**: 889.
11 Fermand JP *et al.* (1990) Danazol-induced hepatocellular adenoma. *American Journal of Medicine*. **88**: 529–530.
12 Boue F *et al.* (1986) Danazol and cholestatic hepatitis. *Annals of Internal Medicine*. **105**: 139–140.
13 Silva MO *et al.* (1989) Danazol-induced cholestasis. *American Journal of Gastroenterology*. **84**: 426-428.
14 Elsharkawy AM *et al.* (2012) Cholestasis secondary to anabolic steroid use in young men. *British Medical Journal*. **344**: e468.
15 Piekarska A and Wojcik K (2009) Modern anabolics and anticatabolics: The scope of the hepatologist's knowledge. *Experimental and Clinical Hepatology*. **5**: 7-11.
16 Lloyd-Thomas H and Sherlock S (1952) Testosterone therapy for the pruritus of obstructive jaundice. *British Medical Journal*. **2**: 1289–1291.
17 Fernandez L *et al.* (1994) Stanozolol and danazol, unlike natural androgens, interact with the low affinity glucocorticoid-binding sites from male rat liver microsomes. *Endocrinology*. **134**: 1401–1408.
18 Feldman S *et al.* (1942) Treatment of senile pruritus with androgens and estrogens. *Archives of Dermatology and Syphilology Chicago*. **46**: 112–127.
19 Johns KKJ *et al.* (2005) Anabolic steroids for the treatment of weight loss in HIV-infected individuals. *Cochrane Database of Systematic Reviews*. **4**: CD005483. www.thecochranelibrary.com
20 Sunesen VH *et al.* (2005) Effect of liquid volume and food intake on the absolute bioavailability of danazol, a poorly soluble drug. *European Journal of Pharmaceutical Sciences*. **24**: 297–303.
21 Hsieh CY and Chen CH (2008) Rhabdomyolysis and pancreatitis associated with coadministration of danazol 600 mg/d and lovastatin 40 mg/d. *Clinical Therapeutics*. **30**: 1330-1335.
22 Andreou ER and Ledger S (2003) Potential drug interaction between simvastatin and danazol causing rhabdomyolysis. *Canadian Journal of Clinical Pharmacology*. **10**: 172-174.
23 Twycross RG and Zylicz Z (2004) Systemic therapy: making rational choices. In: Z Zylicz *et al.* (eds) *Pruritus in advanced disease*. Oxford University Press, London, pp. 161–178.
24 Sherlock S and Dooley J (1993) *Diseases of the Liver and Biliary System* (9e). Blackwell Scientific, Oxford.

Updated August 2016

*THALIDOMIDE

Class: Biologic response modifier.

Indications: Multiple myeloma, †lepromatous leprosy (erythema nodosum leprosum), †graft versus host disease (GVHD), †prevention of graft rejection, †recurrent aphthous stomatitis (e.g. HIV-related, connective tissue disease (Behcet's syndrome)), †paraneoplastic sweating, †paraneoplastic pruritus, †cachexia in HIV and cancer, †intractable GI bleeding, †intractable **irinotecan**-induced diarrhoea, †discoid lupus erythematosus.[1–3]

Contra-indications: Because it causes severe congenital abnormalities (absent or shortened limbs), thalidomide is contra-indicated in pregnant women and in women with childbearing potential unless strict contraception is implemented (see Dose and use).[4]

Pharmacology

Thalidomide is an immunomodulator with anticytokine, anti-integrin, and anti-angiogenic properties.[3,5,6] It was withdrawn from use as a non-barbiturate hypnotic with anti-emetic properties in the early 1960s after it emerged that it was teratogenic (via binding cereblon, an E3 ligase protein).[3] Subsequently, it has been found to have immunomodulatory properties with potential for the treatment of various conditions.[7] However, its use is closely monitored and it is prohibitively expensive (see Supply).

Thalidomide inhibits the synthesis of the pro-inflammatory cytokine tumour necrosis factor α (TNF-α) by monocytes,[8] and stimulates interleukin-2 and interferon-γ production (thereby stimulating human T lymphocytes).[9] It also inhibits chemotaxis of neutrophils and monocytes. Thalidomide antagonizes PGE_2, PGF_2, histamine, serotonin, and acetylcholine.[10] It also affects several other mechanisms associated with inflammation and immunomodulation.[11] These properties probably account for the prevention of **irinotecan**-induced diarrhoea,[12] and the amelioration of paraneoplastic sweating,[13] paraneoplastic pruritus (also see p.757),[14–16] and cough in idiopathic pulmonary fibrosis.[17] This could also explain the beneficial effect of thalidomide in Crohn's disease and ulcerative colitis.[18]

An anti-inflammatory effect is also likely to explain benefit in the cachexia-anorexia syndrome in patients with cancer or HIV,[19–21] although high-quality evidence is limited.[22] Two small RCTs of thalidomide 100–200mg in patients with cancer found no overall benefit on body composition.[23,24] About half the patients experienced undesirable effects with the 200mg dose, particularly rash and drowsiness,[24] suggesting that a lower starting dose is advisable, e.g. 50–100mg at bedtime.

Despite promising case reports suggesting that thalidomide and its analogues (see below) may have an analgesic effect, a large RCT in complex regional pain syndrome (n=184) failed to show any benefit.[25–27]

The main antiproliferative and pro-apoptotic effects of thalidomide (and its analogues) in cancer cells are downstream consequences of binding cereblon.[3] Consistent benefit has been shown in several haematological cancers, but not solid tumours. It also inhibits angiogenesis by suppressing vascular endothelial growth factor (VEGF), a potent angiogenic factor secreted by cancer cells in response to hypoxia. This property also provides the rationale underlying the use of thalidomide in refractory GI bleeding and epistaxis associated with underlying angiodysplasia.[28–32]

Analogues of thalidomide with similar anti-angiogenic, immunomodulatory and anti-inflammatory properties have been developed, e.g. **lenalidomide**, **pomalidomide**.[3] **Lenalidomide** is authorized in the treatment of multiple myeloma, certain myelodysplastic syndromes which cause transfusion-dependent anaemia and mantle cell lymphoma (see SPC). It is also used in relapsed/refractory chronic lymphocytic leukaemia.[33] However, the analogues are also likely to carry serious teratogenic risk, are restricted in their availability, and are very expensive. Further, there is a dearth of experience with the analogues in symptom management and palliative care, and no obvious advantage over thalidomide.

The metabolism of thalidomide is almost completely by non-enzymatic hydrolysis in the plasma. Elimination is primarily via the kidneys with <3% of the dose as unchanged thalidomide. Hepatic and renal impairment appear to have minimal effect on the metabolism and pharmacokinetics of thalidomide. However, because active metabolites are eliminated via the urine, patients with severe renal impairment should be carefully monitored for undesirable effects.

Bio-availability 67–93% PO in animals, no data in humans.
Onset of action varies from 2 days for lepromatous leprosy and paraneoplastic sweating to 1–2 months for GVHD and 2–3 months for rheumatoid arthritis.
Time to peak plasma concentration 2–6h, delayed by food.
Plasma half-life 6h (200mg/24h)–18h (800mg/24h).[11]
Duration of action 24h.

Cautions

Treat as a 'cytotoxic' when handling. Thalidomide potentiates the sedative properties of barbiturates and alcohol, and increases the likelihood of extrapyramidal effects with **chlorpromazine** and **reserpine**.[10] Thalidomide should be used cautiously with other drugs which cause drowsiness, neuropathy or reduce the effectiveness of oral contraception (e.g. HIV protease inhibitors, **rifampicin**, **rifabutin**, **phenytoin**, **carbamazepine**).[10,34]

Undesirable effects

Neuropathy

Low grade peripheral neuropathy occurs in >80% of patients receiving thalidomide, and severe neuropathy in 3–5%, generally after treatment lasting >6 months.[35,36] The incidence is higher in elderly patients, women, and in patients with pre-existing neuropathy or who are treated with neurotoxic chemotherapy, e.g. **vincristine**, **cisplatin**, **paclitaxel**.[36] Generally, the peripheral neuropathy presents as distal paraesthesia or dysaesthesia with or without sensory loss. Physical examination may be normal or show mildly decreased sensation in the distal limbs. Strength is usually preserved, but reflexes, particularly ankle jerks, may be depressed or absent. These symptoms, which are progressive, typically begin in the distal lower limbs and extend proximally and into the upper limbs.[37]

Although some studies have found a relationship between the cumulative dose and the occurrence of neuropathy,[38] others have not.[39] Nerve conduction studies typically show results consistent with a sensory axonal neuropathy. If a patient develops neuropathy, dose reduction or cessation may be required to decrease the likelihood of chronic painful neuropathy (see Dose and use).[40,41]

Some 80% of patients experience a mild decrease in bowel motility; this may reflect autonomic dysfunction, and can exacerbate constipation.[42]

Cardiovascular

Thalidomide and **lenalidomide** increase the risk of VTE in patients with multiple myeloma, particularly when used in combination with high-dose corticosteroids and/or chemotherapy, and thromboprophylaxis is recommended.[43] Both thalidomide and **lenalidomide** increase the risk of arterial thrombosis, e.g. myocardial infarction, stroke.[44] The MHRA recommends thromboprophylaxis for patients at increased thrombotic risk for the first five months of treatment.[44] Generally this is with **LMWH** or **warfarin**. Although **aspirin** has been used, UK guidelines advocate this only in patients with no other risk factors for VTE.[45,46]

Thalidomide is associated with arrhythmia, hypotension, and oedema. Sinus bradycardia, generally mild, has been reported in ≤25% of patients.[47] Severe sinus bradycardia occurs in only 1–3% of patients.[47] Mild peripheral oedema has been reported in 15%. Orthostatic hypotension and dizziness also have been reported with thalidomide.[48] A dose-dependent decrease in supine systolic and diastolic pressures is seen up to 2h after dosing.[49] However, symptom control doses should not affect blood pressure.

Skin

A pruritic and maculopapular rash may occur 10–14 days after starting treatment, starting on the trunk and extending to the back and proximal limbs. This is generally mild and resolves with the use of an emollient and dose reduction.[50] Severe skin reactions, such as Stevens-Johnson syndrome and toxic epidermal necrolysis, may also occur.[51] Skin complications seem more likely when thalidomide is combined with corticosteroids.

Other

These include drowsiness, seizures,[48] altered temperature sensitivity, pulmonary hypertension,[52] irregular menstrual cycles, and hypothyroidism. Thalidomide can increase HIV viral load. Reactivation of varicella zoster (resulting in disseminated herpes zoster) and hepatitis B virus (resulting in acute hepatic failure) have occurred.[52,53] Myelosuppression is rare.

Tumour flare (a temporary increase in size of a cancerous lesion) may occur. When thalidomide is used to treat chronic lymphocytic leukaemia, some patients have experienced increased lymphadenopathy, enlargement of the spleen, and an increased lymphocyte count.[54]

Abnormal LFTs are common with **lenalidomide**. Serious (including fatal) instances of drug-related hepatitis have been reported in <1%, resulting in the recommendation for routine monitoring of LFTs (weekly for the first 8 weeks and monthly thereafter).[55] Patients with multiple myeloma treated with thalidomide or **lenalidomide** have a small increased risk of a second primary malignancy.[56,57]

Dose and use

Thalidomide is prohibitively expensive and cost alone will severely limit its use. In palliative care, thalidomide should *never* be considered as a first-line treatment. Its use should be considered only when more conventional treatments have failed and a full review of the potential benefits and harms has been undertaken with specialist colleagues.

There are several potential uses for thalidomide in palliative care (Table 1).[58] Female patients prescribed thalidomide must be counselled about the need for contraception, and male patients must use a condom. Written consent should be obtained.[59] Contraception should be used for ≥4 weeks before starting, during, and for 4 weeks after stopping treatment. Regular pregnancy testing is advised throughout treatment. Because thalidomide is present in the semen of men treated with the drug, even after vasectomy a latex condom must be used during sexual intercourse with women of childbearing potential.[60]

Table 1 Potential uses of PO thalidomide in palliative care[a]

Indication	*Dose*
Aphthous ulcers in HIV+ disease	100–200mg at bedtime for 10 days[61]
Paraneoplastic sweating	100–200mg at bedtime[62,63]
Paraneoplastic pruritus[b]	100–200mg at bedtime[14–16]
Cachexia-anorexia in HIV+ disease and cancer	50–200mg at bedtime[19–21]
GI bleeding (associated with angiodysplasia/ radiation proctitis/cancer)	100–300mg at bedtime[31]
Intractable irinotecan-induced diarrhoea	400mg at bedtime[12,64]

a. thalidomide is *not* the first-line treatment for any of these indications
b. also see p.757.

7

For dose modifications if peripheral neuropathy occurs (i.e. paraesthesia, weakness and/or loss of reflexes), see Table 2.[4]

Table 2 Dose changes in thalidomide-related neuropathy[a]

Grade	*Impact of neuropathy*	*Dose modification*[b]
1	No loss of function	Consider reducing dose if symptoms worsen
2	Interfering with function but not with activities of daily living	Reduce dose or interrupt treatment. If no improvement or further deterioration, stop treatment. If improves to grade 1 or better, restart treatment (if the benefit/risk ratio remains favourable)
3	Interfering with activities of daily living	Stop treatment
4	Disabling	Stop treatment

a. based on first-line use in multiple myeloma
b. monitor the patient regularly during treatment, e.g. monthly in women of child-bearing potential, otherwise every 3 months.

Supply

In the UK, thalidomide is available through a strictly monitored Thalidomide Celgene pregnancy prevention programme (http://www.celgene.co.uk/content/uploads/sites/3/Thalidomide_Celgene_Healthcare_Professional_Booklet.pdf). Both prescribers and pharmacies must be registered with the programme to prescribe, order and supply thalidomide.

Lenalidomide is similarly monitored through the Revlimid pregnancy prevention programme (http://celgene.co.uk/content/uploads/sites/3/Revlimid_Healthcare_Professional_Information_Pack.pdf).

Thalidomide Celgene® (Celgene)
Capsules 50mg, 28 days @ 50mg at bedtime = £299.

Lenalidomide
Revlimid® (Celgene)
Capsules 2.5mg, 5mg, 7.5mg, 10mg, 15mg, 20mg, 25mg, 28 days @ 5mg at bedtime = £4,760.

1 Chen M *et al.* (2010) Innovative uses of thalidomide. *Dermatologic Clinics.* **28**: 577–586.
2 Hello M *et al.* (2010) Use of thalidomide for severe recurrent aphthous stomatitis: a multicenter cohort analysis. *Medicine (Baltimore).* **89**: 176–182.
3 Millrine D and Kishimoto T (2017) A brighter sde to thalidomide: its potential use in immunological disorders. *Trends in Molecular Medicine.* **23**: 348–361.

4 Celgene (2017) Thalidomide Celgene 50mg Hard Capsules. *SPC*. www.medicines.org.uk

5 Jacobson J (2000) Thalidomide: a remarkable comeback. *Expert Opinion in Pharmacotherapy*. **1**: 849–863.

6 De Sanctis JB *et al.* (2010) Pharmacological properties of thalidomide and its analogues. *Recent Patents on Inflammation and Allergy Drug Discovery*. **4**: 144–148.

7 Peuckmann V *et al.* (2000) Potential novel uses of thalidomide: focus on palliative care. *Drugs*. **60**: 273–292.

8 Sampaio E *et al.* (1991) Thalidomide selectively inhibits tumour necrosis factor alpha production by stimulated human monocytes. *Journal of Experimental Medicine*. **173**: 699–703.

9 Corral LG and Kaplan G (1999) Immunomodulation by thalidomide and thalidomide analogues. *Annals of the Rheumatic Diseases*. **58 (Suppl 1)**: I107–I13.

10 Radomsky C and Levine N (2001) Thalidomide. *Dermatologic Clinics*. **19**: 87–103.

11 Bousvaros A and Mueller B (2001) Thalidomide in gastrointestinal disorders. *Drugs*. **61**: 777–787.

12 Govindarajan R *et al.* (2000) Effect of thalidomide on gastrointestinal toxic effects of irinotecan. *Lancet*. **356**: 566–567.

13 Deaner P (2000) The use of thalidomide in the management of severe sweating in patients with advanced malignancy: trial report. *Palliative Medicine*. **14**: 429–431.

14 Smith J *et al.* (2002) Use of thalidomide in the treatment of intractable itch. Poster abstract 21. In: *Palliative Care Congress*; Sheffield, UK.

15 Lowney AC *et al.* (2014) Thalidomide therapy for pruritus in the palliative setting--a distinct subset of patients in whom the benefit may outweigh the risk. *Journal of Pain and Symptom Management*. **48**: e3–5.

16 Goncalves F (2010) Thalidomide for the control of severe paraneoplastic pruritus associated with Hodgkin's disease. *American Journal of Hospice and Palliative Care*. **27**: 486–487.

17 Horton MR *et al.* (2012) Thalidomide for the treatment of cough in idiopathic pulmonary fibrosis: a randomized trial. *Annals of Internal Medicine*. **157**: 398–406.

18 Bramuzzo M *et al.* (2016) Thalidomide for inflammatory bowel disease: Systematic review. *Medicine*. **95**: e4239.

19 Gordon JN *et al.* (2005) Thalidomide in the treatment of cancer cachexia: a randomised placebo controlled trial. *Gut*. **54**: 540–545.

20 Davis M *et al.* (2012) A Phase II dose titration study of thalidomide for cancer-associated anorexia. *Journal of Pain and Symptom Management*. **43**: 78–86.

21 Reyes-Teran G *et al.* (1996) Effects of thalidomide on HIV-associated wasting syndrome: a randomized, double-blind, placebo-controlled clinical trial. *AIDS*. **10**: 1501–1507.

22 Reid J *et al.* (2012) Thalidomide for managing cancer cachexia. *Cochrane Database of Systematic Reviews*. **4**: CD008664. www.thecochranelibrary.com

23 Yennurajalingam S *et al.* (2012) The role of thalidomide and placebo for the treatment of cancer-related anorexia-cachexia symptoms: results of a double-blind placebo-controlled randomized study. *Journal of Palliative Medicine*. **15**: 1059–1064.

24 Wilkes EA *et al.* (2011) Poor tolerability of thalidomide in end-stage oesophageal cancer. *European Journal of Cancer Care (Engl)*. **20**: 593–600.

25 Song T *et al.* (2015) Involvement of peripheral TRPV1 channels in the analgesic effects of thalidomide. *Neurochemistry International*. **85-86**: 40–45.

26 Asher C and Furnish T (2013) Lenalidomide and thalidomide in the treatment of chronic pain. *Expert Opinion in Drug Safety*. **12**: 367–374.

27 Manning DC *et al.* (2014) Lenalidomide for complex regional pain syndrome type 1: lack of efficacy in a phase II randomized study. *Journal of Pain*. **15**: 1366–1376.

28 Engelen ET *et al.* (2015) Thalidomide for treatment of gastrointestinal bleedings due to angiodysplasia: a case report in acquired von Willebrand syndrome and review of the literature. *Haemophilia*. **21**: 419–429.

29 Craanen ME *et al.* (2006) Thalidomide in refractory haemorrhagic radiation induced proctitis. *Gut*. **55**: 1371–1372.

30 Karajeh MA *et al.* (2006) Refractory bleeding from portal hypertensive gastropathy: a further novel role for thalidomide therapy? *European Journal of Gastroenterology and Hepatology*. **18**: 545–548.

31 Lambert K and Ward J (2009) The use of thalidomide in the management of bleeding from a gastric cancer. *Palliative Medicine*. **23**: 473–475.

32 Franchini M *et al.* (2012) Novel treatments for epistaxis in hereditary hemorrhagic telangiectasia: a systematic review of the clinical experience with thalidomide. *Journal of Thrombosis and Thrombolysis*.

33 Liang L *et al.* (2016) Efficacy of lenalidomide in relapsed/refractory chronic lymphocytic leukemia patient: a systematic review and meta-analysis. *Annals of Hematology*. **95**: 1473–1482.

34 Thomas D and Kantarjian H (2000) Current role of thalidomide in cancer treatment. *Current Opinion in Oncology*. **12**: 564–573.

35 Dimopoulos MA and Eleutherakis-Papaiakovou V (2004) Adverse effects of thalidomide administration in patients with neoplastic diseases. *American Journal of Medicine*. **117**: 508–515.

36 Mileshkin L *et al.* (2006) Development of neuropathy in patients with myeloma treated with thalidomide: patterns of occurrence and the role of electrophysiologic monitoring. *Journal of Clinical Oncology*. **24**: 4507–4514.

37 Wulff CH *et al.* (1985) Development of polyneuropathy during thalidomide therapy. *British Journal of Dermatology*. **112**: 475–480.

38 Fullerton P and O'Sullivan D (1968) Thalidomide neuropathy: a clinical, electrophysiological, and histological follow up study. *Journal of Neurology, Neurosurgery and Psychiatry*. **31**: 543–551.

39 Chapon F *et al.* (1985) [Neuropathies caused by thalidomide]. *Revue Neurologique (Paris)*. **141**: 719–728.

40 Gardner-Medwin J *et al.* (1994) Clinical experience with thalidomide in the management of severe oral and genital ulceration in conditions such as Behcet's disease. *Annals of Rheumatic Diseases*. **128**: 443–450.

41 Ochonisky S *et al.* (1994) Thalidomide neuropathy incidence and clinico-electrophysiologic findings in 42 patients. *Archives of Dermatology*. **130**: 66–69.

42 Grover JK *et al.* (2002) The adverse effects of thalidomide in relapsed and refractory patients of multiple myeloma. *Annals of Oncology*. **13**: 1636–1640.

43 Carrier M *et al.* (2011) Rates of venous thromboembolism in multiple myeloma patients undergoing immunomodulatory therapy with thalidomide or lenalidomide: a systematic review and meta-analysis. *Journal of Thrombosis and Haemostasis*. **9**: 653–663.

44 MHRA (2011) Thalidomide: risk of arterial and venous thromboembolism. *Drug safety update*. **(4) 12**: www.mhra.gov.uk/Safetyinformation

45 Palumbo A *et al.* (2011) Aspirin, warfarin, or enoxaparin thromboprophylaxis in patients with multiple myeloma treated with thalidomide: a phase III, open-label, randomized trial. *Journal of Clinical Oncology*. **29**: 986–993.

46 Bird JM *et al.* (2011) Guidelines for the diagnosis and management of multiple myeloma *British Journal of Haematology*. **154**: 32-75 www.bcshguidelines.com

47 Kaur A *et al.* (2003) Thalidomide-induced sinus bradycardia. *Annals of Pharmacotherapy*. **37**: 1040–1043.

48 Clark T *et al.* (2001) Thalidomid (Thalidomide) capsules: A review of the first 18 months of spontaneous postmarketing adverse event surveillance, including off-label prescribing. *Drug Safety*. **24**: 87–117.
49 Noormohamed F *et al.* (1999) Pharmacokinetics and hemodynamic effects of single oral doses of thalidomide in asymptomatic human immunodeficiency virus-infected subjects. *AIDS Research and Human Retroviruses*. **15**: 1047–1052.
50 Ng SS *et al.* (2002) Thalidomide, an antiangiogenic agent with clinical activity in cancer. *Biomedical and Pharmacology Journal*. **56**: 194–199.
51 Rajkumar SV *et al.* (2000) Life-threatening toxic epidermal necrolysis with thalidomide therapy for myeloma. *New England Journal of Medicine*. **343**: 972–973.
52 MHRA (2016) Thalidomide celgene: new important advice regarding viral reactivation and pulmonary hypertension. *Direct Healthcare Professional Communication*. www.gov.uk/drug-safety-update
53 Marriott J *et al.* (1997) A double-blind placebo-controlled phase II trial of thalidomide in asymptomatic HIV-positive patients: clinical tolerance and effect on activation markers and cytokines. *AIDS Research and Human Retroviruses*. **13**: 1625–1631.
54 Chanan-Khan A *et al.* (2005) Results of a phase I clinical trial of thalidomide in combination with fludarabine as initial therapy for patients with treatment-requiring chronic lymphocytic leukemia (CLL). *Blood*. **106**: 3348–3352.
55 MHRA (2013) Lenolidomide (Revlimid): risk of serious hepatic adverse drug reactions - routine monitoring of liver function now recommended. *Drug Safety Update*. **(6) 6**: www.mhra.gov.uk/Safetyinformation
56 MHRA (2011) Lenolidomide (Revlimid): risk of a second primary malignancy - update. *Drug Safety Update*. **(5) 4**: www.mhra.gov.uk/Safetyinformation
57 MHRA (2013) Thalidomide: risk of second primary malignancies. *Drug Safety Update*. **(6) 10**: www.mhra.gov.uk/Safetyinformation
58 Davis M and Dickerson E (2001) Thalidomide: dual benefits in palliative medicine and oncology. *American Journal of Hospice and Palliative Care*. **18**: 347–351.
59 Powell R and Gardner-Medwin J (1994) Guideline for the clinical use and dispensing of thalidomide. *Postgraduate Medical Journal*. **70**: 901–904.
60 Teo SK *et al.* (2001) Thalidomide is distributed into human semen after oral dosing. *Drug Metabolism and Disposition*. **29**: 1355–1357.
61 Jacobson J *et al.* (1997) Thalidomide for the treatment of oral aphthous ulcers in patients with human immunodeficiency virus infection. *New England Journal of Medicine*. **336**: 1487–1493.
62 Deaner P (1998) Thalidomide for distressing night sweats in advanced malignant disease. *Palliative Medicine*. **12**: 208–209.
63 Calder K and Bruera E (2000) Thalidomide for night sweats in patients with advanced cancer. *Palliative Medicine*. **14**: 77–78.
64 Govindarajan R (2000) Irinotecan and thalidomide in metastatic colorectal cancer. *Oncology (Williston Park)*. **14 (Suppl 13)**: 29–32.

Updated September 2017

8: URINARY TRACT DISORDERS

8

TAMSULOSIN

Class: Uroselective α_1-adrenergic receptor antagonist (α_1 antagonist).[1]

Indications: Symptoms associated with benign prostatic hypertrophy (BPH), †radiation-induced urethritis, †before trial without catheter inserted for acute urinary retention in men,[2] †medical management of urinary stones.[3]

Contra-indications: Symptomatic postural hypotension.

Pharmacology

Tamsulosin is a selective competitive antagonist at post-synaptic α_{1A}- and α_{1D}-adrenergic receptors, causing smooth muscle relaxation in the prostate gland, bladder neck, and possibly the detrusor (i.e. the bladder itself).[4,5] Tamsulosin is metabolized in the liver, primarily by CYP2D6 and CYP3A4; <10% is excreted unchanged in the urine.

In BPH, smooth muscle hyperplasia is estimated to be responsible for nearly half of the obstructive component. Tamsulosin is prescribed for men with moderate–severe voiding lower urinary tract symptoms (voiding LUTS, e.g. urinary hesitancy, poor urinary stream, incomplete bladder emptying, terminal dribble) and a moderately enlarged prostate gland (<30g). Tamsulosin reduces functional prostatic obstruction and increases maximum urinary flow rate. RCTs show that tamsulosin improves LUTS by 20–50%, compared to 20–30% for placebo.[6]

Other less specific α_1 antagonists are available, e.g. **prazosin** (taken b.d.). Symptomatic and urodynamic efficacy is similar when taken at the highest dose possible without unacceptable undesirable effects. Tamsulosin causes less postural hypotension than **prazosin** when given alone or with commonly used antihypertensive drugs, e.g. **atenolol**, **enalapril** and **nifedipine**.[7,8] However, even with tamsulosin there is a risk of severe hypotension necessitating hospital admission in the first 4 weeks after starting treatment.[9]

For men with troublesome moderate–severe LUTS, a greater degree of prostatic enlargement (>30g) or a PSA >1.4nanogram/mL (surrogate marker for a prostate gland >30g)[10] and at risk of progressive obstruction, a 5α-reductase inhibitor, e.g. **dutasteride** or **finasteride**, should be considered. Whereas tamsulosin generally improves symptoms within days with a full response by 6 weeks, 5α-reductase inhibitors improve symptoms only after 3–6 months.[10,11] Combined treatment with α_1 antagonist and a 5α-reductase inhibitor is more effective than either agent alone but has higher incidence of undesirable effects than monotherapy, and generally is neither necessary nor appropriate in patients with a prognosis of only 2–3 months.[12]

15% of men with voiding LUTS associated with BPH also have significant storage LUTS (e.g. frequency, urgency and incontinence). Because tamsulosin may relax bladder smooth muscle, it may reduce detrusor instability and storage LUTS. However, if storage LUTS persist following a trial of tamsulosin, consider adding an anti-muscarinic (see **Oxybutynin** p.567). This has not been demonstrated to increase the risk of acute urinary retention, particularly in men with a post-voiding residual volume of <250mL.[13,14]

An alternative approach to the management of urinary hesitancy when urinary obstruction has been excluded is to use either a muscarinic drug, e.g. **bethanechol** 10–25mg PO t.d.s., or an anticholinesterase, e.g. **distigmine bromide** (not UK) 5mg PO each morning (30min before breakfast) to stimulate bladder contraction. Because of different mechanisms of action, they can be used concurrently with tamsulosin.

Tamsulosin 400–800microgram/24h reduces external beam radiotherapy-induced LUTS (voiding, storage and mixed types) in patients with prostate cancer. When started at least 5 days before prostate radiation brachytherapy, tamsulosin also reduces short-term LUTS.[15]

Bio-availability m/r ~100% PO fasting, reduced by 30% after food.;[4] Flomaxtra® XL 55–59%, not affected by food.

Onset of action m/r 4–8h; maximum benefit 4–8 weeks.

Time to peak plasma concentration 1h; m/r 4h fasting, 6h after food;[4] Flomaxtra® XL 4–6h, not affected by food.

Plasma halflife 5–7h; m/r 9–13h (healthy volunteers), 14–15h (elderly);[4] Flomaxtra® XL 19h (single dose), 15h (steady-state).

Duration of action <24h.

Cautions

Severe hepatic or renal impairment.

Drug interactions

Concurrent use with epidural **morphine**, **sildenafil** or other α_1 antagonist increases the risk of postural hypotension.

Tamsulosin is metabolized mainly by CYP2D6, and CYP3A4. Caution should be taken with concurrent use of drugs which inhibit or induce these enzymes, e.g. **erythromycin**, particularly in those who are poor CYP2D6 metabolizers (see p.725).

Undesirable effects

Very common (>10%): dizziness, orthostatic hypotension, ejaculatory impairment[11]

Common (<10%, >1%): headache, asthenia, drowsiness or insomnia, amblyopia, chest pain, rhinitis, sinusitis, pharyngitis, cough, bitter taste, nausea, abdominal discomfort, diarrhoea, back pain, reduced libido, impotence or erectile dysfunction.

Uncommon (<1%, >0.1%): syncope, palpitations, vomiting, constipation, rash, pruritus, gynaecomastia.

Very rare (<0.01%, >0.001%): priapism.

Dose and use

Hesitancy of micturition

- m/r tamsulosin 400microgram PO once daily (because absorption is significantly affected by food, take at the same time each day with respect to meals)
- if necessary, increase to 800microgram m/r once daily after 2–4 weeks.[4]

Trial without catheter in men with acute retention

- m/r tamsulosin 400microgram PO once daily for 1–3 days before catheter removal.[2]

Supply

Tamsulosin (generic)

Capsules m/r 400microgram, 28 days @ 400microgram once daily = £4.

Tablets m/r 400microgram, 28 days @ 400microgram once daily = £9.

1 Hieble JP *et al.* (1995) International Union of Pharmacology. X. Recommendation for nomenclature of alpha 1-adrenoceptors: consensus update. *Pharmacological Reviews*. **47**: 267–270.

2 Zeif HJ and Subramonian K (2009) Alpha blockers prior to removal of a catheter for acute urinary retention in adult men. *Cochrane Database of Systematic Reviews*. CD006744. www.thecochranelibrary.com

3 Lu Z *et al.* (2012) Tamsulosin for ureteral stones: a systematic review and meta-analysis of a randomized controlled trial. *Urologica Internationalis*. **89**: 107–115.
4 Lyseng-Williamson KA *et al.* (2002) Tamsulosin: an update of its role in the management of lower urinary tract symptoms. *Drugs*. **62**: 135–167.
5 Yamada S *et al.* (2011) alpha1-Adrenoceptors and muscarinic receptors in voiding function - binding characteristics of therapeutic agents in relation to the pharmacokinetics. *British Journal of Clinical Pharmacology*. **72**: 205–217.
6 Wilt TJ *et al.* (2003) Tamsulosin for benign prostatic hyperplasia. *Cochrane Database of Systematic Reviews*. **1**: CD002081. www.thecochranelibrary.com
7 Lowe FC (1997) Coadministration of tamsulosin and three antihypertensive agents in patients with benign prostatic hyperplasia: pharmacodynamic effect. *Clinical Therapeutics*. **19**: 730–742.
8 Michel MC *et al.* (1998) Tamsulosin: real life clinical experience in 19,365 patients. *European Urology*. **34 (Suppl 2)**: 37–45.
9 Bird ST *et al.* (2013) Tamsulosin treatment for benign prostatic hyperplasia and risk of severe hypotension in men aged 40–85 years in the United States: risk window analyses using between and within patient methodology. *British Medical Journal*. **347**: f6320.
10 NICE (2010) Lower urinary tract symptoms. The managment of lower urinary tract symptoms in men. *Clinical Guideline*. **CG97**: www.nice.org.uk
11 NHS (2010) Clinical knowledge summaries. LUTS in men, age related (prostatism). http://cks.nice.org.uk
12 Roehrborn CG *et al.* (2010) The effects of combination therapy with dutasteride and tamsulosin on clinical outcomes in men with symptomatic benign prostatic hyperplasia: 4-year results from the CombAT study. *European Urology*. **57**: 123–131.
13 Sarma AV and Wei JT (2012) Clinical practice. Benign prostatic hyperplasia and lower urinary tract symptoms. *New England Journal of Medicine*. **367**: 248–257.
14 MacDiarmid SA *et al.* (2008) Efficacy and safety of extended-release oxybutynin in combination with tamsulosin for treatment of lower urinary tract symptoms in men: randomized, double-blind, placebo-controlled study. *Mayo Clinic Proceedings*. **83**: 1002–1010.
15 Crawford ED and Kavanagh BD (2006) The role of alpha-blockers in the management of lower urinary tract symptoms in prostate cancer patients treated with radiation therapy. *American Journal of Clinical Oncology*. **29**: 517–523.

Updated (minor change) August 2017

8

OXYBUTYNIN

Class: Antimuscarinic (anticholinergic).

Indications: Symptoms of an overactive bladder: urgency (with or without urge incontinence), frequency (>8 times/day) and/or nocturia (waking more than once at night to void);[1] †bladder spasm.

Contra-indications: Bladder outflow obstruction, GI obstruction including paralytic ileus, severe ulcerative colitis, predisposition to narrow-angle glaucoma, and myasthenia gravis.

Pharmacology

Bladder muscle (detrusor) contains all subtypes of muscarinic receptor. M_2 and M_3 predominate, with M_2 outnumbering M_3 3:1. M_3 receptors are particularly important in relation to detrusor contraction; the function of M_2 receptors is less clear.

Oxybutynin hydrochloride has an antimuscarinic effect on bladder innervation. It is relatively selective for M_1 and M_3 receptor subtypes (see p.5). It also has a direct papaverine-like antispasmodic effect on the detrusor.[2] It inhibits bladder contraction, relieves spasm induced by various stimuli, increases bladder capacity, and delays the desire to void in patients with a neurogenic bladder. Oxybutynin also has a topical anaesthetic effect on the bladder mucosa.[3] Oxybutynin has an active metabolite, N-desethyloxybutynin. It is not clear what proportion of its total effects are due to the metabolite. The plasma halflife of oxybutynin increases in the elderly, generally allowing smaller doses to be given.

Urinary antimuscarinics reduce frequency by 15–20% (vs. 10% with placebo); leakage episodes 45–75% (vs. 20–45%); urgency 40% (vs. 35%), and have subjective improvement rates of 40–70% (vs. 20–50%).[4,5] The absolute probability of continence after 4 weeks of treatment is 15–30%.[6]

Newer antimuscarinics, e.g. **solifenacin, darifenacin**, have higher M_3 receptor selectivity than older ones, e.g. oxybutynin and **tolterodine**.[7] They cause fewer undesirable effects and may have greater efficacy. In fact, compared with immediate-release oxybutynin, all other urinary antimuscarinics, and m/r and TD formulations of oxybutynin, are better tolerated.[5] However, although there is some evidence suggesting that m/r formulations and higher doses of some newer drugs (e.g. **fesoterodine** and **solifenacin**) have greater efficacy than oxybutynin,[1] this is not reflected in recent NICE guidelines.[6]

Oxybutynin (a tertiary amine) enters the CNS relatively easily, whereas **trospium** (a quaternary ammonium compound) does not. The M_1 receptor plays a significant role in modulating cognitive function. Thus, if an antimuscarinic with significant affinity for the M_1 receptor (as does oxybutynin) crosses the blood-brain barrier, it may cause cognitive impairment and delirium.

Newer antimuscarincs which are more M_3 selective should have fewer undesirable CNS effects.[8] In one of very few RCTs to examine this aspect, findings suggested that m/r oxybutynin causes greater cognitive dysfunction in elderly patients compared with **darifenacin.**[9]

Because of the low cost of generic immediate-release oxybutynin, it is still first-line treatment for overactive bladder, but ideally should not be prescribed for the frail elderly. If immediate-release oxybutynin is not tolerated, consider m/r or TD oxybutynin. Alternatively (and in the frail elderly), use one of the newer more selective antimuscarinics, e.g. **fesoterodine** or **darifenacin** (a once daily product).[6,10–12]

It may take four weeks to see the full response to treatment, thus the antimuscarinic should be reviewed after that, and then every 6 months to determine whether it is still needed.[13] For other options, see Box A and B.

Bio-availability 2–11% PO (immediate-release); increased by 50% with m/r tablets (with a corresponding reduction in the amount of N-desethyloxybutynin).[14]

Onset of action 30–60min PO (immediate-release).

Time to peak plasma concentration 30–60min PO (immediate-release); 4–6h (m/r, after first dose);[14,15] 24–48h TD.

Plasma halflife 2–3h PO (immediate-release); 4–5h in the elderly (immediate-release); 12–14h (m/r).[14,15]

Duration of action 6–10h PO (immediate-release); >24h (m/r); >4 days TD.

Box A Alternative drugs for urinary frequency, urgency, urge incontinence

If an antimuscarinic is contra-indicated, poorly tolerated or ineffective, consider a β_3 agonist, e.g. mirabegron 50mg PO once daily; dose adjustments are required with hepatic or renal impairment and concurrent use of a strong CYP3A4 inhibitor.[16]

For postmenopausal women with vaginal atrophy, consider short-term topical intravaginal oestrogen.[11]

For persistent nocturia without daytime urgency or frequency, consider:
- a loop diuretic, e.g. furosemide 40mg PO once daily around 1700–1800h
- a vasopressin analogue, e.g. desmopressin (p.528), although hyponatraemia is a possible complication.[10]

Box B Alternative drugs for bladder spasm

When relatively selective antimuscarinics are inadequate or inappropriate, consider less selective ones, e.g.:
- amitriptyline 10mg PO at night (see p.210)
- hyoscine *hydrobromide* 300microgram SL b.d–q.d.s. (e.g. Kwells®)
- hyoscine *butylbromide* 60–120mg/24h CSCI & 20mg SC p.r.n. (see p.16).

If the above are inadequate, consider intravesical treatments:
- morphine (10–20mg t.d.s or diamorphine 10mg t.d.s. diluted in 0.9% saline to 20mL); instil through an indwelling catheter and clamp for 30min[17]
- bupivacaine t.d.s. (0.5% bupivacaine 10mL diluted in 0.9% saline to 20mL) used alone or with intravesical morphine.[18]

Cautions

See Antimuscarinics, p.5; renal and hepatic impairment, Parkinson's disease.

Drug interactions

Concurrent treatment with ≥2 antimuscarinic drugs (including antihistamines, phenothiazines and TCAs; see Antimuscarinics, Box B, p.6) will increase the likelihood of undesirable effects, and (when centrally acting) of central toxicity, i.e. restlessness, agitation, delirium (see Antimuscarinics, Box C, p.7). Children, the elderly, and patients with renal or hepatic impairment are more susceptible to the central effects of antimuscarinics.

Oxybutynin is metabolized extensively by CYP3A4 hepatic enzyme. Concurrent use of drugs which are strong inhibitors of this enzyme (see Chpater 19. Table 8, p.725) could potentially cause toxicity, and necessitate a reduction in the dose of oxybutynin.

Undesirable effects

Antimuscarinic effects are common, including dry mouth, cognitive impairment and delirium, particularly in the frail and elderly (see Antimuscarinics, Box C, p.7); nausea and abdominal discomfort. Skin reactions are common with TD oxybutynin.

Dose and use

Immediate-release

- start with 5mg PO b.d.
- if necessary, increase progressively to 5mg q.d.s.[11]
- in the over 60s and the very frail, these doses should be halved.

If not tolerated, consider m/r or TD oxybutynin (more expensive options).

Modified-release

- start with 5mg m/r PO once daily
- if necessary, increase in 5mg/day steps at weekly intervals
- maximum recommended dose 20mg once daily.

Remains of m/r tablets may appear in the patient's faeces ('ghost tablets'), but these are inert residues, and do not affect the efficacy of the products.

TD patches

- apply 1 patch (3.9mg/24h) twice weekly to clean, dry skin on abdomen, hip or buttock; avoid application to same site within 1 week.

Similar considerations apply as for other medical transdermal products, e.g. skin hair should be clipped rather than shaved, fold plasters in half and dispose of safely, remove before MRI scans (see p.831).

Supply

Oxybutynin (generic)
Tablets 2.5mg, 3mg, 5mg, 28 days @ 5mg b.d. = £1.50.
Oral solution 2.5mg/5mL, 5mg/5mL, 28 days @ 5mg b.d. = £372.

Modified-release products
Lyrinel® XL (Janssen-Cilag)
Tablets m/r 5mg, 10mg, 28 days @ 10mg once daily = £27.

Transdermal products
Kentera® (Orion)
TD patches 36mg (releasing 3.9mg/24h), 28 days @ 1 patch twice weekly = £27.

---

1 Madhuvrata P *et al.* (2012) Which anticholinergic drug for overactive bladder symptoms in adults. *Cochrane Database of Systematic Reviews.* **1**: CD005429. www.thecochranelibrary.com
2 Andersson KE (2011) Antimuscarinic mechanisms and the overactive detrusor: an update. *European Urology.* **59**: 377–386.
3 Robinson T and Castleden C (1994) Drugs in focus: 11. Oxybutynin hydrochloride. *Prescribers' Journal.* **34**: 27–30.

4 Novara G *et al.* (2008) A systematic review and meta-analysis of randomized controlled trials with antimuscarinic drugs for overactive bladder. *European Urology*. **54**: 740–763.
5 Chapple CR *et al.* (2008) The effects of antimuscarinic treatments in overactive bladder: an update of a systematic review and meta-analysis. *European Urology*. **54**: 543–562.
6 NICE (2013) Urinary incontinence: The management of urinary incontenence in women. *Clinical Guideline*. **CG171**: www.nice.org.uk
7 Abrams P *et al.* (2006) Muscarinic receptors: their distribution and function in body systems, and the implications for treating overactive bladder. *British Journal of Pharmacology*. **148**: 565–578.
8 Callegari E *et al.* (2011) A comprehensive non-clinical evaluation of the CNS penetration potential of antimuscarinic agents for the treatment of overactive bladder. *British Journal of Clinical Pharmacology*. **72**: 235–246.
9 Kay G *et al.* (2006) Differential effects of the antimuscarinic agents darifenacin and oxybutynin ER on memory in older subjects. *European Urology*. **50**: 317–326.
10 NICE (2010) The management of lower urinary tract symptoms in men *Clinical Guideline* **CG97**: www.nice.org.uk
11 NICE (2009) Urinary tract infection (lower) - women. *Clinical Knowledsge Summaries*. http://cks.nice.org.uk
12 NHS (2010) LUTS in men, age related (prostatism). *Clinical knowledge summaries*. http://cks.nice.org.uk
13 Marinkovic SP *et al.* (2012) The management of overactive bladder syndrome. *British Medical Journal*. **344**: e2365.
14 Gupta SK and Sathyan G (1999) Pharmacokinetics of an oral once-a-day controlled-release oxybutynin formulation compared with immediate-release oxybutynin. *Journal of Clinical Pharmacology*. **39**: 289–296.
15 Janssen-Cilag (2009) Lyrinel XL prolonged release tablet. *PSPC*. www.medicines.org.uk
16 NICE (2013) Mirabegron for treating symptoms of overactive bladder. *Technology Appraisal* 290. www.nice.org.uk
17 McCoubrie R and Jeffrey D (2003) Intravesical diamorphine for bladder spasm. *Journal of Pain and Symptom Management*. **25**: 1–3.
18 Chiang D *et al.* (2005) Management of post-operative bladder spasm. *Journal of Paediatrics and Child Health*. **41**: 56–58.

Updated August 2017

METHENAMINE HIPPURATE

Class: Urinary antiseptic.

Indications: Prophylaxis against UTI.

Contra-indications: Methenamine hippurate should not be used in severe renal impairment (creatinine clearance <10mL/min; eGFR <10mL/min/1.73m^2), infection of the *upper* urinary tract (pyelonephritis), metabolic acidosis, hepatic impairment, severe dehydration, or gout.

Pharmacology

Unlike most antibacterials, methenamine does *not* act by impairing bacterial protein synthesis. Methenamine hippurate dissociates into methenamine and hippuric acid in an acid environment (pH <5.5). Methenamine is then converted to formaldehyde which is responsible for the bactericidal effect.[1,2] Most bacteria are sensitive to formaldehyde at concentrations of ≥20microgram/mL, and acquired resistance does not appear to develop.

Urea-splitting bacteria, e.g. *Pseudomonas aeruginosa*, produce ammonia which increases the alkalinity of urine. This could inhibit the formation of formaldehyde, and thereby reduce the effect of methenamine. However, hippuric acid helps maintain an acidic environment.

Prophylaxis against UTIs

Oral antibacterials are more effective than methenamine hippurate for prophylaxis.[3] However, caution must be exercised with antibacterials because of the risk of acquired resistance.

Evidence supporting the use of methenamine hippurate in treating or preventing symptomatic UTIs is limited. It may be more effective in patients with a normal renal tract (e.g. patients without bladder stones or neuropathic bladder).[4] However, trials have been conducted in disparate patient populations, using variable doses and follow up, making results difficult to generalize. As such, efficacy, indications, dose, and length of treatment, are unclear.[4]

An RCT in people after spinal cord injury (some with indwelling urethral or suprapubic catheters, some using intermittent self-catheterization, and some reflex voiding) compared prophylactic methenamine hippurate with **cranberry juice** and placebo for 6 months or until first symptomatic UTI, and found that the incidence of symptomatic UTIs was the same in all three groups.[5]

Prophylaxis against Catheter-associated UTI (CAUTI) or blockage

Bacterial colonization of indwelling catheters is common, occurring in ≤30% of patients catheterized for >7 days and almost 100% in those catheterized for >28 days. An intrinsic limitation of using urinary antiseptics to prevent CAUTI is that some urine-colonizing bacteria produce secretions which eventually thicken enough to form a protective biofilm attached to the catheter surface. This can embed both the bacteria and phosphate crystals in a matrix which is impervious to urinary antiseptics or acidifying catheter patency solutions.

In catheterized patients, formaldehyde remains in the bladder only for a short time. Intermittent clamping may increase the effectiveness of methenamine hippurate, although this has not been tested in an RCT. (Note. Catheter clamping should be avoided in patients with spinal cord compression above spinal cord level T7, because of the risk of autonomic dysreflexia).

Methenamine hippurate given to patients catheterized for ≤7 days following gynaecological surgery and for several days after catheter removal is effective in preventing CAUTI.[4,6] However, benefit from urinary antiseptics for CAUTI in patients with long-term urethral catheters or who undergo regular intermittent catheterisation has not been established in an RCT.[3,6]

Although not recently investigated, methenamine hippurate may reduce the frequency of catheter blockage with long-term indwelling catheters. In an RCT published in 1980, methenamine hippurate doubled the interval between catheter changes from 1 to 2 weeks.[7] However, catheter technology has progressed since then, and much longer intervals are now expected between catheter changes, e.g. 2–3 months.

8

Bio-availability readily absorbed.
Onset of action >2h.
Plasma halflife 4h.
Duration of action no data.

Cautions

Methenamine hippurate should *not* be administered concurrently with:

- sulfonamides because of the risk of crystalluria
- alkalinizing agents (e.g. **acetazolamide, potassium or sodium citrate, sodium bicarbonate**) because of the need for an acid urinary environment.

Undesirable effects

Occasionally causes dyspepsia, nausea and vomiting, rash, pruritus.

With chronic use, the formaldehyde produced from methenamine may irritate and inflame the bladder mucosa, and lead to painful and frequent voiding, haematuria and proteinuria.

Dose and use

The optimum dose for a urinary antiseptic in patients with an indwelling catheter has not been determined. The recommended dose at some centres is methenamine hippurate 1g PO b.d.–t.d.s.[2,6] The tablets may be crushed and taken with milk or fruit juice (see p.785).

Supply

Hiprex® (Meda)
Tablets 1g, 28 days @ 1g b.d. = £19.

1 Strom JJ and Jun H (1993) Effect of urine pH and ascorbic acid on the rate of conversion of methenamine to formaldehyde. *Biopharmaceutics and Drug Disposition*. **14**: 61–69.

2 Sweetman S.C. *Martindale: The Complete Drug Reference*. London: Pharmaceutical Press www.medicinescomplete.com (accessed January 2014).

3 Grabe. M *et al.* (2013) European Association of Urology. Guidelines on urological infections. Available from: http://www.uroweb.org/guidelines

4 Lee BS *et al.* (2012) Methenamine hippurate for preventing urinary tract infections. *Cochrane Database of Systematic Reviews*. **10**: CD003265. www.thecochranelibrary.com

5 Lee BB *et al.* (2007) Spinal-injured neuropathic bladder antisepsis (SINBA) trial. *Spinal Cord*. **45**: 542–550.

6 Hooton TM *et al.* (2010) Diagnosis, prevention, and treatment of catheter-associated urinary tract infection in adults: 2009 International Clinical Practice Guidelines from the Infectious Diseases Society of America. *Clinical Infectious Diseases*. **50**: 625–663.

7 Norberg A *et al.* (1980) Randomized double-blind study of prophylactic methenamine hippurate treatment of patients with indwelling catheters. *European Journal of Clinical Pharmacology*. **18**: 497–500.

Updated (minor change) August 2017

CATHETER PATENCY SOLUTIONS

Indications: Catheter blockage.

General considerations

Catheters can block because of blood clots, bladder mucosal debris, small calculi and/or phosphate encrustations on the surface of an indwelling catheter. Encrustations are associated with colonization of the urine by urease-producing bacteria, e.g. *Proteus mirabilis*, *Pseudomonas aeruginosa* and *Klebsiella*. Urease breaks down urea to form ammonia, increasing the alkalinity of the urine and leading to the deposition of mainly phosphate crystals on the surface of the catheter.

Some bacteria produce secretions which eventually thicken enough to form a protective biofilm attached to the catheter surface. This can embed both bacteria and phosphate crystals in a matrix which is impervious to acidifying solutions or urinary antiseptics. Thus, repeated blockage with encrustation generally means that the catheter needs to be changed.[1,2]

The main purpose of a catheter patency solution is to reduce the frequency of catheter blockage. Although a Cochrane review found insufficient evidence to make firm recommendations,[3] the BNF states that **sodium chloride** 0.9% is generally adequate as a mechanical flush for removing mucosal debris or small blood clots, and that solutions containing **citric acid** 3% (e.g. **solution G**) may be helpful in dissolving retained blood clots.

In a palliativedrugs.com survey, **sodium chloride** 0.9% was most commonly used for both flushing out cell debris or blood clots (75% of respondents) and treating or preventing encrustation (>50%). **Solution G** was next most popular for these indications (<10% and 20–25% respectively). Few respondents used other solutions.[4]

Irrigation does *not* cure catheter-associated urinary tract infection (CAUTI).[5,6] Although the BNF states that **chlorhexidine** 0.02% irrigation can be used in the management of common bladder infections, it is ineffective against most *Pseudomonas* species, and may irritate the bladder mucosa, and cause a burning sensation or haematuria.

Use of irrigations or prophylactic antibacterials to prevent CAUTI is *not* recommended by NICE or current European nursing guidelines.[7,8] Consideration should be given to the long-term use of a PO urinary antiseptic to acidify the urine and to reduce the frequency of infection (see **Methenamine hippurate**, p.570).

Dose and use

To reduce the likelihood of encrustations causing a blockage, latex catheters should be changed:

- uncoated every 2 weeks
- teflon-coated every 4 weeks
- silicone-coated or hydrogel-coated, up to every 6 weeks, depending on manufacturer's instructions.[8]

If the catheter is to be left for longer periods, a silicone catheter should be used with a catheter patency solution. These catheters are designed to remain in place for up to 3 months.[8]

Some patients are more prone to recurrent encrustation than others. If encrustations regularly cause blockage, keep a diary over ≥3 recatheterizations, calculate the average time for which a catheter remains patent, then schedule a catheter change before a blockage is likely.[2]

For flushing out blockages caused by mucosal debris or small blood clots:

- start with **sodium chloride** 0.9% p.r.n.
- if necessary, use routinely every few days or even every day[4]
- if this is inadequate for dissolving retained clots, change to **solution G**.

For prevention of phosphate encrustations or calculi:[1,4]

- start with **sodium chloride** 0.9% p.r.n. or **solution G** once or twice a week
- if necessary, increase frequency.

Commercially available sachets are preferable to using a bladder syringe, because they are less likely to force encrusted material (which contains bacteria) higher up the urinary tract.

Supply

This is not a complete list; see BNF for additional options.

Sodium chloride 0.9%
OptiFlo S® (Bard)
Sachet 50mL, 100mL = £3.25 for both sizes.

Uriflex S® (Coloplast)
Sachet 100mL = £3.50.

Uro-Tainer sodium chloride® (B. Braun Medical)
Sachet 50mL, 100mL = £3.50 for both sizes.

Solution G containing **citric acid** 3.23% with magnesium oxide, sodium bicarbonate and disodium edetate
OptiFlo G® (Bard)
Sachet 50mL, 100mL = £3.50 for both sizes.

Uriflex G® (Coloplast)
Sachet 100mL = £2.50.

Uro-Tainer Twin Suby G® (B. Braun Medical)
Dual-chamber sachet (each chamber contains 30mL) = £5.

1 Williams C and Tonkin S (2003) Blocked urinary catheters: solutions are not the only solution. *British Journal of Community Nursing*. **8**: 321–326.
2 Getliffe K (2002) Managing recurrent urinary catheter encrustation. *British Journal of Community Nursing*. **7**: 574, 576, 578–580.
3 Hagen S (2010) Washout policies in long-term indwelling urinary catheterisation in adults. *Cochrane Database of Systematic Reviews*. **3**: CD004012. www.thecochranelibrary.com
4 Palliativedrugs.com Ltd. Urinary catheter patency solutions - do you use them? *Latest additions: Survey results (December 2010)*. www.palliativedrugs.com
5 Getliffe K (1996) Bladder instillations and bladder washouts in the management of catheterized patients. *Journal of Advanced Nursing*. **23**: 548–554.
6 Pomfret I *et al.* (2004) Using bladder instillations to manage indwelling catheters. *British journal of Nursing*. **13**: 261–267.
7 NICE (2012) Infection control. Prevention of healthcare-associated infections in primary and community care. *Clinical Guideline*. **CG139**: www.nice.org.uk
8 Geng A (2012) Evidence-based guidelines for best practice in urological health care. Catheterisation. Indwelling catheters in adults, urethral and suprapubic. *European Association of Urology Nurses*. http://nurses.uroweb.org

Updated July 2015

DISCOLOURED URINE

Patients need to be warned about drugs and other substances which can discolour urine (Box A). If the urine is red, it may be assumed to be blood, and cause alarm.

The colour-banding in Box A is approximate, i.e. a drug listed under 'brown/orange/yellow' will most likely cause discolouration at some point in that range. Sometimes the colour is pH dependent.

Note. Urine colour will vary according to the concentration or dilution of the urine. Colouring agents in processed food can also affect urine colour.

Purple urine bag syndrome is caused by the breakdown of dietary tryptophan metabolites by bacteria in urine, ultimately producing indigo (blue) and indirubin (red) in alkaline urine.[3–5] Chronic urinary tract infection, long-term catheterization, constipation and immobility are the main risk factors. Although harmless, purple urine bag syndrome causes the urine to develop a strong, unpleasant odour, which becomes more noticeable over time and in warm conditions. This distresses patients more than the discolouration. Changing the drainage bag more frequently, e.g. every 3 days rather than every 5–7 days, helps to avoid the build-up of the odour. Indwelling long-term catheters may also need changing more often than normal.[5]

Box A Selected causes of discoloured urine[a]

Black/dark brown
Iron (ferrous salts)

Brown/orange/yellow
Aloe
Carrots
Dantrolene
Heparin
Nitrofurantoin
Paprika
Quinine
Retinol (vitamin A)
Riboflavin (vitamin B2)
Rifampicin
Senna (pH dependent)
Sulfasalazine
Sulfonamides
Warfarin

Brown/red/pink
Beetroot (alkaline urine)
Blackberries (acid urine)
Dantron
Ibuprofen
Levodopa-containing medicines, e.g. co-beneldopa (levodopa + benserazide) and co-careldopa (levodopa + carbidopa)
Metronidazole (acid urine)
Napthalene-based dyes in foods and medicines, e.g. Ponceau 4R
Nefopam
Phenothiazines
Phenytoin
Rhubarb (pH dependent)
Senna (alkaline urine)

Purple
Degradation of tryptophan by urinary bacteria (see text)

Blue/green
Amitriptyline[1]
Chlorophyll breath mints
FD & C Dye No. 1 (used in foods and medicines)
Promethazine (injection)
Propofol[2]
Pseudomonas aeruginosa (pyocyanin; alkaline urine)
Triamterene

Milky colour
Diffuse glomerular nephritis
Lipids
Neutrophils
Phosphates
Radiographic dyes
Urates

a. excludes discolouration which occurs only when urine is left 'on standing' and causes unlikely to be encountered in palliative care.

1 Beeley L (1986) What drugs turn urine green? *British Medical Journal*. **293**: 750.
2 Leclercq P *et al.* (2009) Green urine. *Lancet*. **373**: 1462.
3 Al-Jubouri MA and Vardhan MS (2001) A case of purple urine bag syndrome associated with Providencia rettgeri. *Journal of Clinical Pathology*. **54**: 412.
4 Ribeiro JP *et al.* (2004) Case report: purple urine bag syndrome. *Critical Care (London, England)*. **8**: R137.
5 Robinson J (2003) Purple urinary bag syndrome: a harmless but alarming problem. *British Journal of Community Nursing*. **8**: 263–266.

Updated July 2015

9: NUTRITION AND BLOOD

9

ANAEMIA

Anaemia is defined as a haemoglobin (Hb) concentration:

- <130g/L in men >15 years old
- <120g/L in non-pregnant women >15 years old.[1]

The normal range for Hb varies between populations. It is acceptable to use the lower limit of the normal range in the laboratory performing the test to define anaemia.

Anaemia is common in chronic disease. In patients with cancer, 30–60% are anaemic at diagnosis, with its prevalence and severity increasing with more advanced disease.[2] The main causes are:

- anaemia of chronic disease
- iron deficiency
- chemotherapy-induced anaemia
- vitamin B_{12} deficiency
- folate deficiency
- malignant infiltration of the marrow
- haemolytic anaemia
- renal failure.

The commonest form in cancer, and in other diseases associated with chronic inflammation, is anaemia of chronic disease (ACD). ACD is caused by cytokine-mediated disturbance of iron homeostasis. This includes overproduction by hepatocytes of hepcidin, a peptide hormone and key regulator of iron homeostasis. Hepcidin reduces iron absorption from the duodenum and iron mobilization from stores in the reticulo-endothelial system. The result is a *functional* iron deficiency, i.e. insufficient iron is available for erythropoiesis, despite generally normal or increased iron stores. (In contrast, iron deficiency anaemia is caused by low iron stores, an *absolute* iron-deficiency). Novel treatments for functional iron-deficiency anaemia are in development, e.g. monoclonal anti-hepcidin antibodies.[3]

It is important to distinguish between the various types of anaemia because treatment differs. There is no simple test to diagnose ACD. When clinically suspected, several parameters can be taken into account (Table 1).[4] Further, it is difficult to diagnose IDA in the presence of ACD because red cell indices are less reliable when there is systemic inflammation, indicated by a raised CRP. When patients have both ACD and IDA, the anaemia may be more severe and microcytic. Alternative methods of diagnosing IDA in the presence of ACD, such as hepcidin assays and serum transferrin receptor assays, remain experimental.[5–7]

Treatment

In addition to trying to correct the underlying cause(s), there are three potential treatment options for anaemia due to IDA and/or ACD:

- **iron** (oral or IV)
- blood transfusion
- SC **erythropoietin**.

Table 1 Anaemia of chronic disease (ACD) vs. iron-deficiency anaemia (IDA)

	ACD	*IDA*	*ACD and IDA*
Red cell appearance	Normochromic, normocytic[a]	Hypochromic, microcytic	Hypochromic, microcytic
Plasma ferritin (microg/L) Normal values Men 40–300 Women 20–200	High/high-normal (>100)	Low[b] (<10)	Intermediate-normal (<100)
Transferrin saturation[c]	Low-normal	Low/very low	Low-normal
Reticulocyte count	Low	Low	Low
Plasma iron	Low	Low	Low

a. anaemia may become microcytic if long standing

b. ferritin reflects iron stores but rises during acute an phase response, e.g. to trauma, infection and some cancers; thus ferritin may be normal or elevated in patients with IDA and cancer or inflammatory illness

c. measurement derived from plasma total iron binding capacity (TIBC) and plasma iron. Reflects availability of iron to erythropoetic cells.

The most appropriate choice is influenced by the severity of symptoms, likelihood of benefit, specific circumstances, and patient preference. Although IM **iron** is available, its use is discouraged; the injections are painful, may cause permanent skin staining and are no safer than IV **iron**.

Iron deficiency anaemia (IDA)

Where IDA alone is diagnosed, **ferrous sulfate** PO is generally prescribed (p.578). There is no inherent advantage to using the IV route, providing PO **iron** is tolerated and absorbed sufficiently to exceed any ongoing loss. The Hb should rise by about 20g/L over 3–4 weeks, and thus full benefit can take weeks–months.

IV **iron** is indicated when PO **iron** is poorly tolerated, ineffective or a more reliable response is required in specific circumstances, e.g. patients with renal failure receiving haemodialysis, and those undergoing surgery or myelosuppressive chemotherapy.[8–10] In some palliative care centres, IV **iron** is used because replacement can be given in 1–2 infusions, thereby reducing tablet burden. Compared to older IV **iron** preparations, the newer preparations are safer. Some have expressed concerns about the potential for IV **iron** to increase the growth of bacteria and cancer cells.[11,12] Thus, some centres avoid IV **iron** when there is active infection (also see **Ferrous sulfate**, Box A, p.579).[13]

Blood transfusion is the treatment of choice in severe IDA causing cardiovascular symptoms, e.g. angina or CHF, because it provides almost immediate benefit.

Anaemia of chronic disease (ACD)

In the palliative care setting, blood transfusion remains the treatment of choice for patients with symptomatic ACD, although its effectiveness is difficult to determine.[14] Blood transfusion can cause transfusion reactions and anaphylaxis, and may increase the risk of stroke, myocardial infarction, acute renal failure and cancer recurrence.[15] Threshold Hb concentration to trigger blood transfusion, and target Hb concentration following transfusion, should be determined on an individual patient basis, taking symptomatic benefit and risks into account.[8,16]

Erythropoetin can be considered in patients with cancer-related anaemia but *only when receiving chemotherapy*. This is because in the initial studies **erythropoietin** increased cancer progression and reduced survival in patients not receiving chemotherapy. Some of the excess deaths related to CVS complications and VTE, associated with high target Hb concentrations (>120g/L).[17,18] Subsequently, the MHRA changed the marketing authorization to stipulate that **erythropoietin** should only be given to patients receiving chemotherapy with a Hb concentration ≤100g/L, using a target Hb of ≤120g/L; further, it should be used with caution in patients receiving potentially curative treatment.[19]

In more recent studies adhering to these parameters, about 60% of patients on chemotherapy respond to **erythropoietin**, increasing to 80% when IV **iron** is also given.[20] Mean increase in

Hb is 16g/L, and mean reduction in transfusion is 1 unit of blood. No differences in survival during erythropoietin treatment, or overall, are seen. However, an increased risk of VTE remains (about 1.5-fold increased risk).[21] NICE recommends **erythropoietin** is used for cancer-related anaemia in patients receiving chemotherapy. In the USA, use of **erythropoietin** is generally restricted to those receiving palliative chemotherapy.[13,22]

Currently, there is insufficient evidence to support the use of IV **iron** alone for ACD, although studies are underway.[20]

Anaemia of chronic disease (ACD) and iron deficiency anaemia (IDA)

Generally, in patients with ACD and suspected IDA, a therapeutic trial of PO **iron** can be considered. If PO **iron** is poorly tolerated or ineffective, IV **iron** can be used.[23–26]

However, in patients with cancer, IV **iron** is more effective than PO **iron** peri-operatively, or when given to those receiving chemotherapy ± **erythropoetin**.[27,28] Although formal data are lacking, anecdotally IV **iron** may also be more effective in cancer patients with ACD and IDA in the palliative care setting, and is increasingly used.

For patients who have very symptomatic ACD and IDA, blood transfusion provides the most rapid improvement.[7,8]

1 WHO (2008) Worldwide prevalence of anaemia. 19932–19005.

2 Maccio A *et al.* (2015) The role of inflammation, iron, and nutritional status in cancer-related anemia: results of a large, prospective, observational study. *Haematologica*. **100**: 124–132.

3 Fraenkel PG (2015) Understanding anemia of chronic disease. *Hematology*. **2015**: 14–18.

4 Thomas DW *et al.* (2013) Guideline for the laboratory diagnosis of functional iron deficiency. *British Journal of Haematology*. **161**: 639–648.

5 Camaschella C (2015) Iron-deficiency anemia. *New England Journal of Medicine*. **372**: 1832–1843.

6 Kelly AU *et al.* (2017) Interpreting iron studies. *British Medical Journal*. **357**: j2513.

7 Cullis JO (2011) Diagnosis and management of anaemia of chronic disease: current status. *British Journal of Haematology*. **154**: 289–300.

8 NICE (2015) Blood transfusion. *National Guideline* **NG24**. www.nice.org.uk

9 Lopez A *et al.* (2016) Iron deficiency anaemia. *Lancet*. **387**: 907–916.

10 Gurusamy KS *et al.* (2014) Iron therapy in anaemic adults without chronic kidney disease. *Cochrane Database of Systematic Reviews*. **12**: CD010640. wwwthecochranelibrary.com

11 Beguin Y *et al.* (2014) Epidemiological and nonclinical studies investigating effects of iron in carcinogenesis--a critical review. *Critical Reviews in Oncology/Hematology*. **89**: 1–15.

12 Litton E *et al.* (2013) Safety and efficacy of intravenous iron therapy in reducing requirement for allogeneic blood transfusion: systematic review and meta-analysis of randomised clinical trials. *British Medical Journal*. **347**: f4822.

13 National Comprehensive Cancer Network Practice Guidelines in Oncology (2016) Cancer and chemotherapy induced anemia. Version 2.2017. www.nccn.org (accessed June 2017).

14 Preston NJ *et al.* (2012) Blood transfusions for anaemia in patients with advanced cancer. *Cochrane Database of Systematic Reviews*. **2**: CD009007. www.thecochranelibrary.com

15 Aapro M *et al.* (2012) Prevalence and management of cancer-related anaemia, iron deficiency and the specific role of i.v. iron. *Annals of Oncology*. **23**: 1954–1962.

16 Carson JL *et al.* (2016) Transfusion thresholds and other strategies for guiding allogeneic red blood cell transfusion. *Cochrane Database of Systematic Reviews*. **10**: CD002042. www.thecochranelibrary.com

17 Steensma DP (2007) Erythropoiesis stimulating agents. *British Medical Journal*. **334**: 648–649.

18 Bohlius J (2009) Recombinant human erythropoiesis-stimulating agents and mortality in patients with cancer: a met-analysis of randomized trails. *Lancet*. **373**: 1532–1542.

19 MHRA (2007) Epoetins for the management of anaemia associated with cancer: risk of tumour progression and mortality. www.mhra.gov.uk

20 Auerbach M *et al.* (2010) Darbepoetin alfa 300 or 500 mug once every 3 weeks with or without intravenous iron in patients with chemotherapy-induced anemia. *American Journal of Hematology*. **85**: 655–663.

21 Tonia T *et al.* (2012) Erythropoietin or darbepoetin for patients with cancer. *Cochrane Database of Systematic Reviews*. **12**: CD003407. www.thecochranelibrary.com

22 NICE (2014) Erythropoiesis-stimulating agents (epoetin and darbepoetin) for treating anaemia in people with cancer having chemotherapy. *Technology Appraisal Guideline* TA323. www.nice.org.uk

23 Lindgren S *et al.* (2009) Intravenous iron sucrose is superior to oral iron sulphate for correcting anaemia and restoring iron stores in IBD patients: A randomized, controlled, evaluator-blind, multicentre study. *Scandinavian Journal of Gastroenterology*. **44**: 838–845.

24 Albaramki J *et al.* (2012) Parenteral versus oral iron therapy for adults and children with chronic kidney disease. *Cochrane Database of Systematic Reviews*. **1**: CD007857. www.thecochranelibrary.com

25 Onken JE *et al.* (2014) A multicenter, randomized, active-controlled study to investigate the efficacy and safety of intravenous ferric carboxymaltose in patients with iron deficiency anemia. *Transfusion*. **54**: 306–315.

26 Bregman DB *et al.* (2013) Hepcidin levels predict nonresponsiveness to oral iron therapy in patients with iron deficiency anemia. *American Journal of Hematology*. **88**: 97–101.

27 Gafter-Gvili A *et al.* (2013) Intravenous iron supplementation for the treatment of chemotherapy-induced anaemia - systematic review and meta-analysis of randomised controlled trials. *Acta Oncologica*. **52**: 18–29.

28 Lebrun F *et al.* (2017) Intravenous iron therapy for anemic cancer patients: a review of recently published clinical studies. *Supportive Care in Cancer*. **25**: 2313–2319.

Updated September 2017

FERROUS SULFATE

Class: Elemental salt.

Indications: Prevention and treatment of iron deficiency anaemia.

Contra-indications: Anaemia not caused by iron deficiency; haemosiderosis, haemochromatosis.

Pharmacology

Ferrous salts are better absorbed than ferric salts. Because there are only marginal differences in terms of efficiency of iron absorption, the choice of ferrous salt is based mainly on the incidence of undesirable effects and cost. Some undesirable effects relate directly to the amount of elemental iron, and improved tolerance after switching to another salt may be because the elemental iron content is less (Table 1). M/r formulations are designed to reduce undesirable effects by releasing iron gradually as the tablet or capsule passes down the GI tract.[1] However, these products are likely to carry most of the iron past the first part of the duodenum into parts of the intestine where iron absorption is poor. Such products have little therapeutic advantage and should not be used.[2]

Dietary accessible (non-haem) iron absorption may be increased by a high intake of red meat, poultry, fish or **ascorbic acid** (e.g. from fruits) but reduced by a high intake of phytates (e.g. in whole-grain cereals), polyphenols (e.g. in tea and coffee), and **calcium** (e.g. in dairy products).[3]

Table 1 Elemental ferrous iron content of different iron salts

Iron salt	*Amount (mg)*	*Ferrous content (mg)*
Ferrous fumarate	200	65
Ferrous sulfate, dried (anhydrous)	200	65
Ferrous sulfate	300	60
Ferrous gluconate	300	35

Some oral formulations contain **ascorbic acid** or chelated iron. These modifications have been shown experimentally to produce a modest increase in the absorption of iron. However, the therapeutic advantage is minimal, and the cost may be increased.[2] Further, **ascorbic acid** may increase GI irritation. There is no clinical justification for the inclusion of other therapeutically active ingredients such as the B group of vitamins (except **folic acid** for pregnant women).

When treating iron deficiency, Hb should rise by about 20g/L over 3–4 weeks. Epithelial tissue changes such as atrophic glossitis and koilonychia also improve but generally more slowly.

Drug interactions

Because of decreased absorption of iron, the other drug or both, ferrous sulfate should not be administered concurrently with antacids, bisphosphonates, **calcium** salts, **colestyramine**, **demeclocycline**, **levodopa**, **levothyroxine**, **penicillamine**, quinolone antibacterials, tetracyclines, and **zinc**.

Undesirable effects

Dyspepsia, nausea, epigastric pain, constipation and diarrhoea. Nausea and epigastric pain are dose-related but the relationship between dose and altered bowel habit is not so clear.[2] Elderly patients are more likely to develop constipation, occasionally leading to faecal impaction; m/r products are more likely to cause diarrhoea, particularly in patients with inflammatory bowel disease.

Note. Liquid formulations may stain teeth. Urine and stools are discoloured (black), and this may result in a false positive faecal occult blood test.

Dose and use

The diagnosis of iron deficiency should be confirmed before iron supplements are prescribed (see Anaemia, p.575).

Oral

The PO dose of **elemental iron** for iron-deficiency anaemia is 100–200mg/24h. This can be provided, for example, as dried (anhydrous) ferrous sulfate 200mg b.d.–t.d.s (= elemental iron 130–195mg/24h). After the Hb has risen to normal, treatment should be continued for a further 3 months to replenish the iron stores.[4]

Doses >600mg/24h of dried (anhydrous) ferrous sulfate exceed the maximal absorption capacity and increase undesirable effects. If undesirable GI effects occur:

- reduce the dose
- take with food (but may reduce absorption by up to 50%)
- switch to an alternative iron salt with a lower elemental iron content
- switch to a liquid formulation (may be less damaging to GI mucosa)[5]
- dilute liquid formulations and swallow through a straw to prevent discolouration of the teeth.

Consider prophylaxis in patients at high risk of iron deficiency, e.g. those with a poor diet, malabsorption, and after total or sub-total gastrectomy; for example, prescribe dried (anhydrous) ferrous sulfate 200mg once daily (elemental iron 65mg).

9

IV iron

Generally, IV iron (Box A) is reserved for when PO iron is not tolerated or ineffective. However, it is the preferred option in several specific circumstances (also see Anaemia, p.575).

Box A IV Iron

For an overview of the role of IV iron in iron deficiency anaemia, anaemia of chronic disease, or when both co-exist, see Anaemia, p.575.

Several IV iron products are available.

Indications: Authorized indications vary between products, see SPCs for details. Iron deficiency anaemia in inflammatory bowel disease, chronic kidney disease, otherwise when PO iron is ineffective, not tolerated, or there is a need to deliver iron rapidly; †cancer-related anemia in patients receiving chemotherapy and erythropoietin; †patients with NYHA stage III–IV heart failure.[6]

Contra-indications: Risk factors for hypersensitivity reactions to IV iron, including asthma, eczema, history of allergic disorders, active rheumatoid arthritis. Use in hepatic or renal impairment varies between preparations, see SPCs for details.

Cautions

Active infection (may aid bacterial growth).

Undesirable effects

Common (<10%, >1%): Nausea.
Uncommon (<1%, ≥0.1%): Severe hypersensitivity reactions including, seizures, malaise, dizziness, tremor, chest pain, tachycardia, arrhythmias, myalgia, arthralgia, sweating.
Rare (<0.1%, ≥0.01%): Anaphylaxis.

The newer IV iron preparations are less likely to cause hypersensitivity reactions than the older high molecular weight iron dextran, now withdrawn from use. Nonetheless, rarely, severe hypersensitivity reactions including anaphylaxis occur, even after previous IV doses have been tolerated. Thus, *IV iron should only be given where resuscitation facilities are immediately available* and patients should be monitored during and for at least 30min after the infusion.[7,8]

Dose and use

There are four IV iron products available in the UK: ferric carboxymaltose, iron dextran, iron isomaltoside 1000 and iron sucrose. The dose, expressed as mg of elemental iron, is calculated from the Ganzoni formula:

Iron dose (mg) = body weight (kg)[a] x (target Hb[b] – actual Hb (g/dL)) x 0.24 + iron for stores (mg)[c]

a. use ideal body weight, e.g. by calculating weight at BMI 25kg/m²
b. determined individually and according to underlying cause of anaemia
c. if body weight >35kg, required iron stores are ≥50mg; some guidelines calculate them using 10–15mg iron/kg body weight.

continued

Box A Continued

Most IV iron products can be given as a total dose infusion over 1–2 treatments (see individual SPCs). The exception is iron sucrose, which has to be given in divided doses of 100–200mg, 1–3 times/week, extending the treatment over several weeks.

For administration procedures see individual SPCs.

In iron-deficiency anaemia, check Hb after 4 weeks; when severe, consider checking ferritin to monitor iron stores. If anaemia has not corrected, confirm diagnosis of iron-deficiency anaemia and repeat IV iron. To monitor treatment of concurrent iron-deficiency anaemia and anaemia of chronic disease, seek haematology advice.

Supply

See below.

Supply

Oral products

Ferrous sulfate, dried (generic)
Tablets 200mg (65mg iron), 28 days @ 200mg t.d.s. (195mg elemental iron/24h) = £3.

Ferrous sulfate
Ironorm® (Wallace)
Oral drops 125mg (25mg iron)/mL, 28 days @ 4mL b.d. (200mg elemental iron/24h) = £448.

Ferrous *fumarate* (generic)
Tablets 210mg (68mg iron), 28 days @ 210mg t.d.s. (204mg elemental iron/24h) = £3.50.
Tablets 322mg (100mg iron), 28 days @ 322mg b.d. (200mg elemental iron/24h) = £2.
Capsules 305mg (100mg iron), 28 days @ 305mg b.d. (200mg elemental iron/24h) = £1.50.
Oral solution 140mg (45mg iron)/5mL, 28 days @ 280mg (10mL) b.d. (180mg elemental iron/24h) = £10.

Ferrous *gluconate* (generic)
Tablets 300mg (35mg iron), 28 days @ 600mg t.d.s. (210mg elemental iron/24h) = £12.

Parenteral products

Ferric carboxymaltose
Ferinject® (Vifor)
Injection 50mg/mL, 2mL, 10mL and 20mL vial = £16, £81 and £154; *contains sodium 0.24mmol/mL.*

Iron dextran
Cosmofer® (Pharmacosmos)
Injection 50mg/mL, 2mL and 10mL amp = £8 and £40.

Iron isomaltoside
Diafer® (Pharmacosmos)
Injection 50mg/mL, 2mL amp= £17.

Monofer® (Pharmacosmos)
Injection 100mg/mL, 1mL, 5mL, 10mL vial = £17, £84, £170.

1 Cancelo-Hidalgo MJ *et al.* (2013) Tolerability of different oral iron supplements: a systematic review. *Current Medical Research and Opinion.* **29**: 291–303.
2 British National Formulary Section 9.1.1.1 Oral Iron. London: BMJ Group and Pharmaceutical Press. www.bnf.org (accessed June 2017).
3 Heath AL and Fairweather-Tait SJ (2002) Clinical implications of changes in the modern diet: iron intake, absorption and status. *Best Practice and Research Clinical Haematology.* **15**: 225–241.
4 Lopez A *et al.* (2016) Iron deficiency anaemia. *Lancet.* **387**: 907–916.

5 Ji H and Yardley JH (2004) Iron medication-associated gastric mucosal injury. *Archives of Pathology and Laboratory Medicine*. **128**: 821–822.
6 Drozd M *et al.* (2017) Iron therapy in patients with heart failure and iron deficiency: review of iron preparations for practitioners. *American Journal of Cardiovascular Drugs*. **17**: 183–201.
7 MHRA (2013) Intravenous iron and serious hypersensitivity reactions: stengthened recommendations. *Drug Safety Update*. www.gov.uk/drug-safety-update
8 Rampton D *et al.* (2014) Hypersensitivity reactions to intravenous iron: guidance for risk minimization and management. *Haematologica*. **99**: 1671–1676.

Updated September 2017

ASCORBIC ACID (VITAMIN C)

Class: Vitamin.

Indications: Scurvy, †decubitus ulcers, †urinary infection.

Pharmacology

Ascorbic acid (vitamin C) is a powerful reducing agent. It is obtained from dietary sources of fresh fruit and vegetables, e.g. blackcurrants, kiwifruit, broccoli, red pepper and oranges. It cannot be synthesized by the body. It is involved in the hydroxylation of proline to hydroxyproline, which is necessary for the formation of collagen. The failure of this accounts for most of the clinical effects found in deficiency (scurvy), e.g. keratosis of hair follicles with 'corkscrew hair', perifollicular haemorrhages, swollen spongy infected and bleeding gums, loose teeth, spontaneous bruising and haemorrhage, anaemia and failure of wound healing. Repeated infections are also common. In healthy adults, a dietary intake of about 30–60mg/24h is necessary; in scurvy, a rapid clinical response is seen with ≥250mg/24h in divided doses.

Absorption occurs mainly from the proximal small intestine by a saturable process. In health, body stores of ascorbic acid are about 1.5g, although larger stores may occur with intakes higher than 200mg/24h. It is excreted as oxalic acid, unchanged ascorbic acid and small amounts of dehydro-ascorbic acid. Ascorbic acid is used to acidify urine in patients with alkaline urine and recurrent urinary infections.

A beneficial effect of megadose ascorbic acid therapy has been claimed for many conditions,[1] including the common cold, asthma, atherosclerosis, cancer, psychiatric disorders, increased susceptibility to infections related to abnormal leucocyte function, infertility and osteogenesis imperfecta. Ascorbic acid has also been tried in the treatment of wound healing, pain in Paget's disease and opioid withdrawal. There are few RCTs to substantiate these claims. Systematic reviews of vitamin C for the prevention and treatment of cancer have found no conclusive evidence of benefit.[2,3] However, vitamin C deficiency is common in cancer patients and low plasma concentrations have been associated with shorter survival.[4] Further, dietary vitamin C intake and supplement use following a diagnosis of breast cancer are associated with a reduced mortality risk for cancer and other causes.[5]

Vitamin C alone or with β-carotene and vitamin E does not prevent the development of colorectal adenoma.[6] However, ascorbic acid does reduce the severity of a cold but not its incidence.[7] On the other hand, enthusiasm for high-dose ascorbic acid for HIV+ people waned after many died from disease progression.[8] Although it has been postulated that ascorbic acid might help prevent ischaemic heart disease, in contrast to other anti-oxidant vitamins, little benefit is seen in RCTs.[9,10] Of more concern are data which indicate that a total daily dose as small as 500mg has a pro-oxidant effect which could result in genetic mutation.[11]

Drug interactions

Aspirin reduces the absorption of ascorbic acid by up to a third. In patients with renal impairment, because of an increased risk of aluminium toxicity, avoid concurrent use of ascorbic acid and **aluminium**-containing products.

Undesirable effects

GI symptoms may occur at doses of >1g/24h.[12] Doses of >3g/24h may result in diarrhoea, acidosis, glycosuria, oxaluria, and renal stones. Tolerance may occur with prolonged use of large doses, resulting in symptoms of deficiency if intake is reduced.

In the past, some centres used undissolved effervescent ascorbic acid tablets (available OTC) for debriding the tongue. However, such use has fallen out of favour because the acidity may:

- exacerbate a sore or inflamed mouth
- contribute to the demineralization of teeth
- predispose to oral infections (see p.615).

Further, if not completely dissolved or swallowed when lying down, the tablets could cause localized oesophagitis.

Dose and use

Ascorbic acid is generally given PO; if this is not feasible or malabsorption is suspected, it can be given by SC or IM injection or IVI.

Vitamin C deficiency

- for florid scurvy, give 100mg PO t.d.s. (or 250mg once daily–b.d. parenterally) for 4 weeks
- otherwise, give 100mg PO once daily; continue indefinitely in undernourished patients, particularly the elderly.

Enhancement of healing

- give 100mg PO b.d. for 4 weeks.

Acidification of urine

- give 100–200mg PO b.d.; test urine with litmus paper until a constant acid result is obtained. Note. May alter the excretion of some drugs.

Supply

Ascorbic acid (generic)

Tablets 50mg, 100mg, 200mg, 500mg, 28 days @ 100mg o.d. = £14.

Injection 100mg/mL, 5mL amp = £4.50.

1 Ovesen L (1984) Vitamin therapy in the absence of obvious deficiency. What is the evidence? *Drugs*. **27**: 148–170.

2 Coulter ID *et al.* (2006) Antioxidants vitamin C and vitamin E for the prevention and treatment of cancer. *Journal of General Internal Medicine*. **21**: 735–744.

3 Jacobs C *et al.* (2015) Is there a role for oral or intravenous ascorbate (vitamin C) in treating patients with cancer? A systematic review. *Oncologist*. **20**: 210–223.

4 Mayland CR *et al.* (2005) Vitamin C deficiency in cancer patients. *Palliative Medicine*. **19**: 17–20.

5 Harris HR *et al.* (2014) Vitamin C and survival among women with breast cancer: a meta-analysis. *European Journal of Cancer*. **50**: 1223–1231.

6 Greenberg E *et al.* (1994) A clinical trial of antioxidant vitamins to prevent colorectal adenoma. Polyp Prevention Study Group. *New England Journal of Medicine*. **331**: 141–147.

7 Hemila H (1994) Does vitamin C alleviate the symptoms of the common cold? a review of current evidence. *Scandinavian Journal of Infectious Diseases*. **26**: 1–6.

8 Abrams D (1990) Alternative therapies in HIV infection. *AIDS*. **4**: 1179–1187.

9 Rimm E (1993) Vitamin E consumption and the risk of coronary heart disease in men. *New England Journal of Medicine*. **328**: 1450–1456.

10 Stampfer M (1993) Vitamin E consumption and the risk of coronary disease in women. *New England Journal of Medicine*. **328**: 1444–1449.

11 Podmore I *et al.* (1998) Vitamin C exhibits pro-oxidant properties. *Nature*. **392**: 559.

12 Beveridge C (2002) Basic Nutrition. In: C Repchinsky and C LeBlanc (eds) *Patient Self Care* (1e). Canadian Pharmacists Association, Ottawa, pp. 339–358.

Updated July 2015

PHYTOMENADIONE (VITAMIN K_1)

Class: Vitamin.

Indications: Vitamin K deficiency, reversal of anticoagulant effects of **warfarin** and other coumarins, †bleeding tendency in patients with hepatic impairment, †hypoprothrombinaemia induced by salicylates, sulfonamides, **quinidine**, **quinine** and antibacterials.

Pharmacology

Vitamin K is a fat-soluble vitamin. Phytomenadione (vitamin K_1) is the active form, and is present in green vegetables, dairy products and soya bean oil. In addition, vitamin K is synthesized by bacteria in the terminal ileum and colon.

Phytomenadione is necessary for the synthesis of coagulation factors II, VII, IX and X, and of proteins involved in bone calcification. Oral coumarins block the recycling of vitamin K metabolites in the liver, and thus block the synthesis of the coagulation factors. This block is circumvented by exogenous vitamin K.

Hepatic stores of vitamin K are depleted in <3 days of dietary restriction. In patients with advanced cancer, >20% are vitamin K deficient.[1] Patients who are malnourished, have fat malabsorption (e.g. in biliary obstruction or liver disease) or are having prolonged courses of antibacterials which sterilize the GI tract are at risk of deficiency and a rapid rise in prothrombin time (PT) and activated partial thromboplastin time (APTT).

Menadiol sodium phosphate is a water-soluble synthetic vitamin K analogue. It can be given PO to prevent vitamin K deficiency in patients with fat malabsorption or to correct dietary deficiency. (Note. Phytomenadione and vitamin K analogues do *not* reverse heparin-induced anticoagulation, see p.91).

9

Hepatic failure

Phytomenadione is *not* indicated routinely in chronic hepatic failure because blood coagulation is 'rebalanced' by a reduction of both procoagulant and anticoagulant factors.[2] If a patient with hepatic failure develops surface bleeding (e.g. petechiae, purpura, multiple bruising, epistaxis, gum bleeding, bleeding from GI tract), PT should be checked, and if prolonged, phytomenadione is indicated. However, its use should be limited to conscious patients with a reasonable performance status for whom other supportive measures are deemed appropriate (e.g. blood transfusion). Phytomenadione should not be used in moribund patients in an attempt to prevent an imminent inevitable death.

Because vitamin K deficiency is rarely the primary cause of coagulopathy in hepatic failure, phytomenadione may only partially correct the PT. A persistently prolonged PT following administration of phytomenadione may indicate the existence of a clotting factor deficiency caused by impaired hepatic synthesis. Other underlying conditions may also contribute to the bleeding tendency, e.g. renal failure, sepsis.[2]

Plasma halflife 1.5–3h.

Cautions

Unless there is major bleeding, phytomenadione should generally not be given to patients with a prosthetic heart valve; fresh frozen plasma or **dried prothrombin complex** should be used instead.

Oral absorption of **menadiol sodium phosphate** is reduced by concurrent administration with **colestyramine** or **liquid paraffin (mineral oil)**.

Undesirable effects

Rarely, anaphylaxis after IV use.

Dose and use

Phytomenadione (Konakion® MM) is given by slow IV injection over at least 30sec, generally 3–5min, or by IVI diluted in 50mL of 5% glucose over 20–30min (protect from light).
Konakion® MM formulation must not be given IM.

Reversal of warfarin anticoagulation

Use the British Society for Haematology guidelines.[3,4]

Major bleeding

- stop **warfarin** *and*
- give reconstituted **dried prothrombin complex** (factors II, VII, IX, X) 25–50 Units/kg IV *and*
- phytomenadione 5mg slow IV; check INR after 3h

- repeat the dose if necessary; re-check INR after 3h
- maximum dose = 40mg/24h.

Note. Recombinant factor VIIa is *not* recommended for emergency reversal of anticoagulation. Fresh frozen plasma produces suboptimal anticoagulation reversal and should be used only if **dried prothrombin complex** is not available.

Minor bleeding INR >5
- stop **warfarin** *and*
- give phytomenadione 1–3mg slow IV.

No bleeding but prolonged INR
- INR >5, withhold 1–2 doses of **warfarin** and reduce maintenance dose
- INR ≥8, give phytomenadione 1–5 mg *by mouth* using the injection formulation, and recheck INR after 24h
- restart **warfarin** when INR <5.

Vitamin K deficiency in malabsorption
Prevention:
- give **menadiol phosphate** 10mg PO once daily
- check PT after 3 days and, if still raised, increase the dose progressively up to 40mg once daily (rarely necessary) until maximal PT correction is achieved
- once maximal PT correction is achieved, give a maintenance dose of **menadiol phosphate** 10mg PO once daily and monitor PT regularly.[5]

If serious bleeding:
- phytomenadione injection (Konakion® MM) 10mg IV (see above)
- if IV access difficult, consider using the Konakion® *MM Paediatric formulation* 10mg which can be administered IM
- **dried prothrombin complex** IV may also be necessary.

Correction of a bleeding tendency in hepatic failure
- give **menadiol phosphate** 10mg PO once daily
- check prothrombin time after 3 days and, if still raised, increase the dose progressively up to 40mg once daily (rarely necessary) until maximal PT correction is achieved
- if **menadiol phosphate** unavailable, consider giving phytomenadione 2.5–10mg *by mouth* using the injection formulation.

If serious bleeding:
- give phytomenadione injection (Konakion® MM) 10mg IV (see above)
- then as for malabsorption above.

When maximal PT correction is achieved, stop **menadiol phosphate** and recheck PT if signs of surface bleeding return. In patients with hepatic impairment, the risk of venous thrombosis is often paradoxically increased. Thus, in this situation, **dried prothrombin complex** should be used only in emergency situations after specialist advice and with regular coagulation monitoring.

Note. **Desmopressin** may improve haemostasis in patients with hepatic platelet dysfunction (see p.528).

Supply
Phytomenadione
Konakion® MM (Roche)
Injection (colloidal) phytomenadione 10mg/mL in a mixed micelles vehicle, 1mL (10mg) amp = £0.50. *For IV or IVI use only, do not use IM.* PO use is off-label.

Konakion® MM Paediatric (Roche)
Injection (colloidal) phytomenadione 10mg/mL in a mixed micelles vehicle, 0.2mL (2mg) amp = £1. *Konakion® MM Paediatric may be administered PO, IM, IV.*

Menadiol phosphate (generic)
Tablets menadiol sodium phosphate equivalent to 10mg of menadiol phosphate, 7 days @ 10mg once daily = £13.

Oral suspension 5mg/5mL, 30mL = £78; unauthorized, available as a special order (see p.751). *Note price based on specials tariff applied in community.*

1 Harrington DJ *et al.* (2008) A study of the prevalence of vitamin K deficiency in patients with cancer referred to a hospital palliative care team and its association with abnormal haemostasis. *Journal of Clinical Pathology.* **61**: 537–540.
2 Tripodi A and Mannucci PM (2011) The coagulopathy of chronic liver disease. *New England Journal of Medicine.* **365**: 147–156.
3 British National Formulary Section 2.8.2. Oral anticoagulants. London: BMJ Group and Pharmaceutical Press. www.bnf.org (accessed January 2014).
4 Makris M *et al.* (2012) Guideline on the management of bleeding in patients on antithrombotic agents. *British Journal of Haematology.* **160**: 35–46.
5 Jagannath VA *et al.* (2013) Vitamin K supplementation for cystic fibrosis. *Cochrane Database of Systematic Reviews.* **4**: CD008482. www.thecochranelibrary.com

Updated (minor change) August 2017

9

POTASSIUM

Class: Elemental salt.

Indications: Hypokalaemia (<3.5mmol/L).

Pharmacology

In palliative care, hypokalaemia is most common in patients receiving non-potassium-sparing diuretics, particularly if also taking a corticosteroid. Hypokalaemia is also associated with chronic diarrhoea and persistent vomiting. Correction of hypokalaemia is important in patients taking **digoxin** or other anti-arrhythmic drugs because of the risk of an arrhythmia. Potassium supplements are seldom required with small doses of diuretics given to treat hypertension.

When larger doses of thiazide or loop diuretics are given to eliminate oedema, potassium-sparing diuretics (e.g. **amiloride**, **spironolactone**) rather than potassium supplements are preferable. Dietary supplements also help to maintain plasma potassium; 10mmol of potassium is contained in a large banana and in 250mL of orange juice.

When treating hypokalaemia, potassium chloride is generally the salt of choice because of associated hypochloraemia. However, occasionally, hypokalaemia is associated with a hyperchloraemic metabolic acidosis, and an alkalinizing salt will be preferable, e.g. potassium *bicarbonate* or potassium *citrate* (not UK). Co-existing hypomagnesaemia should always be corrected (see p.588).

Drugs are a common cause of hyperkalaemia in hospitalized patients (see Drug interactions), particularly in association with pre-existing or new renal impairment. When *mild–moderate* (i.e. 5.5–6.5mmol/L, with no ECG changes or symptoms), dose reduction or stopping the causal drug may be all that needs to be done. However, other causes may need to be considered, e.g. hypo-aldosteronism, tumour lysis syndrome, **digoxin** toxicity. Spurious results can also occur, e.g. as a result of haemolysis, marked leukocytosis or thrombocytosis. Repeating the sample and/or obtaining advice from the clinical chemistry laboratory may be necessary. For the treatment of *severe* hyperkalaemia, see below.

Cautions

Use smaller doses of potassium when there is renal impairment.

Drug interactions

Hyperkalaemia may result if used concurrently with drugs which increase the plasma potassium concentration, e.g. ACE inhibitors, angiotensin II receptor antagonists, **ciclosporin**, potassium-sparing diuretics, potassium-containing laxatives (e.g. Movicol®), **tacrolimus** and **trimethoprim**.

Undesirable effects

Oesophageal or GI ulceration, nausea and vomiting. Liquid or effervescent formulations are distasteful.

Dose and use

The normal adult daily requirement and the typical dietary intake of potassium is 40–80mmol. Whenever possible, orange juice and bananas should be used as a palatable source of potassium (see Pharmacology above).

To minimize nausea and vomiting, potassium supplements are best taken during or after a meal. Effervescent or liquid products are preferable; modified-release formulations, e.g. Slow-K®, are not recommended because of a greater risk of gastric irritation.

Prevention of hypokalaemia

- potassium *chloride*, e.g. Sando-K® 1–2 tablets b.d. (24–48mmol/24h K^+) *or*
- prescribe a potassium-sparing diuretic, e.g. **amiloride** 5–10mg once daily (maximum 20mg once daily) or **spironolactone** 25–200mg/24h.

Treatment of hypokalaemia

- potassium *chloride*, e.g. Sando-K® 2 tablets t.d.s. (72mmol/24h K^+)
- if the patient is hyperchloraemic, prescribe potassium *bicarbonate* effervescent tablets instead
- if hypokalaemia persists, investigate for possible magnesium deficiency (see p.586).

Emergency treatment of hyperkalaemia

Stop and think! Are you justified in correcting a potentially fatal complication in a moribund patient?

Urgent treatment is required when hyperkalaemia is severe (≥6.5mmol/L) or with any level ≥5.5mmol/L accompanied by ECG changes (e.g. reduced or absent P waves, PR prolongation, QRS widening) and/or symptoms (e.g. muscle weakness, paraesthesia, palpitation). An approach is summarized in Box A. However, this is only part of the management of hyperkalaemia and specialist advice should be obtained as necessary.

Box A Emergency treatment of severe hyperkalaemia[1–3]

Stop potentially contributory or antagonistic drugs

These include ACE inhibitors, angiotensin II receptor antagonists, potassium-sparing diuretics, potassium-containing laxatives (e.g. Movicol®), NSAIDs and trimethoprim.

β-blockers and digoxin should also be stopped as they antagonize the effect of insulin and β_2 agonists (see below).

Reduce the risk of cardiac arrhythmia

This is always the first step.

Give calcium gluconate 10mL of 10% solution IV over 2min; any improvement in ECG abnormalities will be seen in <3min; *stop if bradycardia develops.*

If necessary, repeat the same dose every 10min until improvement is obtained; some patients require up to 50mL.

Duration of action is 30–60min, and further doses may be required.

Note. Calcium gluconate can precipitate digoxin toxicity; give in 100mL of 5% dextrose IV over 20min in patients using digoxin (seek specialist advice).

Shift potassium into cells

When hyperkalaemia is severe (≥6.5mmol/L), insulin is generally given.

β_2 agonists (e.g. salbutamol) can be as effective.

Both reduce the plasma potassium concentration by about 0.5–1mmol/L.

Some guidelines do not recommend β_2 agonists as a sole treatment because some patients, e.g. those who are dialysis dependent or using β-blockers or digoxin, are less likely to respond.

The combination of insulin with nebulized salbutamol is more effective than either alone, with the latter helping to reduce the hypoglycaemic effect of the insulin.

These interventions do not remove potassium from the body, but buy time for more definitive treatment to be carried out.

continued

Box A Continued

Insulin

- add 10 units soluble insulin (e.g. Actrapid®) to 50mL dextrose 50% and give IV over 5min
- onset of effect 15min, duration of action at least 1h and commonly 4–6h
- if it becomes necessary to repeat the dose of insulin, additional glucose is not required if plasma glucose is ≥15mmol/L.

β_2 *agonist*

- give salbutamol 10–20mg nebulized over 10–30min (10mg in patients with ischaemic heart disease)
- when a nebulizer is not available, use salbutamol 1,200microgram (12 puffs) inhaled over 2min via a spacer device
- onset of effect 15–30min, duration of action 2h or more.

Monitoring treatment

- recheck urea and electrolytes after 30min; 1h and then q2h for 6h
- when insulin used, check blood glucose after 15min, 30min and then q1h for 6h, as delayed hypoglycaemia can occur.

Other measures

If the combined approach above fails to work, emergency dialysis may be necessary to remove potassium from the body (if appropriate to the patient's overall circumstances).

Calcium polystyrene sulphonate resin (Calcium Resonium®) 15g PO q.d.s. is also used together with regular lactulose to increase potassium loss from the GI tract. However, it is *not* an emergency treatment because it has a slow onset of action (4–24h); it can also be poorly tolerated.

Supply

Potassium *chloride*

Sando-K® (HK Pharma)

Tablets effervescent potassium bicarbonate and chloride equivalent to potassium 470mg (12mmol K^+) and chloride 285mg (8mmol Cl^-), 7 days @ 2 t.d.s. (72mmol/24h K^+ and 48mmol/24h Cl^-) = £3.25.

Kay-Cee-L® (Geistlich)

Oral syrup potassium chloride 7.5% (1mmo/mL K^+ and 1mmol/mL Cl^-), 7 days@ 20mL t.d.s. (60mmol/24h K^+) = £6.

Potassium *bicarbonate*

Tablets effervescent potassium bicarbonate 500mg, potassium acid tartrate 300mg (6.5mmol K^+), 7 days @ 2 q.d.s. (52mmol/24h K^+) = £92; dose depends on acid-base balance as well as plasma potassium concentration.

1 GAIN (Guidelines and Audit Implementation Network) (2014) Guidelines for the treatment of hyperkalaemia in adults. Availabe from: www.gain-ni.org/index.php/audits/guidelines.

2 Mahoney BA (2009) Emergency interventions for hyperkalaemia. *Cochrane Database of Systematic Reviews*. **3**: CD003235 www.thecochranelibrary.com.

3 Mandelberg A *et al.* (1999) Salbutamol metered-dose inhaler with spacer for hyperkalemia: how fast? How safe? *Chest*. **115**: 617–622.

Updated July 2015

MAGNESIUM

Class: Metal element.

Indications: Hypomagnesaemia, constipation (see p.53), †arrhythmia, †eclampsia, †asthma (nebulized), †myocardial infarction.

Pharmacology

Magnesium is the second most abundant intracellular ion after potassium. It is involved in >600 enzymatic reactions and is a co-factor for many biological processes, most of which use ATP. It is important for bone mineralization, cell growth and proliferation, glycolysis, muscular relaxation, protein synthesis (including DNA synthesis, stability and repair) and neurotransmission. About half of the total body magnesium is in soft tissue and the other half in bone. Less than 1% is in blood; thus serum magnesium concentration is a poor predictor of overall body stores.[1–3] Intracellular magnesium is mostly bound to ribosomes, phospholipids and nucleotides.[3]

The recommended total daily intake is about 6–12mmol/24h. However, magnesium intake is falling as the use of processed and fast-foods increases, and increasingly, people are failing to meet this requirement.[2,4] Thus, the incidence of chronic magnesium deficiency is probably increasing, with possible health implications, but is unrecognized because of the diagnostic limitations of serum magnesium (see below).[2,4]

Magnesium competes with calcium for absorption in the small intestine, probably by active transport. The normal serum magnesium is 0.7–1.1mmol/L. However, some have argued that for optimal health, the lower limit for serum magnesium should be considered to be 0.85mmol/L.[2] This is based on a progressive increase in the frequency of magnesium deficiency seen with serum levels between 0.85mmol/L and 0.75mmol/L (from <10% to 90%) which is associated with an increased risk of morbidity, e.g. impaired glucose tolerance, type 2 diabetes mellitus, and mortality, e.g. sudden cardiac death.[2,4] Most of the serum magnesium is in the ionized, active form, with about 30% bound to albumin and inactive. Hypo-albuminaemia may lead to artificially low serum magnesium levels.

Magnesium is excreted by the kidneys, 3–12mmol/24h. Magnesium and calcium share the same transport system in the renal tubules and there is a reciprocal relationship between the amounts excreted.

Magnesium deficiency can result from:

- *reduced intake*, e.g. an inadequate dietary intake (common)
- *reduced absorption*, e.g. small bowel resection, cholestasis, pancreatic insufficiency, diarrhoea, stoma, fistula, PPI (rare and generally with prolonged use, i.e. >1 year, see p.30)
- *increased excretion*, e.g. alcoholism, diabetes mellitus, interstitial nephritis, diuretic phase of acute tubular necrosis, hyperthyroidism, hyperparathyroidism, hyperaldosteronism, drug-induced (aminoglycosides, **amphotericin**, anti-epidermal growth factor receptor monoclonal antibodies, **cisplatin**, **ciclosporin**, loop diuretics).

Cisplatin accumulates within renal tubular cells resulting in cellular injury/death which manifests as hypomagnesaemia ± acute kidney injury. **Cisplatin** accumulation and kidney damage is enhanced by magnesium deficiency and reduced by magnesium replacement.[5,6] The risk of hypomagnesaemia with **cisplatin** is dose-dependent and increases with cumulative doses (40% cycle 1 → 100% cycle 6).[7] It can persist for 4–5 months, and sometimes years, after completing treatment.[8,9] Although generally mild and asymptomatic, it can be severe and symptomatic.

Hypomagnesaemia is an emerging toxicity of anti-epidermal growth factor receptor monoclonal antibodies, e.g. **cetuximab**, **panitumumab**.[10,11] The risk increases in the elderly, in those with a higher baseline serum magnesium, and with duration of treatment (e.g. 5% <3 months → 50% >6 months of **cetuximab**).[10] It is reversible, with magnesium levels returning to normal 4–6 weeks after discontinuation of treatment.[10]

When magnesium deficiency develops acutely, the symptoms may be obvious and severe, particularly muscle cramps, which aids diagnosis (Box A). In chronic deficiency, symptoms may be insidious in onset, less severe and non-specific.

In animal studies, magnesium deficiency results in an increased release of substance P and other mediators from nerve endings. These activate immune cells to release histamine and cytokines, producing a pro-inflammatory state and increased levels of oxygen-derived free radicals and nitric oxide. Manifestations include:[12–14]

- cutaneous vasodilatation → erythema and oedema
- leukocytosis
- inflammatory lesions in cardiac muscle
- atherogenesis
- increased levels of oxidative stress
- hyperalgesia.

In humans, the incidence of magnesium deficiency increases with aging (due to poor diet, reduced intestinal absorption, increased urinary loss etc.) and obesity. Magnesium deficiency, aging and obesity are all associated with low-grade inflammation and increased oxidative stress. This has led some to postulate that magnesium deficiency is a contributing factor to age- and obesity-related diseases such as diabetes mellitus, cardiac failure, some cancers (e.g. breast, colon), and hypertension.[13,15–18] In support of this, there is an inverse relationship between serum magnesium and CRP, and also risk of metabolic syndrome.[19,20] Magnesium supplementation has attenuated the elevated CRP in some patient groups, e.g. cardiac failure, older adults, but not others, e.g. obese adults.[19] The underlying mechanisms remain to be clarified, but in part may relate to magnesium acting as a natural 'calcium antagonist'.[3] Thus, in magnesium deficiency, intracellular calcium levels increase, activating processes which contribute to inflammation.[17]

9

Serum magnesium is associated with muscle performance, e.g. in the elderly[21] and in patients with coronary artery disease.[22] In both of these groups, the use of magnesium supplements can improve exercise capacity.[22,23] However, results are mixed, e.g. in patients with diabetes, the use of magnesium supplements or the correction of mild magnesium deficiency is of inconsistent benefit.[1]

Hypomagnesaemia (and hypokalaemia) are risk factors for drug-induced *torsade de pointes* arrhythmia. Thus, when using a drug known to prolong the QT interval, e.g. **methadone**, monitoring of serum electrolytes is generally recommended in patients with cardiac disease or other risk factors for prolonged QT, and in those at risk of electrolyte imbalance, e.g. because of vomiting, diarrhoea or diuretics (see Chapter 20, p.731).[24]

Hypermagnesaemia is rare and is seen most often in patients with renal impairment who take OTC medicines containing magnesium. Serum concentrations >4mmol/L produce drowsiness, vasodilation, slowing of atrioventricular conduction and hypotension. Over 6mmol/L there is profound CNS depression and muscle weakness (Box A). Calcium gluconate IV is used to help reverse the effects of hypermagnesaemia.

Box A Symptoms and signs of magnesium deficiency and excess

Magnesium deficiency	**Magnesium excess**
Muscle	Muscle
weakness	weakness
tremor	hypotonia
twitching	loss of reflexes
cramps	Sensation of warmth (IV)
tetany (positive Chvostek's sign)	Flushing (IV)
Paraesthesia	Drowsiness
Apathy	Slurred speech
Depression	Double vision
Delirium	Delirium
Choreiform movements	Hypotension
Nystagmus	Cardiac arrhythmia
Seizures	Respiratory depression
Prolonged QT interval	Nausea and vomiting
Cardiac arrhythmia, including *torsade de pointes*	Thirst
Increased pain (?)	Hypermagnesaemia
Hypomagnesaemia (not always)	
Hypokalaemia	
Hypocalcaemia	
Hypophospataemia	

Generally, the clinical history will indicate the most likely cause of hypomagnesaemia. When this is not the case, if necessary, the distinction between renal and non-renal causes can be made by measuring urinary magnesium excretion (Box B).

Box B Distinguishing between renal and non-renal causes of hypomagnesaemia

In hypomagnesaemia caused by renal wasting, renal excretion of magnesium is increased. The converse is true in non-renal causes of deficiency, e.g. poor intake, increased GI loss, because the kidney conserves magnesium.

$$\text{FEMg} = \left[\frac{\text{urine Mg (mmol/L) x plasma Cr (micromol/L)}}{\text{(0.7 X plasma Mg (mmol/L)) x urinary Cr (micromol/L)}} \right] \text{x 100}$$

Either a 24h urine collection can be used to measure total magnesium excretion, or a random urine specimen used to calculate the fractional excretion of magnesium (FEMg):

In a patient with hypomagnesaemia and normal renal function:
- total excretion >4mmol/24h or FEMg >2% indicates renal wasting
- total excretion <4mmol/24h or FEMg <2% indicates a non-renal cause.

Urinary magnesium excretion is a less reliable indicator in the presence of diabetes, renal impairment and drugs which increase renal excretion of magnesium, e.g. diuretics.

In deficiency states which develop more insidiously the serum magnesium is an insensitive guide to total body stores and hypomagnesaemia is not always present.[25,26] In this situation, the finding of a low urinary excretion of magnesium (Box B) may help the diagnosis. Currently, the best method for detecting magnesium deficiency is the magnesium loading test (Box C).[25,27,28]

Box C The magnesium loading test[27]

Collect pre-infusion urine sample for urinary magnesium (Mg)/creatinine (Cr) ratio. Measure Mg and Cr in mmol/L; divide the Mg value by the Cr value to calculate the Mg/Cr ratio.

By IVI over 4h, give 0.1mmol/kg of elemental magnesium, using magnesium sulfate 50% (contains elemental magnesium 2mmol/mL; see Supply) diluted to 50mL with 5% glucose.

Simultaneously, start a 24h urine collection for magnesium and creatinine. Measure the total amounts of magnesium and creatinine excreted in mmol (*not* the concentrations in mmol/L).

Calculate % magnesium retention:

$$1 - \left[\frac{\text{24h urinary Mg (mmol)} - \text{(pre-infusion urinary Mg/Cr ratio (mmol/L) x 24h urinary Cr (mmol))}}{\text{dose of elemental magnesium infused (mmol)}} \right] \text{x 100}$$

>50% retention implies definite deficiency.

If it is not possible to perform a magnesium loading test, hypokalaemia (± hypocalcaemia) not responding to potassium (± calcium) supplementation should raise the possibility of magnesium deficiency, and a trial of magnesium replacement therapy should be considered.[1] Magnesium deficiency results in hypokalaemia via increased potassium loss in the urine, and hypocalcaemia by reducing the release of and tissue sensitivity to PTH.[3]

Magnesium blocks calcium channels including the NMDA-receptor-channel and this probably accounts for its analgesic effect (Box D).[29–32] However, despite the overall positive outcome from numerous RCTs, the role of magnesium as an analgesic in palliative care is yet to be determined and ideally such use should be in the setting of a clinical trial.

Cancer cells preferentially accumulate magnesium, which is used to activate or inhibit various metabolic and genetic pathways in order to promote cell survival and proliferation.[42] Animal studies suggest that magnesium deficiency inhibits the growth of the primary cancer but exacerbates metastatic disease, possibly by enhancing inflammation.[42] The relevance of these findings for patients is unknown.

Box D Magnesium as an analgesic

A number of studies have explored the effects of magnesium, mostly as an adjuvant analgesic for postoperative pain.

A meta-analysis of 27 RCTs concluded that peri-operative IV magnesium reduces postoperative pain and analgesic requirements in patients undergoing cardiovascular, orthopaedic and urogenital surgery.[32]

Further, 8 RCTs of spinal magnesium have all reported lower pain scores and decreased analgesic requirements.[33–40]

In a RCT of PO magnesium in patients with neuropathic pain, although the frequency of pain paroxysms and the emotional component of behaviour improved, there was no overall difference in pain intensity or quality of life.[41]

Cautions

Generally, parenteral magnesium should not be given to patients with heart block or severe renal impairment. Risk of hypermagnesaemia in patients with renal impairment.

Undesirable effects

Flushing, sweating and sensation of warmth IV; diarrhoea PO. Also see features of magnesium excess in Box A.

Dose and use

Severe (serum magnesium <0.5mmol/L) and symptomatic hypomagnesaemia generally necessitates >1mmol/kg of magnesium; the route of choice is IV, given in divided doses over 3–5 days.[1,43]

Mild or asymptomatic hypomagnesaemia may be treated PO. If the cause of the magnesium deficiency persists, PO maintenance therapy will be needed.

In mild–moderate renal impairment reduce IV replacement doses by 50% and monitor plasma magnesium daily. In severe renal impairment, avoid IV replacement if possible.

Prevention of deficiency

- magnesium-rich foods, e.g. meat, seafood, green leafy vegetables, cereals and nuts
- potassium-sparing diuretics also preserve magnesium, e.g. **amiloride**.

IV correction of chronic deficiency

Because the degree of deficiency is difficult to determine from the plasma magnesium, replacement is empirical, guided by symptoms, plasma magnesium and renal function. Guidelines vary widely in their recommended doses, duration of infusion and need for monitoring, e.g. heart rate/rhythm, blood pressure and respiratory rate; as a minimum these should be checked at baseline and if the patient feels unwell during an infusion. The infusion should be through a dedicated line into a central or peripheral vein. The following are examples.

Serum magnesium <0.5mmol/L with symptoms (life-threatening), e.g. arrhythmia, seizure

- give 8mmol IV over 10–15min
- give as 4mL of magnesium sulfate injection 50% (elemental magnesium 2mmol/mL) diluted to 10mL with 0.9% saline or 5% dextrose
- follow with IVI replacement as below.

Serum magnesium <0.5mmol/L with symptoms (not life-threatening)

- on the first day give about 0.5mmol/kg IVI, then 0.25mmol/kg IVI daily for 2–5 days until the deficiency is corrected
- give as an appropriate dose of magnesium sulfate injection 50% (elemental magnesium 2mmol/mL) added to 250mL 0.9% saline or 5% dextrose (maximum concentration 0.2mmol/mL)
- infuse over a convenient time interval, e.g. 1.5h; ensure the infusion rate is restricted to ≤0.6mmol/min to avoid exceeding the maximum renal tubular resorption capacity for magnesium

- if undesirable effects occur, e.g. hypotension, increase the infusion time, e.g. up to 4h
- check serum magnesium levels daily during replacement; there may be artificially high serum levels until equilibration occurs with the intracellular compartment.

IV is the parenteral route of choice. If PO and IV routes are not feasible, options include (in order of preference):

- IM magnesium sulfate: in severe deficiency, give 0.25–0.5mmol/kg/24h as above in divided doses, e.g. multiple injections q4–6h of magnesium sulfate injection 50% (elemental magnesium 2mmol/mL); can be painful. Although dilution to 0.8mmol/mL is recommended by some, this further reduces the practicality of this approach
- CSCI magnesium sulfate: data are limited, but use of an isotonic solution is recommended, i.e. 25mmol of magnesium sulfate in 100mL WFI.[44,45]

Serum magnesium >0.5mmol/L and <0.75mmol/L without symptoms

Begin with a trial of PO replacement. The main limiting factor is diarrhoea, as magnesium salts are generally poorly absorbed PO and have a laxative effect. It is uncommon with doses <40mmol/24h, and the risk is reduced by a gradual introduction and by taking magnesium with or after food.

Several magnesium PO products are now authorized for the treatment and prevention of magnesium deficiency, but are expensive:

- magnesium *aspartate* oral powder sachets (magnesium 10mmol/sachet):
  - ▷ give 1–2 sachets once daily dissolved in 50–200mL water, orange juice or tea (10–20mmol/24h)
- magnesium *glycerophosphate* chewable tablets (magnesium 4mmol/tablet):
  - ▷ give 1–2 tablets t.d.s. (12–24mmol/24h)
- magnesium *glycerophosphate* oral solution (magnesium 5mmol/5mL):
  - ▷ give 5mL q.d.s. (20mmol/24h).

Traditionally, other PO magnesium products, either unauthorized or authorized for other indications, e.g. laxatives, have been used.[46]

Although plasma magnesium levels may respond immediately to PO replacement, generally, 6–12months is required to *fully* correct a deficiency.[47] If poorly tolerated or ineffective, and in patients with a shorter prognosis, use IV replacement as above.

PO maintenance

To prevent recurrence of the deficit, prescribe magnesium ~24mmol/24h in divided doses with food. PO is used unless poorly tolerated or ineffective, e.g. malabsorption.

Supply

Magnesium *aspartate*
Magnaspartate (KoRa Healthcare)
Oral powder elemental magnesium 10mmol sachets, 28 days @ 2 sachets once daily = £50.

Magnesium *glycerophosphate* (generic)
Oral solution elemental magnesium 5mmol/5mL, 28 days @ 5mL q.d.s. (20mmol/24h) = £106.

Neomag® (Neoceuticals)
Tablets (chewable) elemental magnesium 4mmol tablets, 28 days @ 2 tablets t.d.s. (24mmol/24h) = £77.

Magnesium *sulfate*
Injection 10% (100mg/mL), elemental magnesium 0.4mmol/mL, 10mL amp = £6.
Injection 50% (500mg/mL), elemental magnesium 2mmol/mL, 2mL, 5mL, 10mL amps = £1.50, £3 and £1.50 respectively; 20mL and 50mL vials = £4.50 and £6 respectively.

1 Martin KJ *et al.* (2009) Clinical consequences and management of hypomagnesemia. *Journal of the American Society of Nephrology.* **20**: 2291–2295.
2 Elin RJ (2010) Assessment of magnesium status for diagnosis and therapy. *Magnesium Research.* **23**: 1–5.
3 de Baaij JH *et al.* (2015) Magnesium in man: implications for health and disease. *Physiological Reviews.* **95**: 1–46.
4 Rosanoff A *et al.* (2012) Suboptimal magnesium status in the United States: are the health consequences underestimated? *Nutrition Reviews.* **70**: 153–164.

5 Yamamoto Y *et al.* (2016) Hydration with 15 mEq magnesium is effective at reducing the risk for cisplatin-induced nephrotoxicity in patients receiving cisplatin (>/=50 mg/m2) combination chemotherapy. *Anticancer Research.* **36**: 1873–1877.

6 Romani AM (2015) Cisplatin-induced renal toxicity magn...ified: role of magnesium deficiency in AKI onset. *American Journal of Physiology Renal Physiology.* **309**: F1005–1006.

7 Hodgkinson E *et al.* (2006) Magnesium depletion in patients receiving cisplatin-based chemotherapy. *Clinical Oncology.* **18**: 710–718.

8 Schilsky RL *et al.* (1982) Persistent hypomagnesemia following cisplatin chemotherapy for testicular cancer. *Cancer Treatment Reports.* **66**: 1767–1769.

9 Buckley JE *et al.* (1984) Hypomagnesemia after cisplatin combination chemotherapy. *Archives of Internal Medicine.* **144**: 2347–2348.

10 Costa A *et al.* (2011) Hypomagnesaemia and targeted anti-epidermal growth factor receptor (EGFR) agents. *Target Oncology.* **6**: 227–233.

11 Cao Y *et al.* (2010) Meta-analysis of incidence and risk of hypomagnesemia with cetuximab for advanced cancer. *Chemotherapy.* **56**: 459–465.

12 Mazur A *et al.* (2007) Magnesium and the inflammatory response: Potential physiopathological implications. *Archives of Biochemistry and Biophysics.* **458**: 48–56.

13 Tejero-Taldo MI *et al.* (2006) The nerve-heart connection in the pro-oxidant response to Mg-deficiency. *Heart Failure Reviews.* **11**: 35–44.

14 Maier JA (2012) Endothelial cells and magnesium: implications in atherosclerosis. *Clinical Science.* **122**: 397–407.

15 Barbagallo M *et al.* (2009) Magnesium homeostasis and aging. *Magnesium Research.* **22**: 235–246.

16 Nielsen FH (2010) Magnesium, inflammation, and obesity in chronic disease. *Nutrition Reviews.* **68**: 333–340.

17 King DE (2009) Inflammation and elevation of C-reactive protein: does magnesium play a key role? *Magnesium Research.* **22**: 57–59.

18 Song Y *et al.* (2005) Magnesium intake, C-reactive protein, and the prevalence of metabolic syndrome in middle-aged and older U.S. women. *Diabetes Care.* **28**: 1438–1444.

19 Dibaba DT *et al.* (2014) Dietary magnesium intake is inversely associated with serum C-reactive protein levels: meta-analysis and systematic review. *European Journal of Clinical Nutrition.* **68**: 510–516.

20 Dibaba DT *et al.* (2014) Dietary magnesium intake and risk of metabolic syndrome: a meta-analysis. *Diabetic Medicine.* **31**: 1301–1309.

21 Dominguez LJ *et al.* (2006) Magnesium and muscle performance in older persons: the InCHIANTI study. *American Journal of Clinical Nutrition.* **84**: 419–426.

22 Pokan R *et al.* (2006) Oral magnesium therapy, exercise heart rate, exercise tolerance, and myocardial function in coronary artery disease patients. *British Journal of Sports Medicine.* **40**: 773–778.

23 Veronese N *et al.* (2014) Effect of oral magnesium supplementation on physical performance in healthy elderly women involved in a weekly exercise program: a randomized controlled trial. *American Journal of Clinical Nutrition.* **100**: 974–981.

24 Al-Khatib SM *et al.* (2003) What clinicians should know about the QT interval. *Journal of the American Medical Association.* **289**: 2120–2127.

25 Dyckner T and Wester P (1982) Magnesium deficiency - guidelines for diagnosis and substitution therapy. *Acta Medica Scandinavica.* **661**: 37–41.

26 Ismail Y and Ismail AA (2010) The underestimated problem of using serum magnesium measurements to exclude magnesium deficiency in adults; a health warning is needed for "normal" results. *Clinical Chemistry and Laboratory Medicine.* **48**: 323–327.

27 Ryzen E *et al.* (1985) Parenteral magnesium testing in the evaluation of magnesium deficiency. *Magnesium.* **4**: 137–147.

28 Crosby V *et al.* (2000) The importance of low magnesium in palliative care. *Palliative Medicine.* **14**: 544.

29 Zeng C *et al.* (2016) Analgesic effect and safety of single-dose intra-articular magnesium after arthroscopic surgery: a systematic review and meta-analysis. *Scientific Reports.* **6**: 38024.

30 Crosby V *et al.* (2000) The safety and efficacy of a single dose (500mg or 1g) of intravenous magnesium sulfate in neuropathic pain poorly responsive to strong opioid analgesics in patients with cancer. *Journal of Pain and Symptom Management.* **19**: 35–39.

31 Chiu HY *et al.* (2016) Effects of intravenous and oral magnesium on reducing migraine: a meta-analysis of randomized controlled trials. *Pain Physician.* **19**: E97–112.

32 Guo BL *et al.* (2015) Effects of systemic magnesium on post-operative analgesia: is the current evidence strong enough? *Pain Physician.* **18**: 405–418.

33 Bilir A *et al.* (2007) Epidural magnesium reduces postoperative analgesic requirement. *British Journal of Anaesthesia.* **98**: 519–523.

34 Arcioni R *et al.* (2007) Combined intrathecal and epidural magnesium sulfate supplementation of spinal anesthesia to reduce post-operative analgesic requirements: a prospective, randomized, double-blind, controlled trial in patients undergoing major orthopedic surgery. *Acta Anaesthesiologica Scandinavica.* **51**: 482–489.

35 Farouk S (2008) Pre-incisional epidural magnesium provides pre-emptive and preventive analgesia in patients undergoing abdominal hysterectomy. *British Journal of Anaesthesia.* **101**: 694–699.

36 Ghatak T *et al.* (2010) Evaluation of the effect of magnesium sulphate vs. clonidine as adjunct to epidural bupivacaine. *Indian Journal of Anaesthesia.* **54**: 308–313.

37 Yousef AA and Amr YM (2010) The effect of adding magnesium sulphate to epidural bupivacaine and fentanyl in elective caesarean section using combined spinal-epidural anaesthesia: a prospective double blind randomised study. *International Journal of Obstetrics and Anesthesia.* **19**: 401–404.

38 Ouerghi S *et al.* (2011) The effect of adding intrathecal magnesium sulphate to morphine-fentanyl spinal analgesia after thoracic surgery. A prospective, double-blind, placebo-controlled research study. *Annales Francaises d'Anesthethesie et de Reanimation.* **30**: 25–30.

39 Khalili G *et al.* (2011) Effects of adjunct intrathecal magnesium sulfate to bupivacaine for spinal anesthesia: a randomized, double-blind trial in patients undergoing lower extremity surgery. *Journal of Anesthesia.* **25**: 892–897.

40 Khezri MB *et al.* (2012) Comparison of postoperative analgesic effect of intrathecal magnesium and fentanyl added to bupivacaine in patients undergoing lower limb orthopedic surgery. *Acta Anaesthesiol Taiwan.* **50**: 19–24.

41 Pickering G *et al.* (2011) Oral magnesium treatment in patients with neuropathic pain: a randomized clinical trial. *Magnesium Research.* **24**: 28–35.

42 Castiglioni S and Maier JA (2011) Magnesium and cancer: a dangerous liason. *Magnesium Research.* **24**: S92–100.

43 Miller S (1995) Drug-induced hypomagnesaemia. *Hospital Pharmacy.* **30**: 248–250.

44 UK Medicines Information (2015) How is acute hypomagnesaemia treated in adults *Medicines Q&A.* **350.4**: www.evidence.nhs.uk

45 UK Medicines Information (2016) Can magnesium sulphate be given subcutaneously? *Medicines Q&A.* **14.6**: www.evidence.nhs.uk

46 UK Medicines Information (2015) What oral magnesium preparations are available in the UK and which preparation is preferred for the treatment and prevention of hypomagesaemia? *Medicines Q&A* **111.6**: www.evidence.nhs.uk

47 Zang X (2016) The circulating concentration and 24-h urine excretion of magnesium dose- and time- dependently respond to oral magnesium supplementation in a meta-analysis. *Journal of Nutrition.* **146**: 595–602.

Updated September 2017

ZINC

Class: Metal element.

Indications: Zinc deficiency (zinc sulfate), Wilson's disease (zinc acetate), †anorexia due to taste changes, †wound healing.

Pharmacology

Zinc is an essential trace element with multiple functions. It is present in >300 enzymes, and has catalytic, structural and regulatory functions (Box A).[1-3] It occurs in all tissues, particularly muscle and bone, and to a lesser extent in skin and liver. Most is intracellular, and much is intranuclear. Plasma contains only 0.1% of the body's zinc, mostly bound to albumin.[4]

Box A Physiological functions of zinc

Gene expression and cellular stability
Zinc-dependent RNA and DNA polymerases and reverse transcriptase
Cell proliferation and differentiation
Regulation of apoptosis (cell-specific; either increases or decreases)
Zinc-fingers transcription factors
Structural maintenance of biomembranes

Homeostasis and metabolism
Cellular signal and transmission
Hormone storage, synthesis and action, e.g. sex and thyroid hormones
Metabolism of proteins, carbohydrates and lipids
Tissue growth and repair
Neurosensory (cognition, behavioural response, taste, smell, appetite)

Anti-oxidant
Protects from free radical reactions
Component of super oxide dismutase (SOD)
Induces metal-binding protein production
Membrane stabilization

Anti-inflammatory
Inhibits expression of pro-inflammatory cytokines (IL-4, IL-6, and TNF-α)

Immune response
Thymulin activity
T-cell maturation and differentiation
Regulates cytokine production
Natural killer cell activity
T-lymphocyte activation
Direct effect on DNA for immune cell proliferation

Homeostasis is achieved primarily through regulation of the intestinal absorption. When dietary zinc is high, intestinal metal-binding proteins increase, and these slow absorption.[3] With a very high intake, secondary homeostatic mechanisms operate, e.g. increased renal excretion and redistribution of tissue zinc.[4]

There are no significant stores of zinc in the body and a constant dietary intake is essential. The UK reference nutrient intake (RNI) for daily dietary (elemental) zinc is 5.5–9.5mg in men and 4–7mg for women.[2,5] In contrast, the EU recommended daily allowance is 15mg.[2,6] Sources include meat, sea food, dairy products, wholegrain cereals, legumes and nuts. Bio-availability of dietary zinc is about 20–30%, and is lower from plant sources because of phytate-binding.[2]

Excessive intake is generally safe. However, acute and chronic poisoning has been reported.[3,7] Prolonged ingestion of high doses (50–300mg/24h elemental zinc) is associated with impaired immune function with leucopenia and neutropenia, sideroblastic anaemia and reduced ferritin levels. It can lead to secondary copper deficiency with increased LDL:HDL cholesterol ratio and HbA_{1c}.[3,7] The safe upper levels for elemental zinc intake recommended in the UK are 25mg/day from supplements and 42mg/day in total (i.e. from supplements and diet combined).[6,7]

In the brain, the main effect of zinc is to reduce neuronal excitability.[8] However, as a consequence of various insults (e.g. trauma, ischaemia, hypoglycaemia) zinc may accumulate to toxic levels and cause neural damage and apoptosis. Zinc also appears to have a role in the pathogenesis of neurodegenerative disease. Thus, zinc-dependent proteins have been implicated in MND/AML, and zinc induces amyloid deposition in Alzheimer's disease.[8] It is concentrated in and around plaques, and metal protein-attenuating compounds, which interact with zinc and promote solubilization of amyloid, are undergoing clinical trials.[9]

Zinc concentrations can be measured in the cellular components of blood (RBC, mononuclear cells and platelets), plasma, urine, faeces, skin, hair and saliva. Cellular zinc is sensitive but measurement is complex.[10] Consequently, plasma concentration is widely used instead, with zinc deficiency defined as <15micromol/L.[11] However, plasma zinc may not reflect total body zinc, and is influenced by various factors, e.g. plasma protein, drugs (see Cautions), infection, and inflammation.[2,7,10,12] Thus, when zinc deficiency is clinically suspected, even if the plasma zinc concentration is within the normal range, a therapeutic trial of replacement therapy should be considered.

9

Zinc deficiency can occur relatively rapidly as a result of inadequate dietary intake, poor intestinal absorption or increased loss due to conditions such as cancer, malabsorption, alcoholism, renal disease, sickle cell anaemia and AIDS. Metal-binding proteins, in addition to binding zinc and other heavy metals such as copper, have a protective role scavenging toxic metals and free radicals, and improving immunity. However, in stressful states, e.g. inflammation and with increasing age, levels increase and bind more intracellular zinc. Consequently, the persistent sequestration of zinc leads to reduced bio-availability and a relative deficiency state.[3,13] The effects of zinc deficiency are numerous and reflect its multifunctional role and importance in gene expression, protein synthesis and enzyme function (Box B).[2,3,13]

Box B Consequences of zinc deficiency

Immunological
Increased risk of infections due to impaired cellular immunity
Reduced neutrophils, monocytes, natural killer cells
Reduced T-helper$_1$ cytokines (IL-2 and IFN-γ)
Reduced thymulin activity
Increased inflammation secondary to increased pro-inflammatory cytokines, NO, COX-2 and NF-κB

Other cellular effects
Increased apoptosis
Increased oxidative stress with lipid peroxidation of mitochondrial membranes

Haematological
Defective platelet aggregation
Iron-deficiency anaemia

Neuropsychological
Impaired smell, taste and vision
Impaired cognition
Behavioural disturbance
Depression

Gastro-intestinal
Anorexia
Diarrhoea
Gastric acid and pepsin secretion causing mucosal damage

continued

Box B Continued

Hormonal
Thyroid hormone function
Hypogonadism and infertility

Dermatological
Dermatitis
Alopecia
Nail dystrophy
Delayed wound healing

There are conflicting reports regarding the relationship between zinc and cancer. Some studies show no effect, others a protective effect and some an increased risk. A possible explanation is that the proliferative and apoptotic actions of zinc are cell-specific. In prostate, ovarian, oesophageal, and hepatocellular cancers, for example, malignant cells are unable to accumulate zinc and this results in a loss of zinc-induced apoptosis. In these cancers, zinc deficiency would lead to an increased risk, and supplementation could have an anti-cancer effect.[14] In contrast, in breast and pancreatic cancers, malignant cells have a high zinc concentration which enhances cell proliferation.[15]

Zinc may have a contributory role in cachexia. Systemic inflammation affects zinc transporters in cell membranes, leading to zinc accumulation in the liver and also skeletal muscle where, it is suggested, it could enhance protein catabolism and inhibit protein synthesis.[16] Further, this redistribution is also proposed to cause a deficiency of zinc elsewhere, resulting in systemic features of zinc deficiency, e.g. anorexia, hypogonadism and impaired immunity, which are common features of cachexia.[16]

Zinc supplements are of benefit in the common cold. A Cochrane review concluded that, in otherwise healthy people, zinc lozenges and syrup reduce the severity and duration of symptoms if started within 24h of the onset of symptoms. Studies have used different doses (30–190mg/24h) for different lengths of time. However, lozenges have been widely studied with benefit from doses ≥75mg/24h continued throughout the cold. Prophylactic supplementation cannot be recommended because of insufficient data.[17] Another systematic review concluded a dose-dependant effect and found zinc acetate to be more effective than other formulations.[18] Patients with impaired immunity have not been investigated.

In zinc-deficient patients, supplements promote wound healing.[2] However, a Cochrane review (based on poor quality studies) found no strong evidence of benefit on leg ulcer healing.[19] There is inconclusive or insufficient evidence regarding zinc's effectiveness as a treatment for male infertility.[2] It may be of benefit in slowing the progression of age-related macular degeneration.[20]

Supplementation improves zinc deficiency, dry mouth (xerostomia) and disturbances of taste and smell.[21–23] Evidence is limited, but improvement in taste is also reported in idiopathic and radiotherapy-induced taste disorders[23–25] but not if drug-induced.[11] The beneficial effect on zinc-related anorexia is linked to an increase in leptin levels and by influencing the hypothalamic neuropeptides which regulate appetite.[26] The effect on leptin possibly involves increased cytokine production.[27] Zinc is also used to prevent the absorption of copper in Wilson's disease.

Cautions

Acute renal impairment (zinc may accumulate). If taken for prolonged periods, monitor zinc and copper plasma concentrations, FBC and plasma cholesterol to detect incipient zinc toxicity and copper deficiency.

Drug interactions

PO zinc decreases GI absorption of PO bisphosphonates, chelating agents (**penicillamine**, **trientine**), **iron**, and quinolone and tetracycline antimicrobials. Absorption of PO zinc is decreased by **calcium** and **iron** supplements, chelating agents (**penicillamine**, **trientine**), phosphorus-containing products, and tetracyclines. Separating administration times by 2–3h avoids these interactions.

Thiazides and loop diuretics increase the urinary excretion of zinc which, if used long-term, may lead to deficiency.

Undesirable effects

More common: gastric irritation, gastritis, dyspepsia, abdominal pain, nausea, vomiting, diarrhoea; these can be reduced by giving PO zinc with or after food.
Less common: headache, lethargy and irritability.

Dose and use

Zinc deficiency

- elemental zinc ≤50mg PO t.d.s., e.g. zinc sulfate (Solvazinc®) 1 tablet (elemental zinc 45mg) dissolved in water once daily–t.d.s. with or after food, *or*
- zinc sulfate 14.6mg/mL injection: give 2mL IVI once daily (elemental zinc 6.5mg).

Wilson's disease

Zinc *acetate* ± chelating agents (**penicillinamine**, **trientine**) under specialist supervision to decrease copper absorption from the GI tract in Wilson's disease.[2] See BNF section 9.8.1.

Supply

Zinc sulfate (generic)
Injection 14.6mg/mL (elemental zinc 3.25mg/mL), 10mL vial = £2.50.

Solvazinc® (Galen)
Tablets effervescent zinc sulfate monohydrate 125mg (elemental zinc 45mg), 28 days @ 1 tablet t.d.s. = £12.

Many zinc products are available OTC (citrate, gluconate, glycinate, oxide and sulfate salts) as dietary supplements and as symptomatic treatment for the common cold.

1 Frassinetti S *et al.* (2006) The role of zinc in life: a review. *Journal of Environmental Pathology, Toxicology and Oncology.* **25**: 597–610.
2 Mason P (2006) Physiological and medicinal zinc. *Pharmaceutical Journal.* **276**: 271–274.
3 Stefanidou M *et al.* (2006) Zinc: a multipurpose trace element. *Archives of Toxicology.* **80**: 1–9.
4 King JC *et al.* (2000) Zinc homeostasis in humans. *Journal of Nutritrion.* **130**: 1360S–1366S.
5 COMA (1991) Committee on Medical Aspects of Food and Nutrition Policy. Dietary reference values for food energy and nutrients for the United Kingdom. Report of the panel on dietary reference values. HMSO, London.
6 Mason P (2003) Upper safety limits for vitamins - why have different authorities set different guidance? *Pharmaceutical Journal.* **271**: 55–57.
7 EVM (2003) Expert Group on Vitamins and Minerals. Risk assessment: zinc: In: Safe upper levels for vitamins and minerals. pp253–262. Food Standards Agency, London. Available from: www.food.gov.uk
8 Frederickson CJ *et al.* (2005) The neurobiology of zinc in health and disease. *Nature Reviews Neuroscience.* **6**: 449–462.
9 Sampson E *et al.* (2014) Metal protein attenuating compounds for the treatment of Alzheimers Disease. *Cochrane Database of Systematic Reviews.* **2**: CD005380. www.thecochranelibrary.com.
10 Hambridge M (2003) Biomarkers of trace mineral intake and status. *Journal of Nutritrion.* **133**: 948S–955S.
11 Heyneman CA (1996) Zinc deficiency and taste disorders. *Annals of Pharmacotherapy.* **30**: 186–187.
12 Alpers DH (1994) Zinc and deficiencies of taste and smell. *Journal of the American Medical Association.* **272**: 1233–1234.
13 Vasto S *et al.* (2007) Zinc and inflammatory/immune response in aging. *Annals of the New York Academy of Sciences.* **1100**: 111–122.
14 Prasad AS *et al.* (2009) Zinc in cancer prevention. *Nutrition and Cancer.* **61**: 879–887.
15 Franklin RB and Costello LC (2009) The important role of the apoptotic effects of zinc in the development of cancers. *Journal of Cellular Biochemistry.* **106**: 750–757.
16 Siren PM and Siren MJ (2010) Systemic zinc redistribution and dyshomeostasis in cancer cachexia. *Journal of Cachexia Sarcopenia Muscle.* **1**: 23–33.
17 Singh M and Das RR (2011) Zinc for the common cold. . *Cochrane Database of Systematic Reviews.* **2**: CD001364 www.thecochranelibrary.com.
18 Science M *et al.* (2012) Zinc for the treatment of the common cold: a systematic review and meta-analysis of randomized controlled trials. *Canadian Medical Association Journal.* **184**: E551–561.
19 Wilkinson EA (2014) Oral zinc for arterial and venous leg ulcers. *Cochrane Database of Systematic Reviews.* **9**: CD001273 www.thecochranelibrary.com.
20 Evans JR (2006) Antioxidant vitamin and mineral supplements for slowing the progression of age-related macular degeneration. *Cochrane Database of Systematic Reviews.* **2**: CD000254 www.thecochranelibrary.com.
21 Tanaka M (2002) Secretory function of the salivary gland in patients with taste disorders or xerostomia: correlation with zinc deficiency. *Acta Otolaryngolica Supplementum.* 134–141.
22 Henkin RI *et al.* (1999) Efficacy of exogenous oral zinc in treatment of patients with carbonic anhydrase VI deficiency. *American Journal of Medical Sciences.* **318**: 392–405.
23 Nagraj SK *et al.* (2014) Interventions for the management of taste disturbances. *Cochrane Database of Systematic Reviews.* **11**: CD010470 www.thecochranelibrary.com.
24 Heckmann SM *et al.* (2005) Zinc gluconate in the treatment of dysgeusia–a randomized clinical trial. *Journal of Dental Research.* **84**: 35–38.

25 Ripamonti C *et al.* (1998) A randomized, controlled clinical trial to evaluate the effects of zinc sulfate on cancer patients with taste alterations caused by head and neck irradiation. *Cancer.* **82**: 1938–1945.
26 Shay NF and Mangian HF (2000) Neurobiology of zinc-influenced eating behavior. *Journal of Nutritrion.* **130**: 1493S–1499S.
27 Mantzoros CS *et al.* (1998) Zinc may regulate serum leptin concentrations in humans. *Journal of American College of Nutrition.* **17**: 270–275.

Updated May 2015

10: MUSCULOSKELETAL AND JOINT DISEASES

10

DEPOT CORTICOSTEROID INJECTIONS

Indications: Inflammation of joints and soft tissues, †pain in superficial bones (e.g. rib, scapula, iliac crest), †intractable pain caused by spinal metastases, †malignant (peritoneal) ascites.

Contra-indications: Untreated local or systemic infection. Must not be given IV or IT.

Pharmacology

Corticosteroids have an anti-inflammatory effect; they reduce the concentration of algesic substances present in inflammation which sensitize nerve endings.[1] Further, in animal studies, when injected locally around an injured nerve, corticosteroids have been shown to have a direct inhibitory effect on the spontaneous activity associated with nerve injury.[2]

For many years depot injections of corticosteroids have been given epidurally in selected patients with non-malignant radicular (nerve root) compression pain associated with spinal pathology, e.g. lumbar disc herniation, sciatica.[3] However, a systematic review found only weak RCT evidence for their efficacy.[4] Even so, in patients with spinal metastases and intractable radicular pain, clinical experience indicates that ED depot corticosteroids are sometimes helpful.

Cautions

Also see Systemic corticosteroids, p.513. History of severe affective disorders (e.g. depression, bipolar disorder) or steroid-induced psychosis, epilepsy, glaucoma, myasthenia gravis, hypertension, CHF, predisposition to thrombophlebitis, peptic ulceration, diverticulitis, ulcerative colitis, severe hepatic impairment, renal impairment, hypothyroidism, osteoporosis.

Depot formulations may result in symptomatic hyperglycaemia for several days in patients with diabetes mellitus and suppression of the hypothalamic-pituitary-adrenal axis for up to 4 weeks. Injection under a rib may be complicated by a pneumothorax.

Corticosteroids may mask or alter the presentation of infection in immunocompromised patients; such patients should not receive live vaccines and, if exposed to chickenpox, should receive *Varicella zoster* immunoglobulin.

Drug interactions

Pharmacodynamic interactions include antagonism of antihypertensive, antidiabetic and diuretic drugs, and increased risk of hypokalaemia if used concurrently with β_2 agonists (e.g. **salbutamol, terbutaline**) or other potassium-wasting drugs.

Undesirable effects

Undesirable effects associated with systemic corticosteroids can also occur with depot injections (see Systemic corticosteroids, p.517), including adrenal suppression; patients should carry a steroid card (see p.519).

Occasionally, a patient develops lipodystrophy (local fat necrosis) which results in an indentation of the overlying skin.

ED injection of **methylprednisolone *acetate*** (unauthorized route) has been associated with wound dehiscence and with loss of sphincter control.

Dose and use

Injection into and/or over painful bone secondary[5]

- infiltrate the skin and SC tissues overlying the point of maximal bone tenderness with local anaesthetic
- with the tip of the needle pressing against the tender bone, inject depot **methylprednisolone *acetate*** 80mg in 2mL
- if there are 2 painful bones, inject 40mg at each spot; generally limit the total amount given at any one time to 80mg.

Also, for rib lesions, reposition the needle under the rib and inject 5mL of **bupivacaine** 0.5% to anaesthetize the intercostal nerve. Complete or good relief occurs in about 70% of patients. If of benefit, injections can be repeated if the pain returns but not within 2 weeks.

Epidural injection[3]

Depot **methylprednisolone *acetate*** 80mg in 2mL (unauthorized route). A single ED injection is given, followed if necessary by a further 1–2 injections at 3–4 week intervals. The effect of ED corticosteroids is unpredictable and may not peak until 1 week after an injection. Depot corticosteroids cannot be injected through an epidural bacterial filter. In some countries, depot **triamcinolone** or a *non-depot* formulation of **dexamethasone sodium phosphate** is used for ED injection.

Malignant (peritoneal) ascites

After a preliminary paracentesis, inject intra-abdominally:

- **triamcinolone *acetonide*** 8mg/kg, to a maximum of 520mg (13 vials of the 40mg/mL depot injection) *or*
- **methylprednisolone *acetate*** 10mg/kg, to a maximum of 640mg (8 vials of the 80mg/2mL depot injection).

In an open study, the mean interval between paracentesis doubled to 18 days.[6] When neither of the above are available, another alternative is **triamcinolone *hexacetonide*** 10mg/kg, to a maximum of 640mg (32 ampoules of the 20mg/mL depot injection); however, it is more expensive.

Supply

Methylprednisolone *acetate*

Depo-Medrone® (Pfizer)

Depot injection (aqueous suspension) 40mg/mL, 1mL vial = £3.50, 2mL vial = £6, 3mL vial = £9.

Triamcinolone *acetonide*

Adcortyl® Intra-articular/Intradermal (Squibb)

Depot injection (aqueous suspension) 10mg/mL, 1mL amp = £1, 5mL vial = £3.50. *Contains benzyl alcohol.*

Kenalog® Intra-articular/Intramuscular (Squibb)

Depot injection (aqueous suspension) 40mg/mL, 1mL vial = £1.50. *Contains benzyl alcohol.*

Triamcinolone *hexacetonide* (generic)

Depot injection (aqueous suspension) 20mg/mL, 1mL amp = £12. *Contains benzyl alcohol.*

1 Pybus P (1984) Osteoarthritis: a new neurological method of pain control. *Medical Hypothesis.* **14**: 413–422.

2 Devor M *et al.* (1985) Corticosteroids reduce neuroma hyperexcitability. In: HL Fields *et al.* (eds) *Advances in Pain Research and Therapy* Vol 9. Raven Press, New York, pp. 451–455.

3 McLain RF *et al.* (2004) Epidural steroids for back and leg pain: mechanism of action and efficacy. *Cleveland Clinic Journal of Medicine.* **71**: 961–970.

4 Armon C *et al.* (2007) Assessment: use of epidural steroid injections to treat radicular lumbosacral pain: report of the Therapeutics and Technology Assessment Subcommittee of the American Academy of Neurology. *Neurology.* **68**: 723–729.

5 Rowell NP (1988) Intralesional methylprednisolone for rib metastases: an alternative to radiotherapy? *Palliative Medicine*. **2**: 153–155.
6 Mackey J *et al.* (2000) A phase II trial of triamcinolone hexacetanide for symptomatic recurrent malignant ascites. *Journal of Pain and Symptom Management*. **19**: 193–199.

Updated (minor change) August 2017

RUBEFACIENTS AND OTHER TOPICAL PRODUCTS

Indications: Soft tissue pains (rubefacients, topical NSAIDs), pain relief in osteo-arthritis of the hand or knee (**capsaicin** cream 0.025%, topical NSAIDs),[1] post-herpetic neuralgia (after lesions have healed) and diabetic neuralgia (**capsaicin** cream 0.075%), peripheral neuropathic pain (**capsaicin** TD patch 8%), †notalgia paraesthetica, †severe skin reaction to an indwelling SC cannula and/or phlebitis (**kaolin** poultice).

Contra-indications: Inflamed or broken skin.
Capsaicin TD patch 8%: do not apply to the face or head.
Topical NSAIDs: if nasal polyps or history of asthma, angioedema, urticaria or acute rhinitis precipitated by aspirin or another NSAID.

10

Pharmacology

Rubefacients act by counter-stimulation of the skin, closing the pain 'gate' in the dorsal horn of the spinal cord.[2,3] Further benefit is obtained by the inclusion of **levomenthol** (**menthol**). This cools the skin for several hours by acting on heat-sensitive transient receptor potential (TRP) channels expressed on sensory nerve endings.[4,5] **Levomenthol**-containing rubefacients have been used as 'home remedies' for tension headache, muscle spasm, and joint pain. (**Levomenthol** is also an ingredient in several topical antipruritic products, see p.635.) Warm **kaolin** poultices also act by counter-stimulation, substituting the pleasure of warmth for the stinging/burning of the inflamed skin.

Capsaicin

Capsaicin is a naturally occurring alkaloid found in the fruits of various species of *Solanaceae* (the nightshade family) and in pepper plants of the genus *Capsicum* (chilli peppers).[6] It acts by depleting substance P (SP) at sensory nerve endings. In animals, **capsaicin** has also been shown to be neurotoxic, particularly for nociceptive C fibres.[7]

Application of **capsaicin** causes an initial release of SP from C fibres which manifests as a burning or stinging sensation (see Undesirable effects below) with subsequent depletion on continued use. Axonal transport of SP to synaptic terminals is reduced and synthesis inhibited.[8] **Capsaicin** may also elevate the thresholds for the release of SP and other neurotransmitters. Reduced availability of SP diminishes pain transmission. After stopping topical **capsaicin**, SP stores revert to pretreatment levels and neuronal sensitivity returns to normal.[9–11]

In an open study of topical **capsaicin** cream 0.025% in post-axillary dissection pain, 12/18 women reported benefit after 1 month, eight of whom had good or excellent responses; and, after 6 months, most still had good relief.[12] An RCT of **capsaicin** cream 0.075% for 6 weeks gave comparable results: 8/13 patients had ≥50% improvement, five of whom had a good or excellent result.[13] Benefit was mainly in relation to stabbing pain.

In an RCT in 99 patients with persistent neuropathic pain after cancer surgery, **capsaicin** cream 0.075% produced a mean reduction in pain scores of >50%, compared with <20% for placebo. Improvement was seen most often in women with post-mastectomy pain.[14]

However, a systematic review was unable to reach a firm conclusion about benefit from 0.075% **capsaicin** cream in neuropathic pain generally[15]. NICE no longer recommends 0.075% **capsaicin** cream for post-herpetic neuralgia in primary care.[16]

A TD patch containing **capsaicin** 8% is available for diabetic and non-diabetic painful neuropathy, e.g. post-herpetic or HIV. This was developed to deliver high-concentration **capsaicin** to the cutaneous nociceptors in a single application, thereby achieving rapid 'knock-out' of their function, as opposed to the periods of enhanced sensitivity and slow desensitization seen after repeated application of 0.025% and 0.075% creams. A systematic review found that TD **capsaicin** provided long-term pain relief after a single application. There was moderate quality evidence for post-herpetic neuralgia with NNTs of 8.8 and 7 for patients grading themselves as 'much or very much better' at 8 and 12 weeks respectively. NNT values for reductions in pain intensity of ≥30% and ≥50% at 8 and 12 weeks were between 10 and 12. The quality of evidence was very low in other conditions. In HIV-related neuropathy, the NNT for reduction in pain intensity of ≥30% at 12 weeks was 11. In diabetic neuropathy, compared to placebo, about 10% and 3% more patients obtained a reduction in pain intensity of ≥30% and ≥50% at 12 weeks, respectively.[17] Their use is generally restricted to specialist pain clinics, when more usual options are either ineffective or not tolerated.

Capsaicin cream is of benefit in histamine-related pruritus, aquagenic pruritus, and pruritus associated with uraemia, nodular prurigo, psoriasis and post-axillary dissection syndrome (see Topical antipruritics, p.635).[5,18] Benefit is also seen with pruritus caused by notalgia paraesthetica (nerve injury, often caused by entrapment, of the dorsal ramus of the T2–T6 thoracic nerves which causes pruritus and/or altered sensation in the areas of skin between or below the shoulder blade on either side of the back).[19,20]

Topical NSAIDs

Topical NSAIDs are of value for the relief of pain associated with soft tissue trauma, e.g. strains and sprains, inflammation of superficial joints, early osteo-arthritis of the hand or knee.[1,21] Topically applied salicylates and some other NSAIDs can achieve local high SC concentrations and therapeutically effective concentrations within synovial fluid and peri-articular tissues similar to those seen after PO administration.[22–25]

A Cochrane review compared topical NSAIDs with placebo in *acute* musculoskeletal pain over about 1 week and found using moderate-high quality evidence that the NNT for a 50% reduction in pain were lowest for **diclofenac** Emulgel® (1.8) and **ketoprofen** gel (2.5).[21] In *chronic* musculoskeletal pain (mostly hand and knee osteoarthritis) assessed over 6–12 weeks, NNTs for the same outcome were higher, i.e. **diclofenac** gel (9.8) and **ketoprofen** gel (6.9).[21] The evidence for all other topical salicylate or NSAID therapies was considered low/very-low.

Pharmacokinetic details for **capsaicin** products and topical NSAIDs are shown in Table 1.

Table 1 Pharmacokinetic details for capsaicin products and topical NSAIDs

	Capsaicin cream 0.025% and 0.075%	*Capsaicin TD patch 8%*	*Topical NSAIDs*
Onset of action	Counter-stimulation generally immediate. 1 week in osteo-arthritis but full effect may not be seen for ≤2 months. 2–4 weeks in neuralgia	1–14 days in peripheral neuropathy	Product- and drug-dependent
Duration of action	No data; manufacturers advise applying q4–6h	≥12 weeks in peripheral and HIV-related neuropathy; manufacturers advise a 3-month gap between applications	Product and drug dependent; manufacturers advise applying b.d.–q.d.s.

Cautions

General

Avoid contact with eyes, mucous membranes, and inflamed or broken skin; discontinue if rash develops. Do not cover with occlusive dressings or tight bandages.

Capsaicin cream 0.025% and 0.075%

Avoid hot baths or showers immediately before application because this can enhance the burning sensation. Avoid inhaling the vapour from the cream. Wash hands immediately after application (unless treating the hands, in which case, wash them 30min after application).

**Capsaicin TD patch 8%*

Unstable or poorly controlled blood pressure, heart disease (see Undesirable effects). The painful burning sensation may necessitate local cooling (e.g. with a cold compress) or systemic analgesia. Avoid inhaling the vapour from the patch. Special precautions are required for handling (see Dose and use).

Topical NSAIDs

History of peptic ulcer, renal disease or asthma. Wash hands immediately after application (unless treating the hands, in which case, wash them 30min after application). May cause photosensitivity, particularly **ketoprofen**. Avoid exposing the treated area to sunlight when using topical **ketoprofen** and for 2 weeks afterwards.

Provided very large amounts are not applied, because plasma concentrations are much lower, undesirable effects and drug interactions are much less likely with topical NSAIDs than with systemic NSAIDs. Conversely, skin reactions (e.g. rash) occur more commonly with topical NSAIDS.[1]

Undesirable effects

The commonest undesirable effect of **capsaicin** cream is tingling, stinging or burning at the site of application. This effect is thought to be related to the initial release of SP from C fibres. The stinging and burning generally decreases with continued applications, often clearing in a few days but sometimes persisting for >4 weeks. Some patients discontinue treatment because of this. Runny eyes and respiratory tract irritation, causing coughing and sneezing, may result from rubbing the eyes and/or inhaling **capsaicin** vapour when applying the cream. Breathlessness and exacerbation of asthma have occurred occasionally.

Almost all patients experience local erythema and a burning sensation with **capsaicin** TD patches, unless the area is pretreated with local anaesthetic (see Dose and use). Other common local effects (1–10% of patients) are itching, blistering, swelling and dryness. Uncommon symptoms (1–10 per 1,000 patients) include eye irritation, raised blood pressure, arrhythmia including atrioventricular block, palpitations, cough, throat irritation, loss of taste sensation, muscle spasm, reduced sensation in limbs, local wheals, prickling sensation and bruising.

Large quantities of topical NSAIDs have been associated with systemic effects (e.g. hypersensitivity, rash, asthma, renal impairment[26]) and potentiation of **warfarin**, occasionally leading to bleeding.[27] Local reactions include drying, reddening, burning sensations, and contact dermatitis. A Cochrane review found that, in short-term studies, topical NSAIDs and placebo produced a similar incidence of local reactions and systemic undesirable effects (about 6% and 3% respectively).[21]

Dose and use

Capsaicin cream 0.025–0.075%

- apply a pea-sized amount t.d.s.–q.d.s. (the manufacturers specify q.d.s. initially for the 0.025% cream), leaving at least 4h between applications.

The burning sensation associated with the application of **capsaicin** cream is intensified and/or prolonged when larger quantities are applied (particularly with the higher-strength) or if initially applied less frequently than t.d.s.–q.d.s. If the burning is severe, topical **lidocaine** or another local anaesthetic can be applied before **capsaicin** in the first few weeks of treatment.

Because heat and humidity influence dysaesthesia, patients should avoid excessive sweating and not take a hot bath immediately before application. Occlusion and tight bandaging should also be avoided.

Patients should apply the cream using gentle massage, avoiding contact with eyes, mucous membranes and broken/inflamed skin. *Patients must wash their hands after applying the cream to avoid subsequent unintentional contact with the eyes (unless treating the hands, in which case, wash them 30min after application).*

**Capsaicin TD patch 8%*

Health professionals should wear nitrile gloves when handling the patches and cleansing solution; latex gloves do *not* provide adequate protection. Also consider using protective masks and safety glasses to avoid accidental contact of aerosolized **capsaicin** particles with the eyes and mucous membranes, particularly when removing the patch:

- mark out the most painful areas with ink
- depending on the size of the painful areas, up to 4 patches may be applied simultaneously, or a patch may be cut to fit
- wash the skin in the treatment area with soap and water and dry thoroughly; any hair may be clipped but not shaved

- because most patients experience a burning sensation when the patches are applied, pre-treat the area with topical **lidocaine** or another local anaesthetic 1h before applying the patches; wash off the local anaesthetic cream/ointment and thoroughly dry the skin before applying the **capsaicin** patch
- leave patches in place for:
  - ▷ 30min if applied to the feet
  - ▷ 1h if applied elsewhere
  - ▷ if necessary, disposable socks or an open-weave bandage can be used to keep the patch in place
- when removing patches, roll them inwards to enclose the remaining **capsaicin**
- use the cleansing gel supplied to remove any traces of **capsaicin** from the patient's skin, both after any accidental contact and after removing the patches; leave the gel on the skin for 1min, then wipe off
- wash the skin with soap and water after using the cleansing gel
- treatment can be repeated after 3 months if necessary.

Used patches, gloves, wipes, socks and bandages should be placed in a plastic bag and disposed of safely.

Topical NSAIDs

- generally apply b.d.–q.d.s.

Kaolin poultice

- warm the poultice before use
- generally apply b.d.

Supply

Capsaicin
Zacin® (Teva)
Cream 0.025%, 45g = £18.

Axsain® (Teva)
Cream 0.075%, 45g = £15.

Qutenza® (Astellas)
TD patch 8% (contains 179mg **capsaicin**), 1 patch (with cleansing gel) = £210.

Diclofenac
Voltarol Emulgel® (GlaxoSmithKline)
Gel 1.16%, 30g, 50g, 100g = £3.50, £5 and £8; 2.32% 30g, 50g, 100g = £4.25, £6.50 and £11; *also available OTC.*

Ketoprofen (generic)
Gel 2.5%, 50g, 100g = £1.75 and £3.25.

Kaolin (generic)
Poultice 200g = £3.

For **levomenthol** products, see Topical antipruritics, p.635.

---

1 NICE (2013) Osteoarthritis. *Clinical Knowledge Summaries*. http://cks.nice.org.uk
2 Melzack R and Wall P (1965) Pain mechanisms: a new theory. *Science*. **150**: 971–979.
3 Melzack R (1991) The gate control theory 25 years later: new perspectives on phantom limb pain. In: M Bond *et al.* (eds) *Proceedings of the VIth World Congress on Pain*. Elsevier Science, Amsterdam, pp. 9–21.
4 Peier AM *et al.* (2002) A TRP channel that senses cold stimuli and menthol. *Cell*. **108**: 705–715.
5 Patel T *et al.* (2007) Menthol: a refreshing look at this ancient compound. *Journal of the American Academy of Dermatology*. **57**: 873–878.
6 Towlerton GR and Rice AS (2003) Topical analgesics for chronic pain. In: AS Rice *et al.* (eds) *Clinical Pain Management: Chronic Pain*. Arnold, London, pp. 213–226.

7 Chung JM *et al.* (1993) Chronic effects of topical application of capsaicin to the sciatic nerve on responses of primate spinothalamic neurons. *Pain.* **53**: 311–321.
8 Gamse R *et al.* (1982) Capsaicin applied to peripheral nerve inhibits axoplasmic transport of substance P and somatostatin. *Brain Research.* **239**: 447–462.
9 Gamse R *et al.* (1981) Differential effects of capsaicin on the content of somatostatin, substance P, and neurotensin in the nervous system of the rat. *Naunyn Schmiedebergs Archives of Pharmacology.* **317**: 140–148.
10 Fitzgerald M (1983) Capsaicin and sensory neurones: a review. *Pain.* **15**: 109–130.
11 LaMotte RH *et al.* (1988) Hypothesis for novel classes of chemoreceptors mediating chemogenic pain and itch. In: R Dubner *et al.* (eds) *Proceedings of the Vth World Congress on Pain.* Elsevier, New York, pp. 529–535.
12 Watson C *et al.* (1989) The postmastectomy pain syndrome and the effect of topical capsaicin. *Pain.* **38**: 177–186.
13 Watson CPN and Evans RJ (1992) Post-mastectomy pain syndrome and topical capsaicin: a randomized trial. *Pain.* **51**: 375–379.
14 Ellison N *et al.* (1997) Phase III placebo-controlled trial of capsaicin cream in the management of surgical neuropathic pain in cancer patients. *Journal of Clinical Oncology.* **15**: 2974–2980.
15 Derry S and Moore RA (2012) Topical capsaicin (low concentration) for chronic neuropathic pain in adults. *Cochrane Database of Systematic Reviews.* CD010111. www.thecochranelibrary.com
16 NICE (2013) Post-herpetic neuralgia. *Clinical Knowledge Summaries.* http://cks.nice.org.uk
17 Derry S *et al.* (2017) Topical capsaicin (high concentration) for chronic neuropathic pain in adults. *Cochrane Database of Systematic Reviews.* **1**: CD007393. www.thecochranelibrary.com
18 Xander C *et al.* (2013) Pharmacological interventions for pruritus in adult palliative care patients. *Cochrane Database of Systematic Reviews.* **6**: CD008320. www.thecochranelibrary.com
19 Bernstein JE (1988) Capsaicin in dermatologic disease. *Seminars in Dermatology.* **7**: 304–309.
20 Breneman D *et al.* (1992) Topical capsaicin for treatment of hemodialysis-related pruritus. *Journal of the American Academy of Dermatology.* **26**: 91–94.
21 Derry S *et al.* (2017) Topical analgesics for acute and chronic pain in adults - an overview of Cochrane Reviews. *Cochrane Database of Systematic Reviews.* **5**: CD008609. www.thecochranelibrary.com
22 Mondino A *et al.* (1983) Kinetic studies of ibuprofen on humans. Comparative study for the determination of blood concentrations and metabolites following local and oral administration. *Medizinische Welt.* **34**: 1052–1054.
23 Chlud K and Wagener H (1987) Percutaneous nonsteroidal anti-inflammatory drug (NSAID) therapy with particular reference to pharmacokinetic factors. *EULAR Bulletin.* **2**: 40–43.
24 Peters H *et al.* (1987) Percutaneous kinetics of ibuprofen (German). *Aktuelle Rheumatologie.* **12**: 208–211.
25 Dominkus M *et al.* (1996) Comparison of tissue and plasma levels of ibuprofen after oral and topical administration. *Arzneimittelforschung.* **46**: 1138–1143.
26 O'Callaghan C *et al.* (1994) Renal disease and use of topical NSAIDs. *British Medical Journal.* **308**: 110–111.
27 Makris UE *et al.* (2010) Adverse effects of topical nonsteroidal antiinflammatory drugs in older adults with osteoarthritis: a systematic literature review. *Journal of Rheumatology.* **37**: 1236–1243.

Updated September 2017

10

SKELETAL MUSCLE RELAXANTS

Skeletal muscle relaxants are used to relieve painful chronic muscle spasm and spasticity associated with neural injury, e.g. paraplegia, post-stroke, multiple sclerosis, and sometimes motor neurone disease/amyotrophic lateral sclerosis (MND/AML),[1] and also troublesome cramp. †**Baclofen** is also used to relieve hiccup.

Spasticity

All skeletal muscle relaxants may reduce voluntary muscle power. This can be a disadvantage in people with hemiplegia or paraplegia if increased spastic muscle tone is what enables them to walk or function more independently. Thus, generally, dose escalation should be spread out over 4–8 weeks to balance the benefits of reduced spasticity with possible loss of functional performance and independence.

In contrast, in patients unable to use their limbs because of severe spasticity or paralysis or motor weakness, the dose can be escalated more rapidly. For these patients, sedation is likely to be the dose-limiting factor.[2]

There is low level evidence that spasticity in multiple sclerosis can be improved by exercise programmes, magnetic stimulation and electromagnetic therapies.[3]

Cramp

Cramp has many causes (Box A), including drugs (Box B). With diuretics, it relates to volume depletion ± electrolyte imbalance, i.e. loss of sodium and magnesium (see p.588). Cramp with **cisplatin** possibly relates to both hypomagnesaemia and peripheral neuropathy. In many cases, the mechanism is not known.

Box A Causes of cramp[4]

Idiopathic
Exercise
Old age (nocturnal leg cramps)

Acute extracellular volume depletion
Diuretics
Excessive sweating ('heat cramps')
Haemodialysis
GI fluid loss (diarrhoea, vomiting)

Drugs (Box B)

Endocrine
Hypo-adrenalism
Hypothyroidism
Pregnancy

Lower motor neurone disorders
MND/ALS
Neuropathy
Radiculopathy

Metabolic
Cirrhosis
Hypomagnesaemia
Renal impairment

Miscellaneous
Autoimmune disease
(antibodies to voltage-gated potassium channels)
Hereditary disorders

Box B Drug-induced cramps[4]

ACE inhibitors
- enalapril
- ramipril

Amitriptyline
Amphotericin B
β_2-agonists
- salbutamol
- terbutaline

Bisphosphonates
- pamidronate
- zoledronic acid

Celecoxib
Chemotherapy
- cisplatin
- vincristine

Cimetidine
Clofibrate (not UK)
Diuretics
Lithium
Statins
Steroids
- beclometasone (by inhaler)
- medroxyprogesterone acetate
- prednisolone

As always, it is important to consider correcting the correctable. Cramp cannot be induced or sustained in a stretched muscle, and calf stretching movements (both active and passive) and exercise are useful non-drug measures particularly before going to bed,[4] despite the lack of a strong evidence base.[5,6]

Drug treatment of lower limb muscle cramp is similar to that of spasticity.[7] The use of **quinine** to relieve nocturnal cramp is now discouraged (Box C).

Box C Quinine and cramp

Quinine is more effective than placebo in reducing the frequency and intensity of cramp at doses of 200–500mg/24h, most commonly 300mg.[8]

The most common undesirable effects were GI or headache (quinine 13% vs. placebo 9%).[8] After 2 months, the incidence of major undesirable effects and withdrawal was not significantly greater for quinine than for placebo (1.5% vs. 1.4%).[8]

continued

Box C Continued

Even so, various regulatory agencies consider that, because alternatives are available, the collective risks associated with using quinine for cramp are too high to permit continued routine use:

- rare but serious undesirable effects:
  - ▷ thrombocytopenia → severe bleeding (several deaths have been reported)
  - ▷ haemolytic-uraemic syndrome → permanent renal damage
- toxicity in overdose → permanent blindness or death
- serious drug interactions with, e.g. digoxin, warfarin.[9,10]

Consequently, the MHRA advises that quinine should not be used for nocturnal cramp unless the following criteria are all met:

- treatable causes have been ruled out
- non-drug measures have failed
- they regularly cause loss of sleep
- they are very painful or frequent.[9]

Further, a case control study of patients with idiopathic cramp or restless legs found a small but significant increased risk of all-cause mortality in those receiving quinine ≥100mg/24h for at least one year compared with those not receiving quinine. There was a dose and age effect; mortality was greater in those *under* 50.[11]

Typical doses of quinine are:

- quinine *sulfate* 200mg at bedtime, increased if necessary to 300mg at bedtime
- quinine *bisulfate* (not UK) 300mg at bedtime (equivalent to *sulfate* 200mg).

During the early stages of treatment, patients should be monitored for signs of thrombocytopenia, e.g. unexplained petechiae, bruising or bleeding.

Treatment should be discontinued after 4 weeks if there is no benefit, and interrupted approximately every 3 months to re-evaluate benefit.[5,9]

In people with MND/ALS, NICE guidelines recommend quinine as first-line treatment for cramp because it is considerably cheaper than baclofen and other drugs.[12]

10

Choice of drug

Baclofen, **dantrolene**, **tizanidine** and **diazepam** are all authorized for use in spasticity. **Baclofen**, **tizanidine** and **diazepam** act principally on spinal and supraspinal sites within the CNS; **dantrolene** (and **quinine**) acts on muscle. There is no clear evidence that any one drug is superior to the others.[13–15]

If there is no concurrent indication for a benzodiazepine, **baclofen** is generally a good first-line choice, particularly if long-term treatment is likely. For the use of **diazepam** as a muscle relaxant, see p.158.

Use in renal impairment

Skeletal muscle relaxants differ in their potential to cause toxicity when renal function is impaired. For information on their use in ESRF, see Chapter 17, p.695.

Other options

Anti-epileptics are used to treat cramp unresponsive to more conventional approaches (Table 1). Indeed, NICE guidelines specifically mention the use of **gabapentin** for the management of spasticity in MND/ALS.[12]

Table 1 Anti-epileptics for treating cramp[a,4]

Drug	*Dose*
Gabapentin	300mg at bedtime[16]; up to 900mg t.d.s.[17,18]
Carbamazepine	100–200mg at bedtime[4]
Phenytoin	100–200mg once daily[4]

a. also see p.256

More invasive treatments for spasticity include IT **phenol**. This is neurotoxic and can cause urinary and faecal incontinence. The use of indwelling devices to deliver IT **baclofen** has generally superseded the use of **phenol**.[7,18]

Botulinum toxin (BTX) injections are largely reserved for treatment of contractures. The BTX-type A light chain acts as a zinc endopeptidase and interferes with acetylcholine release.[19] The toxin is injected into each spastic muscle separately and reduces spasticity in a dose-dependent manner.[20] Its use is rarely relevant in palliative care. It has been used in people with neurodegenerative disorders, e.g. MND/ALS to manage drooling and, less commonly, dysphagia secondary to upper oesophageal sphincter dysfunction.[21,22]

1 Zafonte R *et al.* (2004) Acute care management of post-TBI spasticity. *Journal of Head Trauma Rehabilitation*. **19**: 89–100.
2 Noth J and Fink GR (2004) Spasticity. In: R Voltz *et al.* (eds) *Palliative care in neurology* (No. 69). Oxford University Press, Oxford, p. 154.
3 Amatya B *et al.* (2013) Non pharmacological interventions for spasticity in multiple sclerosis. *Cochrane Database of Systematic Reviews*. **2**: CD009974. www.thecochranelibrary.com
4 Miller TM and Layzer RB (2005) Muscle cramps. *Muscle Nerve*. **32**: 431–442.
5 NHS (2012) Clinical knowledge summary. Leg cramps. https://cks.nice.org.
6 Blyton F *et al.* (2012) Non-drug therapies for lower limb muscle cramps. *Cochrane Database of Systematic Reviews*. **1**: CD008496. www.thecochranelibrary.com
7 Kita M and Goodkin D (2000) Drugs used to treat spasticity. *Drugs*. **59**: 487–495.
8 El Tawil S *et al.* (2010) Quinine for muscle cramps. *Cochrane Database of Systematic Reviews*. **12**: CD005044. www.thecochranelibrary.com
9 MHRA (2010) Quinine: not to be used routinely for nocturnal leg cramps. *Drug Safety Update*. **3**: www.gov.uk/drug-safety-update.
10 FDA (2010) Qualaquin (quinine sulfate): new risk evaluation and mitigation strategy - risk of serious hematological reactions. www.fda.gov/Safety/MedWatch
11 Fardet L *et al.* (2017) Association between long-term quinine exposure and all-cause mortality. *JAMA*. **317**: 1907–1909.
12 NICE (2016) Motor neurone disease: assessment and management. *Clinical guideline*. NG42. www.nice.org.uk
13 Shakespeare DT *et al.* (2003) Anti-spasticity agents for multiple sclerosis. *Cochrane Database of Systematic Reviews*. **4**: CD001332. www.thecochranelibrary.com
14 Chou R *et al.* (2004) Comparative efficacy and safety of skeletal muscle relaxants for spasticity and musculoskeletal conditions: a systematic review. *Journal of Pain and Symptom Management*. **28**: 140–175.
15 Baldinger R *et al.* (2012) Treatment for cramps in amyotrophic lateral sclerosis/motor neuron disease. *Cochrane Database of Systematic Reviews*. **4**: CD004157. www.thecochranelibrary.com
16 Serrao M *et al.* (2000) Gabapentin treatment for muscle cramps: an open-label trial. *Clinical Neuropharmacology*. **23**: 45–49.
17 Paisley S *et al.* (2002) Clinical effectiveness of oral treatments for spasticity in multiple sclerosis: a systematic review. *Multiple Sclerosis*. **8**: 319–329.
18 Royal College of Physicians (2004) Multiple Sclerosis: National clinical guidelines for diagnosis and management in primary and secondary care. Available from: http://shop.rcplondon.ac.uk
19 Brin M (1997) Dosing, administration and a treatment algorithm for use of botulinum toxin A for adult-onset of spasticity. *Muscle and Nerve*. **20 (Suppl 6)**: 208–220.
20 Royal College of Physicians of London (2009) Spasticity in adults: management using botulinum toxin. National guidelines. Available from: http://shop.rcplondon.ac.uk
21 Young CA *et al.* (2011) Treatment for sialorrhea (excessive saliva) in people with motor neuron disease/amyotrophic lateral sclerosis. *Cochrane Database of Systematic Reviews*. **5**: CD00698. www.thecochranelibrary.com
22 Regan J *et al.* (2014) Botulinum toxin for upper oesophageal sphincter dysfunction in neurological swallowing disorders. *Cochrane Database of Systemstic Reviews*. **7**: CD009968. www.thecochranelibrary.com

Updated (minor change) July 2017

BACLOFEN

Class: Skeletal muscle relaxant.

Indications: Spasticity ± painful flexor muscle spasms of voluntary (skeletal) muscle resulting from spinal or CNS lesions, †hiccup.

Contra-indications: PO: Active peptic ulcer (baclofen stimulates gastric acid secretion). **IT:** treatment-resistant epilepsy.

Pharmacology

Baclofen is a chemical congener of the naturally occurring neurotransmitter, GABA.[1] It acts upon the GABA-receptor, inhibiting the release of the excitatory amino acids glutamate and aspartate, principally at the spinal level and also at supraspinal sites, thereby decreasing spasm in skeletal muscle.[2,3] It is preferable to **diazepam** for long-term use (e.g. in patients with chronic neurological disease such as multiple sclerosis[4]) because it avoids the problem of **diazepam** dependence. Further, its use is not associated with tolerance; it retains its antispasmodic effects even after many years of continued use.[5] Baclofen relieves hiccup, possibly by a direct effect on the diaphragm.

In patients with severe chronic spasticity in whom PO treatment is ineffective or poorly tolerated, baclofen can be given IT. However, a neurologist must be consulted before using this route. An overdose can cause rostral progression of hypotonia, respiratory depression, coma, and occasionally seizures.[6] Symptoms of underdosing are generally limited to a return of the patient's baseline spasticiy and rigidity. A life-threatening withdrawal syndrome can occur if IT baclofen is abruptly discontinued (see below).

Baclofen is predominantly excreted unchanged in the urine (70–80%); accumulation and toxicity can occur in renal impairment (see below).

Bio-availability >90% PO.

***Onset of action* PO:** for hiccup 4–8h, for muscle spasm 1–2 days, for spasticity 3–4 days. **IT:** for spasticity bolus 30–60min, infusion 6–8h.

Time to peak plasma concentration 0.5–3h.

Plasma halflife 3.5h; 4.5h in the elderly.

Duration of action 6–8h.[7]

10

Cautions

Withdrawal: abrupt withdrawal of PO baclofen may precipitate serious psychiatric reactions, e.g. agitation, confusion, hallucinations, paranoia, delusions, psychosis. Thus, discontinue by gradual dose reduction over 1–2 weeks, or longer if withdrawal symptoms occur.[8] Sudden withdrawal of IT baclofen or failure of the IT pump may lead to a potentially fatal withdrawal syndrome (Box A).

Box A IT baclofen withdrawal syndrome[6,9]

Cause

Sudden cessation of IT baclofen (e.g. delivery device failure).
Reported with a wide range of doses (50–1,500microgram/24h).

Clinical features

Symptoms evolve over 1–3 days:

- prodromal pruritus or paraesthesia; ± priapism
- seizures (early and/or late onset)
- tachycardia, hypotension or labile blood pressure
- fever (→ hyperthermia)
- dysphoria and malaise → decreased level of consciousness
- spasticity and rigidity greater than patient's baseline
- rhabdomyolysis → hepatic and renal failure, DIC
- coma (→ death).

Management

Restart the IT baclofen infusion as soon as possible.
Cardiopulmonary support as necessary.
High-dose baclofen PO or by enteral feeding tube (up to 120mg/24h), see Chapter 28, Table 2, p.793.
If necessary, give a benzodiazepine by CSCI/CIVI (e.g. midazolam) titrated to achieve muscle relaxation, normothermia, stabilization of blood pressure and cessation of seizures.

Use with caution in patients with severe psychiatric disorders, epilepsy, Parkinson's disease, respiratory impairment, stroke, history of peptic ulceration, renal impairment (see Dose and use and also Chapter 17, p.695), liver impairment (monitor LFTs), diabetes mellitus, hesitancy of micturition (may precipitate urinary retention), patients who use spasticity to maintain posture or to aid function. Drowsiness may affect skilled tasks and driving; effects of alcohol enhanced.

Because PO baclofen can increase gastric acid secretion, use is cautioned against in patients with a previous peptic ulcer (and contra-indicated in those with an active peptic ulcer). However, data are limited and the clinical relevance of this is unknown, e.g. one study found an overall *increase* in gastric pH.[10]

Undesirable effects

Very common (>10%): sedation, drowsiness, nausea.
Common (<10%, >1%): dizziness, fatigue, muscle hypotonia, pain or weakness, ataxia, tremor, insomnia, headache, visual disturbances, nystagmus, psychiatric disturbances, hypotension, respiratory depression, dry mouth, vomiting, constipation or diarrhoea, urinary frequency or incontinence, dysuria, hyperhidrosis, rash.
Uncommon, rare or very rare (<1%, >0.001%): paradoxical increase in spasticity, seizures (particularly in known epileptics), joint pain, hypothermia, paraesthesia, taste disturbance, abdominal pain, hepatic impairment, urinary retention, impotence.

Dose and use

The starting dose intervals and titration steps given here are more cautious than those in the SPC.

Starting doses are the same for muscle spasm, spasticity and hiccup:

- start with 5mg PO once daily–t.d.s.; the risk of GI irritation is less if taken after food (see Chapter 14, Box B, p.661)
- if necessary, increase by 5mg b.d.–t.d.s. every 3 days but more slowly if troublesome undesirable effects, particularly in the elderly
- effective doses for hiccup are often relatively low, e.g. 5–10mg t.d.s. but it may be necessary to increase to 20mg t.d.s.
- for spasticity, the typical effective dose is generally ≤20mg q.d.s. (maximum 100mg/24h)
- effective doses for muscle spasm fall somewhere in between.

With spasticity, if no improvement with maximum tolerated dose after 6 weeks, *withdraw gradually over 1–2 weeks.*

An undesirable degree of hypotonia may occur, but generally can be relieved by reducing the daytime dose and increasing the evening dose.

Parenteral administration

Baclofen CSCI has been used to prevent a withdrawal reaction when PO and enteral tube administration became impossible.[11] The solution for IT infusion was used for several days at a dose of 10mg/24h. However, this is expensive and, if used, should be short-term (e.g. 4–5 days) to prevent a potential withdrawal reaction.

IT administration is restricted to specialist use.

Renal impairment

In moderate–severe renal impairment, baclofen toxicity (particularly reduced level of consciousness) will occur[12] unless the total daily dose is reduced:

- for patients with creatinine clearance (Cl_{cr}) 10–20mL/min, start with 5mg PO once daily–b.d. and titrate to response
- for patients with Cl_{cr} <10mL/min, avoid if possible but, if unavoidable, start with 5mg PO once daily and titrate to response.[13]

Also see Chapter 17, Miscellaneous drugs, p.695.

Supply

Baclofen (generic)
Tablets 10mg, 28 days @ 10mg t.d.s. = £3.
Oral solution (sugar-free) 5mg/5mL, 28 days @ 10mg t.d.s. = £9.
****IT injection*** (for test dose) 50microgram/mL, 1mL amp = £2.50.
****IT solution for infusion*** (for use with implantable pump) 500microgram/mL, 20mL amp = £50; 2mg/mL, 5mL and 20mL amp = £50 and £240 respectively.

1 Zafonte R *et al.* (2004) Acute care management of post-TBI spasticity. *Journal of Head Trauma Rehabilitation.* **19**: 89–100.
2 Ramirez FC and Graham DY (1992) Treatment of intractable hiccup with baclofen: results of a double-blind randomized, controlled, crossover study. *American Journal of Gastroenterology.* **87**: 1789–1791.
3 Guelaud C *et al.* (1995) Baclofen therapy for chronic hiccup. *European Respiratory Journal.* **8**: 235–237.
4 NICE (2014) Multiple sclerosis in adults: management. *Clinical Guideline.* CG186. www.nice.org.uk
5 Gaillard JM (1977) Comparison of two muscle relaxant drugs on human sleep: diazepam and parachlorophenylgaba. *Acta Psychiatrica Belgica.* **77**: 410–425.
6 Coffey RJ *et al.* (2002) Abrupt withdrawal from intrathecal baclofen: recognition and management of a potentially life-threatening syndrome. *Archives of Physical Medicine and Rehabilitation.* **83**: 735–741.
7 Kochak GM *et al.* (1985) The pharmacokinetics of baclofen derived from intestinal infusion. *Clinical Pharmacology and Therapeutics.* **38**: 251–257.
8 CSM (Committee on Safety of Medicines and Medicines Control Agency) (1997) Reminder! Severe withdrawal reactions with baclofen can be prevented by gradual dose reduction. *Current Problems in Pharmacovigilance.* **23**: 6.
9 Mohammed I and Hussain A (2004) Intrathecal baclofen withdrawal syndrome - a life-threatening complication of baclofen pump: a case report. *BMC Clinical Pharmacology.* **4**: 6.
10 Ciccaglione AF and Marzio L (2003) Effect of acute and chronic administration of the GABA B agonist baclofen on 24 hour pH metry and symptoms in control subjects and in patients with gastro-oesophageal reflux disease. *Gut.* **52**: 464–470.
11 Remi C and Albrecht E (2014) Subcutaneous use of baclofen. *Journal of Pain and Symptom Management.* **48**: e1–3.
12 Su W *et al.* (2009) Reduced level of consciousness from baclofen in people with low kidney function. *British Medical Journal.* **339**: b4559.
13 Ashley C and Dunleavy A (2014). *The Renal Drug Database.* Oxon: CRC Press, UK. http//renaldrugdatabase.com (accessed March 2017).

Updated April 2017

DANTROLENE SODIUM

Class: Skeletal muscle relaxant.

Indications: Chronic severe spasticity of skeletal muscle.

Contra-indications: Hepatic impairment, particularly active liver disease, e.g. hepatitis or cirrhosis (may cause severe liver damage); acute muscle spasm or where spasm is useful in maintaining posture, balance or walking.

Pharmacology

Unlike **baclofen** and **diazepam**, dantrolene acts directly on skeletal muscle by binding to ryanodine receptors, thereby reducing the amount of intracellular calcium available for contraction.[1] It produces fewer central undesirable effects than **baclofen** and **diazepam** and, if necessary, can be used concurrently with these drugs in an attempt to produce a better balance between muscle relaxation and undesirable effects, e.g. unacceptable drowsiness.[2]

Dantrolene is metabolized in the liver mainly to the active hydroxylated metabolite, which is nearly as potent as the parent drug, and the acetamide metabolite, which has weak muscle relaxant activity. It is excreted in the urine, mainly as metabolites with a small amount of unchanged dantrolene; some is excreted in the bile.

Bio-availability 35% PO.
Onset of action up to 1 week.
Time to peak plasma concentration up to 3h.
Plasma halflife 5–9h.
Duration of action no data.

Cautions

Compromised pulmonary function, particularly COPD; predisposition to or actual cardiovascular impairment. Avoid concurrent use with other hepatotoxic drugs (see Chapter 18, p.704).

Undesirable effects

Drowsiness, dizziness, muscle weakness, general malaise, fatigue and diarrhoea (all generally transient). However, diarrhoea may be severe and may necessitate stopping dantrolene temporarily or permanently.

Common (>1%): Seizure, visual disturbances, speech disturbances, headache, pericarditis, pleural effusion, respiratory depression, nausea, vomiting, abdominal pain, anorexia, fever, skin rash, elevation of LFTs.

Severe hepatotoxicity develops rarely, most often after 1–12 months, and is more likely in people over 30 years old, women (particularly those taking oral contraceptives), and with doses >400mg/24h.[3] Fatalities have occurred only with doses >200mg/24h.[4,5]

Dose and use

Because of the risk of hepatotoxicity with long-term use, discontinue if no benefit is observed after 6 weeks of treatment. Perform LFTs before starting treatment and then at regular intervals, e.g. monthly, throughout treatment.

The dose of dantrolene should be built up slowly:
- start with 25mg once daily
- initially increase by no more than 25mg/24h weekly
- above 100mg/24h, larger increments are permissible (see SPC)
- usual effective dose 75mg t.d.s.
- maximum recommended dose 100mg q.d.s.

Supply

Dantrium® (Norgine)
Capsules 25mg, 100mg, 28 days @ 75mg t.d.s. = £43.

Dantrolene (generic)
Oral suspension 25mg/5mL, 100mg/5mL 28 days @ 75mg t.d.s. = £120 (unauthorized; available as a special order, see Chapter 24, p.751); *price based on specials tariff in the community.*

1 Zafonte R *et al.* (2004) Acute care management of post-TBI spasticity. *Journal of Head Trauma Rehabilitation.* **19**: 89–100.
2 Krause T *et al.* (2004) Dantrolene–a review of its pharmacology, therapeutic use and new developments. *Anaesthesia.* **59**: 364–373.
3 Kim JY *et al.* (2011) Safety of low-dose oral dantrolene sodium on hepatic function. *Archives of Physical Medicine and Rehabilitation.* **92**: 1359–1363.
4 Utili R *et al.* (1977) Dantrolene-associated hepatic injury. Incidence and character. *Gastroenterology.* **72**: 610–616.
5 Wilkinson S *et al.* (1979) Hepatitis from dantrolene sodium. *Gut.* **20**: 33–36.

Updated June 2017

TIZANIDINE

Class: Skeletal muscle relaxant.

Indications: Spasticity in multiple sclerosis, spinal cord injury or disease.

Contra-indications: Severe hepatic impairment, patients for whom spasm is useful in maintaining posture, balance or walking, concurrent use with potent CYP1A2 inhibitors, e.g. **ciprofloxacin**, **fluvoxamine**.

Pharmacology

Tizanidine, like **clonidine**, is a central α_2 agonist within the CNS at supraspinal and spinal levels.[1] It inhibits spinal polysynaptic reflex activity. This reduces the sympathetic outflow which in turn reduces muscle tone. Tizanidine has no direct effect on skeletal muscle, neuromuscular junctions or monosynaptic spinal reflexes. Tizanidine reduces pathologically increased muscle tone, including resistance to passive movements, and alleviates painful spasms and clonus.[2] In spasticity, tizanidine is comparable in efficacy to **diazepam** and **baclofen**,[3] and has superior tolerability.[4]

Tizanidine is well absorbed but undergoes extensive first-pass metabolism in the liver to inactive metabolites which are mostly excreted by the kidneys. Wide interindividual variability in the effective plasma concentration means that the optimal dose must be titrated slowly over 2–4 weeks. Maximum effects occur within 2h of administration.[5]

Bio-availability 40% PO.
Onset of action 1–2h; peak response 8 weeks.
Time to peak plasma concentration 1.5h.
Plasma halflife 2.5h; up to 14h ± 10h in renal failure.[6]
Duration of action 'relatively short' (SPC).

Cautions

Elderly; renal impairment (see Chapter 17, p.695); cardiovascular disorders. Drowsiness may affect performance of skilled tasks, e.g. driving.

If possible, avoid concurrent use in high doses with other drugs which can cause QT interval prolongation.

In patients taking ≥12mg/24h, LFTs should be monitored monthly for the first 4 months because of a risk of hepatotoxicity (see Chapter 18, p.704); discontinue if LFTs remain persistently raised >3 times the upper limit of normal.

Avoid abrupt withdrawal, particularly after long-term use or high doses (risk of rebound hypertension and tachycardia); monitor blood pressure during withdrawal.

10

Drug interactions

Tizanidine plasma concentrations are increased by CYP1A2 inhibitors, potentially leading to severe hypotension. Avoid concurrent use with potent CYP1A2 inhibitors, e.g. **ciprofloxacin** (and possibly **enoxacin** (not UK)), **fluvoxamine**. Use with caution with other CYP1A2 inhibitors, e.g. **cimetidine**, **norfloxacin**, **oestrogens**, **progestogens** (see Chapter 19, p.717).

Concurrent administration with antihypertensive drugs may potentiate hypotension; with **digoxin** may potentiate bradycardia.

Undesirable effects

Drowsiness, weakness and dry mouth in more than two thirds of those taking it,[7] drowsiness and weakness may be less than with **diazepam** and **baclofen**.[8]

Hypotension and dizziness, nausea and other GI disturbances. Less frequently insomnia, bradycardia, hallucinations and hepatotoxicity (rare if dose ≤12mg/24h).

Dose and use

Slow upward titration helps to reduce undesirable effects:

- start with 2mg PO once daily
- if necessary, increase by 2mg every 3–4 days; build up to 2mg q.d.s. before increasing individual doses
- effective dose generally ≤24mg/24h
- maximum recommended dose 36mg/24h.

In elderly patients and in those with severe renal impairment (creatinine clearance <25mL/min) an even slower titration is recommended. Because of the prolonged plasma halflife in renal impairment, the manufacturer recommends slow titration with a *single* daily dose (also see Chapter 17, p.695).

Avoid abrupt withdrawal; if possible, taper higher doses over several weeks (see Cautions).

Supply

Tizanidine (generic)
Tablets 2mg, 4mg, 28 days @ 8mg t.d.s. = £49.
Oral solution or suspension 2mg/5mL, 28 days @ 8mg t.d.s. = £116 or £258, respectively (unauthorized; available as a special order, see Chapter 24, p.751); *price based on specials tariff in community.*

1 Zafonte R *et al.* (2004) Acute care management of post-TBI spasticity. *Journal of Head Trauma Rehabilitation*. **19**: 89–100.
2 Wallace J (1994) Summary of combined clinical analysis of controlled clinical trials with tizanidine. *Neurology*. **44 (11 Suppl 9)**: s60–s69.
3 Lataste X *et al.* (1994) Comparative profile of tizanidine in the management of spasticity. *Neurology*. **44 (11 Suppl 9)**: s53–s59.
4 Kamen L *et al.* (2008) A practical overview of tizanidine use for spasticity secondary to multiple sclerosis, stroke, and spinal cord injury. *Current Medical Research and Opinion*. **24**: 425–439.
5 Wagstaff A and Bryson H (1997) Tizanidine. A review of its pharmacology, clinical efficacy and tolerability in the management of spasticity associated with cerebral and spinal disorders. *Drugs*. **53**: 435–452.
6 Keyser E and Ohnhaus E (1986) *Data on file*. Pharmacokinetic study with Sirdalud (tizanidine, DS 103–282) in patients with renal insufficiency.
7 Nance P *et al.* (1997) Relationship of the antispasticity effect of tizanidine to plasma concentration in patients with multiple sclerosis. *Archives of Neurology*. **54**: 731–736.
8 Smith H and Barton A (2000) Tizanidine in the management of spasticity and musculoskeletal complaints in the palliative care population. *American Journal of Hospice and Palliative Care*. **17**: 50–58.

Updated June 2017

11: EAR, NOSE AND OROPHARYNX

MOUTHWASHES

Cleaning and freshening the mouth

Lemon glycerine mouth swabs should not be used because the lemon flavouring has a drying effect.[1]

For home use, one of the following rinses made in tepid water is generally satisfactory:

- mix 1/4 teaspoon of **sodium chloride** (table salt) in 1 cup (approximately 250mL)
- mix 1 teaspoon of **sodium bicarbonate** (baking soda) in 1 cup
- mix 1/2 teaspoon of **sodium chloride** and 2 tablespoons of **sodium bicarbonate** in 4 cups.[2]

Some centres use less **sodium bicarbonate**, e.g. 1/2 teaspoon each of **sodium chloride** and **sodium bicarbonate**. In hospital, **compound sodium chloride mouthwash BP** (containing both **sodium chloride** and **sodium bicarbonate**) is often used. **Sodium bicarbonate** is widely used as symptomatic treatment for mild oral mucositis.

Chlorhexidine mouthwashes are used to prevent/treat various oral infections (e.g. periodontal disease, oral candidosis),[3,4] and to sterilize dentures and other prostheses.[5] **Chlorhexidine** inhibits the formation of plaque on teeth, and thus is useful when toothbrushing is not possible. However, **chlorhexidine** does not remove established plaque; this requires professional dental cleaning.

Note. **Chlorhexidine** is inactivated by ingredients in some toothpastes. Thus, if a patient is using both, the use of the mouthwash should be delayed for ≥30min after using toothpaste. Further, because **chlorhexidine** binds to **nystatin** and leads to inactivation of both drugs, it is important to delay giving **nystatin** oral suspension for ≥30min after using **chlorhexidine** mouthwash.[6]

Most brands of **chlorhexidine** mouthwash contain alcohol which may cause discomfort; diluting the mouthwash with an equal amount of water may reduce this;[5] however, an alcohol-free product is available. **Chlorhexidine** can stain the teeth and tongue, and this is exacerbated by drinking tea and coffee. The staining can be removed by professional dental cleaning.

Debridement

Generally, a coated ('furred') tongue is indicative of inadequate salivary gland function (most likely drug-induced). Initial treatment is thus frequent routine mouth care, e.g. sips or sprays of cold water, sucking ice-cubes. When inadequate, consider the use of artificial saliva and/or saliva stimulant (see p.616 and p.618). Specific debridement is achieved by gentle brushing with a baby's soft toothbrush several times per day until the tongue is clean.

In the past, some centres used effervescent **ascorbic acid** tablets or pineapple for debriding. However, such use is now considered poor practice. Both agents are acidic, and thus may exacerbate a sore or inflamed mouth, contribute to the demineralization of teeth, and predispose to oral infections (see p.616).

Cautions

MHRA has issued an alert for products or medical devices containing **chlorhexidine** following reports of anaphylaxis, including one precipitated by the use of a **chlorhexidine** skin wipe.[7]

Use

Rinse the mouth with the recommended volume, generally 10mL, for about 30–60sec and then spit out:

- **sodium chloride** or **sodium bicarbonate** mouthwashes can be used p.r.n.; dilute **compound sodium chloride BP** mouthwash with an equal volume of warm water
- **chlorhexidine** has a prolonged duration of action, and generally needs to be used only b.d., either undiluted or diluted with an equal volume of warm water
- use **hydrogen peroxide** mouthwash undiluted after meals and at bedtime.

Supply

Sodium chloride mouthwash, compound BP
Mouthwash containing **sodium chloride** 1.5%, **sodium bicarbonate** 1% in peppermint-flavoured chloroform water; can be prepared locally.

Chlorhexidine gluconate (generic)
Mouthwash 0.2% (2mg/mL), 300mL = £3; *original or mint flavour.*
Mouthwash (alcohol-free) 0.2% (2mg/mL), 300mL = £4.

Hydrogen peroxide
Peroxyl® (Colgate Palmolive)
Mouthwash 1.5% (15mg/mL), 300mL = £3.

1 Poland JM *et al.* (1987) Comparing Moi-Stir to lemon-glycerin swabs. *American Journal of Nursing*. **87**: 422–424.
2 National Cancer Institute (2016) Oral complications of chemotherapy and head/neck radiation (PDQ). Available from: www.cancer.gov
3 Chow A (2010) Oral bacterial infections. In: AN Davies and JB Epstein (eds) *Oral Complications of Cancer and its Management*. Oxford University Press, Oxford, pp. 185–193.
4 Finlay I and Davies A (2005) Fungal Infections. In: A Davies and I Finlay (eds) *Oral Care in Advanced Disease*. Oxford University Press, Oxford, pp. 55–71.
5 Sweeney P (2005) Oral hygiene. In: A Davies and I Finlay (eds) *Oral Care in Advanced Disease*. Oxford University Press, Oxford, pp. 21–35.
6 Barkvoll P and Attramadal A (1989) Effect of nystatin and chlorhexidine digluconate on Candida albicans. *Oral Surgery Oral Medicine and Oral Pathology*. **67**: 279–281.
7 MHRA (2012) All medical devices and medicinal products containing chlorhexidine. *Medical Devices Alert*. MDA/2012/2075 www.mhra.gov.uk/Safetyinformation

Updated April 2017

ARTIFICIAL SALIVA

Dry mouth (xerostomia) is managed by saliva stimulants or substitutes. Although 99% of saliva is water, the remaining 1% comprises a wide range of electrolytes and molecules which are important for saliva's many roles, e.g. lubricant, cleansing, antimicrobial, taste, digestion, buffering, and mineralization of teeth.[1] This may explain why sipping water gives only short-lived relief.

Artificial saliva is a poor substitute for natural saliva. Thus, *unless a main salivary duct is blocked*, a saliva stimulant is preferable. Chewing gum acts as a saliva stimulant and is as effective as, and preferred to, mucin-based artificial saliva.[2] The gum should be sugar-free and, in patients with dentures, low-tack, e.g. Orbit®.

If dry mouth remains a problem, **pilocarpine** or **bethanechol** should be considered (see p.618). Acidic products should *not* be used as saliva stimulants because they predispose to oral infection (e.g. dental caries, oral candidosis) and cause demineralization of the teeth (leading to dental erosion and dental pain). For patients who do not respond to, or cannot tolerate saliva stimulants, artificial saliva is an option.

The ideal artificial saliva should be easy to use, pleasant, effective and well tolerated.[3] Further, it should have a neutral pH and contain fluoride (to enhance remineralization of the teeth).[4]

Generally, RCTs indicate that mucin-based products are better tolerated and more effective than cellulose-based ones,[5–7] with some patients finding cellulose-based products no better than frequent sips of fluid.

The mucin comes from the stomach of pigs, and this may be an issue for some patients (e.g. Jews, Muslims, vegetarians). There is no good evidence that gels are more effective or last longer than sprays.

Undesirable effects

Unpleasant taste, irritation of the mouth, nausea and/or diarrhoea in ≤30% of patients.[2,8]

Dose and use

PCF regards sugar-free chewing gum as the saliva stimulant of choice for most patients. For patients with dentures, it should be low-tack, e.g. Orbit®.

Artificial salivas with a neutral pH are preferred for long-term use. Artificial salivas or saliva stimulants with an acidic pH should be avoided.

The duration of effect of artificial salivas is relatively short, due to a combination of swallowing and evaporation. Thus, artificial salivas may need to be taken every 10–30min, and also before (and sometimes during) meals. Proprietary artificial salivas with a neutral pH include:

- AS Saliva Orthana® (mucin-based sprays and lozenges); lozenges are ACBS classified (see supply)
- Biotène Oralbalance® gel
- BioXtra® gel; ACBS classified (see supply).

Supply

Some products, e.g. AS Saliva Orthana® lozenges and BioXtra® gel, are classified in the UK as borderline substances and have ACBS approval only for dry mouth associated with radiotherapy or sicca syndrome. The prescriber must endorse an NHS FP10 prescription for one of these products with 'ACBS', otherwise the Prescription Pricing Authority will investigate whether it has been issued for an approved indication.

Mucin-based (porcine)
AS Saliva Orthana® (AS Pharma)
Oral spray 50mL bottle = £5; 500mL refill = £34.
Lozenges 30 = £3.50 (ACBS).

Cellulose-based
Biotène Oralbalance® (GSK Consumer Health)
Saliva replacement gel 50g = £4.50.

BioXtra® (RIS Products)
Saliva replacement gel 40mL tube = £4, 50mL spray = £4 (ACBS).

1 Davies A (2005) Salivary gland dysfunction. In: A Davies and I Finlay (eds) *Oral Care in Advanced Disease*. Oxford University Press, Oxford, pp. 97–114.

2 Davies AN (2000) A comparison of artificial saliva and chewing gum in the management of xerostomia in patients with advanced cancer. *Palliative Medicine*. **14**: 197–203.

3 Epstein JB and Stevenson-Moore P (1992) A clinical comparative trial of saliva substitutes in radiation-induced salivary gland hypofunction. *Special Care Dentistry*. **12**: 21–23.

4 Davies A (2010) Salivary gland dysfunction. In: AN Davies and JB Epstein (eds) *Oral Complications of Cancer and its Management*. Oxford University Press, Oxford, pp. 203–223.

5 S'Gravenmade E *et al.* (1974) The effect of mucin-containing artificial saliva on severe exerostomia. *International Journal of Oral Surgery*. **3**: 435–439.

6 Vissink A *et al.* (1983) A clinical comparison between commercially available mucin- and CMC-containing saliva substitutes. *International Journal of Oral Surgery*. **12**: 232–238.

7 Visch L et *al.* (1986) A double-blind crossover trial of CMC- and mucin-containing saliva substitutes. *International Journal of Oral and Maxillofacial Surgery*. **15**: 395–400.

8 Davies A *et al.* (1998) A comparison of artificial saliva and pilocarpine in the management of xerostomia in patients with advanced cancer. *Palliative Medicine*. **12**: 105–111.

Updated September 2017

PILOCARPINE

Class: Parasympathomimetic.

Indications: Xerostomia (dry mouth) after radiotherapy for head and neck cancer, dry mouth (and dry eyes) in Sjögren's syndrome and †drug-induced dry mouth.

Contra-indications: Intestinal or urinary obstruction, or when increased intestinal or urinary tract motility could be harmful (e.g. after recent surgery); when miosis could be harmful (e.g. narrow-angle glaucoma, acute iritis); unstable asthma.

Pharmacology

Pilocarpine is a parasympathomimetic (predominantly muscarinic) drug with mild β-adrenergic activity which stimulates secretion from exocrine glands, including salivary glands. A systematic review suggests that about 40–50% of patients with radiotherapy-induced dry mouth respond to pilocarpine, with a time to response of up to 12 weeks.[1] However, undesirable effects are common, and were the main reason for withdrawal from studies (≤15% of patients taking 5mg t.d.s.).

About 90% of patients with drug-induced dry mouth respond to pilocarpine with benefit seen in <24h.[2] In an RCT, half of the patients preferred pilocarpine because it was more effective, and half preferred the comparator **mucin**-based artificial saliva, mainly because it was a spray and not a tablet.[2] Undesirable effects were much more common in patients receiving pilocarpine (84% vs. 22%), which resulted in about a quarter of the patients withdrawing from the study.

Alternatives to pilocarpine are used at some centres, e.g. **bethanechol**.[3,4] Pharmacokinetic data for **bethanechol** are limited. Because of poor GI absorption, it is recommended to be taken on an empty stomach. Although cheaper than pilocarpine, it has a slower onset of action (30–90min), and a shorter duration of action (possibly only 1–2h).[5]

Bio-availability 96% PO.
Onset of action 20min (drug-induced dry mouth); up to 3 months (after radiation).
Time to peak plasma concentration 1h.
Plasma halflife 1h.
Duration of action 3–5h (single dose).

Cautions

Pilocarpine may antagonize the effects of antimuscarinic drugs, e.g. inhaled **ipratropium bromide**. Concurrent use with β antagonists (β-blockers) may cause cardiac conduction disturbances.

Cognitive or psychiatric disorder, epilepsy, parkinsonism. Miosis may affect vision and driving ability, particularly at night. Cardiovascular disease (changes in haemodynamics or heart rhythm), hyperthyroidism, COPD (increased bronchial smooth muscle tone, airway resistance and bronchial secretions). Peptic ulcer (increased acid secretion), gallstones or biliary tract disease (increased biliary smooth muscle contraction). Renal impairment (no reliable human data on metabolism and excretion), kidney stones (potential for renal colic).

Reduce dose in moderate–severe hepatic impairment (see p.714). Increased sweating may exacerbate dehydration in patients unable to drink sufficient fluids.

Undesirable effects

Very common (>10%): headache, flu-like syndrome, nausea, urinary frequency, sweating.
Common (<10%, >1%): dizziness, asthenia, chills, blurred vision, eye pain, conjunctivitis, flushing, palpitations, hypertension (after initial hypotension), rhinitis, abdominal pain, dyspepsia, vomiting, diarrhoea or constipation, rash, pruritus.

Undesirable effects with **bethanechol** are similar to pilocarpine but generally less severe.

Dose and use

The manufacturer recommends t.d.s. during or directly after meals but, given its duration of action (3–5h), there is scope for greater flexibility. Adding a dose at bedtime reduces the likelihood of the patient waking in the night with an excessively dry mouth.[6]

In drug-induced dry mouth 5mg PO q.d.s. is generally effective, but after radiotherapy 10mg q.d.s. may be needed:

- start with 5mg PO t.d.s. and at bedtime
- if necessary and if tolerated, increase the dose to 10mg q.d.s. after 2 days if the dry mouth is drug-induced, and after 4 weeks if radiation-induced
- if no improvement with 10mg q.d.s., stop after 4 days if the dry mouth is drug-induced, and after 12 weeks if radiation-induced.

In patients with moderate–severe hepatic impairment, start on a lower total daily dose, e.g. 5mg b.d., and increase to 5mg q.d.s. if well tolerated.

Some centres use the eyedrop formulation PO: 3 drops of a 4% solution contains 6mg. It is cheaper than tablets (see supply), but is no more effective and is not always acceptable to patients.[7]

If **bethanechol** is used instead for drug-induced dry mouth:

- start with 25mg PO t.d.s. on an empty stomach, e.g. 30min before meals
- reduce to 10mg t.d.s. if patients experience excessive salivation.

Supply

Pilocarpine (generic)
Eyedrops 4% (40mg/mL), 10mL, 28 days @ 3 drops (6mg) PO q.d.s. = £26. (10mL lasts approximately 15 days).

Salagen® (Merus Labs)
Tablets 5mg, 28 days @ 5mg q.d.s. = £55.

Bethanechol
Myotonine® (Cheplapharm)
Tablets *(scored)* 10mg, 25mg, 28 days @ 25mg t.d.s. = £23.

1 Davies AN and Thompson J (2015) Parasympathomimetic drugs for the treatment of salivary gland dysfunction due to radiotherapy. *Cochrane Database of Systematic Reviews*. **10**: CD003782. www.thecochranelibrary.com
2 Davies A *et al.* (1998) A comparison of artificial saliva and pilocarpine in the management of xerostomia in patients with advanced cancer. *Palliative Medicine*. **12**: 105–111.
3 Epstein J *et al.* (1994) A clinical trial of bethanechol in patients with xerostomia after radiation therapy. A pilot study. *Oral Surgery, Oral Medicine and Oral Pathology*. **77**: 610–614.
4 Davies A (2005) Salivary gland dysfunction. In: A Davies and I Finlay (eds) *Oral Care in Advanced Disease*. Oxford University Press, Oxford, pp. 97–114.
5 McEvoy GK. *American Hospital Formulary Service*. Maryland, USA: American Society of Health-System Pharmacists www.medicinescomplete.com (accessed April 2017).
6 Davies A (2014) *Personal communication.*
7 Nikles J *et al.* (2015) Testing pilocarpine drops for dry mouth in advanced cancer using n-of-1 trials: A feasibility study. *Palliative Medicine*. **29**: 967–974.

Updated June 2017

DRUGS FOR ORAL INFLAMMATION AND ULCERATION

'Oral stomatitis' is a term applied to diffuse inflammatory, erosive and ulcerative conditions affecting the mucous membranes of the mouth, whereas 'oral mucositis' tends to be restricted to stomatitis caused by local radiotherapy, chemotherapy or other anti-cancer modalities.

The causes of oral ulceration include trauma (physical, chemical), recurrent aphthous ulceration, infection, cancer, skin conditions, nutritional deficiencies, GI conditions, haematopoietic disorders and drug treatment (Box A). It is important to determine the cause so that, if appropriate, specific treatment is given as well as symptomatic treatment. For example, ill-fitting dentures which cause traumatic ulceration (and/or mucosal hyperplasia) should be relined, or ideally replaced.[1]

Box A Drug-related oral ulceration

Alimentary
Pancreatin

Analgesics
NSAIDs

Antibiotics
Aztreonam
Clarithromycin
Proguanil
Vancomycin
Zalcitabine

Cardiac
Captopril
Isoprenaline (not UK)
Losartan
Nicorandil
Phenindione

Chemotherapy
Bleomycin
Doxorubicin
5-Fluoro-uracil
Melphalan
Mercaptopurine
Methotrexate

Corticosteroids
Flunisolide (not UK)

Psychotropics
Carbamazepine
Olanzapine
Phenytoin
Sertraline

Other
Alendronic acid
Allopurinol
Emepronium (not UK)
Gold
Interferons
Interleukin-2
Molgramostim
Penicillamine
Potassium chloride

Management strategy

The symptomatic management of oral inflammation and ulceration involves measures which:

- maintain oral hygiene
- relieve pain
- protect ulcerated mucosa
- treat secondary infection
- reduce inflammation.

Advice should be sought from an oral medicine specialist if unexplained ulceration persists for >3 weeks.

Maintain oral hygiene

Simple mouthwashes, e.g. water or 0.9% **saline**, can be soothing, help to maintain oral hygiene, and prevent secondary infection (see p.615). The temperature of the mouthwash appears to be important, with tepid ones being more soothing than cold or warm ones.

Pain relief

Topical analgesics

These include:

- local anaesthetics
- NSAIDs
- antihistamines
- opioids.

Local anaesthetics

The efficacy of topical local anaesthetics depends on the formulation, duration of application (at least 5min is required) and site of application. There are limited data to support their use in oral mucositis, and any effect is of short duration.[2] They are less effective in more keratinized areas of the mouth, e.g. the palate.[3]

Some systemic absorption of the local anaesthetic occurs, which is increased by mucosal inflammation. However, plasma concentrations are generally low, and toxicity has been reported only in exceptional circumstances (see p.71). With all topical local anaesthetics, care must be taken not to produce pharyngeal anaesthesia before meals because this could lead to aspiration and choking:

- **lidocaine** ointment 5% (has a water-miscible base), rubbed gently onto the affected areas before food and p.r.n.
- **lidocaine** spray 10% (Xylocaine®), applied thinly to the ulcer using a cotton bud before food and p.r.n. (unauthorized use)
- **oxetacaine** in combination with **aluminium hydroxide-magnesium hydroxide** oral suspension (available as a special order), is used for post-radiation oesophagitis and candidosis which is causing painful swallowing (see p.1)
- **cocaine hydrochloride** 2% has been used as a mouthwash in cases unresponsive to standard treatment (available as a special order); use 10mL (200mg) q4h p.r.n., rinse around the mouth for a few minutes and then *spit out.* It should *not* be swallowed as this can lead to agitation and hallucinations. *Avoid concurrent use with mouthwashes containing sodium bicarbonate because this enhances transmucosal absorption of cocaine.*

Various OTC products are also available.

NSAIDs

Benzydamine, an NSAID, also has local anaesthetic and antimicrobial effects.[4,5] It is available as an oral rinse or spray, and can ease the discomfort associated with oral stomatitis. It is recommended for the prevention of oral mucositis secondary to radiotherapy:

- **benzydamine** 0.15% mouthwash, rinse or gargle 15mL for 20–30sec before spitting out, repeat q3h–q1.5h p.r.n. Dilute with an equal volume of water if stinging occurs.[6,7]

Excessive use of **choline salicylate** dental gel or confinement under a denture can result in oral irritation and/or ulceration. Remove any dentures before use and wait ≥30min before re-inserting:

- **choline salicylate** 8.7% oromucosal gel (e.g. Bonjela®), apply 1–2cm by gentle massage q3h p.r.n.; maximum recommended dose 6 applications/day.

Other options include **flurbiprofen** lozenges (can also result in oral ulceration).

Antihistamines

Diphenhydramine (not UK) is an antihistamine with a topical analgesic effect. It has been used for decades for oral mucositis, particularly in the USA,[8] as a locally prepared oral rinse. It is spread around the mouth and then swallowed or spat out after 2min, e.g.:

- **diphenhydramine** 25mg/5mL and **magnesium hydroxide** in equal parts, up to 30mL q2h
- **diphenhydramine** 12.5mg/5mL, **lidocaine** viscous 2% and an antacid in equal parts[8]
- **diphenhydramine** 12.5mg/5mL and **kaopectate** in equal parts (the latter helps mixture to adhere to the oral mucosa).

Some centres use **doxepin** (a TCA and a potent H_1- and H_2-receptor antagonist) instead. It is given as an oral rinse containing **doxepin** 25mg/5mL (not UK) up to six times per day.[9] It must *not* be swallowed: a dose of this size several times per day would cause drowsiness and possibly other toxicity (also see p.635).

Opioids

Opioids have a topical analgesic effect on inflamed tissue and can be used as a mouthwash. Some recommend that the mouthwash is subsequently swallowed in order to combine a systemic analgesic effect with the topical one:

- special order **morphine sulfate** 2mg/mL solution, take 10mg in 5mL q4h–q3h, hold in the mouth for 2min *and then spit out or swallow*; some patients need higher doses, occasionally 30mg q4h–q3h.[10,11] Note. The commercially available products contain alcohol and should *not* be used
- locally prepared **morphine sulfate** 1–5mg/mL gel, initially 3mL q8h–q4h, hold in mouth for 10min *and then spit out or swallow.*

Also see **morphine**, p.380.

Systemic analgesics

Systemic analgesics include non-opioids and opioids given as for other pains, balancing benefit against undesirable effects. For severe mucositis (patient unable to eat ± unable to drink) with inadequate pain relief from topical measures, a parenteral opioid should be administered either by patient-controlled analgesia, continuous infusion with p.r.n. boluses as required, or transdermal administration (e.g. **fentanyl**).[6] Chemotherapy patients often have a permanent IV access which can be used.

Protect the ulcerated areas

Coating agents are of limited value because they can be difficult to apply and they do not relieve persistent oral inflammatory pain. However, by adhering to and coating the denuded surface, they may help to reduce contact pain, e.g. from eating or drinking. Available agents include:

- **carmellose (carboxymethylcellulose) sodium** (Orabase® paste, Orahesive® powder) apply the paste to, or sprinkle the powder onto, the sore area after food
- **polyvinylpyrrolidine** and **sodium hyaluronate** oral gel (Gelclair®) t.d.s. p.r.n., ideally 30–60min before eating; mix contents of 1 sachet with 40mL water, rinse around mouth for at least 1min, gargle and then spit out; an expensive option
- **sucralfate** is *not* of benefit in radiation-induced oral mucositis,[12] but may help in other types of oral stomatitis; it can be given in a suspension 1g/5mL q.d.s. (not UK).

Treat secondary infection

Antiseptic and antibacterial mouthwashes may help prevent or treat secondary infection, particularly with multiple ulcers not easily accessible to covering pastes:

- *prevention*: **chlorhexidine gluconate** mouthwash 0.2%, ideally alcohol-free (see p.615)
- *treatment*: **doxycycline** suspension 100mg in 10mL q.d.s. for 3 days (unauthorized use; prepared by mixing a dispersible tablet or the contents of a capsule with a small quantity of water) rinse around the mouth for 2–3min and then spit out.

Alternatively if available, **tetracycline** suspension 250mg in 10mL[13] *or* **minocycline** suspension 10mg in 5mL[14] can be prepared from capsules in the same way (not UK).

For oral candidosis, see p.475.

Reduce the inflammation

Topical corticosteroids are useful in the management of certain types of oral ulceration, e.g. recurrent aphthous ulceration (Box B). However, corticosteroids do *not* feature in the management of oral mucositis. Systemic corticosteroids are generally reserved for severe ulcerative conditions, e.g. pemphigus vulgaris.

Box B Treatment of aphthous ulcers

Corticosteroids

Corticosteroids are the mainstay of treatment. Use as soon as symptoms/ulcers appear; avoid in oral infections:

- hydrocortisone oromucosal tablets 2.5mg q.d.s. for up to 5 days; tablets are placed at the site of the ulcers and left to dissolve
- beclometasone metered-dose aerosol inhaler 50 or 100microgram sprayed into the mouth b.d., when a more potent corticosteroid is needed for difficult-to-reach sites such as the soft palate and oropharynx (unauthorized use)
- betamethasone soluble tablets 500microgram, dispersed in 20mL water and rinsed around the mouth q.d.s.; also suitable when a more potent corticosteroid is needed for difficult-to-reach sites (unauthorized use).

Supply

The following list is selective.

Topical analgesics
Lidocaine (generic)
Ointment 5% in a water-miscible base, 15g = £6.

Xylocaine® (AstraZeneca)
Spray 10%, 50mL = £6. Apply thinly to ulcer using cotton bud (unauthorized use).

Cocaine hydrochloride
Mouthwash 2%, 200mL = £50 (Schedule 2 **CD**; unauthorized, available as a special order from St Thomas Pharmacy Manufacturing Unit 0207 188 4992).

For **oxetacaine** with **aluminium hydroxide-magnesium hydroxide** oral suspension see p.1.

Benzydamine (generic)
Oral rinse (mouthwash) 0.15%, 300mL = £6.
Oromucosal spray 0.15%, 30mL = £4.

Choline salicylate dental gel BP
Bonjela® (Reckitt Benckiser)
Oral gel 8.7%, 15g = £2.50; also available OTC.

Flurbiprofen
Strefen® (Reckitt Benckiser)
Lozenges 8.75mg, 16 = £2.50.

Also see **Morphine**, p.380.

Coating agents
Orabase® (ConvaTec)
Oral paste containing **carmellose sodium** 16.7%, **gelatin** 16.7% and **pectin** 16.7%, 30g = £2.

Orahesive® (ConvaTec)
Powder containing **carmellose sodium**, **gelatin** and **pectin**, equal parts, 25g = £2.50.

11

Gelclair® (Cambridge Laboratories)
Oral gel containing **polyvinylpyrrolidine** and **sodium hyaluronate**, 28 days @ one 15mL sachet t.d.s. = £134.

Antiseptic and antibacterial mouthwashes
For **chlorhexidine gluconate** mouthwashes, see p.615.

Doxycycline (generic)
Capsules 100mg (as hyclate), 3 days @ 100mg q.d.s. = £1.25.

Vibramycin-D® (Pfizer)
Dispersible tablets 100mg, 3 days @ 100mg q.d.s. = £7.50.

Corticosteroids
Hydrocortisone (generic)
Oromucosal tablets 2.5mg (as sodium succinate), 5 days @ 2.5mg q.d.s. = £7.

Beclometasone (generic)
Aerosol inhalation 50microgram/metered dose, 200-dose inhaler = £4; 100microgram/metered dose, 200-dose inhaler = £7.

Betamethasone (generic)
Tablets soluble 500microgram, 5 days @ 500microgram q.d.s. = £8.50.

1 Walls A (2005) Domiciliary dental care. In: A Davies and I Finlay (eds) *Oral Care in Advanced Disease*. Oxford University Press, Oxford, pp. 37–45.
2 Saunders DP *et al.* (2013) Systematic review of antimicrobials, mucosal coating agents, anesthetics, and analgesics for the management of oral mucositis in cancer patients. *Supportive Care in Cancer*. **21**: 3191–3207.
3 Meecham J (2005) Oral pain. In: A Davies and I Finlay (eds) *Oral Care in Advanced Disease*. Oxford University Press, Oxford, pp. 134–143.
4 Turnbull RS (1995) Benzydamine Hydrochloride (Tantum) in the management of oral inflammatory conditions. *Journal Canadian Dental Association*. **61**: 127–134.
5 Fanaki NH and el-Nakeeb MA (1992) Antimicrobial activity of benzydamine, a non-steroid anti-inflammatory agent. *Journal of Chemotherpy*. **4**: 347–352.
6 MASCC Oral mucsositis guidelines. www.mascc.org/mucositis-guidelines
7 Kim J *et al.* (1985) A clinical study of benzydamine for the treatment of radiotherapy induced mucositis of the orpharynx. *International Journal of Tissue Reaction*. **7**: 215–218.
8 NIH Consensus Development Conference Statement (1989) Oral complications of cancer therapies, prevention and treatment. *NIH Consensus Statement*. **7**: 1–11.

9 Epstein JB *et al.* (2007) Management of pain in cancer patients with oral mucositis: follow-up of multiple doses of doxepin oral rinse. *Journal of Pain and Symptom Management.* **33**: 111–114.
10 Cerchietti LC *et al.* (2002) Effect of topical morphine for mucositis-associated pain following concomitant chemoradiotherapy for head and neck carcinoma. *Cancer.* **95**: 2230–2236.
11 Cerchietti L and Cerchietti L (2007) Morphine mouthwashes for painful mucositis. *Supportive Care in Cancer.* **15**: 115–116.
12 Keefe DM *et al.* (2007) Updated clinical practice guidelines for the prevention and treatment of mucositis. *Cancer.* **109**: 820–831.
13 Barrons RW (2001) Treatment strategies for recurrent oral aphthous ulcers. *American Journal of Health-System Pharmacy.* **58**: 41–50.
14 Gorsky M *et al.* (2007) Topical minocycline and tetracycline rinses in treatment of recurrent aphthous stomatitis: a randomized cross-over study. *Dermatology Online Journal.* **13**: 1.

Updated September 2017

CERUMENOLYTICS

Indications: Impacted earwax (cerumen).

Contra-indications: perforated ear drum, presence of myringotomy tubes (grommets), recent ear surgery.

Pharmacology

Cerumen impaction is defined as an accumulation of earwax which causes symptoms, prevents adequate examination of the ear, or both; it does not necessarily imply complete obstruction.[1,2] Symptoms associated with impacted earwax include deafness, tinnitus, fullness, itching, otalgia, discharge, and chronic cough. Asymptomatic earwax does *not* need to be removed.

Earwax is secreted to provide a protective film on the skin of the external ear canal. It is generally expelled naturally. The risk of impaction is increased in children, the elderly, people with learning disabilities, and when natural expulsion is obstructed, e.g. by anatomical abnormalities of the ear canal, hearing aids, or inappropriate use of 'cotton buds' to clean the ears.[1,3]

Cerumenolytics are classified as either water-based (e.g. water, 0.9% saline, 5% **sodium bicarbonate**), oil-based (e.g. **almond oil**, **olive oil**), or non-water/non-oil based (e.g. **urea-hydrogen peroxide**).[4] Water-based products are true cerumenolytics (i.e. break up keratin within earwax),[5] whereas oil-based products lubricate and soften the earwax. The mechanism of action of non-water/non-oil-based products is unclear.

Evidence is too limited to indicate if one type of cerumenolytic is more effective than any other.[1,6] Systematic reviews suggest that cerumenolytics can clear earwax in about one third of cases in 4 days, thereby obviating the need for syringing.[4,6] For these patients, self-treatment with clean tap water will be the most cost-effective treatment.

Syringing without pre-treatment with a cerumenolytic is effective in about three quarters of patients.[3,4,6] After pre-treatment, success approaches 100%.[1] Pre-treatment with water 15–30min before syringing is as effective as applying drops b.d. for several days.[4,7] It works in 'nearly all cases' and is more convenient for patients.[8]

Syringing can cause undesirable effects, including pain, minor damage to the external ear canal, and otitis externa; less commonly perforation of the tympanic membrane and vertigo (the latter generally if the water is too cold).[1]

In those few cases where syringing fails to remove the wax, common sense dictates that drops should be continued for several more days before a further attempt.[3,8]

There is limited evidence to support any type of manual removal of earwax.[2] However, many practitioners consider manual techniques to be standard practice.

Management strategy

PCF regards water (tap or sterile) or 0.9% saline as cerumenolytics of choice.

- use drops alone for at least 4 days (e.g. 3–4 drops b.d.)
- if this fails, proceed to syringing
- if this fails, use drops for 3–4 more days and syringe again
- if syringing fails on the second occasion, proceed to manual removal using curette, probe, forceps, suction or hook.

To minimize the risk of damaging the ear canal and tympanic membrane, manual removal after failed syringing is best undertaken by those with specialist training.[1,3]

Supply

Although OTC products are available, their relative effectiveness is unproven and they appear to be no better than water or 0.9% saline. Thus, none is recommended.
Some proprietary products contain potentially irritant constituents.[2]

0.9% Saline (generic)
Injection (use as ear drops) 5mL = £0.50.
Nasal drops (use as ear drops), 10mL = £1; available OTC.

1 Wright T (2015) Ear wax. *BMJ Clincial Evidence*. http://clinicalevidence.bmj.com
2 Roland PS *et al.* (2008) Clinical practice guideline: cerumen impaction. *Otolaryngology - Head and Neck Surgery*. **139 (3 Suppl 2)**: S1–S21.
3 McCarter DF *et al.* (2007) Cerumen impaction. *American Family Physician*. **75**: 1523–1528.
4 Hand C and Harvey I (2004) The effectiveness of topical preparations for the treatment of earwax: a systematic review. *British Journal of General Practice*. **54**: 862–867.
5 Chalishazar U and Williams H (2007) Back to basics: finding an optimal cerumenolytic (earwax solvent). *British Journal of Nursing*. **16**: 806–808.
6 Burton MJ and Doree CJ (2009) Ear drops for the removal of ear wax. *Cochrane Database of Systematic Reviews*. **1**: CD004326. www.thecochranelibrary.com
7 Pavlidis C and Pickering JA (2005) Water as a fast acting wax softening agent before ear syringing. *Australian Family Physician*. **34**: 303–304.
8 Eekhof JA *et al.* (2001) A quasi-randomised controlled trial of water as a quick softening agent of persistent earwax in general practice. *British Journal of General Practice*. **51**: 635–637.

Updated April 2017

12: SKIN

EMOLLIENTS

Indications: Dry or rough skin.

Introduction

Emollients soften and increase the hydration of the outermost layer of the epidermis (stratum corneum). This increases the integrity and resilience of the skin and so helps to protect the skin from irritants, allergens, and microbes.[1] Emollients also hydrate skin by preventing loss of water. Older patients are particularly likely to develop dry skin (asteotic dermatitis). Other common causes include:

- varicose (stasis) dermatitis
- drying environments
- excessive washing
- diuretics
- drug reactions
- radiotherapy.

Types of emollients

Emollients vary in greasiness depending on the amount of oil and water they contain (Table 1). Creams and ointments are most commonly used. However, other formulations may be used for specific indications. The choice of emollient depends on many factors.

Ointments are greasy because of their structure, even when their water content is high. Anhydrous ointments provide an occlusive film of oil over the surface of the skin. The water trapped under the ointment passes back into the stratum corneum which then swells up, improving skin barrier function.

Some creams contain **propylene glycol** which gives a smoother texture, and facilitates application. The properties of oily lotions are comparable to creams but, because they are more liquid, they can be applied more easily to large areas and are easier to apply to hairy skin. Both creams and oily lotions have a cooling effect on the skin (heat lost by evaporation of the water content).

Humectants are substances which attract moisture to, and retain it in, the stratum corneum, e.g. **urea**, **glycerol**, **lactic acid**, **alpha-hydroxy acids, propylene glycol** and **sodium pidolate**.[2] Adequate hydration is generally obtained with creams containing **urea** 5–10%[3,4] and, for patients with only mild–moderate dryness, this may be more cosmetically acceptable than using an ointment. **Urea** at higher concentrations of 20–30% is antipruritic, breaks down keratin, decreases the thickness of the stratum corneum, and is used in scaling conditions such as ichthyosis.[3] However, humectants may be irritating, particularly on inflamed skin, when humectant-free creams or ointments may be preferable.

Table 1 Emollient formulations

	Description	*Features*	*Potential limitations*
Ointments	Grease-based	Increased absorption	Messy Difficult to apply to hairy areas May occlude hair follicles Perspiration can be trapped under the ointment, causing discomfort from excessive body heat and moisture Avoid applying to large areas
Creams	Emulsions of water and oil; vary between greasy (water-in-oil, 'rich creams') to aqueous (oil-in-water, 'light creams')	Cosmetically acceptable Suitable for face and flexures May be used for large areas	May contain fragrances or preservatives
Lotions	Solutions, suspensions or emulsions from which water evaporates leaving a thin coating of powder or oil	Suitable for wet rashes and hairy areas Spread well Useful for soaks or wet dressings	Only emulsions containing oil have an emollient effect; other lotions are drying Often contain alcohol which will sting broken skin
Sprays	Oil in volatile silicone	Spray on, so application is quick No touching the skin No contamination from the hands	Make skin and surfaces slippery
Soap substitutes	Available as creams, lotions or ointments	Unlike soaps, no detergent properties	
Bath additives	Oil; often contain an antimicrobial or antipruritic	Widely used despite the absence of scientific evidence of benefit	Make skin and surfaces slippery; particular care needed when bathing Additives can cause contact dermatitis if used excessively

Cautions

Clothing and dressings in contact with paraffin-based emollients, e.g. **emulsifying ointment BP** or **liquid paraffin and white soft paraffin ointment NPF (liquid paraffin** in **white soft paraffin** 50/50), are easily ignited by a naked flame. The risk is increased when the products are applied to large areas of the body, and clothing or dressings become soaked with them. Patients should keep away from fire or flames, and not smoke when using these products, particularly if applying large quantities.

Undesirable effects

Proprietary emollients often contain additives and fragrances (perfumes) which are potentially allergenic (Table 2). Concern about **lanolin** is largely misplaced; many emollients contain refined ('hypo-allergic') **lanolin** which is rarely responsible for contact dermatitis.[5]

Official advice states that emollients containing **arachis** (peanut) **oil** should not be used by patients with peanut or soya allergy.[6] However, unlike *crude* **arachis oil**, the *refined* oil used in pharmaceutical products is not allergenic, and thus is highly unlikely to cause allergic reactions in people with (whole) peanut allergy.[7,8]

Aqueous cream sometimes causes burning/stinging ± erythema when used as an emollient, rather than just as a soap substitute, particularly in children with atopic dermatitis (eczema).[9] This has been linked to sodium lauryl sulfate (SLS), an ingredient of the emulsifying wax BP used to prepare **aqueous cream**, but may be caused by other sensitizing ingredients. The reaction generally occurs within 20min of applying the cream, but is rarely severe. Should it occur, another proprietary emollient which does not contain SLS or emulsifying wax BP can be substituted, e.g. Diprobase® cream (also see Table 4).[10]

12

Table 2 Potential skin allergens in topical emollient products

Allergen	*Comment*
Fragrances (perfumes)[a,3,11]	
Preservatives (particularly parabens and cresols)[a,3,11]	In many creams, lotions, and some ointments
Emulsifying agents and ointment bases (particularly sodium lauryl sulfate and cetostearyl alcohols)[a,3,11]	In many creams, lotions and ointments
Wool fat derivatives (includes lanolin)[a,3,11]	In many creams and ointments
Topical local anaesthetics	
Neomycin	
Ethyl alcohol	In some products and skin wipes
Chlorhexidine[12]	In antimicrobial products
Rubber additives (plasticizers, preservatives)	Undersheets, elastic stockings, etc.
Paraphenylenediamine, chromates	In leather
Tea tree oil[13]	

a. the BNF lists potential sensitizers which mainly fall into these categories.

Dose and use

In hairy patients prone to folliculitis, to reduce the risk of further episodes, creams and ointments should be applied using downward strokes in the direction of hair growth, particularly on the legs.[14]
Choice of emollient involves consideration of:

- patient preference
- area to be treated, e.g. ointments are generally acceptable for the legs and trunk but not the face, and ointment may be necessary for the thicker skin of the palms and soles
- ingredients; does it contain known or potential allergens?
- degree of dryness; very dry skin often requires an ointment initially
- packaging, e.g. patients with weak hands may find removing screw-top lids or squeezing tubes difficult
- patient's lifestyle

- season; ointments are less well tolerated in the summer
- cost-effectiveness; **aqueous cream BP** is the cheapest product but does not suit everyone (see above).

Emollients should be applied as frequently as needed to keep the skin well hydrated. This is generally twice daily. Very dry skin may require more frequent applications. Enough emollient should be applied to make the skin glisten.[14] However, if the emollient is applied too thickly, it may make the patient uncomfortable, hot or itchy, and may stain clothing.

The emollient should be applied immediately after a bath or shower when the skin is most hydrated. The patient should shake off excess water or lightly dab dry with a soft towel, and then apply the emollient to the damp skin. Emollients are essential for maintaining skin condition and should continue to be used at least once daily even when the dryness has improved/resolved.

It is helpful to demonstrate the use of the recommended emollient (or one of comparable consistency) to the patient and the family or carers. This is particularly useful in patients with unsightly skin who may feel ostracized, and for whom physical contact (touch) generally provides real psychological benefit.

In practice, *the best emollient is the one which a patient is happy to use*. This implies that it is both cosmetically acceptable and effective, and preferably should not be expensive. For example, many patients like the silky feel of **colloidal oatmeal** (e.g. Aveeno®), particularly on their hands and face. Average quantities required for b.d. application for 1 week are shown in Table 3.

Table 3 Quantities required for b.d. application for 1 week

	Creams and ointments (g)	*Lotions (mL)*
Face	15–30	100
Groins and genitalia	15–25	100
Both hands	25–50	200
Scalp	50–100	200
Both arms or both legs	100–200	200
Trunk	400	500

A light cream (e.g. **aqueous cream BP**, Cetraben®, Diprobase®) or emollient lotion b.d. generally suffices with mild–moderate degrees of dryness (Table 4). For severe dryness an ointment will be needed (e.g. Hydromol®, Epaderm®).

Soap should *not* be used because of its drying effect on the skin. It contributes to the breakdown of the skin barrier by raising the pH; this enhances protease activity, inhibts lipid synthesis, and promotes bacterial colonization. Use instead a soap substitute (e.g. **aqueous cream BP**, **emulsifying ointment BP**, Cetraben® cream, Dermol® cream or lotion) or a proprietary soap-free cleanser (e.g. E45® Emollient Wash Cream or Oilatum® Shower Gel). Also see Table 4.

An emollient bath additive, such as Dermalo® or E45® Emollient Bath Oil, can also be used when bathing. It is advisable to use a bath mat to prevent slipping when using such products in the bath or shower.

If emollient-related contact dermatitis is suspected, patch testing with the standard set of potential allergens may identify an allergen. If allergy is confirmed, a product which does not contain the allergen (and, ideally, any other added preservatives or fragrances) should be prescribed. However, not all contact dermatitis is allergic; sometimes it is caused by direct chemical irritation.

When there is an active inflammatory skin condition causing redness and eroded or scaly skin, apply a topical corticosteroid b.d. to the affected area for 3–7 days or until the inflammation settles. Apply the corticosteroid 30–60min before or after any emollient has been applied. In practice, topical corticosteroids are prescribed mostly for dermatoses of the face and hands. Mild topical corticosteroids, e.g. **hydrocortisone** 1%, are generally used for the face. For the trunk, hands, feet or limbs, choose a moderately potent topical corticosteroid, e.g. **clobetasone butyrate** 0.05% or **betamethasone valerate** 0.025% ointment.

If the inflamed skin is deeply cracked and secondary infection is suspected, a topical corticosteroid + a topical antifungal and/or antibacterial should be prescribed; various combination products are available. *To minimize the risk of developing resistance, products containing antimicrobials must not be used p.r.n. but as a full course for 7 days.*

Lymphoedema

Skin care is just one component of multimodal lymphoedema management.[15,16] The following advice must be applied within the broader management context.

The choice depends on the state of the skin but also on current fashion and local contracts:[17]

- if not obviously dry and flaky, a light cream, can be applied once daily–b.d. as a prophylactic measure, e.g. **aqueous cream BP** or an alternative (see Table 4)
- if the skin is dry ± cracked, apply **liquid and white soft paraffin ointment NPF** (**liquid paraffin** in **white soft paraffin** 50/50)
- if there is a build-up of scales wash the affected area with a light cream (see Table 4) using a circular motion in order to soften and lift off the scales; then apply **liquid and white soft paraffin ointment NPF**, and cover with a hydrocolloid dressing (e.g. Granuflex®) and bandage; repeat every 1–3 days until the skin condition is good
- if there are toe web fissures, take scrapings to look for fungus and, if present, treat appropriately, e.g. **clotrimazole** 1% or **terbinafine** 1% cream b.d. for 2 weeks.

Note:

- ointments are generally needed for only 1–2 weeks
- some people prefer coconut oil because it has a skin-cooling effect.

Antipruritic emollients

If pruritus is caused by dry skin, rehydration of the skin will correct it. Thus, all emollients are antipruritic in this sense. However, some products have a specific antipruritic agent added, and can provide extra benefit in some patients (see p.635).

Supply

This is not a complete list; see BNF for additional options.

Pharmaco-economics

Before prescribing a relatively expensive proprietary product, check to see whether, content for content, there is a cheaper essentially equivalent product.

Mild topical corticosteroid
Hydrocortisone (generic)
Cream 1%, 15g = £1, 30g = £1.75, 50g = £3.
Ointment 1%, 15g = £1, 30g = £2, 50g = £3.25.

Moderately potent topical corticosteroids
Betamethasone valerate
Betnovate-RD® (GSK)
Cream 0.025%, 100g = £3.25; *this is 1/4 of the strength of Betnovate® cream. Excipients include cetostearyl alcohol, chlorocresol.*
Ointment 0.025%, 100g = £3.25; *this is 1/4 of the strength of Betnovate® ointment.*

Clobetasone butyrate
Eumovate® (GSK)
Cream 0.05%, 30g = £2, 100g = £5.50. *Excipients include beeswax substitute, cetostearyl alcohol, chlorocresol.*
Ointment 0.05%, 30g = £2, 100g = £5.50.

Antifungal creams
Clotrimazole (generic)
Cream 1%, 20g = £1.25.

Terbinafine (generic)
Cream 1%, 15g = £1.50, 30g = £3.

For more antifungal products, see Barrier products, p.638 and the *BNF*.

Table 4 Emollient and additive content of selected topical products[a]

	Emollient base	*Additional ingredients*	*Sensitizing excipients*[b]	*Supply*
Ointments				
Emulsifying ointment BP[c]	White soft paraffin 50% Emulsifying wax 30% Liquid paraffin 20%		Cetostearyl alcohol Sodium lauryl sulfate	500g = £3
White *or* Yellow soft paraffin BP	Petroleum jelly (white or yellow)			500g = £3.50
Liquid paraffin and white soft paraffin ointment NPF	Liquid paraffin 50% White soft paraffin 50%			500g = £4.50
Hydromol®	Liquid paraffin 40% Emulsifying wax 30% Yellow soft paraffin 30%		Cetostearyl alcohol Sodium lauryl sulfate	125g = £3, 500g = £5, 1kg = £9
Oils				
Coconut oil BP	Coconut oil			OTC
Water-in-oil (rich) creams				
Hydrous ointment BP	Wool alcohols ointment 50%	Magnesium sulfate 0.5% Phenoxyethanol 1%		500g = £5
Aquadrate®	White soft paraffin	Urea 10%		100g = £4.50
Lipobase®	Light liquid paraffin White soft paraffin		Cetostearyl alcohol Hydroxybenzoates (parabens)	50g = £1.50
Unguentum M®	Saturated neutral oil Liquid paraffin White soft paraffin		Cetostearyl alcohol Polysorbate 40 Propylene glycol Sorbic acid	50g = £1.50, 100g = £2.75, 200g = £5.50, 500g = £8.50
Oil-in-water (light) creams				
Aqueous cream BP[c]	Emulsifying ointment 30%	Phenoxyethanol[d] 1%	Cetostearyl alcohol Sodium Lauryl Sulfate	100g = £1, 500g = £4.50
Aveeno® cream	Emollient basis	Colloidal oatmeal	Benzyl alcohol Cetyl alcohol Isopropyl palmitate	ACBS, 100mL = £4, 300mL = £7, 500mL = £7

continued

Table 4 Continued

	Emollient base	*Additional ingredients*	*Sensitizing excipients*[b]	*Supply*
Cetraben®,[c]	White soft paraffin 13.2% Light liquid paraffin 10.5%		Cetostearyl alcohol Hydroxybenzoates (parabens)	50g = £1.50, 150g = £4, 500g = £6, 1kg = £12
Dermol®,[c] cream	Liquid paraffin 10% Isopropyl myristate 10%	Benzalkonium chloride 0.1% Chlorhexidine hydrochloride 0.1%	Cetostearyl alcohol	100g = £3, 550g = £6.50
Diprobase® cream	White soft paraffin 15% Liquid paraffin 6% Cetomacrogol 2.25%		Cetostearyl alcohol Chlorocresol	50g = £1.25, 500g = £6.50
E45® cream	White soft paraffin 14.5% Liquid paraffin 12.6% Lanolin[e] 1%		Cetyl alcohol Hydroxybenzoates (parabens)	50g = £1.50, 125g = £3, 350g = £5, 500g = £5.50
E45® Itch relief	Lauromacrogols 3% Liquid paraffin Octyldodecano Cetyl palmitate Dimeticone	Glycerol 85% Urea 5%	Benzyl alcohol Polysorbates	50g = £2.75, 100g = £3.75, 500g = £15
Hydromol® cream	Liquid paraffin 13.8%	Sodium pidolate 2.5%	Cetostearyl alcohol Hydroxybenzoates (parabens)	50g = £2.25, 100g = £4, 500g = £12
Zerobase®	Liquid paraffin 11%		Cetostearyl alcohol Chlorocresol	50g = £1, 500g = £5.50
Lotions				
Aveeno® lotion	Emollient basis	Colloidal oatmeal	Benzyl alcohol, Cetyl alcohol, Isopropyl palmitate	ACBS 500mL = £7
Dermol® 500 lotion	Liquid paraffin 2.5% Isopropyl myristate 2.5%	Benzalkonium chloride 0.1% Chlorhexidine hydrochloride 0.1%	Cetostearyl alcohol	500mL = £6
E45® lotion	White soft paraffin 10% Light liquid paraffin 4% Lanolin[e] 1% Cetomacrogol Glyceryl monostearate		Isopropyl palmitate Hydroxybenzoates (parabens) Benzyl alcohol	200mL = £2.50, 500mL = £4.50

continued

Table 4 Continued

	Emollient base	*Additional ingredients*	*Sensitizing excipients*[b]	*Supply*
Bath/shower preparations				
Dermalo® bath oil	Liquid paraffin 65% Acetylated wool alcohols 5%			500mL = £3.50
Dermol 200 shower emollient *or* Dermol Wash cutaneous emulsion	Liquid paraffin 2.5% Isopropyl myristate 2.5%	Benzalkonium chloride 0.1% Chlorhexidine hydrochloride 0.1%	Cetostearyl alcohol	200mL = £3.50
E45 emollient wash cream	Liquid paraffin White soft paraffin Ceresin wax Carauba wax	Zinc oxide Dimeticone	Cetostearyl alcohol, polysorbates	ACBS 250mL = £3.50
E45 bath oil	Liquid paraffin	Dimeticone	Cetostearyl alcohol, polysorbates	ACBS 250mL = £3.50, 500mL = £5.50,
Hydromol® bath/shower	Light liquid paraffin 37.8% Isopropyl myristate 13%			350mL = £3.75, 500mL = £4.50, 1L = £9
Oilatum® shower gel (fragrance free)	Light liquid paraffin 70%			150g = £5.50

a. list is not exhaustive; see BNF for alternative products
b. excipients which are associated, rarely, with sensitization
c. can be used as a soap substitute
d. or other antimicrobial
e. hypoallergenic anhydrous wool fat (hypoallergenic lanolin).

1 Cork MJ and Danby S (2009) Skin barrier breakdown: a renaissance in emollient therapy. *British Journal of Nursing*. **18**: 872, 874, 876–877.
2 Kraft JN and Lynde CW (2005) Moisturizers: what they are and a practical approach to product selection. *Skin Therapy Letter*. **10**: 1–8.
3 Sibbald D (2002) Dermatitis. In: C Repchinsky (ed) *Patient Self-care (2e)*. Canadian Pharmacists Association, Ottawa, pp. 479–505.
4 Fluhr JW *et al.* (2008) Emollients, moisturizers, and keratolytic agents in psoriasis. *Clinics in Dermatology*. **26**: 380–386.
5 Hoppe U (ed) (1999) The Lanolin Book. Beierdorf AG, Hamburg.
6 MHRA (2003) Medicines containing peanut (arachis) oil. *Current Problems in Pharmacovigilance*. **29**: 5.
7 Hourihane JO *et al.* (1997) Randomised, double blind, crossover challenge study of allergenicity of peanut oils in subjects allergic to peanuts. *British Medical Journal*. **314**: 1084–1088.
8 Keating MU *et al.* (1990) Immunoassay of peanut allergens in food-processing materials and finished foods. *Journal of Allergy and Clinical Immunology*. **86**: 41–44.
9 Cork MJ *et al.* (2003) An audit of adverse drug reactions to aqueous cream in children with atopic eczema. *The Pharmaceutical Journal*. **271**: 747–748.
10 MHRA (2013) Aqueous cream: may cause skin irritation, particularly in children with eczema, possibly due to sodium lauryl sulphate content. *Drug Safety Update*. **6**: www.gov.uk/drug-safety-update
11 Voegeli D (2008) Care or harm: exploring essential components in skin care regimens. *British Journal of Nursing*. **17**: 24–30.
12 MHRA (2012) All medical devices and medicinal products containing chlorhexidine. Risk of anaphylactic reaction due to chlorhexidine allergy. *Medical Devices Alert*. MDA/2012/2075 www.gov.uk/drug-device-alerts
13 Rubel DM *et al.* (1998) Tea tree oil allergy: what is the offending agent? Report of three cases of tea tree oil allergy and review of the literature. *Australasian Journal of Dermatology*. **39**: 244–247.
14 Lawton S (2009) Practical issues for emollient therapy in dry and itchy skin. *British Journal of Nursing*. **18**: 978–984.
15 Twycross R and Wilcock A (eds) (2016) *Introducing Palliative Care* (5e). palliativedrugs.com Ltd, Nottingham, pp. 131–135.
16 Twycross R *et al.* (2000) *Lymphoedema*. Radcliffe Medical Press, Oxford.
17 Linnitt N (2000) Skin management in lymphoedema. In: RG Twycross *et al.* (eds) *Lymphoedema*. Radcliffe Medical Press, Oxford, pp. 118–129.

Updated September 2017

12

TOPICAL ANTIPRURITICS

Indications: Pruritus which fails to respond to an emollient and/or specific treatment.

Background

Pruritus may be caused by systemic disease (such as drug hypersensitivity, obstructive jaundice, endocrine disease, malignant disease), skin disease (e.g. eczema, urticaria, psoriasis, scabies) or drugs (e.g. opioids).

Dryness of the skin (xerosis) is the commonest cause of pruritus without an accompanying rash, and an emollient is the first-line treatment (see p.627). Dryness is associated with normal ageing, inflammatory skin conditions (e.g. atopic dermatitis), systemic disease (e.g. hypothyroidism, renal failure), and cachexia and general debility in advanced cancer.

Whenever possible, the treatment of pruritus should be cause-specific.[1,2] For example, in skin disorders:

- scabies → treat patient and the whole family with topical **permethrin** (preferred) or **malathion**[3,4]
- atopic dermatitis → topical corticosteroid (+ emollient)[5]
- contact dermatitis → topical corticosteroid, identify causal substance and avoid further contact.

In systemic disorders or when caused by opioids, a range of options exist (see Chapter 26, p.757). A topical antipruritic should be considered only if a bland emollient and cause-specific treatment fail to relieve.

Although topical products are not convenient to apply regularly to the whole body, many patients with generalized pruritus have patches of more intense discomfort, and may benefit from more limited application.

Pharmacology

Traditional topical antipruritics include **phenol**, **levomenthol** (**menthol**) and **camphor**. **Phenol** 0.5–3% acts by anaesthetizing cutaneous nerve endings. **Levomenthol** 0.5–2% and **camphor** 0.5–3% may relieve pruritus by cooling the skin by acting on heat-sensitive transient receptor potential (TRP) channels expressed on sensory nerve endings.[6,7] Cooling the skin is known to reduce the intensity of histamine-induced pruritus, and patients who suffer from chronic pruritic conditions such as atopic dermatitis, psoriasis and uraemic pruritus often find that cold showers reduce the pruritus.

Capsaicin is a naturally occurring alkaloid found in the fruits of various species of *Solanaceae* (the nightshade family) and in pepper plants of the genus *Capsicum* (chilli peppers).[8] It acts by depleting substance P at sensory nerve endings. **Capsaicin** products are useful in relieving neuropathic pain (see p.601). Benefit has also been reported in histamine-related pruritus, aquagenic pruritus, and pruritus associated with uraemia, nodular prurigo, psoriasis and post-axillary dissection syndrome.[6]

A Cochrane review of pruritus in adult palliative care patients also found benefit in uraemic pruritus, but the methodological quality of the studies was low, introducing a risk of bias and thus preventing meaningful interpretation of the results.[9] **Capsaicin** has also been used successfully in the treatment of intractable pruritus ani.[10]

In practice, **capsaicin** will be applied to relatively limited areas of the skin. It often initially causes localized burning and stinging. This irritation subsides with repeated use but patients may have difficulty continuing treatment. Patients should initially use **capsaicin** cream t.d.s.–q.d.s. (leaving at least 4h between applications; the manufacturers specify q.d.s. for the 0.025% cream) to overcome the irritation, after which the frequency of applications can be reduced. The topical anaesthetic **EMLA** (**eutectic mixture of local anaesthetics, lidocaine** 2.5% and **prilocaine** 2.5%), used in conjunction with **capsaicin**, may reduce the initial irritation.[11] Excessive use of **EMLA** may result in acute transient systemic local anaesthetic neurotoxicity.[12]

Polidocanol (**macrogol lauryl ether**) is an anionic detergent with local anaesthetic properties.[13] Benefit has been reported in patients with pruritus associated with atopic dermatitis, non-atopic dermatitis and psoriasis, with the regular application of a cream containing 5% **urea** and 3% **polidocanol** (E45® Itch Relief Cream).[14,15] Benefit has also been reported in patients with pruritus associated with chronic renal failure who regularly used a **polidocanol**-containing bath oil (Balneum Plus®).[16]

Crotamiton 10% lotion (Eurax®) has a mild antiscabetic effect which is probably the reason for its reputation as an antipruritic. However, in an RCT in patients with chronic pruritic dermatoses, **crotamiton** lotion was no more effective than its vehicle.[17]

Topical H_1 antihistamines, e.g. **diphenhydramine**, are of benefit only when the pruritus is cutaneous in origin and related to histamine release.[1] Topical **diphenhydramine** can cause contact dermatitis and photosensitivity; if used, limit to 3 days. Oral sedating H_1 antihistamines, e.g. **alimemazine**, **chlorphenamine**, **hydroxyzine** may be helpful if sedation is desirable in intractable pruritus, e.g. if itch is disturbing sleep (see Chapter 26, p.757).

A **coal tar**-based shampoo, e.g. Polytar®, has a long tradition of use with scalp pruritus.

Calamine lotion has traditionally been used for pruritus, and generally also contains **phenol** 0.5%. However, proprietary formulations are very drying and, because it is unsightly, **calamine** is unlikely to be acceptable except on a short-term basis, e.g. in acute contact dermatitis.

Doxepin

Doxepin is a TCA which is a potent H_1- and H_2-receptor antagonist. Its affinity for H_2-receptors is 6 times that of **cimetidine**.[18] It is also antimuscarinic, and may antagonize the pruritic effects of substance P at skin receptors.

Doxepin 5% cream is reported to be of benefit in some patients with atopic dermatitis[18–20] but long-term independent studies are lacking.[21] It is not generally suitable for children. It is possible that the benefit is systemic rather than topical. About 15% of patients complain initially of localized stinging or burning, and a similar proportion complain of drowsiness, secondary to systemic absorption.[19] The sedation may help the antipruritic effect.

Doxepin cream is less effective than systemic treatment[22] (see Chapter 26, p.757) and allergic contact dermatitis may occur.[19] However, PO capsules are expensive (see Supply). Patients with contact allergy should not take the drug by mouth.[23]

Cautions

Because of:

- the risk of contact dermatitis, *discourage* the use of topical H_1 antihistamines and of local anaesthetics
- their drying effect, *discourage* the use of products containing **calamine** unless they contain oil (e.g. **calamine oily lotion BP**).

Calamine oily lotion BP (only available as a special order product) contains *refined* **arachis** (peanut) **oil**, and official advice states that emollients containing **arachis** (peanut) **oil** should not be used by patients with peanut or soya allergy.[24,25] However, unlike *crude* **arachis oil**, the *refined* oil is not allergenic, and is highly unlikely to cause allergic reactions in people with (whole) peanut allergy.[26,27]

Polytar® products also contain traces of **arachis** (peanut) **oil** from the **coal tar** extraction process, and thus might cause allergic reactions in people with peanut or soya allergy.

Patients prescribed **doxepin**, either systemically or topically, should avoid the concurrent use of drugs which inhibit cytochrome P450, e.g. **cimetidine**, imidazole antifungals and macrolide antibacterials (see Chapter 19, Table 8, p.725). As with other TCAs, MAOIs should be discontinued ≥2 weeks before starting treatment with **doxepin**. Monitor carefully in patients with glaucoma, severe heart disease, cardiac arrhythmias, urinary hesitancy, severe liver disease or a history of mania. Because of the possibility of undesirable systemic effects, e.g. dizziness, antimuscarinic effects, headache, GI disturbances, avoid applying the cream to large areas of skin. The manufacturer recommends a maximum of 3g per application, covering no more than 10% of the body area.

Use

Because pruritus is commonly associated with dry skin, an emollient (moisturizer) should be tried first (see p.627). A light cream (oil-in-water), e.g. Cetraben®, Diprobase®, or an emollient lotion often suffices with mild–moderate degrees of dryness. **Aqueous cream BP** is an option but at many centres is used only as a soap substitute. Products containing **colloidal oatmeal** (Aveeno®) are popular because of their silky feel (see p.631). Storing creams and lotions in a refrigerator may increase benefit.

Levomenthol 0.5–5% is available as a proprietary product authorized for pruritus, e.g. Dermacool®. When unavailable or unsuitable, **levomenthol** 0.5%–2% (or **camphor** 0.5–3%) in a bland emollient base can be obtained as a special order (see Chapter 24, p.751) and applied topically t.d.s.–q.d.s.

12

Supply

Several OTC products contain **levomenthol** and **camphor** (with contents as high as 11%). These are marketed for rheumatic aches and pains, sprains or minor sports injuries, e.g. Tiger Balm Red®. Others are mainly intended for use on insect bites and the unit size is small.

Levomenthol

Dermacool® (Pern Consumer Products)
Cream 0.5%, 1%, 2%, 5%, 100g tube = £4.40, 500g pump pack = £17.

Polidocanol (macrogol lauryl ether)

Balneum Plus® (Almirall)
Bath oil containing **soya oil** 83%, mixed **lauromacrogols** 15%, 500mL = £7.

E45 Itch Relief® (Crookes)
Cream (oil-in-water) containing **urea** 5%, **macrogol lauryl ether** 3%, 100g = £3.75; 500g pump-pack = £15.

Doxepin

Doxepin (generic)
Capsules 25mg, 50mg, 28 days @ 25mg, 50mg, 75mg at bedtime = £97, £154 and £251 respectively.

Xepin® (CHS)
Cream 5%, 30g = £12.

Also see Rubefacients and other topical products for **capsaicin.**

1 Zylicz Z *et al.* (2004). *Pruritus in Advanced Disease.* Oxford University Press, Oxford.
2 Twycross R and Wilcock A (eds) (2016) *Introducing Palliative Care* (5e). palliativedrugs.com Ltd., Nottingham, pp. 228–232.
3 British National Formulary 13.2. Parasiticidal preparations. London: BMJ Group and Pharmaceutical Press. www.medicinescomplete.com (accessed June 2017).
4 Strong M and Johnstone P (2007) Interventions for treating scabies. *Cochrane Database of Systematic Reviews.* **3**: CD000320. www.thecochranelibrary.com

5 Cork MJ (1999) Taking the itch out of eczema: how careful use of emollients can break the itch-scratch cycle of atopic eczema. *Asthma Journal*. **4**: 16–20.
6 Patel T *et al.* (2007) Menthol: a refreshing look at this ancient compound. *Journal of the American Academy of Dermatology*. **57**: 873–878.
7 Peier AM *et al.* (2002) A TRP channel that senses cold stimuli and menthol. *Cell*. **108**: 705–715.
8 Towlerton GR and Rice AS (2003) Topical analgesics for chronic pain. In: AS Rice *et al.* (eds) *Clinical Pain Management: Chronic Pain*. Arnold, London, pp. 213–226.
9 Xander C et *al.* (2013) Pharmacological interventions for pruritus in adult palliative care patients. *Cochrane Database of Systematic Reviews*. **6**: CD008320. www.thecochranelibrary.com
10 Lysy J et *al.* (2003) Topical capsaicin--a novel and effective treatment for idiopathic intractable pruritus ani: a randomised, placebo controlled, crossover study. *Gut*. **52**: 1323–1326.
11 Yosipovitch G and Hundley JL (2004) Practical guidelines for relief of itch. *Dermatology Nursing*. **16**: 325-328; quiz 329.
12 Brosh-Nissimov T *et al.* (2004) Central nervous system toxicity following topical skin application of lidocaine. *European Journal of Clinical Pharmacology*. **60**: 683–684.
13 Vieluf D *et al.* (1992) Dry and itching skin - therapy with a new preparation, containing urea and polidocanol. *Zeitschrift fur Hautkrankheiten*. **67**: 816–821.
14 Hauss H *et al.* (1993) Comparative study of a formulation containing urea and polidocanol and a greasy cream containing linoleic acid in the treatment of dry, pruritic skin lesions [in German]. *Dermatosen in Beruf und Umwelt Occupational and Environmental Dermatoses*. **41**: 184–188.
15 Freitag G and Hoppner T (1997) Results of a postmarketing drug monitoring survey with a polidocanol-urea preparation for dry, itching skin. *Current Medical Research and Opinion*. **13**: 529–537.
16 Wasik F *et al.* (1996) Relief of uraemic pruritus after balneological therapy with a bath oil containing polidocanol (Balneum Hermal Plus). An open clinical study. *Journal of Dermatological Treatment*. **7**: 231–233.
17 Smith E *et al.* (1984) Crotamiton lotion in pruritus. *International Journal of Dermatology*. **23**: 684–685.
18 Drake L *et al.* (1994) Relief of pruritus in patients with atopic dermatitis after treatment with topical doxepin cream. The Doxepin Study Group. *Journal of the American Academy of Dermatology*. **31**: 613–616.
19 DTB (2000) Doxepin cream for eczema? *Drug and Therapeutics Bulletin*. **38**: 31.
20 Breneman D *et al.* (1997) Doxepin cream relieves eczema-associated pruritus within 15 minutes and is not accompanied by a risk of rebound upon discontinuation. *Journal of Dermatological Treatment*. **8**: 161–168.
21 Hoare C *et al.* (2000) Systematic review of treatments for atopic eczema. *Health Technology Assessment*. **4**: 1–191.
22 Smith P and Corelli R (1997) Doxepin in the management of pruritus associated with allergic cutaneous reactions. *Annals of Pharmacotherapy*. **31**: 633–635.
23 Bonnel RA *et al.* (2003) Allergic contact dermatitis from topical doxepin: Food and Drug Administration's postmarketing surveillance experience. *Journal of the American Academy of Dermatology*. **48**: 294–296.
24 MHRA (2003) Medicines containing peanut (arachis) oil. *Current Problems in Pharmacovigilance*. **29**: 5.
25 Anonymous (2003) Peanut allergy research is published. *Pharmaceutical Journal*. **270**: 391.
26 Keating MU *et al.* (1990) Immunoassay of peanut allergens in food-processing materials and finished foods. *Journal of Allergy and Clinical Immunology*. **86**: 41–44.
27 Hourihane JO *et al.* (1997) Randomised, double blind, crossover challenge study of allergenicity of peanut oils in subjects allergic to peanuts. *British Medical Journal*. **314**: 1084–1088.

Updated September 2017

BARRIER PRODUCTS

Indications: Skin protection, napkin rash.

Introduction

Barrier products contain water-repellent substances which help to protect the skin, and prevent maceration and infection. They can be used around stomas and in the perineal and peri-anal areas in patients with urinary or faecal incontinence as long as the skin is intact. Once skin damage is present, typical barrier preparations generally have a limited role. However, a barrier product such as Cavilon No-Sting Barrier Film® coats damaged skin with a protective film for ≤72h and thereby protects it from urine, faeces and other body fluids, and reduces friction and adhesive trauma from dressings.

A cream is less greasy than an ointment and is easier to apply and wash off. Most barrier creams and ointments are **silicone-**, **titanium-** or **zinc oxide**-based.[1] Some products contain *refined* **arachis** (peanut) **oil**. However, unlike *crude* **arachis oil**, the *refined* oil is not allergenic, and thus is highly unlikely to cause allergic reactions in people with (whole) peanut allergy.[2,3]

Cautions

If the damaged skin is infected, because barrier products prevent topical antimicrobials from penetrating the skin, delay their use until the infection has been treated.

Use

Ensure that infection is treated promptly with topical antifungals (more common) and/or antibacterials (less common).

Intertrigo

Intertrigo is an inflammatory dermatosis of skin folds primarily caused by skin on skin friction. Exacerbating factors cause skin maceration and inflammation, e.g. obesity, lack of air, heat and moisture. Secondary fungal or bacterial infection is common. The wet component is the most easily modified, and drying the involved skin is essential. Initial treatment may comprise:

- cleanse with a soap substitute (e.g. Cetraben®) or a proprietary soap-free cleanser (e.g. Dermol® Shower Emollient or Wash Emulsion, E45® Emollient Wash Cream or Oilatum® Shower Gel; see Emollients, Table 4, p.631)
- dry well; blow-drying with a hand-held hair dryer can be used if necessary
- avoid tight clothing and non-breathable fabrics; change dressings and incontinence pads before they become saturated
- if infection is likely and because fungal infection is more common, a topical broad-spectrum antifungal should be prescribed, e.g. **clotrimazole**
- if inflammation or pruritus are problematic, add a mild topical corticosteroid for 7–14 days, e.g. **hydrocortisone** 1% cream (see p.627); combination products containing both an antifungal and **hydrocortisone** 1% are available
- when infection is widespread, the patient is immunocompromised, or topical treatment ineffective, give PO antifungal treatment, e.g. **fluconazole** 50mg PO once daily for 14 days
- when the wetness and infection has settled, then begin to use a barrier product.

Protection around a stoma

Many products designed to protect the skin around a stoma from liquid effluent are available; a stoma-care nurse can advise on product selection. Sprays or wipes which dry to form a protective film are commonly used. An alcohol-free formulation is preferable because it is less likely to sting or irritate the skin.

Stoma therapists frequently use Comfeel® barrier cream prophylactically if the stoma effluent is liquid or if the stoma bag is being changed more than once daily. It is gently rubbed in and any excess wiped off. If the skin becomes red and sore, Cavilon No-Sting Barrier Film® is used instead.

A topical corticosteroid can be used short-term to treat moderate–severe inflammation. Foam products are well tolerated, e.g. Bettamousse® (off-label use). Topical application of **beclomethasone** dry powder inhaler has been reported successfully (also off-label use), without compromising the adhesion of the stoma bag, which can occur with creams and lotions.[4]

Incontinence

After cleansing with a soap substitute and gently drying, apply a barrier product to the affected area whenever the dressing or padding is changed.[1] Avoid excessive amounts of cream that could coat the pad and thereby interfere with its ability to absorb fluids.

Painful malignant wounds

An unauthorized topical product, containing **lidocaine** 2% in Lutrol gel, has been used up to b.d. with dressing changes for patients with pain from malignant wounds, especially in areas where dressings are difficult to apply and keep in place or are exposed to body fluids such as urine.[5,6] Benefit is from the barrier properties of the Lutrol gel in addition to the **lidocaine** (also see **lidocaine** medicated plasters, p.71). A fact sheet with further information can be obtained from the Document library of palliativedrugs.com.

For the use of topical **morphine** in wounds, see p.375.

Supply

The following is only a selection of the available products.

Cavilon Durable Barrier Cream® (3M)
Cream 2g sachet, 20 = £7.50, 28g tube = £4, 92g tube = £8.

Cavilon No-Sting Barrier Film® (3M)
Foam applicator 5 × 1mL = £5; 5 × 3mL = £8.
Pump spray 28mL = £6.

Comfeel® barrier cream (Coloplast)
Cream 60g = £5.

Conotrane® (Leo)
Cream containing **dimeticone 350** 22% and **benzalkonium chloride** 0.1%, 100g = £1, 500g = £3.50.

Zinc and castor oil (generic)
Ointment containing **zinc oxide** 7.5% in a **castor oil**, **arachis** (peanut) **oil**, **white beeswax** and **cetostearyl alcohol** base, 100g = £1.50, 500g = £5.50.

Lidocaine
Topical gel **lidocaine** 2% in Lutrol gel, 5mL = £16 (unauthorized product, available as a special order from St Thomas Pharmacy Manufacturing Unit, London 0207 188 4992); *there is a lead-time of several days from order.*

Antifungal products
Clotrimazole (generic)
Cream 1%, 20g = £1.25.

Canesten® (Bayer Consumer Care)
Solution 1%, 20mL = £2.50.
Spray 1%, 40mL = £5; *contains isopropyl alcohol.*

Miconazole (generic)
Daktarin® (Janssen-Cilag)
Cream 2%, 15g or 30g = £2.
Powder spray (Daktarin Aktiv®) 0.16%, 100g = £3.

Topical corticosteroids
For **hydrocortisone** 1%, see p.627.

Bettamousse® (Focus)
Foam (scalp application) containing **betamethasone valerate** 0.12%, 100g = £10.

Combined antifungal and topical corticosteroid products
Canestan HC® (Bayer Consumer Care)
Cream containing **clotrimazole** 1% and **hydrocortisone** 1%, 30g = £2.50.

Daktacort® (Janssen-Cilag)
Cream containing **miconazole** 2% and **hydrocortisone** 1%, 30g = £2.50.

1 Nazarko L (2007) Managing a common dermatological problem: incontinence dermatitis. *British Journal of Community Nursing*. **12**: 358–363.
2 Hourihane JO *et al.* (1997) Randomised, double blind, crossover challenge study of allergenicity of peanut oils in subjects allergic to peanuts. *British Medical Journal*. **314**: 1084–1088.
3 Keating MU *et al.* (1990) Immunoassay of peanut allergens in food-processing materials and finished foods. *Journal of Allergy and Clinical Immunology*. **86**: 41–44.
4 Boland J and Brooks D (2012) Topical application of a beclometasone steroid inhaler for treatment of stoma inflammation. *Palliative Medicine*. **26**: 1055–1056.
5 MacGregor K *et al.* (1994) Symptomatic relief of excoriating skin conditions using a topical thermoreversible gel. *Palliative Medicine*. **8**: 76–77.
6 Beynon T *et al.* (2003) Lutrol gel: a potential role in wounds? *Journal of Pain and Symptom Management*. **26**: 776–780.

Updated September 2017

13: ANAESTHESIA

*KETAMINE

The use of ketamine is associated with neuropsychiatric, urinary tract and hepatobiliary toxicity. Although most reports involve long-term recreational abusers, it has also arisen after only 1–2 weeks of therapeutic use (Box A). Accordingly, the use of ketamine should be restricted to specialists in pain or palliative care for patients who have failed to obtain relief from standard drug and non-drug treatments.

Class: General anaesthetic.

Indications: Induction and maintenance of anaesthesia; †neuropathic, inflammatory, ischaemic limb and procedure-related pain unresponsive to standard treatments.[1,2]

13

Contra-indications: Any situation in which an increase in blood pressure would constitute a hazard.

Pharmacology

Ketamine, a derivative of phencyclidine (PCP), is a dissociative anaesthetic which has analgesic properties in sub-anaesthetic doses.[2,3] Ketamine is the most potent NMDA-receptor-channel blocker available for clinical use, binding to the PCP site when the channels are in the open activated state (Figure 1).[3] It also binds to a second membrane-associated site which decreases the frequency of channel opening.[3]

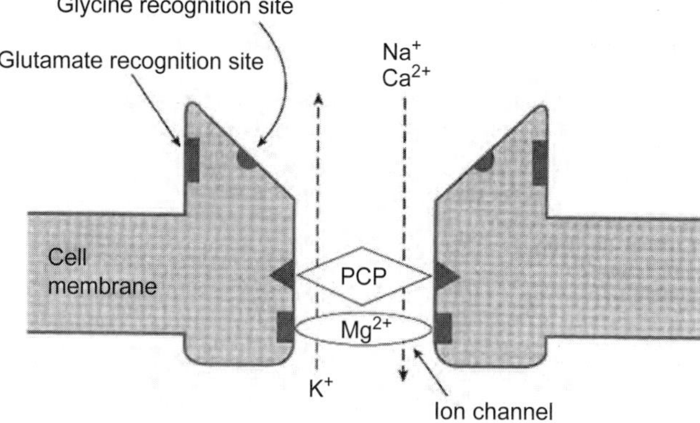

Figure 1 Diagram of the NMDA (excitatory) receptor-channel complex. The channel is blocked by magnesium (Mg^{2+}) when the membrane potential is at resting level (*voltage-dependent block*) and by drugs which act at the phencyclidine (PCP) binding site in the glutamate-activated channel, e.g. dextromethorphan, ketamine, methadone (*use-dependent block*).[4]

The NMDA receptor-channel complex is composed of four subunits, generally two GluN1 in combination with two GluN2 (rarely GluN3) subunits, with binding of agonists (e.g. glutamate and glycine or serine) to all four units necessary for activation. There are several forms of the GluN2 (i.e. A–D) and GluN3 (i.e. A–B) subunits. This variation influences localization to synaptic or extrasynaptic sites and may partly explain the differences in clinical effects between NMDA receptor-channel blocking drugs, e.g. ketamine and **memantine**.[5] Drugs are in development with greater selectivity for the various types of subunit.

The NMDA receptor-channel complex is closely involved in the development of central sensitization of dorsal horn neurons which transmit pain signals.[4] At normal resting membrane potentials, the channel is blocked by magnesium and is inactive.[3] When the resting membrane potential is changed as a result of prolonged excitation, the channel unblocks and calcium moves into the cell. This leads to neuronal hyperexcitability and results in hyperalgesia and allodynia, and a reduction in opioid-responsiveness. These effects are probably mediated by the intracellular formation of nitric oxide and cyclic guanosine monophosphate.[3]

The reduction in opioid-responsiveness arises from cross-talk between opioid receptors and the NMDA receptor-channel. Opioid receptor activation results in phosphorylation and opening of the NMDA receptor-channel leading to a cascade of events which ultimately down-regulates the opioid receptor and its effects, thereby contributing towards tolerance and hyperalgesia.[3]

In addition to blocking the NMDA receptor-channel, ketamine has other actions, some of which may contribute to its analgesic effect.[2] These include opioid-like and anti-inflammatory effects,[6] and interactions with, e.g.:

- other calcium, potassium and sodium channels, e.g. hyperpolarisation-activated cyclic nucleotide, AMPA
- cholinergic, dopaminergic and noradrenergic transmission
- descending inhibitory pathways.

Resultant changes in cellular processes, e.g. in gene expression and protein regulation, could explain ongoing benefit even after discontinuation of ketamine.[7]

Ketamine is generally administered PO or SC/CSCI.[8,9] It can also be administered IM, IV, SL, intranasally, PR and spinally (preservative-free formulation, not UK).[10–17] However, for spinal routes, concerns have been raised about the potential for neurotoxicity.[18] Ketamine has been given by CIVI in adults and children in combination with opioids (**fentanyl, morphine**) ± **midazolam** to control intractable pain and agitation.[19–21]

Although in some countries both racemic ketamine and the *S*-enantiomer are available for clinical use, in the UK only the racemic mixture is marketed. However, it is possible to import the preservative-free *S*-enantiomer (see Supply). Because of its greater affinity and selectivity for the NMDA-receptor, the *S*-enantiomer as a parenteral analgesic is about 4 times more potent than the *R*-enantiomer, and twice as potent as the racemic mixture.[22–24] When equi-analgesic doses are compared, the *S*-enantiomer is also associated with lower levels of undesirable effects, e.g. anxiety, tiredness, cognitive impairment.[23,25]

About 90% of a parenteral dose of ketamine is excreted in the urine, mostly as conjugates of hydroxylated metabolites. Less than 5% is excreted unchanged via the faeces and urine. Ketamine undergoes hepatic metabolism by CYP2B6 and CYP3A4, mainly to norketamine.[26] There is wide variation in clearance of ketamine, which is mostly explained by genetic polymorphism in the activity of CYP2B6 together with increasing age.[27] Because of extensive first-pass metabolism, a greater proportion of a PO dose of ketamine is converted to norketamine compared to one administered by injection.[28] Norketamine has a lower affinity for the NMDA-receptor-channel than ketamine. Although norketamine (particularly *S*-norketamine) is analgesic in rodents, this remains to be clarified in humans.[29,30] Norketamine is further metabolized to the inactive dehydronorketamine.

Ketamine causes hepatic enzyme induction and enhances its own metabolism. The implications of this for the efficacy or tolerability of therapeutic ketamine is unknown. However, in abusers, it may contribute towards the relatively rapid tolerance to the desired 'high', with those taking it most days of the week reporting about a 7-fold increase in dose after the first 2 months of use.[31]

Ketamine increases sympathetic nervous system activity and causes tachycardia and intracranial hypertension. When ketamine is used for procedural anaesthesia, a quarter of patients experience vivid dreams, misperceptions, hallucinations and alterations in body image and mood as emergent (psychotomimetic) phenomena, i.e. as the effects of a bolus dose wear off. The incidence is reduced to <10% by the concurrent use of **midazolam**.[32] Emergent phenomena occur to a lesser extent with the sub-anaesthetic analgesic doses given PO or CSCI, and generally can be controlled by concurrent administration of a benzodiazepine (e.g. **diazepam**, **midazolam**) or **haloperidol**.[14,33,34] Sub-anaesthetic doses of ketamine are associated with impaired attention, memory and judgement, and it is used as a pharmacological model for acute schizophrenia.[3]

Although ketamine is widely used as a short-term analgesic in various clinical settings (including peri-operatively where it reduces pain and opioid requirements),[35,36] the potential for neuropsychiatric, urinary tract and hepatobiliary toxicity (Box A) must be considered when contemplating its long-term use. In palliative care, ketamine should generally be reserved for pain which has failed to respond to standard analgesic drugs, including opioids and adjuvants (see Adjuvant analgesics, p.299).

Chronic non-cancer pain

A review of sub-anaesthetic doses of ketamine for chronic non-cancer pain (mostly neuropathic but also ischaemic, fibromyalgia, post-whiplash, etc.) identified 29 RCTs and concluded that:

- ketamine provides relief
- undesirable effects can limit its use
- long-term use should be restricted to a controlled trial.[37]

A systematic review of analgesics for phantom limb pain reached similar conclusions.[38] A systematic review concluded there was only weak evidence of benefit in complex regional pain syndrome.[39]

Cancer pain

A systematic review of ketamine as an adjunct to opioids in cancer pain found only two studies of sufficient quality[14,40] and concluded that there is insufficient robust evidence to assess potential benefits and harms.[41] Thus, in patients with cancer, evidence of ketamine's efficacy as an analgesic is mostly from case reports, retrospective surveys or uncontrolled studies in patients with refractory neuropathic, bone, and mucositis-related pain.[8,9,14,40,42–53] Results from a large RCT of PO racemic ketamine in cancer-related neuropathic pain are pending.[54] 13

Short-term 'burst' treatment with ketamine sometimes has a relatively long-lasting effect (i.e. several days to weeks and occasionally for months).[55,56] For example, ketamine 100mg/24h by CIVI for 2 days in a cancer patient, repeated a month later, reduced opioid requirements by 70%.[57] Similarly, in non-cancer patients taking regular strong opioids for ischaemic limb pain, a single 4h IV infusion of ketamine 600microgram/kg reduced opioid requirements during the next week.[58]

However, in a large case series, about a quarter of patients experienced severe undesirable effects from higher-dose 'burst' CSCI ketamine involving rapid dose escalation 100 → 300 → 500mg/24h over 3–5 days.[55] Further, in a 5-day RCT in cancer patients using the same regimen, there was no difference in the proportion responding in the ketamine and placebo arms (about 50% in each, based on average pain score).[59] There were fewer treatment failures at the maximum dose (25 vs. 50%) but more undesirable effects and withdrawals due to toxicity (19 vs. 2%).[59] *These results suggest that rapid titration involving such doses of CSCI ketamine is generally inadvisable.*

Miscellaneous

Ketamine (generally IV, in combination with **morphine** or **midazolam**) can provide analgesia in severe acute pain due to trauma and other causes in patients presenting to emergency departments,[60] severe cancer treatment-related mucositis,[61] and during painful procedures, e.g. change of dressings, reduction of fractures and dislocations.[62–65] There are reports of its successful use in children and adolescents with pain of various causes.[66]

Topical ketamine has been applied to the skin in various non-cancer pains,[67,68] and used as an oral rinse in cancer treatment-related mucositits.[69,70]

Ketamine has a rapid antidepressant effect in patients with major depression and bipolar disorder, including a reduction in suicidal ideation.[71–73] Following a single IV dose (typically 500microgram/kg over 40–60min), up to 70% of patients respond, with improvements seen within hours. However, duration of benefit is generally ≤1 week.[71,73] Serial treatments (e.g. 6 doses given on alternate days) improves and maintains the response, but following completion most relapse within 1–6 weeks.[71] The exact mechanism is unclear but includes the release of brain-derived neurotrophic factor which helps to restore neuroplasticity, e.g. through the formation of new synapses, more rapidly than seen with conventional antidepressants (see Antidepressants, p.193).[71] Although case reports of benefit are emerging from the palliative care setting,[74–78] the use of ketamine to treat major depression is experimental, and should ideally be restricted to RCTs.[71] Other drugs which act on the NMDA receptor-channel complex are undergoing clinical trials in depression.[79] There are preliminary reports of similar rapid but short-lasting benefit from ketamine in refractory anxiety.[80]

CIVI ketamine appears effective in refractory status epilepticus, but its place in clinical practice remains to be determined.[81]

Bio-availability 93% IM; 45% nasal; 30% SL; 30% PR; 20% PO.[82,83]
Onset of action 5min IM; 15–30min SC; 30min PO.
Time to peak plasma concentration no data SC; 30min PO; 1h norketamine.[84]
Plasma halflife 1–3h IM; 3h PO; 12h norketamine.[85]
Duration of action 30min–2h IM; 4–6h PO, sometimes longer.[86]

Cautions

History of psychiatric disorder; epilepsy, glaucoma, hypertension, heart failure, ischaemic heart disease, CVAs, acute intermittent porphyria.[87] Hyperthyroidism (increased risk of hypertension and tachycardia). Conditions causing excessive upper airway secretions; ketamine both increases salivation and sensitizes the gag reflex, leading on rare occasions to laryngospasm. Severe hepatic impairment (consider dose reduction).

Because of reports of ketamine increasing CSF pressure, raised intracranial pressure (e.g. as a result of head injury, intracranial tumour, hydrocephalus) is a traditional caution. However, systematic reviews report no such concerns in ventilated patients with traumatic or non-traumatic brain injury.[88,89]

Drug interactions

Reports involving the CYP450 enzyme system are mostly limited to PO *S*-ketamine:

- **clarithromycin** and grapefruit juice (potent CYP3A4 inhibitors) increase the plasma concentration of *S*-ketamine and reduce that of norketamine[90,91]
- **ticlopidine** (potent CYP2C19 and weak CYP2B6 inhibitor) increases the area under the plasma concentration-time curve[92]
- **rifampicin** and **St John's wort** (potent CYP3A4 inducers) decrease the plasma concentration of *S*-ketamine; **rifampicin** also following IV *S*-ketamine.[93,94]

The clinical relevance of these interactions is unclear. Other potent inhibitors or inducers of these enzymes could have similar effects (see Chapter 19, Table 8, p.725).

Undesirable effects

Ketamine can be abused or diverted; careful monitoring is essential.

Dose-related psychotomimetic phenomena occur in about 40% of patients with CSCI ketamine, less with PO: euphoria, dysphasia, blunted affect, psychomotor retardation, vivid dreams, nightmares, impaired attention, memory and judgement, illusions, hallucinations, altered body image.

Delirium, drowsiness, dizziness, diplopia, blurred vision, nystagmus, altered hearing, hypertension, tachycardia, hypersalivation, nausea and vomiting. At higher anaesthetic doses, tonic-clonic movements are very common (>10%) but these have not been reported after PO use or with analgesic parenteral doses.

Erythema and pain at injection site. Neuropsychiatric, urinary and hepatobiliary toxicity (Box A).

Box A Ketamine and neuropsychiatric, urinary and hepatobiliary toxicity

Neuropsychiatric

There are no studies of neuropsychiatric effects in patients receiving therapeutic ketamine long-term. Most participants in the studies below took ketamine in much larger doses and also abused multiple other drugs.

A study of long-term ketamine abusers (mostly regular users of ~3.5g/24h for 3 years) suggested a high incidence of moderate–severe depression (75%) and anxiety (50%), and only a low incidence of, at most, mild psychosis (<10%).[95] The relevance is uncertain; no definite link exists between ketamine abuse and mood disorder or psychosis.

continued

Box A Continued

In frequent abusers of ketamine (≥5 days/week), both short- and long-term memory are affected with dose-related impairments in visual recognition memory (tested by remembering patterns) and spatial working memory (tested by remembering which boxes contained hidden tokens).[96,97]

MRI changes were evident with *total estimated lifetime doses* of ≤3g.[98,99] Functional MRI showed dose-related alterations in the anterior cingulate cortex (decrease) and in the left precentral frontal gyrus (increase).[98]

These effects may be the consequence of long-term NMDA-receptor-channel blockade. Dopamine depletion in the prefrontal cortex, a key area involved in working memory, is also reported in those abusing ≥200mg/week.[100] Ketamine is also directly neurotoxic, with dose-related MRI changes suggestive of disruption or damage to the white matter in the frontal and left temporoparietal regions.[99]

Memory impairments appear to improve with abstinence, but former abusers continue to score higher than controls on delusional symptoms.[97]

Urinary tract

In three patients with chronic pain, urinary symptoms developed after receiving ketamine 650–800mg/24h PO for 5–18 months.[101] In another patient, severe damage necessitated cystectomy after three years of ketamine 240mg/24h PO for chronic back pain.[102] However, urinary symptoms developed after only 9 *days* in a 16 year-old receiving ketamine 8mg/kg/24h PO.[103]

13

Urinary symptoms have been reported in abusers of 'street' ketamine, generally taken as powdered ketamine via nasal insufflation. The risk appears related to both dose and frequency of use.[104]

Symptoms include frequency, urgency, urge incontinence, dysuria, haematuria and lower abdominal pain.[104–106] The exact cause of the inflammation is unclear, but possible triggers include a direct irritant effect, disruption of the bladder epithelial barrier, and IgE-mediated hypersensitivity.[107]

Investigations (e.g. cystoscopy and biopsy, CT urogram) may show inflammation and ulceration of the mucosa, detrusor overactivity, decreased bladder capacity, vesico-ureteric reflux, hydronephrosis, papillary necrosis, and renal impairment. Irreversible damage leading to renal failure has occurred.

Animal studies have found an increased expression of P2X1 purinergic receptors (activated by ATP) but not muscarinic receptors on bladder smooth muscle, which may explain the reports of limited benefit from antimuscarinic antispasmodics.[108]

Consequently, when patients receiving therapeutic ketamine experience urinary symptoms without evidence of bacterial infection, practitioners should consider stopping the ketamine and seeking the advice of a urologist.

Symptoms generally settle several weeks after stopping ketamine. However, in some abusers, symptoms have persisted despite abstinence.[104,109]

Hepatobiliary

Abnormal LFTs have been associated with both ketamine abuse and therapeutic use, e.g. IV for maintenance anaesthesia (>10h) or infusions for pain relief (≥4 days).[110–113] In the latter, although abnormal LFTs were sometimes apparent after 4–5 days, in others it occurred only with a second infusion some 2 weeks later.[113]

In abusers, abdominal pain has been reported and, in some, dilation or strictures of the common bile duct.[111,114,115]

The cause is unknown, but possibilities include a direct toxic effect of ketamine or a metabolite, or ketamine-related dysfunction of the sphincter of Oddi.[110,116]

With abstinence, the LFTs, abdominal pain and biliary duct dilation generally improve. Some recommend regular monitoring of LFTs during the long-term therapeutic use of ketamine.[113]

Dose and use

Because of the undesirable effects profile of ketamine, which includes neuropsychiatric, urinary tract and hepatobiliary toxicity, prescription of ketamine as an analgesic should be restricted to specialists in pain or palliative care for patients who have failed to obtain adequate relief from standard non-drug and drug treatments, including the optimal use of opioids, non-opioids and adjuvant analgesics (see Adjuvant analgesics, p.299). A toxicity monitoring form is available.[117]

In patients with a prognosis of more than a few weeks, once analgesia has been obtained, an attempt should be made to withdraw ketamine over 2–3 weeks. Benefit from a short course can last for weeks or even months, and can be repeated if necessary.[54] Thus, apart from patients with a prognosis of just days–weeks, long-term continuous ketamine should be used only as a last resort, i.e. in those patients with unsatisfactory analgesia from a short course approach.

Note. Whole body hyperalgesia and allodynia may occur if ketamine is abruptly stopped after ≥3 weeks of use.[118]

Ketamine is included in a new law in England and Wales relating to driving with certain drugs above specified plasma concentrations (see Chapter 22, p.743).

All doses in this section relate to racemic ketamine.

Dose recommendations vary widely, but ketamine is often started low dose PO (see below). In some centres, an initial test dose is given to assess tolerability and efficacy. The prophylactic concurrent administration of a benzodiazepine or an antipsychotic is also routine in some but not all centres, where it is reserved for more select circumstances (see below). Long-term success, i.e. both pain relief and tolerable undesirable effects, varies from <20% to about 50%.[11,12,47,119]

Some practitioners routinely reduce the background opioid dose by 25–50% when starting parenteral ketamine. If the patient becomes drowsy, the dose of opioid should be reduced. If a patient experiences dysphoria or hallucinations, the dose of ketamine should be reduced and a benzodiazepine prescribed, e.g. **diazepam** 5mg PO stat & at bedtime, **lorazepam** 1mg PO stat & b.d., **midazolam** 5mg SC stat and 5–10mg CSCI, or **haloperidol**, e.g. 2–5mg PO stat & at bedtime, or 2–5mg SC stat and 2–5mg CSCI.[34] In patients at greatest risk of dysphoria (those with high anxiety levels), these measures may be more effective if given before starting ketamine.

When switching from CSCI to PO after just a few days, a conversion ratio of 1:1 should be used.[48,120] However, after weeks–months of use, some have found that a *smaller* total daily dose (25–50% of the parenteral dose) can maintain a similar level of analgesia, e.g. 400mg/24h CSCI → 150mg/24h PO.[46] In both instances, the patient should be monitored closely and the dose titrated accordingly. When switching from PO to CSCI or CIVI, it is advisable to commence on a small dose and titrate as required.

By mouth[8,9,121–123]

In the UK, an oral solution can be obtained as a special order (see Supply). When this option is not available, use direct from a vial or dilute for convenience (immediately before administration) to 50mg/5mL; add a flavouring of the patient's choice, e.g. fruit cordial, to mask the bitter taste:

- start with 10–25mg t.d.s.–q.d.s. and p.r.n.
- if necessary, increase dose in steps of 10–25mg up to 100mg q.d.s.
- maximum reported dose 200mg q.d.s.[121,123]
- give a smaller dose more frequently if psychotomimetic phenomena or drowsiness occurs which does not respond to a reduction in opioid.

Unauthorized capsules can be obtained as a special order, however these are expensive. Where the 100mg/mL vial is available (not UK), an oral solution can be prepared by a local pharmacy (see Box B).

Subcutaneous[9]

- typically 10–25mg p.r.n., some use 2.5–5mg
- if necessary, increase dose in steps of 25–33%.

CSCI[8,33,42,43,45,124]

Because ketamine is irritant, dilute to the largest volume possible, and consider the use of 0.9% saline as the diluent (see Chapter 29, p.819). Consider the use of prophylactic **diazepam**, **lorazepam**, **midazolam** or **haloperidol** (see text above).

- start with 1–2.5mg/kg/24h
- if necessary, increase by 50–100mg/24h
- continue to titrate until adequate pain relief
- usual maximum 500mg/24h
- maximum reported dose 3.6g/24h.

CSCI compatibility with other drugs: There are 2-drug compatibility data for ketamine in WFI with **metoclopramide, midazolam** and **morphine sulfate**. For more details and 3-drug compatibility charts see Appendix 3.

There are 2-drug compatibility data for ketamine in 0.9% saline with **alfentanil, clonazepam, dexamethasone** (low-dose), **diamorphine, haloperidol, hydromorphone, levomepromazine, metoclopramide, midazolam, morphine sulfate** and **oxycodone**. For more details and 3-drug compatibility charts see the extended Appendix 3 of the on-line *PCF* on *www.palliativedrugs.com.*

Intravenous[9,125]

For cancer pain:

- typically 2.5–5mg p.r.n.

To cover procedures which may cause severe pain:

- give 500microgram–1mg/kg (typically 25–50mg; some start with 5–10mg), over 1–2min preceded by, e.g. **lorazepam** 1mg IV or **midazolam** 100microgram/kg IV (typically 5–10mg; some start with 1–2mg) to reduce emergent phenomena
- use a maximum concentration of ketamine 50mg/mL; 0.9% saline or 5% glucose are suitable diluents.

The right dose should provide analgesia within 1–5min lasting for 10–20min. 13

There is a risk of marked sedation when ketamine and a benzodiazepine are given concurrently. Use only if competent in airway management and the patient can be adequately monitored.

Procedures of longer duration may require ketamine CIVI; obtain advice from an anaesthetist.

CIVI[21,126,127]

Dilute to a concentration of 1mg/mL with 0.9% saline or 5% glucose.

- give a single 'burst' of 600microgram/kg up to a maximum of 60mg over 4h (reduce dose by 1/3–1/2 in elderly/frail patients); monitor blood pressure at baseline and then hourly:
  - ▷ if necessary, repeat daily for up to 5 days
  - ▷ if *no* analgesic response to an infusion, increase the dose of the next one by 30%
  - ▷ further dose titrate according to response and/or undesirable effects
  - ▷ repeat the above if the pain subsequently recurs.[54]

Or

- start with 50–150microgram/kg/h (typically 50–100mg/24h) and titrate as necessary (typical increments 25–50mg/24h)
- in one series of 46 patients with cancer:
  - ▷ 20% responded to ≤100mg/24h
  - ▷ typical dose 100–300mg/24h
  - ▷ no psychotomimetic effects were seen with doses <300mg/24h.

Supply

All products are Schedule 2 **CD**.

Ketamine (generic)
Capsules 10mg, 40mg, 28 days @ 40mg q.d.s. = £223 (unauthorized, available as a special order from NHS Oxford store, see Chapter 24, p.751).
Oral solution or suspension (sugar-free) 50mg/5mL, 28 days @ 50mg q.d.s. = £142 (unauthorized, available as a special order see Chapter 24, p.751; *price based on community specials tariff*).
Injection 50mg/mL, 10mL vial = £7.

Ketalar® (Pfizer)
Injection 10mg/mL, 20mL vial = £5; 50mg/mL, 10mL vial = £9.

Although use as an analgesic is unauthorized, ketamine injection can be prescribed both in hospitals and in the community. Community pharmacies can order ketamine injection through their usual Alliance Healthcare wholesale account. To initiate an account, contact head office (Tel: 020 8391 2323).

Box B Preparation of ketamine 50mg/5mL oral solution: pharmacy guidelines

Note. An option when 100mg/mL vials are available (not UK).

Use ketamine 100mg/mL, 10mL vials because this is the cheapest concentration. Raspberry Syrup BP can be used for dilution but this is too sweet for some patients. Alternatively, use purified water as the diluent and ask patients to add their own flavouring, e.g. fruit cordial, just before use to disguise the bitter taste.

To prepare 100mL of 50mg/5mL ketamine oral solution:
- mix 10mL vial of ketamine 100mg/mL for injection with 90mL purified water.

Store in a refrigerator with an expiry date of 1 week from manufacture.

S-ketamine (esketamine)

S-ketamine is about *twice* as potent as the racemic mixture (see Pharmacology); thus, an equivalent dose of S-ketamine is about *half that of the racemic mixture.*

Ketanest S®
***Injection (preservative-free)* S-ketamine hydrochloride** (esketamine hydrochloride) *equivalent to S-ketamine base* 5mg/mL, 10 x 5mL amp = £90; (unauthorized, available to import via IDIS, see Chapter 24, p.751); a doctor's letter with the reason why the preservative-free formulation is needed, GMC number and patient's initials is required.

Note. There is a long-term supply problem with Ketanest S®. Further, because this is a Schedule 2 CD, it is not held as a stock item and can take over 6 weeks to obtain.

1 Persson J *et al.* (1998) The analgesic effect of racemic ketamine in patients with chronic ischemic pain due to lower extremity arteriosclerosis obliterans. *Acta Anaesthesiologica Scandinavica*. **42**: 750–758.
2 Iacobucci GJ *et al.* (2017) Ketamine: an update on cellular and subcellular mechanisms with implications for clinical practice. *Pain Physician*. **20**: e285–301.
3 Mion G and Villevieille T (2013) Ketamine pharmacology: an update (pharmacodynamics and molecular aspects, recent findings). *CNS Neuroscience and Therapeutics*. **19**: 370–380.
4 Richens A (1991) The basis of the treatment of epilepsy: neuropharmacology. In: M Dam (ed) *A Practical Approach to Epilepsy*. Pergamon Press, Oxford, pp. 75–85.
5 Johnson JW et *al.* (2015) Recent insights into the mode of action of memantine and ketamine. *Current Opinions in Pharmacology*. **20**: 54–63.
6 De Kock M *et al.* (2013) Ketamine and peripheral inflammation. *CNS Neuroscience and Therapeutics*. **19**: 403–410.
7 Sleigh J (2014) Ketamine - more mechanisms of action than just NMDA blockade. *Trends in Anaesthesia and Critical Care*. **4**: 76–81.
8 Luczak J *et al.* (1995) The role of ketamine, an NMDA receptor antagonist, in the management of pain. *Progress in Palliative Care*. **3**: 127–134.
9 Kotlinska-Lemieszek A and Luczak J (2004) Subanesthetic ketamine: an essential adjuvant for intractable cancer pain. *Journal of Pain and Symptom Management*. **28**: 100–102.
10 Lin T *et al.* (1998) Long-term epidural ketamine, morphine and bupivacaine attenuate reflex sympathetic dystrophy neuralgia. *Canadian Journal of Anaesthesia*. **45**: 175–177.
11 Haines D and Gaines S (1999) N of 1 randomised controlled trials of oral ketamine in patients with chronic pain. *Pain*. **83**: 283–287.
12 Batchelor G (1999) Ketamine in neuropathic pain. *The Pain Society Newsletter*. **1**: 19.
13 Beltrutti D *et al.* (1999) The epidural and intrathecal administration of ketamine. *Current Review of Pain*. **3**: 458–472.
14 Mercadante S *et al.* (2000) Analgesic effect of intravenous ketamine in cancer patients on morphine therapy: a randomized, controlled, double-blind, crossover, double-dose study. *Journal of Pain and Symptom Management*. **20**: 246–252.
15 Carr DB *et al.* (2004) Safety and efficacy of intranasal ketamine for the treatment of breakthrough pain in patients with chronic pain: a randomized, double-blind, placebo-controlled, crossover study. *Pain*. **108**: 17–27.
16 Mercadante S *et al.* (2005) Alternative treatments of breakthrough pain in patients receiving spinal analgesics for cancer pain. *Journal of Pain and Symptom Management*. **30**: 485–491.
17 Yeaman F *et al.* (2013) Sub-dissociative dose intranasal ketamine for limb injury pain in children in the emergency department: a pilot study. *Emergency Medicine Australasia*. **25**: 161–167.
18 Vranken JH *et al.* (2005) Neuropathological findings after continuous intrathecal administration of S(+)-ketamine for the management of neuropathic cancer pain. *Pain*. **117**: 231–235.
19 Berger J *et al.* (2000) Ketamine-fentanyl-midazolam infusion for the control of symptoms in terminal life care. *American Journal of Hospice and Palliative Care*. **17**: 127–132.
20 Enck R (2000) A ketamine, fentanyl, and midazolam infusion for uncontrolled terminal pain and agitation. *American Journal of Hospice and Palliative Care*. **17**: 76–77.

21 Conway M *et al.* (2009) Use of continuous intravenous ketamine for end-stage cancer pain in children. *Journal of Pediatric Oncology Nursing*. **26**: 100–106.
22 Oye I *et al.* (1991) The chiral forms of ketamine as probes for NMDA receptor function in humans. In: T Kameyama (ed) *NMDA receptor Related Agents: biochemistry, pharmacology and behavior*. NPP, Ann Arbor, Michigan, pp. 381–389.
23 White PF *et al.* (1980) Pharmacology of ketamine isomers in surgical patients. *Anesthesiology*. **52**: 231–239.
24 Mathisen L *et al.* (1995) Effect of ketamine, an NMDA receptor inhibitor, in acute and chronic orofacial pain. *Pain*. **61**: 215–220.
25 Pfenninger EG *et al.* (2002) Cognitive impairment after small-dose ketamine isomers in comparison to equianalgesic racemic ketamine in human volunteers. *Anesthesiology*. **96**: 357–366.
26 Hijazi Y *et al.* (2002) Contribution of CYP3A4, CYP2B6, and CYP2C9 isoforms to N-demethylation of ketamine in human liver microsomes. *Drug Metabolism & Disposition*. **30**: 853–858.
27 Li Y *et al.* (2015) CYP2B6*6 allele and age substantially reduce steady-state ketamine clearance in chronic pain patients: impact on adverse effects. *British Journal of Clinical Pharmacology*. **80**: 276–284.
28 Clements JA *et al.* (1982) Bio-availability, pharmacokinetics and analgesic activity of ketamine in humans. *Journal of Pharmaceutical Sciences*. **71**: 539–542.
29 Olofsen E *et al.* (2012) Estimation of the contribution of norketamine to ketamine-induced acute pain relief and neurocognitive impairment in healthy volunteers. *Anesthesiology*. **117**: 353–364.
30 Holtman JR, Jr. *et al.* (2008) Effects of norketamine enantiomers in rodent models of persistent pain. *Pharmacology, Biochemistry and Behavior*. **90**: 676–685.
31 Muetzelfeldt L *et al.* (2008) Journey through the K-hole: phenomenological aspects of ketamine use. *Drug Alcohol Dependence*. **95**: 219–229.
32 Sener S *et al.* (2011) Ketamine with and without midazolam for emergency department sedation in adults: a randomized controlled trial. *Annals of Emergency Medicine*. **57**: 109–114.
33 Hughes A *et al.* (1999) Ketamine. *CME Bulletin Palliative Medicine*. **1**: 53.
34 Giannini A *et al.* (2000) Acute ketamine intoxication treated by haloperidol: a preliminary study. *American Journal of Therapeutics*. **7**: 389–391.
35 Assouline B *et al.* (2016) Benefit and harm of adding ketamine to an opioid in a patient-controlled analgesia device for the control of postoperative pain: systematic review and meta-analyses of randomized controlled trials with trial sequential analyses. *Pain*. **157**: 2854–2864.
36 Bell RF *et al.* (2006) Perioperative ketamine for acute postoperative pain. *Cochrane Database of Systematic Reviews*. CD004603. www.thecochranelibrary.com
37 Bell RF (2009) Ketamine for chronic non-cancer pain. *Pain*. **141**: 210–214.
38 Alviar MJM (2011) Pharmacological interventions for treating phantom limb pain. *Cochrane Database of Systematic Reviews*. CD006380. www.thecochranelibrary.com
39 Connolly SB *et al.* (2015) A systematic review of ketamine for complex regional pain syndrome. *Pain Medicine*. **16**: 943–969.
40 Yang CY *et al.* (1996) Intrathecal ketamine reduces morphine requirements in patients with terminal cancer pain. *Canadian Journal of Anaesthesia*. **43**: 379–383.
41 Bell RF *et al.* (2012) Ketamine as an adjuvant to opioids for cancer pain. *Cochrane Database Systematic Reviews*. **11**: CD003351. www.thecochranelibrary.com
42 Oshima E *et al.* (1990) Continuous subcutaneous injection of ketamine for cancer pain. *Canadian Journal of Anaesthetics*. **37**: 385–392.
43 Cherry DA *et al.* (1995) Ketamine as an adjunct to morphine in the treatment of pain. *Pain*. **62**: 119–121.
44 Mercadante S (1996) Ketamine in cancer pain: an update. *Palliative Medicine*. **10**: 225–230.
45 Bell R (1999) Low-dose subcutaneous ketamine infusion and morphine tolerance. *Pain*. **83**: 101–103.
46 Fitzgibbon EJ *et al.* (2002) Low dose ketamine as an analgesic adjuvant in difficult pain syndromes: a strategy for conversion from parenteral to oral ketamine. *Journal of Pain and Symptom Management*. **23**: 165–170.
47 Kannan TR *et al.* (2002) Oral ketamine as an adjuvant to oral morphine for neuropathic pain in cancer patients. *Journal of Pain and Symptom Management*. **23**: 60–65.
48 Benitez-Rosario M *et al.* (2003) A retrospective comparison of the dose ratio between subcutaneous and oral ketamine. *Journal of Pain and Symptom Management*. **25**: 400–402.
49 Fitzgibbon EJ and Viola R (2005) Parenteral ketamine as an analgesic adjuvant for severe pain: development and retrospective audit of a protocol for a palliative care unit. *Journal of Palliative Medicine*. **8**: 49–57.
50 Lauretti G *et al.* (1999) Oral ketamine and transdermal nitroglycerin as analgesic adjuvants to oral morphine therapy and amitriptyline for cancer pain management. *Anesthesiology*. **90**: 1528–1533.
51 Lossignol DA *et al.* (2005) Successful use of ketamine for intractable cancer pain. *Support Care Cancer*. **13**: 188–193.
52 James PJ *et al.* (2010) The addition of ketamine to a morphine nurse- or patient-controlled analgesia infusion (PCA/NCA) increases analgesic efficacy in children with mucositis pain. *Paediatric Anaesthesia*. **20**: 805–811.
53 Cheng HW *et al.* (2015) Successful analgesic use of ketamine infusion in malignant cord compression. *Pain Medicine*. **16**: 2045–2047.
54 Fallon M (2017) Personal communication.
55 Jackson K *et al.* (2010) The effectiveness and adverse effects profile of "burst" ketamine in refractory cancer pain. *Journal of Palliative Care*. **26**: 176–183.
56 Jackson K *et al.* (2001) 'Burst' ketamine for refractory cancer pain: an open-label audit of 39 patients. *Journal of Pain and Symptom Management*. **22**: 834–842.
57 Mercadante S *et al.* (2003) Burst ketamine to reverse opioid tolerance in cancer pain. *Journal of Pain and Symptom Management*. **25**: 302–305.
58 Mitchell AC and Fallon MT (2002) A single infusion of intravenous ketamine improves pain relief in patients with critical limb ischaemia: results of a double blind randomised controlled trial. *Pain*. **97**: 275–281.
59 Hardy J *et al.* (2012) Randomized , double-blind, placebo-controlled study to assess the efficacy and toxicity of subcutaneous ketamine in the management of cancer pain. *Journal of Clinical Oncology*. **30**: 11–17.
60 Lee EN and Lee JH (2016) The effects of low-dose ketamine on acute pain in an emergency setting: a systematic review and meta-analysis. *PLoS ONE*. **11**: e0165461.
61 White MC *et al.* (2011) Pain management in 100 episodes of severe mucositis in children. *Peadiatric Anesthesia*. **21**: 411–416.
62 Arroyo-Novoa CM *et al.* (2011) Efficacy of small doses of ketamine with morphine to decrease procedural pain responses during open wound care. *Clinical Journal of Pain*. **27**: 561–566.
63 Celik GE *et al.* (2013) Are drug provocation tests still necessary to test the safety of COX-2 inhibitors in patients with cross-reactive NSAID hypersensitivity? *Allergologia et Immunopathologia (Madr)*. **41**: 181–188.

13

64 Kundra P *et al.* (2013) Oral ketamine and dexmedetomidine in adults' burns wound dressing--A randomized double blind cross over study. *Burns.* **39**: 1150–1156.
65 Norambuena C *et al.* (2013) Oral ketamine and midazolam for pediatric burn patients: a prospective, randomized, double-blind study. *Journal of Pediatric Surgery.* **48**: 629–634.
66 Sheehy KA *et al.* (2017) Subanesthetic ketamine for pain management in hospitalized children, adolescents, and young adults: a single-center cohort study. *Journal of Pain Research.* **10**: 787–795.
67 Finch PM *et al.* (2009) Reduction of allodynia in patients with complex regional pain syndrome: A double-blind placebo-controlled trial of topical ketamine. *Pain.* **146**: 18–25.
68 Gammaitoni A *et al.* (2000) Topical ketamine gel: possible role in treating neuropathic pain. *Pain Medicine.* **1**: 97–100.
69 Slatkin NE and Rhiner M (2003) Topical ketamine in the treatment of mucositis pain. *Pain Medicine.* **4**: 298–303.
70 Shillingburg A *et al.* (2017) Treatment of severe mucositis pain with oral ketamine mouthwash. *Supportive Care in Cancer.* **25**: 2215–2219.
71 Bobo WV *et al.* (2016) Ketamine for treatment-resistent unipolar and bipolar major depression: Critical review and implications for clinical practice. *Depression and Anxiety.* **33**: 698–710.
72 Bartoli F *et al.* (2017) Ketamine as a rapid-acting agent for suicidal ideation: A meta-analysis. *Neuroscience and Biobehavioral Reviews.* **77**: 232–236.
73 Caddy C *et al.* (2015) Ketamine and other glutamate receptor modulators for depression in adults. *Cochrane Database of Systematic Reviews.* **9**: CD011612. www.thecochranelibrary.com
74 Irwin SA *et al.* (2013) Daily oral ketamine for the treatment of depression and anxiety in patients receiving hospice care: a 28-day open-label proof-of-concept trial. *Journal of Palliative Medicine.* **16**: 958–965.
75 Stefanczyk-Sapieha L *et al.* (2008) Intravenous ketamine "burst" for refractory depression in a patient with advanced cancer. *Journal of Palliative Medicine.* **11**: 1268–1271.
76 Irwin SA and Iglewicz A (2010) Oral ketamine for the rapid treatment of depression and anxiety in patients receiving hospice care. *Journal of Palliative Medicine.* **13**: 903–908.
77 Zanicotti CG *et al.* (2012) Mood and pain responses to repeat dose intramuscular ketamine in a depressed patient with advanced cancer. *Journal of Palliative Medicine.* **15**: 400–403.
78 Grott Zanicotti C *et al.* (2013) Case report: long-term mood response to repeat dose intramuscular ketamine in a depressed patient with advanced cancer. *Journal of Palliative Medicine.* **16**: 719–720.
79 Dolgin E (2013) Rapid antidepressant effects of ketamine ignite drug discovery. *Nature Medicine.* **19**: 8.
80 Glue P *et al.* (2017) Ketamine's dose-related effects on anxiety symptoms in patients with treatment refractory anxiety disorders. *Journal of Psychopharmacology.* (Epub ahead of print).
81 Fang Y and Wang X (2015) Ketamine for the treatment of refractory status epilepticus. *Seizure.* **30**: 14–20.
82 Chong CC *et al.* (2006) Bioavailability of ketamine after oral or sublingual administration. *Pain Medicine.* **7**: 469–469.
83 Yanagihara Y *et al.* (2003) Plasma concentration profiles of ketamine and norketamine after administration of various ketamine preparations to healthy Japanese volunteers. *Biopharmacentrics and Drug Disposition.* **24**: 37–43.
84 Grant IS *et al.* (1981) Pharmacokinetics and analgesic effects of IM and oral ketamine. *British Journal of Anaesthesia.* **53**: 805–810.
85 Domino E *et al.* (1984) Ketamine kinetics in unmedicated and diazepam premedicated subjects. *Clinical Pharmacology and Therapeutics.* **36**: 645–653.
86 Rabben T *et al.* (1999) Prolonged analgesic effect of ketamine, an N-methyl-D-aspartate receptor inhibitor, in patients with chronic pain. *Journal of Pharmacology and Experimental Therapeutics.* **289**: 1060–1066.
87 Ward J and Standage C (2003) Angina pain precipitated by a continuous subcutaneous infusion of ketamine. *Journal of Pain and Symptom Management.* **25**: 6–7.
88 Zeiler FA *et al.* (2014) The ketamine effect on ICP in traumatic brain injury. *Neurocritical Care.* **21**: 163–173.
89 Zeiler FA *et al.* (2014) The ketamine effect on intracranial pressure in nontraumatic neurological illness. *Journal of Critical Care.* **29**: 1096–1106.
90 Peltoniemi MA *et al.* (2012) S-ketamine concentrations are greatly increased by grapefruit juice. *European Journal of Clinical Pharmacology.* **68**: 979–986.
91 Hagelberg N *et al.* (2010) Clarythromycin, a potent inhibitor of CYP3A, greatly increases exposure to oral S-ketamine. *European Journal of Pain.* **14**: 625–629.
92 Peltoniemi MA *et al.* (2011) Exposure to oral S-ketamine is unaffected by itraconazole but greatly increased by ticlopidine. *Clinical Pharmacology and Therapeutics.* **90**: 296–302.
93 Peltoniemi MA *et al.* (2012) Rifampicin has a profound effect on the pharmacokinetics of oral S-Ketamine and less on intravenous S-ketamine. *Basic and Clinical Pharmacology and Toxicology.* **111**: 325–332.
94 Peltoniemi MA *et al.* (2012) St John's wort greatly decreases the plasma concentrations of oral S-ketamine. *Fundamental and Clinical Pharmacology.* **26**: 743–750.
95 Fan N *et al.* (2016) Profiling the psychotic, depressive and anxiety symptoms in chronic ketamine users. *Psychiatry Research.* **237**: 311–315.
96 Morgan CJ *et al.* (2010) Consequences of chronic ketamine self-administration upon neurocognitive function and psychological wellbeing: a 1-year longitudinal study. *Addiction.* **105**: 121–133.
97 Morgan CJ and Curran HV (2012) Ketamine use: a review. *Addiction.* **107**: 27–38.
98 Liao Y *et al.* (2012) Alterations in regional homogeneity of resting-state brain activity in ketamine addicts. *Neuroscience Letters.* **522**: 36–40.
99 Liao Y *et al.* (2010) Frontal white matter abnormalities following chronic ketamine use: a diffusion tensor imaging study. *Brain.* **133**: 2115–2122.
100 Narendran R *et al.* (2005) Altered prefrontal dopaminergic function in chronic recreational ketamine users. *American Journal of Psychiatry.* **162**: 2352–2359.
101 Storr TM and Quibell R (2009) Can ketamine prescribed for pain cause damage to the urinary tract? *Palliative Medicine.* **23**: 670–672.
102 Shahzad. K *et al.* (2012) Analgesic ketamine use leading to cystectomy: a case report. *British Journal of Medical and Surgical Urology.* **5**: 188–191.
103 Gregoire MC *et al.* (2008) A pediatric case of ketamine-associated cystitis. *Urology.* **71**: 1232–1233.
104 Winstock AR *et al.* (2012) The prevalence and natural history of urinary symptoms among recreational ketamine users. *British Journal of Urology International.* **110**: 1762–1766.
105 Chu PS *et al.* (2008) The destruction of the lower urinary tract by ketamine abuse: a new syndrome? *British Journal of Urology International.* **102**: 1616–1622.

106 Shahani R *et al.* (2007) Ketamine-associated ulcerative cystitis: a new clinical entity. *Urology.* **69**: 810–812.
107 Jhang JF *et al.* (2015) Possible pathophysiology of ketamine-related cystitis and associated treatment strategies. *International Journal of Urology.* **22**: 816–825.
108 Meng E *et al.* (2011) Involvement of purinergic neurotransmission in ketamine induced bladder dysfunction. *Journal of Urology.* **186**: 1134–1141.
109 Cheung RY *et al.* (2011) Urinary symptoms and impaired quality of life in female ketamine users: persistence after cessation of use. *Hong Kong Medical Journal.* **17**: 267–273.
110 Ng SH *et al.* (2010) Emergency department presentation of ketamine abusers in Hong Kong: a review of 233 cases. *Hong Kong Medical Journal.* **16**: 6–11.
111 Wong SW *et al.* (2009) Dilated common bile ducts mimicking choledochal cysts in ketamine abusers. *Hong Kong Medical Journal.* **15**: 53–56.
112 Dundee JW *et al.* (1980) Changes in serum enzyme levels following ketamine infusions. *Anaesthesia.* **35**: 12–16.
113 Noppers IM *et al.* (2011) Drug-induced liver injury following a repeated course of ketamine treatment for chronic pain in CRPS type I patients: a report of 3 cases. *Pain.* **152**: 2173–2178.
114 Ng SH *et al.* (2009) Dilated common bile ducts in ketamine abusers. *Hong Kong Med J.* **15**: 157.
115 Seto WK *et al.* (2011) Ketamine-induced cholangiopathy: a case report. *American Journal of Gastroenterology.* **106**: 1004–1005.
116 Lee ST *et al.* (2009) Apoptotic insults to human HepG2 cells induced by S-(+)-ketamine occurs through activation of a Bax-mitochondria-caspase protease pathway. *British Journal of Anaesthesia.* **102**: 80–89.
117 Palliativedrugs.com (2013) Ketamine monitoring chart. *Document Library.* Pain (neuropathic). www.palliativedrugs.com
118 Mitchell AC (1999) Generalized hyperalgesia and allodynia following abrupt cessation of subcutaneous ketamine infusion. *Palliative Medicine.* **13**: 427–428.
119 Enarson M *et al.* (1999) Clinical experience with oral ketamine. *Journal of Pain and Symptom Management.* **17**: 384–386.
120 Benitez-Rosario MA *et al.* (2011) A strategy for conversion from subcutaneous to oral ketamine in cancer pain patients: efficacy of a 1:1 ratio. *Journal of Pain and Symptom Management.* **10**: 1098–1105.
121 Clark JL and Kalan GE (1995) Effective treatment of severe cancer pain of the head using low-dose ketamine in an opioid-tolerant patient. *Journal of Pain and Symptom Management.* **10**: 310–314.
122 Broadley K *et al.* (1996) Ketamine injection used orally. *Palliative Medicine.* **10**: 247–250.
123 Vielvoye-Kerkmeer A (2000) Clinical experience with ketamine. *Journal of Pain and Symptom Management.* **19**: 3.
124 Lloyd-Williams M (2000) Ketamine for cancer pain. *Journal of Pain and Symptom Management.* **19**: 79–80.
125 Mason KP *et al.* (2002) Evolution of a protocol for ketamine-induced sedation as an alternative to general anesthesia for interventional radiologic procedures in pediatric patients. *Radiology.* **225**: 457–465.
126 Hocking G *et al.* (2007) Ketamine: does life begin at 40? *Pain Clinical Updates IASP.* **XV.** Issue 3.
127 Okamoto Y *et al.* (2012) Can gradual dose titration of ketamine for management of neuropathic pain prevent psychotomimetic effects in patients with advanced cancer? *American Journal of Hospice and Palliative Medicine.* **30**: 450–454.

Updated August 2017

*PROPOFOL

Class: General anaesthetic.

Indications: Induction and maintenance of general anaesthesia, conscious sedation (diagnostic or therapeutic procedures, e.g. radiation therapy in children),[1] continuous sedation of intubated and mechanically ventilated patients ≥16 years on intensive care units, †refractory agitated delirium or intolerable distress in the imminently dying, †intractable nausea and vomiting.[2]

Contra-indications: Continuous sedation in children ≤16 years; when used for sedation in children in intensive care, the death rate increased 2–3 times.[3] Propofol 0.5% is contra-indicated for maintenance of general anaesthesia or continuous sedation in intensive care in adults and children, and maintenance of conscious sedation in children (diagnostic or therapeutic procedures).

Allergy to eggs, soya or peanuts (the available products contain purified egg phosphatide as an emulsifying agent and soya bean oil).[4]

Pharmacology

Propofol is an ultrafast-acting IV anaesthetic agent. It is rapidly metabolized, mainly in the liver, to inactive compounds which are excreted in the urine. The incidence of untoward haemodynamic changes is low. Propofol reduces cerebral blood flow, cerebral metabolism and, less consistently, intracranial pressure.[5] The reduction in intracranial pressure is greater if the baseline pressure is raised. On discontinuation patients rapidly regain consciousness (10–30min) without residual drowsiness.

In palliative care, propofol is occasionally used, when other approaches have failed, to relieve agitated delirium or intolerable distress in the imminently dying.[6] Careful titration generally permits 'conscious sedation', i.e. patients open their eyes on verbal command, possess intact autonomic reflexes, and tolerate mild noxious stimuli.[2] Such use has also been described in children at the end of life, and algorithms to assist physicians considering initiation of palliative sedation therapy in children have been suggested.[7,8]

Propofol also has an anti-emetic effect resulting in less postoperative vomiting compared with other anaesthetic agents.[9–11] Specific postoperative anti-emetic regimens have been designed.[12–14] Chemotherapy-related nausea and vomiting is also helped by adjunctive propofol.[15] In patients receiving non-platinum regimens who were refractory to a combination of **dexamethasone** and a $5HT_3$-receptor antagonist, propofol was of benefit in ≥80%.[16] Propofol has also been used to relieve refractory nausea and vomiting in other settings, including palliative care.[2,17] In the group of patients with bowel obstruction, propofol was more effective in relieving nausea than vomiting.

Animal studies suggest that the mechanism of action of propofol as an anti-emetic is by inhibition of serotonin release by enhancing GABA activity, possibly by direct GABA-mediated action on $5HT_3$-receptors in the area postrema/chemoreceptor trigger zone.[18]

Propofol also has antipruritic, anxiolytic, bronchodilator, muscle relaxant and anti-epileptic properties. A possible role in refractory status epilepticus requires further clarification.[19–21] Transient excitatory phenomena are seen occasionally (e.g. myoclonus, opisthotonus, tonic-clonic activity), during induction or recovery when blood levels are low, and presumably at a time when inhibitory centres but not excitatory centres have been depressed.[5,22,23]

Onset of action 30 seconds.

Time to peak effect 5min.

Plasma halflife 2–4min initial distribution phase; 30–60min slow distribution and initial elimination phase; 3–12h terminal elimination phase. The terminal elimination halflife may increase with prolonged use.

Duration of action 3–10min after single IV bolus.[24,25]

Cautions

Risk of cardiorespiratory depression. Propofol clearance will reduce if cardiac output falls. Involuntary movements and seizures have been reported, particularly in epileptics, during induction or recovery.[22,26] With prolonged use in intensive care, the following have been reported: ECG changes, including prolongation of the QT interval (see Chapter 20, p.731), cardiac arrhythmia, heart failure, hepatomegaly, renal failure, rhabdomyolysis, metabolic acidosis, hyperkalaemia and hyperlipidaemia; when these occur in combination, it is termed a propofol infusion syndrome.

Although in intensive care use it is good practice to check plasma lipid levels in patients receiving propofol for ≥3 days, it is unnecessary in patients whose expected prognosis is only days.

Diprivan® contains disodium edetate (EDTA), a chelating agent which can reduce circulating concentrations and increase urinary losses of trace metals, e.g. zinc. Supplements should be considered for patients who are not imminently dying and who are likely to receive prolonged propofol treatment, particularly those at particular risk of deficiency, e.g. from fluid loss, catabolic states or infection.

Undesirable effects

Very common (>10%): local pain at the injection site.

Common (<10%, >1%): headache, hypotension, bradycardia, transient apnoea.

Uncommon (<1%, >0.1%): thrombosis, phlebitis.

Rare: epileptiform movements, propofol infusion syndrome, euphoria during recovery, misuse resulting in addiction and/or death. Concerns over a growing incidence among medical staff with access to propofol, e.g. anaesthetists, has prompted moves to designate propofol a controlled drug, particularly in the USA.[27–29]

Dose and use

Propofol is an emulsion of oil-in-water. This gives it a white appearance and makes it a potential growth medium. Diprivan® contains EDTA, a chelating agent which binds to divalent metal ions and reduces their availability for bacterial growth, replication and cell wall integrity. However, the concentration (0.005%) is sufficient only to *retard* microbial growth for up to 12h in the event of accidental contamination.[30] Propofol-Lipuro® contains no preservatives. Thus, with all propofol products, strict aseptic technique must be employed to prevent microbial contamination *and the container and IV line renewed every 6–12h, in accordance with the individual manufacturer's instructions.* The propofol products available in the UK must not be infused through a microbiological filter.

The use of propofol in palliative care should be restricted to units with access to the necessary expertise and equipment.

Undiluted propofol requires a computer-controlled volumetric infusion pump or IV syringe pump (see manufacturer's SPC for full details). It is given by CIVI as a 1% (10mg/mL) or 2% (20mg/mL) solution, using the antecubital vein (or a large vein in the fore-arm) to minimize the risk of pain.[31,32] Pain at the IV injection site appears rare with undiluted propofol CIVI as used in palliative care practice. If problematic, seek the advice of an anaesthetist; options include:

- injecting *preservative-free* **lidocaine** prior to the propofol infusion
- mixing *preservative-free* **lidocaine** with propofol 0.5% or 1% immediately before administration; see specific SPC for details. Note. *Propofol 2% injection should not be mixed with* ***lidocaine*** *or any other drug*
- using propofol 0.5% (5mg/mL; Propofol-Lipuro®) for induction of anaesthesia or sedation for infusions of a maximum duration of 1h.

Diluted propofol 1% injection can be administered through a less sensitive infusion control device, e.g. an in-line burette or drop counter, after dilution with 5% glucose (Diprivan®; see SPC for details). Dilution is advised with less sensitive infusion control devices because the weaker concentration reduces the risk of severe overdose if the infusion runs fast. The concentration of propofol in the diluted solution must not be less than 2mg/mL because this can disrupt the emulsion. Diluted propofol should be used within 6h. *Propofol 2% injection should not be diluted.*

Compatibility: See the specific SPC for full details; formulations of propofol differ between manufacturers and compatibility data cannot be extrapolated from one product to another.

Propofol 1% injection is compatible with certain concentrations of **alfentanil** (Diprivan® only) and **lidocaine**, and can be diluted with 5% glucose before use. *Propofol 2% injection should not be diluted or mixed with any other drugs.*

Both propofol 1% and 2% can be added through a Y-connector to a running infusion of 5% glucose, 0.9% saline or 4% glucose + 0.18% saline; the Y-connector should be placed as close to the injection site as possible.

13

Refractory agitated delirium or intolerable distress in the imminently dying

Consider propofol only if standard treatments have failed, i.e. a sedative antipsychotic + a benzodiazepine (Figure 1).[2,6,33–35] However, generally, **phenobarbital** should be used in preference to propofol because it is less complicated for clinical staff to titrate and monitor (see p.289).

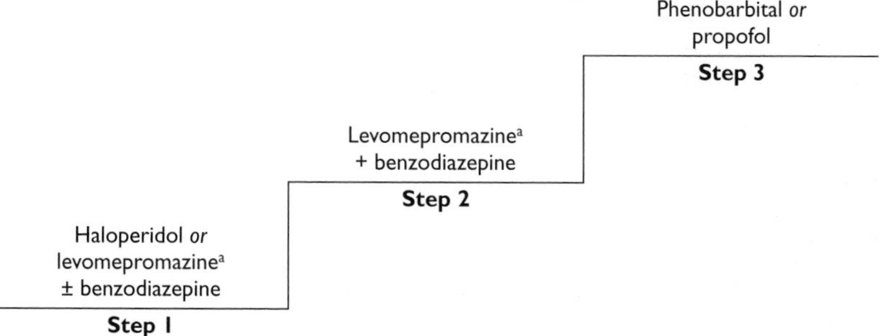

Figure 1 Drug treatment used at some centres for irreversible agitated delirium or intolerable distress in the imminently dying.

a. in countries where levomepromazine is not available, e.g. the USA, chlorpromazine is used instead.

Aim to titrate the dose until *conscious sedation* is achieved, i.e. patients open their eyes on verbal command but are not distressed by nursing interventions (e.g. mouth care, turning):

- remain with the patient throughout the initial titration process to ensure an effective and safe dose is found
- generally start with propofol 1mg/kg/h CIVI

- if necessary, increase by 0.5mg/kg/h every 5–10min until a satisfactory level of sedation is achieved; smaller dose steps can be used to fine-tune the treatment; most patients respond well to 1–2mg/kg/h
- to increase the level of sedation quickly, a bolus dose can be given by increasing the rate to 1mg/kg/*min* for a maximum of 1–2*min*
- monitor the patient closely during the first hour of treatment with respect to symptom relief and/or level of sedation, and then after 2, 6, and 12h
- continue to monitor the effect of propofol and the level of sedation at least twice daily
- if the patient is too sedated (i.e. does not respond to a verbal command to open their eyes, shows no response to noxious stimuli) and/or there is evidence of drug-induced respiratory depression, the infusion should be turned off for 2–3min and restarted at a lower rate; occasionally this leads to a progressive reduction in dose because the patient has become unconscious as a result of their disease
- tolerance can develop, necessitating a dose increase, but generally not within 1 week
- long-term use of doses >4mg/kg/h is not recommended because of increasing risk of undesirable effects
- if the patient does not respond to propofol 4mg/kg/h alone, supplement with **midazolam** by CSCI, starting with 10–30mg/24h
- it is important to replenish the infusion quickly when a container empties, because the effect of an infusion of propofol wears off after 10–30min
- *because propofol has no definite analgesic properties, analgesics should be continued.*

Intractable nausea and vomiting

The use of propofol as an anti-emetic should be considered only if all other treatments have failed (see QCG: Nausea and vomiting, p.240).[2] Dose titration is generally slower for intractable nausea and vomiting than for terminal agitation:

- remain with the patient for at least 10min following any dose change to ensure that excessive sedation does not occur
- generally start with propofol 0.5mg/kg/h CIVI
- if necessary, increase by 0.25–0.5mg/kg/h every 30–60min until a satisfactory response is obtained; smaller dose steps can be used to fine-tune the treatment
- most patients respond well to 0.5–1mg/kg/h; doses >1mg/kg/h may result in sedation
- monitor the patient closely during the first hour of treatment with respect to symptom relief and/or level of sedation and then after 2, 6, and 12h
- continue to monitor the effect of propofol and level of sedation at least twice daily
- if the patient is too sedated, the infusion should be turned off for 2–3min and then restarted at a lower rate
- if the patient responds well, reduce the infusion rate on a trial basis after 18–24h
- tolerance can develop, necessitating a dose increase, but generally not within 1 week
- it is important to replenish the infusion quickly when a container empties, because the effect of an infusion of propofol wears off after 10–30min
- when used solely for its anti-emetic effect in the last days of life, some centres reduce the dose of, or even discontinue, propofol when the patient becomes unconscious.

Supply

Propofol (generic; Propofol-Lipuro®)

Injection (emulsion) 5mg/mL (0.5%), 20mL amp = £3; *restricted to induction of general anaesthesia or induction of conscious sedation for diagnostic and therapeutic procedures in adults and children, and short-term sedation in adults (1h maximum duration of infusion).*

Diprivan® (AstraZeneca)

Injection (emulsion) 10mg/mL (1%), 20mL amp = £3, 50mL pre-filled siringe = £11.

Injection (emulsion) 20mg/mL (2%), 50mL pre-filled syringe = £15.

1 Harris EA (2010) Sedation and anesthesia options for pediatric patients in the radiation oncology suite. *International Journal of Pediatrics*. EPUB article ID 870921.

2 Lundstrom S *et al.* (2005) When nothing helps: propofol as sedative and antiemetic in palliative cancer care. *Journal of Pain and Symptom Management*. **30**: 570–577.

3 Anonymous (2001) Propofol (Diprivan) infusion: sedation in children aged 16 years or younger contraindicated. *Current Problems in Pharmacovigilance*. **27**: 10.
4 Hofer KN *et al.* (2003) Possible anaphylaxis after propofol in a child with food allergy. *Annals of Pharmacotherapy*. **37**: 398–401.
5 Mirenda J and Broyles G (1995) Propofol as used for sedation in the ICU. *Chest*. **108**: 539–548.
6 McWilliams K *et al.* (2010) Propofol for terminal sedation in palliative care: a systematic review. *Journal of Palliative Medicine*. **13**: 73–76.
7 Hooke MC *et al.* (2007) Propofol use in pediatric patients with severe cancer pain at the end of life. *Journal of Pediatric Oncology Nursing*. **24**: 29–34.
8 Anghelescu DL *et al.* (2012) Pediatric palliative sedation therapy with propofol: recommendations based on experience in children with terminal cancer. *Journal of Palliative Medicine*. **15**: 1082–1090.
9 Tramer M *et al.* (1997) Meta-analytic comparison of prophylactic antiemetic efficacy for postoperative nausea and vomiting: propofol anaesthesia vs omitting nitrous oxide vs total i.v. anaesthesia with propofol. *British Journal of Anaesthesia*. **78**: 256–259.
10 Sneyd JR *et al.* (1998) A meta-analysis of nausea and vomiting following maintenance of anaesthesia with propofol or inhalational agents. *European Journal of Anaesthesiology*. **15**: 433–445.
11 DeBalli P (2003) The use of propofol as an antiemetic. *International Anesthesiology Clinics*. **41**: 67–77.
12 Fujii Y *et al.* (2001) Small doses of propofol, droperidol, and metoclopramide for the prevention of postoperative nausea and vomiting after thyroidectomy. *Otolaryngology - Head and Neck Surgery*. **124**: 266–269.
13 Gan TJ *et al.* (1997) Determination of plasma concentrations of propofol associated with 50% reduction in postoperative nausea. *Anesthesiology*. **87**: 779–784.
14 Gan TJ *et al.* (1999) Patient-controlled antiemesis: a randomized, double-blind comparison of two doses of propofol versus placebo. *Anesthesiology*. **90**: 1564–1570.
15 Scher C *et al.* (1992) Use of propofol for the prevention of chemotherapy-induced nausea and emesis in oncology patients. *Canadian Journal of Anaesthesia*. **39**: 170–172.
16 Borgeat A *et al.* (1994) Adjuvant propofol enables better control of nausea and emesis secondary to chemotherapy for breast cancer. *Canadian Journal of Anaesthesia*. **41**: 1117–1119.
17 Hunter-Johnson L and Wheeler WL (2016) Use of propofol to manage nonmalignant intractable nausea and vomiting: a case study. *Journal of Palliative Medicine*. **19**: 252–253.
18 Cechetto DF *et al.* (2001) The effects of propofol in the area postrema of rats. *Anesthesia and Analgesia*. **92**: 934–942.
19 Rossetti AO (2007) Which anesthetic should be used in the treatment of refractory status epilepticus? *Epilepsia*. **48 (Suppl 8)**: 52–55.
20 Garcia Penas JJ *et al.* (2007) Status epilepticus: evidence and controversy. *Neurologist*. **13 (6 Suppl 1)**: S62–73.
21 Dulin JD *et al.* (2014) Management of refractory status epilepticus in an actively dying patient. *Journal of Pain and Palliative Care Pharmacotherpy*. **28**: 243–250.
22 Sneyd JR (1999) Propofol and epilepsy. *British Journal of Anaesthesia*. **82**: 168–169.
23 Meyer S *et al.* (2009) Propofol: pro- or anticonvulsant drug? *Anesthesia and Analgesia*. **108**: 1993–1994.
24 Jungheinrich C *et al.* (2002) Pharmacokinetics of the generic formulation Propofol 1 Fresenius in comparison with the original formulation (Disoprivan 1). *Clinical Drug Investigation*. **22**: 417–427.
25 Fechner J *et al.* (2004) Comparative pharmacokinetics and pharmacodynamics of the new propofol prodrug GPI 15715 and propofol emulsion. *Anesthesiology*. **101**: 626–639.
26 AstraZeneca (2006) *Data on file*.
27 Wilson C *et al.* (2010) The abuse potential of propofol. *Clinical Toxicology*. **48**: 165–170.
28 Charatan F (2009) Concerns mount over misuse of anaesthetic propofol among US health professionals. *British Medical Journal*. **339**: b3673.
29 Monroe T *et al.* (2011) The misuse and abuse of propofol. *Substance Use and Misuse*. **46**: 1199–1205.
30 AstraZeneca (2010) *Personal communication*.
31 Wijeysundera DN and Kavanagh BP (2011) Prevention of pain from propofol injection. *British Medical Journal*. **342**: d1102.
32 Jalota L *et al.* (2011) Prevention of pain on injection of propofol: systematic review and meta-analysis. *British Medical Journal*. **342**: d1110.
33 Cheng C *et al.* (2002) When midazolam fails. *Journal of Pain and Symptom Management*. **23**: 256–265.
34 Moyle J (1995) The use of propofol in palliative medicine. *Journal of Pain and Symptom Management*. **10**: 643–646.
35 Mercadante S *et al.* (1995) Propofol in terminal care. *Journal of Pain and Symptom Management*. **10**: 639–642.

Updated (minor change) August 2016

14: PRESCRIBING IN PALLIATIVE CARE

In recent years, both national drug regulatory authorities and the general public have become increasingly concerned about the possibility of dangerous/life-threatening adverse drug reactions. Official documents and drug manufacturers' information often include a warning along the lines of:

'Use the lowest effective dose for the shortest possible time in order to reduce the risk of serious adverse events.'

This is, of course, one of the foundational principles of therapeutic drug use; it simply emphasises 'good practice'. Official documents and drug manufacturers' information also highlight when caution is necessary in relation to, for example, hepatic and renal impairment.

In palliative care, many patients are elderly and debilitated, and many have impaired organ function. Accordingly, in *PCF*, it is assumed that prescribers will adopt an appropriately cautious approach in relation to both dose and duration of treatment (also see *Getting the most out of PCF*, p.xiv).

For information about prescribing for children or in patients with significant renal or hepatic impairment, see p.675, p.681 and p.703 respectively. For information about anticipatory prescribing in the community, see p.671.

GENERAL PRINCIPLES

Drugs should be used only within the context of a systematic approach, which is encapsulated in the acronym ***EEMMA***:

- ***E****valuation* of the impact of the illness on the patient and family, and of the causes of the patient's symptoms (often multifactorial)
- ***E****xplanation* to the patient before starting treatment about what is going on, and what is the most appropriate course of action
- ***M****anagement*: correct the correctable, non-drug treatment, drug treatment
- ***M****onitoring:* frequent review of the impact of treatment; optimizing the doses of symptom relief drugs to maximize benefit and minimize undesirable effects
- ***A****ttention to detail:* do not make unwarranted assumptions; listen actively to the patient, respond to non-verbal and verbal cues.

In palliative care, the axiom *diagnosis before treatment* is still relevant. Even when cancer is responsible, a symptom may be caused by different mechanisms. For example, in lung cancer, vomiting may be caused by hypercalcaemia or by raised intracranial pressure (to name just two possible causes). Treatment often varies with the cause. Further, for many symptoms, the concurrent use of non-drug measures is equally important, and sometimes more important.

Attention to detail

Precision in taking a drug history

If a patient says, 'I take morphine every 4 hours', the doctor should ask, 'Tell me, when do you take your first dose?' 'And the second dose?' etc. It often turns out that the patient is taking morphine q.d.s. rather than q4h, and possibly p.r.n. rather than prophylactically.

A 90 year-old woman interpreted 'paracetamol four times a day' as meaning 0800h, 1200h, 1600h, and 2000h. She was pain-free during the day but regularly woke between 0200h and 0300h in excruciating pain – so much so that she dreaded going to bed at night. Retiming her medication, so that the doses were more equally spaced out around the clock (on waking, 1200h, 1800h, bedtime), resulted in a pain-free night.

"Think before you ink"

Consider non-drug options, but when prescribing any drug, it is important for doctors to ask themselves:

'What is the treatment goal?'
'How can it be monitored?'
'What is the risk of undesirable effects?'
'What is the risk of drug interactions?'
'Can I stop any of the patient's other drugs?'

Safe prescribing

Safe prescribing is a skill, and is crucial to success in symptom management. It extends to considering size, shape and taste of tablets and solutions, and avoiding doses which force patients to take more tablets, and/or open more containers, than would be the case if doses were 'rounded up' to a more convenient tablet size. For example, m/r **morphine** 100mg (one tablet, one container) is easier for the patient than 90mg (two tablets and two containers: 60mg + 30mg).

Safe prescribing requires good communication with patients, carers, and other professionals. Poor communication contributes to about half of preventable drug errors.[1] A lack of information and involvement may leave patients dissatisfied.[2]

Good communication includes clear documentation (e.g. allergies, co-morbidities, prescription writing).[3–5] The use of a patient's 'logbook' is to be encouraged; this would include important contact names and telephone numbers.

Safe prescribing practice is particularly important in palliative care. Polypharmacy, debility, co-morbidities (e.g. renal and/or hepatic impairment), involvement of multiple professionals, and the use of higher risk drugs are among the many factors which make patients particularly vulnerable to problems with adherence (compliance), medication errors, undesirable effects, and drug interactions.

Keep it simple!

Polypharmacy in palliative care is the norm. In one study of patients receiving opioids, >25% were taking 10 or more different drugs concurrently.[6] Patients with diabetes and those with COPD or heart failure are likely to be among these. Drugs should be reviewed to see whether they are still necessary, e.g. long-term prophylactic medication such as statins, antihypertensives and oral hypoglycaemics, and stopped if possible.[7]

Clear written instructions

A home medicines chart is essential to prevent chaotic drug administration, e.g. one drug or other being taken in succession 'on the hour' throughout the day with hardly any respite, and also to facilitate adherence.

Drug regimens should be written out in full for patients and/or families to work from. The recommendations published by the Royal Pharmaceutical Society[8] about the information to be recorded in writing when a patient transfers from one care provider to another also serve as a guide in relation to patients:

- name of drug (generic and, if appropriate, also brand)
- formulation and strength
- reason for use ('for pain', 'for bowels', etc.)
- dose (x mL, y tablets)
- frequency and times to be taken (Figures 1 and 2).

Details about how to obtain further supplies should be included. An alternative system will be necessary if both the patient and the immediate family cannot read.

Hospice Home Care

Name *Linda Barton* **Age** *58* **Date** *7 July 2017*

Tablets/Medicines	2am	On waking	10am	2pm	6pm	Bed time	Purpose
MORPHINE (Oramorph 2mg in 1mL)		*10mL*	*10mL*	*10mL*	*10mL*	*20mL*	*pain relief*
METOCLOPRAMIDE (10mg tablet)		*1*	*1*		*1*	*1*	*anti-sickness*
NAPROXEN (500mg tablet)			*1*			*1*	*pain relief*
LANSOPRAZOLE (30mg capsule)			*1*				*to protect stomach*
SENNA (7.5mg/5mL liquid)			*10mL*			*10mL*	*for bowels*
TEMAZEPAM (20mg tablet)						*1*	*for sleep*

If troublesome pain: take an extra 10mL of MORPHINE between regular doses.
If bowels remain constipated: increase SENNA to 15mL twice a day.

[Use this space for adding additional information, e.g. further advice about 'rescue' medication]

- Keep this chart with you so you can show your doctor or nurse this list of what you are taking.
- Ask for a fresh supply of your medication 2–3 days before you need it.
- Sometimes your medication may be supplied in different strengths or presentations. If you have any concerns about this, check with your pharmacist.
- In an emergency, phone ____________________ and ask to speak to ____________________

Figure 1 Example of a patient's home medication chart (q4h).

Hospice Home Care

Name *Nicolas Crowthorne* **Age** *65* **Date** *7 July 2017*

Tablets/Medicines	*Breakfast*	*Midday meal*	*Evening meal*	*Bedtime*	Purpose
MORPHINE (MST 100mg tablet)	*1*			*1*	*pain relief*
NAPROXEN (500mg tablet)	*1*			*1*	*pain relief*
LANSOPRAZOLE (30mg capsule)	*1*				*to protect stomach*
SENNA (7.5mg/5mL liquid)	*10mL*			*10mL*	*for bowels*
HALOPERIDOL (1.5mg tablet)				*1*	*anti-sickness*

If troublesome pain: take MORPHINE SOLUTION (2mg in 1mL) 10mL, up to every hour.

If bowels remain constipated: increase SENNA to 15mL twice a day.

[Use this space for adding additional information, e.g. further advice about 'rescue' medication]

- Keep this chart with you so you can show your doctor or nurse this list of what you are taking.
- Ask for a fresh supply of your medication 2–3 days before you need it.
- Sometimes your medication may be supplied in different strengths or presentations. If you have any concerns about this, check with your pharmacist.
- In an emergency, phone ______________ and ask to speak to ______________

Figure 2 Example of a patient's home medication chart (q.d.s.).

Generally, the drug which needs to be taken most frequently should act as the 'anchor' drug and, as far as possible, other drugs linked to its administration times. Although the SPC may indicate that an antibacterial should be given 'every 8 hours' or 'every 6 hours', for PO administration there is generally no need to be so exact. Further, although patients with opioid-induced nausea are sometimes advised to take **metoclopramide** 30min before the opioid, in practice this is *rarely necessary*.

Antacids physically interact with many drugs, e.g. azithromycin, e/c products, quinolone antibacterials, itraconazole, and tetracyclines, and reduce absorption. Accordingly, antacids should ideally be taken 2h before or after these drugs (see p.1, p.475 and p.524).

Drugs and food

Some SPC and PIL indicate 'before food' (e.g. **lansoprazole**, p.31), or 'with/just after food' (e.g. NSAIDs, p.312) when this is not always necessary. Only when absolutely necessary should patients be asked to separate out drugs in relation to food. For example:

- when drug absorption is significantly affected by food. Box A lists drugs featured in *PCF* which, for maximal absorption, need to be taken either on an empty stomach or after food
- drugs which are known GI irritants. Box B lists those drugs featured in *PCF* for which food may reduce the risk or severity of undesirable GI effects.

Box A Optimal absorption of drugs in relation to food[a] [9,10]

Take on an *empty* stomach[b]	**Take *with or just after* food**
Antibacterials	Cefuroxime
demeclocycline[c]	Itraconazole *capsules*[d]
doxycycline[c]	Nitrofurantoin
flucloxacillin	
itraconazole *liquid*[d]	
phenoxymethylpenicillin	
tetracycline[c]	
rifampicin	
voriconazole	
Bisphosphonates[c]	
ibandronic acid[c]	
sodium clodronate[c]	
Propantheline	

a. these lists are limited to drugs featured in *PCF*
b. generally 30min before first food or drink of the day or 1h before and 2h after food at other times of the day
c. also avoid antacids, iron, zinc or milk for 2h before or after each dose to improve absorption
d. itraconazole liquid requires an empty stomach for full absorption, whereas food significantly improves the absorption of itraconazole capsules.

Box B Drugs for which food *may* reduce the risk of nausea/vomiting or GI irritation[a]

Baclofen	Iron
Corticosteroids	Potassium
Etamsylate (not UK)	Spironolactone
Metronidazole	Tinidazole
Misoprostol	Venlafaxine
NSAIDs[b]	Zinc

a. this list is limited to drugs which feature in the *PCF*
b. no substantial evidence.

In addition:

- drugs for diabetes and **pancreatin** should always be taken as recommended in relation to food/meal times
- in order to increase the contact time of the drug with the mucosa, food should *not* be taken immediately after drugs have been administered via the buccal mucosa (e.g. transmucosal **fentanyl**) or those used topically to treat oral ulceration or oral candidosis.

Monitoring medication

It is often difficult to predict the optimum dose of a symptom relief drug, particularly opioids, laxatives and psychotropics. Further, undesirable effects put drug adherence in jeopardy. Thus, arrangements must be made for monitoring the effects of medication. The responsibility for monitoring must be clearly stated; shared care is a definite risk factor for medication errors and problematic polypharmacy.[2,11]

Albumin binds acidic drugs, e.g. **phenytoin**, **warfarin**, **digoxin**, **naproxen** and **lorazepam**. When the albumin level is reduced by malnutrition, cirrhosis, nephrotic syndrome, and/or end-stage renal disease, the proportion of unbound (active) drug increases. This increases the probability of toxicity with standard drug doses and normal total plasma drug concentrations, particularly with highly protein-bound drugs.

Most measured drug concentrations reflect the total drug concentration in the plasma (i.e. bound and unbound). Measuring free (unbound) levels of highly protein-bound drugs is not always possible but formulas to 'correct' for low plasma protein concentrations are available for some drugs, e.g. **phenytoin** (see p.263).

Compromise is sometimes necessary

It may be necessary to compromise on complete relief in order to avoid unacceptable undesirable effects. Antimuscarinic effects, e.g. dry mouth and visual disturbance, may limit dose escalation. Also, with inoperable bowel obstruction, it may be better to aim to reduce the incidence of vomiting to once or twice a day rather than to seek complete control.

Rescue ('as needed') medication

Patients need advice about what to do for intermittent symptoms, particularly break-through pain. Generally, it is good practice to err on the side of generosity in relation to the recommended frequency of p.r.n. medication. However, it does depend on the class and formulation of the drug in question, and whether the patient is an inpatient or at home.

In all circumstances, it is important that the dose and permitted frequency is stated clearly on the patient's medication chart (see Figure 1and Figure 2), and also verbally explained to the patient and the family.

Patients taking regular m/r strong opioid medication at home

The *corresponding* immediate-release opioid analgesic formulation should also be prescribed q1h p.r.n. in an appropriate dose (see p.297).

Patients taking regular immediate-release strong opioid medication at home

The *same* immediate-release opioid analgesic formulation should also be prescribed routinely q1h p.r.n. in an appropriate dose (see p.297).

With regular immediate-release strong opioids, if a patient needs an *occasional* rescue dose, say, 40min or less before the next regular dose is due, it may suffice to give the next regular dose early. However, opinion is divided. Some specialists say that a p.r.n. dose should be given, followed in due course by the regular dose.

Patients taking regular analgesic medication other than a strong opioid

If receiving the maximum recommended dose of **paracetamol** or NSAID, a low dose of an immediate-release strong opioid/morphine can be prescribed *q2h p.r.n.* Recommendations for anti-emetics, laxatives, and psychotropics are given in their respective sections.

Inpatients

Recommendations can be more generous because there are trained personnel to monitor the effect of any additional medication, and thus prevent serious toxicity. For example, prescribing a range of permitted doses allows nurses to increase the amount given on their own initiative.

Example: Patient taking m/r **morphine** 100mg b.d.
Expected p.r.n. dose = 1/10–1/6 of total 24h dose, i.e. 20–30mg
Prescribe **morphine** immediate-release tablets/suspension 20–30mg q1h p.r.n.

In practice, nurses tend to start with the lower dose, but increase to the top of the range if necessary. If two consecutive top-of-the-range doses at the maximum permitted frequency are insufficient, medical advice should be obtained and alternative measures considered, e.g. rapid titration with IV **morphine** (see p.375 and Boxes B and C, p.381), with a subsequent upward adjustment of the regular PO dose.

REVIEWING MEDICATION WHEN A PATIENT IS CLOSE TO DEATH

When a patient is clearly approaching death:

- *simplify medication:* stop long-term prophylactic medication if not already done so, e.g. statins, antihypertensives, oral hypoglycaemics, **warfarin**
- *when the patient is moribund:* stop antidepressants and laxatives
- *anticipate and prescribe drugs p.r.n.* for common end-of-life problems, e.g. pain, breathlessness, vomiting, agitation, delirium, myoclonus, death rattle (see below)
- *prescribe all drugs both PO and SC/IV*
- *insulin-dependent diabetes:* reduce the dose of **insulin** as intake decreases (see p.533).
- *review need for IV hydration:* is it still appropriate? Can it be stopped?

For advice about stopping **dexamethasone** in patients with intracranial malignancy, see p.521.

In the last days, some nursing procedures normally regarded as essential may be discontinued. For example, standard care of pressure areas may cause a moribund patient to become distressed. If so, such care should be reduced or stopped.

'As needed' medication

Because patients close to death may well have increasing difficulty in swallowing, non-PO p.r.n. drugs should be prescribed (in addition to any existing PO p.r.n. drugs) in case of new distressing symptoms.

In some countries, SL, PR and TD products are preferred but, in the UK, SC injections are generally used. A typical pre-emptive regimen would include:

- **morphine** SC q1h p.r.n. (*dose depends on regular dose*) for pain, breathlessness, cough
- **haloperidol** 1–5mg SC q1h p.r.n. for nausea and vomiting, delirium
- **midazolam** 2.5–5mg SC q1h p.r.n. for anxiety, breathlessness; and, if seizures are likely, 10mg SC q1h p.r.n. (also see Anti-epileptic drugs, Box B, p.265)
- **hyoscine *butylbromide*** 20mg SC q1h p.r.n. for bowel colic, death rattle.

Note. Charting all these drugs 'q1h p.r.n.' facilitates rapid dose titration. However, if after several q1h doses there is no benefit or any benefit is short-lived, it is important to consider if an alternative or an additional drug is needed (also see Chapter 15, p.671).

Other drugs may be necessary in various circumstances, e.g. renal failure (see p.681), heart failure (see p.665), and Parkinson's disease (see p.667).

PRESCRIBING FOR THE ELDERLY

Elderly patients taking five or more drugs have a significantly increased risk of delirium and falls, the latter possibly related to postural hypotension.

The majority of patients receiving palliative care are elderly (≥65 years old). They are more likely to be receiving multiple drugs for existing comorbid conditions. The addition of more drugs for symptom relief may adversely affect adherence, and increases the risk of drug interactions (see Chapter 19, p.717) and adverse reactions.[6]

Presentation of adverse drug reactions in the elderly may be atypical and non-specific, and wrongly be attributed to a new medical problem. Drugs should be reviewed regularly and any of doubtful benefit should be stopped.[12,13] These include drugs for primary and secondary prevention which become irrelevant for a patient with a poor prognosis, e.g. statins, and drugs which do not treat symptoms caused by an underlying disease.[14,15]

Drug formulation and administration

Frail elderly patients may have difficulty swallowing tablets. They should be instructed to take tablets or capsules with fluid in an upright position to minimize the possibility of them remaining in the mouth or oesophagus, and causing ulceration (e.g. NSAIDs, **temazepam**). Alternative formulations (e.g. liquid) or routes of administration (e.g. SC) may be preferable (see Chapter 28, p.785).

Pharmacokinetics

With increasing age, several changes occur which influence the pharmacokinetics of many drugs. The most important of these is the progressive decline in renal function. Drugs are excreted more slowly and a lower dose may suffice, particularly those with a narrow therapeutic ratio, e.g. **digoxin** (also see p.681). Acute illness, particularly accompanied by dehydration, can lead to a rapid further reduction in renal clearance.

Reduction in liver size and blood flow may reduce hepatic metabolism (also see p.700). Drugs with significant first-pass metabolism, e.g. **amitriptyline**, **glyceryl trinitrate**, **morphine**, may have higher bio-availability and a faster onset, necessitating starting with lower doses and/or at less frequent intervals.

Box C Examples of risks when prescribing for the elderly

Antidepressants
Postural hypotension, sedation, delirium, falls and femoral fracture.

Antimuscarinics
Falls, delirium, urinary retention, constipation.

Antihypertensives, digoxin, psychotropics
Undesirable effects more common; use smaller doses and monitor closely.

Hypoglycaemics
Chlorpropamide (not UK) and glibenclamide are best avoided because of their long halflives and consequential risk of hypoglycaemia.

Night sedatives (hypnotics), including Z drugs
Cognitive impairment, delirium, falls, fractures; use a short course of a drug with a short halflife.

Nitrofurantoin
Lack of efficacy in patients with creatinine clearance <60mL/min because of inadequate urinary drug concentration.

NSAIDs
Serious GI bleeding is more common; may exacerbate fluid retention in patients with heart disease or renal impairment.

Reduction in lean body mass and increase in body fat will alter distribution of lipophilic drugs, e.g. benzodiazepines and **fentanyl**. When first given, these drugs will be stored in body fat, reducing their initial effect, but repeated administration may lead to prolonged release and significantly increased drug plasma concentrations.[14]

Pharmacodynamics

The ageing body has an increased sensitivity to drugs, notably centrally-acting psychotropics and opioids (Box C).[16]

END-STAGE HEART FAILURE

In some *cancer patients*, congestive heart failure (CHF) is a significant cause of breathlessness. It is important to recognize this, and treat appropriately.

More detailed guidance about the care of patients with end-stage CHF is available from NICE[17] and elsewhere.[18–20] Resources include:

- *Supportive Care in Heart Failure*[21]
- *Heart Failure: from Advanced Disease to Bereavement*[22]
- *Heart Failure and Palliative Care: a team approach.*[23]

This section provides guidance about which drugs can be stopped to ease a patient's 'tablet burden' without adversely affecting the level of comfort.[24] In end-stage CHF, it is important *not* to stop 'disease control' medication which also has an important contribution in symptom relief. Unlike cancer, where disease-specific treatment tends to become increasingly burdensome and futile (and possibly counterproductive), the continued disease-specific treatment of CHF generally continues to be essential for symptom management even when end-stage (Figure 3). If in doubt, and for patients with CHF and preserved systolic ejection fraction, obtain advice from the patient's cardiologist or specialist heart failure nurse.

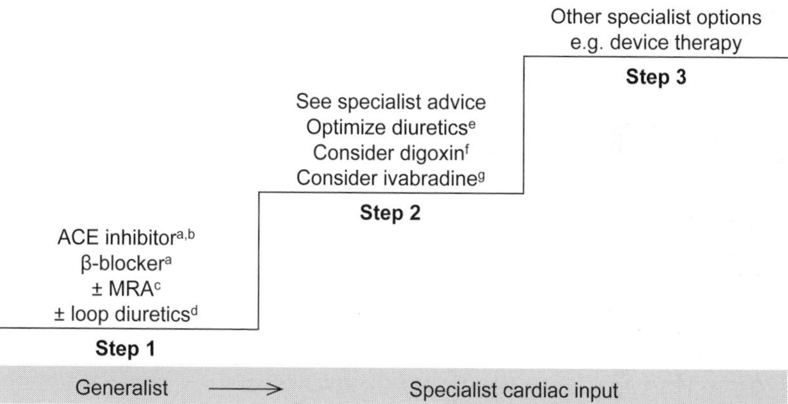

Figure 3 Synopsis of guidance for drug treatment of CHF with reduced systolic ejection fraction.

a. in all patients who are stable, i.e. minimal or no signs of fluid overload or depletion, even if asymptomatic
b. if an ACE inhibitor is not tolerated, substitute an adrenoreceptor blocker (ARB), e.g. losartan
c. MRAs (mineralocorticoid antagonists) include spironolactone and eplerenone
d. in patients with signs of fluid overload
e. thiazide diuretics and those affecting the renal distal tubule may be added, e.g. bendroflumethiazide, metolozone
f. digoxin can be considered irrespective of presence or absence of arrhythmias
g. ivabradine is used to slow heart rate to <75 beats per minute for those in sinus rhythm.

Drugs that improve survival and symptoms

Aldosterone antagonists, angiotensin-converting enzyme (ACE) inhibitors; angiotensin receptor blockers; β-blockers

These should generally be continued because there is good evidence that in CHF with a reduced systolic ejection fraction they slow progression, prolong survival, and improve symptom control.[25–31] Indications for considering a dose reduction or discontinuation on either a temporary or permanent basis are:

- symptomatic hypotension
- deteriorating renal function
- excessive tablet burden.

The patient's clinical condition, electrolytes and renal function should be monitored closely, and further dose adjustments made (up or down) as necessary (also see p.67).

Drugs that primarily improve symptoms in advanced disease

Loop diuretics

Furosemide (see p.61) and **bumetanide** are widely used.[32,33] In very end-stage disease, the increasing dose necessary for symptom control may exacerbate renal dysfunction. However, unless the patient becomes anuric or clinically hypovolaemic, a loop diuretic should be continued for symptom management. **Furosemide** by CSCI may reduce the need for hospital admission (see p.65).[34,35]

Anti-arrhythmic drugs

Anti-arrhythmic drugs can generally be considered for discontinuation at a relatively early stage. Most anti-arrhythmics lower blood pressure and can contribute to fatigue. However, if *symptomatic* tachycardias are present, or rate control is also helping angina symptoms, it may be best to continue. **Amiodarone** has a very long halflife (some 6 months) and thus can generally be stopped in end-stage CHF.

Anti-anginal agents

These can be discontinued if the patient has no angina. However, low-dose **isosorbide mononitrate**, with an 8h nitrate-free interval/24h, may help breathlessness.

Simplify long-term medication

Drugs for long-term prophylaxis and for co-morbid conditions need to be reviewed as in any other end-stage disease, bearing in mind the likely impact of discontinuation, e.g. **warfarin** (see p.87), thyroid replacement therapy.

This is particularly important for NSAIDs because of evidence regarding increased risk of hospitalization when used in CHF.[36] As always, an individual value judgement will be necessary. Consideration should be given to the undesirable effects of other drugs which may exacerbate symptom burden in CHF, particularly those with antimuscarinic effects (e.g. cyclizine), renal toxicity (e.g. NSAIDs), cardiac arrhythmias (e.g. TCAs) or those which may result in fluid retention (e.g. steroids, antihistamines, NSAIDs, gabapentinoids).

Statins

Cholesterol-lowering drugs can generally be the first to be discontinued because they have no symptom-relieving properties.[37]

Antihypertensive drugs

These are generally inappropriate in end-stage disease.

Digoxin

In atrial fibrillation, **digoxin** may be important for rate control. Uncontrolled fast atrial fibrillation may be unpleasant for the patient and exacerbate symptoms. In patients in sinus rhythm, symptoms are less likely to worsen if digoxin is stopped.[38] If renal failure develops as the heart failure progresses, accumulation could lead to toxicity.

END-STAGE IDIOPATHIC PARKINSON'S DISEASE

Patients with idiopathic Parkinson's disease (IPD) can die directly from IPD or from a concurrent condition (e.g. cancer). Consequently, patients with IPD can be at differing stages as they approach death, and thus may have different degrees of dopamine responsiveness.

Even at the end of life, dopamine can be important for the control of rigidity, bradykinesia, tremor, and pain in these patients. Thus, one of the key challenges is to assess and optimize dopamine treatment as they deteriorate. A further challenge is trying to avoid centrally acting D_2 antagonists (e.g. antipsychotics, **metoclopramide**) because they exacerbate IPD, particularly rigidity and the associated pain.

Although predicting prognosis in idiopathic IPD is often difficult, a progressive decline in physical status, continuing weight loss, recurrent infections, cognitive impairment, swallowing problems, and episodes of aspiration pneumonia strongly suggest that the patient may be at the end-stage. Given the unreliability of prognostication, frequent review is necessary. When deterioration is rapid, this may need to be daily (see p.663). Each patient requires careful individual evaluation; and, when possible, there should be ongoing liaison with an IPD specialist.

A rapid decline from diagnosis (within 3–5 years) with a poor response to **levodopa** could indicate a 'PD plus syndrome' (e.g. progressive supranuclear palsy, multisystem atrophy). Most of these patients die some 6–9 years after diagnosis. The approach to palliative care in these conditions is the same as for IPD, namely, determining dopamine responsiveness (often poorer in these groups) and avoiding drugs which may exacerbate symptoms (e.g. **haloperidol** and **metoclopramide**).

In the last few days of life the patient with IPD is likely *not* to be able to swallow.[39] An attempt to continue dopaminergic drugs should be made in patients dying with concurrent IPD (see below). On the other hand, in patients dying from IPD, withdrawal of dopaminergic drugs is sometimes appropriate because of loss of efficacy and/or increased undesirable effects, e.g. agitation, delirium, hallucinations.[40]

Rigidity

Rigidity is not always a major issue for patients with end-stage IPD, and many tolerate a reduction in their often complex IPD drug regimens. On the other hand, important causes of rigidity towards the end of life are:

- not getting dopaminergic drugs on time
- an inability to swallow medication
- worsening IPD which is less dopamine-responsive.

Thus, if the patient can still swallow, ensure that medication is given on time, and consider prescribing p.r.n. doses of dispersible Madopar®, e.g. 62.5mg (= **benserazide** 12.5mg + **levodopa** 50mg).

If the patient is not able swallow, consider giving previous dopaminergic medication via an existing PEG or an NG tube. Alternatively, discuss the use of one of the following parenteral dopamine agonists with a PD specialist:

- TD **rotigotine**:
  - ▷ start with a 2mg/24h patch; use a fresh site each day
  - ▷ if necessary, after 1 week, increase to 4mg/24h
  - ▷ maximum recommended dose = 8mg/24h
- SC **apomorphine**; also prescribe prophylactic **domperidone** to prevent almost inevitable nausea.[41]

Relieving rigidity without causing delirium or hallucinations can be difficult. Both **rotigotine** and **apomorphine** can cause delirium ± agitation; generally use only with guidance from a PD specialist.

If dopaminergic medication is stopped, **midazolam** 5–10mg/24h by CSCI may help relieve rigidity. Optimal nursing care and gentle physiotherapy are also crucial.

Pain

Careful evaluation is needed to determine if pain is related to rigidity or to some other cause. Different pains often require different approaches to management:

- if related to rigidity, see above
- If not, consider:
  - ▷ non-drug treatment, e.g. positioning, nursing care, physiotherapy, massage, heat, TENS
  - ▷ drug treatment (see p.295).

Nausea and vomiting

Metoclopramide, **haloperidol** and **prochlorperazine** are D_2 antagonists (see p.235), and ideally should be avoided in IPD because they will exacerbate rigidity and bradykinesia. Despite being D_2 antagonists, it may sometimes be necessary to prescribe small doses of **levomepromazine** (e.g. 2.5–5mg PO/SC at bedtime, see p.184) or **olanzapine** (e.g. 1.25–2.5mg PO at bedtime, see p.187) if all else fails.

Anecdotal reports suggest that **cyclizine** may also exacerbate IPD. Anti-emetics *least* likely to exacerbate IPD are:

- **domperidone** (see p.247)
- **ondansetron** (see p.253)
- **hyoscine *hydrobromide*** (see p.19), but may exacerbate delirium.

Delirium and agitation

Remember: both **rotigotine** and **apomorphine** can cause delirium ± agitation.

There may well be need for a 'trade-off' between increased rigidity (and the consequential pain) and the relief of an agitated delirium. However, there are many potential causes for delirium and agitation in end-stage IPD and, as always, a systematic approach is necessary:

- if feasible, treat any obvious underlying cause, e.g. constipation and/or urinary retention
- review dopaminergic drugs; discuss with the PD team the best order for stopping these
- this generally results in **levodopa** monotherapy, and perhaps reducing the dose of this as well
- if the patient can swallow, consider **quetiapine** (e.g. 25mg PO once daily–b.d.), an atypical antipsychotic available only as an oral product but the one least likely to cause extrapyramidal movement disorders
- if the patient cannot swallow, consider a benzodiazepine (see p.149) *but be aware that this sometimes exacerbate delirium*, e.g.:
  - ▷ **midazolam** 2.5mg SC p.r.n.
  - ▷ **lorazepam** 0.5–1mg SL p.r.n.
- if the situation remains unsatisfactory, prescribe an injectable antipsychotic, e.g. **levomepromazine** 6.25–12.5mg SC p.r.n. (see p.184).

The use of **levomepromazine** will generally result in a reduction in the patient's level of consciousness, but will exacerbate PD less than **haloperidol**.

Some patients with PD also have dementia, commonly Alzheimer's or dementia with Lewy bodies (DLB).[42,43] Extra care needs to be taken in DLB. About 50% of such patients are oversensitive to antipsychotics and, if used, they will experience a marked exacerbation of the PD, reduced level of consciousness, increased delirium, and possibly neuroleptic (antipsychotic) malignant syndrome (see p.173).

1 Rothschild JM *et al.* (2002) Analysis of medication-related malpractice claims: causes, preventability, and costs. *Archives of Internal Medicine*. **162**: 2414–2420.
2 Spinewine A *et al.* (2005) Appropriateness of use of medicines in elderly inpatients: qualitative study. *British Medical Journal*. **331**: 935.
3 Kanjanarat P *et al.* (2003) Nature of preventable adverse drug events in hospitals: a literature review. *American Journal of Health System Pharmacy*. **60**: 1750–1759.
4 Jones TA and Como JA (2003) Assessment of medication errors that involved drug allergies at a university hospital. *Pharmacotherapy*. **23**: 855–860.
5 Neale G *et al.* (2001) Exploring the causes of adverse events in NHS hospital practice. *Journal of the Royal Society of Medicine*. **94**: 322–330.
6 Kotlinska-Lemieszek A *et al.* (2014) Polypharmacy in patients with advanced cancer and pain: a European cross-sectional study of 2282 patients. *Journal of Pain and Symptom Management*. **48**: 1145–1159.
7 Duerden M *et al.* (2013) Polypharmacy and medicines optimisation:making it safe and sound. Kings Fund, London. www.kingsfund.org.uk
8 Royal Pharmaceutical Society (2012) Keeping patients safe when they transfer between care providers - getting the medicines right. www.rpharms.com
9 British National Formulary Appendix 3: Cautionary and advisory lables for dispensed medicines London: BMJ Group and Pharmaceutical Press www.bnf.org (accessed April 2013).
10 Sweetman S.C. *Martindale: The Complete Drug Reference*. London: Pharmaceutical Press www.medicinescomplete.com
11 Dean B *et al.* (2002) Causes of prescribing errors in hospital inpatients: a prospective study. *Lancet*. **359**: 1373–1378.
12 Cruz-Jentoft AJ *et al.* (2012) Drug therapy optimization at the end of life. *Drugs Aging*. **29**: 511–521.
13 Milton JC *et al.* (2008) Prescribing for older people. *British Medical Journal*. **336**: 606–609.

14 Hubbard RE *et al.* (2013) Medication prescribing in frail older people. *European Journal of Clinical Pharmacology*. **69**: 319–326.
15 Petrovic M *et al.* (2012) Adverse drug reactions in older people: detection and prevention. *Drugs & Aging*. **29**: 453–462.
16 O'Mahony D *et al.* (2015) STOPP/START criteria for potentially inappropriate prescribing in older people: version 2. *Age and Ageing*. **44**: 213–218.
17 NICE (2010) Chronic heart failure in adults: management. *Clinical Guideline* CG108. www.nice.org.uk
18 Arnold JM *et al.* (2006) Canadian Cardiovascular Society consensus conference recommendations on heart failure 2006: diagnosis and management. *Canadian Journal of Cardiology*. **22**: 23–45.
19 Hunt SA *et al.* (2005) Guideline update for the diagnosis and management of chronic heart failure in the adult. *Circulation*. **112**: e154–235.
20 Ponikowski P *et al.* (2016) 2016 ESC Guidelines for the diagnosis and treatment of acute and chronic heart failure: The Task Force for the diagnosis and treatment of acute and chronic heart failure of the European Society of Cardiology (ESC). Developed with the special contribution of the Heart Failure Association (HFA) of the ESC. *European Journal of Heart Failure*. **18**: 891–975.
21 Beattie J and Goodlin S (2008). *Supportive care in heart failure*. Supportive Care Series, Oxford University Press.
22 Johnson MJ (2012). *Heart Failure: from advanced disease to bereavement*. End of Life Series, Oxford University Press, Oxford.
23 Johnson MJ and Lehman R (2006). *Heart failure and palliative care: a team approach*. Radcliffe Publishing Ltd, Oxford.
24 Cleland JG *et al.* (2000) Polypharmacy (or polytherapy) in the treatment of heart failure. *Heart Failure Monitor*. **1**: 8–13.
25 Jong P *et al.* (2002) Angiotensin receptor blockers in heart failure: meta-analysis of randomized controlled trials. *Journal of the American College of Cardiology*. **39**: 463–470.
26 Shibata MC *et al.* (2001) Systematic review of the impact of beta blockers on mortality and hospital admissions in heart failure. *European Journal of Heart Failure*. **3**: 351–357.
27 The SOLVD Investigators (1991) Effect of enalapril on survival in patients with reduced left ventricular ejection fractions and congestive heart failure. The SOLVD Investigators. *New England Journal of Medicine*. **325**: 293–302.
28 Consensus Trial Study Group (1987) Effects of enalapril on mortality in severe congestive heart failure. Results of the Cooperative North Scandinavian Enalapril Survival Study (CONSENSUS). *New England Journal of Medicine*. **316**: 1429–1435.
29 Pitt B *et al.* (2003) Eplerenone, a selective aldosterone blocker, in patients with left ventricular dysfunction after myocardial infarction. *New England Journal of Medicine*. **348**: 1309–1321.
30 Pitt B *et al.* (1999) The effect of spironolactone on morbidity and mortality in patients with severe heart failure. Randomized Aldactone Evaluation Study Investigators. *New England Journal of Medicine*. **341**: 709–717.
31 The RALES Investigators (1996) Effectiveness of spironolactone added to an angiotensin-converting enzyme inhibitor and a loop diuretic for severe chronic congestive heart failure (the Randomized Aldactone Evaluation Study [RALES]). *American Journal of Cardiology*. **78**: 902–907.
32 McMurray JJ and Pfeffer MA (2005) Heart failure. *Lancet*. **365**: 1877–1889.
33 Faris R *et al.* (2006) Diuretics for heart failure. *Cochrane Database of Systematic Reviews*. CD003838. www.thecochranelibrary.com
34 Zacharias H *et al.* (2011) Is there a role for subcutaneous furosemide in the community and hospice management of end-stage heart failure? *Palliative Medicine*. **26**: 658–663.
35 Zatarain-Nicolas E *et al.* (2013) Subcutaneous infusion of furosemide administered by elastomeric pumps for decompensated heart failure treatment: initial experience. *Revista Espanola de Cardiologica (English Ed)*. **66**: 1002–1004.
36 Arfe A *et al.* (2016) Non-steroidal anti-inflammatory drugs and risk of heart failure in four European countries: nested case-control study. *British Medical Journal*. **354**: i4857.
37 McGowan MP and Treating to New Target Study G (2004) There is no evidence for an increase in acute coronary syndromes after short-term abrupt discontinuation of statins in stable cardiac patients. *Circulation*. **110**: 2333–2335.
38 Digitalis Invesitgation Group (1997) The effect of digoxin on mortality and morbidity in patients with heart failure. *New England Journal of Medicine*. **336**: 525–533.
39 Goy ER *et al.* (2008) Neurologic disease at the end of life: caregiver descriptions of Parkinson disease and amyotrophic lateral sclerosis. *Journal of Palliative Medicine*. **11**: 548–554.
40 National Council of Palliative Care Neurological Conditions Group (2011) Consensus statement for the management of symptoms in idiopathic Parkinsons's Disease (PD) and related conditions in the last few days of life. http://www.ncpc.org.uk
41 Dewhurst F *et al.* (2009) The pragmatic use of apomorphine at the end of life. *Palliative Medicine*. **23**: 777–779.
42 McKeith IG *et al.* (2005) Diagnosis and management of dementia with Lewy bodies: third report of the DLB Consortium. *Neurology*. **65**: 1863-1872.
43 McKeith I (2002) Dementia with Lewy bodies. *British Journal of Psychiatry*. **180**: 144–147.

Updated April 2017

15: ANTICIPATORY PRESCRIBING IN THE COMMUNITY

15

Anticipatory prescribing enables professional and informal carers to respond rapidly to an actual or potential symptom crisis in terminally ill patients at home. Drugs are prescribed to manage likely or foreseeable symptoms when treating reversible causes is no longer possible or desirable, including injections for when the PO route is no longer feasible.[1]

The drugs are often kept in an easily identified container (e.g. 'Just in Case' boxes; 'Breathing Space' boxes) along with clear guidance about their intended use, administration authorization and record, and a stock balance sheet.[2]

Prescribing is only one component of planning for symptom crises.[3] Planning must integrate training, written guidance, and rapid access to relevant patient information (e.g. an Advance Care Plan) so that staff can respond confidently and effectively.[4] Good communication between daytime and out-of-hours services is essential.[2,5]

CHOICE OF DRUGS

The choice of medicines must be sufficient to respond to the more common symptoms while also minimizing wastage. Thus, consider familiar drugs suitable for more than one indication (Table 1), bearing in mind relative costs.

However, fixed lists of recommended drugs are unlikely to be suitable for all patients. Choice should be adapted to individual circumstances:

- co-morbid conditions
  - ▷ Parkinson's disease: consider alternatives to antipsychotic anti-emetics (see p.667)
  - ▷ renal impairment: modify doses and perhaps choice of opioid (see p.683)
- present medication
  - ▷ if taking PO **oxycodone**, parenteral **oxycodone** generally preferable to **morphine**
- specific foreseeable problems
  - ▷ seizures or major haemorrhage: modify dose of **midazolam** prescribed (see p.154).

Table 1 Examples of drugs used for more than one symptom

Medication	*Indication*
Morphine	Pain Breathlessness Cough
Midazolam	Anxiety Seizures
Hyoscine *butylbromide*	Colic Respiratory secretions
Haloperidol, levomepromazine	Nausea Agitated delirium

ACCESSING ADDITIONAL DRUGS

Because not all symptoms are foreseeable, anticipatory prescribing is generally combined with one or both approaches below.

Palliative care emergency kits

These contain a wider range of drugs and equipment (e.g. syringe driver) which can be kept in an out-of-hours (OOH) service provider's base or car. Local guidelines, contact numbers for specialist advice, and guidance on relevant local arrangements should be included with the kit or be easily accessible, remembering the wide range of care settings an OOH service provider may cover. To carry CDs, they must be able to demonstrate compliance with Home Office regulations.[6]

Extended pharmacy schemes

These generally involve networks of community pharmacies able to offer extended opening hours, and carrying a locally agreed palliative care stock list.[7] Some schemes reduce wastage by keeping less frequently used medicines in a smaller number of locations, typically close to OOH or community nursing teams (Table 2). Some also agree to provide palliative care information, advice and an emergency contacts list for patients, carers and clinicians.[8] Examples of local practice are available in the Document library on www.palliativedrugs.com, filed under Medication issues (Out of hours issues).

Table 2 Isle of Wight community pharmacy palliative care stock list

Drug	*Form*	*Strength*	*Quantity stocked*
Commonly used medicines kept by all late opening community pharmacies			
Cyclizine	Injection	50mg/mL	10
Dexamethasone	Injection	3.3mg/mL	10
Fentanyl	Injection	100microgram/2mL	10
Haloperidol	Injection	5mg/mL	10
Hyoscine butylbromide	Injection	20mg/mL	10
Levomepromazine	Injection	25mg/mL	10
Lorazepam	Tablets	1mg	28
Metoclopramide	Injection	10mg/2mL	2 x 12
Midazolam	Injection	10mg/2mL	2 x 10
Morphine sulfate	Oral solution	10mg/5mL	1 x 300mL
	Oral solution	20mg/1mL	1 x 120mL
	Injection	10mg/mL	10
	Injection	30mg/mL	10
Oxycodone hydrochloride	Injection	20mg/2mL	10
Water	Injection	20mL	10
Infrequently used medicines kept by a single central pharmacy			
Levetiracetam	Injection	500mg/5mL	10
Methadone	Injection	10mg/mL	10
Octreotide	Injection	500microgram/mL	5
Ondansetron	Injection	4mg/2mL	10
Phenobarbital	Injection	200mg/mL	10
Ranitidine	Injection	50mg/2mL	10

INTERMITTENT SC DRUG ADMINISTRATION BY INFORMAL CARERS

Injections are regularly given by relatives and other informal carers to children or adults with, for example, diabetes mellitus or cystic fibrosis. In palliative care, there are occasions when it is helpful to train one or more relative, or other informal carer, to give intermittent SC injections (including CDs):

- regular medication which cannot be taken by a less invasive route
- emergency medication for symptoms which may develop particularly during a patient's last days.

This may include insertion and priming of a cannula and/or preparation and administration of drugs via a previously inserted cannula.[9] Clear procedures are necessary to ensure the safety of the patient, support for the carer, and to comply with Nursing and Midwifery Council standards for medicines management (Box A).[10,11] Examples of procedures and documentation are available on www.palliativedrugs.com Document library, filed under Medication issues (Subcutaneous administration).

Some emergency medication can be given SL, rather than by injection. The same procedures and safeguards are needed when delegating the administration of any medicinal product to a relative or other informal carer.[11]

Box A Procedures and safeguards for informal carers giving SC injections[6,9,12,13]

Careful evaluation of the situation by the healthcare team.

Informed consent obtained from the patient for administration by a named carer (signed if feasible).

Informal carers, particularly if qualified nurses or doctors, must not be pressured to give injections.

Both the patient and the carer should be able to opt out of the care arrangement at any time.

Carer's fears must be explored, including the possibility of the patient dying shortly after an injection.

Carers must:

- be trained and assessed as competent, and documented in the patient's notes (together with the reason for using this approach)
- be provided with written information for each drug, including the name, dose, indication, common undesirable effects, interval before a repeat dose is permitted, maximum number of injections/24h
- keep a record of all injections given, including date, time, drug strength, formulation and dose, and name of person giving the injection
- be provided with contact telephone numbers for both in- and out-of-hours.

Regular support and review of the situation must be carried out by a named health professional.

Close liaison with the primary health care team, and all out-of-hours services.

1 NICE (2015) *Care of dying adults in the last days of life*. www.nice.org.uk/guidance/ng31

2 Gold Standards Framework (2006) Check list of contents for "Just in Case Boxes". Available from: www.goldstandardsframework.org.uk

3 Finucane AM *et al.* (2014) Anticipatory prescribing at the end of life in Lothian care homes. *British Journal of Community Nursing*. **19**: 544–547.

4 Wilson E *et al.* (2015) Administering anticipatory medications in end-of-life care: a qualitative study of nursing practice in the community and in nursing homes. *Palliative Medicine*. **29**: 60–70.

5 Faull C *et al.* (2013) Anticipatory prescribing in terminal care at home: what challenges do community health professionals encounter? *BMJ Supportive and Palliative Care*. **3**: 91–97.

6 NHS National Prescribing Centre (2009) A guide to good practice in the management of controlled drugs in primary care (England) 3rd Edition.

7 Wanklyn S (2016) Improving the quality of care in the last days of life. A practical guide to getting the medications right. *NHS London Clinical Networks*. www.londonscn.nhs.uk/
8 Allanson H (2008) Medicines in unplanned care toolkit. NHS Medicines Management Network Northwest and Department of Health. Available from: www.palliativedrugs.com document library
9 NHS Lothian (2009) Patients and or carers administration of subcutaneous drugs by intermittent injections: adult palliative care. Protocol, procedure and teaching guideline version 2.
10 Nursing and Midwifery Council (2007) Standards for medicines management. Available from: www.nmc-uk.org
11 Lau DT *et al.* (2012) Hospice providers' key approaches to support informal caregivers in managing medications for patients in private residences. *Journal of Pain and Symptom Management*. **43**: 1060–1071.
12 Bradford and Airedale NHS Trust (2006) Subcutaneous drug administration by carers (adult palliative care). Available from: www.palliativedrugs.com document library
13 Lincolnshire Community Health Services NHS Trust (2015) The Lincolnshire policy for informal carer's administration of as required subcutaneous injections in community palliative care. (version 8) St Barnabas Lincolnshire Hospice.

Updated March 2017

16: PRESCRIBING FOR CHILDREN

INTRODUCTION

Worldwide, there are about 20 million children who could benefit from palliative care.[1] In England, the prevalence rate is estimated to be 32 per 10,000 population aged 0–19.[2] There are about 50,000 children in the United Kingdom living with a life-limiting or life-threatening condition. About 2,500 children die from such a condition in England and Wales each year.[2]

Although cancer, after trauma, is the second most common condition causing death in children, most children needing palliative care have diagnoses other than cancer. The largest group have neurological or neuromuscular disorders, e.g. hypoxic brain injury or inherited progressive metabolic, muscle or degenerative disease.

The need for palliative care may extend over many years, sometimes from the time of diagnosis, and is commonly needed in parallel with ongoing treatment of the underlying condition and of any intercurrent illness. Evaluation is inherently more difficult than in most adults. Further, in children with life-limiting conditions, it is often difficult to identify the end-stage, particularly with disorders other than cancer.

Common problems include cerebral irritability, intractable seizures, skeletal muscle spasm, dystonia, pain, swallowing and feeding difficulties, gastro-oesophageal reflux, breathlessness and troublesome secretions. Symptom evaluation is particularly difficult in children with cognitive impairment.[3,4]

When possible, use self-reporting tools appropriate to the child's age and ability.[5-8] A parent's report and observation by staff are important, particularly for assessment of symptoms in children who are preverbal, non-verbal or cognitively impaired. Symptom scales and diaries may aid continuity between different carers, and across different settings, e.g. home, school, hospital, hospice, and respite centre.

Ongoing care should be under the direction of a multiprofessional team,[9,10] including specialist paediatric palliative care,[10,11] ideally with advice from a paediatric pharmacist. Written individualized symptom management plans facilitate communication and consistency of care across different settings.

GENERAL CONSIDERATIONS

The general comments in relation to prescribing for adults in palliative care (see Chapter 14, p.657) apply equally to children.

Extra care is required when prescribing for children:

- prescribe only if there is a definite indication; always consider non-drug options
- become familiar with a limited range of drugs and their effects in children
- simplify regimens as much as possible
- try to avoid the need to administer drugs at school or when the child should be sleeping
- check dose calculations (often based on weight or surface area)
- round down to the nearest practical dose
- involve children in decisions about their medication (at a level appropriate to their age and understanding).

Children are at increased risk of medication errors because of:

- lack of evidence-based data
- the diversity and rarity of their conditions
- the need to calculate and adjust the dose for the age and/or weight of the child
- the lack of suitable dose formulations
- variations in recommended doses and administration regimens
- inconsistent presentation of recommended dose information (e.g. microgram/kg per dose, microgram/kg/h, mg per dose, total 24h dose).

Particular care is required when prescribing in the neonatal period (<1 month) because of immature renal and liver function, immature reticular activating systems, and higher volumes of distribution.

Flexible personalized regimens make it easier for the child, increasing adherence and minimizing disruption to schooling and sleep. However, regular timing is important for some drugs, e.g. IV antibacterials.

As far as possible, drugs should be prescribed within the terms of their marketing authorization. However, historically most drugs have been developed and tested in adults. Few are authorized for use in children, or for indications for which they are regularly used. Many are not marketed in suitable dose form or strength, and there is little age-related information about adverse reactions.[12] As in adult palliative care, there are many occasions when it is necessary to prescribe 'off-label', i.e. beyond a drug's authorized indications and/or routes of administration (see p.xix).[13]

Fortunately, there are several respected sources providing guidance about prescribing medication for children generally[14-16], via enteral feeding tubes[17] (also see Chapter 28, p.785), for neonates[18], and in paediatric palliative care.[1,19,20] A Master Formulary is available from the Association for Paediatric Palliative Medicine.[21]

There is still a dearth of paediatric data for pharmacokinetics, pharmacodynamics, and drug safety,[22] and practice has often evolved from personal experience and case series. To increase the body of knowledge, significant undesirable effects in children should be reported:

- in UK:
  - ▷ through the Yellow Card website or App, https://yellowcard.mhra.gov.uk/
  - ▷ through the PaedPalCare electronic care forum, www.togetherforshortlives.org.uk/professionals/care_provision/care_forum
- other countries have similar national and specialist reporting schemes, e.g.:
  - ▷ FDA Medwatch, http://www.fda.gov/Safety/MedWatch/ (USA)
  - ▷ Medeffect, www.hc-sc.gc.ca/dhp-mps/medeff/index-eng.php (Canada)
  - ▷ Canadian Network of Palliative Care for Children, http://cnpcc.ca/
  - ▷ pediatric pain mailing list, http://pediatric-pain.ca/pediatric-pain-mailing-list (Canada)
- to www.palliativedrugs.com.

PHARMACOKINETICS AND PHARMACODYNAMICS

Compared with adults, children under 12 years tend to absorb and metabolize drugs differently. In general, paediatric dosing based on weight alone may result in too small a dose in infants and children (because elimination does not change in direct proportion to weight), and too large a dose in neonates (who have immature drug elimination pathways).[23]

Neonates (<1 month)

Relatively low renal and hepatic clearances, and higher volumes of distribution, result in a *longer halflife* for many drugs. This may necessitate lower doses at longer intervals. Neonates also have less fat and muscle, and increased bio-availability. Drugs primarily metabolized by the liver should be administered with extreme care in those under 2 months.[24] There is a higher risk of respiratory depression with opioids (see below).

Immaturity also affects pharmacodynamics, e.g. paradoxical reactions to benzodiazepines have been observed in neonates, particularly in premature infants, probably due to the delayed maturation of $GABA_A$ receptors.[25,26]

Infants and children (1 month–12 years)

Relatively high drug clearances, and normal volumes of distribution result in a *shorter halflife* for many drugs. This may necessitate relatively higher doses at shorter intervals compared with adults. However, in infants, liver enzyme systems may still not be fully developed, and metabolic pathways may differ from those in older children. For example, **alfentanil, midazolam, morphine** all have *longer halflives* in infants (also in neonates).[24]

Monitoring drug concentrations

Monitoring plasma drug concentrations is distressing for children and generally of limited value, so should be used only when dose adjustment on a clinical basis is insufficient, e.g. **gentamicin, phenobarbital, phenytoin, teicoplanin**.

DECIDING THE DOSE

Appropriate paediatric dosing is guided by the physiological characteristics of the child and the pharmacokinetics of the drug.[16,24] Factors which need to be taken into account include the child's size, organ maturation, body composition, impact of disease at different stages, route of administration, and interactions with other drugs.

Dosing by age may be particularly misleading in palliative care where, because of underlying disease, children are unlikely to be close to the mean weight for their age. Thus, generally, the dose is better determined by *body weight* than by age.

Body surface area tends to mirror physiological processes more closely, and this should be used to calculate doses for certain drugs, e.g. cytotoxics. Generally, doses in children should not exceed the maximum adult dose.

DRUG FORMULATION AND ADMINISTRATION

Most children are able to take medicines orally, and many continue to do so throughout their illness. An oral liquid may be easier to administer than tablets or capsules, particularly for young children who are very unwell and/or have dysphagia. An oral syringe should be used for accurate measurement of oral liquids. However, some oral liquids may not be suitable because of unacceptable amounts of sugar or excipients, e.g. ethanol, propylene glycol, sorbitol. The taste of unpleasant oral liquids/tablets can sometimes be masked by adding *small* quantities of food or fruit juice immediately before administration. However, medication should not be added to a feeding bottle or left mixed with food or fruit juice.

Tablets or capsules may be preferable to large volumes of unpleasant tasting oral liquids. Many tablets or capsules can be modified to aid administration, e.g. opening capsules, dispersing tablets, splitting or crushing tablets. However, this is not a safe option for all formulations, e.g. do *not* split or crush m/r formulations, (also see Chapter 28, Box B) (p.788)

For advice on suitable alternative formulations, see Chapter 28 (p.785) and discuss with a clinical pharmacist. The use of alternative routes of administration (EFT, buccal, intranasal, inhaled, PR, TD, SC, IV) is common in children.

Many seriously ill children are fed by nasogastric tube or gastrostomy, and these provide an alternative route of drug administration (see Chapter 28, p.785). However, close to death, GI absorption may be impaired. There is also the risk that drugs may continue to be administered via a feeding tube, even when no longer necessary or appropriate. Regular review is essential.

Buccal and intranasal administration are often used in children's palliative care because of ease of administration and rapid systemic absorption. Such routes avoid degradation by gastric acid, hepatic first-pass metabolism, and the need for injections.[27] However, absorption can be affected by other factors, e.g. drug concentration and venous drainage of mucosal tissue, which result in significant inter-patient variation in response. Some swallowing of the drug is also possible, with delayed absorption.[15]

Although not recommended by the manufacturers, some TD matrix (but *not* reservoir) patches can be cut.[21]

IM administration is particularly distressing for children, and should generally be avoided. SC administration may be appropriate and acceptable for children, and is the route of choice for continuous infusions, particularly if there is no permanent central venous access.

SPECIFIC PRESCRIBING ADVICE

Analgesics, opioids

Codeine, effectively a pro-drug of **morphine**, is *not* recommended in children because of genetic variation in metabolism affecting efficacy, undesirable effects, and safety (see p.349).[28,29] Ultrafast metabolizers are particularly at risk of fatal respiratory depression. Current WHO guidance recommends a 2-step analgesic ladder for children rather than a 3-step one, by removing the original second (weak opioid) step.[30]

Strong opioids can generally be used safely in children, although this may require careful explanation to parents and carers to allay fears. The transmucosal route (buccal, SL) is often used for p.r.n. doses of **morphine**, **diamorphine** or **fentanyl** to relieve break-through pain. As in adults, doses of transmucosal **fentanyl** products should be titrated against the child's pain. The needed dose may not correlate closely with background opioid requirements, although these should be taken into account.

When a convenient strength is available, **fentanyl** and **buprenorphine** TD patches are often used as a convenient long-acting opioid formulation for children. Because of the risk of respiratory depression, TD medications should be used only after initial dose titration with an oral opioid. Extra care is necessary if a child becomes pyrexial because this can accelerate the rate of diffusion from the patch (see Chapter 30, p.831).

Other than when used inappropriately, there is little evidence of TD opioids causing serious respiratory depression in children when the dose is individually titrated against the child's pain, *except in neonates* (<1 month). In the latter, late respiratory depression has been reported, >4h after immediate-release **morphine**.[31] Compared with children aged 2–12 years, the recommended doses per kg in those under 2 years are lower, and much lower in neonates.

Of the undesirable effects of opioids, pruritus and urinary retention are possibly more common, and nausea less common, than in adults.[32] Prophylactic anti-emetics are not provided routinely when opioids are prescribed for children.

Anti-emetics

Children probably have an age-related increased risk of dystonic reactions with D_2 antagonists, e.g. phenothiazines and **metoclopramide** (see Chapter 21, p.739). Such drugs should be used with caution in those <20 years.[33,34] **Metoclopramide** (p.244) has restricted indications and generally should not be used for more than 5 days, and not used at all in infants under 1 year.[35]

Domperidone (p.247) use in children is also under review because of concerns about undesirable cardiac effects. It should be used only at the lowest dose and for the shortest time possible.[36]

Anti-epileptics

Many children with life-limiting or life-threatening conditions are on complicated anti-epileptic regimens. Interactions are common between anti-epileptics, and are mostly caused by liver enzyme induction or inhibition. They are variable and unpredictable and may increase toxicity without a corresponding increase in anti-epileptic effect.

Anti-epileptics also have significant interactions with other drugs (see Anti-epileptics, p.256 and Chapter 19, p.717). Specialist paediatric neurology advice is recommended when titrating or reducing anti-epileptics in children.

Generally, anti-epileptic drugs should *not* be stopped when a child is close to death. An alternative route of administration, and the addition or substitution of SC **midazolam** or **phenobarbital** may be necessary.

Some anti-epileptics (**carbamazepine, clonazepam, diazepam, lorazepam, phenobarbital** and **valproate**) can be given PR, but may require dose adjustment.[37] For example, the dose of **carbamazepine** should be increased by 25% when converting from PO to PR.[38] Rectal administration may also be possible for **lamotrigine**[39] and **vigabatrin**, but strong evidence is lacking.

Corticosteroids

In paediatric palliative care, the commonest reason for prescribing a corticosteroid is headache and vomiting caused by raised intracranial pressure associated with an intracranial tumour. Compared with adults, children seem to experience a more rapid onset of relatively severe undesirable effects (particularly cushingoid facies, proximal myopathy, weight gain, changes in mood and behaviour).

Accordingly, short courses of corticosteroids should be the norm, e.g. **dexamethasone** ≤500microgram/kg/day for 3–5 days for symptoms of raised intracranial pressure.[21] This approach often provides adequate symptom relief with less toxicity than continuous dosing. Following a review of treatment goals, this can be repeated as necessary.[40]

Occasionally, continuous dosing may be required. Because of increased undesirable effects and increased difficulty in weaning a child off corticosteroids, continuous dosing should be at the lowest effective dose and for the shortest time possible.[41,42]

1 International Children's Palliative Care Network (2008). Available from: www.icpcn.org.uk

2 Fraser LK *et al.* (2012) Rising national prevalence of life-limiting conditions in children in England. *Pediatrics.* **129**: e923–929.

3 Regnard C *et al.* (2007) Understanding distress in people with severe communication difficulties: developing and assessing the Disability Distress Assessment Tool (DisDAT). *Journal of Intellectual Disability Research.* **51**: 277–292.

4 Regnard C *et al.* (2003) Difficulties in identifying distress and its causes in people with severe communication problems. *International Journal of Palliative Nursing.* **9**: 173–176.

5 Herr K *et al.* (2006) Pain assessment in the nonverbal patient: position statement with clinical practice recommendations. *Pain Management Nursing.* **7**: 44–52.

6 Wong D and Baker C (1988) Pain in children: comparison of assessment scales. *Pediatric Nursing.* **14**: 9017.

7 von Baeyer CL and Spagrud LJ (2007) Systematic review of observational (behavioral) measures of pain for children and adolescents aged 3 to 18 years. *Pain.* **127**: 140–150.

8 von Baeyer CL (2009) Children's self-report of pain intensity: what we know, where we are headed. *Pain Res Manag.* **14**: 39–45.

9 EAPC Taskforce (2007) IMPaCCT: Standards for paediatric palliative care in Europe. *European Journal of Palliative Care.* **14**: 109–114.

10 NICE (2016) End of life care for infants, children and young people with life-limiting conditions. *Clinical Guideline.* CG61. www.nice.org.uk

11 Department of Health (2008) Better Care. Better Lives. Available from: http://www.dh.gov.uk/en/Publicationsandstatistics/Publications/PublicationsPolicyAndGuidance/DH_083106 (archived).

12 Jamieson L *et al.* (2016) Palliative medicines for children - a new frontier in paediatric research. *Journal of Pharmacy and Pharmacology.* **69**: 377–383.

13 AAP (American Academy of Pediatrics) (2014) Off-label use of drugs in children. *Pediatrics.* **133**: 563–567.

14 General Medical Council (GMC) (2007) 0-18. Guidance for all doctors. Available from: www.gmc-uk.org

15 Ballantine N and Bing Daglish E (2012) Chapter 17. Using Medications in Children. In: A Goldman et al. (eds) *Oxford Textbook of Palliative Care for Children* 2e. Oxford University Press, Oxford.

16 Pharmaceutical Press. BMJ Group, RCPCH Publications Ltd (2016) British National Formulary for Children (2016-17). wwwbnf.org (accessed January 2017).

17 White R and Bradnam V (2015). *Handbook of Drug Administration via Enteral Feeding Tubes 3e.* London: Pharmaceutical Press www.medicinescomplete.com

18 Wiley Blackwell BMJ Books (2014) Neonatal Formulary 7th edition (NNF7). www.neonatalformulary.com

19 Hain R and Jassal S (2016) Paediatric Palliative Medicine (2nd edition), Oxford Specialist Handbooks in Paediatrics. Oxford University Press, Oxford.

20 Jassal S (2016) Basic symptom control in paediatric palliative care: the Rainbows Children's Hospice Guidelines (edition 9.5). Available from: http://www.togetherforshortlives.org.uk

21 Association for Paediatric Medicine Master Formulary 2017 (4th edition). Available from: www.appm.org.uk (accessed January 2017).

22 Stephenson T (2005) How children's responses to drugs differ from adults. *British Journal of Clinical Pharmacology.* **59**: 670–673.

23 Anderson BJ and Holford NH (2013) Understanding dosing: children are small adults, neonates are immature children. *Archives of Disease in Childhood.* **98**: 737–744.

24 Bartelink IH *et al.* (2006) Guidelines on paediatric dosing on the basis of developmental physiology and pharmacokinetic considerations. *Clinical Pharmacokinetics.* **45**: 1077–1097.

25 Waisman D *et al.* (1999) Myoclonic movements in very low birth weight premature infants associated with midazolam intravenous bolus administration. *Pediatrics*. **104**: 579.
26 Ng E *et al.* (2002) Safety of benzodiazepines in newborns. *Annals of Pharmacotherapy*. **36**: 1150–1155.
27 Anderson BJ (2013) Goodbye to needles. *Archives of Disease in Childhood*. **98**: 718–719.
28 MHRA (2013) Codeine: restricted use as an analgesic in children and adolescents after European safety review. *Drug Safety Update*. www.gov.uk/drug-safety-update
29 European Medicines Agency (2013) PRAC (Pharmacovigilance Risk Assessment Committee) recommends restricting the use of codeine when used for pain relief in children.
30 World Health Organisation (2012) WHO guidelines on the pharmacological treatment of persisting pain in children with medical illnesses. Available from: www.who.int
31 Zernikow B *et al.* (2006) Paediatric cancer pain management using the WHO analgesic ladder-results of a prospective analysis from 2265 treatment days during a quality improvement study. *European Journal of Pain*. **10**: 587–595.
32 Hain RDW (2006) Pharmacodynamics of morphine and M6G in children with cancer: analgesia and adverse effects. *International Conference in Paediatric Palliative Care*.
33 Grosset KA and Grosset DG (2004) Prescribed drugs and neurological complications. *Journal of Neurology, Neurosurgery, and Psychiatry*. **75 (Suppl 3)**: iii2–8.
34 van Harten PN *et al.* (1999) Acute dystonia induced by drug treatment. *British Medical Journal*. **319**: 623–626.
35 MHRA (2013) Metoclopramide: risk of neurological adverse effects. *Drug Safety Update*. www.gov.uk/drug-safety-update
36 MHRA (2014) Domperidone: risk of cardiac side effects. *Drug Safety Update*. www.gov.uk/drug-safety-update
37 Smith S *et al.* (2001) Guidelines for rectal administration of anticonvulsant medication in children. *Paediatric and Perinatal Drug Therapy*. **4**: 140–147.
38 Arvidsson J *et al.* (1995) Replacing carbamazepine slow-release tablets with carbamazepine suppositories: a pharmacokinetic and clinical study in children with epilepsy. *Journal of Child Neurology*. **10**: 114–117.
39 Birnbaum AK *et al.* (2000) Rectal absorption of lamotrigine compressed tablets. *Epilepsia*. **41**: 850–853.
40 Harrop E and Sen G (2010) The use of dexamethasone in children referred to a tertiary palliative care service who died from inoperable brain tumours over a 2 year period. What can we learn? Presented at. *Cardiff International Conference for Paediatric Palliative Care*.
41 Waterson G (2006) Corticosteroids in the palliative phase of brain tumours. *Archives of Disease in Childhood*. **86 (Suppl 1)**: A76.
42 Glaser AW *et al.* (1997) Corticosteroids in the management of central nervous system tumours. Kids Neuro-Oncology Workshop (KNOWS). *Archives of Disease in Childhood*. **76**: 76–78.

Updated April 2017

17: RENAL IMPAIRMENT

INTRODUCTION

Palliative care services are increasingly involved in the care of patients with chronic kidney disease, either alone or as a comorbid condition. Because renal impairment often changes the pharmacokinetic and/or pharmacodynamic effects of a drug, this presents a challenge for prescribers.

Pharmacologically, the most important consequence of renal impairment is increased toxicity as a result of accumulation of a renally excreted drug ± active metabolites. Renal impairment also has many other consequences which may alter the effect of a drug, whether or not accumulation occurs, e.g. an enhanced sedative effect of a centrally-acting drug (Box A).

Box A Drug-related consequences of renal impairment[1]

Pharmacokinetic

Absorption

↑ gastric pH, ↑ gut wall oedema → ↓ PO absorption

Distribution

↑ oedema/ascites → ↑ volume of distribution → ↓ effect of water soluble drugs
↑ cachexia or dehydration → ↓ volume of distribution → ↑ effect of water soluble drugs
↓ drug removal transporters in the blood-brain barrier, e.g. p-glycoprotein → ↑ CNS effects
↓ albumin levels and binding capacity → ↑ unbound (active) fraction of highly protein-bound drugs → ↑ effect (and metabolism)
↓ tissue binding → ↓ volume of distribution → ↑ effect

Metabolism

↓ hepatic enzyme function, particularly CYP450 → ↓ metabolism → variable effect depending on drug, e.g. pro-drug, active metabolite

Elimination

↓ GFR and ↓ tubular secretion → ↓ elimination of parent drug/active metabolite → ↑ effect, ↑ risk of toxicity
↓ drug removal transporters, e.g. p-glycoprotein → ↓ biliary and GIT elimination → ↓ elimination of parent drug/active metabolite → ↑ effect, ↑ risk of toxicity

Pharmacodynamic

Uraemia can alter the clinical response to certain drugs:
↑ sensitivity to drugs acting on the CNS
↑ risk of hyperkalaemia with potassium-sparing-drugs
↑ risk of GI bleeding or oedema with NSAIDs
↓ efficacy or ↑ toxicity of drugs such as warfarin or statins (due to altered physiological or pathological processes involved in other conditions)
Electrolyte imbalance can increase the risk of cardiac arrhythmia with QT prolonging drugs

Hypo-albuminaemia can lead to an increase in the proportion of free drug in highly protein-bound drugs, resulting in a greater therapeutic effect and, if the serum drug concentration is used to monitor treatment, difficulty in interpreting the results, see Chapter 14, p.662. In addition, there may be:

- reduced efficacy of some drugs acting on the kidneys, e.g. diuretics
- increased nephrotoxic effect of a drug, e.g. **allopurinol**, aminoglycosides, **ciclosporin**, **lithium**, NSAIDs; this may be particularly important for patients with mild–moderate renal impairment which is made worse by such drugs.

Some of these problems can be overcome by:

- avoiding drugs which are nephrotoxic
- using alternative drugs which are not renally excreted
- reducing the total daily maintenance dose of a renally excreted drug, either by reducing the size of the individual doses or by increasing the interval between doses, see Dose adjustment in renal impairment (p.683)
- taking special care with drugs with a narrow therapeutic index, where undesirable effects are likely with accumulation of the drug or its metabolites.

ASSESSING RENAL FUNCTION

The glomerular filtration rate (GFR) is the best overall measure of renal function, but the most accurate ways of measuring GFR are impractical for routine use. Serum creatinine concentration has traditionally been used as a proxy but is only a rough guide because a significant proportion of renal function may be lost before creatinine levels rise above the upper limit of normal, particularly in patients with a low body muscle mass or low protein intake. One approach is to use a formula-based *estimation* of GFR (eGFR), which takes into account some of the factors that complicate serum creatinine interpretation, e.g. Modification of Diet in Renal Disease (MDRD) study formula.[2]

The 4-variable (serum creatinine, age, sex, and ethnic origin) MDRD study formula is the nationally adopted standard in England.[3] It is more accurate than the Cockcroft-Gault formula with 90% of estimates <60mL/min/1.73m^2 within 30% of the true value. Changes in MDRD eGFR are more reliable than single estimates, with a decrease of ≥15% likely to represent a true change in renal function.[2] Five stages of renal disease are categorized according to MDRD eGFR (Table 1).[4]

Table 1 Diagnostic stages of renal disease

Stage	*eGFR (mL/min/1.73m^2)*	*Description*[a]
1	>90	Normal renal function but renal disease based on urine findings, or presence of structural abnormalities or genetic trait
2	60–89	Mildly reduced renal function in the presence of renal disease (as above); in the absence of renal disease, an eGFR ≥60mL/min/1.73m^2 is considered normal
3	30–59	Moderately reduced renal function
4	15–29	Severely reduced renal function
5	<15	Very severe, established, end-stage renal failure (ESRF)

a. evidence of damage or a reduced eGFR must be present for >3 months.

The MDRD eGFR is expressed as a normalized value, i.e. what that individual's GFR would be if they had a body surface area of 1.73m^2. *Thus, the MDRD eGFR is not generally considered appropriate for considering drug clearance and dose adjustment because this should be based on an individual's absolute GFR.* For example, for individuals with a body surface area <1.73m^2, the MDRD eGFR could overestimate renal function and potentially lead to drug overdosing, with the converse being true for individuals with a body surface area >1.73m^2. The MDRD formula may also be misleading in situations where creatinine production, volume of distribution or excretion rate are altered, and in patients with a clearance of <50mL/min.[5] Further, it has not been validated for use in:

- children <18 years old
- pregnancy
- acute renal impairment
- oedematous states
- malnourished patients
- muscle wasting disease states
- amputees.

Thus, in palliative care patients who are elderly, malnourished, cachectic and/or oedematous, renal impairment may exist even when the serum creatinine or the MDRD eGFR are within normal limits, and it may be prudent to assume that there is at least mild renal impairment in such patients. Even when abnormal, the serum creatinine or the MDRD eGFR may both underestimate the actual degree of renal impairment.

DOSE ADJUSTMENT IN RENAL IMPAIRMENT

The need for dose reduction in renal impairment depends on the extent to which the drug and any active metabolite are renally excreted and how serious any undesirable effects of the drug may be:

- for drugs with minimal undesirable effects, a simple scheme for dose reduction is sufficient, i.e. start low and monitor for efficacy and toxicity
- for drugs with a small safety margin, dose adjustments should be based on a measure of renal function, e.g. creatinine clearance, often estimated using the Cockcroft-Gault formula (see below)
- for drugs where both efficacy and/or toxicity are closely related to serum concentration, ongoing treatment must be adjusted according to clinical response and serum concentration, e.g. **gentamicin, phenytoin** (see p.683).

For dose adjustment in patients on dialysis, see Patients on diaylsis, p.685.

Modifying drug dose based on renal function

In patients known to have chronic renal impairment or those at high risk of renal impairment, e.g. the elderly, and those with hypertension or diabetes, renal function should be checked before prescribing a drug which may need dose modification. A baseline serum creatinine and MDRD eGFR (bearing in mind the above limitations) can help to indicate the need for dose modification and serial measurements used to monitor the effect of the drug on renal function.

However, *when considering dose adjustment guidelines, creatinine clearance or an absolute MDRD eGFR should be calculated.* Because most dose adjustment guidelines are currently based on an estimated creatinine clearance using the Cockcroft-Gault formula, this should be used in preference. Alternatively, the MDRD eGFR can be converted to an absolute value:

Cockcroft-Gault formula

$$\text{Creatinine clearance} = \frac{F \times [140 - \text{age}] \times [\text{weight (kg)}]}{\text{serum creatinine (micromol/L)}}$$

F = 1.23 (male) or 1.04 (female)

Converting the MDRD eGFR to an absolute value:

Absolute eGFR (mL/min) = MDRD eGFR (mL/min/1.73m^2) × (body surface area/1.73) (m^2)

Body surface area (m^2) = $\sqrt{((\text{height (cm)} \times \text{weight (kg)})/3600)}$

The Cockcroft-Gault formula, by taking weight rather than body surface area into account, tends to overestimate or underestimate creatinine clearance in obese and underweight patients respectively. As with the MDRD eGFR, it can be misleading in situations where creatinine production, volume of distribution or excretion rate are altered and similar precautions regarding the interpretation of results in palliative care patients will apply. It is not appropriate to use when renal function is changing rapidly.

Dose adjustment can then be made using the advice given in *PCF* or other resources such as the manufacturer's SPC, *The Renal Drug Handbook / Database,*[6] *Drug Prescribing in Renal Failure*[7] and the *BNF*. It should be noted that the advice will vary.[8] For example, the *BNF* advice on dose adjustment is now generally expressed in terms of MDRD eGFR. Nonetheless, it points out that this:

- should not be used to adjust doses of nephrotoxic drugs or drugs with a narrow therapeutic index; use instead serum drug concentrations or creatinine clearance calculated using the Cockcroft-Gault formula
- should not be used to adjust drug doses in patients at both extremes of weight; use instead the absolute GFR or creatinine clearance calculated using the Cockcroft-Gault formula
- is not validated for use in children under 18 years.

Given the limitations of the estimates of creatinine clearance, any guidance should be regarded only as useful approximations of a safe starting dose. Subsequent further adjustments are then based on response and undesirable effects, with monitoring of serum drug concentrations undertaken when appropriate.[9]

For *prescribing purposes*, renal impairment is generally arbitrarily divided into mild, moderate and severe, corresponding to creatinine clearances of 20–50mL/min, 10–20mL/min and <10mL/min respectively. However, the cut-off points vary slightly between sources.

Monitoring drugs in renal impairment

When a drug dose modification has been necessary, or for drugs known to cause renal impairment, a clinical review and evaluation of renal function should be carried out within 2 weeks, or at any time if drug-induced nephrotoxicity is suspected, e.g. symptoms such as rash, arthralgia, oedema.[2]

For drugs with a narrow therapeutic range, e.g. **digoxin**, **gentamicin**, **phenytoin**, **warfarin**, plasma levels must be measured and, where necessary, adjusted for hypo-albuminaemia using the formula modified for ESRF, e.g. **phenytoin** (see ch14, p.662 and p.263).

PALLIATIVE CARE DRUGS FOR CHRONIC USE IN END-STAGE RENAL FAILURE

Where necessary, the individual drug monographs contain specific information regarding dose adjustments for mild–moderate renal impairment.

This section provides guidance for prescribing drugs commonly used for palliative care symptom relief in patients with end-stage renal failure (ESRF) ± dialysis *with a prognosis of weeks–months or longer*. For patients in the last days of life see the separate section below, p.698.

Tables 2–8 and the accompanying text were developed to provide user-friendly summaries to guide rational and safe prescribing in patients with ESRF (± dialysis), by raising awareness of:

- suitable drugs and their starting doses
- suitable alternatives when patients experience undesirable effects
- the potential risks of using a less renally safe drug.

The tables cover the most common symptom relief drug classes, and highlight, when possible, the most, intermediate and least 'renally safe' drugs for *chronic use*. Because it is generally good practice to become experienced in using relatively few drugs well, the list is purposely limited.

The tables should be used in conjunction with the accompanying text which highlights any general considerations for that class of drug and provides a commentary to help inform choice.

As far as possible, specific prescribing advice is given. Even when a drug appears to be 'renally safe', because of the other effects of renal impairment (Box A), smaller starting doses and a slower titration than usual is generally advisable, particularly in the elderly and/or frail patient. Thus, the adage 'start low, go slow' will generally apply to the use of *any* drug, and particularly those with CNS effects.

In addition to the impact of ESRF and familiarity, the selection of the most appropriate symptom relief drug in ESRF also requires the prescriber to consider any relevant additional factors such as the presence of concurrent symptoms, co-morbidities (e.g. cardiovascular disease, liver impairment), other drugs (e.g. in relation to risk of a drug–drug interaction, QT prolongation) and patient preference.

Sometimes the cautious use of a familiar drug may be preferable to an unfamiliar (albeit 'renally safer') one. Similarly, we do *not* advocate the automatic switching of patients to a 'renally safer' drug when an alternative is proving satisfactory. This section aims to complement and not replace specialist renal unit guidance.

Additional notes on the use of the tables:

- drugs are categorized as 'generally safe', 'use cautiously' and 'avoid if possible' from a *purely renal perspective*, according to their risk of accumulation with chronic use in ESRF
- although ESRF is defined as an eGFR <15mL/min/1.73m^2, most sources of *prescribing* information use creatinine clearance to guide drug dosing, with slight variation in the values reflecting ESRF; in the tables, a creatinine clearance of <10mL/min has been adopted
- consensus dosing guidelines are presented (for methodology behind their development, see reference.[10] These include off-label use. However, it is impractical to highlight all cases of off-label use because this can vary according to country, brand, indication, formulation, dose, route of administration or patient population. Prescribers should be aware of the implications of off-label use, see p.xix.

Patients on dialysis

Generally, seek specialist renal advice. The dialysis column in Tables 2–8 provide information on whether the effect of dialysis is sufficient to require a further change in the ESRF dosing regimen specified for that drug. Unless specified otherwise, the information is relevant for both peritoneal dialysis (PD; continuous ambulatory or automated) and thrice weekly conventional haemodialysis (HD). However, because information is often limited and HD regimens are variable, some renal units adjust drug regimens for HD patients so that administration is timed to occur after the dialysis procedure.

Specialist advice should be sought for those patients on more frequent conventional HD, high flux dialysis or haemodiafiltration; drug removal is more likely and closer monitoring is required.[6]

Antidepressants[6,11–24]

Low starting doses and cautious titration are required for *all* antidepressants, regardless of whether they (± any active metabolites) are renally excreted. In ESRF there is an increased sensitivity to drugs acting on the CNS coupled with a risk of enhanced central depressant effects from the variable pharmacokinetic changes (Box A), e.g.:

- all the featured antidepressants (apart from **venlafaxine**) are highly protein bound
- all the featured antidepressants are dependent on one or more of CYP3A4, CYP2D6, CYP2C19 and CYP1A2
- metabolism will be further impaired in constitutionally poor metabolizers, e.g. **amitriptyline**, **nortriptyline** (CYP2D6), **amitriptyline**, **citalopram** and **sertraline** (CYP2C19), and the risk of toxicity increased from a pharmacokinetic drug–drug interaction involving an inhibitor of the CYP450 enzyme(s).

Concurrent use of other drugs with CNS depressant activity, e.g. opioids, increases the risk of toxicity.

Because of the time taken to accumulate, undesirable effects may become apparent only after days or weeks of regular use for those antidepressants with long halflives, e.g. **amitriptyline, citalopram, mirtazapine, nortriptyline** and **sertraline**.

Table 2 Antidepressants and ESRF. Before use, see introductory and class specific text above

Antidepressant[a]	*Halflife in normal renal function (h)*	*Active metabolite(s)*[b]	*Accumulation in renal impairment*[c]	*Removed by dialysis*[d]	*Dose and comment*
Generally safe					
Sertraline[e]	26	No	No	No	Dose unchanged PO: start with 25mg each morning
Use cautiously					
Amitriptyline[e]	9–25	Yes	Possible	No	Lower doses may be sufficient PO: start with 10mg at night *Not a first-line treatment for depression*
Citalopram[e]	36	Yes	Possible	No	Dose unchanged; lower doses may be sufficient PO: start with 10mg each morning
Nortriptyline[e]	15–39	Yes	Possible	No	Lower doses may be sufficient PO: start with 10mg at night *Not a first-line treatment for depression*
Trazodone	5–13	Yes	Possible	No	Lower doses may be sufficient PO: start with 25–50mg at night *Not a first-line treatment for depression*
Avoid if possible					
Duloxetine	8–17	No	Yes	No	If unavoidable, use lower doses PO: start with ≤30mg at night
Mirtazapine[e]	20–40	Yes	Yes	No	If unavoidable PO: start with 15mg at night
Venlafaxine	5 (11[f])	Yes	Yes	No	If unavoidable PO: start with 37.5mg daily, maximum 112.5mg/24h in divided doses *For HD patients* PO: dose after HD session to minimise undesirable effects

a. whichever antidepressant is used, because ESRF can have general effects on the pharmacokinetics and/or pharmacodynamics of a drug (see text), a slower than usual titration and close monitoring of the patient is required
b. of actual or potential clinical relevance in ESRF
c. of drug and/or active metabolite(s); 'possible' has been used when definitive data are lacking, but accumulation likely on clinical or theoretical grounds
d. sufficient to require a change in dosing regimen with PD or HD; for other forms of dialysis seek specialist advice
e. because of a long half-life and time taken to reach steady state, undesirable effects with these antidepressants may only become apparent after several days or weeks of regular use
f. active metabolite.

Choice of antidepressant

From a renal perspective, the first-line antidepressant of choice for the treatment of depression in ESRF is **sertraline**. **Citalopram** can be used cautiously, but has a risk of prolongation of the QT interval (and increased risk of ventricular arrhythmia), e.g. as a result of possible accumulation, electrolyte imbalance, drug-drug interaction or concurrent use of other QT prolonging drugs.

If an SSRI is not suitable, some renal units favour the cautious use of **mirtazapine** for depression, despite it being extensively excreted unchanged by the kidney and known to accumulate in ESRF.

Amitriptyline and **nortriptyline** may be used with caution for neuropathic pain, but starting doses in ESRF should be low. The presence of cardiac co-morbidity may limit their use.

For patients on PD or HD, none of the drugs in Table 2 require any additional changes to the ESRF dosing regimen.

Anti-emetics[6,11–13,20–26]

In addition to any specific advice because of reduced elimination, for any individual anti-emetic, lower starting doses should be used, and then cautiously titrated to response. This is because patients are at risk of an enhanced central depressant effect as a result of reduced hepatic clearance (reduced CYP450 activity), reduced protein binding (increased unbound (active) fraction), and increased CNS levels and sensitivity (Box A). All of the featured anti-emetics are affected by one or more of these general consequences of renal impairment, albeit variably, e.g. **domperidone** does not cross the blood-brain barrier.

The risk of toxicity is also greater from a pharmacokinetic drug–drug interaction involving an inhibitor of the CYP450 enzyme. For example, CYP3A4 inhibitors will lead to reduced metabolism of **domperidone**.

The risk of prolongation of the QT interval (and the consequential increased risk of ventricular arrhythmia) is higher with **domperidone**, **haloperidol**, **levomepromazine** and **ondansetron**. The risk may be increased as a result of, e.g. drug accumulation, drug–drug interaction, concurrent use of other drugs that either prolong the QT interval or cause electrolyte imbalance.

Because of the time taken to accumulate, undesirable effects may become apparent only after days or weeks of regular use, for those anti-emetics with a long halflife, e.g. **cyclizine**, **haloperidol** and **levomepromazine**. Concurrent use of other drugs with CNS depressant activity, e.g. opioids, increases the risk of toxicity of anti-emetics with central effects.

Choice of anti-emetic

Generally, all the anti-emetics used commonly in palliative care can be used in ESRF. Even those listed as 'use cautiously' are regularly used, in reduced doses, on renal units. Thus, choice should be primarily guided by the likely cause of the nausea and vomiting along with co-morbid conditions.

For patients on PD or HD, none of the drugs in Table 3 require any additional changes to the ESRF dosing regimen.

Table 3 Anti-emetics and ESRF. Before use, see introductory and class specific text above

Anti-emetics[a]	*Halflife in normal renal function (h)*	*Active metabolite(s)*[b]	*Accumulation in renal impairment*[c]	*Removed by dialysis*[d]	*Dose and comment*
Generally safe					
Cyclizine[e]	20	No	No	No	Dose unchanged; lower doses may be sufficient
Granisetron	4–11	No	No	No	Dose unchanged
Ondansetron	3–6	No	No	No	Dose unchanged
Prochlorperazine[e]	6–20	No	No	No	Lower doses may be sufficient

continued

Table 3 Continued

Anti-emetics[a]	*Halflife in normal renal function (h)*	*Active metabolite(s)*[b]	*Accumulation in renal impairment*[c]	*Removed by dialysis*[d]	*Dose and comment*
Use cautiously					
Domperidone[f]	7–9	No	Possible	No	PO: maximum 10mg daily–b.d.
Haloperidol	12–38	Yes	Possible	No	For occasional use, dose unchanged For regular use, halve the usual dose *Also see Antipsychotics Table 5, p.691*
Levomepromazine[e]	15–30	Yes	Possible	No	PO/SC: start with 6–6.25mg at night and p.r.n. up to q8h; lower doses may be sufficient, e.g. 2.5mg–3mg
Metoclopramide[f]	4–6	No	Yes	No	PO/SC: start with 5mg t.d.s., maximum 10mg t.d.s.
Promethazine hydrochloride	5–14	No	No	No	PO: start with 10mg b.d., maximum 25mg t.d.s.

a. whichever anti-emetic is used, because ESRF can have general effects on the pharmacokinetics and/or pharmacodynamics of a drug (see text), a slower than usual titration and close monitoring of the patient is required
b. of actual or potential clinical relevance in ESRF
c. of drug and/or active metabolite(s); 'possible' has been used when definitive data are lacking, but accumulation likely on clinical or theoretical grounds
d. sufficient to require a change in dosing regimen with PD or HD; for other forms of dialysis seek specialist advice
e. because of a long half-life and time taken to reach steady state, undesirable effects with these anti-emetics may only become apparent after several days or weeks of regular use
f. domperidone and metoclopramide should be used at the lowest effective dose for the shortest possible time because of concerns over prolonged QT interval or drug-induced movement disorders respectively.

Anti-epileptics[6,11–13,20–24,27–31]

In addition to any specific advice because of reduced elimination, for any anti-epileptic, lower starting doses should be used, and then cautiously titrated to response. This is because patients are at risk of an enhanced central depressant effect as a result of reduced hepatic clearance (reduced CYP450 activity), reduced protein-binding (increased unbound (active) fraction) and increased CNS levels and sensitivity (Box A). All the featured anti-epileptics are affected by one or more of these general consequences of renal impairment, albeit variably, e.g.:

- reduced protein-binding affects the most highly protein-bound, e.g. **phenytoin** and **valproate** (for monitoring purposes, or when toxicity is suspected, the free fraction plasma concentration should be measured)
- all but **levetiracetam**, **oxcarbazepine** and **gabapentin/pregabalin** are dependent on CYP450
- the risk of toxicity is also greater from a pharmacokinetic drug–drug interaction involving an inhibitor of CYP450 or other enzymes responsible for metabolism of the anti-epileptic. For example:
  - ▷ CYP3A4 inhibitors will lead to reduced metabolism of **carbamazepine**; CYP2C9 inhibitors, of **phenobarbital** and **phenytoin**; and CYP2C19 inhibitors, of **phenytoin**
  - ▷ **valproate**, by inhibiting epoxide hydrolase may reduce the metabolism of **carbamazepine**.

Concurrent use of other drugs with CNS depressant activity, e.g. opioids, increases the risk of toxicity.

Because of the time taken to accumulate, undesirable effects may become apparent only after days or weeks of regular use for those anti-epileptics with a long halflife, e.g. **carbamazepine**, **clonazepam**, **phenobarbital** and **phenytoin**.

Table 4 Anti-epileptics and ESRF. Before use, see introductory and class specific text above

Antiepileptic[a]	*Halflife in normal renal function (h)*	*Active metabolite(s)*[b]	*Accumulation in renal impairment*[c]	*Removed by dialysis*[d]	*Dose and comment*
Generally safe					
Carbamazepine[e]	16–36	No	No	No	Dose unchanged
Valproate	6–20	No	Possible	No	Dose unchanged; lower doses may be sufficient
Use cautiously					
Clonazepam[e]	20–60	Yes	Possible	No	Lower doses may be sufficient PO: start with 500microgram/24h *Also see Benzodiazepines Table, p.692*
Gabapentin	5–7	No	Yes	Yes	*For non-dialysis or PD patients* PO: start with 100mg on alternate nights and titrate slowly *For HD patients with a urine output >100mL/24h* PO: start with 100mg at night; consider either a supplementary dose after each HD session or timing the daily dose post HD *For anuric HD patients* PO: start with 100mg stat and 100mg after every HD session; a regular maintenance dose is generally not required
Levetiracetam	6–8	No	Yes	Yes	*For non-dialysis patients* PO/IV: start with 250mg b.d., maximum dose 500mg b.d. If <50kg, dose on a mg/kg basis (see SPC) *For PD or HD patients* PO/IV: start with 750mg stat and give the maintenance dose (above) as a once daily dose, consider either a supplementary dose of 250–500mg after each HD session or timing the daily dose post HD
Oxcarbazepine	1–3 (9[f])	Yes	Yes	Unknown	PO: maximum starting dose 150mg b.d., lower doses may be sufficient, e.g. 75mg b.d., titrate by 75mg at weekly intervals

continued

Table 4 Continued

Antiepileptic[a]	*Halflife in normal renal function (h)*	*Active metabolite(s)*[b]	*Accumulation in renal impairment*[c]	*Removed by dialysis*[d]	*Dose and comment*
Pregabalin	5-9	No	Yes	Yes	*For non-dialysis or PD patients* PO: start with 25mg once daily, maximum dose 75mg once daily *For HD patients* PO: consider either a supplementary dose of 25–100mg after each HD session or timing the daily dose post HD
Avoid if possible					
Phenobarbital[d]	75–120	No	Possible	No	If unavoidable, use only under specialist neurological advice
Phenytoin[d]	20–60	No	A clinically significant increase in the free (unbound fraction) can occur; high risk of toxicity due to narrow therapeutic range	No	If unavoidable, dose as in normal renal function. Monitor plasma levels adjusted for hypo-albuminaemia in ESRF, see text and phenytoin, p.263

a. whichever antiepileptic is used, because ESRF can have general effects on the pharmacokinetics and/or pharmacodynamics of a drug (see text), a slower than usual titration and close monitoring of the patient is required
b. of actual or potential clinical relevance in ESRF
c. of drug and/or active metabolite(s); 'possible' has been used when definitive data are lacking, but accumulation likely on clinical or theoretical grounds
d. sufficient to require a change in dosing regimen with PD or HD; for other forms of dialysis seek specialist advice
e. because of a long half-life and time taken to reach steady state, undesirable effects with these anti-epileptics may only become apparent after several days or weeks of regular use
f. active metabolite.

Choice of anti-epileptic

From a renal perspective, the first-line anti-epileptic of choice in ESRF is **valproate**. Although **carbamazepine** is also 'renally clean', it is disadvantaged by drug–drug interactions. There does not appear to be any good evidence to support the commonly quoted advice to avoid modified-release formulations of anti-epileptics in ESRF.

Levetiracetam is increasingly used and the availability of a parenteral formulation is an advantage. It is primarily renally excreted, and thus accumulates in renal impairment. However, in reduced doses, it is authorized for use in ESRF (± dialysis), as are **gabapentin** and **pregabalin**. **Gabapentin** is used for pruritus and restless legs syndrome associated with ESRF,[32] and this may make its use for neuropathic pain a sensible multiple-purpose option.

There is an increased risk of toxicity from **phenytoin**; further, it is disadvantaged by drug–drug interactions. If it cannot be avoided, monitor plasma levels corrected for hypo-albuminaemia using the formula modified for ESRF, see p.263.[33]

Phenobarbital is not generally used except in conjunction with specialist neurological advice.

For patients on PD or HD, specific changes to the dosing regimens are required for **gabapentin**, **levetiracetam** and **pregabalin**. The clinical effect should be monitored carefully for **valproate**, as the effect of dialysis may be variable.

Antipsychotics[6,11–13,20–24]

In addition to any specific advice because of reduced elimination, for any individual antipsychotic, lower starting doses should be used, and then cautiously titrated to response. This is because patients are at risk of an enhanced central depressant effect as a result of reduced hepatic clearance (reduced CYP450 activity), reduced protein-binding (increased unbound (active) fraction) and increased CNS levels and sensitivity (Box A). All of the featured antipsychotics are affected by one or more of these general consequences of renal impairment, albeit variably, e.g.:

- all the featured antipsychotics are highly protein bound
- all the featured antipsychotics are dependent on one or more of CYP3A4, CYP2D6, and CYP1A2; the risk of toxicity is greater from a pharmacokinetic drug-drug interaction with inhibitors of the relevant CYP450, e.g. **haloperidol**, **quetiapine**, **risperidone** (CYP3A4), **haloperidol** and **risperidone** (CYP2D6), and **olanzapine** (CYP1A2).

Undesirable effects may become apparent only after days or weeks of regular use for those antipsychotics with long halflives, e.g. **haloperidol, olanzapine, risperidone**. Concurrent use of other drugs with CNS depressant activity, e.g. opioids, increases the risk of toxicity.

Table 5 Antipsychotics and ESRF. Before use, see introductory and class specific text above

Antipsychotic[a]	*Halflife in normal renal function (h)*	*Active metabolite(s)*[b]	*Accumulation in renal impairment*[c]	*Removed by dialysis*[d]	*Dose and comment*
Generally safe					
Olanzapine[e]	34 (52 elderly)	No	No	No	Lower doses may be sufficient PO: maximum starting dose 5mg/24h
Use cautiously					
Haloperidol[e]	12–38	Yes	Possible	No	For occasional use, dose unchanged. For regular use, halve the usual dose *Also see Anti-emetics Table 3, p.688*
Quetiapine	6–14	Yes	Possible	No	Lower doses may be sufficient PO: maximum starting dose 25mg/24h
Avoid if possible					
Risperidone[e]	20[f]	Yes	Yes	Yes	If unavoidable, use lower doses PO: start with 500microgram b.d. and titrate in steps of 500microgram b.d. every 3–4 days *For PD or HD patients* Avoid due to unpredictable drug removal

a. whichever antipsychotic is used, because ESRF can have general effects on the pharmacokinetics and/or pharmacodynamics of a drug (see text), a slower than usual titration and close monitoring of the patient is required

b. of actual or potential clinical relevance in ESRF

c. of drug and/or active metabolite(s); 'possible' has been used when definitive data are lacking, but accumulation likely on clinical or theoretical grounds

d. sufficient to require a change in dosing regimen with PD or HD; for other forms of dialysis seek specialist advice

e. because of a long half-life and time taken to reach steady state, undesirable effects with these antipsychotics may only become apparent after several days or weeks of regular use

f. total for the parent drug and active metabolite.

The risk of prolongation of the QT interval (and increased risk of ventricular arrhythmia) may be higher with **haloperidol** and lowest for **quetiapine**. The risk may be increased as a result of, e.g. drug accumulation, drug–drug interaction, concurrent use of other drugs that either prolong the QT interval or cause electrolyte imbalance.

Choice of antipsychotic

From a renal perspective, **olanzapine** is a good first-line choice in ESRF; it is also least dependent on CYP450 for its metabolism. **Haloperidol** can also be used cautiously, halving the dose for chronic use. For the use of **levomepromazine** as an anti-emetic, see Table 3.

For patients on PD or HD, **haloperidol**, **olanzapine** and **quetiapine** do not require any additional changes to the ESRF dosing regimen. **Risperidone** should be avoided due to unpredictable drug removal.

Benzodiazepines[6,11–13,20–24,34–36]

In addition to any specific advice because of reduced elimination, for any individual benzodiazepine, lower starting doses should be used, and then cautiously titrated to response. This is because patients are at risk of an enhanced central depressant effect as a result of reduced hepatic clearance (reduced CYP450 activity), reduced protein-binding (increased unbound (active) fraction) and increased CNS levels and sensitivity (Box A). All of the featured benzodiazepines are affected by one or more of these general consequences of renal impairment, albeit variably, e.g. **lorazepam** elimination is not dependent on CYP450.

The risk of toxicity is also greater from a pharmacokinetic drug–drug interaction involving an inhibitor of the CYP450 enzyme mostly responsible for metabolism of the benzodiazepine, e.g. **clonazepam** and **diazepam** (CYP3A4), and **diazepam** (CYP2C19).

All the featured benzodiazepines have a long halflife and thus take time to accumulate. Undesirable effects may become apparent only after days or weeks of regular use. Concurrent use of other drugs with CNS depressant activity, e.g. opioids, increases the risk of toxicity.

Table 6 Benzodiazepines and ESRF. Before use, see introductory and class specific text above

Benzodiazepine[a]	*Halflife in normal renal function (h)*	*Active metabolite(s)*[b]	*Accumulation in renal impairment*[c]	*Removed by dialysis*[d]	*Dose and comment*
Generally safe					
Lorazepam[e]	10–20	No	No	No	Lower doses may be sufficient SL/PO: start with 500microgram/24h
Use cautiously					
Clonazepam[e]	20–60	Yes	Possible	*No*	*Lower doses may be sufficient* *PO: start with 500microgram/24h* *Also see Anti-epileptics Table 4, p.689*
Avoid if possible					
Diazepam[e]	25–50 (≤200[f])	Yes	Yes	No	If unavoidable, use half the usual dose

a. whichever benzodiazepine is used, because ESRF can have general effects on the pharmacokinetics and/or pharmacodynamics of a drug (see text), a slower than usual titration and close monitoring of the patient is required
b. of actual or potential clinical relevance in ESRF
c. of drug and/or active metabolite(s); 'possible' has been used when definitive data are lacking, but accumulation likely on clinical or theoretical grounds
d. sufficient to require a change in dosing regimen with PD or HD; for other forms of dialysis seek specialist advice
e. because of a long half-life and time taken to reach steady state, undesirable effects with these benzodiazepines may only become apparent after several days or weeks of regular use
f. active metabolite.

Choice of benzodiazepine

From a renal point of view, **lorazepam** is a good first-line choice. **Clonazepam** can also be used cautiously and is used by some renal units for restless legs syndrome associated with ESRF. **Diazepam** should be avoided if possible due to the risks of accumulation from an active metabolite with a very long half-life. Even so, some patients with ESRF tolerate it.

For patients on PD or HD, none of the drugs in Table 6 require any additional changes to the ESRF dosing regimen.

Opioids [6,9,11–13,20–23,37–43]

In severe renal impairment, opioids differ in their potential for toxicity. The evidence base is limited,[41] and recommendations need to be made partly on the basis of 'expert opinion'.

In addition to specific advice because of reduced elimination, lower starting doses should be used for all opioids, and cautiously titrated to response, not least because of the possibility of an enhanced central depressant effect. This is because of the impact of severe renal impairment on hepatic function, e.g. reduced hepatic clearance (reduced CYP450 activity), reduced protein-binding (increased unbound (active) fraction) and increased CNS levels and sensitivity (Box A). All opioids are affected variably by one or more of these general consequences of renal impairment, e.g.:

- **alfentanil, buprenorphine, fentanyl** and **methadone** are highly protein-bound
- **alfentanil, buprenorphine, codeine, dihydrocodeine, fentanyl, methadone, oxycodone** and **tramadol** are dependent on one or more of CYP3A4, CYP2D6, and CYP2B6; the risk of toxicity is greater from a pharmacokinetic drug-drug interaction with inhibitors of the relevant CYP450.

Undesirable effects may become apparent only after days or weeks of regular use for those opioids with long halflives, e.g. **methadone**. Concurrent use of other drugs with CNS depressant activity increases the risk of toxicity.

Choice of opioid

Because of the risks associated with using an unfamiliar opioid, a pragmatic approach is important. Thus, the cautious use of a familiar opioid (including **morphine**) may be preferable to switching to an unfamiliar (albeit 'renally safer') one. The ease of obtaining, administrating and titrating the opioid are also important considerations, particularly in a community setting.

In *mild–moderate renal impairment*, weak and strong opioids with active metabolites (e.g. **codeine, hydromorphone, morphine, oxycodone, tramadol**) can be used with caution.

In *severe renal impairment and failure*, it is generally preferable to use a strong opioid which has no clinically relevant active metabolite, e.g. **alfentanil, buprenorphine, fentanyl, methadone**. However, there are practical limitations to their use (see below).

Clinical experience and limited objective data suggests that more familiar opioids (e.g. **hydromorphone, oxycodone, tramadol**) can still be used with caution in this setting by:

- starting with low doses
- reducing the frequency of administration
- titrating more cautiously/slowly
- reducing the upper dose limit, e.g. **tramadol**.[38,41,44–46]

Current practice includes progression from:

- **tramadol** →
- **hydromorphone** or **oxycodone** →
- **fentanyl** or **alfentanil**.

However, some centres start with, and continue **oxycodone** as long as tolerated. For dose information, see Table 7.

When the PO route is unavailable, **hydromorphone** or **oxycodone** can be given SC/CSCI. **Fentanyl** can be administered TD or CSCI. TD is a useful long-term option when the pain is stable and opioid requirements are at least equivalent to the lowest strength **fentanyl** TD patch.

Fentanyl SC p.r.n. is a good choice when titration is required in acute pain. SL, buccal and nasal **fentanyl** products are also suitable for p.r.n. use, although authorized only for break-through cancer pain (see p.409).

Buprenorphine could become a popular choice in patients with renal impairment.[39,43,47,48] It does have an active metabolite (norbuprenorphine) with similar opioid receptor-binding affinities to **buprenorphine**, but this does not normally cross the blood-brain barrier and thus has little, if any, central effect (see p.397).[49,50] However, because renal impairment increases the permeability of the blood-brain barrier, more experience is required with **buprenorphine** in this setting.[41]

Although it has no active metabolites, **methadone** is for specialist use only because of the unpredictable accumulation and risk of toxicity even in the absence of renal impairment (see p.437).

At the end of life, consensus guidelines[37] favour **fentanyl** for analgesia in patients with *severe renal impairment or failure* (GFR <30mL/min), see Box B, p.699 (also see p.409). **Alfentanil** has also been used in this setting, but when used as a rescue analgesic, its short duration of action may necessitate frequent p.r.n. use (see p.390).

However, an automatic switch to an alternate, unfamiliar (albeit 'renally safer') opioid may *not* be desirable. Continuing with the existing opioid is appropriate when symptoms are relieved without unacceptable undesirable effects, particularly when the prognosis is hours–days.

For patients on PD or HD, generally none of the drugs in Table 7 require any additional changes to the ESRF dosing regimen. However, caution is still necessary, particularly with **buprenorphine**, **fentanyl**, **hydromorphone** and **tramadol**. If loss of analgesia occurs before or soon after dialysis, give an additional dose of the opioid.

Table 7 Opioids and ESRF. Before use, see introductory and class specific text above

Opioid[a]	*Halflife in normal renal function (h)*	*Active metabolite(s)*[b]	*Accumulation in renal impairment*[c]	*Removed by dialysis*[d]	*Dose and comment*
Generally safe					
Alfentanil	1.5	No	No	No	Lower doses may be sufficient SC: start with 50–100microgram p.r.n. CSCI: start with 0.5–1mg/24h
Buprenorphine[e]	3–16 (IV) 20–25 (SL) 30 (TD)	No	Possible	Possible	SL/SC/CSCI: reduce initial dose by 25–50% TD: only use when pain is stable; start with 5microgram/h or a dose equivalent to previous opioid use
Fentanyl	4–16 (injection) 13–22 (TD)	No	Possible	Possible (HD)	Lower doses may be sufficient SC: start with 12.5–25microgram p.r.n. CSCI: start with 100–150microgram/24h TD: only use when pain is stable; use a dose equivalent to previous opioid use Certain dialysis membranes adsorb fentanyl variably
*Methadone[e]	5–130	No	Possible	No	Use only under specialist palliative care advice Start with 50% of the usual dose; requires careful and *very slow* titration; accumulation occurs even without renal impairment (see p.437)

continued

Table 7 Continued

Opioid[a]	*Halflife in normal renal function (h)*	*Active metabolite(s)*[b]	*Accumulation in renal impairment*[c]	*Removed by dialysis*[d]	*Dose and comment*
Use cautiously					
Hydromorphone	2.5	Yes	Yes	Possible (HD)	PO: start with 1.3mg q6h and p.r.n. SC: start with 0.25–0.5mg q6h and p.r.n. CSCI: start with 1mg/24h
Oxycodone	2–4	Yes	Yes	No	PO: start with 1–2mg q6–8h and p.r.n. Once pain is controlled consider switching to equivalent dose of TD fentanyl
Tramadol	6	Yes	Yes	Possible (HD)	PO: start with 50mg q8–12h, maximum dose 200mg/24h
Avoid if possible					
Codeine	3–4	Yes	Yes	No	If unavoidable PO: maximum 30mg q6h
Diamorphine	3min (IV); ≤5h[f]	Yes	Yes	No	If unavoidable SC: start with 2.5mg q8h
Dihydrocodeine	3.5–5	Yes	Yes	No	If unavoidable PO: start with 30mg q6h
Morphine	2–5	Yes	Yes	No	If unavoidable PO/SC: start with 1.25–2.5mg p.r.n. and once pain is controlled consider switching to an equivalent dose of fentanyl TD

a. whichever opioid is used, because ESRF can have general effects on the pharmacokinetics and/or pharmacodynamics of a drug (see text), a slower than usual titration and close monitoring of the patient is required
b. of actual or potential clinical relevance in ESRF
c. of drug and/or active metabolite(s); 'possible' has been used when definitive data are lacking, but accumulation likely on clinical or theoretical grounds
d. sufficient to require a change in dosing regimen with PD or HD; for other forms of dialysis seek specialist advice
e. because of a long half-life and time taken to reach steady state, undesirable effects with these opioids may only become apparent after several days or weeks of regular use
f. active metabolite.

Miscellaneous[6,11–13,20–24,51,52]

The relative safety and dose adjustments for other common palliative care drugs in ESRF are shown in Table 8.

Full data have not been included for corticosteroids or laxatives. Corticosteroids, e.g. **dexamethasone**, **fludrocortisone**, **hydrocortisone**, **methylprednisolone**, **prednisolone**, can be used in normal doses. Similarly, commonly used laxatives, e.g. **bisacodyl**, **docusate**, **lactulose**, **macrogols** (polyethylene glycols), **senna**, are also generally safe in ESRF with doses unchanged. However, because of the amount of water required for their administration, **macrogols** should be used with caution and bulking agents, e.g. **ispaghula** (psyllium) husk, avoided completely.

Loperamide is highly protein bound, extensively metabolised by CYP3A4 and is a substrate for p-glycoprotein. In ESRF, lower doses may be sufficient, particularly in the presence of CYP3A4 and p-glycoprotein inhibitors, the latter potentially increasing the amount of loperamide within the CNS and the risk of central opioid effects.

Hyoscine *butylbromide* is generally safe in ESRF, and **glycopyrronium** can be used cautiously. However, for both, there is potential for greater CNS penetration due to the changes to the blood brain barrier.

Table 8 Miscellaneous drugs and ESRF. Before use, see introductory and class specific text above

Drug[a]	*Halflife in normal renal function (h)*	*Active metabolite(s)*[b]	*Accumulation in renal impairment*[c]	*Removed by dialysis*[d]	*Relative safety*	*Dose and comments*
Antidiarrhoeals						
Loperamide	9–14	No	No	No	**Use cautiously**	Dose unchanged; lower doses may be sufficient
Antimuscarinics						
Glycopyrronium	1–1.5	Yes	Yes	Unknown	**Use cautiously**	SC: Start with 200micorgram p.r.n.; lower doses may be sufficient PO: dose unchanged
Hyoscine *butylbromide*	5–10	No	No	No	**Generally safe**	CSCI or PO: dose unchanged
Bisphosphonates and denosumab						
Denosumab	624	No	No	No	**Generally safe**	Dose unchanged; see text
Ibandronic acid	10–72	No	Yes	No	**Use cautiously**	For prevention of skeletal-related events in patients with bone metastases in breast cancer: PO: 50mg once weekly IVI : 2mg in 500mL 0.9% saline or 5% glucose over 1h every 3–4 weeks For tumour-induced hypercalcaemia, seek specialist renal unit advice
Pamidronate disodium	1–27	No	Yes	No	**Avoid if possible**	For tumour-induced hypercalcaemia, seek specialist renal unit advice
Zoledronic acid	146	No	Yes	No	**Avoid if possible**	See text

continued

17

Table 8 Continued

Drug[a]	*Halflife in normal renal function (h)*	*Active metabolite(s)*[b]	*Accumulation in renal impairment*[c]	*Removed by dialysis*[d]	*Relative safety*	*Dose and comments*
Corticosteroids					**Generally safe**	See text
Laxatives					**Generally safe**	See text
Non-opioids						
Paracetamol	1–4	Yes	Possible	No	**Use cautiously**	PO: start with 500mg q6–q8h; maximum 3g/24h IV: see SPC; minimum interval 6h
Nefopam	4 (10–15)[e]	Yes	Possible	No	**Use cautiously**	PO: maximum 30mg t.d.s.
NSAIDs					**Avoid if possible**	See text
Skeletal muscle relaxants						
Baclofen	3–4	No	Yes	Yes	**Avoid if possible**	If unavoidable PO: maximum 5mg once daily *For HD patients* Dose after HD session
Tizanidine	3	No	Yes	No	**Use cautiously**	PO: start with 2mg once daily; if necessary, slowly titrate in 2mg steps. Only increase the frequency of administration if a single daily dose is inadequate

a. whichever drug is used, because ESRF can have general effects on the pharmacokinetics and/or pharmacodynamics of a drug (see text), a slower than usual titration and close monitoring of the patient is required
b. of actual or potential clinical relevance in ESRF
c. of drug and/or active metabolite(s); 'possible' has been used when definitive data are lacking, but accumulation likely on clinical or theoretical grounds
d. sufficient to require a change in dosing regimen with PD or HD; for other forms of dialysis seek specialist advice
e. for active metabolite.

Of the bisphosphonates, **pamidronate disodium** and **zoledronic acid** are both nephrotoxic, whereas the risk of renal toxicity with **ibandronic acid** is no greater than placebo.[53] Thus, for the reduction of skeletal-related events in cancer, the risk-benefit balance favours the use of **ibandronic acid** over other bisphosphonates. An alternative in this setting is **denosumab**, which is authorized for use in renal impairment and does not require dose adjustment.

The management of tumour-induced hypercalcaemia can be complex in ESRF, because of the need for caution with fluid administration and presence of other potentially contributing factors, e.g. tertiary hyperparathyroidism, use of vitamin D analogues, calcium-based phosphate binders. Thus, specialist renal unit advice should be sought.

For non-opioid analgesics, a reduced dose of **paracetamol** or **nefopam** is preferable to NSAIDs which should be avoided due to their nephrotoxicity. However, in anuric patients on dialysis, NSAIDs can be used in normal doses.

The choice of skeletal muscle relaxant in ESRF is not straightforward; for all, changes in the integrity of the blood brain barrier may result in increased penetration into the CNS. **Baclofen** and **diazepam** (also see Table 6) are best avoided because of the risks of accumulation. Even so, many renal units report that patients can tolerate low doses of **diazepam**. However, the better long-term option may be the cautious use of **tizanidine** in reduced doses. CYP1A2 inhibitors can significantly reduce the metabolism of **tizanidine**, and the concurrent use of **ciprofloxacin** and **fluvoxamine** is contra-indicated.

For patients on PD or HD, apart from baclofen for which dosing is recommended after HD, none of the featured drugs in Table 8 require any additional changes to the ESRF dosing regimen.

SIMPLIFYING LONG-TERM RENAL DRUGS

Patients with ESRF typically take numerous drugs to manage the various aspects of their kidney disease and co-morbidities. These drugs can be divided into categories according to function (see below). When to stop drugs as the end of life approaches will depend on:

- how close to death they are
- the purpose of the drug
- likely effects from stopping it
- the burden of taking tablets.

The guidance below should be used in conjunction with specialist renal advice.

Drugs for mineral and bone disease

Calcium and vitamin D preparations should be continued while the patient is swallowing or until they stop dialysis because of the risk of hypocalcaemia. This is particularly important for the patient who has had a parathyroidectomy. However, for those who have not and are taking **cinacalcet**, a calcimimetic, this may generally be stopped earlier. Phosphate binders can be reduced or stopped as intake reduces because their effect is on the food which is eaten.

Drugs for anaemia

For as long as it is desirable to maintain the haemoglobin for optimal symptom relief, **iron** (given as an infusion at dialysis) can be continued, as can **epoetin** until the final weeks.

Diuretics for fluid control

Patients may be taking high doses of diuretics, these should be continued if stopping them is likely to exacerbate symptoms.

Drugs for cardiovascular disease

End-stage kidney patients may be taking **aspirin** and antihypertensives. These are often continued until dialysis is stopped.

Drugs to maintain dialysis access

Warfarin should be continued until dialysis stops.

LAST DAYS OF LIFE

The two groups of patients for consideration in the last days of life are:

- those already on dialysis in whom a decision to stop dialysis has been made
- those with ESRF being treated with maximum conservative management (i.e. all renal care except dialysis), who are now approaching death.

For the patient who stops dialysis the mean survival is 8–10 days, whereas the duration of survival in the conservatively managed group is very variable, ranging from weeks to more than a year. Indicators that death may be approaching are similar to other non-malignant conditions:

- declining physical function
- increasing dependence
- increasing number of symptoms.[54]

Patients with ESRF experience more symptoms than patients with advanced cancer, with a mean of 20 symptoms in the last month of life.[55] Common symptoms in the last days include:

- breathlessness (may relate to fluid overload and acidosis)
- myoclonic jerks and seizures (relate to both increased drug toxicity and uraemia)
- delirium (also relates to both increased drug toxicity and uraemia).

Other symptoms particularly associated with ESRF may continue to be a major problem, e.g. pruritus (see p.757) and restless legs. **Clonazepam** in low doses (see Table 6) is often helpful in relieving restless legs; myoclonus, and also neuropathic pain.

Occasionally, with severe fluid overload, if the patient still has a dialysis line in place, it may be appropriate to have a few hours of ultra-filtration to correct the overload.

Anticipatory prescribing in the last days of life

The general principles for anticipatory prescribing in the last days of life apply, see p.663. However, for patients with ESRF, specific additional considerations apply (Box B).

Box B Anticipatory prescribing in patients with ESRF in the last days of life. Adapted from references[13,37]

Starting doses given below take into account the risk of accumulation and thus may be lower than used in other circumstances, see individual drug monographs and Chapter 14, p.662. All p.r.n. doses should be prescribed q1h.

Pain

Some centres prescribe fentanyl or alfentanil SC instead of morphine or oxycodone; their lack of active metabolites is theoretically advantageous but it is uncertain if this outweighs the advantages of more cautious use of more familiar opioids, see Opioids section (p.693). Starting doses in opioid-naïve patients:

- alfentanil 50–100microgram SC p.r.n.
- fentanyl 12.5–25microgram SC p.r.n.
- morphine 1.25–2.5mg SC p.r.n.
- oxycodone 1–2mg SC p.r.n.

Breathlessness

The prescribed strong opioid can be used for breathlessness as well as pain; when there is concurrent anxiety combine with midazolam, e.g. 2.5mg SC p.r.n.

Nausea and vomiting

Haloperidol 0.5–1mg SC p.r.n. If ≥3 doses/24h, consider 1.5–3mg/24h CSCI.
Alternatively, levomepromazine 6.25mg SC p.r.n. or 6.25mg/24h CSCI.

Agitation, restlessness

Midazolam 2.5mg SC p.r.n. If ≥3 doses/24h, consider 5–10mg/24h CSCI.

Delirium

Haloperidol or levomepromazine ± midazolam, starting with similar doses to above.

Noisy rattling breathing

Hyoscine *butylbromide* 20mg SC p.r.n. If ≥3 doses/24h, consider 40–120mg/24h CSCI.
Also see QCG: Death rattle (noisy rattling breathing), p.12.

1 UK Medicines Information (2016) What factors need to be considered when dosing patients with renal impairment? *Medicines Q&A*. **167.6**: www.evidence.nhs.uk
2 Anonymous (2006) The patient, the drug and the kidney. *Drug and Therapeutics Bulletin*. **44**: 89–95.
3 DoH (2001) *National Service Framework for Older People*. HMSO, London.
4 Royal College of Physicians of London and Renal Association (2006) Chronic kidney disease in adults: UK guidelines for identification, management and referral. Available from: www.renal.org
5 Holweger K *et al.* (2008) Novel algorithm for more accurate calculation of renal function in adults with cancer. *Annals of Pharmacotherapy*. **42**: 1749–1757.
6 Ashley C and Dunleavy A. *The Renal Drug Database*. Oxon: CRC Press, UK. http://renaldrugdatabase.com (accessed May 2016).
7 Brier M and Aronoff G (2007) *Drug Prescribing in Renal Failure (5e)*. ACP Press, Philadelphia.
8 Vidal L *et al.* (2005) Systematic comparison of four sources of drug information regarding adjustment of dose for renal function. *British Medical Journal*. **331**: 263.
9 Davison SN *et al.* (2010) Management of pain in renal failure. In: EJ Chambers *et al.* (eds) *Supportive Care for the Renal Patient* (2e). Oxford University Press, Oxford, pp. 139–188.
10 Wilcock A *et al.* (2017) Therapeutic review: prescribing non-opioid drugs in end-stage kidney disease. *Journal of Pain and Symptom Management*. (In press).
11 McEvoy GK. *American Hospital Formulary Service*. Maryland, USA: American Society of Health-System Pharmacists www.medicinescomplete.com
12 Sweetman SC (2012). *Martindale: The Complete Drug Reference*. London: Pharmaceutical Press www.medicinescomplete.com
13 Brown *et al.* (2012) Kidney disease from advanced disease to bereavement. *Oxford Specialist Handbook* (2e). Oxford University Press.
14 Dawling S *et al.* (1982) Nortriptyline metabolism in chronic renal failure: metabolite elimination. *Clinical Pharmacology and Therapeutics*. **32**: 322–329.
15 Nagler EV *et al.* (2012) Antidepressants for depression in stage 3-5 chronic kidney disease: a systematic review of pharmacokinetics, efficacy and safety with recommendations by European Renal Best Practice (ERBP). *Nephrology Dialysis Transplant Perspectives*. **27**: 3736–3745.
16 Taylor D *et al.* (2012) Use of psychotropics in special patient groups: Renal Impairment. *The Maudsley Prescribing Guidelines, (11e)*. The South London and Maudsley NHS Foundation Trust, Oxleas NHS Foundation Trust. London: Informa Healthcare.
17 UK Medicines Information (2014) What is the first choice antidepressant for patients with renal impairment? *Medicines Q&A* 369.2. www.evidence.nhs.uk
18 Bayer AJ *et al.* (1983) Pharmacokinetic and pharmacodynamic characteristics of trazodone in the elderly. *British Journal of Clinical Pharmacology*. **16**: 371–376.
19 Nilsen OG *et al.* (1993) Pharmacokinetics of trazodone during multiple dosing to psychiatric patients. *Pharmacology and Toxicology*. **72**: 286–289.
20 Marie Curie Palliative Care Institute (2008) Guidelines for the LCP drug prescribing in advanced chronic kidney disease. *Liverpool Care Pathway for the dying patient*. National LCP Steering Group. Liverpool.
21 NHS Lothian (2011) Symptom control in patients with chronic kidney disease/renal impairment. *Palliative Care Guidelines*.
22 Royal Melbourne Hospital. *Nephrology Symptom Management Guidelines*. Australia. www.thermh.org.au (accessed July 2016).
23 Yorkshire Palliative Medicine Guidelines Group (2006) Clinical guidelines for the use of palliative care drugs in renal failure.
24 Micromedex Solution Truven Health Analytics, Inc. Ann Arbor, MI. www.micromedexsolutions.com (accessed January 2017).
25 Dahl SG *et al.* (1982) Plasma and erythrocyte levels of methotrimeprazine and two of its nonpolar metabolites in psychiatric patients. *Therapeutic Drug Monitoring*. **4**: 81–87.
26 Finn A *et al.* (2005) Bioavailability and metabolism of prochlorperazine administered via the buccal and oral delivery route. *Journal of Clinical Pharmacology*. **45**: 1383–1390.
27 Vulliemoz S *et al.* (2009) Levetiracetam accumulation in renal failure causing myoclonic encephalopathy with triphasic waves. *Seizure*. **18**: 376–378.
28 Tsanaclis LM *et al.* (1984) Effect of valproate on free plasma phenytoin concentrations. *British Journal of Clinical Pharmacology*. **18**: 17–20.
29 Sakkas GK *et al.* (2015) Current trends in the management of uremic restless legs syndrome: a systematic review on aspects related to quality of life, cardiovascular mortality and survival. *Sleep Medicine Reviews*. **21**: 39–49.
30 Asconape JJ (2014) Use of antiepileptic drugs in hepatic and renal disease. *Handbook of Clinical Neurology*. **119**: 417–432.
31 Gunal AI *et al.* (2004) Gabapentin therapy for pruritus in haemodialysis patients: a randomized, placebo-controlled, double-blind trial. *Nephrology, Dialysis, Transplantation*. **19**: 3137–3139.
32 Cheikh Hassan HI *et al.* (2015) Efficacy and safety of gabapentin for uremic pruritus and restless legs syndrome in conservatively managed patients with chronic kidney disease. *Journal of Pain and Symptom Management*. **49**: 782–789.
33 Winter ME (2009). *Basic Clinical Pharmacokinetics* (5e). Lippincott Williams & Wilkins; Wolters Kluwer Health. Philadelphia.
34 Kangas L *et al.* (1976) The protein binding of diazepam and N-demethyldiazepam in patients with poor renal function. *Clinical Nephrology*. **5**: 114–118.
35 Morrison G *et al.* (1984) Effect of renal impairment and hemodialysis on lorazepam kinetics. *Clinical Pharmacology and Therapeutics*. **35**: 646–652.
36 Verbeeck R *et al.* (1976) Biotransformation and excretion of lorazepam in patients with chronic renal failure. *British Journal of Clinical Pharmacology*. **3**: 1033–1039.
37 Douglas C *et al.* (2009) Symptom management for the adult patient dying with advanced chronic kidney disease: a review of the literature and development of evidence-based guidelines by a United Kingdom Expert Consensus Group. *Palliative Medicine*. **23**: 103–110.
38 UK Medicines Information (2016) Which opioids can be used in renal impairment? *Medicines Q&A* 402.3. www.evidence.nhs.uk
39 Caraceni A *et al.* (2012) Use of opioid analgesics in the treatment of cancer pain: evidence-based recommendations from the EAPC. *Lancet Oncology*. **13**: e58–68.
40 Sande TA *et al.* (2017) The use of opioids in cancer patients with renal impairment-a systematic review. *Supportive Care in Cancer*. **25**: 661–675.
41 King S *et al.* (2011) A systematic review of the use of opioid medication for those with moderate to severe cancer pain and renal impairment: A European palliative care research collaborative opioid guidelines project. *Palliative Medicine*. **25**: 525–552.
42 Dean M (2004) Opioids in renal failure and dialysis patients. *Journal of Pain and Symptom Management*. **28**: 497–504.
43 Niscola P *et al.* (2010) The use of major analgesics in patients with renal dysfunction. *Current Drug Targets*. **11**: 752–758.
44 Clemens KE and Klaschik E (2009) Morphine and hydromorphone in palliative care patients with renal impairment. *Anasthesiologie und Intensivmedizin*. **50**: 70–76.

45 Lee MA *et al.* (2001) Retrospective study of the use of hydromorphone in palliative care patients with normal and abnormal urea and creatinine. *Palliative Medicine.* **15**: 26–34.
46 Ferro CJ *et al.* (2004) Management of pain in renal failure. In: EJ Chambers *et al.* (eds) *Supportive Care for the Renal Patient.* Oxford University Press, Oxford, UK, pp. 105–153.
47 Murtagh FE *et al.* (2007) The use of opioid analgesia in end-stage renal disease patients managed without dialysis: recommendations for practice. *Journal of Pain and Palliative Care Pharmacotherapy.* **21**: 5–16.
48 Boger RH (2006) Renal impairment: a challenge for opioid treatment? The role of buprenorphine. *Palliative Medicine.* **20 Suppl 1**: s17–23.
49 Hand CW *et al.* (1990) Buprenorphine disposition in patients with renal impairment: single and continuous dosing, with special reference to metabolites. *British Journal of Anaesthesia.* **64**: 276–282.
50 Elkader A and Sproule B (2005) Buprenorphine: clinical pharmacokinetics in the treatment of opioid dependence. *Clinical Pharmacokinetics.* **44**: 661–680.
51 Cervelli MJ (2007). *The renal drug reference guide, (1e).* Adelaide, South Australia Kidney Health.
52 Mimoz O *et al.* (2010) Nefopam pharmacokinetics in patients with end-stage renal disease. *Anaesthesia and Analgesia.* **111**: 1146–1153.
53 Geng CJ *et al.* (2015) Ibandronate to treat skeletal-related events and bone pain in metastatic bone disease or multiple myeloma: a meta-analysis of randomised clinical trials. *British Medical Journal Open.* **5**: 1–10.
54 Murtagh F and Sheerin N (2010) Conservative management of end-stage renal disease. In: Chambers EJ *et al.* (eds) *Supportive Care for the Renal Patient* (2e). Oxford University Press, Oxford.
55 Murtagh FE *et al.* (2010) Symptoms in the month before death for stage 5 chronic kidney disease patients managed without dialysis. *Journal of Pain and Symptom Management.* **40**: 342–352.

Added April 2017

18: HEPATIC IMPAIRMENT

The recommendations in this chapter are *not* comprehensive, more a direction of travel than a detailed road map. Specific recommendations are limited to analgesics, anti-emetics, psychotropics, and anti-epileptics. For other drugs, see the relevant monograph and the manufacturer's SPC. However, some SPCs are unnecessarily restrictive.[1]

There will be occasions when hard evidence is not available, and clinicians may have to *prescribe and proceed with caution*, e.g.:

- reduce polypharmacy as much as possible
- use a low starting dose
- reduce frequency of administration
- titrate upwards slowly
- monitor for both early and late onset toxicity (accumulation more likely if the plasma halflife is prolonged)
- ensure that the patient does not become constipated (may → encephalopathy)
- beware of sedation (may → encephalopathy; see Box A).

When deciding drug doses in moderate–severe hepatic impairment, it is important to take the patient's overall clinical condition and rate of deterioration into account, and *not* rely solely on LFTs.

CLASSIFICATION OF LIVER DISEASE

In palliative care, liver metastases, chronic liver disease, alcohol and/or drugs are responsible for most instances of hepatic impairment. When severe, this affects the pharmacokinetics and pharmacodynamics of most drugs.

Unlike renal impairment, there is no one parameter which indicates the extent to which drug clearance will be affected by hepatic impairment. However, the Child-Pugh score, designed as a *prognostic aid in cirrhosis*, gives a general indication of the degree of hepatic impairment (Table 1).[2]

Table 1 Child-Pugh score: see footnote for interpretation

Factor	*Units*	*Score of 1*	*Score of 2*	*Score of 3*
Serum bilirubin	micromol/L mg/dL	<34 <2	34–51 2–3	>51 >3
Serum albumin	g/L g/dL	>35 >3.5	30–35 3–3.5	<30 <3
Prothrombin time (*or* INR)	%	>70 <1.7	40–70 1.7–2.3	<40 >2.3
Ascites		None	Easily controlled	Poorly controlled
Hepatic encephalopathy (see Box A)	Grade	None	1–2 (subtle changes)	3–4 (drowsy–deep coma)

a. Child-Pugh A = score of 5–6 (well compensated liver function)
b. Child-Pugh B = score of 7–9 (moderate functional impairment)
c. Child-Pugh C = score of 10–15 (severe impairment, hepatic decompensation).

Box A Hepatic encephalopathy[3]

A neuropsychiatric disorder caused by effects on the CNS of toxins which accumulate in the blood because of inadequate hepatic detoxification.

It manifests as a spectrum of abnormalities affecting cognition, attention, functional ability, personality and intellect, and ranges from mild alteration of cognition ± drowsiness to coma. It is also characterized by neuromuscular symptoms, such as flapping tremor (asterixis), and hyperreflexia.

It is often episodic (not persistent, fluctuating), and can be precipitated by constipation, sedatives, GI bleeding, dietary protein, uraemia, metabolic alkalosis and infections. Most of these result in an increase in blood levels of ammonia, the putative cause of the neuropsychiatric symptoms.

Grade 1
Minimal lack of awareness
Euphoria or anxiety
Shortened attention span
Impaired performance of addition

Grade 2
Lethargy or apathy
Minimal disorientation of time or place
Subtle personality changes
Inappropriate behaviour
Impaired performance of subtraction

Grade 3
Somnolence–stupor (but responsive to verbal stimuli)
Confusion
Gross disorientation

Grade 4
Coma (unresponsive to verbal or noxious stimuli)

The drug literature generally refers to grades of hepatic impairment or to hepatic failure, and not to Child-Pugh scores. Even so, pragmatically, one can regard Child-Pugh categories as roughly equivalent to mild, moderate and severe impairment.

Drug-induced impairment can be directly hepatocellular or secondary to biliary stasis (bile salts are hepatotoxic), or a combination of both. Progressive liver disease tends to cause fibrosis, leading to cirrhosis, a condition in which the disorganized anatomy results in portal hypertension and complications such as oesophageal varices and the risk of major (sometimes fatal) haemorrhage.

Portal hypertension leads to splanchnic vasodilation and a 'splanchnic steal syndrome' resulting in reduced arterial blood volume. Compensatory mechanisms initially maintain the systemic circulation but, when these fail, it can result in renal vasoconstriction, oliguria, and functional renal insufficiency (hepatorenal syndrome).[4] This carries a prognosis of weeks to a few months.

DRUG-INDUCED HEPATOTOXICITY

Hepatotoxic drug reactions can be divided into predictable (*dose-dependent*) and idiosyncratic (*dose-independent*). The predictable group is obviously small because recommended doses are at levels known to be safe from early phase drug studies. Thus, predictable toxicity is associated with predisposing factors such as high doses and co-morbidity (alcoholism, malnutrition, genetic variation). Although not completely clear-cut, the following are potential causes of predictable hepatotoxicity:

- **paracetamol**, generally with doses >4g/24h *but toxicity has been reported with normal doses in the presence of additional risk factors* (see p.303)
- **dantrolene** particularly with doses ≥400mg/24h (see p.611) and **tizanidine** ≥12mg/24h (see p.612)
- **fluconazole** and **itraconazole**, particularly if prolonged course and high dose
- **rifampicin**, used to treat cholestatic pruritus (see p.481)
- **valproate**, toxicity mostly limited to children <3 years (see p.282).[5]

LFTs should be monitored when using high doses of these drugs and in patients with pre-existing hepatic impairment.

On the other hand, most drugs at recommended doses can cause idiosyncratic (*dose-independent*) liver injury, with a frequency ranging from 1/1,000–1/100,000 patients, and with a female preponderance of 3:1.[6] Latency ranges from a few days to 6 months, occasionally longer.[7,8] Fatalities have been reported.[7]

The mechanism underlying drug-induced liver injury varies, but clinically it often resembles viral hepatitis: rapid onset malaise and jaundice with raised plasma aminotransferase concentrations.[6] Raised alkaline phosphatase and bilirubin concentrations predominate in cholestasis.

Drug-induced mild elevation of liver enzymes is relatively common and, by itself, does *not* necessitate immediate discontinuation of the drug; the situation should be monitored. The enzymes often spontaneously revert to normal but occasionally increasing concentrations will subsequently necessitate discontinuation.

Only a small minority of hepatotoxic drug reactions have a suggestive allergic component. For example, **phenytoin** can cause fever, rash, lymphadenopathy, and severe hepatocyte injury; sulfa drugs may induce fever, rash and eosinophilia; and **chlorpromazine**-related cholestasis may also be associated with fever and eosinophilia.

Hepatitis B and C increase the risk of drug-induced hepatotoxicity, as do antiretrovirals. Drugs used in palliative care most likely to cause *idiosyncratic (dose-independent)* drug-induced liver injury include:

- NSAIDs, notably **diclofenac** (5/100,000 users/year)[9]
- antimicrobials, notably **amoxicillin** and **co-amoxiclav**.

In patients with hepatic impairment, drugs causing *predictable (dose-dependent)* toxicity do so at lower doses; but there is *not* a uniform increase in the risk of *idiosyncratic (dose-independent)* toxicity.[6]

The use of hepatotoxic drugs in a patient with cirrhosis increases the risk of hepatic encephalopathy. Because patients with cirrhosis are prone to renal injury, aminoglycosides and NSAIDs should be used with caution. However, this does not mean that essential drugs should be withheld, but that high-risk patients should be closely monitored.[5]

PHARMACOLOGICAL IMPACT OF SEVERE HEPATIC IMPAIRMENT

The liver is the main site for the metabolism of most drugs. Hepatic reserve is large and, generally, impairment must be severe for drug metabolism to be altered to a clinically important extent. Hepatic metabolism includes:

- *phase I (modification) reactions:* particularly oxidation catalysed by CYP450 enzymes in the endoplasmic reticulum, (see Chapter 19, p.717)
- *phase II (conjugation) reactions:* particularly glucuronidation catalysed by glucuronyl transferases in the endoplasmic reticulum and cytosol.

In liver disease, drug metabolism is not uniformly affected; thus, it is *not* possible to predict from routine LFTs the degree to which the metabolism of any given drug will be altered. Severe impairment leads to changes in both pharmacokinetics and pharmacodynamics (Box B). In severe cirrhosis, the pharmacodynamics of centrally-acting drugs are also altered because of changes in the blood-brain barrier.

Further, *moderate–severe hepatic impairment reduces renal clearance*, necessitating a reduction in the dose of renally-excreted drugs (see Chapter 17, p.717). Thus, when hepatic and renal impairment occur concurrently, extra caution is necessary.

Box B Drug-related consequences of severe hepatic impairment

Pharmacokinetic (*see also main text below*)

Absorption
↓ intestinal bile salts in cholestasis → ↓ absorption of lipid-soluble drugs
Ascites → ↓ absorption

Distribution
Ascites → ↑ volume of distribution of water-soluble drugs
Hypo-albuminaemia → ↑ active unbound drug for highly protein-bound drugs

Metabolism
Accumulation of pro-drugs, drugs and/or metabolites
↓ hepatic blood flow → ↓ first-pass metabolism → ↑ bio-availability, ↑ halflife
Active drugs: ↓ enzymatic function (e.g. CYP450) → ↑ bio-availability, ↑ halflife
Pro-drugs: ↓ enzymatic function (e.g. CYP450) → ↓ bio-availability

Elimination
Cholestasis → ↓ elimination of drugs excreted in bile, e.g. rifampicin, fusidic acid

Pharmacodynamic
Altered sensitivity to the effects of drugs
Anticoagulants → ↑ risk of bleeding
Antihypertensives → ↑ risk of hypotension
Benzodiazepines, psychotropics, opioids → ↑ sedation → ↑ encephalopathy
Diuretics → reduced response
Hypoglycaemics → ↑ risk of hypoglycaemia
NSAIDs → ↑ risk of GI bleeding; fluid retention

Secondary phenomena necessitating extra caution
Ascites: drugs with a high sodium content and salt and water-retaining drugs
Coagulopathy: anticoagulants and NSAIDs
Disruption of the blood-brain barrier → higher CNS concentrations of some drugs
Encephalopathy:
- increased sensitivity to sedatives and CNS depressants, including opioids
- diuretics, corticosteroids (if these cause hypokalaemia)
- drugs which constipate (increased bowel transit time → increased ammonia absorption).

Pharmacokinetic considerations

Absorption

Bile salts facilitate the absorption of lipid-soluble drugs. Thus, in cholestasis, absorption will be decreased, leading to reduced plasma concentrations and decreased efficacy, e.g. **ibuprofen**.[10] Cholestasis will also decrease the absorption of lipid-soluble vitamins A, D, E, and K.

Indometacin undergoes enterohepatic circulation (and biliary excretion), and its halflife and duration of action will be increased by cholestasis.

Hepatic extraction

In severe hepatic impairment, drugs can be grouped according to the extent of their hepatic extraction:
- low extraction (*high bio-availability in healthy subjects*): bio-availability is not affected by liver disease. For such drugs, only the maintenance dose has to be reduced to allow for associated decreased hepatic clearance

- intermediate extraction (*moderate bio-availability in healthy subjects not due to poor GI absorption*): initial PO doses should be in the low range of normal, and maintenance doses should be reduced likewise
- high extraction (*low bio-availability in healthy subjects not due to poor GI absorption*) bio-availability increases, sometimes dramatically, with associated decreased hepatic clearance: the initial dose (if administered PO) and the maintenance dose (by any route) of such drugs need to be reduced (Box C), sometimes dramatically.[11]

Box C Example of drug toxicity because of changes in drug extraction in severe hepatic impairment[11]
A patient with alcoholic cirrhosis is given clomethiazole as a prophylaxis against delirium tremens. After a standard dose, he goes into respiratory failure which necessitates assisted ventilation. Prophylaxis is switched to IV midazolam and then to PO oxazepam for several days; both are well tolerated. In healthy subjects, the bio-availability of clomethiazole is 10% but, in cirrhosis, this may increase to 100%.

Distribution and protein-binding

With highly protein-bound drugs, the proportion of free drug is greater in hypo-albuminaemia. Bilirubin also binds to plasma proteins, and hyperbilirubinaemia leads to displacement of highly protein-bound drugs (e.g. most NSAIDs), thereby increasing the free fraction.

Water-soluble drugs will distribute into ascites and, in theory, could reduce systemic availability. Larger loading doses could be required but, in practice, this is unlikely to be a problem if the ascites is treated successfully or drained.

Metabolism

The liver typically converts active lipophilic drugs into inactive hydrophilic metabolites for excretion by the kidneys. However, pro-drugs such as **codeine**, **tramadol**, and **oxcarbazepine** are metabolized by the liver into their active forms. Thus, severe hepatic impairment will reduce their efficacy to a variable extent.

High bio-availability means little first-pass metabolism, and less need to consider a dose reduction. However, low bio-availability may not necessarily mean high first-pass metabolism because low bio-availability can also relate to poor absorption from the GI tract.

In severe hepatic impairment, drugs predominantly metabolized in the liver will accumulate, with a greater likelihood of toxicity. Phase II enzymes (conjugation reactions) are generally less affected than phase I enzymes (CYP450-mediated reactions), which are also affected to different degrees, e.g. CYP1A2, 2C19>2A6, 3A4>2C9, 2E1.[12]

Impaired hepatic metabolic capacity may well go hand in hand with impaired hepatic synthetic functions, reflected in an elevated prothrombin time/INR and hypo-albuminaemia, and also by encephalopathy (see Box A). These can be used as pointers to the need to reduce maintenance doses.

Elimination

In cholestasis, the clearance of drugs with predominant biliary elimination will be impaired. Guidelines for dose reduction in cholestasis exist for many antineoplastic drugs, but are mostly lacking for other drugs with biliary elimination. Drugs which undergo enterohepatic circulation will be affected, but to an unpredictable extent.[10]

The dose of drugs with predominant renal elimination may also have to be adjusted in patients with liver disease. Because of reduced muscle mass, patients with cirrhosis (or cachexia) may have a normal plasma creatinine concentration despite impaired renal function. Thus, in cirrhosis, *creatinine clearance* should be used to determine the dose of drugs with predominant renal elimination (see Chapter 17, p.681). Further, because the creatinine clearance tends to overestimate glomerular filtration in cirrhosis, the dose may still be too high.

APPROACH TO PRESCRIBING IN LIVER DISEASE

As a general rule, the safest drugs are those with a normally high PO bio-availability, low–moderate protein-binding, and/or a short halflife.

Recommendations for dose adjustment can only be approximate, and cannot replace careful clinical monitoring, including factors such as:
- rate of disease progression
- changes in LFTs/Child-Pugh score
- overall goals of care.

If in doubt, start with a low dose, and titrate slowly to response (Box D).

Box D 'Red flags' for considering dose reduction in severe hepatic impairment[13]

Consider dose reduction if prescribing a drug which normally:
- has low systemic PO bio-availability because of high first-pass hepatic extraction
- is highly protein-bound and the patient has hypo-albuminaemia (<30g/L) ± elevated plasma bilirubin
- is cleared mainly by phase I hepatic metabolism, i.e. CYP1A2, 2C19, 2D6 or 3A4 (see Chapter 19, Table 8, p.725) and has:
  - ▷ a narrow therapeutic range *or*
  - ▷ a long halflife.

Other factors indicative of severe hepatic impairment and possible need for dose reduction:
- prothrombin time >130% of normal
- bilirubin >100micromol/L
- severe cirrhosis ± encephalopathy
- ascites.

DOSE RECOMMENDATIONS

Specific recommendations are limited to analgesics, anti-emetics, anti-epileptics and antipsychotics. In Tables 2–8, drugs are categorized as 'generally safe', 'use cautiously' and 'avoid if possible' according to the risk of toxicity with chronic use in cirrhosis/severe hepatic impairment.

Sometimes the cautious use of a familiar drug may be preferable to an unfamiliar (albeit 'safer') one. Similarly, *PCF* does *not* advocate the automatic switching of patients to a 'safer' drug when an alternative is proving satisfactory.

Generally, whatever drug is used, because hepatic impairment can have general effects on pharmacokinetics and/or pharmacodynamics, *a slower than usual titration and close monitoring of the patient is advisable*. Drugs with a long halflife may reach steady-state only after 1–2 weeks or more of regular use, and undesirable effects may consequently be 'late onset'. *Remember: recommendations can only be approximate, and cannot replace clinical monitoring.*

Analgesics

Non-opioids (Table 2)

In severe hepatic impairment, PO **paracetamol** can still be used with appropriate caution *provided there are no additional risk factors for toxicity* (see Box A, p.303).[14] Because its halflife is nearly doubled,[15] start with 500mg PO q8h; monitor LFTs if dose increased above 500mg q6h and limit to an absolute maximum of 1g PO q8h, particularly in patients weighing <50kg. IV **paracetamol** should *not* be used.

Patients with hepatic impairment are more susceptible to NSAID-related renal impairment. Thus, most SPCs for NSAIDs include active liver disease or moderate–severe hepatic impairment as a contra-indication. However, particularly in cancer, the potential analgesic benefit may well outweigh the risk.

Most NSAIDs are highly protein-bound, and the proportion of free drug will be greater in hypo-albuminaemia and hyperbilirubinaemia. However, regardless of any pharmacokinetic changes,

Table 2 Non-opioid analgesics in cirrhosis or severe hepatic impairment. Before use, see introductory and class specific text above

Drug	*PO bio-availability (%)*	*Protein-binding (%)*	*Halflife in normal liver function (h)*	*Active metabolite(s)*	*Increase in halflife in severe hepatic impairment (h)*	*Dose and comments*
Use cautiously						
Paracetamol[a]	<90	20–30	1–4	Toxic metabolite	<50%	PO: start with 500mg q8h; monitor LFTs if increased above 500mg q6h; maximum 1g q8h
Diclofenac	50	>99	1–2	No	No data	Dose unchanged; check LFTs after 1–2 months to screen for hepatotoxicity
Ibuprofen	90	90–99	2–3	No	No	Dose unchanged
Naproxen	95	99	12–15	No	<50%	PO: maximum 250mg b.d.
Avoid if possible						
Celecoxib	22–40	97	11	No	Yes	See text

a. use only when no additional risk factors for toxicity (see Box A, p.304); IV paracetamol should *not* be used.

non-selective NSAIDs are high risk in severe hepatic impairment (→ prolonged prothrombin time) because they inhibit platelet aggregation (COX-1 inhibition).

Non-selective NSAIDs, but *not* **celecoxib,** double the risk of bleeding from oesophageal varices.[16] However, because it is eliminated almost entirely by hepatic excretion, the SPC recommends that **celecoxib** is *not* prescribed if Child-Pugh class C, and the dose halved if Child-Pugh class B.

Cholestasis may reduce the elimination of NSAIDs excreted in bile (e.g. **indometacin**), and may reduce or delay absorption of fat-soluble NSAIDs, e.g. **ibuprofen.**[10] However, in the absence of cholestasis, the halflife of **ibuprofen** is little changed in moderate–severe liver disease (and the dose does not need to be altered),[17] whereas the halflife of **naproxen** is increased some 50% (and the dose should be halved).[18] The pharmacokinetics of **diclofenac** are unchanged in hepatic impairment.

Hepatotoxicity is a rare unpredictable effect seen with most NSAIDs, including coxibs. **Diclofenac** may have the highest risk and **ibuprofen** the least.[1]

Opioids (Table 3)

Except for **morphine** and **buprenorphine**, the major metabolic pathway for most opioids is oxidation. This is reduced in patients with cirrhosis, resulting in increased oral bio-availability because of decreased first-pass metabolism. However, for pro-drugs such as **codeine** and **tramadol** (activated by hepatic metabolism), bio-availability will be decreased. Accordingly, they are best avoided in moderate–severe liver impairment. **Dihydrocodeine** is also best avoided because of lack of data and the limited range of immediate-release products. Thus, *the use of all weak opioids is best avoided in severe hepatic impairment.*

Morphine has a PO bio-availability of 35% (range 15–64), which increases to almost 100% in patients with severe cirrhosis.[19] The plasma halflife is also increased, enabling a decreased frequency of administration of immediate-release products.[19,20]

Table 3 Opioid analgesics in cirrhosis or severe hepatic impairment. Before use, see introductory and class specific text above

Drug	*PO bio-availability (%)*	*Protein-binding (%)*	*Halflife in normal liver function (h)*	*Active metabolite(s)*	*Increase in halflife in severe hepatic impairment (h)*	*Dose and comments*
Generally safe						
Fentanyl	–	80–85	4–16 (injection) 30 (TD)	No	No	TD/SC: dose unchanged
Use cautiously						
Alfentanil	–	92	1.5	No	Yes	SC: lower doses may be sufficient
Buprenorphine	50 (SL)	96	3–16 (injection) 13–35 (TD)	No	Probably ↑	See text
Diamorphine	No data	–	3min (IV)	Yes	No	*Pro-drug:* see text; prescribe as for morphine
*Methadone	40–100	60–90	5–130	No	No data	*Use only with specialist palliative care advice* Requires careful and *very slow* titration; accumulation occurs even without hepatic impairment (see p.437)
Morphine	15–64	20–35	2–5	Yes	<100%	Titrate slowly; decrease frequency of PO/SC immediate-release products to q6h–q8h
Avoid if possible						
Codeine	12–84	7	3–4	Yes	Yes	*Pro-drug:* reduced bio-transformation and thus reduced effect
Dihydrocodeine	20	No data	3.5–5	Yes	Probably ↑	See text
Hydromorphone	32	<10	2.5	No	Probably ↑	If unavoidable: decrease frequency of PO/SC immediate release products to q8h
Oxycodone	60–87	45	2–4	No	<400%	If unavoidable: decrease frequency of PO/SC immediate release products to q8h
Tramadol	90 (multiple doses)	20	6	Yes	<300%	*Pro-drug:* reduced bio-transformation and thus reduced effect

Diamorphine (di-acetylmorphine) is, in effect, a pro-drug for **morphine** which is de-acetylated by digestive juices and body fluids (see p.387). Thus, *advice for **morphine** applies equally to **diamorphine***.

Buprenorphine can also be used with caution in severe hepatic impairment. Two thirds are eliminated unchanged in the faeces and one third eliminated renally after hepatic glucuronidation of unchanged or dealkylated **buprenorphine** (norbuprenorphine). There is some enterohepatic recirculation. Its stated halflife (after removal of a patch) varies between TD products.

Although norbuprenorphine has similar opioid receptor-binding affinities to **buprenorphine**, it does not normally cross the blood-brain barrier and thus has little, if any, central effect. However, in severe hepatic impairment, this could change as the blood-brain barrier becomes more permeable.

The SPC for **hydromorphone** lists hepatic impairment as a contra-indication. In *moderate* hepatic impairment, because of increased bio-availability, both C_{max} and the AUC are quadrupled, although surprisingly the halflife is unchanged. Thus, if used, low starting doses at standard time intervals are advisable.[21,22] With severe liver impairment, the halflife will almost certainly increase, and the frequency of dosing should be reduced.

In severe cirrhosis, **oxycodone** has severely impaired hepatic elimination,[23] and is best avoided. In contrast, **fentanyl** pharmacokinetics are *not* altered.[24] This may be because of its large volume of distribution, with only a small fraction in the central compartment for hepatic uptake. In this case, its terminal halflife would reflect its slow release from tissue depots more than its hepatic elimination.[24] **Fentanyl** may be the opioid of choice in patients with moderate–severe liver failure.

Anti-emetics (Table 4)

Domperidone is the anti-emetic of choice in many liver centres even though SPC states that it is contra-indicated in moderate–severe impairment.[25] However, because the bio-availability in healthy subjects is low (and thus will increase in hepatic impairment), the starting dose should be halved.

In severe hepatic impairment, the halflife of **metoclopramide** increases by >100%; reduce daily dose by 50%.[26,27] Clearance of **ondansetron** is progressively reduced with increasing hepatic impairment; in severe hepatic impairment, limit PO/SC dose to 8mg/24h.[28]

Table 4 Anti-emetics in cirrhosis or severe hepatic impairment. Before use, see introductory and class specific text above

Drug	*PO bio-availability (%)*	*Protein-binding (%)*	*Halflife in normal liver function (h)*	*Active metabolite(s)*	*Increase in halflife in severe hepatic impairment (h)*	*Dose and comments*
Use cautiously						
Domperidone	12–18	>90	7–9	No	50%	PO: start with 5mg b.d., maximum 10mg t.d.s.
Cyclizine	No data	No data	20	No	No data	Dose unchanged
Haloperidol	45–75	92	12–38	Yes	No data	Start with low dose, titrate slowly
Levomepromazine	20–40	No data	15–30	No	No data	Start with low dose, titrate slowly
Metoclopramide	50–80	13–22	4–6	No	>100%	PO/SC: start with 5mg b.d., maximum 10mg b.d.
Ondansetron	56–71	70–76	3–6	No	>300%	PO/SC: maximum 8mg/24h
Prochlorperazine	6	96	15–20	No	Probably ↑	Start with low dose, titrate slowly

Benzodiazepines and Z-drugs (Table 5)

Sedatives have been implicated as common precipitants of coma in patients with severe hepatic impairment, even in usual doses.[29,30] However, possibly because they are eliminated by glucuronidation as well as CYP450 oxidation, the halflives of **lorazepam** and **temazepam** are little changed in cirrhosis.[30,31]

Midazolam is extensively metabolized in the liver via CYP3A4 oxidation.[32] Elimination is significantly reduced in cirrhosis. However, the hypnotic effects were reported to be similar in both cirrhosis and healthy controls. Even so, in advanced cirrhosis, it is best to start with a reduced dose, and titrate carefully.[32]

The halflife of **diazepam** in cirrhosis more than doubles.[33] Given its long halflife in healthy subjects (≤5 days, with an active metabolite with a halflife of ≤8 days), it should be avoided if possible, or used only p.r.n. **Clonazepam** also has a long halflife in healthy subjects and thus is best avoided in severe hepatic impairment.

Table 5 Benzodiazepines and Z-drugs in cirrhosis and severe hepatic impairment. Before use, see introductory and class specific text above

Drug	*PO bio-availability (%)*	*Protein-binding (%)*	*Halflife in normal liver function (h)*	*Active metabolite(s)*	*Increase in halflife in severe hepatic impairment (h)*	*Dose and comments*
Generally safe						
Lorazepam	90	85	10–20	No	<50%	Dose unchanged
Temazepam	90	96	8–15	No	No	Dose unchanged
Use cautiously						
Midazolam	–	96–98	4	Yes	<100%	SC: start with low dose (see p.149)
Zopiclone	75	45–80	5	Yes	<50%	PO: start with 3.75mg at bedtime
Avoid if possible						
Clonazepam	90	86	20–60	No	No data	See text
Diazepam	90	95–99	25–50 (nordiazepam ≤200)	Several	>100%	See text

Antipsychotics (Table 6)

There are limited data on antipsychotics. Dose reductions are recommended for most antipsychotics. Because all phenothiazines cause sedation and constipation, they may precipitate hepatic encephalopathy. Thus, they should be avoided if possible.[34] **Chlorpromazine** appears more hepatotoxic than other antipsychotics, and is associated with cholestasis.

Antidepressants (Table 7)

All antidepressants should be used with caution. TCAs vary in their propensity to cause sedation and constipation, and thus the likelihood of precipitating hepatic encephalopathy. Seemingly based on clinical experience, The Maudsley Prescribing Guidelines recommend that **imipramine** may be the safest; **amitriptyline, dosulepin** and **trimipramine** are best avoided; and **lofrepramine** definitely avoided.[34]

Other sources indicate that the halflife of:

- **amitriptyline** is unchanged; and could be used with caution
- **duloxetine** more than doubles in *moderate* hepatic impairment, and the AUC almost quadruples; the dose should be halved in *mild* impairment
- **venlafaxine** is prolonged even in *mild* hepatic impairment but with a large degree of inter-subject variation, and the dose should be halved.

Of the SSRIs, **citalopram** is probably the best choice; **sertraline** is best avoided.

Table 6 Antipsychotics in cirrhosis and severe hepatic impairment. Before use, see introductory and class specific text above

Drug	*PO bio-availability (%)*	*Protein-binding (%)*	*Halflife in normal liver function (h)*	*Active metabolite(s)*	*Increase in halflife in severe hepatic impairment (h)*	*Dose and comments*
Use cautiously						
Haloperidol	45–75	92	12–38	Yes	No data	Start with low dose, titrate slowly
Olanzapine	60	93	34 (52 elderly)	No	No data	Start with low dose, titrate slowly
Quetiapine	100	83	6–14	Yes	Probably ↑	PO: start with 25mg/24h; increase daily by 25–50mg/24h
Risperidone	99	90	20	Yes	No data	Start with low dose, titrate slowly
Avoid if possible						
Chlorpromazine	10–25	95–98	30	No	No data	See text

Table 7 Antidepressants in cirrhosis and severe hepatic impairment. Before use, see introductory and class specific text above

Drug	*PO bio-availability (%)*	*Protein-binding (%)*	*Halflife in normal liver function (h)*	*Active metabolite(s)*	*Increase in halflife in severe hepatic impairment (h)*	*Dose and comments*
Use cautiously						
Amitriptyline	45	96	9–25	Yes	No	PO: start with 10mg at bedtime, titrate slowly
Citalopram	80	<80	36	Yes	>200%	PO: start with 10mg once daily; maximum dose 20mg once daily
Mirtazapine	50	85	20–40	Yes	No data	PO: start with 15mg once daily, maximum dose 30mg once daily
Nortriptyline	60	95	15–39	Yes	No data	PO: start with 10mg at bedtime, titrate slowly
Trazodone	65	89–95	5–13 (doubles in elderly)	Yes	Probably ↑	Not a first-line treatment for depression
Avoid if possible						
Duloxetine	90	96	8–17	No	>200%	See text
Sertraline	>44	98	26	No	>300%	See text
Venlafaxine	13 (45 m/r)	27	5	Yes	Yes	See text

Anti-epileptics (Table 8)

Oxcarbazepine is a pro-drug which is rapidly converted in the liver to an active metabolite (see p.256). The pharmacokinetics of **oxcarbazepine** and the metabolite are unchanged in mild–moderate hepatic impairment, but reduced biotransformation should be anticipated in severe impairment.

The halflife of **valproate** is significantly prolonged in cirrhosis and in acute hepatitis, but generally it is not necessary to adjust the dose.[35] **Gabapentin** and **pregabalin** are not affected by hepatic impairment but still proceed cautiously.

Because **phenytoin** is highly protein-bound, there is a danger of toxicity if the dose is not adjusted if the patient is hypo-albuminaemic (see p.263) or is jaundiced.

Clonazepam has a long halflife in healthy subjects and is best avoided in severe hepatic impairment.

Table 8 Anti-epileptics in cirrhosis or severe hepatic impairment. Before use, see introductory and class specific text above

Drug	*PO bio-availability (%)*	*Protein-binding (%)*	*Halflife in normal liver function (h)*	*Active metabolite(s)*	*Increase in halflife in cirrhosis or hepatic impairment (h)*	*Dose and comments*
Generally safe						
Levetiracetam	≥95	<10	6–8	No	Probably ↑	Dose unchanged
Oxcarbazepine	≥95	40–60 metabolite	1–3 (metabolite 9)	Yes	No data	Pro-drug: reduced bio-transformation and thus reduced effect
Use cautiously						
Carbamazepine	85–100	70–80	16–36	Yes	No data	Start with low dose, titrate slowly
Gabapentin	30–75	<3	5–7	No	No data	Start with low dose, titrate slowly
Pregabalin	≥90	0	5–9	No	No data	Start with low dose, titrate slowly
Valproate	95	90–95	6–20	No	No data	Start with low dose, titrate slowly
Avoid if possible						
Clonazepam	90	86	20–60	No	No data	See text
Phenobarbital	≥90	45–60	75–120	No	No data	If unavoidable, use only with specialist neurological advice
Phenytoin	90–95	90	20–60	No	No data	If unavoidable, monitor plasma levels adjusted for hypo-albuminaemia (see p.263)

1 Gupta NK and Lewis JH (2008) Review article: The use of potentially hepatotoxic drugs in patients with liver disease. *Alimentary Pharmacology and Therapeutics*. **28**: 1021–1041.

2 Albers I *et al.* (1989) Superiority of the Child-Pugh classification to quantitative liver function tests for assessing prognosis of liver cirrhosis. *Scandinavian Journal of Gastroenterology*. **24**: 269–276.

3 Mullen KD (2007) Review of the final report of the 1998 Working Party on definition, nomenclature and diagnosis of hepatic encephalopathy. *Alimentary Pharmacology and Therapeutics*. **25 (Suppl 1)**: 11–16.

4 Low G *et al.* (2015) Hepatorenal syndrome: aetiology, diagnosis, and treatment. *Gastroenterology Research and Practice.* **15**: Article ID 207012.

5 Schenker S *et al.* (1999) Antecedent liver disease and drug toxicity. *Journal of Hepatology.* **31**: 1098–1105.

6 Lee WM (2003) Drug-induced hepatotoxicity. *New England Journal of Medicine.* **349**: 474–485.

7 Banks AT *et al.* (1995) Diclofenac-associated hepatotoxicity: analysis of 180 cases reported to the Food and Drug Administration as adverse reactions. *Hepatology.* **22**: 820–827.

8 Carrillo-Jimenez R and Nurnberger M (2000) Celecoxib-induced acute pancreatitis and hepatitis: a case report. *Archives of Internal Medicine.* **160**: 553–554.

9 Hernandez-Diaz S and Garcia-Rodriguez LA (2001) Epidemiologic assessment of the safety of conventional nonsteroidal anti-inflammatory drugs. *American Journal of Medicine.* **110 (Suppl 3A)**: 20s–27s.

10 North-Lewis P (ed) (2008) *Drugs and the Liver.* Pharmaceutical Press, London, pp. 178–187.

11 Delco F *et al.* (2005) Dose adjustment in patients with liver disease. *Drug Safety.* **28**: 529–545.

12 North-Lewis P (ed.) (2008). *Drugs and the Liver.* Pharmacuetical Press, London. pp. 324.

13 UK Medicines Information (2014) What pharmacokinetic and pharmacodynamic factors need to be considered when prescribing drugs for patients with liver disease? *Medicines Q&A* 170.3. www.evidence.nhs.uk

14 Hayward KL *et al.* (2016) Can paracetamol (acetaminophen) be administered to patients with liver impairment? *British Journal of Clinical Pharmacology.* **81**: 210–222.

15 Forrest JA *et al.* (1979) Paracetamol metabolism in chronic liver disease. *European Journal of Clinical Pharmacology.* **15**: 427–431.

16 Lee YC *et al.* (2012) Non-steroidal anti-inflammatory drugs use and risk of upper gastrointestinal adverse events in cirrhotic patients. *Liver International.* **32**: 859–866.

17 Juhl RP *et al.* (1983) Ibuprofen and sulindac kinetics in alcoholic liver disease. *Clinical Pharmacology and Therapeutics.* **34**: 104–109.

18 Williams RL *et al.* (1984) Naproxen disposition in patients with alcoholic cirrhosis. *European Journal of Clinical Pharmacology.* **27**: 291–296.

19 Hasselstrom J *et al.* (1990) The metabolism and bioavailability of morphine in patients with severe liver cirrhosis. *British Journal of Clinical Pharmacology.* **29**: 289–297.

20 Tegeder I *et al.* (1999) Pharmacokinetics of opioids in liver disease. *Clinical Pharmacokinetics.* **37**: 17–40.

21 Bosilkovska M *et al.* (2012) Analgesics in patients with hepatic impairment: pharmacology and clinical implications. *Drugs.* **72**: 1645–1669.

22 Durnin C *et al.* (2001) Pharmacokinetics of oral immediate-release hydromorphone (Dilaudid IR) in subjects with renal impairment. *Proceedings of the Western Pharmacology Society.* **44**: 83–84.

23 Tallgren M *et al.* (1997) Pharmacokinetics and ventilatory effects of oxycodone before and after liver transplantation. *Clinical Pharmacology and Therapeutics.* **61**: 655–661.

24 Haberer JP *et al.* (1982) Fentanyl pharmacokinetics in anaesthetized patients with cirrhosis. *British Journal of Anaesthesia.* **54**: 1267–1270.

25 North-Lewis P (ed.) (2008). *Drugs and the Liver.* Pharmaceutical Press, London. pp. 211.

26 Albani F *et al.* (1991) Kinetics of intravenous metoclopramide in patients with hepatic cirrhosis. *European Journal of Clinical Pharmacology.* **40**: 423–425.

27 Magueur E *et al.* (1991) Pharmacokinetics of metoclopramide in patients with liver cirrhosis. *British Journal of Clinical Pharmacology.* **31**: 185–187.

28 Figg WD *et al.* (1996) Pharmacokinetics of ondansetron in patients with hepatic insufficiency. *Journal of Clinical Pharmacology.* **36**: 206–215.

29 Shull HJ *et al.* (1976) Normal disposition of oxazepam in acute viral hepatitis and cirrhosis. *Annals of internal medicine.* **84**: 420–425.

30 Kraus JW *et al.* (1978) Effects of aging and liver disease on disposition of lorazepam. *Clinical Pharmacology and Therapeutics.* **24**: 411–419.

31 Ghabrial H *et al.* (1986) The effects of age and chronic liver disease on the elimination of temazepam. *European Journal of Clinical Pharmacology.* **30**: 93–97.

32 Pentikainen PJ *et al.* (1989) Pharmacokinetics of midazolam following intravenous and oral administration in patients with chronic liver disease and in healthy subjects. *Journal of Clinical Pharmacology.* **29**: 272–277.

33 Klotz U *et al.* (1975) The effects of age and liver disease on the disposition and elimination of diazepam in adult man. *Journal of Clinical Investigation.* **55**: 347–359.

34 Taylor D and Paton C (eds) (2015) Hepatic impairment In: *The Maudsley Prescribing Guidelines in Psychiatry*, (11ed). Wiley Blackwell, London, pp 590–597.

35 Klotz U *et al.* (1978) Disposition of valproic acid in patients with liver disease. *European Journal of Clinical Pharmacology.* **13**: 55–60.

Added July 2017

19: VARIABILITY IN RESPONSE TO DRUGS

19

VARIABILITY IN RESPONSE TO DRUGS

There is great inter-individual variability in the way people respond to a drug (Box A). Some of this variability is predictable in the presence of clinical factors known to impact upon the pharmacokinetics and/or pharmacodynamics of a drug. For example, an age-related decrease in overall metabolic capacity of the liver, because of reductions in liver mass, liver enzyme activity and hepatic blood flow, results in the elderly being at a significantly higher risk of toxicity from drugs metabolized in the liver. Similarly, an age-related decline in renal function can reduce the excretion of active drugs and metabolites, e.g., morphine-6-glucuronide and morphine-3-glucuronide, increasing the risk of toxicity from morphine (see p.681).

Genetic variations also contribute towards differences in drug response. Clinically, these are less predictable, although some may be detected with specific testing. They are particularly important for drugs metabolized by cytochrome P450 (CYP450) with the rate of metabolism either reduced or increased. Examples of how these manifest include:

- reduced or no response because of
  - ▷ the failure to convert a pro-drug to its active form
  - ▷ increased metabolism of an active drug to an inactive metabolite
- increased toxicity because of
  - ▷ more rapid conversion to the active form or to a metabolite which is more active than the parent drug
  - ▷ failure to metabolize an active drug to inactive metabolite(s).

Other genetic variations, such as genes coding for receptors or drug transporters also can influence overall response, e.g., the μ-opioid receptor or P-glycoprotein transporter and the response to opioids. Induction or inhibition of CYP450 activity also can result from a drug–drug or drug–food interaction causing similar manifestations to those resulting from genetic variation. Each of these factors is considered in more detail below.

VARIABILITY IN RESPONSE TO OPIOIDS

Many factors contribute to the inter-individual variation in response to opioids.[1–4]

μ-Opioid receptor

This is the key receptor mediating opioid analgesia.[5] Genetic variation in the μ-opioid receptor gene has been associated with variation in opioid response in acute post-operative pain,[6–8] chronic non-cancer pain,[9,10] and cancer pain.[11,12] However, meta-analysis of opioid pain studies showed no overall association with pain and only weak associations with **morphine** dose or undesirable effects.[13]

Box A Common factors affecting response to drugs

Adherence
Whether drug regimen adhered to or not

Genetic variation/polymorphism
Sequence variation including single nucleotide polymorphisms, gene deletions, gene duplications resulting in altered protein function, e.g. receptors, enzymes, drug transporters

Pharmacokinetics
Absorption
Distribution
Metabolism
Drug–drug and drug–food interactions
Excretion

Pharmacodynamics
Receptor–drug interaction and effect
Drug–drug and drug–food interactions
Decreased/increased receptor affinity due to concurrent disease state

Physiological factors
Gender
Age
Ethnicity
Hormonal changes
Circadian and seasonal factors

Environmental factors
Diet
Environmental toxins
Alcohol and recreational drugs
Smoking

Potential specific associations/concomitant disease
Diabetes mellitus
GI microbiology
Hypoalbuminaemia
Liver failure
Malabsorption
Malnutrition
Obesity
Renal failure

P-glycoprotein

The membrane-bound drug transporter P-glycoprotein influences drug absorption and drug excretion.[14,15] It limits the uptake of compounds from the GI tract, regulates the transfer of various drugs across the blood–brain barrier,[16] and influences drug excretion by the liver and kidneys. It is encoded by the ATP-binding cassette subfamily B member 1 (ABCB1) gene.

P-glycoprotein modulation of opioid CNS concentrations varies substantially between opioids, with **morphine**, **fentanyl**, and **methadone** being among those most affected.[17,18] In animals, removal ('knockout' mice) or inhibition (by **ciclosporin**) of P-glycoprotein activity enhances absorption and increases CNS concentrations of **fentanyl** and **morphine**, resulting in prolonged analgesia.[19] Thus, inhibitors of P-glycoprotein (e.g. **ciclosporin**, **clarithromycin**, **erythromycin**, **itraconazole**, **ketoconazole**, **quinidine** (not UK), **verapamil**) could increase CNS effects of opioids.

Variation in ABCB1 has been associated with increased pain relief with **morphine** in cancer pain[11] and decreased opioid requirements in mixed chronic pain.[10] Studies have shown conflicting results in relation to opioid-induced nausea and vomiting and other undesirable effects.[20–22]

Catechol-O-methyltransferase

Catechol-O-methyltransferase (COMT) is an enzyme which has a significant impact on the metabolism of several important neurotransmitters: dopamine, adrenaline (epinephrine) and noradrenaline (norepinephrine). The COMT gene is polymorphic, and <25% of Caucasians have low activity variants.

One common variant in which the amino acid valine is substituted for methionine results in a 3–4 times decrease in COMT activity. It has been associated with increased pain sensitivity and higher μ-opioid system activation in experimental pain,[23,24] and increased **morphine** dose requirements in cancer patients.[25] Other variants of the COMT gene are associated with increased undesirable opioid effects, e.g. nausea and vomiting.[20,26,27]

Hepatic metabolism

Opioid metabolism takes place primarily in the liver. Opioids are metabolized via two main pathways, cytochrome P450 (CYP450) and uridine diphosphate glucuronosyltransferase (UGT; Table 1). Two phases of metabolism are generally described: phase 1 metabolism (modification reactions) and phase 2 metabolism (conjugation reactions).

The most important phase 1 reaction is oxidation, catalysed by CYP450. The most important phase 2 reaction is glucuronidation, catalysed by UGT. Glucuronidation produces molecules which are highly hydrophilic and thus easily excreted by the kidneys.[28] Drug–drug interactions can occur from changes in CYP450 or UGT activity, although the latter are less well documented.[29]

Table 1 Major opioid enzyme pathways

Drug	*Pathway*[a]			
	CYP2D6	*CYP3A4/5*	*CYP2B6*	*UGT*
Alfentanil		++		
Buprenorphine		++		+
Codeine	++			+
Dihydrocodeine	+			+
Fentanyl		++		
Hydrocodone	+			
Hydromorphone				++
Methadone		++	+	
Morphine				++
Oxycodone	+	++		
Oxymorphone		+		+
Sufentanil		++		
Tapentadol				++
Tramadol	++	++		

a. ++ for CYP pathways may result in clinically important drug–drug interactions (see Table 8).

GENETIC POLYMORPHISM IN CYTOCHROME P450 (CYP450)

About 75% of all drugs are metabolized partly or completely by cytochrome P450 (Box B). Thus, variation in activity of the cytochrome P450 system can have a major impact on drug action.

Box B Cytochrome P450 (CYP450)[30,31]

CYP450 is a super-family of numerous enzymic proteins responsible for the oxidative metabolism of many drugs and some endogenous substances (e.g. fatty acids, eicosanoids, steroids, bile acids).

The root symbol used in naming the individual enzymes is CYP, followed by:
- a number designating the enzyme family (18 in humans)
- a capital letter designating the subfamily (44 in humans)
- a number designating the individual enzyme.

CYP450 enzymes exist in virtually all tissues, but their highest concentration is in the liver.

The enzymes concerned with drug metabolism are mostly CYP1–CYP3; these account for about 70% of the total CYP450 content of the liver.

The most important enzyme is CYP3A4, followed by CYP2D6 and CYP2C9.

The presence of CYP3A4 in the wall of the GI tract is important; it probably acts in conjunction with P-glycoprotein, and together determine the extent of the intestinal metabolism of CYP3A4 substrates.

Some 20–25% of drugs are affected by genetic variants of drug-metabolizing enzymes.[32] The bulk of the population will manifest a normal distribution in terms of the rate of drug metabolism, with activity ranging from well below-average to well above-average, but generally lumped together as extensive metabolizers (EM).[33] In addition, there are discrete genetic populations of individuals who fall beyond the ends of the spectrum. These are designated poor (PM) and ultra-rapid metabolizers (URM). More recently, intermediate metabolizers have been identified for some enzymes (Table 2).[30]

Table 2 Metabolizer status[34]

Category	*Description*	*Possible impact*
Poor (PM) *or* slow	Lacks functional enzyme (deletion of gene or non-functional variant)	Increased toxicity due to slower drug metabolism (e.g. flecainde, phenytoin) *or* Therapeutic failure due to poor metabolism of a pro-drug to its active form (e.g. codeine) or a parent drug to an active metabolite (e.g. tamoxifen, tramadol)
Intermediate	Has two decreased-function enzymes or one decreased, one non-functional	Comparable to slow metabolizer but less marked
Extensive (EM) *or* rapid	Has at least one fully-functional enzyme	This is the norm
Ultra-rapid (URM)	Increased enzyme activity (duplication of gene or other mutation); relatively rare	Therapeutic failure due to faster drug metabolism *or* Increased toxicity due to faster conversion of parent drug to more active metabolite (e.g. tramadol) *or* pro-drug to active form (e.g. codeine)

As a general rule, an URM may need a higher dose to obtain a therapeutic effect, and a PM a lower dose to prevent increased undesirable effects (Table 3).[32] Exceptions are 'pro-drugs' where metabolites are mainly responsible for the effect of the drug (see below). The effects of such genetic variations can be further modified by the co-administration of the relevant CYP450 inhibitor or inducer.

Table 3 Genetic polymorphism and PM/URM status[a,28,30,35-37]

Pathway	*A selection of affected drugs*	*Population affected*
CYP2C9	NSAIDs Phenytoin Sulfonylureas (glipizide, tolbutamide) Warfarin	Caucasians 35% Asian/African <1%
CYP2C19	Antidepressants (imipramine, sertraline) Clopidogrel[b] Diazepam PPIs	Asians 10–35% Africans 15% Caucasians 2–5%
CYP2D6 (debrisoquine hydroxylase)	β-Blockers (metoprolol)[c] Codeine[b] Flecainide Oxycodone SSRIs (some, e.g. paroxetine) Tamoxifen[b] TCAs (imipramine, nortriptyline)[d] Tramadol[b]	Africans 0–34% Caucasians 5–10% Asians ≤1%

a. there is roughly a similar number of URM as PM

b. enzyme conversion produces active or more active metabolite

c. 70% dose reduction recommended in PM; note also that co-administration with paroxetine (2D6 inhibitor) increases plasma concentrations four times

d. TCAs most likely to need a lower dose.

Of particular note is **codeine**, for which most of its analgesic effect results from partial conversion to morphine by O-demethylation catalysed by CYP2D6 (see p.349).[38,39] Compared with the general population (EM), a PM produces little or no **morphine** from **codeine**, and obtains little or no pain relief. On the other hand, undesirable effects are comparable in both categories.[40,41] At the other extreme, URM produce more **morphine**; this can lead to life-threatening opioid toxicity which, rarely, has been fatal in children (following adenoidectomy/tonsillectomy; altered respiratory drive due to obstructive sleep apnoea was a probable contributing factor).[42–46]

Genetic variation involving CYP2D6 is also important in relation to **tramadol** for which the (+) O-desmethyltramadol metabolite is responsible for the opioid analgesic effect. A PM produces little or none and thus obtains little or no analgesic benefit;[47] conversely, an URM produces higher levels with a potential to cause opioid toxicity (see p.354).[48]

Polymorphism in CYP3A4/5 may be of less clinical significance when considering opioid response.[49] Nonetheless, CYP3A4 activity varies up to 10 times and could be partly responsible for different dose requirements.[50] Opioids potentially affected are the fentanils, **methadone**, **oxycodone** and, to a lesser extent, **buprenorphine**.

Although genetic variation can result in serious consequences, pharmacogenetic testing is not routine, partly because it is not cost-effective, e.g. the impact of testing in relation to **warfarin** dosing.[51,52] Thus, generally, close clinical monitoring is recommended for drugs with a major metabolic enzyme pathway affected by genetic polymorphism (see Tables 3 and 8). However, in some settings, e.g. oncology, testing has been used to determine if an individual is likely to respond to a specific drug, e.g. **cetuximab** (colorectal cancer), **trastuzumab** (breast cancer), and **dasatinib** (acute lymphoblastic leukaemia).

CYP450 DRUG–DRUG INTERACTIONS

Pharmacokinetic drug–drug interactions mediated through increased or decreased activity of CYP450 enzymes are common, but the resultant clinical impact is difficult to predict.[30,53–55] Some drugs (inducers) increase the activity of specific CYP450 enzymes and others (inhibitors) decrease enzyme activity (see Table 7, and Table 8 p.725).

When CYP450 inhibitors or inducers are co-administered with drugs which are already affected by genetic polymorphisms they will either augment or mitigate the clinical effects of the genetic variation.

Induction

Onset and offset of enzyme induction is gradual, possibly 2–3 weeks, because:

- onset depends on drug-induced synthesis of new enzyme
- offset depends on elimination of the enzyme-inducing drug and the decay of the increased enzyme stores.

Induction of the rate of drug biotransformation generally leads to a decrease in the parent drug plasma concentration, and thus a *decreased effect*. However, if the substrate drug is an inactive pro-drug or metabolism produces a more active metabolite, induction will result in an *increased effect* and possible toxicity.

The impact of enzyme induction depends on the relative importance of the induced pathway to the substrate's metabolism, whether active metabolites are present, and on the concentration (dose) of the inducer. Sequential dose adjustments, either up or down, may be necessary to maintain the desired clinical effect of the affected drug.[30] Converse dose adjustments may be required if the inducer is discontinued, e.g. **methadone** toxicity has occurred following discontinuation of **carbamazepine**, an inducer.[56]

Some anti-epileptics (e.g. **carbamazepine**, **phenobarbital**, **phenytoin**) and some other drugs (e.g. **rifampicin, St John's wort**) induce members of the CYP3A subfamily (Table 4). **Rifampicin** is the most potent clinically used inducer of cytochrome CYP3A. Some oestrogens are metabolized by CYP3A4/5, and induction by **rifampicin** (or another enzyme inducer) can cause oral contraceptive failure.

Chronic alcohol consumption can induce CYP450 enzymes, mostly CYP2E1 and possibly CYP3A. However, in cirrhosis, overall enzyme activity is reduced.

Table 4 Examples of drug interactions based on enzyme induction of CYP3A4/5

Substrate	*Inducers*	*Outcome*
Carbamazepine	Phenytoin	Metabolism ↑, effect ↓
Methadone	Carbamazepine, phenobarbital, phenytoin, rifampicin, St John's wort	Metabolism ↑, effect ↓ (possible recurrence of pain ± withdrawal symptoms)[57]
Midazolam	Carbamazepine, phenytoin	Metabolism ↑, effect ↓[58]
Phenytoin	Rifampicin	Metabolism ↑, halflife halved, effect ↓[59]
Protease inhibitors (for HIV)	St John's wort	Metabolism ↑, treatment failure[60-62]

Inhibition

Inhibition of drug biotransformation begins *within a few hours* of the administration of the inhibitor drug. For most drugs, inhibition leads to an increase in the plasma concentration and effect of the substrate drug, and increased risk of toxicity. However, the converse is true with *pro-drugs*, e.g. **clopidogrel**, where the plasma concentration of the active metabolite is reduced, increasing the risk of therapeutic failure. Table 5 gives examples of altered drug effects resulting from enzyme inhibition.

The mechanism of enzymatic inhibition is either reversible or irreversible. In reversible inhibition, the inhibitor drug (e.g. azole antifungals) binds to the P450 enzyme and prevents the metabolism of the substrate drug.[74,75] The extent of inhibition of one drug by another depends on their relative affinities for the P450 enzyme, and the respective doses. In irreversible inhibition, the enzyme is destroyed or inactivated by the inhibitor drug or its metabolites (e.g. **clarithromycin**, **erythromycin**).

Table 5 Examples of drug interactions based on enzyme inhibition

Substrate	*Inhibitors*	*Outcome*
Codeine	Quinidine (not UK) (CYP2D6)	Biotransformation to morphine ↓, analgesic effect ↓[63]
Clopidogrel	Esomeprazole, omeprazole (CYP2C19)	Biotransformation to active metabolite ↓, antithrombotic effect ↓[64–67]
Diazepam	Cimetidine (multiple CYP)	Metabolism ↓, effect ↑[68]
Lovastatin (not UK), simvastatin	Clarithromycin, erythromycin (CYP3A4/5)	Metabolism ↓, risk of undesirable effects ↑ (e.g. raised CK plasma concentration, muscle pain, rhabdomyolysis)
Theophylline	Ciprofloxacin (CYP1A2)	Metabolism ↓ (18–113%), effect ↑[69]
TCAs	SSRIs (multiple CYP)	Metabolism ↓ (plasma concentrations ↑ 50–350%), effect ↑[70–72]
Warfarin	Fluvoxamine (multiple CYP)	Metabolism ↓ (plasma concentration ↑ 65%), effect ↑[73]

CYP450 DRUG–DRUG INTERACTIONS IN PALLIATIVE CARE

It can be challenging to determine the likelihood of a clinically relevant drug–drug interaction in practice. Many patients receiving palliative care are elderly and have several chronic conditions, resulting in the use of numerous drugs, typically 7–8 (range 1–20).[76,77] This polypharmacy increases the likelihood of drug interactions involving CYP450, with possibly 10–20% of patients receiving a combination likely to produce a clinically relevant CYP-mediated interaction (Table 6).[76,77] For a longer list of commonly used drugs which are moderate-to-potent enzyme inhibitors or inducers, also see Table 8.

Table 6 Common drug combinations likely to produce clinically important CYP-mediated interactions in palliative care patients.[76,77]

Drug combination	*Likely outcome of the interaction*[a]
Benzodiazepines[b]+ CYP3A4 inhibitor e.g. diazepam + itraconazole	Diazepam ↑
Benzodiazepines[b] + CYP3A4 inducer e.g. midazolam + carbamazepine	Midazolam ↓
Corticosteroids + CYP3A4 inhibitor e.g. dexamethasone + clarithromycin	Dexamethasone ↑
Corticosteroids + CYP3A4 inducer e.g. dexamethasone + phenytoin	Dexamethasone ↓
Diazepam + omeprazole[c]	Diazepam ↑
Opioids[b] + CYP3A4 inhibitor e.g. oxycodone + fluconazole	Oxycodone ↑
Opioids[b] + CYP3A4 inducer e.g. fentanyl + carbamazepine	Fentanyl ↓

a. ↑ = drug effect increased; ↓ = effect decreased
b. which are full or part substrates of CYP3A4 (see Table 8, p.727)
c. inhibitor of CYP2C19 (see Table 8, p.726).

In one series, about 50% of the interactions involved corticosteroids, and 25% analgesics.[76] In a second series, the most frequently used inducers or inhibitors of CYP450 (and/or P-glycoprotein, or UGT) were **dexamethasone**, **esomeprazole**, **omeprazole**, **fluconazole**, **ciprofloxacin**, **carbamazepine**, **carvedilol** and **verapamil** (also see Table 8, p.725).[77] Interactions may be missed, e.g. recurrence of pain may be interpreted as disease progression rather than altered analgesic metabolism. The BNF has a comprehensive list of drug interactions and their significance.

Serotonin toxicity (see p.200) is generally a pharmacodynamic interaction resulting from the combination of two or more serotonergic drugs. However, in some circumstances, a pharmacokinetic interaction may contribute to an increase in serotonergic transmission, e.g. **fluoxetine** (a CYP2D6 and CYP2C19 inhibitor) and **amitriptyline**.

The addition of a CYP450 inhibitor to a drug known to prolong the QT interval may result in increased plasma levels, QT prolongation and risk of *torsade de pointes*, e.g. **itraconazole** (a CYP3A4 inhibitor) and **methadone**.

CYP450 DRUG–FOOD INTERACTIONS

An important interaction associated with CYP450 inhibition is a food–drug interaction involving grapefruit juice and CYP3A substrates administered PO, including some benzodiazepines (**diazepam**, **midazolam**, **triazolam** (not UK)), some statins (**atorvastatin**, **lovastatin** (not UK), **simvastatin**), **buspirone**, **ciclosporin**, **felodipine**, **nifedipine** and **saquinavir**.[30,78–80]

Grapefruit juice contains several bioflavonoids (naringenin, naringin, kaempferol and quercetin) and furanocoumarins (bergamottin) which non-competitively inhibit oxidation reactions mediated by CYP3A enzymes in the wall of the GI tract.[79,81,82] The effect is unpredictable because the quantity of these components in grapefruit products varies considerably.[83,84]

The effect is maximal when grapefruit juice is ingested 30–60min before the drug. A single 250mL glass of grapefruit juice can inhibit CYP3A for 24–48h and regular intake continually suppresses GI CYP3A.[30,79] Thus, patients taking drugs metabolized by CYP3A are warned to avoid grapefruit juice, particularly if the drug has a narrow therapeutic index, e.g. **ciclosporin**. Pomelo, Seville orange and lime juices may also inhibit CYP3A;[85,86] apple juice has not been implicated.

Besides inhibiting CYP3A, naringin (and thus grapefruit juice) inhibits organic anion-transporting polypeptide 1A2 (OATP1A2), a carrier protein in the wall of the GI tract which is responsible for the uptake of several drugs. Orange juice (through its major flavonoid, hesperidin) has a similar effect[87] and possibly apple juice.[88] Drugs which may have their absorption reduced by this inhibition include some β-blockers (**atenolol**, **celiprolol**), **ciclosporin**, **etoposide**, **fexofenadine**, **itraconazole**, and quinolone antibacterials (**ciprofloxacin**, **levofloxacin**).[87,88]

Case reports of serious adverse events related to grapefruit-drug interactions include:

- **amiodarone** → *torsade de pointes*
- **atorvastatin** and **simvastatin** → rhabdomyolysis.

Other drugs which may be affected by grapefruit include novel oral anticoagulants (**apixaban**, **rivaroxaban**), calcium channel blockers (**amlodipine**, **felodipine**, **verapamil**), CNS drugs (**quetiapine**, **buspirone**), cytotoxics (**nilotinib**, **lapatinib**), and immunosuppressants (**ciclosporin**, **tacrolimus**, **sirolimus**).[89] Interactions are generally drug-specific, not a class effect, and the BNF or SPC should be referred to for more information.

There is also concern that ingestion of cranberry juice may also modify drug action, mediated through flavonoids which specifically inhibit CYP2C9 (see p.489). **Warfarin** is an example of a drug which might be affected by this interaction and, indeed, early reports linked cranberry juice with adverse events associated with **warfarin**.[90–93] However, recent reports suggest that this interaction is unlikely to occur with the amounts of cranberry juice recommended for prophylaxis against UTIs.[94–97]

Nonetheless, an interaction with **warfarin** cannot be ruled out, particularly when large volumes of cranberry juice are drunk regularly, or when cranberry products other than juice are taken.[94,95,98] Thus, the INR should be monitored more closely in patients on **warfarin** if they consume large amounts of cranberry juice or take other cranberry supplements for prophylaxis against UTIs.[94]

QUANTIFYING THE EFFECTS OF CYP450 INHIBITION AND INDUCTION

Quantification of the effects of CYP450 inhibitors and inducers is still evolving. The more important enzymes for drug metabolism have generally accepted 'probe' substrates and potent inhibitors and inducers (Table 7), and these are used to determine reliable results, e.g. for new drugs in development. Increasingly, data are becoming available which predict the clinical importance of drug–drug interactions. However, there is still much to be determined and, in palliative care where polypharmacy is the norm, in addition to understanding the pharmacokinetics of any drug used, a general awareness of potential interactions is important (Table 8).

Table 7 Examples of *in vivo* probe substrates and potent inhibitors and inducers used for evaluation (all PO)[99]

Enzyme	*Substrate*	*Inhibitor*	*Inducers*
CYP1A2	Caffeine Theophylline	Fluvoxamine	Tobacco smoking
CYP2B6	Efavirenz		
CYP2C8	Repaglinide	Gemfibrozil	Rifampicin
CYP2C9	Tolbutamide Warfarin	Amiodarone Fluconazole	Rifampicin
CYP2C19	Esomeprazole Lansoprazole Omeprazole Pantoprazole	Fluvoxamine Omeprazole	Rifampicin
CYP2D6	Dextromethorphan	Fluoxetine Paroxetine Quinidine (not UK)	None known
CYP3A4	Midazolam	Clarithromycin Itraconazole Ketoconazole Ritonavir	Carbamazepine Rifampicin

Table 8 Examples of enzyme or transporter protein substrates, inhibitors and inducers which may result in clinically significant drug interactions[a,29,77,99]

Enzyme or transporter protein	*Substrates*	*Moderate or potent inhibitors*	*Moderate or potent inducers*
CYP1A2	Amitriptyline Clomipramine Duloxetine Flecainide Imipramine Melatonin Mirtazapine Olanzapine Propranolol Ramelteon (not UK) Theophylline Tizanidine Trimipramine	Cimetidine[b] Ciprofloxacin Fluvoxamine	Phenytoin Rifampicin Tobacco smoking
CYP2B6	Methadone		Rifampicin

continued

Table 8 Continued

Enzyme or transporter protein	*Substrates*	*Moderate or potent inhibitors*	*Moderate or potent inducers*
CYP2C8	Loperamide Pioglitazone Repaglinide Rosiglitazone (not UK)		Rifampicin
CYP2C9[c]	Celecoxib Chlorpropamide (not UK) Diclofenac Flurbiprofen Fluvastatin Glibenclamide (glyburide) Gliclazide Glimepiride Glipizide Ibuprofen Irbesartan Losartan Nateglinide Phenytoin Tolbutamide Torasemide (torsemide) Warfarin	Amiodarone Fluconazole	Carbamazepine Rifampicin
CYP2C19[c]	Amitriptyline Citalopram Clomipramine Clopidogrel Diazepam Fluoxetine Imipramine Lansoprazole Omeprazole Pantoprazole Phenytoin Sertraline	Esomeprazole Fluconazole Fluoxetine Fluvoxamine Omeprazole Ticlopidine Voriconazole	Rifampicin
CYP2D6[c]	Amitriptyline Carvedilol Codeine Desipramine (not UK) Dextromethorphan Dihydrocodeine Duloxetine Flecainide Fluoxetine Hydrocodone (not UK) Imipramine Metoprolol Mirtazapine Nebivolol Nortriptyline Ondansetron Oxycodone	Cimetidine[b] Duloxetine Fluoxetine Paroxetine	

continued

Table 8 Continued

Enzyme or transporter protein	*Substrates*	*Moderate or potent inhibitors*	*Moderate or potent inducers*
CYP2D6[c] (continued)	Paracetamol Paroxetine Pindolol Propranolol Risperidone Sertraline Tamoxifen Timolol Tolterodine Tramadol Trazodone Trimipramine Venlafaxine		
CYP3A4/5[d,e]	Alfentanil Alprazolam Amiodarone Aprepitant Atorvastatin Budesonide (PO) Buprenorphine Carbamazepine Clarithromycin Clonazepam Clorazepate Codeine Dexamethasone Diazepam Diltiazem Domperidone Erythromycin Estradiol Ezopiclone (not UK) Felodipine Fentanyl Haloperidol Imipramine Itraconazole Ketamine Loperamide Losartan Lovastatin (not UK) Methadone Methylprednisolone Midazolam Mirtazapine Nifedipine Omeprazole Oxybutynin Oxycodone Paracetamol (acetaminophen) Phenytoin	Cimetidine[b] Ciprofloxacin Clarithromycin Diltiazem Erythromycin Fluconazole Grapefruit juice Itraconazole Verapamil Voriconazole	Carbamazepine Modafinil Phenobarbital (and other barbiturates) Phenytoin Rifampicin St John's wort

continued

Table 8 Continued

Enzyme or transporter protein	*Substrates*	*Moderate or potent inhibitors*	*Moderate or potent inducers*
CYP3A4/5[d,e] (continued)	Quetiapine Risperidone Sertraline Simvastatin Tamoxifen Tolterodine Tolvaptan Toremifene Tramadol Trazodone Venlafaxine Verapamil Voriconazole Warfarin Zolpidem Zopiclone		
P-glycoprotein[e]	Digoxin Loperamide	Amiodarone Carvedilol Clarithromycin Diltiazem Erythromycin Felodipine Itraconazole Verapamil	Carbamazepine Dexamethasone Phenytoin Rifampicin St John's wort

a. *not* an exhaustive list; limited to drugs most likely to be encountered in palliative care and *excludes* anticancer, HIV and immunosuppressive drugs (seek specialist advice)
b. cimetidine is classified as a weak inhibitor of multiple CYP enzymes
c. enzyme can also be subject to genetic polymorphism, see Table 3
d. CYP3A enzyme is also expressed in the GI mucosa resulting in substantial first-pass metabolism of some drugs during absorption
e. there is a large overlap between the substrates, inhibitors and inducers of P-glycoprotein and CYP3A.

1 Droney J *et al.* (2011) Evolving knowledge of opioid genetics in cancer pain. *Clinical Oncology.* **23**: 418–428.
2 Lloyd RA et al. (2016) Pharmacogenomics and patient treatment parameters to opioid treatment in chronic pain: A focus on morphine, oxycodone, tramadol and fentanyl. *Pain Medicine.* **0**: 1–19.
3 Ross JR *et al.* (2006) Clinical pharmacology and pharmacotherapy of opioid switching in cancer patients. *Oncologist.* **11**: 765–773.
4 Somogyi AA *et al.* (2007) Pharmacogenetics of opioids. *Clinical Pharmacology & Therapeutics.* **81**: 429–444.
5 Matthes H *et al.* (1996) Loss of morphine-induced analgesia, reward effect and withdrawal symptoms in mice lacking the mu-opioid-receptor gene. *Nature.* **383**: 819–823.
6 Chou WY *et al.* (2006) Association of mu-opioid receptor gene polymorphism (A118G) with variations in morphine consumption for analgesia after total knee arthroplasty. *Acta Anaesthesiologica Scandinavica.* **50**: 787–792.
7 Chou WY *et al.* (2006) Human opioid receptor A118G polymorphism affects intravenous patient-controlled analgesia morphine consumption after total abdominal hysterectomy. *Anesthesiology.* **105**: 334–337.
8 Sia AT *et al.* (2008) A118G single nucleotide polymorphism of human mu-opioid receptor gene influences pain perception and patient-controlled intravenous morphine consumption after intrathecal morphine for postcesarean analgesia. *Anesthesiology.* **109**: 520–526.
9 Janicki PK *et al.* (2006) A genetic association study of the functional A118G polymorphism of the human mu-opioid receptor gene in patients with acute and chronic pain. *Anesthesia and Analgesia.* **103**: 1011–1017.
10 Lotsch J *et al.* (2009) Cross-sectional analysis of the influence of currently known pharmacogenetic modulators on opioid therapy in outpatient pain centers. *Pharmacogenetics and Genomics.* **19**: 429–436.
11 Campa D *et al.* (2008) Association of ABCB1/MDR1 and OPRM1 gene polymorphisms with morphine pain relief. *Clinical Pharmacology and Therapeutics.* **83**: 559–566.
12 Klepstad P *et al.* (2004) The 118A > G polymorphism in the human mu-opioid receptor gene may increase morphine requirements in patients with pain caused by malignant disease. *Acta Anaesthesiologica Scandinavica.* **48**: 1232–1239.
13 Walter C and Lotsch J (2009) Meta-analysis of the relevance of the OPRM1 118A>G genetic variant for pain treatment. *Pain.* **146**: 270–275.

14 Schinkel AH (1997) The physiological function of drug-transporting P-glycoproteins. *Seminars in Cancer Biology.* **8**: 161–170.
15 Marzolini C *et al.* (2004) Polymorphisms in human MDR1 (P-glycoprotein): recent advances and clinical relevance. *Clinical Pharmacology and Therapeutics.* **75**: 13–33.
16 Davis MP *et al.* (eds) (2009) Pharmacogenetics and opioids. In: *Opioids in Cancer Pain* (2e). OUP, Oxford, pp. 287–299.
17 Dagenais C *et al.* (2004) Variable modulation of opioid brain uptake by P-glycoprotein in mice. *Biochemical Pharmacology.* **67**: 269–276.
18 Barratt DT *et al.* (2012) ABCB1 haplotype and OPRM1 118A > G genotype interaction in methadone maintenance treatment pharmacogenetics. *Pharmgenomics and Personalized Medicine.* **5**: 53–62.
19 Thompson SJ *et al.* (2000) Opiate-induced analgesia is increased and prolonged in mice lacking P-glycoprotein. *Anesthesiology.* **92**: 1392–1399.
20 Ross JR *et al.* (2008) Genetic variation and response to morphine in cancer patients: catechol-O-methyltransferase and multidrug resistance-1 gene polymorphisms are associated with central side effects. *Cancer.* **112**: 1390–1403.
21 Zwisler ST *et al.* (2010) The antinociceptive effect and adverse drug reactions of oxycodone in human experimental pain in relation to genetic variations in the OPRM1 and ABCB1 genes. *Fundamental and Clinical Pharmacology.* **24**: 517–524.
22 Coulbault L *et al.* (2006) Environmental and genetic factors associated with morphine response in the postoperative period. *Clinical Pharmacology and Therapeutics.* **79**: 316–324.
23 Kim H *et al.* (2006) Genetic polymorphisms in monoamine neurotransmitter systems show only weak association with acute post-surgical pain in humans. *Molecular Pain.* **2**: 24.
24 Zubieta JK *et al.* (2003) COMT val158met genotype affects mu-opioid neurotransmitter responses to a pain stressor. *Science.* **299**: 1240–1243.
25 Rakvag TT *et al.* (2005) The Val158Met polymorphism of the human catechol-O-methyltransferase (COMT) gene may influence morphine requirements in cancer pain patients. *Pain.* **116**: 73–78.
26 Laugsand EA *et al.* (2011) Clinical and genetic factors associated with nausea and vomiting in cancer patients receiving opioids. *European Journal of Cancer.* **47**: 1682–1691.
27 Kolesnikov Y *et al.* (2011) Combined catechol-O-methyltransferase and mu-opioid receptor gene polymorphisms affect morphine postoperative analgesia and central side effects. *Anesthesia and Analgesia.* **112**: 448–453.
28 Smith HS (2009) Opioid metabolism. *Mayo Clinic Proceedings.* **84**: 613–624.
29 Baxter K, Preston CL *Stockley's Drug Interactions.* London: Pharmaceutical Press www.medicinescomplete.com (accessed July 2014).
30 Wilkinson GR (2005) Drug metabolism and variability among patients in drug response. *N Engl J Med.* **352**: 2211–2221.
31 Sim SC (2005) Human Cytochrome P450 (CYP). Allele Nomenclature Committee. Available from: www.CYPalleles.ki.se
32 Stamer UM *et al.* (2010) Personalized therapy in pain management: where do we stand? *Pharmacogenomics.* **11**: 843–864.
33 Meyer U (1991) Genotype or phenotype: the definition of a pharmacogenetic polymorphism. *Pharmacogenetics.* **1**: 66–67.
34 Sajantila A *et al.* (2010) Pharmacogenetics in medico-legal context. *Forensic Science International.* **203**: 44–52.
35 Poulsen L *et al.* (1996) The hypoalgesic effect of tramadol in relation to CYP2D6. *Clinical Pharmacology and Therapeutics.* **60**: 636–644.
36 Riddick D (1997) Drug biotransformation. In: H Kalant and W Roschlau (eds) *Principles of Medical Pharmacology* (6e). Oxford University Press, New York.
37 Williams DG *et al.* (2002) Pharmacogenetics of codeine metabolism in an urban population of children and its implications for analgesic reliability. *British Journal of Anaesthesia.* **89**: 839–845.
38 Persson K *et al.* (1992) The postoperative pharmacokinetics of codeine. *European Journal of Clinical Pharmacology.* **42**: 663–666.
39 Findlay JWA *et al.* (1978) Plasma codeine and morphine concentrations after therapeutic oral doses of codeine-containing analgesics. *Clin Pharmacol Ther.* **24**: 60–68.
40 Eckhardt K *et al.* (1998) Same incidence of adverse drug events after codeine administration irrespective of the genetically determined differences in morphine formation. *Pain.* **76**: 27–33.
41 Susce MT *et al.* (2006) Response to hydrocodone, codeine and oxycodone in a CYP2D6 poor metabolizer. *Progress in Neuropsychopharmacology and Biological Psychiatry.* **30**: 1356–1358.
42 Gasche Y *et al.* (2004) Codeine intoxication associated with ultrarapid CYP2D6 metabolism. *New England Journal of Medicine.* **351**: 2827–2831.
43 Koren G *et al.* (2006) Pharmacogenetics of morphine poisoning in a breastfed neonate of a codeine-prescribed mother. *Lancet.* **368**: 704.
44 Kirchheiner J *et al.* (2007) Pharmacokinetics of codeine and its metabolite morphine in ultra-rapid metabolizers due to CYP2D6 duplication. *Pharmacogenomics Journal.* **7**: 257–265.
45 Racoosin JA *et al.* (2013) New evidence about an old drug - risk with codeine after adenotonsillectomy. *New England Journal of Medicine.* **368**: 2155–2157.
46 MHRA (2013) Codeine: restricted use as an analgesic in children and adolescents after European safety review. *Drug Safety Update.* www.gov.uk/drug-safety-update
47 Stamer UM *et al.* (2007) Concentrations of tramadol and O-desmethyltramadol enantiomers in different CYP2D6 genotypes. *Clinical Pharmacology and Therapeutics.* **82**: 41–47.
48 Stamer UM *et al.* (2008) Respiratory depression with tramadol in a patient with renal impairment and CYP2D6 gene duplication. *Anesthesia and Analgesia.* **107**: 926–929.
49 Pirmohamed M and Park BK (2003) Cytochrome P450 enzyme polymorphisms and adverse drug reactions. *Toxicology.* **192**: 23–32.
50 Haddad A *et al.* (2007) The pharmacological importance of cytochrome CYP3A4 in the palliation of symptoms: review and recommendations for avoiding adverse drug interactions. *Supportive Care in Cancer.* **15**: 251–257.
51 Kimmel SE *et al.* (2013) A pharmacogenetic versus a clinical algorithm for warfarin dosing. *New England Journal of Medicine.* **369**: 2283–2293.
52 Pirmohamed M *et al.* (2013) A randomized trial of genotype-guided dosing of warfarin. *New England Journal of Medicine.* **369**: 2294–2303.
53 Aeschlimann J and Tyler L (1996) Drug interactions associated with cytochrome P-450 enzymes. *Journal of Pharmaceutical Care in Pain and Symptom Control.* **4**: 35–54.
54 Johnson MD *et al.* (1999) Clinically significant drug interactions. *Postgraduate Medicine.* **105**: 193–222.
55 Samer CF *et al.* (2013) Applications of CYP450 testing in the clinical setting. *Molecular Diagnosis and Therapy.* **17**: 165–184.
56 Benitez-Rosario MA *et al.* (2006) Methadone-induced respiratory depression after discontinuing carbamazepine administration. *Journal of Pain and Symptom Management.* **32**: 99–100.
57 Kreek MJ *et al.* (1976) Rifampin-induced methadone withdrawal. *New England Journal of Medicine.* **294**: 1104–1106.
58 Backman J *et al.* (1996) Concentrations and effects of oral midazolam are greatly reduced in patients treated with carbamazepine or phenytoin. *Epilepsia.* **37**: 253–257.
59 Kay L *et al.* (1985) Influence of rifampicin and isoniazid on the kinetics of phenytoin. *British Journal of Clinical Pharmacology.* **20**: 323–326.

60 Piscitelli SC *et al.* (2000) Indinavir concentrations and St John's wort. *Lancet.* **355**: 547–548.
61 Henderson L *et al.* (2002) St John's wort (Hypericum perforatum): drug interactions and clinical outcomes. *British Journal of Clinical Pharmacology.* **54**: 349–356.
62 Flexner C (2000) Dual protease inhibitor therapy in HIV-infected patients: pharmacologic rationale and clinical benefits. *Annual Review of Pharmacology and Toxicology.* **40**: 649–674.
63 Sindrup S *et al.* (1992) The effect of quinidine on the analgesic effect of codeine. *European Journal of Clinical Pharmacology.* **42**: 587–591.
64 MHRA (2010) Clopidogrel and proton pump inhibitors: interaction - updated advice. *Drug Safety Update.* www.gov.uk/drug-safety-update
65 Society for Cardiovascular Angiography and Interventions (2009) A national study of the effect of individual proton pump inhibitors on cardiovascular outcomes in patients treated with clopidogrel following coronary stenting: The Clopidrogrel Medco Outcomes Study.: Available from: www.scai.org
66 Juurlink DN *et al.* (2009) A population-based study of the drug interaction between proton pump inhibitors and clopidogrel. *Canadian Medical Association Journal.* **180**: 713–718.
67 Ho M *et al.* (2009) Risk of adverse outcomes associated with concomitant use of clopidogrel and proton pump inhibitors following acute coronary syndrome. *Journal of the American Medical Association.* **301**: 937–944.
68 Klotz U and Reimann I (1980) Delayed clearance of diazepam due to cimetidine. *New England Journal of Medicine.* **302**: 1012–1014.
69 Nix D *et al.* (1987) Effect of multiple dose oral ciprofloxacin on the pharmacokinetics of theophylline and indocyanine green. *Journal of Antimicrobial Chemotherapy.* **19**: 263–269.
70 Vandel S *et al.* (1992) Tricyclic antidepressant plasma levels after fluoxetine addition. *Neuropsychobiology.* **25**: 202–207.
71 Finley P (1994) Selective serotonin reuptake inhibitors: pharmacologic profiles and potential therapeutic distinctions. *Annals of Pharmacotherapy.* **28**: 1359–1369.
72 Pollock B (1994) Recent developments in drug metabolism of relevance to psychiatrists. *Harvard Reviews of Psychiatry.* **2**: 204–213.
73 Tatro D (1995) Fluvoxamine drug interactions. *Drug Newsletter.* **14**: 20ff.
74 Monaham B (1990) Torsades de Pointes occurring in association with terfenadine. *Journal of the American Medical Association.* **264**: 2788–2790.
75 Honig P *et al.* (1993) Terfenadine-ketoconazole interaction. Pharmacokinetic and electrocardiographic consequences. *Journal of the American Medical Association.* **269**: 1513–1518.
76 Wilcock A *et al.* (2005) Potential for drug interactions involving cytochrome P450 in patients attending palliative day care centres: a multicentre audit. *British Journal of Clinical Pharmacology.* **60**: 326–329.
77 Kotlinska-Lemieszek A *et al.* (2014) Polypharmacy in patients with advanced cancer and pain: a European cross-sectional study of 2282 patients. *Journal of Pain and Symptom Management.* **48**: 1145–1159.
78 Maskalyk J (2002) Grapefruit juice: potential drug interactions. *Canadian Medical Association Journal.* **167**: 279–280.
79 Dahan A and Altman H (2004) Food-drug interaction: grapefruit juice augments drug bioavailability-mechanism, extent and relevance. *European Journal of Clinical Nutrition.* **58**: 1–9.
80 MHRA (2008) Statins: interactions, and updated advice for atorvastatin. *Drug Safety Update.* www.gov.uk/drug-safety-update
81 Rouseff RL (1988) Liquid chromatographic determination of naringin and neohesperidin as a detector of grapefruit juice in orange juice. *Journal - Association of Official Analytical Chemists.* **71**: 798–802.
82 Gibaldi M (1992) Drug interactions. Part II. *Annals of Pharmacotherapy.* **26**: 829–834.
83 Tailor S *et al.* (1996) Peripheral edema due to nifedipine-itraconazole interaction: a case report. *Archives of Dermatology.* **132**: 350–352.
84 Fukuda K *et al.* (2000) Amounts and variation in grapefruit juice of the main components causing grapefruit-drug interaction. *Journal of Chromatography B, Biomedical Sciences and Applications.* **741**: 195–203.
85 Savage I (2008) Forbidden fruit: interactions between medicines, foods and herbal products. *Pharmaceutical Journal.* **281**: f17.
86 Baxter K (2008) Drug interactions and fruit juices. *Pharmaceutical Journal.* **281**: 333.
87 Bailey DG *et al.* (2007) Naringin is a major and selective clinical inhibitor of organic anion-transporting polypeptide 1A2 (OATP1A2) in grapefruit juice. *Clinical Pharmacology and Therapeutics.* **81**: 495–502.
88 Sampson M (2008) New reasons to avoid grapefruit and other juices when taking certain drugs. Report from the 236th National Meeting of the American Chemical Society. Philadelphia, August 19th 2008. Available from: www.eurekalert.org/pub_releases/2008-08/acs-nrt072308.php
89 Bailey DG *et al.* (2013) Grapefruit-medication interactions: forbidden fruit or avoidable consequences? *Canadian Medical Association Journal.* **185**: 309–316.
90 Grant P (2004) Warfarin and cranberry juice: an interaction? *Journal of Heart Valve Disease.* **13**: 25–26.
91 MHRA (2004) Interaction between warfarin and cranberry juice: new advice. *Current Problems in Pharmacovigilance.* **30**: 10 (Archived).
92 MHRA (2003) Possible interaction between warfarin and cranberry juice. *Current Problems in Pharmacovigilance.* **29**: 8 (Archived).
93 Suvarna R *et al.* (2003) Possible interaction between warfarin and cranberry juice. *British Medical Journal.* **327**: 1454.
94 O'Mara N (2007) Does a cranberry juice-warfarin interaction really exist? *Pharmacist's Letter/Prescriber's Letter.* **23**: 1–3.
95 Aston JL *et al.* (2006) Interaction between warfarin and cranberry juice. *Pharmacotherapy.* **26**: 1314–1319.
96 Lilja JJ *et al.* (2007) Effects of daily ingestion of cranberry juice on the pharmacokinetics of warfarin, tizanidine, and midazolam–probes of CYP2C9, CYP1A2, and CYP3A4. *Clinical Pharmacology and Therapeutics.* **81**: 833–839.
97 Li Z *et al.* (2006) Cranberry does not affect prothrombin time in male subjects on warfarin. *Journal of the American Dietetic Society.* **106**: 2057–2061.
98 Welch J and Forster K (2007) Probable elevation in international normalized ratio from cranberry juice. *Journal of Pharmacy Technology.* **23**: 104–107.
99 FDA (2006) Drug development and drug interactions: table of substrates, inhibitors and inducers. www.fda.gov (accessed July 2014).

Updated May 2015

20: PROLONGATION OF THE QT INTERVAL IN PALLIATIVE CARE

20

The QT interval has attained greater clinical significance since it became apparent that various factors which prolong the QT interval, particularly drugs, predispose to a potentially fatal ventricular arrhythmia, *torsade de pointes*.

An accurate diagnosis of *torsade de pointes* is important because its management differs from other forms of ventricular tachycardia. Indeed, conventional drug treatments for ventricular tachycardia can exacerbate the underlying electrochemical derangement and perpetuate *torsade de pointes*.

Palliative care clinicians caring for patients with cardiac disease, or using **methadone**, need to be particularly aware of this phenomenon.

The QT interval lies on the electrocardiograph (ECG) between the beginning of the QRS complex (which marks the start of ventricular depolarization) and the end of the T wave (which marks the end of ventricular repolarization) (Figure 1).

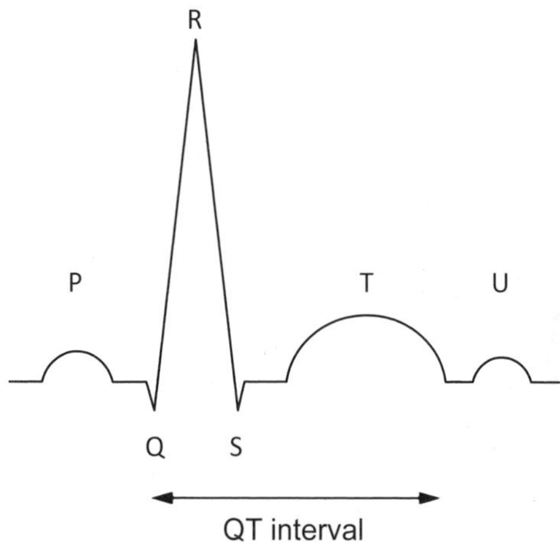

Figure 1 The QT interval.

The QT interval tends to be longer with slower heart rates. For comparative purposes, it is important to adjust ('correct') the observed QT interval to take account of this. The corrected value is designated QTc. Some ECG machines automatically calculate QTc, and this is a useful guide. However, automatic calculations can be inaccurate, particularly in the presence of atrial fibrillation, frequent ventricular ectopics, or a noisy trace. Thus, manual calculation of QTc is more accurate (Box A).[1] There are several ways of doing this, and local practice varies.[1,2]

Box A Measuring the QT interval and calculating QTc[1]

ECG

A 12-lead ECG at 25mm/sec at 10mm/mV amplitude is generally adequate, taken after the patient has rested supine for about 5min.

Measure the QT interval together with the preceding RR interval in 3–5 heart beats from leads II and V5/V6.

Calculate the mean QT and RR interval from these 3–5 measurements.

Calculate QTc using one of the following formulas:

- Bazett's (exponential square root):

$$QTc = \frac{QT\ (sec)}{\sqrt{RR\ (sec)}}$$

- Fridericia's (exponential cube root):

$$QTc = \frac{QT\ (sec)}{\sqrt[3]{RR\ (sec)}}$$

Although Bazett's formula is the most widely used, Fridericia's may be more accurate at the extremes of heart rate.

Interpretation

QTc (msec)	*Male*	*Female*
Normal	<430	<450
Borderline	430–450	450–470
Abnormal	>450	>470

Note. These limits are to a certain extent arbitrary, and given a lack of international consensus, they vary between sources.

Obtain advice

Obtain cardiology advice if:

- the end of the T wave is difficult to determine, e.g. because of a U wave
- there is bundle branch block
- there is atrial fibrillation.

A prolonged QT interval is a pro-arrhythmic state associated with an increased risk of ventricular arrhythmia, particularly *torsade de pointes* (Figure 2); this is a form of polymorphic ventricular tachycardia of varying polarity which appears to wind around the baseline and hence its name. Short runs may cause palpitation or dizziness, longer ones syncope (generally without warning) or seizure-like activity; it can settle spontaneously within seconds or degenerate into fatal ventricular fibrillation.[3] Treatment includes cardioversion when haemodynamically compromised and **magnesium sulfate** IV (2g bolus followed by an infusion of 2–4mg/min).[3]

Additional premonitory ECG signs of *torsade de pointes* include T-U wave distortion (more exaggerated in a beat after a pause), T-wave alternans (marked alternate variation in size), new ventricular ectopics or couplets, and nonsustained polymorphic ventricular tachycardia initiated in the beat after a pause.[4]

The risk of *torsade de pointes* grows as the QT interval increases, particularly >500msec. A drug which leads to an increase in QTc interval of 20–60msec should also raise concern and, if by >60msec, serious concern about the risk of arrhythmia.[5]

Drugs prolong the QT interval mainly through potassium-channel blockade (particularly I_{Kr} 'rapid' subtype) by interfering with potassium currents in (enhanced) and out (reduced) of the cardiac myocytes, modifying their repolarization and prolonging the duration of the action potential.[6] The resulting dispersion of intramural repolarization may promote triggered activity and re-entry, the electrophysiological substrate for *torsade de pointes*. Several drugs have been definitely linked with *torsade de pointes* (Box B). Concerns about safety have resulted in some drugs

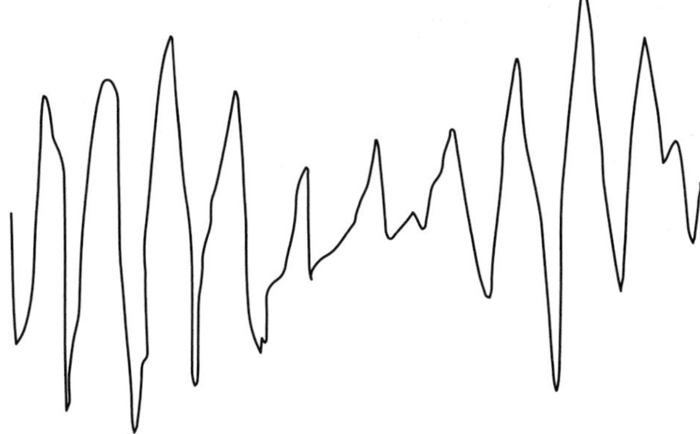

Figure 2 *Torsade de pointes.* Twisting complexes of ventricular tachycardia.

either having dose restrictions applied, e.g. **domperidone** (p.247), **citalopram/escitalopram** (p.212), and **ondansetron** (p.253), or being withdrawn completely from the UK market, e.g. **astemizole**, **cisapride**, **sertindole, terfenadine**, **thioridazine**.

Apart from providing a list of drugs with a known risk of prolonged QT and *torsade de pointes*, the website www.crediblemeds.org also identifies drugs considered 'possible risk' (insufficient evidence that authorized use causes arrhythmia) and 'conditional risk' (arrhythmia has occurred only under certain conditions, e.g. excessive dose, drug–drug interaction). The website also includes a list of drugs to be avoided by patients with congenital long QT syndrome.

Box B Drugs available in the UK with a known risk of prolonged QT interval and *torsade de pointes*[a]

Anti-arrhythmic drugs
Amiodarone
Disopyramide
Dronedarone
Flecainide
Sotalol

Antidepressant drugs
Citalopram
Escitalopram

Antimicrobial drugs
Fluconazole
Macrolides: azithromycin, clarithromycin, erythromycin
Quinolones: ciprofloxacin, levofloxacin, moxifloxacin
Pentamidine

Antimalarial drugs
Chloroquine

Psychotropic drugs
Chlorpromazine
Droperidol
Haloperidol
Levomepromazine
Pimozide
Sulpiride

Miscellaneous
Anagrelide
Arsenic trioxide
Cilostazol
Cocaine
Domperidone
Donepezil
Methadone
Ondansetron
Oxaliplatin
Propofol
Saquinavir
Sevoflurane
Toremifene
Vandetanib

a. for a full list, including those considered a possible or conditional risk, see www.crediblemeds.org

The incidence of *torsade de pointes* is greatest with cardiac anti-arrhythmics, particularly those with class Ia or III activity. For some drugs, the risk becomes significant only with:[7,8]

- high doses
- IV administration
- a pharmacokinetic drug interaction (see Chapter 19, p.717)
- impaired metabolism:
  - ▷ congenital, e.g. CYP2D6 poor metabolizers may be exposed to dangerously high plasma concentrations of risk-related drugs which are substrates for CYP2D6, even with normal doses, e.g. **flecainide**
  - ▷ acquired, e.g. hepatic or renal impairment.

The risk of drug-induced *torsade de pointes* is increased by the concurrent use of two or more drugs which prolong the QT interval, and is more likely to occur in the presence of other risk factors (Box C).[8] Some patients have a subclinical congenital long QT syndrome unmasked by a QT-prolonging drug.[3] Thus, the degree of prolongation of the QT interval is not only dose-related.

An additional contributory factor may be central sleep apnoea, which is associated with bradycardia and QT prolongation, and is reported to occur in 30% of patients on **methadone** maintenance.[9]

Box C Main additional risk factors in drug-induced *torsade de pointes*

Female gender

Congenital long QT syndrome

Baseline prolonged QT interval

Electrolyte imbalance:
- hypokalaemia
- hypomagnesaemia

Cardiac disease, e.g.:
- bradycardia <50 beats/min
- left ventricular hypertrophy
- heart failure
- recent conversion from atrial fibrillation
- ventricular arrhythmia

Implications for practice

General recommendations to guide practice are given in Box D.[2]

Box D A clinical approach to drug-induced QT prolongation

When using drugs known to prolong the QT interval, a prescriber needs to:

- understand the pharmacology of the drug, in particular factors which may lead to accumulation, e.g. drug–drug interaction, impaired elimination
- whenever possible, avoid the concurrent use of more than one drug which prolongs the QT interval
- use the lowest effective dose of the QT-prolonging drug
- evaluate and balance the potential benefit against the potential risk, taking into account the specific circumstances of the patient and the presence of other risk factors (see Box C), e.g.:
  - ▷ in patients with a known (pre-existing) prolonged QT interval, avoid the use of all QT-prolonging drugs except under specialist guidance (see Box B)
  - ▷ in patients with cardiac disease, drugs which prolong the QT interval should generally be avoided unless no suitable alternative exists
  - ▷ in patients with cardiac disease, if a cardiac anti-arrhythmic known to prolong the QT interval is prescribed, consider undertaking an ECG before and after starting the drug, and regular monitoring of plasma potassium and magnesium concentrations to ensure these remain well within their normal ranges
  - ▷ in patients without cardiac disease but with other risk factors, consider similar monitoring to above when using a QT-prolonging drug
  - ▷ for advice about patients at the end of life and also methadone, see text
- explain to the patient (and family) the risk involved and the reasons for using the drug in question, to allow an informed decision to be made
- report instances of drug-related QT prolongation to the MHRA through the yellow card scheme at www.mhra.gov.uk/index.htm
- consider *torsade de pointes* as a possible cause of palpitations, syncope or seizure-like activity.

Palliative care patients in general may be at higher risk of a prolonged QT interval given the high prevalence of multiple drug use and metabolic disturbance. Polypharmacy is the norm in palliative care,[10] and using more than one drug concurrently increases the risk of drug interactions.[11-13] However, of 300 patients referred to a specialist palliative care unit who were not imminently dying, although 48 (16%) had a prolonged QT interval, only 2 (0.7%) had a severely prolonged uncorrected QT interval of >500msec (Figure 3).[5,14] Both patients had ischaemic heart disease and, if being considered for a QT-prolonging drug such as **methadone**, would have been identified by following the guidance to undertake an ECG in patients with one or more risk factors.

Nonetheless, a commonsense approach should prevail and the benefit of certain drugs used in the last days of life, e.g. **haloperidol**, **levomepromazine**, is likely to far outweigh any risk, and an ECG is not required.[15]

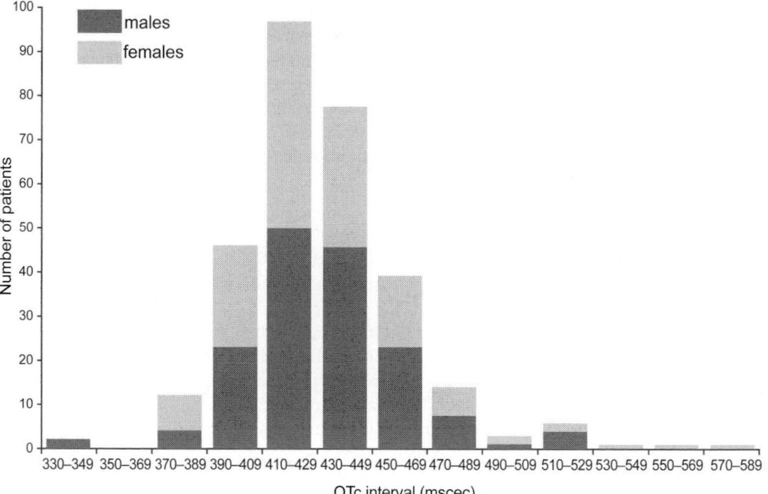

Figure 3 Distribution of the QT interval in 300 palliative care patients.[14]

Methadone

There have been longstanding concerns relating to the occurrence of serious adverse events with **methadone**, including deaths, from apparent unintentional overdose, particularly in the first 2 weeks of administration. As the use of **methadone** has increased, for both **methadone** maintenance and chronic pain, so has the number of deaths, disproportionately more than with other opioids, resulting in the US FDA issuing an alert to health professionals in 2006.[9] A major factor is considered to be a lack of knowledge among clinicians about the need to carefully monitor the use of **methadone**, particularly during the first 2–4 weeks (see **Methadone**, p.437). Although many of these deaths are likely to be a result of respiratory depression, *torsade de pointes* may be a contributing factor (Box E).

Guidelines to minimize the risk of cardiac toxicity with **methadone** are based largely on expert opinion, and recommendations vary.[15,18] Although some suggest routine ECG screening, this is debatable.[29,30] However, most advise an ECG in the presence of other risk factors for QT interval prolongation.[15,18] For example, since 2006, the SPC for **methadone** has recommended that it is used with caution in patients with any of the following risk factors for QT prolongation:

- a history of cardiac conduction abnormalities
- advanced heart disease or ischemic heart disease
- liver disease
- a family history of sudden death
- electrolyte abnormalities
- concurrent treatment with drugs which:
  - ▷ may cause electrolyte abnormalities
  - ▷ have a potential to prolong QT
  - ▷ inhibit CYP3A4 (see p.717).

Box E Methadone, prolonged QT and *torsade de pointes*

The association between methadone and prolonged QT was first reported in 1973.[16] The link with *torsade de pointes* was made in 2002 when it was described in 17 patients receiving a median dose of methadone of 330mg/day PO; all had QT >500msec and most had other risk factors.[17]

Subsequently, methadone has been found to block ion channels associated with QT prolongation, and to increase the QT interval and the risk of *torsade de pointes* generally in a dose-dependent manner.[18]

However, although some found QTc unaltered by doses <100mg/24h PO,[19] QTc >500msec and *torsade de pointes* have been reported with daily doses as low as 30–40mg PO.[20] A review of 21 patients on methadone with confirmed prolonged QT and *torsade de pointes* found generally higher daily doses (median 130mg, range 40–700mg). However, multiple risk factors were common including female gender, heart disease, hypokalaemia, hypomagnesaemia, drug interaction, multiple QT-prolonging drugs, hepatic impairment, sinus bradycardia and cocaine misuse.[21] The frequent co-existence of other risk factors makes it difficult to quantify the risk from methadone alone and may explain the inconsistent dose-relationship seen between methadone and QT prolongation.

Although slight prolongation of the QT interval by methadone appears to be common, the clinical significance of this is unclear. A marked increase in QTc to >500msec is seen in a small proportion of patients given methadone (generally about ≤5%, but 16% in one report).[18,20-24] The incidence of *torsade de pointes* and of *fatal torsade de pointes* is hard to quantify, but both are likely to be rare, e.g.:

- of the 400 adverse drug events for methadone reported to the MHRA between 1964 and 2009, 13 (3 fatal) were classified as cardiac; these included only one report each of *torsade de pointes* or ventricular fibrillation, both non-fatal; the deaths occurred after cardiopulmonary arrest or an unspecified fatal arrhythmia[25]
- the incidence of *non-fatal torsade de pointes* is estimated at 3 episodes/day per 1 million patients receiving methadone maintenance[26]
- the maximum mortality attributable to prolonged QT has been estimated to be 6 per 10,000 patient-years, based on the examination of deaths of patients receiving methadone maintenance therapy in Norway.[27]

IV methadone has been considered high-risk. In cancer patients receiving median IV doses of 430mg/day (range 2.4mg–2.4g):[28]

- two patients with prolonged QT died suddenly (although a definite link with *torsade de pointes* was not proven)
- QTc >500msec occurred in a patient receiving as little as 10mg/day.

However, the formulation of methadone contained the QT-prolonging preservative chlorbutanol; this works synergistically with methadone to prolong the QT interval. Note. None of the methadone injections marketed in the UK contain chlorbutanol.

ECG monitoring is recommended in such patients before starting **methadone** and repeated when the dose is stabilized. Some guidelines suggest an annual ECG thereafter.[18] ECG monitoring is also recommended in patients without recognized risk factors for QT prolongation, before dose titration above 100mg/day PO and 1 week after such up-titration (an arbitrary dose, based on expert opinion; others suggest 120mg/day).[18] Monitoring of serum electrolytes, e.g. potassium, magnesium, is generally recommended in patients taking diuretics or at risk of hypokalaemia, e.g. because of vomiting or diarrhoea.

Other guidelines also recommend an ECG if other risk factors or cardiac symptoms (e.g. palpitation, dizziness, fainting spells, seizures) develop during treatment and highlight the importance of educating patients taking **methadone** to avoid where possible the use of other drugs which can prolong QT or inhibit **methadone** metabolism, and to urgently report cardiac symptoms.[31]

Guidance specific for palliative care is limited. In the USA, an expert group has developed a guideline for the use of *parenteral* **methadone** for chronic pain and in the palliative/hospice setting. Partly because of the increased risk presented by the preservative **chlorbutanol** (Box E), an ECG is recommended:

- before starting IV therapy and after 1 and 4 days of treatment
- when the dose is significantly increased
- if an additional risk factor for QT prolongation develops.[32]

Monitoring serum electrolytes in high risk patients and discussing the potential risks of prolonged QT and *torsade de pointes* with the patient and carers are also recommended. However, consideration of burden vs. benefit is paramount and, in those with life-limiting illness, the potential benefit of controlling otherwise refractory pain may far outweigh the risks, even when monitoring for arrhythmia is impractical.[32] A commonsense approach should prevail: ECG monitoring is generally irrelevant in the last days of life.[15]

On the other hand, for a patient with a reasonable prognosis, it may be appropriate to identify any risk factors for QT prolongation and consider ECG monitoring as recommended in the SPC. Nonetheless, research is required to establish the magnitude of the risk of *torsade de pointes* with **methadone** and the overall value of adopting such an approach in the palliative care setting.

If the baseline QT is prolonged, an alternative opioid should be considered. Further, if the QT interval increases to >500msec when on **methadone**, generally it should be discontinued and an alternative used, e.g. SL **buprenorphine**. However, there has been a report of the successful use of parenteral **methadone** for analgesia in a patient with a prolonged QT interval.[33] Implantable cardioverter-defibrillators have also been used in addicts with *torsade de pointes* who needed to remain on **methadone**.[34]

Generally, **methadone** is available only as a racemic mixture. *S*–**methadone** is a more potent blocker of the potassium channels in the cardiac myocytes than *R*–**methadone**. CYP2B6 also displays stereoselectivity for the metabolism of *S*–**methadone**, and initial findings suggest that CYP2B6 poor metabolizers (found in about 6% of Caucasians and African-Americans) have higher levels of *S*–**methadone** and may thus be at greater risk of prolonged QTc.[35] The use of *R*–**methadone** may thus be safer in this respect but, at present, it is available only in Germany.[36,37]

1 Goldenberg I *et al.* (2006) QT interval: how to measure it and what is "normal". *Journal of Cardiovascular Electrophysiology*. **17**: 333–336.
2 Al-Khatib SM *et al.* (2003) What clinicians should know about the QT interval. *Journal of the American Medical Association*. **289**: 2120–2127.
3 Gupta A *et al.* (2007) Current concepts in the mechanisms and management of drug-induced QT prolongation and torsade de pointes. *American Heart Journal*. **153**: 891–899.
4 Drew BJ *et al.* (2010) Prevention of torsade de pointes in hospital settings: a scientific statement from the American Heart Association and the American College of Cardiology Foundation. *Circulation*. **121**: 1047–1060.
5 Committee for Proprietary Medicinal Products (1996) Points to consider: the assessment of the potential for QT interval prolongation by non-cardiovascular medicinal products. *European Agency for the Evaluation of Medicinal Products (EMEA)*. CPMP/986/996.
6 Haverkamp W *et al.* (2000) The potential for QT prolongation and proarrhythmia by non-antiarrhythmic drugs: clinical and regulatory implications. Report on a policy conference of the European Society of Cardiology. *European Heart Journal*. **21**: 1216–1231.
7 Idle JR (2000) The heart of psychotropic drug therapy. *Lancet*. **355**: 1824–1825.
8 Zipes DP *et al.* (2006) ACC/AHA/ESC 2006 guidelines for management of patients with ventricular arrhythmias and the prevention of sudden cardiac death: a report of the American College of Cardiology/American Heart Association Task Force and the European Society of Cardiology Committee for Practice Guidelines (Writing Committee to Develop guidelines for management of patients with ventricular arrhythmias and the prevention of sudden cardiac death) developed in collaboration with the European Heart Rhythm Association and the Heart Rhythm Society. *Europace*. **8**: 746–837.
9 Andrews CM *et al.* (2009) Methadone-induced mortality in the treatment of chronic pain: role of QT prolongation. *Cardiology Journal*. **16**: 210–217.
10 Twycross RG *et al.* (1994) Monitoring drug use in palliative care. *Palliative Medicine*. **8**: 137–143.
11 Bernard SA and Bruera E (2000) Drug interactions in palliative care. *Journal of Clinical Oncology*. **18**: 1780–1799.
12 Davies SJ *et al.* (2004) Potential for drug interactions involving cytochromes P450 2D6 and 3A4 on general adult psychiatric and functional elderly psychiatric wards. *British Journal of Clinical Pharmacology*. **57**: 464–472.
13 Wilcock A *et al.* (2005) Potential for drug interactions involving cytochrome P450 in patients attending palliative day care centres: a multicentre audit. *British Journal of Clinical Pharmacology*. **60**: 326–329.
14 Walker G *et al.* (2003) Prolongation of the QT interval in palliative care patients. *Journal of Pain and Symptom Management*. **26**: 855–859.
15 Wilcock A and Beattie JM (2009) Prolonged QT interval and methadone: implications for palliative care. *Current Opinion in Supportive and Palliative Care*. **3**: 252–257.
16 Stimmel B *et al.* (1973) Electrocardiographic changes in heroin, methadone and multiple drug abuse: a postulated mechanism of sudden death in narcotic addicts. *Proceedings of the National Conference on Methadone Treatment*. **1**: 706–710.
17 Krantz MJ *et al.* (2002) Torsade de pointes associated with very-high-dose methadone. *Annals of Internal Medicine*. **137**: 501–504.
18 Martin JA *et al.* (2011) QT interval screening in methadone maintenance treatment: report of a SAMHSA expert panel. *Journal of Addictive Diseases*. **30**: 283–306.
19 Stallvik M *et al.* (2013) Corrected QT interval during treatment with methadone and buprenorphine--relation to doses and serum concentrations. *Drug and Alcohol Dependence*. **129**: 88–93.

20 Stringer J *et al.* (2009) Methadone-associated QT interval prolongation and torsades de pointes. *American Journal of Health System Pharmacy*. **66**: 825–833.
21 Vieweg WV *et al.* (2013) Methadone, QTc interval prolongation and torsade de pointes: Case reports offer the best understanding of this problem. *Therapeutic Advances in Psychopharmacology*. **3**: 219–232.
22 Reddy S *et al.* (2010) The effect of oral methadone on the QTc interval in advanced cancer patients: a prospective pilot study. *Journal of Palliative Medicine*. **13**: 33–38.
23 Price LC *et al.* (2014) Methadone for pain and the risk of adverse cardiac outcomes. *Journal of Pain and Symptom Management*. **48**: 333–342.
24 Huh B and Park CH (2010) Retrospective analysis of low-dose methadone and QTc prolongation in chronic pain patients. *Korean Journal Anesthesiology*. **58**: 338–343.
25 MHRA (2009) Personal communication.
26 Hanon S *et al.* (2010) Ventricular arrhythmias in patients treated with methadone for opioid dependence. *Journal of Interventional Cardiac Electrophysiology*. **28**: 19–22.
27 Anchersen K *et al.* (2009) Prevalence and clinical relevance of corrected QT interval prolongation during methadone and buprenorphine treatment: a mortality assessment study. *Addiction*. **104**: 993–999.
28 Kornick CA *et al.* (2003) QTc interval prolongation associated with intravenous methadone. *Pain*. **105**: 499–506.
29 Haigney MC (2011) First, do no harm: QT interval screening in methadone maintenance treatment. *Journal of Addictive Diseases*. **30**: 309–312.
30 Bart G (2011) CSAT's QT interval screening in methadone report: outrageous fortune or sea of troubles? *Journal of Addictive Diseases*. **30**: 313–317.
31 Office of Alcoholism and Substance Abuse Services (2009 March) Medical advisory panel position on QTc interval screening in methadone treatment. Available from: https://www.oasas.ny.gov
32 Shaiova L *et al.* (2008) Consensus guideline on parenteral methadone use in pain and palliative care. *Palliative and Supportive Care*. **6**: 165–176.
33 Sekine R *et al.* (2007) The successful use of parenteral methadone in a patient with a prolonged QTc interval. *Journal of Pain and Symptom Management*. **34**: 566–569.
34 Patel AM *et al.* (2008) Role of implantable cardioverter-defibrillators in patients with methadone-induced long QT syndrome. *American Journal of Cardiology*. **101**: 209–211.
35 Eap CB *et al.* (2007) Stereoselective block of hERG channel by (S)-methadone and QT interval prolongation in CYP2B6 slow metabolizers. *Clin Pharmacol Ther*. **81**: 719–728.
36 Gaertner J *et al.* (2008) Methadone: a closer look at the controversy. *Journal of Pain and Symptom Management*. **36**: e4-7.
37 Ansermot N *et al.* (2010) Substitution of (R,S)-methadone by (R)-methadone: Impact on QTc interval. *Archives of Internal Medicine*. **170**: 529–536.

Updated (minor change) June 2016

21: DRUG-INDUCED MOVEMENT DISORDERS

Drug-induced movement disorders (DIMD) include:

- extrapyramidal reactions
  - ▷ onset ≤weeks: acute akathisia, dystonia and Parkinsonism (Box A)
  - ▷ onset ≥months: tardive akathisia, dyskinesia and dystonia (Box B)
- cerebellar ataxia (Box C)
- postural (essential) tremor (Box D)
- disorders with concurrent non-motor symptoms
  - ▷ acute dopamine depletion (neuroleptic/antipsychotic malignant syndrome, Box A, p.175)
  - ▷ serotonin toxicity (see Box A, p.200)
  - ▷ antidepressant withdrawal syndrome (see Box B, p.206)

The risk is associated with dose, pre-existing neurological disease and a genetic predisposition.[1–3]

Most DIMD develop within days or weeks of starting or increasing one of the drugs described below. However, many other drugs are implicated and symptom onset can be delayed by months or even years, or arise as a result of a drug interaction. Thus DIMD should be considered in any unexplained movement disorder; if in doubt, seek advice from a clinical pharmacist.

Pharmacology

Most extrapyramidal reactions are caused by drugs which block dopamine receptors in the CNS; these include all antipsychotics and **metoclopramide**. Antipsychotic drugs differ in their propensity for causing extrapyramidal reactions. A lower risk is associated with lower affinity for the D_2-receptor, D_2-receptor partial agonism, $5HT_{1A}$-receptor partial agonism and/or $5HT_2$-receptor antagonism (see p.168). Thus, the risk is a spectrum (in descending order):

- **haloperidol** (the highest risk)
- phenothiazines (e.g. **levomepromazine**)
- **risperidone**
- **olanzapine**
- **quetiapine**, **clozapine** (the lowest risk).[4]

However, their overall tolerability is comparable because lower rates of extrapyramidal reactions are offset by increased rates of sedation and/or undesirable metabolic effects (see p.168).[5]

Although the above risk spectrum still applies, akathisia remains a more common problem with atypical antipsychotics than dystonia and Parkinsonism.

Serotonin modulating drugs affect both the extrapyramidal system and spinal motor neurones. Extrapyramidal dopaminergic neurones are inhibited by $5HT_{2A}$- and $5HT_{2C}$-receptors.[6] Spinal serotonin release correlates with motor activity, stimulating spinal motor neurones at low levels and inhibiting them at higher levels.[7]

Box A Acute extrapyramidal reactions[1,8–15]

Causes

- dopamine modulators (antipsychotics, metoclopramide, levodopa)
- serotonin modulators (SSRIs, $5HT_3$ antagonists, 5-hydroxytryptophan)
- anti-epileptic drugs (carbamazepine, valproate)
- miscellaneous (diltiazem, lithium).

Classification

Parkinsonism

Generally occurs within weeks of starting the causal drug:

- resting tremor (suppressed during voluntary movements)
- muscular rigidity
- bradykinesia (e.g. shuffling gait, expressionless face).

Acute dystonia

Abnormal positioning or spasm of one or more muscle group, occurring within days of starting the causal drug:

- dysphagia
- dysphonia
- jaw (trismus, gaping, grimacing)
- tongue (dysarthria, protrusion)
- head and neck (retrocollis, torticollis)
- laryngopharyngeal spasm
- limbs or trunk
- fixed direction of gaze (oculogyric crisis).

Acute akathisia

Motor restlessness, occurring within days–weeks of starting the causal drug:

- pacing to relieve restlessness
- inability to sit or stand still
- fidgety movements or swinging of legs
- rocking from foot to foot when standing.

Treatment

Reduce or stop causal drug, or switch to an alternative with a lower risk, e.g.:

- metoclopramide → domperidone
- antipsychotic → quetiapine (see text).

If distressed, treat symptomatically while waiting for the causal drug to be cleared:

- *parkinsonism*: start an antimuscarinic, e.g. procyclidine 2.5–5mg PO t.d.s. or 5–10mg IV/IM
- *dystonia*: start an antimuscarinic (as above). If ineffective or contra-indicated, benzodiazepines are an alternative (e.g. diazepam 5mg IV then PO)
- *akathisia:* start propranolol[a] 10mg PO t.d.s.; increase if necessary every few days to a maximum daily dose of 120mg; further benefit above this level is unlikely. Alternatives include:
  - ▷ mirtazapine 15mg PO nocte
  - ▷ antimuscarinics, particularly if concurrent parkinsonism
  - ▷ benzodiazepines (as above).

a. because selective β_1-adrenergic receptor antagonists such as **atenolol** penetrate the blood-brain barrier less readily, they are less effective for akathisia.

Box B Tardive (delayed onset) extrapyramidal reactions[1,13–16]

Causes

Long-term (>3 months) treatment with antipsychotics or metoclopramide, particularly in the elderly, those on high doses, and those receiving 'typical' antipsychotics (see p.168). Also seen following reduction or cessation of treatment (withdrawal-emergent dyskinesia).

Clinical features (may co-exist)

- *tardive dyskinesia*: involuntary athetoid (writhing) and choreiform movements of the tongue, jaw and extremities, exacerbated by anxiety and reduced by drowsiness and during sleep
- *tardive dystonia*: abnormal positioning of the limbs and tonic contractions of the neck and trunk muscles causing torticollis, lordosis or scoliosis
- *tardive akathisia*: motor restlessness.

Treatment

- reduce or stop causal drug, or switch to an alternative with a lower risk, e.g.:
  - ▷ metoclopramide → domperidone
  - ▷ antipsychotic → quetiapine (see text)
- withdraw antimuscarinics (these exacerbate tardive dyskinesia)
- seek specialist advice before initiating other drug treatments (e.g. benzodiazepines).

Box C Drug-induced cerebellar ataxia[2]

Causes

Generally occurs within days or weeks of starting the causal drug, occasionally seen after using causal drug for months-years (particularly lithium, phenytoin, and valproate). Typically resolves, but can persist indefinitely, particularly when caused by lithium, phenytoin or cytarabine.

- anti-epileptic drugs
- benzodiazepines
- cytotoxics (cytarabine, irinotecan)
- immunosuppressants (cyclosporine, tacrolimus)
- miscellaneous (lithium, metronidazole).

Clinical features

- intention tremor, past pointing
- clumsy, poorly co-ordinated movements (dysdiadochokinesis)
- nystagmus.

Treatment

Reduce or stop causal drug.

Box D Drug-induced postural tremor[1,17]

Causes

- anti-epileptics (valproate)
- antidepressants
- antipsychotics
- bronchodilators (salbutamol, theophylline)
- psychostimulants (caffeine, methylphenidate)
- lithium.

Clinical features

Tremor with frequency of 8–12 cycles per second, best observed with hands held outstretched.

Treatment

Reduce or stop causal drug.

1 DSM-5 (Desk reference to the diagnostic criteria from DSM-5. The American Psychiatric Association. Chapter: medication -induced movement disorders and other adverse effects of medication).
2 van Gaalen J *et al.* (2014) Drug-induced cerebellar ataxia: a systematic review. *CNS Drugs*. **28**: 1139–1153.
3 Barnes TR (2011) Evidence-based guidelines for the pharmacological treatment of schizophrenia: recommendations from the British Association for Psychopharmacology. *Journal of Psychopharmacology*. **25**: 567–620.
4 Rummel-Kluge C *et al.* (2012) Second-generation antipsychotic drugs and extrapyramidal side effects: a systematic review and meta-analysis of head-to-head comparisons. *Schizophrenia Bulletin*. **38**: 167–177.
5 Lieberman JA *et al.* (2005) Effectiveness of antipsychotic drugs in patients with chronic schizophrenia. *New England Journal of Medicine*. **353**: 1209–1223.
6 Stahl SM (2013) Chapter 4: Psychosis and schizophrenia. In: *Essential Psychopharmacology: Neuroscientific Basis and Practical Applications* (4e). Cambridge University Press, USA. 79–128.
7 Perrier JF and Cotel F (2015) Serotonergic modulation of spinal motor control. *Current Opinion in Neurobiology*. **33**: 1–7.
8 Poyurovsky M (2010) Acute antipsychotic-induced akathisia revisited. *British Journal of Psychiatry*. **196**: 89–91.
9 Laoutidis ZG and Luckhaus C (2014) 5-HT2A receptor antagonists for the treatment of neuroleptic-induced akathisia: a systematic review and meta-analysis. *International Journal of Neuropsychopharmacology*. **17**: 823–832.
10 Lima AR *et al.* (2002) Benzodiazepines for neuroleptic-induced acute akathisia. *Cochrane Database of Systematic Reviews*. **1**: CD001950. www.thecochranelibrary.com
11 Gagrat D *et al.* (1978) Intravenous diazepam in the treatment of neuroleptic-induced acute dystonia and akathisia. *American Journal of Psychiatry*. **135**: 1232–1233.
12 Bondon-Guitton E *et al.* (2011) Drug-induced parkinsonism: a review of 17 years' experience in a regional pharmacovigilance center in France. *Movement Disorders*. **26**: 2226–2231.
13 The ICD-10 Classification of mental and behavioural disorders. http://apps.who.int/classifications/icd10/
14 Taylor D *et al.* (2015). *The Maudsley Prescribing Guidelines in Psychiatry, (12th edition)*. Publisher: Wiley-Blackwell; chapter 2 (schizophrenia), 15–185.
15 Anderson I and McAllister-Williams H (2016). *Fundamentals of Clinical Psychopharmacology*. (4th edition). Published by CRC Press, chapter 3 (antipsychotics); 47-76.
16 Bhidayasiri R *et al.* (2013) Evidence-based guideline: treatment of tardive syndromes: report of the Guideline Development Subcommittee of the American Academy of Neurology. *Neurology*. **81**: 463–469.
17 Morgan JC and Sethi KD (2005) Drug-induced tremors. *Lancet Neurolology*. **4**: 866–876.

Updated April 2017

22: DRUGS AND FITNESS TO DRIVE

This chapter summarizes the evidence regarding the effect of centrally-acting drugs of most relevance to palliative care, i.e. opioids, anti-epileptics, antidepressants, benzodiazepines and cannabinoids, on driving performance and the risk of a road traffic accident. Although impaired driving performance from stable doses of centrally-acting drugs is not inevitable, doctors have a duty of care to inform patients of the risk of impairment, particularly during initial titration, and advise them appropriately. As a minimum, patients should be informed that:

- it is their legal responsibility to drive only if they feel 100% safe to do so
- drugs should be taken in accordance with the advice of the PIL or of a health professional; this has specific implications relating to the use of certain drugs and the potential for prosecution (see below).

The presence of other factors which can impair driving performance must also be taken into account, e.g. pain, depression, insomnia, anxiety, frailty, visual disturbance. Conversely, treatment of some of these factors, e.g. pain, depression, with an appropriate centrally-acting drug can reverse the impaired driving performance. Thus, the advice given must be tailored to the individual circumstances of the patient.[1–5]

22

Evaluating the effect of drugs on driving performance

The evidence relating to the impact of centrally-acting drugs on driving can be conflicting and difficult to interpret. For example, although epidemiological studies of road traffic accidents generally find higher rates of use of centrally-acting drugs, the underlying conditions requiring their use can also impair driving performance.[1,2,6] Such confounding factors can be controlled for by studying actual or simulated driving, or surrogate laboratory markers of such skills, before and after drug administration. However, this approach may not capture all influences on driving performance, from altered attention and reaction time to impaired judgment and risk taking.[1,2,7] Thus, in this chapter, the methodology underlying the evidence is indicated for each drug class.

Guidance for patients

In the UK, drivers are liable to prosecution if driving or attempting to drive while impaired by drugs, *whether prescribed or illicit.*[3] Thus, it is important to remind patients of this when prescribing drugs which could impair their driving performance (see Box A).

Further, a recent addition to the Road Traffic Act[4] in England and Wales has specified levels for certain drugs (Box B) above which drivers are liable to prosecution, *even when driving is not impaired,* unless following the directions of a PIL or health professional. The main focus of this new law is the *illicit* use of drugs.

The evidence for sedative drugs most relevant to palliative care practice, summarized in Table 1, suggests that patients should be warned not to drive after starting and when titrating potentially sedating medication, or after taking a dose for break-through pain. They should be warned that sedation will be increased by the concurrent use of alcohol (even within normal alcohol driving limits) or other sedating medication, whether obtained by prescription, over-the-counter or illicitly.

More specifically, patients receiving opioids, anti-epileptics and antidepressants can consider driving once a stable dose is achieved if they are not affected by drowsiness, nor impaired by the disease itself. If possible, use a less sedating drug, e.g. consider the use of an SSRI rather than a TCA when treating depression. For benzodiazepines, particularly if taken in the daytime and/or those with a long halflife, the risk is more persistent, and consideration should be given to using a less sedating alternative, e.g. an SSRI for anxiety, or not driving. The risk with stable doses of prescribed cannabinoids is unclear.

Providing the patient with written information also helps (Box A). Other examples of information leaflets are available on the www.palliativedrugs.com Document library under Prescribing issues (Driving on medication).

continued

Box A Example of a patient advice leaflet: Medicines, drowsiness and driving (based on references[4,8–10])

The medicines you are taking do not automatically disqualify you from driving in the United Kingdom. *However, it is illegal to drive if medicines are reducing the speed of your reactions or general alertness.* Both the label and the Patient Information Leaflet will warn you about possible drowsiness. If so, it is important that you take the following precautions:

Do not drive

- unless you feel 100% safe to do so
- after starting or increasing the dose of any drug which may make you drowsy (whether prescribed for you or bought from a pharmacist); wait until the drowsiness fully wears off (for painkillers this takes about 5 days, sometimes longer)
- after taking an extra dose of a sedative medicine, e.g. for at least 3 hours after a 'rescue' dose of morphine for pain
- if you feel drowsy or dizzy; or your thinking, reactions, co-ordination or eyesight are impaired
- after drinking alcohol.

Restarting driving

You may try driving when you feel 100% safe to do so and you no longer feel drowsy. Begin by making a short trip:

- on roads that are quiet and familiar
- at a quiet time of day when the light is good
- with a companion who may take over driving if required.

If you and your companion are happy with your attentiveness, reactions and general ability, then you may start to drive.

Do not exhaust yourself by driving long distances. If in doubt, discuss with your doctor or other health professional.

Who to inform if you are planning to drive

- *your doctor*, who can warn you about medicines which might affect your general alertness or the speed of your reactions
- *your insurance company*, to be sure that you are covered (Note. It may help if you send the company a copy of this leaflet).

Although you do not automatically need to inform the DVLA that you are taking regular painkillers, in practice insurance companies generally advise this.

In relation to cancer, you must inform the DVLA if you have a brain tumour, a secondary tumour in your brain or if you have had a fit or problems with eyesight.

If in doubt, discuss with your doctor or the DVLA medical advisory helpline (0870 600 0301, and have your driving licence number ready).

Be prepared!

If you are taking any of the following medicines, it is recommend that, when driving, you carry evidence with you to confirm that they have been prescribed for you, e.g. a repeat prescription together with your doctor's contact details:

- *benzodiazepines;* clonazepam, diazepam, lorazepam, oxazepam, temazepam
- *opioids;* diamorphine, methadone, morphine
- *others;* amfetamine, cannabis-based medicines, ketamine

The police use roadside tests to look for illicit use of these medicines. Carrying evidence that you are taking legitimately supplied medicines is not a legal requirement but may minimise inconvenience if stopped.

However, it *is* a legal requirement that you are taking them *as advised*: do not change the dose without first discussing it with your doctor or other health professional.

Box B Drugs relevant to palliative care with specific limits set for prosecution under Section 5a of the Road Traffic Act[4,a]

Benzodiazepines
Clonazepam
Diazepam
Lorazepam
Oxazepam
Temazepam

Opioids
Diamorphine
Methadone
Morphine

Psychostimulants
Amfetamine

Miscellaneous
Δ^9-tetrahydrocannabinol
Ketamine

a. cocaine, Ecstasy, flunitrazepam (not UK), lysergic acid diethylamide (LSD) and methylamfetamine are also included on the full Department for Transport list, which is based on commonly misused drugs.

Table 1 Drugs and driving: a summary of the evidence available for sedative drugs relevant to palliative care practice

Class of drug	*Impact on risk of road traffic accidents*	*Comments*[a]
Opioids	No increased risk with chronic use of a stable dose carefully titrated to avoid drowsiness and cognitive impairment[1,2]	Cognition and driving performance impaired for about 1 week after the start of treatment or after dose increments. The risk is shared by weak opioids. Additional transient impairment with doses for break-through pain[1,2]
Anti-epileptics	No increased risk with chronic use of a stable dose carefully titrated to avoid drowsiness and cognitive impairment[11]	Cognition impaired by multiple, high-dose anti-epileptics; marginally less with newer drugs (e.g. gabapentin) compared with older drugs (e.g. carbamazepine)[12,13]
Antidepressants	Possible increased risk in the elderly (>60 years); unclear if related to the drug or underlying reason for their use, e.g. depression[2,6,14]	Sedative antidepressants impair performance for about 1 week after the start of treatment (mianserin ≥2 weeks). SSRIs appear to cause less impairment[2,3,6,14]
Benzodiazepines	60–80% increase in risk[2]	Risk only partially decreases with time and is related to dose, halflife and concurrent alcohol. Risk from nocturnal use of shorter halflife hypnotic benzodiazepines is unclear[2]
Cannabinoids	Risk likely to be increased initially. The degree of tolerance to chronic use of stable doses of prescribed cannabinoids is uncertain	Most studies deal with illicit use, frequently confounded by alcohol consumption and risk-taking behaviours[15–18]

a. advice should also take into account the presence of any comorbid conditions known to impair driving performance, e.g. pain, depression, insomnia.

Risk from specific drug classes

Opioids

Driving performance does not appear to be affected by stable doses of appropriately titrated strong opioids:[1,2]

- cognition returns to normal about 1 week after the start of treatment or after dose increments
- long-term opioid analgesia for cancer pain and non-cancer pain has little or no impact on surrogate laboratory measures of driving performance compared with:
  - ▷ healthy volunteers
  - ▷ cancer patients not taking opioids
  - ▷ patients with various causes of cerebral impairment who had passed a standardized fitness-to-drive test
- patients with non-cancer pain taking opioids at stable doses for ≥1 week do not differ from those not taking opioids or from healthy volunteers in tests of actual driving performance.

The results of epidemiological studies are mixed.[2,14,19] However, an increased risk of road traffic accidents among drivers using opioid analgesics appears unlikely if confounding variables are taken into account:

- new vs. long-term use
- opioids vs. other psychotropics taken concurrently
- prescription vs. illicit use
- opioids vs. anxiety, depression and insomnia, and the pain itself.[1]

The optimal interval between dose initiation or increase and returning to driving is unclear and may vary between individuals and formulation used, e.g. steady-state plasma concentrations of TD **fentanyl** are generally achieved after 36–48h but, according to the manufacturers, this is sometimes achieved only after 6–12 days (see p.409).

Anti-epileptics

The use of multiple or high-dose anti-epileptics, particularly **phenobarbital** is associated with marked cognitive impairment. Newer drugs, e.g. **gabapentin**, may cause marginally less impairment than older drugs, e.g. **carbamazepine**, **valproate**.[12,13] The results of epidemiological studies are mixed. However, patients with epilepsy who adhere strictly to their anti-epileptic regimen are less likely to have road traffic accidents than those patients who do not.[20]

Antidepressants

In standard on-the-road tests, sedating antidepressants (e.g. **amitriptyline**, **doxepin**, **imipramine**, **mirtazapine**, **mianserin**) impair driving performance. However, performance returns to baseline within 1 week, except for **mianserin** where impairment persists at least 2 weeks (the study endpoint). In similar studies, driving performance is unaffected by non-sedating antidepressants (e.g. SSRIs, **venlafaxine**), and on this basis they are the preferred choice in patients wanting to drive.[2,3,6] However, results of epidemiological studies suggest that both sedating and non-sedating antidepressants are associated with an increased risk of road traffic accidents, particularly in those >60 years. Depression *per se* impairs driving performance and may help explain these findings.[2,6,14] Nonetheless, caution appears necessary regardless of age and choice of antidepressant.

Benzodiazepines

In epidemiological studies, benzodiazepines increase the risk of road traffic accidents by 60–80%. The risk is highest in those taking higher doses, drugs with a longer halflife, or concurrent alcohol. The risk only partially decreases with time.[2]

Simulated driving tests show impaired reaction times, tracking and co-ordination with the acute use of benzodiazepines. In multiple-dose studies the degree of attenuation of impairment over time was variable.[2]

The risk from a bedtime dose of a hypnotic benzodiazepine with a short halflife is unclear; studies of airline pilots suggest that shorter-acting benzodiazepines do not cause a detectable sedating effect the following morning.[3] However, the results of epidemiological studies examining the risk of road traffic accidents are conflicting. Z-drugs, e.g. **zopiclone** are *not* a safer alternative.[21]

Cannabinoids

Most epidemiological studies consider the risk from the illicit use of the whole cannabis plant. Interpretation is hampered by associated alcohol consumption, risk-taking behaviour (potentially a cause and/or effect of cannabis use), and methodological limitations. However, when taken together, these studies suggest that cannabis causes dose-dependent impairment of driving ability.[3,15–18] The risk of road traffic accidents is approximately doubled, and is further increased by concurrent alcohol consumption.[15] Some studies suggest a degree of insight into the impairment, and an ability to compensate partially for it (e.g. by driving more cautiously).[22]

These studies are unlikely to reflect the risk associated with the use of stable doses of prescribed cannabinoids (see p.229). Stable doses may allow tolerance to impairment to develop, as with many psychotropics. For example, patients with multiple sclerosis and painful spasticity showed no change in surrogate markers of driving ability after receiving **nabilone** 2mg/day for 4 weeks (n=6)[23] or Sativex® for 6 weeks (n=31).[24]

However, caution remains necessary and it is sensible to advise against driving during initial dose titration. Once on a stable dose, and having evaluated the degree of psychomotor impairment caused by cannabinoids, restarting driving can be discussed. The impact of the underlying condition should also be taken into account, e.g. in one study, half of participants with multiple sclerosis had evidence of driving impairment prior to commencing cannabinoids.[24]

1 Mailis-Gagnon A *et al.* (2012) Systematic review of the quality and generalizability of studies on the effects of opioids on driving and cognitive/psychomotor performance. *Clinical Journal of Pain*. **28**: 542–555.

2 Dassanayake T *et al.* (2011) Effects of benzodiazepines, antidepressants and opioids on driving: a systematic review and meta-analysis of epidemiological and experimental evidence. *Drug Safety*. **34**: 125–156.

3 Carter T (2006) *Fitness to Drive: A Guide for Health Professionals*. Royal Society of Medicine Press, London.

4 Department for Transport (2014) Guideline for healthcare professionals on drug driving. www.gov.uk

5 Department for Transport (2013) At a glance guide to the current medical standards of fitness to drive. www.gov.uk

6 Brunnauer A and Laux G (2013) The effects of most commonly prescribed second generation antidepressants on driving ability: a systematic review. *Journal of Neural Transmission*. **120**: 225–232.

7 Verster JC and Roth T (2012) Predicting psychopharmacological drug effects on actual driving performance (SDLP) from psychometric tests measuring driving-related skills. *Psychopharmacology*. **220**: 293–301.

8 Pease N et al. (2004) Driving advice for palliative care patients taking strong opioid medication. *Palliative Medicine*. **18**: 663–665.

9 Twycross RG (1997) *Oral Morphine in Advanced Cancer* (3e). Beaconsfield Publishers, Beaconsfield.

10 MHRA (2014) New law on driving having taken certain drugs. Information leaflet to give to patients. www.gov.uk

11 Neutel I (1998) Benzodiazepine-related traffic accidents in young and elderly drivers. *Human Psychopharmacology*. **13**(Suppl): s115–s123.

12 Aldenkamp AP *et al.* (2003) Newer antiepileptic drugs and cognitive issues. *Epilepsia*. **44** (Suppl 4): 21–29.

13 Brunbech L and Sabers A (2002) Effect of antiepileptic drugs on cognitive function in individuals with epilepsy: a comparative review of newer versus older agents. *Drugs*. **62**: 593–604.

14 Orriols L *et al.* (2009) The impact of medicinal drugs on traffic safety: a systematic review of epidemiological studies. *Pharmacoepidemiology Drug Safety*. **18**: 647–658.

15 Asbridge M *et al.* (2012) Acute cannabis consumption and motor vehicle collision risk: systematic review of observational studies and meta-analysis. *British Medical Journal*. **344**: e536.

16 Downeya LA (2013) The effects of cannabis and alcohol on simulated driving: Influences of dose and experience. *Accident Analysis and Prevention 50*. 879–886.

17 Department for Transport (2010) A review of evidence related to drug driving in the UK: A report submitted to the North Review Team by P. G. Jackson and C. J. Hilditch. Currently available from http://webarchive.nationalarchives.gov.uk/20100921035225/http:/northreview.independent.gov.uk/docs/NorthReview-Report.pdf

18 Bondallaz P *et al.* (2016) Cannabis and its effects on driving skills. *Forensic Science International*. **268**: 92–102.

19 Gomes T et al. (2013) Opioid dose and risk of road trauma in Canada: a population-based study. *JAMA Internal Medicine*. **173**: 196–201.

20 Hetland A and Carr DB (2014) Medications and impaired driving. *Annals of Pharmacotherapy*. **48**: 494–506.

21 Gunja N (2013) In the Zzz zone: the effects of Z-drugs on human performance and driving. *Journal of Medical Toxicology*. **9**: 163–171.

22 Hartman RL *et al.* (2016) Cannabis effects on driving longitudinal control with and without alcohol. *Journal of Applied Toxicology*. **36**: 1418–1429.

23 Kurzthaler I *et al.* (2005) The effect of nabilone on neuropsychological functions related to driving ability: an extended case series. *Human Psychopharmacology*. **20**: 291–293.

24 Freidel M *et al.* (2015) Drug-resistant MS spasticity treatment with Sativex® add-on and driving ability. *Acta Neurologica Scandinavica*. **131**: 9–16.

Updated March 2017

23: TAKING CONTROLLED AND PRESCRIPTION DRUGS TO OTHER COUNTRIES

Some patients receiving palliative care travel to other countries and need to take medicinal products with them. Two sets of laws need to be considered, those of the country from which they are leaving and those of the country or countries to which they are travelling. Detailed advice can be obtained from the regulatory authorities, embassies or consulates in the relevant countries.[1]

UK Customs regulations

It is advisable to check for the latest Home Office guidance by contacting them directly or visiting the website:

The Home Office
Drugs and Firearms Licensing Unit
5th Floor, Fry Building
2 Marsham Street
London SW1P 4DF
Tel: 020 7035 6330
e-mail: dflu.ie@homeoffice.gsi.gov.uk
https://www.gov.uk/controlled-drugs-licences-fees-and-returns

The UK Customs regulations for travelling with prescribed medicinal products are the same for leaving or entering the UK. For UK residents, the main limitation is likely to be the legislation of the country/countries to which they are travelling (see below).

Although not a legal requirement, when travelling with *any* prescribed medicinal product, the UK Home Office advises that patients carry a covering letter from a doctor because it provides good supporting evidence that they are for the patient's own use and in quantities necessary for that period of travel.[2] The letter should state:

- the patient's name, address and date of birth
- the destination(s) and dates of outward and return travel
- the names, forms, strengths, doses and total amounts of the drugs being carried.

All prescribed medicinal products should be kept in their original packaging and carried in the patient's hand luggage, together with the covering letter ± import/export licence that may be required for controlled drugs (see below) in case Customs want to examine them.

In the UK, a covering letter is sufficient to permit air passengers to carry >100mL of a liquid/gel medicine in their hand luggage. The liquid/gel medicines must be carried in containers that permit examination by airport staff.[3] Note. Countries outside the EU may have different rules on carrying liquids as a transit or transfer passenger.

In the UK, a covering letter is also sufficient to permit essential medical equipment to be carried in hand luggage, e.g. hypodermic syringes, inhalers, TENS machine. Such equipment must be presented at security to be screened separately.

Controlled drugs

If travelling for ≥3 months *and* carrying ≥3 months supply of Schedule 2, 3, 4 part I and part II controlled drugs for personal use into or out of the UK, a personal import/export licence is required. A licence application form can be downloaded from the website above. Once completed, it must be e-mailed to the Home Office Drugs and Firearms Licensing Unit along with a letter (on headed notepaper) from a doctor confirming the patient's name, travel itinerary, names of prescribed controlled drugs, dosages and total amounts of each to be carried. At least 2 weeks should be allowed for processing. Applications from patients who are abroad, to import drugs into the UK, take longer.

If patients are carrying ≤3 months supply of Schedule 2, 3, 4 part I and part II controlled drugs for personal use, a personal import/export licence is *not* needed and a covering letter is sufficient. Thus, for some patients travelling ≥3 months, one option may be to carry ≤3 months supply and seek further supplies from a doctor in the country in which they will be staying.

A list of controlled drug schedules is included in the BNF and on the UK government website.[4,5] The amount being carried must not exceed what is required for personal use for the duration of the travel as specified in the covering letter ± personal import/export licence.

Customs regulations in other countries

It is important to fulfil the prescription and controlled drug import/export requirements for *all* the countries in which the patient will pass through Customs, otherwise entry may be refused.

The International Narcotics Control Board has produced a list of *suggested* maximum quantities of internationally controlled substances beyond which a traveller would require an import/export licence (Table 1). *However, patients should check the exact legal details and the quantities they are allowed to take into the country or countries before travelling with the relevant embassies or consulates, and the procedure for declaration at Customs.* For example, **codeine**, **dihydrocodeine** or **diamorphine** are not allowed in certain countries. A contact list of foreign embassies in the UK is available.[1] It is also advisable to carry a duplicate copy of the prescription, preferably stamped by the pharmacy from which the drugs were obtained.

Table 1 Suggested maximum quantities of controlled substances for international travellers[a,6]

Drug	*Quantity*
Buprenorphine	300mg
Codeine	12g
Diazepam	300mg
Dihydrocodeine	12g
Dronabinol	1g
Fentanyl transdermal patches[b]	100mg
Fentanyl (other formulations)	20mg
Hydromorphone	300mg
Lorazepam	75mg
Methadone	2g
Methylphenidate	2g
Morphine	3g
Oxycodone	1g
Temazepam	600mg

a. this is not a complete list; see referenced source for more details

b. approximately, this adds up to 6 fentanyl 100microgram/h patches, and 8, 12, 24, 48 of the 75, 50, 25, 12microgram/h patches, respectively.

1 Foreign and Commonwealth Office (2016) London diplomatic list: Foreign embassies in the UK. www.gov.uk

2 UK Government Controlled drugs: licences, fees and returns. www.gov.uk (accessed January 2017).

3 UK Government Hand luggage restrictions at UK airports. www.gov.uk (accessed January 2017).

4 British National Formulary Controlled drugs and drug dependence. London: BMJ Group and Pharmaceutical Press. www.medicinescomplete.com (accessed January 2017).

5 UK Government List of the most commonly encountered drugs controlled under the misuse of drugs legislation. www.gov.uk (accessed January 2017).

6 International Narcotics Control Board (2004) International guidelines for national regulations concerning travellers under tratment with internationally controlled drugs. www.incb.org

Updated March 2017

24: OBTAINING SPECIALS

For a full explanation of the authorization process, definitions and general details related to prescribing of medicinal products without a marketing authorization (unauthorized) in the UK see p.xix.

'Specials' encompasses special-order manufactured formulations (Box A) and products that require importation, e.g. ***S*-ketamine** injection, **metolazone** tablets. They do not have a marketing authorization in the UK and are thus unauthorized.

The MHRA maintains a register of manufacturing sites which includes special-order manufacturers, NHS manufacturing units and specialist importing companies (updated monthly).[1] NHS manufacturing units are also listed in the BNF.

Box A Special-order manufactured formulations

A special-order manufactured formulation includes the following:

- a bespoke formulation made by a specials manufacturer holding a manufacturer's specials licence (MS) for an individual patient, *without* end product analytical testing, e.g. a specific strength of an oral solution for a child
- a commonly requested formulation manufactured by a specials manufacturer holding an MS, produced in multiple quantities (batches) *with* end product analytical testing, e.g. some prefilled opioid syringes, ketamine oral solution, alfentanil nasal/buccal spray.

To ensure the quality of the product, the Royal Pharmaceutical Society advises that a certificate of conformity (bespoke products) or a certificate of analysis (batch manufactured specials) should be requested by pharmacists with every product.

A certificate of conformity is a signed statement by the manufacturer that they believe the product complies with the purchaser's specification.

A certificate of analysis is evidence that critical parameters have been confirmed by retrospective physical, chemical or microbiological assay of a sample of the final product.

An MS guarantees the sourcing of ingredients, product development, packaging and labelling, the manufacturing and ex-factory supply processes are to regulatory standards. Unlike a MA, *it does not include formal evaluation of safety or efficacy of the product, and therefore there is no SPC.*

Issues to consider when prescribing and supplying a special[2,3]

Prescribers need to know (or be made aware) if a product is unauthorized.[4] This can be forgotten particularly with readily available batch-made specials for local 'routine' specialist use, e.g. **ketamine** oral solution. Pharmacists have a professional duty to liaise with the prescriber regarding the supply of a special. Royal Pharmaceutical Society guidance is available for prescribers and pharmacists, both underpinned by five principles (Box B).[2,3]

Box B Principles for the prescribing, procurement and supply of a special[2,3]

1. Establish a clinical need.
2. Understand the patient's experience and make a shared decision.
3. Identify medicines and preparations.
4. Monitor and review.
5. Ensure effective prescribing governance.

Product specification

Specials are supplied according to the specification agreed between the purchaser and the manufacturer. Thus, it is important to understand the patient's exact requirements and to specify details relating to dosage, strength or concentration, and formulation, e.g.:

- *tablets*; scored/non-scored, e.g. scored, **levomepromazine** 6mg tablets
- *oral liquid*:
  - ▷ consistency, e.g. solutions rather than suspensions for administration via EFT
  - ▷ alcohol-content, sugar-content, flavouring, e.g. for children
- *injections/nasal or buccal sprays/eye-drops*:
  - ▷ drug salt, e.g. for imported injections when there are UK supply issues
  - ▷ racemic mix or enantiomer, e.g. for **S-ketamine** vs **ketamine** injection
  - ▷ excipients, e.g. propylene glycol content which may not be suitable for all routes of administration
- *creams/ointments*:
  - ▷ type of base, excipients, e.g. to avoid allergens or to prolong shelf-life.

Because the quality and bio-equivalence of the product can vary between manufacturers or imported products, whenever possible, the same supplier should be used.

Availability and shelf-life

Practical issues such as availability and shelf-life can influence the choice of the product, formulation and supplier. Shelf-lives may be short, particularly for preservative-free formulations, which will have implications for quantities prescribed, cost and ordering of repeat prescriptions. Some commonly requested batch-made specials, e.g. **ketamine** oral solution, are kept as stock in some specialist units. However, in the community a supply may not be so readily available and require several days to organise.

Cost

Generally, costs for specials are higher than for authorized products. Some commonly prescribed specials are listed in part VIIIB of the Drug Tariff (Arrangements for payment of specials and imported unlicensed medicines). This standardizes the cost to the prescriber for that product. However, for products not listed in this section, the price can vary significantly depending on which supply route and/or manufacturer is used by the hospital/community pharmacy.

Transfer of care

Close collaboration between primary and secondary care health professionals is essential to ensure continuity of supply and product consistency for the patient.[2,3,5] In the community there may be less familiarity with specials, they make take longer to obtain and cost more. The new prescriber and dispensing pharmacist need to understand the clinical need for the special, the specific formulation details and the practical implications of taking over the prescribing and supply of the special.

Further, the patient/carer should be informed that they have been prescribed a special and given appropriate information about use, product specification and implications for follow up supply.

Record-keeping

Pharmacists should keep records of the source, quantity obtained, batch numbers and the quantity supplied of the unauthorized product, along with prescriber and patient details. They must also record and report any adverse reactions associated with their use.[2,4] Although pharmacists should record patient details (hence the commonly used term 'named patient supply'), there is no legal requirement to provide special-order manufacturers or specialist importing companies with this information[1]. When ordering, most companies require confirmation that the product is being supplied for a definite individual clinical need which cannot be satisfied by an existing authorized product.

In hospitals, some specials, e.g. **ketamine** oral solution, are used as standard supplies and kept as stock at ward level. Thus, they may be used without obtaining patient details; however, this is considered acceptable as long as the hospital formulary committee takes responsibility and appropriate governance is in place, e.g. a risk stratification and management plan.[2,6]

1 MHRA (2016) Human and veterinary medicines: register of licensed manufacturing sites. www.gov.uk
2 Royal Pharmaceutical Society (2015) Professional guidance for the procurement and supply of specials. www.rpharms.com
3 Royal Pharmaceutical Society (2016) Prescribing specials. Guidance for the prescribers of specials. www.rpharms.com
4 MHRA (2014) The supply of unlicensed relevant medicinal products ("specials"). *MHRA Guidance Note 14*. Available from: www.gov.uk
5 Royal Pharmaceutical Society (2012) Keeping patients safe when they transfer between care providers - getting the medicines right. www.rpharms.com
6 Royal Pharmaceutical Society (2016) Personal communication. *Professional support department*. www.rpharms.com

Updated March 2017

25: MANAGEMENT OF POSTOPERATIVE PAIN IN OPIOID-DEPENDENT PATIENTS

Opioid-dependent patients include those using long-term opioids for:

- pain relief (mostly cancer but also non-cancer pain)
- long-term opioid maintenance for opioid dependence
- current substance misuse.

All such patients will require *additional opioids* to relieve *additional pain*. It is thus crucially important that pre-operative, peri-operative and postoperative doses take this into account, and that *extra amounts* of a strong opioid are prescribed. Generally, these will be larger than the typical doses used by non-opioid-dependent patients in these circumstances.[1] For example, if only typical postoperative doses are prescribed (e.g. **morphine** 2.5–10mg IV/SC q1h p.r.n.), patients who are tolerant to higher doses may experience little or no pain relief. However, opioid requirements vary widely and close monitoring is essential.

Because tolerance to undesirable effects, e.g. respiratory depression, develops more rapidly than to analgesia (often within days or 1–2 weeks at most), opioids can be safely titrated to the higher doses required in opioid-dependent patients.

Further, a sudden significant reduction in overall opioid dose may well precipitate an opioid withdrawal syndrome, possibly accompanied by *hyperalgesia*. This will magnify the postoperative pain and any other underlying pain. Thus, under-prescribing can lead to devastating overwhelming pain.

As far as possible, a multidisciplinary approach should be adopted, e.g. pre-operative consultation with the patient's substance misuse team, the anaesthetist and the acute pain team, to develop a pain management plan which should include intra-operative and postoperative monitoring, with dose adjustments made by an experienced anaesthetist. There are no uniform recommendations, but Box A outlines the general approach.[2–9] Addicts receiving maintenance therapy with **methadone** or high-dose SL **buprenorphine**, or **naltrexone** require additional considerations (see below).

Other classes of drugs used for analgesia, e.g. antidepressants, anti-epileptics, should also be continued with as little interruption as possible.[10]

Addicts receiving methadone maintenance therapy

Generally, **methadone** maintenance therapy is administered once daily, which is adequate to prevent opioid withdrawal symptoms, but not pain, for 24h. In acute pain, the maintenance dose should be continued at the same dose but, by giving half the daily dose b.d., it contributes better towards analgesia (e.g. 40mg once daily → 20mg b.d.).[8] When the PO route cannot be used, SC or CSCI are alternative routes of administration (see p.437).

Addicts receiving high-dose SL buprenorphine maintenance therapy

Buprenorphine acts as a partial agonist at the μ-opioid receptor, to which it binds with a higher affinity than other μ-opioid receptor agonists. Thus, when **buprenorphine** is present in sufficient amounts, it will antagonize the analgesic effects of other μ-opioid receptor agonists. This is likely only with the higher doses used SL for opioid maintenance, i.e. ≥16mg/day (see p.397). This has led some to advocate discontinuing high-dose SL **buprenorphine** 5–7 days before elective surgery to avoid compromising postoperative pain relief, and to manage withdrawal symptoms with **methadone** instead.[12] On the other hand, various μ-opioid receptor agonists have been successfully used for postoperative pain in patients on SL **buprenorphine** 2–32mg/day, although higher doses than usual may be required.[13–15]

Box A Management of postoperative pain in opioid-dependent patients

1 Consider local anaesthetic or multimodal approaches to analgesia, e.g. regional blocks, paracetamol, NSAIDs, ketamine, clonidine, etc.

2 Identify the baseline opioid dose: in patients misusing opioids this may mean a 'best guess' estimate.

3 Generally, the baseline opioid dose should be continued as a regular prescription.

4 Reduce the baseline dose if:
- the surgery will improve the pre-operative pain
- the baseline opioid needs to be replaced by an alternative opioid; because of possible incomplete cross-tolerance, reduce the dose calculated from equipotency tables by at least 1/3, particularly when dealing with large doses, e.g. ≥ morphine 1g PO/24h or equivalent (see p.371).

5 Patients on m/r opioids PO can take them (and other analgesics) on the day of surgery, even if fasting, unless there is a specific contra-indication.[8]

6 If PO is not possible pre- or immediately postoperatively, an alternative route, e.g. CSCI or CIVI should be used to deliver the baseline dose. This can also be done via IV patient-controlled analgesia (PCA; see point 12).

7 Before restarting m/r opioids PO, ensure that GI function has returned to normal. Gastric stasis can lead to delayed dissolution and drug absorption, followed by 'dose-dumping' when motility improves, with consequential overdose. Conversely, surgery which shortens GI transit time (e.g. small bowel resection) may render the use of m/r products inappropriate.

8 If the surgery is unlikely to lead to major changes in skin perfusion and the ongoing opioid requirements are unlikely to change, it is best to leave TD fentanyl patches in place, and give additional p.r.n. opioid.

9 If TD patches are removed, pain relief will persist for several hours because fentanyl is sequestrated widely throughout the body, particularly in adipose tissue (see p.409). Note. In postoperative patients, after a patch has been removed, the mean time for the plasma fentanyl concentration to drop below the minimum effective level is 16h, with a range of 2–23h.[11]

10 Continue long-term ED or IT pumps unchanged unless the surgery is expected to reduce the pain for which these are being used.

11 Prescribe an appropriate dose of a strong opioid for p.r.n. use; typically equivalent to 1/10–1/6 to of the total daily dose.

12 With IV PCA, a larger bolus dose is generally necessary compared with the typical bolus dose of morphine 1mg. PCA can also be used to continuously deliver part or all of the baseline opioid dose.

Example
Patient on long-term morphine 300mg/day PO = 100mg/day IV = 4mg/h IV.
PCA background infusion = 2–3mg/h IV.
PCA bolus dose = 2mg IV with a 5min lockout period between doses.

With addicts, if there is considerable uncertainty about their opioid intake, it may be safer to underestimate both the background infusion dose and bolus dose required.

13 Close monitoring is required to:
- identify inadequate dosing (unrelieved pain, withdrawal phenomena)
- ensure rapid dose titration
- prevent excessive dosing (sedation, respiratory depression)
- ensure that bolus doses are not being misused.

For someone on high-dose SL **buprenorphine** who experiences acute pain unexpectedly, options include:

- regional anaesthesia
- optimizing the use of non-opioid analgesics (see Box A)
- prescribing a μ-opioid receptor agonist, e.g. IV **morphine**, **fentanyl**; higher doses than usual may be required
- progressively increasing the SL **buprenorphine** dose up to 24–32mg/day, and give in divided doses t.d.s.–q.d.s.[12,14]

Addicts receiving long-term naltrexone therapy

The opioid antagonist **naltrexone** is used to prevent relapse in opioid ex-addicts (by blocking the opioid 'high'), and in the treatment of alcohol dependence. It blocks all types of opioid receptor, and is long-acting. It thus prevents/blocks opioid analgesia. Analgesia for these patients is even more challenging (see Opioid antagonists (therapeutic target within the CNS) Box A, p.460).[16]

1 Rapp SE *et al.* (1995) Acute pain management in patients with prior opioid consumption: a case-controlled retrospective review. *Pain.* **61**: 195–201.

2 Macintyre PE (2001) Safety and efficacy of patient-controlled analgesia. *British Journal of Anaesthesia.* **87**: 36–46.

3 Roberts DM and Meyer-Witting M (2005) High-dose buprenorphine: perioperative precautions and management strategies. *Anaesthesia and Intensive Care.* **33**: 17–25.

4 Alford DP *et al.* (2006) Acute pain management for patients receiving maintenance methadone or buprenorphine therapy. *Annals of Internal Medicine.* **144**: 127–134.

5 British Pain Society (2007) Pain and substance misuse: improving the patient experience. British Pain Society, London. Available from: www.britishpainsociety.org

6 Macintyre PE and Ready LB (2006) *Acute Pain Management - A Practical Guide* (2e). Saunders Ltd., p. 272.

7 Mehta V and Langford RM (2006) Acute pain management for opioid dependent patients. *Anaesthesia.* **61**: 269–276.

8 Huxtable CA *et al.* (2011) Acute pain management in opioid-tolerant patients: a growing challenge. *Anaesthesia and Intensive Care.* **39**: 804–823.

9 British Pain Society (2010) Cancer pain management. British Pain Society, London. Available from: www.britishpainsociety.org

10 Farrell C and McConaghy P (2012) Perioperative management of patients taking treatment for chronic pain. *British Medical Journal.* **345**: e4148.

11 Grond S *et al.* (2000) Clinical pharmacokinetics of transdermal opioids: focus on transdermal fentanyl. *Clinical Pharmacokinetics.* **38**: 59–89.

12 Savage SR *et al.* (2008) Challenges in using opioids to treat pain in persons with substance use disorders. *Addiction Science and Clinical Practice.* **4**: 4–25.

13 Kornfield H and Manfredi L (2010) Effectiveness of full agonist opioids in patients stablized on buprenorphine undergoing major surgery: A case series. *American Journal of Therapeutics.* **17**: 523–528.

14 Heit HA and Gourlay DL (2008) Buprenorphine: new tricks with an old molecule for pain management. *Clinical Journal of Pain.* **24**: 93–97.

15 Macintyre PE *et al.* (2013) Pain relief and opioid requirements in the first 24 hours after surgery in patients taking buprenorphine and methadone opioid substitution therapy. *Anaesthesia and Intensive Care.* **41**: 222–230.

16 Vickers AP and Jolly A (2006) Naltrexone and problems in pain management. *British Medical Journal.* **332** (7534): 7132–7533.

Updated April 2017

25

26: DRUGS FOR PRURITUS

Pathophysiology

Although pruritus is limited to skin, conjunctivae or a mucous membrane (including the upper respiratory tract), the cause is not always peripheral (Box A).

Box A A neuro-anatomical classification of pruritus	
Peripheral causes	**Central causes**
Cutaneous ('pruritoceptive'), e.g.	Neuropathic, e.g.
skin diseases	brain injury[1]
urticaria (most)	brain abscess
stinging nettle rash	brain tumour[1]
insect bite reactions	multiple sclerosis
drug (± rash)	Neurogenic, e.g.
cutaneous mastocytosis (rare)	opioid
Neuropathic, e.g.	cholestasis
post-herpetic neuralgia	paraneoplastic
	Psychogenic
	Mixed peripheral and central causes
	Uraemia

Pruritogens

The afferent nerve fibres associated with peripheral causes of pruritus are a subset of C-fibres.[2,3] Their terminals are more superficial than the nociceptive C-fibres, close to the junction between epidermis and dermis and are stimulated by a wide range of pruritogens (Box B).

Box B Chemical mediators of pruritus (pruritogens)	
Amines, e.g.	Neuropeptides, e.g.
histamine	substance P
serotonin	calcitonin-gene-related peptide (CGRP)
Opioids	bradykinin
Eicosanoids[a]	somatostatin
Cytokines	vaso-active intestinal peptide (VIP)
Proteases	cholecystokinin
Growth factors	

a. collective term for metabolites of arachidonic acid, including prostanoids and leukotrienes.

Studies suggest that there are two peripheral pathways for pruritus; one activated by histamine and the other by alternative pruritogens (e.g. cowhage spicules).[4] This helps to explain why some types of pruritus do not respond, or respond only weakly, to H_1 antihistamines.

Histamine

Histamine is an important chemical mediator of pruritus of cutaneous origin. Endogenous histamine released in the skin is mostly from mast cells and mediates pruritus via H_1-, H_4-[5,6] and possibly H_3-receptors.[7] Further, histamine probably also stimulates the formation of other pruritogens.[8]

H_4-receptors are also found in the spinal cord and brain.[9] Thus, histamine may be involved in some forms of central pruritus.

Proteases

Proteases are released from mast cells and keratinocytes and act on PAR2 receptors expressed on afferent neurones and keratinocytes.[10,11]

Serotonin/5HT

Serotonin/5HT is a weaker pruritogen than histamine.[12] SSRIs relieve pruritus associated with primary biliary cirrhosis,[13,14] cancer[15] and uraemia.[16] **Ondansetron** relieves pruritus related to spinal **morphine**[17] but *not* cholestatic or uraemic pruritus.[18]

Substance P

Substance P is released from mast cells and mediates pruritus via NK_1-receptors. The expression of these receptors is increased on keratinocytes in pruritic skin disease.[19] Aprepitant, an NK_1 antagonist, relieves pruritus in cancer patients receiving targeted anti-cancer drugs.[20]

Pruritus in systemic disease

Pruritus occurs in many systemic conditions (Box C), and may be caused by peripheral or central mechanisms, or both (Box D).

Box C Systemic disease associated with pruritus[20]

Endocrine
Carcinoid syndrome
Diabetes mellitus (associated with genital candidosis)
Hyperparathyroidism (secondary to chronic renal failure)[a]
Hyperthyroidism
Hypothyroidism

Haematological
Leukaemia
Lymphoma
Mastocytosis
Multiple myeloma
Polycythaemia rubra vera

Hepatic
Cholestasis
Hepatitis
Primary biliary cirrhosis

Renal
Chronic renal failure

Other
AIDS
Cancer
Multiple sclerosis

a. correction of hypercalcaemia leads to the rapid relief; in other circumstances, hypercalcaemia is *not* associated with pruritus.

Box D Causal factors in pruritus[a]

Cholestasis
Endogenous opioids ↑
Autotaxin and LPA[b] ↑
Serotonin release ↑

Old age
Dry skin
Mast cell degranulation[22] ↑
Skin sensitivity to histamine[22] ↑

Paraneoplastic
Histamine release from basophils
Serotonin release ↑
Immune response

Renal failure
Cytokines
Substance P release ↑
Skin divalent ions (Ca^{2+}, Mg^{2+}, PO_4^{2-}) ↑
Skin vitamin A ↑
Mast cell proliferation
μ- and κ-opioid receptor imbalance
Peripheral neuropathy

Targeted treatment with anti-EGFR drugs or tyrosine-kinase inhibitors
Secretion of stem-cell factors ↑ and accumulation of dermal mast cells in areas of skin rash
NK_1-receptors in mast cells and keratinocytes in inflamed areas[23] ↑

a. dry skin is often an important concurrent factor
b. plasma concentrations of autotaxin and lysophosphatidic acid (LPA) correlate with pruritus and are reduced by antipruritic treatments, e.g. rifampicin (see p.481).[24]

Drugs

All drugs have the potential to cause an allergic reaction which can cause pruritus, with or without a rash (Box E). The mechanism involves the release of histamine from mast cells. The pruritus responds to H_1 antihistamines (and stopping the offending drug).

Box E Common allergic drug skin reactions

Rashes	**Urticaria**
Cephalosporins	Cephalosporins
Penicillins	Penicillins
Phenytoin	Radio-opaque dyes
Sulfonamides	Sulfonamides

Opioid-induced pruritus

There are two types of opioid-induced pruritus. One is an allergic reaction related to cutaneous histamine release, and possibly occurs in only ~1% of patients receiving an opioid systemically. It responds to H_1 antihistamines and a switch in opioid.

Histamine is also released after an *intradermal* injection of an opioid (and responds to H_1 antihistamines). However, this is probably irrelevant in relation to pruritus associated with systemic opioids because *in vitro* studies indicate that the dose of **morphine** or **methadone** needed to release histamine from mast cells is some 10,000 times greater than the dose needed for μ agonist effects.[25]

The second type is a central reaction to opioids, and is less histamine-dependent.[26–28] In surgical (opioid-naïve) patients who receive spinal opioids pre-operatively, the incidence is ≤80% but, in patients with chronic pain already taking opioids by another route, only 10–15%.[29–31] The incidence also depends on the opioid used; for example, with caesarean section, pruritus is more common with epidural **morphine** than epidural **hydromorphone**.[32]

However, anecdotally in cancer patients receiving palliative care, the incidence of pruritus in such patients appears to be virtually zero,[33] possibly because of the concurrent use of **bupivacaine**.[34,35]

Several hours after spinal injection, pruritus typically spreads rostrally through the thorax from the level of the injection and is typically maximal in the face, but may be limited to the nose (more likely when **bupivacaine** is given concurrently).[36]

Although pruritus induced by either systemic or spinal **morphine** is relieved by **naloxone** or **naltrexone**, this risks reversal of analgesia.[37] Other options are discussed in Chapter 32, p.839.

Management

Correct the correctable

Consider and treat:

- dry skin: very common in advanced cancer. Even when there is a probable endogenous cause, rehydration of the skin may obviate the need for specific measures (see Emollients, p.627)
- review the patient's medication: if a drug is the likely cause (Box E) it should be stopped, and an alternative prescribed if necessary (for opioids, see Table 1 below). With **penicillins** the pruritic rash may not appear until several days after the antibacterial has been stopped
- atopic dermatitis: topical corticosteroid and an emollient (see Emollients, p.627)
- contact dermatitis: topical corticosteroid, identify causal substance, avoid further contact
- scabies: topical **permethrin** or **malathion** (see respective SPCs)
- cholestatic pruritus secondary to obstruction of the common bile duct: this resolves if the jaundice is relieved by inserting an intraductal stent via ERCP or other drainage procedure
- uraemic pruritus in haemodialysis patients: optimise renal support, correct hyperphosphataemia, iron deficiency
- Hodgkin's lymphoma: radiotherapy and/or chemotherapy.

Non-drug treatment

Non-drug treatment includes the following measures:

- avoid soap; use moisturizing soap substitutes
- apply emollient b.d–t.d.s.
- discourage scratching: file finger nails, allow gentle rubbing
- avoid prolonged hot baths
- dry the skin by patting gently with a soft towel or use a hair dryer *on a cool setting*
- avoid overheating and sweating, particularly in bed at night
- increase air humidity in the bedroom to avoid skin drying
- in uraemia: UVB phototherapy.[38]

Drug treatment

Topical applications

Traditional topical antipruritics include **phenol** 0.5–3%, **levomenthol (menthol)** 0.5–2% and **camphor** 0.5–3% (see p.635). Although not practical to apply topical products over the whole body, some patients with generalized pruritus have areas of greater intensity and obtain benefit from the more selective application of a topical antipruritic.

In uraemic pruritus, **capsaicin** cream 0.025–0.075% once daily–q.d.s. may help.[39,40] Some patients find the burning sensation after application unacceptable (see p.601). Transdermal high-dose capsaicin has been reported to be of benefit in localized pruritus, e.g. brachioradial pruritus[41] and notalgia paresthetica.[42]

Although **doxepin** has also been used topically in various conditions, it has several disadvantages which limit such use (see p.635).

Systemic treatment

If the skin is inflamed as a result of scratching (but not infected), consider a corticosteroid, e.g. **dexamethasone** 2–4mg each morning or **prednisolone** 10–20mg each morning for 1 week.

Unless specific treatment is indicated, consider a trial of a sedative antihistamine either at bedtime (pruritus is generally worse at bedtime and through the night) or round the clock, depending on circumstances. Either an H_1-receptor antagonist or a phenothiazine with antihistaminic properties can be used:

- **chlorphenamine** 4mg t.d.s.–12mg q.d.s.; useful for rapid dose escalation to determine if an antihistamine is of benefit
- **promethazine** 25–50mg b.d.
- **hydroxyzine** 10–25mg b.d.–t.d.s.; 25–100mg at bedtime
- **alimemazine (trimeprazine)** 5–10mg b.d.–t.d.s.; 10–30mg at bedtime
- **levomepromazine** 6–25mg PO at bedtime.[43]

For some patients, a benzodiazepine is as effective as a sedative antihistamine.[44]

Doxepin, a TCA and potent H_1- and H_2-receptor antagonist, is a further alternative. Most TCAs have antihistaminic properties but **doxepin** is the most potent in this respect.[45] Some patients with chronic urticaria unresponsive to conventional H_1 antihistamines obtain relief from **doxepin** 10–75mg PO at bedtime.[46] In an RCT, **doxepin** 10mg b.d. PO was effective in patients with uraemic pruritus.[47]

Table 1 provides clinicians with a synopsis of possible treatments of choice. Some are supported by evidence from RCTs but, for others, the evidence is low level ('opinions and/or clinical experiences of respected authorities'). Further information is available elsewhere.[48,49]

Commentary

There appear to be similarities between neuropathic pain, pruritus and cough. The common theme being peripheral and central sensitization of the sensory nervous system. This may explain why a range of anti-epileptics and antidepressants have been reported as effective treatments for these very different symptoms. The persistence of pruritus in patients with myeloproliferative disorders despite disease control suggests central sensitization.

The inclusion of **carbamazepine** as an option for the treatment of pruritus with lymphoma or cancer is based on its successful use in just four patients (three with B-cell lymphoma and one with myeloma).[62] It had previously been used with good effect in three patients with multiple sclerosis.[65]

Table 1 Suggested treatment for specific causes of pruritus (UK)[a,b]

Condition	*Step 1*	*Step 2*	*Step 3*
Cholestasis[c]	Sertraline 50–100mg once daily **A**[14] *or* Rifampicin 150–600mg once daily **A**[50,51]	Alternate Step 1 *or* Danazol 200mg once daily–t.d.s.; if successful, titrate progressively downwards (e.g. to thrice weekly) after 2–3 weeks[52,53]	Naltrexone[d,e] 12.5–250mg once daily **A**[51,54]
Uraemia	If localized, capsaicin cream 0.025–0.075% once daily–q.d.s. **A**[39,40] *or* UVB phototherapy **A**[38]	Gabapentin 100–400mg after haemodialysis **A**[55–57] *or* Doxepin 10mg b.d. **A**[47]	Sertaline 50mg once daily **B**[16] *or* Naltrexone 50mg once daily **A**[e,f 58]
Systemic opioids (for spinal opioids, see Chapter 32, p.839)	Stat dose of H_1-antihistamine, e.g. chlorphenamine 4–12mg; if after 2–3h there is definite benefit, prescribe 4mg t.d.s. (for alternatives, see main text above) *or* a less sedative second generation H_1-antihistamine, e.g. cetirizine 10mg once daily/at bedtime[59]	Switch opioid, e.g. morphine → oxycodone[28,60]	Ondansetron 8mg PO b.d.
Hodgkin's lymphoma	Prednisolone 10–20mg t.d.s.	Cimetidine 800mg/24h[g 61]	Carbamazepine 200mg b.d.[62]
Paraneoplastic, other causes, idiopathic	Sertraline 50–100mg once daily *or* Paroxetine 5–20mg once daily **A**	Mirtazapine 15–30mg at bedtime[63]	Thalidomide (see below *When all else fails*)

a. strength of recommendations: grade **A** is based on evidence from ≥1 RCTs, and grade **B** on well-designed non-randomized studies;[64] where no grade is given, the recommendation is based on case reports and/or expert opinion
b. given PO unless stated otherwise
c. in total bile obstruction, where bile duct stenting is impossible or unwanted
d. this is first-line treatment at some specialist liver centres
e. unsuitable for patients who need opioids for pain relief (for the use of methylnaltrexone in cholestasis, see *Other options* below and p.457)
f. RCTs give contradictory results: much benefit vs. no benefit (see *Commentary* below and p.457)
g. in various haematological cancers, there are anecdotal reports of enhanced benefit when an H_1 antagonist and an H_2 antagonist are used in combination.

Although potentially a class effect, it is unknown if other SSRIs are as equally effective as **fluvoxamine**, **paroxetine** and **sertraline** which improve pruritus in various situations (including solid cancers, haematological cancers, non-cancer disorders and idiopathic). **Sertraline** is a good choice because of a lower risk of drug interactions and discontinuation reactions. The antidepressant **mirtazapine**, an H_1-, $5HT_2$-, $5HT_3$-receptor antagonist, is reported anecdotally to be effective in pruritus associated with cancer and lymphoma.[63] Anecdotally, patients who fail to respond to an SSRI may respond to **mirtazapine**, and sometimes vice versa.

Although **ondansetron**, a $5HT_3$ antagonist, relieves pruritus induced by spinal **morphine**,[17] it does *not* relieve cholestatic or uraemic pruritus.[66]

The classic hepatic enzyme inducer, **rifampicin** (p.481), in a dose of 300–600mg once daily has been shown to be of benefit in two RCTs lasting 1–2 weeks in patients with cholestatic pruritus.[50,51] Because of rare reports of severe hepatotoxicity with **rifampicin** and because of intolerance in cachectic patients, a lower starting dose is advisable, i.e. 150mg.

It has long been known that 17-α alkyl androgens relieve pruritus associated with cholestasis.[52,53] However, because they can be hepatotoxic, cholestasis (and thus the accompanying jaundice) may worsen. In patients with primary biliary cirrhosis this may be unwelcome. Over the decades several of this class of androgens have been withdrawn from the market for commercial reasons. **Danazol** (p.556) is available in the UK but, in some countries, **methyltestosterone** (not UK) 25mg SL once daily will be a more convenient alternative.[52,53]

Significant benefit with **naltrexone** was seen in an RCT of uraemic patients with very severe pruritus[67] but not in patients with only moderate pruritus (also see Opioid antagonists (therapeutic target within the CNS), p.457).[68] Uraemic pruritus is multifactorial in origin (see Box D), and it is possible that μ- and κ-opioid receptor imbalance is significant only in very severe cases. This would fit with the results of a third RCT in which there was a subset of patients with uraemic pruritus who responded 'dramatically well' to **naltrexone**.[69] **Nalfurafine** (a κ agonist, not UK) 5microgram has been shown to be of benefit when given either IV after haemodialysis or PO once daily.[70,71]

Some patients with liver metastases and cholestasis produce endogenous opioids which may cause both pruritus and analgesia.[72] Anecdotally, although pain-free and not requiring opioids beforehand, some patients with cancer and cholestatic pruritus experience pain after treatment with **naltrexone**. Further, transient opioid withdrawal effects are common when PO **nalmefene**, an opioid antagonist, is used in cholestasis.[73]

Pruritus occurs in $\leq$50% of patients with polycythaemia vera. The treatment of choice is aspirin 300mg once daily–b.d. This is usually effective in <30min, and the effect lasts 12–24h.[74] Benefit is also reported with SSRIs.[75]

Other options

In *en cuirass* breast cancer complicated by inflammation, local pruritus and pain, an NSAID may reduce both pruritus and pain.[76] An NSAID can also be helpful whenever there is inflammation present, either primary or secondary to scratching.

Specialist guidelines recommend **colestyramine** for cholestatic pruritus in *incomplete* biliary obstruction, e.g. PBC.[77–79] However, the two RCTs which showed benefit with **colestyramine** (4g once or twice daily) were methodologically poor.[51] Further, many patients find **colestyramine** unpalatable, and it may cause nausea, vomiting and diarrhoea. Because it binds bile salts within the gut, it is ineffective in *complete* biliary obstruction.

Some recommendations are more or less specific to one particular disease. For example, **gabapentin** is a good choice in uraemic pruritus,[55–57] whereas in an RCT in cholestasis it was less effective than placebo.[80] However, there are anecdotal reports of benefit in neuropathic pruritus and in pruritus of unknown origin.[81,82] Dose as for neuropathic pain (see p.272).

Case reports suggest **methylnaltrexone**, a peripherally acting opioid antagonist (see p.466), may be of benefit in cholestatic pruritus. In two jaundiced patients with cancer, pruritus resolved completely 30min–12h after a dose of **methylnaltrexone**, with a duration of benefit ranging from 24h–3 weeks.[83] This avoids the risk of opioid-withdrawal and/or reversal of opioid analgesia, making it a reasonable option to try in patients receiving opioids.

Aprepitant has been used successfully for the management of severe pruritus related to targeted biological cancer treatment with anti-EGFR antibodies and tyrosine-kinase inhibitors.[20] There are also case reports of benefit in other cancer patients.[84,85]

When all else fails

The treatments suggested for pruritus associated with 'other causes or idiopathic' (Table 1, bottom row) should be considered in all cases of intractable pruritus if the more specific options have failed to relieve.

Thalidomide 100–200mg at bedtime has been used successfully in paraneoplastic, Hodgkin's lymphoma and uraemic pruritus.[86–88] However, its cost is prohibitive, and it may cause severe neuropathy when used long-term (see p.558).

Midazolam may be of benefit in intractable central pruritus.[89,90] In one patient with cancer of the pancreas and cholestatic pruritus, CSCI **midazolam** was effective 'within a few hours' (2mg bolus followed by 1mg/h, increasing by 1mg/h every 15min p.r.n.), whereas **lorazepam** 1mg q6h or 2mg at bedtime (and several other psychotropic drugs) was ineffective.[90]

Lidocaine 0.5mg/kg/h CIVI has been used successfully in a patient with cutaneous T-cell lymphoma in the last days of life.[91] No loading dose was given and she was not monitored as per the general norm, e.g. blood pressure, ECG (see p.71). The pruritus settled in 3–4h and she died 3 days later. Previously well-controlled on **gabapentin** 100mg at bedtime, **lidocaine** was introduced when she could no longer swallow.

1 Dey DD *et al.* (2005) Central neuropathic itch from spinal-cord cavernous hemangioma: a human case, a possible animal model, and hypotheses about pathogenesis. *Pain.* **113**: 233–237.
2 Schmelz M *et al.* (1997) Specific C-receptors for itch in human skin. *Journal of Neuroscience.* **17**: 8003–8008.
3 Schmelz M *et al.* (2000) Which nerve fibers mediate the axon reflex flare in human skin? *Neuroreport.* **11**: 645–648.
4 Namer B *et al.* (2008) Separate peripheral pathways for pruritus in man. *Journal of Neurophysiology.* **100**: 2062–2069.
5 Cowden JM *et al.* (2010) The histamine H4 receptor mediates inflammation and pruritus in Th2-dependent dermal inflammation. *Journal of Investigative Dermatology.* **130**: 1023–1033.
6 Dunford PJ *et al.* (2007) Histamine H4 receptor antagonists are superior to traditional antihistamines in the attenuation of experimental pruritus. *Journal of Allergy and Clinical Immunolgy.* **119**: 176–183.
7 Sugimoto Y *et al.* (2004) Pruritus-associated response mediated by cutaneous histamine H3 receptors. *Clinical and Experimental Allergy.* **34**: 456–459.
8 Yao G *et al.* (1992) Histamine-caused itch induces Fos-like immunoreactivity in dorsal horn neurons: effect of morphine pretreatment. *Brain Research.* **599**: 333–337.
9 Strakhova MI *et al.* (2009) Localization of histamine H4 receptors in the central nervous system of human and rat. *Brain Research.* **1250**: 41–48.
10 Steinhoff M *et al.* (2003) Proteinase-activated receptor-2 mediates itch: a novel pathway for pruritus in human skin. *Journal of Neuroscience.* **23**: 6176–6180.
11 Reddy VB *et al.* (2008) Cowhage-evoked itch is mediated by a novel cysteine protease: a ligand of protease-activated receptors. *Journal of Neuroscience.* **28**: 4331–4335.
12 Lowitt M and Bernhard J (1992) Pruritus. *Seminars in Neurology.* **12**: 374–384.
13 Browning J *et al.* (2003) Long-term efficacy of sertraline as a treatment for cholestatic pruritus in patients with primary biliary cirrhosis. *American Journal of Gastroenterology.* **98**: 2736–2741.
14 Mayo MJ *et al.* (2007) Sertraline as a first-line treatment for cholestatic pruritus. *Hepatology.* **45**: 666–674.
15 Zylicz Z *et al.* (2003) Paroxetine in the treatment of severe non-dermatological pruritus: a randomized, controlled trial. *Journal of Pain and Symptom Management.* **26**: 1105–1112.
16 Shakiba M *et al.* (2012) Effect of sertraline on uremic pruritus improvement in ESRD patients. *International Journal of Nephrology.* **2012**: Article ID: 363901.
17 Borgeat A and Stimemann H-R (1999) Ondansetron is effective to treat spinal or epidural morphine-induced pruritus. *Anesthesiology.* **90**: 432–436.
18 Weisshaar E *et al.* (1997) Can a serotonin type 3 (5-HT3) receptor antagonist reduce experimentally-induced itch? *Inflamm Research.* **46**: 412–416.
19 Chang SE *et al.* (2007) Neuropeptides and their receptors in psoriatic skin in relation to pruritus. *British Journal of Dermatology.* **156**: 1272–1277.
20 Santini D *et al.* (2012) Aprepitant for management of severe pruritus related to biological cancer treatments: a pilot study. *Lancet Oncology.* **13**: 1020–1024.
21 Greaves M (1992) Itching-research has barely scratched the surface. *New England Journal of Medicine.* **326**: 1016–1017.
22 Guillet G *et al.* (2000) Increased histamine release and skin hypersensitivity to histamine in senile pruritus: study of 60 patients. *European Academy of Dermatology and Venerology.* **14**: 65–68.
23 Gerber PA *et al.* (2010) Preliminary evidence for a role of mast cells in epidermal growth factor receptor inhibitor-induced pruritus. *Journal of the American Academy of Dermatology.* **63**: 163–165.
24 Kremer AE *et al.* (2012) Serum autotaxin is increased in pruritus of cholestasis, but not of other origin, and responds to therapeutic interventions. *Hepatology.* **56**: 1391–1400.
25 Barke K and Hough L (1993) Opiates, mast cells and histamine release. *Life Sciences.* **53**: 1391–1399.
26 Reisine T and Pasternak G (1996) Opioid analgesics and antagonists. In: J Hardman *et al.* (eds) *Goodman and Gilman's The Pharmacological Basis of Therapeutics* (9e). McGraw-Hill, London, pp. 521–555.
27 Krajnik M (2004) Opioid-induced pruritus. In: Z Zylicz *et al.* (eds) *Pruritus in advanced disease.* Oxford University Press, London, pp. 84–96.
28 Tarcatu D *et al.* (2007) Are we still scratching the surface? A case of intractable pruritus following systemic opioid analgesia. *Journal of Opioid Management.* **3**: 167–170.

29 Paice JA *et al.* (1996) Intraspinal morphine for chronic pain: a retrospective, multicenter study. *Journal of Pain and Symptom Management.* **11**: 71–80.

30 Winkelmuller W et *al.* (1999) Intrathecal opioid therapy for pain: Efficacy and outcomes. *Neuromodulation.* **2**: 67–76.

31 Smith TJ *et al.* (2002) Randomized clinical trial of an implantable drug delivery system compared with comprehensive medical management for refractory cancer pain: impact on pain, drug-related toxicity, and survival. *Journal of Clinical Oncology.* **20**: 4040–4049.

32 Chaplan SR et *al.* (1992) Morphine and hydromorphone epidural analgesia. *Anesthesiology.* **77**: 1090–1094.

33 Lynch L (2014) Personal communication.

34 Asokumar B *et al.* (1998) Intrathecal bupivacaine reduces pruritus and prolongs duration of fentanyl analgesia during labor: a prospective, randomized, controlled trial. *Anaesthesia and Analgesia.* **87**: 1309–1315.

35 Reich A and Szepietowski JC (2010) Opioid-induced pruritus: an update. *Clinical Experimental Dermatology.* **35**: 2–6.

36 Ballantyne J *et al.* (1988) Itching after epidural and spinal opiates. *Pain.* **33**: 149–160.

37 Kjellberg F and Tramer M (2001) Pharmacological control of opioid-induced pruritus: a quantitative systematic review of randomized trials. *European Journal of Anaesthesiology.* **18**: 346–357.

38 Gilchrest B *et al.* (1997) Relief of uremic pruritus with ultraviolet phototherapy. *New England Journal of Medicine.* **297**: 136–138.

39 Breneman D et *al.* (1992) Topical capsaicin for treatment of hemodialysis-related pruritus. *Journal of the American Academy of Dermatology.* **26**: 91–94.

40 Makhlough A (2010) Topical capsaicin therapy for uremic pruritus in patients on hemodialysis. *Iranian Journal of Kidney Disease.* **4**: 137–140.

41 Zeidler C *et al.* (2013) A capsaicin 8% patch for the treatment of brachioradial pruritus. *Acta Dermato-venereologica.* **93**: 599–640.

42 Metz M *et al.* (2011) Treatment of notalgia paraesthetica with an 8% capsaicin patch. *British Journal of Dermatology.* **165**: 1359–1361.

43 Closs S (1997) Pruritus and methotrimeprazine.

44 Muston H *et al.* (1979) Differential effect of hypnotics and anxiolytics on itch and scratch. *Journal of Investigative Dermatology.* **72**: 283.

45 Figge J *et al.* (1979) Tricyclic antidepressants: potent blockade of histamine H_1 receptors of guinea pig ileum. *European Journal of Pharmacology.* **58**: 479–483.

46 Figueiredo A *et al.* (1990) Mechanism of action of doxepin in the treatment of chronic urticaria. *Fundamental and Clinical Pharmacology.* **4**: 147–158.

47 Pour-Reza-Gholi F *et al.* (2007) Low-dose doxepin for treatment of pruritus in patients on hemodialysis. *Iranian Journal of Kidney Diseases.* **1**: 34–37.

48 Misery. L *et al.* (eds) (2016) Pruritus. Springer, London.

49 Siemens W *et al.* (2016) Pharmacological interventions for pruritus in adult palliative care patients. *Cochrane Database of Systematic Reviews.* **11**: CD008320. www.thecochranelibrary.com

50 Ghent C and Carruthers S (1988) Treatment of pruritus in primary biliary cirrhosis with rifampin. Results of a double-blind crossover randomized trial. *Gastroenterology.* **94**: 488–493.

51 Tandon P *et al.* (2007) The efficacy and safety of bile acid binding agents, opioid antagonists, or rifampin in the treatment of cholestasis-associated pruritus. *American Journal of Gastroenterology.* **102**: 1528–1536.

52 Ahrens E *et al.* (1950) Primary biliary cirrhosis. *Medicine.* **29**: 299–364.

53 Lloyd-Thomas H and Sherlock S (1952) Testosterone therapy for the pruritus of obstructive jaundice. *British Medical Journal.* **2**: 1289–1291.

54 Wolfhagen F *et al.* (1997) Oral naltrexone treatment for cholestatic pruritus: a double-blind, placebo-controlled study. *Gastroenterology.* **113**: 1264–1269.

55 Razeghi E *et al.* (2009) Gabapentin and uremic pruritus in hemodialysis patients. *Renal Failure.* **31**: 85–90.

56 Gunal AI *et al.* (2004) Gabapentin therapy for pruritus in haemodialysis patients: a randomized, placebo-controlled, double-blind trial. *Nephrology, Dialysis, Transplantation.* **19**: 3137–3139.

57 Naini AE *et al.* (2007) Gabapentin: a promising drug for the treatment of uremic pruritus. *Saudi J of Kidney Diseases and Translanation.* **18**: 378–381.

58 Quan Phan N (2010) Antipruritic treatment with systemic u-opioid receptor antagonists; a review. *Journal of the American Academy of Dermatology.* **63**: 680–688.

59 Gaudy-Marqueste C (ed) (2016) Antihistimines. In: *Pruritus.* Springer, London. 363–377.

60 Hassenbusch SJ *et al.* (2004) Polyanalgesic Consensus Conference 2003: an update on the management of pain by intraspinal drug delivery-- report of an expert panel. *Journal of Pain and Symptom Management.* **27**: 540–563.

61 Aymard J *et al.* (1980) Cimetidine for pruritus in Hodgkin's disease. *British Medical Journal.* **280**: 151–152.

62 Korfitis C and Trafalis DT (2008) Carbamazepine can be effective in alleviating tormenting pruritus in patients with hematologic malignancy. *Journal of Pain and Symptom Management.* **35**: 571–572.

63 Davis M *et al.* (2003) Mirtazapine for pruritus. *Journal of Pain and Symptom Management.* **25**: 288–291.

64 BMJ Publishing Group (2009) Resources for authors. Checklists and forms: clinical management guidelines. http://www.bmj.com/about-bmj/resources-authors

65 Osterman PO (1976) Paroxysmal itching in multiple sclerosis. *British Journal of Dermatology.* **95**: 555–558.

66 To TH *et al.* (2012) The role of ondansetron in the management of cholestatic or uremic pruritus--a systematic review. *Journal of Pain and Symptom Management.* **44**: 725–730.

67 Peer G *et al.* (1996) Randomised crossover trial of naltrexone in uraemic pruritus. *Lancet.* **348**: 1552–1554.

68 Pauli-Magnus C *et al.* (2000) Naltrexone does not relieve uremic pruritus. *Journal of the American Society of Nephrology.* **11**: 514–519.

69 Legroux-Crespel E *et al.* (2004) A comparative study on the effects of naltrexone and loratadine on uremic pruritus. *Dermatology.* **208**: 326–330.

70 Wikstrom B *et al.* (2005) Kappa-opioid system in uremic pruritus: multicenter, randomized, double-blind, placebo-controlled clinical studies. *Journal of the American Society of Nephrology.* **16**: 3742–3747.

71 Kumagai H *et al.* (2012) Efficacy and safety of a novel k-agonist for managing intractable pruritus in dialysis patients. *American Journal of Nephrology.* **36**: 175–183.

72 Bergasa NV *et al.* (1994) Cholestasis in the male rat is associated with naloxone-reversible antinociception. *Journal of Hepatology.* **20**: 85–90.

73 Thornton J and Losowksy M (1988) Opioid peptides and primary biliary cirrhosis. *British Medical Journal.* **297**: 1501–1504.

74 Jackson N *et al.* (1987) Skin mast cells in polycuthaemia vera: relationship to the pathogenesis and treatment of pruritus. *British Journal of Dermatology.* **116**: 21–29.

75 Tefferi A and Fonseca R (2002) Selective serotonin reuptake inhibitors are effective in the treatment of polycythemia vera-associated pruritus. *Blood.* **99**: 2627.

76 Twycross RG (1981) Pruritus and pain on en cuirass breast cancer. *Lancet.* **2**: 696.
77 EASL (2009) Clinical Practice Guidelines: management of cholestatic liver diseases. *Journal of Hepatology.* **51**: 237–267.
78 Lindor KD (2009) AASLD Practice Guidelines: Primary biliary cirrhosis. *Hepatology.* **50**: 291–308.
79 Hegade VS *et al.* (2015) Drug treatment of pruritus in liver diseases. *Clinical Medicine.* **4**: 351–357.
80 Bergasa NV *et al.* (2006) Gabapentin in patients with the pruritus of cholestasis: a double-blind, randomized, placebo-controlled trial. *Hepatology.* **44**: 1317–1323.
81 Kanitakis J (2006) Brachioradial pruritus: report of a new case responding to gabapentin. *European Journal of Dermatology.* **16**: 311–312.
82 Yesudian PD and Wilson NJ (2005) Efficacy of gabapentin in the management of pruritus of unknown origin. *Archives of Dermatology.* **141**: 1507–1509.
83 Hohl CM *et al.* (2015) Methylnaltrexone to palliate pruritus in terminal hepatic disease. *Journal of Palliative Care.* **31**: 124–126.
84 Vincenzi B *et al.* (2010) Aprepitant against pruritus in patients with solid tumours. *Supportive Care in Cancer.* **18**: 1229–1230.
85 Torres T *et al.* (2012) Aprepitant: Evidence of its effectiveness in patients with refractory pruritus continues. *Journal of the American Academy of Dermatology.* **66**: e14–15.
86 Silva S *et al.* (1994) Thalidomide for the treatment of uremic pruritus: a crossover randomized double-blind trial. *Nephron.* **67**: 270–273.
87 Goncalves F (2010) Thalidomide for the control of severe paraneoplastic pruritus associated with Hodgkin's disease. *American Journal of Hospice and Palliative Care.* **27**: 486–487.
88 Lowney AC *et al.* (2014) Thalidomide therapy for pruritus in the palliative setting--a distinct subset of patients in whom the benefit may outweigh the risk. *Journal of Pain and Symptom Management.* **48**: e3–5.
89 Thomsen JS *et al.* (2002) Suppression of spontaneous scratching in hairless rats by sedatives but not by antipruritics. *Skin Pharmacology and Applied Skin Physiology.* **15**: 218–224.
90 Prieto LN (2004) The use of midazolam to treat itching in a terminally ill patient with biliary obstruction. *Journal of Pain and Symptom Management.* **28**: 531–532.
91 McDonald JC *et al.* (2015) Control of intractable pruritus in a patient with cutaneous T-cell lymphoma using a continuous subcutaneous infusion of lidocaine. *Journal of Pain and Symptom Management.* **49**: e1–3.

Updated (minor change) September 2017

26

27: ORAL NUTRITIONAL SUPPLEMENTS

This section provides an overview of cachexia and the use of oral nutritional supplements in adults with cancer. It does not address nutritional supplements in children, patients with renal or hepatic failure, tube feeding or parenteral nutrition, but indicates where these may be required.

Introduction

Weight loss is a common adverse feature of cancer, associated with increased morbidity, poorer treatment tolerability and outcomes, and reduced survival. It generally occurs in the context of cancer cachexia, a multifactorial syndrome characterized by an ongoing loss of *skeletal muscle* mass (± fat), leading to progressive functional impairment.[1] There is negative protein and energy balance driven by a variable combination of reduced food intake and abnormal metabolism, with no standard treatment available for the latter.[2]

Screening

Whatever the cause of malnutrition, early detection and intervention is preferable and requires a multiprofessional pro-active approach. NICE guidance suggests that all patients should be screened for malnutrition when:

- admitted to hospital, and weekly thereafter
- admitted to care homes, and repeated if there is clinical concern
- first seen in outpatients, and repeated if there is clinical concern
- registering with a general practice.

27

As a minimum, screening should evaluate:

- the body mass index (BMI):

$$\text{BMI} = \frac{\text{weight (kg)}}{\text{height}^2\text{ (m)}}$$

- percentage unintentional weight loss
- time over which nutrient intake has been unintentionally reduced and/or the likelihood of future impaired intake.[3]

Screening tools include the Malnutrition Universal Screening Tool (MUST) and the Nutritional Risk Screening Tool 2002.[4,5] Although not validated specifically for use in patients with cancer, they are easy to complete.[5,6] The Patient Generated Subjective Global Assessment is a specific tool for patients with cancer but requires more training and takes longer to complete.[7,8]

NICE guidance suggests nutritional support should be considered for patients with:

- BMI <18.5kg/m^2
- unintentional weight loss of >10% in the last 3–6 months
- BMI <20kg/m^2 and unintentional weight loss of >5%
- inadequate oral intake for >5 days
- malabsorption, increased nutrient losses, increased catabolism.[3]

Using these criteria, 30% and 60% of patients with thoracic or upper GI cancers respectively are malnourished even at the time of diagnosis.[9,10] Further, it could be argued that the remainder are at risk of malnutrition because of increased catabolism.

Recent cancer-specific recommendations have suggested lower thresholds for the diagnosis of cachexia, i.e. *any* of the following:

- weight loss >5% over past 6 months
- BMI <20kg/m^2 and weight loss >2%
- sarcopenia and weight loss >2%.[1]

Ideally, patients identified by the screening process should then have their nutritional status assessed by an appropriately trained health professional (typically a dietitian) in order to produce an individualized nutrition care plan, which includes monitoring.[6,11] The assessment would take into account the patient's physical condition and prognosis, state of hydration, dietary intake, estimation of nutritional requirements, identification of underlying symptoms contributing to malnutrition (e.g. poor oral health or dentition, nausea, early satiety), and other psychosocial and dietary considerations.

Assessment and management

Box A is mostly based on the European Society for Clinical Nutrition and Metabolism (ESPEN) guidelines on nutrition in cancer patients.[2]

Box A Guidelines on nutrition in cancer patients

Nutritional assessment should be performed and nutritional support started when:

- malnutrition exists *or*
- a patient has inadequate nutritional intake, i.e.:
  - ▷ unable to eat for >1 week *or*
  - ▷ estimated energy intake <60% of requirement for >1–2 weeks.

Daily energy requirement

When energy expenditure cannot be measured, a reasonable estimate of daily total energy expenditure (TEE) is 25–30Kcal/kg/day.
Note. This estimate is less accurate in patients who are severely underweight (underestimates TEE) or obese (overestimates TEE).

Daily protein requirement

Generally 1–1.5g/kg/day; limit to 1 and 1.2g/kg/day in acute and chronic renal failure respectively.

Daily fluid requirement

Generally 30–35mL/kg/day; 30mL/kg/day in patients with cachexia, because of changes in extracellular fluid volumes and reduced fluid clearance.
In addition, account for losses caused by pyrexia, malabsorption, fistulas, high output stomas.

Aims of nutrition therapy

- identify, prevent and treat reversible elements of malnutrition
- maintain/improve food intake and mitigate derangements in protein, carbohydrate and lipid metabolism
- maintain skeletal muscle and physical performance
- improve tolerability of anticancer treatments
- improve quality of life.

General approach

With the exception of patients at the end of life, the aim is to meet patient's energy and substrate requirements by offering interventions step by step, i.e.:

- dietary fortification
- oral nutritional supplements
- artificial enteral or parenteral nutrition.

Nutrition should be introduced slowly over several days when there is risk of refeeding syndrome (see p.782).
Physical therapy (activities of daily living, resistance and aerobic training) should be encouraged to prevent muscle deconditioning and promote muscle anabolism, mass and strength.
Drugs are used in specific circumstances (see below).

Route

In a patient with a functioning GI tract, the enteral route (PO or tube feeding when PO insufficient/not feasible) is preferred to the parenteral route.
Tube feeding can be delivered via transnasal or percutaneous (e.g. gastrostomy, jejunostomy) routes; percutaneous is preferred for long-term use (>30 days).

continued

Box A Continued

Tube feeding is preferable in patients with head and neck or oesophageal cancers causing dysphagia, or when severe radiation therapy-induced oral or oesophageal mucositis is anticipated (when the percutaneous route may need to be used). Patients should be taught how to manage the dysphagia and maintain their swallowing function.

The parenteral route is preferred when there is an increased risk of bleeding or infections from tube placement, e.g. in neutropenic or thrombocytopenic patients, or when the GI tract is not functioning. Generally, it should be avoided in patients with a prognosis of <2 months, when the burden is considered to outweigh the benefit.

Formula

Standard nutrient composition formulas (1–1.5kcal/mL) should generally be used.

For patients with early satiety or increased nutritional requirements, high-energy high-protein formulas may be preferable.

In weight-losing patients with insulin resistance, it is recommended to increase the proportion of energy intake from fat rather than carbohydrate.

Peri-operatively, for upper GI cancer, formulas which provide immune-modulating substrates, e.g. arginine, ω-3 fatty acids, nucleotides, are recommended.

Drug treatment

In patients with advanced cancer and anorexia, corticosteroids and progestogens can enhance appetite, with inconsistent effects on body weight and quality of life. They should be used for short periods only, e.g. 1–3 weeks, weighing their benefits against their undesirable effects, particularly the risk of thrombosis with progestogens (see p.552).

In patients with advanced cancer undergoing chemotherapy at risk of weight loss or who are malnourished, supplementation with long-chain N-3 fatty acids (e.g. eicosapentanoic acid (EPA)), or fish oil can stabilize or improve appetite, lean body mass and body weight. Typical doses are 1–2g N-3 fatty acids/day and 4–6g fish oil/day.

In patients with early satiety due to delayed gastric emptying, the prokinetic drugs domperidone (p.247) and metoclopramide (p.244) can be considered taking their respective risks of undesirable cardiovascular and CNS effects into account.

There is insufficient evidence to recommend the use of androgens, cannabinoids or NSAIDs.

Peri-operative

Patients receiving curative or palliative surgery at risk of malnutrition should receive nutritional support as part of an enhanced recovery after surgery programme. This should extend to ongoing nutritional support following discharge from hospital.

GI cancer patients undergoing surgical resection should receive peri-operative immune-modulating nutrition (see Formula above).

Radiation therapy

Adequate nutritional intake should be maintained during radiation therapy, particularly to the head and neck, thorax and GI tract, using the general approach. Tube feeding is recommended when severe dysphagia is present or anticipated (see Route above).

Anticancer drug treatment

Adequate nutritional intake and physical activity should be maintained. In those receiving potentially curative drug treatments, including stem cell transplant, consider enteral nutrition when counselling + oral nutritional supplements are inadequate. The parenteral route can be considered when there is severe mucositis, intractable vomiting, ileus, severe malabsorption, protracted diarrhoea or symptomatic graft versus host disease affecting the GI tract.

Cancer survivors

A healthy lifestyle is recommended, which includes maintaining a healthy weight (BMI 18.5–25Kg/m^2), being physically active and a diet high on vegetables, fruits and whole grains and low on saturated fat, red meat and alcohol.

continued

27

Box A Continued

Patients with advanced cancer on no anticancer treatment

Those malnourished or at risk should be assessed with a particular focus on improving symptoms impacting on nutrition together with eating- or weight loss-associated psychosocial distress.

Nutritional interventions should be offered only after considering (together with the patient) the likely prognosis, the potential benefit on quality of life and survival, and associated burdens.

End of life

Generally, hunger and the urge to eat are much diminished or absent in the last weeks/days of life.[12,13] There is little or no benefit from nutritional support in this setting and the focus of care is on providing symptom relief, addressing patient and family eating-related distress, and the use of appetite stimulants when appropriate.[1] Small amounts of food can be offered as desired by the patient to alleviate hunger, and for pleasure and social purposes.[14]

Routine artificial hydration has little or no benefit in the imminently dying. It may have a limited role in selected circumstances, e.g. to improve delirium or symptomatic dehydration, and a short trial (e.g. 24h) may be appropriate. It should *not* be used for the palliation of dry mouth or thirst for which regular oral care measures are effective.

Provision of oral nutrition support

Correct the correctable

If oral intake is to be improved, attention must be paid to:

- the ability to obtain and prepare food
- oral problems, e.g. xerostomia, mucositis, oral candidosis
- uncontrolled nausea and vomiting
- dysphagia.

Particularly in relation to neurogenic dysphagia, simple measures such as adding thickeners to liquids and to semi-solid foods may be enough. Generally, patients with swallowing difficulties which put them at risk of aspiration should be assessed by a speech and language therapist (SALT).

General advice

This includes:

- meal patterns, e.g. eat small amounts frequently
- substitute water-based drinks, e.g. tea, coffee with milk-based drinks, e.g. hot chocolate, malted drinks, milky coffee
- dietary fortification, e.g. use full-fat milk and cream, extra butter, margarine, oil and sugar (fats are the most concentrated source of energy)
- consider relaxing pre-imposed dietary restrictions, e.g. diabetic diet; if necessary, adjust drugs for diabetes to maintain adequate glycaemic control
- making use of microwave meals and convenience foods; quick and easy to prepare, often small portions, high in fat and salt. The latter may help patients with a reduced sense of taste.

Generally, weight gain is more likely with dietary advice and nutritional supplements than with dietary advice alone in patients with illness-related malnutrition.[15]

Appetite stimulants

See Progestogens (p.552) and Systemic corticosteroids (p.513).

Oral nutritional supplements

Oral nutritional supplements should be considered when a patient is unable to improve their nutritional intake by diet alone. Generally, they should supplement existing intake rather than replace it, e.g. 1–2 cartons/day of a 1.5kcal/mL milk-based nutritional supplement. However, some products are nutritionally complete and, if ingested in sufficient quantities, can be used as a sole source of nutrition (e.g. see Table 2, p.773).

Oral nutritional supplements are available in liquid, semi-solid or powder formulations. General prescribing guidelines are contained in Box B and product details in Table 1–Table 13, including thickeners and thickened drinks for use in patients with dysphagia. Generally, the supplements are ordered within the tables according to their energy density and protein content.

Box B Guidelines for prescribing oral nutritional supplements

1. Ensure correctable underlying problems are addressed and general nutritional advice has been given (see text).
2. Exclude any food allergies. Advisory Committee on Borderline Substances approved products list potential allergens. If necessary, seek advice from a dietitian.
3. To aid adherence, be guided by the patient's preferences and provide a variety of locally available formulations and flavours either separately or in commercially available starter packs, e.g.:
   - Abbott: Ensure Plus Commence®
   - Nutricia: Complan® Shake, Fortijuce®, Fortisip® Compact, Fortisip® Extra and Fortisip® Range (contains Fortisip®, Fortijuce® and Fortisip® Yoghurt Style).
4. Provide information on how to use the supplements together with any special instructions, e.g.:
   - keep supplements chilled to improve palatability
   - use the straw provided with supplement to minimize unpleasant odour
   - use supplement as a between-meal snack, not as a meal replacement
   - maintenance of good oral hygiene
   - once opened, supplements can be stored in a refrigerator for up to 24h.
5. Review patient after one week:
   - prescribe the required number of cartons/units per day of the formulation and flavour(s) which are acceptable to the patient
   - if none are acceptable, try an alternative, e.g. juice-based or milkshake powder.
6. Review patient after 4 weeks of supplement use. If weight loss continues, seek advice from a dietitian. Monitoring should continue on a monthly basis until supplements are no longer required.

Patients with renal or hepatic failure, malabsorption, dysphagia, or at risk of refeeding syndrome (p.782) should be referred to a dietitian.

Box C Aiding compliance with milk- and juice-based supplements

Milk-based

Serve chilled ± ice

Add extra full-fat milk

Make a smoothie by adding fresh fruit and ice cream

Make into a jelly

Use instead of milk on cereals and in puddings (unflavoured)

Use to make custard/rice pudding (vanilla flavour)

Further recipes are available from:
www.abbottnutrition.co.uk.
www.fresenius-kabi.co.uk
www.nestlehealthscience.co.uk
www.nutricia.co.uk
www.vitaflo.co.uk

Juice-based

Serve chilled ± ice

Add extra fruit juice

Make a spritzer by adding soda water/lemonade/carbonated water

Make into a jelly

Pour over fresh or tinned fruit

Freeze to make an ice lolly or ice cubes

Energy content is given per unit and per mL and the protein content per unit. For other supplements, the nutritional content is given per 100mL or 100g as appropriate. Flavours frequently alter; check availability with the manufacturer. Unless otherwise stated, all products listed are Advisory Committee on Borderline Substances (ACBS) approved for patients with disease-related malnutrition.

The oral nutritional supplements listed are gluten-free and most are suitable for vegetarians. Those containing fish oils (EPA), micronutrients or colourings derived from animal sources may not be acceptable to strict vegetarians, vegans or patients of certain religious & ethnical denominations. If uncertain with patients who have specific dietary restrictions, consult a dietitian or the manufacturers for advice.

Ingesting sufficient quantities orally may be difficult for patients with anorexia or taste changes and various strategies, including recipes suggested by the manufacturers, can be tried to aid compliance (Box C).

continued

Table 1 Milkshake-style nutritional supplements (suitable as a sole source of nutrition)[a,b]
Included for completeness: generally supplements with higher energy and protein content should be used.

Product	*Unit size*	*Energy content*	*Protein content*	*Flavours/comments*
Ensure® (Abbott)	250mL Can	250kcal (1kcal/mL)	10g	Chocolate, coffee, vanilla
Fresubin® Original Drink (Fresenius)	200mL Bottle	200kcal (1kcal/mL)	9g	Blackcurrant, chocolate, mocha, nut, peach, vanilla

a. avoid acidic citrus/tangy flavours in patients with a sore mouth
b. best served chilled.

Table 2 High-energy milkshake-style nutritional supplements (suitable as a sole source of nutrition)[a,b]

Product	*Unit size*	*Energy content*	*Protein content*	*Flavours/comments*
Ensure® Compact (Abbott)	125mL Bottle	300kcal (2.4kcal/mL)	13g	Banana, strawberry, vanilla
Fortisip® Compact (Nutricia)	125mL Bottle	300kcal (2.4kcal/mL)	12g	Apricot, banana, chocolate, forest fruit, mocha, strawberry, vanilla
Ensure® Plus Milkshake Style (Abbott)	220mL Bottle	330kcal (1.5kcal/mL)	14g	Banana, chocolate, coffee, fruits of the forest, neutral, orange, peach, raspberry, strawberry, vanilla
Fortisip® Bottle (Nutricia)	200mL Bottle	300kcal (1.5kcal/mL)	12g	Banana, caramel, chocolate, neutral, orange, strawberry, tropical fruit, vanilla
Fresubin® Energy Drink (Fresenius)	200mL Bottle	300 kcal (1.5kcal/mL)	11g	Banana, blackcurrant, cappuccino, chocolate, lemon, strawberry, tropical fruit, vanilla, unflavoured
Resource® Energy (Nestle Health Science)	200mL Bottle	300kcal (1.5kcal/mL)	11g	Apricot, banana, chocolate, coffee, strawberry-raspberry, vanilla

a. avoid acidic citrus/tangy flavours in patients with a sore mouth
b. best served chilled.

Table 3 Savoury-style nutritional supplements[a,b]

Product	*Unit size*	*Energy content*	*Protein content*	*Flavours/comments*
Ensure® Plus Savoury (Abbott)	220mL Bottle	330kcal (1.5kcal/mL)	14g	Suitable as a sole source of nutrition; chicken, mushroom
Vitasavoury® 300 (Vitaflo)	50g Sachet	309 Kcal (375 Kcal) (6kcal/g)	6g	Reconstitute with hot water/full-fat milk; not for use as a sole source of nutrition; chicken, leak and potato, mushroom, vegetable
Vitasavoury® 200 (Vitaflo)	33g Cup	204kcal (6kcal/g)	4g	Reconstitute with hot water/full-fat milk; chicken, leek and potato, mushroom, vegetable
Meritene® Energis Soup (Nestle Health Science)	50g Sachet	207kcal (4.1kcal/g)	7g	Reconstitute with 150mL hot water/ full-fat milk; contains 3.7g fibre; chicken, vegetable

a. best served warmed, do not boil
b. vitamin and mineral content varies between products.

Table 4 Milkshake-style nutritional supplements with fibre (suitable as a sole source of nutrition)[a,b]

Product	*Unit size*	*Energy content*	*Protein content*	*Flavours/comments*
Fortisip® Compact Fibre (Nutricia)	125mL Bottle	300kcal (2.4kcal/mL)	12g	Contains 4.5g fibre; mocha, strawberry, vanilla
Resource® 2.0 Fibre (Nestle Health Science)	200mL Bottle	400kcal (2.0kcal/mL)	18g	Contains 5g soluble fibre (50:50 FOS:GOS), do not exceed 4 bottles/day; apricot, coffee, strawberry, summer fruit, vanilla, unflavoured
Ensure® Plus Fibre (Abbott)	200mL Bottle	310kcal (1.6kcal/mL)	13g	Contains 5g fibre and fructo-oligosaccharides; banana, chocolate, raspberry, strawberry, vanilla
Fresubin® Energy Fibre Drink (Fresenius)	200mL Bottle	300kcal (1.5kcal/mL)	11g	Contains 4g mixed fibre blend; banana, caramel, cherry, chocolate, strawberry, vanilla

a. useful for patients with constipation
b. shake well before use.

Table 5 Yoghurt-style nutritional supplements (suitable as a sole source of nutrition)[a,b]

Product	*Unit size*	*Energy content*	*Protein content*	*Flavours/comments*
Ensure® Plus Yoghurt Style (Abbott)	200mL Bottle	300kcal (1.5kcal/mL)	13g	Peach, strawberry
Fortisip® Yoghurt Style (Nutricia)	200mL Bottle	300kcal (1.5kcal/mL)	12g	Peach-orange, raspberry, vanilla-lemon

a. can be more palatable in patients with taste change (citrus/tangy flavours vs. sweet)
b. avoid acidic citrus/tangy flavours in patients with a sore mouth.

Table 6 Fruit juice-style nutritional supplements (not suitable as a sole source of nutrition)[a,b]

Product	*Unit size*	*Energy content*	*Protein content*	*Flavours/comments*
Ensure® Plus Juce (Abbott)	220mL Bottle	330kcal (1.5kcal/mL)	11g	Apple, fruit punch, lemon and lime, orange, peach, strawberry
Fortijuce® (Nutricia)	200mL Bottle	300kcal (1.5kcal/mL)	8g	Apple, blackcurrant, forest fruit, lemon, orange, strawberry, tropical
Fresubin® Juicy Drink (Fresenius)	200mL Bottle	300kcal (1.5kcal/mL)	8g	Apple, blackcurrant, cherry, orange, pineapple
Resource® Fruit (Nestle Health Science)	200mL Bottle	250kcal (1.3kcal/mL)	8g	Apple, orange, pear-cherry, raspberry-blackcurrant

a. may be preferable for patients with a dry mouth
b. avoid acidic citrus/tangy flavours in patients with a sore mouth.

Table 7 High protein milkshake-style nutritional supplements (not suitable as a sole source of nutrition)[a]

Product	*Unit size*	*Energy content*	*Protein content*	*Flavours/comments*
Altraplen® Protein (Nualtra)	200mL Bottle	300kcal (2.4kcal/mL)	20g	Strawberry, vanilla
Fortisip® Compact Protein (Nutricia)	125mL Bottle	300kcal (2.4kcal/mL)	18g	Banana, mocha, strawberry, vanilla
Fresubin® 2kcal Drink (Fresenius)	200mL Bottle	400kcal (2kcal/mL)	20g	Apricot-peach, cappuccino, friuits of the forest, toffee, unflavoured, vanilla
Fresubin® 2kcal Fibre Drink (Fresenius)	200mL Bottle	400kcal (2kcal/mL)	20g	Contains 3g fibre; apricot-peach, cappuccino, chocolate, lemon, unflavoured, vanilla
Ensure® TwoCal (Abbott)	200mL Bottle	400kcal (2kcal/mL)	17g	Contains 2g FOS; banana, strawberry, vanilla, unflavoured
Fortisip® Extra (Nutricia)	200mL Bottle	320kcal (1.6kcal/mL)	20g	Chocolate, forest fruit, mocha, strawberry, vanilla
Fresubin® Protein Energy Drink (Fresenius)	200mL Bottle	300kcal (1.5kcal/mL)	20g	Cappuccino, chocolate, strawberry, tropical fruits, vanilla
Resource® Protein (Nestle Health Science)	200mL Bottle	250kcal (1.25kcal/mL)	19g	Apricot, chocolate, forest fruits, strawberry, vanilla
Fortimel® Regular (Nutricia)	200mL Bottle	200kcal (1kcal/mL)	20g	Chocolate, forest fruits, strawberry, vanilla

FOS is a soluble fibre

a. consider in patients with high protein loss or wounds when overall energy intake is adequate.

27

Table 8 Semi-solid nutritional supplements (suitable as a sole source of nutrition)[a]

Product	*Unit size*	*Energy content*	*Protein content*	*Flavours/comments*
Fresubin® Creme (Fresenius)	125g Pot	230kcal (1.8kcal/g)	13g	Cappuccino, chocolate, praline, strawberry, vanilla
Forticreme® Complete (Nutricia)	125g Pot	200kcal (1.6kcal/g)	12g	Banana, chocolate, forest fruit, vanilla
Resource® Dessert Energy (Nestle Health Science)	125g Pot	200kcal (1.6kcal/g)	6g	Caramel, chocolate, vanilla
Resource® Dessert Fruit (Nestle Health Science)	125g Pot	205kcal (1.6kcal/g)	6g	Contains 1.6g fibre; apple, apple-peach, apple-strawberry
Fresubin® YOcreme (Fresenius)	125g Pot	187kcal (1.5kcal/g)	9g	Apricot-peach, biscuit, lemon, raspberry, unflavoured
Ensure® Plus Creme (Abbott)	125g Pot	171kcal (1.4kcal/g)	7g	Banana, chocolate, vanilla, unflavoured
Nutilis® Fruit Stage 3 (Nutricia)	150g Pot	206kcal (1.4kcal/g)	11g	Contains 3.9g fibre; apple, strawberry
ProSource® Jelly (Nutrinovo)	118mL Pot	90kcal (0.75kcal/mL)	20g	Fruit punch, orange

a. useful for patients with dysphagia.

Table 9 Powdered milkshake-style nutritional supplements (not suitable as a sole source of nutrition)[a,b,c]

Product	*Unit size*	*Energy content*	*Protein content*	*Flavours/comments*
Calshake® (Fresenius)	87g Sachet	431kcal (5kcal/g)	4g	600kcal and 12g protein when reconstituted with full-fat milk (240mL); banana, chocolate, strawberry, unflavoured, vanilla, in boxes of 7
Scandishake Mix® (Nutricia)	85g Sachet	430kcal (5kcal/g)	4g	600kcal and 12g protein when reconstituted with full-fat milk (240mL); banana, caramel, chocolate, strawberry, vanilla, unflavoured, in boxes of 6
Enshake® (Abbott)	96.5g Sachet	434kcal (4.5kcal/g)	8g	600kcal and 16g protein when reconstituted with full-fat milk (240mL); banana, chocolate, strawberry, vanilla, in boxes of 6
Ensure® Shake (Abbott)	57g Sachet	253kcal (4kcal/g)	10g	389kcal and 17g protein when reconstituted with full-fat milk (200mL); banana, chocolate, strawberry, vanilla, in boxes of 7
Foodlink Complete (Foodlink)	450g Box	245kcal (4kcal/g)	12g	1 serving = 4 heaped dessert spoons. Reconstitute with full-fat milk or water (200mL); banana, chocolate, strawberry, vanilla with fibre, unflavoured
Aymes® Shake (Aymes)	57g Sachet	389Kcal (1.6Kcal/mL)	16g	When reconstituted with 200mL whole milk; 126Kcal and 5g protein when reconstituted with water; with added vitamins and minerals; banana, chocolate, neutral, strawberry, vanilla
Fresubin® Powder Extra (Fresenius)	62g Sachet	260kcal (4kcal/g)	11g	397kcal and 18g protein when reconstituted with full-fat milk (200mL); with added vitamins and minerals; chocolate, strawberry, vanilla, unflavoured
Complan® Shake (Nutricia)	57g Sachet	250kcal (4kcal/g)	9g	385kcal and 16g protein when reconstituted with full-fat milk (200mL); with added vitamins and minerals; banana, chocolate, strawberry, vanilla, unflavoured

a. high palatability
b. some products are lower in vitamins and minerals compared with other supplements
c. milkshake style should be reconstituted using full-fat milk to optimize energy content.

Table 10 OTC nutritional supplements (not suitable as a sole source of nutrition)

Product	*Unit size*	*Energy content*	*Protein content*	*Flavours/comments*
Complan (Nutricia)	57g Sachet	250kcal (4.4kcal/g)	9g	Reconstitute with 200mL hot or cold water/full-fat milk; banana, chicken, chocolate, strawberry, vanilla, unflavoured, in boxes of 4

continued

Table 10 Continued

Product	*Unit size*	*Energy content*	*Protein content*	*Flavours/comments*
Complan Milkshake (Nutricia)	250mL Carton	214kcal (0.9kcal/mL)	9g	Ready to drink; chocolate, strawberry
Complan Smoothie (Nutricia)	250mL Carton	272kcal (1kcal/mL)	10g	Ready to drink; berry, tropical
Meritene® Energis® Shakes (Nestle Health Science)	30g Sachet	107kcal 3.6 kcal/g)	9g	Reconstitute with 200mL full-fat milk; chocolate, strawberry, vanilla

a. unconstituted.

Table 11 Special application nutritional products[a,b]

Product	*Unit size*	*Energy content*	*Protein content*	*Flavours/comments*
Ensure® Plus Advance (Abbott)	220mL Bottle	330kcal (1.5kcal/mL)	20g	For use in patients over 65 years who have, or are at risk of, malnutrition; contains 13microgram vitamin D and 499mg calcium; banana, chocolate, vanilla
Forti Care® (Nutricia)	125mL Bottle	200kcal (1.6kcal/mL)	11g	For use in patients with cachexia (pancreatic cancer and lung cancer undergoing chemotherapy). Contains eicosapentanoic acid (EPA), fibre and anti-oxidants. Recommended dose 3 bottles/day (providing 2.2g EPA); not nutritionally complete at this dose; cappuccino, orange-lemon, peach-ginger
Supportan® Drink (Fresenius)	200mL Bottle	300kcal (1.5kcal/mL)	20g	For use in patients with cachexia (pancreatic cancer and lung cancer undergoing chemotherapy). Contains eicosapentanoic acid (EPA) and docosahexanoic acid (DHA), anti-oxidants and fibre. Recommended dose 2 bottles/day (providing 2.85g EPA and DHA); cappuccino, tropical fruits
ProSure® (Abbott)	240mL Tetrapak	305kcal (1.3kcal/mL)	16g	For use in patients with cachexia (pancreatic cancer and lung cancer undergoing chemotherapy). Contains eicosapentanoic acid (EPA) and anti-oxidants. An intake of 1.5–2 cartons/day is required for benefit; not nutritionally complete at this dose; vanilla
Oral Impact® (Nestle Health Science)	74g Sachet	303kcal	17g	Contains immune-modulating substrates and soluble fibre (e.g. ω-3 fatty acids, arginine, nucleotides). Pre-operatively, 2–4 sachets a day (dissolved in 250mL of cool boiled water) recommended for 5–7 days; not nutritionally complete at this dose; citrus, coffee, tropical

continued

27

Table 11 Continued

Product	*Unit size*	*Energy content*	*Protein content*	*Flavours/comments*
Respifor® (Nutricia)	125mL Bottle	188kcal (1.5kcal/mL)	9g	For early intervention use in patients with COPD. Recommended dose 125mL t.d.s in combination with activity plan for 3 months; chocolate, strawberry, vanilla
Elemental E028 Extra Liquid® (Nutricia)	250mL Carton	215kcal (0.9kcal/mL)	6g	A liquid elemental feed for patients with intractable malabsorption or radiation enteritis. Protein source is a mixture of essential and non-essential amino acids. Nutritionally complete; grapefruit, orange and pineapple, summer fruits
Elemental E028 Extra Powder® (Nutricia)	100g Sachet	427kcal/100g	13g/100g	An elemental feed for patients with intractable malabsorption or radiation enteritis. Protein source is a mixture of essential and non-essential amino acids. Nutritionally complete. Reconstitute with 100g powder in 500mL water; banana, orange, unflavoured
Vital® (Abbott)	200mL Bottle	300kcal (1.5kcal/mL)	14g	A peptide based sip feed for patients with malabsorption: nutritionally complete; vanilla
Survimed® OPD Drink (Fresenius)	200mL Bottle	200kcal (1kcal/mL)	9g	A peptide based sip feed for patients with malabsorption; nutritionally complete; vanilla
Peptamen® Vanilla Bottle (Nestle Health Science)	200mL Bottle	200kcal (1kcal/mL)	8g	For patients with impaired GI function. Contains protein source as peptides and fat is 70% medium-chain triglycerides to improve digestion and absorption. Nutritionally complete. Can be flavoured with 2 scoops of Nestle Nutrition Flavour Mix/100mL to improve palatability; banana, chocolate, coffee, lemon and lime, strawberry
Resource® OptiFibre® (Nestle Health Science)	250g Tub (5g per scoop) 10g Sachet	–	–	For use with patients who have constipation. Each scoop contains 4g and each sachet 6g of soluble fibre (partially hydrolyzed guar gum) which is mixed into hot or cold liquids and foods. Introduce gradually; begin with 1 scoop or 1/2 sachet and increase by 1 scoop or 1/2 sachet every 3 days. Recommended dose is 2 sachets/3 scoops/day, maximum 32g/day
Forceval® Capsules (Alliance)	15, 30 and 90 Cap pack	–	–	Multivitamin and mineral supplement given as 1 capsule daily. Capsule can be opened and contents mixed, for example, with a teaspoon of jam
Forceval® Soluble (Alliance)	30 Tablet pack			Effervescent multivitamin and mineral supplement given as 1 tablet daily

a. use with dietetic supervision

b. listed according to type.

Table 12 Modular carbohydrate, protein and fat supplements (not suitable as a sole source of nutrition)[a,b]

Product	*Unit size*	*Energy source*	*Energy content*	*Comments*
Caloreen® (Nestle Health Science)	500g Tub	Carbohydrate	385kcal/100g	Glucose polymer powder to add to food and drinks; unflavoured
Polycal® Powder (Nutricia)	400g Tub	Carbohydrate	384kcal/100g	Glucose polymer powder to add to food and drinks; unflavoured
Maxijul® Super Soluble Powder (SHS)	132g Sachet, 200g, 25kg Tub	Carbohydrate	380kcal/100g	Glucose polymer powder to add to food and drinks; recommended dilution 1:2; unflavoured
Vitajoule® (Vitaflo)	500g Tub	Carbohydrate	380kcal/100g	Glucose syrup powder to add to food and drinks; unflavoured
Polycal® Liquid (Nutricia)	200mL Bottle	Carbohydrate	247kcal/100mL	Glucose polymer solution; can be used undiluted or diluted in drinks; orange, unflavoured
Protifar® (Nutricia)	225g Tub	Protein	368kcal/100g 87g protein/100g	High-protein powder to add to food and drinks; unflavoured
Vitapro® (Vitaflo)	250g, 2kg Tub	Protein	378kcal/100g 75g protein /100g	High-biological value powdered protein to add to food and drinks; unflavoured
Fresubin® 5kcal SHOT (Fresenius)	120mL Bottle	Fat	500kcal/100mL	Long and medium-chain triglyceride fat emulsion. Recommended dose 30mL t.d.s– q.d.s; lemon, unflavoured
Liquigen® (Nutricia)	250mL, Bottle	Fat	450kcal/100mL	Medium-chain triglyceride fat emulsion; unflavoured
Calogen® (Nutricia)	200mL, 500mL Bottle	Fat	450kcal/100mL	Long-chain triglyceride fat emulsion. Recommended dose 30mL t.d.s; banana, strawberry,unflavoured
Calogen® Extra (Nutricia)	200mL Bottle, 40mL Cup	Fat, carbohydrate	400kcal/100mL 5g protein/100mL	High energy fat emulsion with protein, carbohydrate, vitamins and minerals. Recommended dose 40mL t.d.s; strawberry, unflavoured
Super Soluble Duocal® (SHS)	400g Tub	Fat, carbohydrate	492kcal/100g	Fat and glucose polymer powder to add to food and drinks; unflavoured
ProSource® Liquid (Nutrinovo)	100x30mL Sachet	Protein and carbohydrate	333kcal/100mL 33g protein/100mL (30mL sachet 100kcal, 10g protein)	Protein and energy liquid to drink as a 'shot' or to add to food and drinks; citrus-berry, lemon, orange, unflavoured

continued

Table 12 Continued

Product	*Unit size*	*Energy source*	*Energy content*	*Comments*
ProSource® Plus (Nutrinovo)	100x30mL Sachet	Protein and carbohydrate	333kcal/100mL 50g protein/100mL (30mL sachet 100kcal, 15g protein)	Protein and energy liquid to drink as a 'shot' or to add to food and drinks; unflavoured
Pro-Cal® Powder (Vitaflo)	15g Sachet 510g, 1.5kg, 12.5kg Tub	Protein, fat, carbohydrate	667kcal/100g 14g protein /100g	Energy and protein powder to add to food and drinks; unflavoured
MCTprocal® (Vitaflo)	16g Sachet	Protein, MCT, carbohydrate	657kcal/100g 13g protein/100g	Energy, protein and MCT powder to add to food and drinks; unflavoured
Pro-Cal Shot® (Vitaflo)	120mL, 250mL Bottle	Protein, fat, carbohydrate	334kcal/100mL 7g protein/100mL	Fat, protein and carbohydrate emulsion; banana, strawberry, unflavoured
Pro-Cal® Singles (Vitaflo)	30mL Pot	Protein, fat, carbohydrate	333kcal/100mL 7g protein/100mL (30mL pot 100kcal, 2g protein)	Fat, protein and carbohydrate emulsion; strawberry, unflavoured

MCT: Medium-chain trigyceride
a. use with dietetic supervision
b. listed according to type.

Table 13 Thickeners and thickened drinks[a,b]

Product	*Unit size*	*Energy content*	*Comments*
Fresubin® Thickened (Fresenius)	200mL Bottle	150kcal/100mL 10g protein/100mL	Texture modified supplement drink in stage 1 and stage 2 consistency; strawberry, vanilla
Resource® Thickened Drinks (Nestle Health Science)	114mL Cup	89kcal/100mL	Ready to use, available in syrup and custard consistency; apple, orange
Nutilis® Complete (Nutricia)	125mL Bottle (Stage 1) 125mL Pot (Stage 2)	245kcal/100mL 10g protein/100mL	Texture modified supplement drink; stage 1 and 2; strawberry, vanilla
Multi-thick® (Abbott)	250g Can	366kcal/100g	Modified maize starch. Can be used to thicken fluids and food
Nutilis® Clear (Nutricia)	175g Can	299kcal/100g	Maltodextrin, xanthangum and guar gum. Can be used to thicken foods and fluids. Fluids remain clear
Nutilis® Powder (Nutricia)	300g Can 12g Sachet	358kcal/100g	Modified maize starch. Can be used to thicken fluids and food
Resource® Thicken Up® (Nestle Health Science)	4.5g Sachet 227g Can	365kcal/100g	Modified maize starch. Can be used to thicken fluids and food
Resource® Thicken Up Clear™ (Nestle Health Science)	1.2g Sachet 125g Can	306kcal/100g	Maltodextrin, xanthangum and potassium chloride. Can be used to thicken fluids and food. Fluids remain clear
Thick and Easy® Instant Food Thickener (Fresenius)	9g Sachet 225g, 4.5kg Tub	373kcal/100g	Modified maize starch. Can be used to thicken fluids and food
Vitaquick® (Vitaflo)	300g, 2kg, Tub	391kcal/100g	Pre-gelatinized modified starch. Can be used to thicken fluids and food

a. for patients with dysphagia

b. listed according to type.

Cautions

Patients with renal or hepatic failure, malabsorption, dysphagia, or at risk of refeeding syndrome (see below) should be referred to a dietitian.

The high sugar content and acidity of some nutritional supplement drinks can encourage dental caries and patients should be advised on good oral hygiene, e.g. ingest the supplement relatively quickly and then clean teeth. However, sipping the supplement over a prolonged period may be unavoidable in patients with early satiety.

Generally, patients with diabetes can use nutritional supplements without problem. However, monitoring of blood sugars may be required when using supplements with a high carbohydrate content, e.g. carbohydrate modular supplements. Rarely, and generally in patients already taking large doses of additional vitamins, nutritional supplements have contributed to ingestion of harmful amounts of vitamins, e.g. vitamin B6 leading to sensory neuropathy. Drug-nutrient interactions may occur with:

- vitamin K, present in significant quantities in the nutritional supplement drinks, and **warfarin** → reduced anticoagulation
- eicosapentanoic acid, in Forticare®, Oral Impact®, Prosure®, and Supportan®, and **warfarin** → enhanced anticoagulation.[16,17]

Also see drug interactions and complications with enteral feeding tubes, p.785).

Refeeding syndrome

Refeeding syndrome is a potentially fatal condition caused by major shifts in fluids and electrolytes in malnourished patients who are started too rapidly on enteral or parenteral nutrition.[18,19] Biochemically, refeeding syndrome is characterized primarily by hypophosphataemia.

During a period of starvation, the body adapts in various ways to cope with the lack of readily available carbohydrate, and switches to using fat and protein as the main source of energy. If malnutrition is prolonged, there are further hormonal and metabolic changes aimed at preventing protein and muscle breakdown. Several intracellular minerals become severely depleted (although plasma concentrations may remain normal).

During refeeding, glycaemia leads to increased insulin secretion and a series of sequential effects, including decreases in the plasma concentrations of phosphate, potassium, magnesium, and thiamine. If unrecognized and untreated, refeeding syndrome can result in life-threatening complications, including cardiac arrhythmia and multi-organ failure.[19] It is thus important that high risk patients should be managed by appropriately trained health professionals.

Although a regimen of rapid refeeding is unlikely in patients with advanced cancer and chronic oligophagia and/or cachexia, palliative care clinicians should be aware of the syndrome, and have a basic understanding of its management (Box D).

Box D Risk factors for and management of refeeding syndrome[20]

Patients who have had very little or no nutritional intake for >5 days are at risk of refeeding syndrome. It is associated with high morbidity and mortality and should be managed by appropriately trained health professionals.

High-risk patients

Those with one or more of the following:

- BMI <16kg/m^2
- unintentional weight loss of >15% in the last 3–6 months
- little or no nutritional intake for >10 days
- low plasma concentrations of PO_4^-, K^+, Mg^{2+} before restarting feeding.

Or two or more of the following:

- BMI <18.5kg/m^2
- unintentional weight loss >10% within the last 3–6 months
- little or no nutritional intake for > 5 days
- a history of alcohol abuse or drugs, including insulin, chemotherapy, antacids and diuretics.

Management

For the first 2 days, patients who have had little or nothing to eat for ≥5 days should only be offered/given nutritional support estimated to meet ≤50% of their ideal requirements. After this, if biochemical parameters are satisfactory, it is safe to provide full nutrition.

If high risk:

- ensure adequate hydration
- before feeding, and for the next 10 days, administer:
  - ▷ thiamine 200–300mg PO once daily
  - ▷ strong compound vitamin B 1–2 tablets t.d.s. (or IV vitamin B once daily)
  - ▷ multivitamin and mineral supplement PO once daily
- start nutritional support at ≤10kcal/kg/day (5kcal/kg/day in extreme cases)
- increase intake progressively to achieve full nutritional requirements after 4–7 days
- if pre-feeding plasma concentrations are low, prescribe biochemical supplements:
  - ▷ magnesium (e.g. 0.2mmol/kg/day IV, 0.4mmol/kg/day PO)
  - ▷ phosphate (e.g. 0.3–0.6mmol/kg/day)
  - ▷ potassium (e.g. 2–4mmol/kg/day).

Monitoring

Daily until stable, and then 2–3 times weekly: fluid balance, nutritional intake, biochemical parameters, and general physical and psychological condition.

1 Fearon K *et al.* (2011) Definition and classification of cancer cachexia: an international consensus. *Lancet Oncology*.
2 Arends J *et al.* (2016) ESPEN guidelines on nutrition in cancer patients. *Clinical Nutrition*. **36**: 11–48.
3 National Collaborating Centre for Acute Care (2006) *Nutrition Support in Adults: Oral nutrition support, enteral tube feeding and parenteral nutrition* (No. 32). National Institute for Clinical Excellence, London.
4 The Malnutrition Universal Screening Tool (MUST). BAPEN, UK. Available from: www.bapen.org.uk
5 Kyle UG *et al.* (2006) Comparison of tools for nutritional assessment and screening at hospital admission: a population study. *Clinical Nutrition*. **25**: 409–417.
6 Davies M (2005) Nutritional screening and assessment in cancer-associated malnutrition. *European Journal of Oncology Nursing*. **9 (Suppl 2)**: S64–73.
7 Ottery FD (1996) Definition of standardized nutritional assessment and interventional pathways in oncology. *Nutrition*. **12**: S15–19.
8 Bauer J *et al.* (2002) Use of the scored Patient-Generated Subjective Global Assessment (PG-SGA) as a nutrition assessment tool in patients with cancer. *European Journal of Clinical Nutrition*. **56**: 779–785.
9 Chauhan A *et al.* (2007) NICE guidance for screening for malnutrition: implications for lung cancer services. *Thorax*. **62**: 835.
10 Halliday V *et al.* (2010) Screening for malnutrition: implications for upper gastrointestinal cancer services. *Journal of Surgical Oncology*. **102**: 543-544.
11 Thoresen L and de Soysa AK (2006) The nutritional aspects of palliative care. *European Journal of Palliative Care*. **13**: 194–197.
12 McCann RM *et al.* (1994) A comfort care for terminally ill patients: the appropriate use of nutrition and hydration. *Journal of the American Medical Association*. **272**: 179–181.
13 Sarhill N *et al.* (2003) Evaluation of nutritional status in advanced metastatic cancer. *Supportive Care in Cancer*. **11**: 652–659.
14 Antoun S *et al.* (2006) Artificial nutrition at the end of life: is it justified? *European Journal of Palliative Care*. **13**: 194–197.
15 Baldwin C and Weekes C (2008) Dietary advice for illness-related malnutrition in adults. *Cochrane Database of Systematic Reviews*. **1**: CD002008. www.thecochranelibrary.com
16 Baxter K and Preston CL. *Stockley's Drug Interactions*. London: Pharmaceutical Press www.medicinescomplete.com (accessed January 2015).
17 Holbrook AM *et al.* (2005) Systematic overview of warfarin and its drug and food interactions. *Archives of Internal Medicine*. **165**: 1095–1106.
18 Mehanna HM *et al.* (2008) Refeeding syndrome: what it is, and how to prevent and treat it. *British Medical Journal*. **336**: 1495-1498.
19 Boateng AA *et al.* (2010) Refeeding syndrome: treatment considerations based on collective analysis of literature case reports. *Nutrition*. **26**: 156-167.
20 NICE (2006) Nutrition support in adults. Clinical guidelines CG32. www.nice.org.uk

Updated April 2017

28

28: DRUG ADMINISTRATION TO PATIENTS WITH SWALLOWING DIFFICULTIES OR ENTERAL FEEDING TUBES

GENERAL PRINCIPLES

Simplifying drug therapy by reducing the number of medications and frequency of administration is particularly important for patients who are not able to swallow solids or for whom administering drugs by an enteral feeding tube (EFT) is being considered.

Modifying a product in a way not specified in the manufacturer's SPC renders its use off-label, e.g. emptying out the contents of a capsule. Thus, if available, appropriate alternative formulations of those drugs still considered necessary should be used, e.g. a soluble tablet or an oral liquid instead of a solid tablet (or an alternative authorized drug).

Administering drugs by EFT is generally off-label, and consideration should also be given to using an alternative authorized route, e.g. PR, SC, IV.[1,2] However, administration by EFT may be preferable from a practical or personal point of view.

Drug therapy, the formulations used, and swallowing ability should be kept under review, particularly before inpatient discharge. Training and detailed written instructions regarding the supply, preparation and administration of each drug should be given to the patient and/or carer and primary care team.[3–5]

Wrong route errors occurring with drugs intended for PO or other enteral routes, are considered by NHS England as 'Never events'.[6] Guidance on minimizing wrong route errors has been published by the UK National Patient Safety Agency (NPSA).[7] Only enteral syringes should be used to draw up and administer oral liquids. Many local guidelines stipulate once only use. NPSA has also produced guidance on testing the position of nasogastric tubes.[8]

The administration of drugs by EFT is considered a level 3 skill for care workers in care homes. Staff must be adequately trained.[9,10] General guidance for the administration of drugs by EFT is given in the Quick Clinical Guide (see p.792).

CHOOSING A SUITABLE FORMULATION

When planning to change to an alternative formulation or administer a drug by EFT, guidance should be obtained from a pharmacist. For those with impaired swallowing a Speech and Language Therapist (SALT) should also be consulted in order to understand the degree of swallowing impairment and perform a risk assessment.[11,12] Taking into account the balance of risks and uncertainties for drug administration to these patients, the choice of formulation in descending order of preference generally comprises:

- authorized soluble tablet or oral liquid
- effervescent tablet or dispersed tablet (authorized or off-label)
- oral liquid prepared by local pharmacy or special order
- dispersed capsule contents or crushed tablet
- injection (given PO or by EFT).

However, there are considerations and disadvantages for each of these options which can vary according to the drug prescribed, the patient's clinical need and the practical situation, particularly in children (see p.675). These issues are summarized in Table 1. Thus, every drug needs to be assessed individually to determine which would be the most appropriate formulation, i.e. do not simply convert all solid dose medication to oral liquids.[1,5] Table 2 contains a list of the formulations available for palliative care drugs with authorized and off-label alternatives for patients with swallowing difficulties and EFT.

Table 1 Summary of the issues to consider when choosing a suitable formulation

Formulation	*Considerations / Disadvantages*
Soluble tablet	Availability Sodium content, may be high Cost
Authorized oral liquid	Excipients causing undesirable effects Bio-availability and dosing frequency Viscosity and particle size Volume and palatability Cost
Effervescent tablet or dispersed tablet (authorized or off-label)	Sodium content, may be high Particle size Practicality Cost of authorized formulations
Locally prepared or special order oral liquid	As for authorized oral liquid *plus*: shelf-life/expiry storage conditions continuity of supply reduced quality assurance variable formulations between special order manufacturers higher cost than authorized oral liquid
Dispersed capsule contents (authorized or off- label) or crushed tablet	Occupational exposure Particle size Practicality Reduced dose (≤20% lost with crushing) Risk of using an inappropriate formulation, e.g. m/r and causing destruction of m/r mechanism, more rapid absorption, and danger to patient
Injection given PO or by EFT	Osmolality/hypertonicity/unsuitable pH Excipients unsuitable for PO administration Risk of wrong route error Continuity of supply in the community Cost

Option 1: Authorized soluble tablet or oral liquid

If available, soluble tablets are generally the preferred option. Soluble tablets dissolve *completely* when placed in 10mL water to give a solution of the drug in contrast to effervescent, dispersible or orodispersible tablets which disperse in water or in the mouth to give particles (see option 2 below).

Liquid formulations are not always suitable as direct substitutes for solid dosage forms for several reasons:

- *excipients e.g. sorbitol, ethanol, glycerol, propylene glycol, causing undesirable effects:* many oral liquid formulations contain excipients which in large volumes can cause osmotic diarrhoea, particularly with jejunal administration, e.g. sorbitol ≥15g/24h. The normal osmolality of GI secretions is 100–400mosm/kg, but many liquid formulations are >1,000mosm/kg.[13,14] Reduce osmolality by diluting with as much water as is practical. Some liquid formulations contain alcohol, e.g. Oramorph®, **loperamide**, **phenobarbital**, **ranitidine**
- *altered bio-availability and/or dosing frequency:* an oral liquid formulation may have a different bio-availability from the corresponding solid formulation, e.g. **citalopram**, **phenytoin**, **sodium fusidate**, necessitating a different dose. When converting from a m/r formulation to an immediate-release oral liquid, the dose and/or frequency may need to be changed
- *viscosity and particle size of suspensions:* patients may be unable to swallow a highly viscous formulation or particulate suspension. EFT are easily blocked by a highly viscous formulation, e.g. **amoxicillin-clavulanate**, mineral oil, syrups or by particles from a suspension, e.g. **ciprofloxacin**, **clarithromycin**. Viscosity may be reduced by diluting with 30–50mL water if practical [14]
- *large volumes:* from high doses or multiple drugs may be impractical, unpalatable and costly.

Option 2: Effervescent tablet or dispersed tablet (authorized or off-label)

Do not administer a formulation by EFT if it has failed to disperse into small, barely visible particles or has an oily residue. Sediment and oily films increase the risk of blocking EFTs (Box A).[14,15]

Effervescent tablets and authorized dispersible tablets disintegrate in water to particle/granule form. Many standard tablets will also disperse or dissolve when mixed with 10mL water even if not marketed as dispersible/soluble. Although off-label, this is often the most practical option for both patients with swallowing difficulties and those with EFT (Box A). However, for any tablets dispersed in water the following should be noted:

- fractional dosing from effervescent or dispersed tablets is not recommended due to inaccuracy
- the resulting particles/granules may be too large for administration by fine-bore EFT
- this option is unsuitable for patients unable to swallow biphasic preparations, i.e. solids and liquids together.

Box A Guidelines for preparation of dispersed formulations for EFT administration[1,3]

Information about the preparation of each medication should be documented on the prescription and in the patient's notes.

Prepare each drug separately.

Place the tablet(s) or capsule contents into the barrel of a 50mL enteral syringe; use a large container/drug pot for effervescent formulations.

Add 10mL of tap water (50mL for effervescent formulations), allow to disperse, then mix well:

- use sterile water for jejunal tubes or immunocompromised patients
- if using a drug pot or other container, once dispersed, draw up the contents using a 50mL enteral syringe; this reduces the risk of rupture of the EFT.

Inspect the contents of the enteral syringe to ensure that there are no large particles that might block the EFT.

Administer each drug separately via the EFT (see QCG: Administration of drugs by enteral feeding tube, p.792).

If using a drug pot or other container, rinse with water, draw up with the same enteral syringe and administer the rinsings through the tube.

To ensure the patient receives the whole dose, use the same enteral syringe to draw up and administer the flush (see QCG: Administration of drugs by enteral feeding tube, p.792).

Thoroughly clean any drug pots/containers/tablet crushers with hot soapy water according to local policy to avoid cross-contamination.

Do not:

- use hot water for drug dispersion as this may alter bio-availability
- leave dispersed medicines lying around unlabelled.

Orodispersible tablets are designed to disperse on the tongue and are generally swallowed with the saliva without water. Some orodispersible formulations may be more suitable than others for patients with swallowing difficulties and may depend on the extent of dysphagia. The formulations, dose equivalences and administration of orodispersible tablets vary depending on the drug concerned. Individual product details should be consulted before using by EFT.

Buccal, sublingual and most oromucosal formulations are designed to be absorbed by the oral mucosa and not the GI tract, thus bypassing first-pass hepatic metabolism. These may be suitable alternatives for patients with swallowing difficulties but are unsuitable for EFT administration. Check if the formulation is intended for buccal or enteral administration to prevent wrong route errors.

Option 3: Locally prepared or special order oral liquid

An oral liquid formulation prepared locally or by special order (see Chapter 24, p.751) may be an alternative if an authorized product is not available or not suitable.[16] The same issues as for authorized oral liquids need to be considered (see Table 1). However, it may be possible for an experienced pharmacist to alter a formulation with careful consideration for quality, storage and shelf-life and thus make it more suitable.[16] Continuity of supply after a patient has returned home, short shelf-life, storage conditions (e.g. refrigeration), differences in formulation between manufacturers and higher cost often make this option impractical.[5]

Option 4: Dispersed capsule contents or crushed tablet

Opening capsules in order to disperse the contents is generally off-label and risks topical and inhaled exposure of the contents to the health professional. It is not recommended for certain drugs, e.g. antibiotics, cytotoxics, prostaglandin analogues or hormone antagonists. There are also risks to the patient if unsuitable formulations are used, e.g. m/r formulations may be harmful if accidentally chewed or crushed, or if the contents are irritant, e.g. **demeclocycline**.[17]

A few capsules contain liquid contents, e.g. **nifedipine**. Because of the small volume of the contents (which varies between brands), it is not recommended that these are used as a source of a drug for swallowing difficulties or EFT administration.

It is sometimes feasible to add the contents of some capsules to water for administration by EFT, or to soft food, fruit juice or other liquids to aid those with swallowing difficulties. The manufacturer's SPC should be consulted to ensure that this will not cause problems with absorption or cause undesirable effects. Small quantities of soft food or liquids, e.g. a tablespoon (15mL), should be used to ensure that the entire dose is administered.

Crushing tablet/capsule contents to facilitate dispersion is *not* generally necessary as many tablets and capsule contents will disperse sufficiently in water without crushing (see option 2). Crushing can be dangerous for certain formulations (Box B) and care must be taken to ensure that this is safe for both the patient and health professionals.[17] There is also significant risk of loss of dose or subsequent cross contamination. Thus, crushing should be considered a last resort and avoided unless specifically recommended by a pharmacist.[1]

Box B Formulations which must not be crushed or chewed

Do not crush

M/r formulations (including m/r capsule contents) because this will destroy the m/r mechanism and result in dangerous dose peaks and troughs.[14,15,18–20]

E/c (gastro-resistant) formulations (including e/c capsule contents) because this will destroy the e/c properties of the formulation, may alter bio-availability, and may block the tube.[14,15,19,20]

Cytotoxics, prostaglandin analogues, hormone antagonists or antibiotics because there are risks to the staff through inhalation and/or topical absorption.[14,15,20]

Buccal or sublingual formulations because their bio-availability may be dramatically reduced if absorbed by the GI tract.[14,15,20]

Option 5: Injection (given PO or by EFT)

Formulations for injection are often unsuitable for enteral administration. This may be for one or more of several reasons:

- high osmolality or hypertonicity; the high solute concentration can cause osmotic diarrhoea
- unsuitable pH of the formulation or acidic conditions of the stomach chemically degrading the drug, e.g. **omeprazole**

- formulation with a different salt of unknown bio-availability
- an additive which is irritant to the GI tract, e.g. polysorbate 80 (Tween® 80) in **amiodarone**[1,21]
- risk of IV administration by mistake[6,7]
- cost.

Generally, all injections suitable for enteral administration should be diluted before administration, e.g. with 30–50mL water by EFT. Bio-availability between the solid dose form and the injection solution may be different and alter clinical response, e.g. more rapid absorption and higher peak levels may occur.

SPECIFIC CONSIDERATIONS FOR EFT

Testing of tube position before drug administration

Fatalities from aspiration have occurred as a result of incorrect placement of nasogastric (NG) tubes.[22,23] Thus, even when placement devices are used, it is essential that correct NG tube position is confirmed *before anything is administered via the tube*. This includes water for activating lubricant to facilitate removal of the placement device. Use specific CE marked pH paper for testing gastric contents to confirm pH is within the 'safe' range of 1–5.5.[8] Radiographic confirmation in accordance with specific NPSA guidance is necessary only when there is doubt.[24]

Correct NG tube position should be confirmed before each feed, before each drug administration and at least once daily. A break in feeding of 1h is required before testing. However, for patients on continuous feeding, multiple drug administration times, or on acid-suppressing drugs (e.g. antacids, H_2 antagonists and PPIs) this is impractical. Providing initial tube placement has been correctly confirmed and there is no reason to suspect displacement, tube position should be confirmed by observation of the external tube length and positioning in accordance with NPSA guidelines.[8]

Nasoduodenal and nasojejunal tubes are usually inserted under some form of guidance (e.g. endoscopic, radiological) to ensure correct tube placement. Initial confirmation of position should be undertaken as per local guidelines. Subsequent confirmation of tube position should be undertaken by observation of the external tube length (see above); testing with pH paper is not appropriate.

Semi-permanent and permanent devices, e.g. gastrostomy tubes, do not require repeated confirmation of position.

Site of drug delivery

The position of the tube may alter bio-availability, e.g. with jejunal tubes, absorption may be unpredictable because of the effects of pH or because the tube may extend beyond the main site of absorption of the drug, e.g. **cephalexin, metronidazole benzoate**.[1,13] Care should also be taken with drugs that have a narrow therapeutic range, e.g. **digoxin, warfarin, phenytoin** and other anti-epileptics.[13] Drugs which undergo extensive first-pass hepatic metabolism may have greater systemic effects because of increased absorption from direct delivery to the jejunum, e.g. opioids, TCAs.[2] Undesirable effects may also be increased because of rapid delivery into the jejunum. The acid barrier of the stomach is bypassed with jejunal tubes, some centres use aseptic technique to reduce the risk of infective diarrhoea.

Function of the tube

Drugs should not be administered if the tube is on free drainage or suction.[14]

Number of lumens

Ensure the correct lumen is used with multilumen tubes; some tubes have one lumen terminating in the stomach and another in the jejunum. *Do not use an aspiration gastric decompression port for drug administration.*

Lumen size

The outer diameter of an EFT is measured by the French gauge (1 French unit = 0.33mm).[2] However, the internal diameter of equivalent French gauge tubes varies between manufacturers. The tube material also affects the internal lumen size, e.g. silicone and latex tubes have thicker walls and therefore narrower internal lumens. Narrow lumen, e.g. 5–12 French, or long tubes, e.g. NJ, are more likely to block, particularly with thick oral syrups and suspensions with large particles. Wide bore tubes require larger flush volumes.

Flushing the tube

This is essential to minimize drug interactions with the feeds. Water is the standard flush; use sterile water for jejunal tubes or immunocompromised patients because the acid barrier in the stomach is bypassed.[1] Tubes should be flushed before, in between drugs, and after drug administration ideally with 30mL water.[1,25] Use a 50mL enteral syringe to reduce the risk of tube rupture which can be caused by smaller syringes. Flush slowly with a push-pause technique to prevent leaving a coating of feed on the internal tube surface. Record the total flush and drug volume administered.

Feeding regimen

With continuous feeding and multiple drug administration periods, it may be necessary to adjust the feeding rate to compensate for the breaks in feed administration. If possible, the drug schedule should be rationalized, aiming for once daily drug administration to allow time for adequate nutrition.[2]

Bulk-forming laxatives

Do not administer by EFT because they may block the tube; use an enteral feed with a high-fibre content instead.[14]

DRUG INTERACTIONS AND COMPLICATIONS WITH EFT

Drugs can interact with food in many ways.[26,27] Enteral feeds can cause different problems associated with bio-availability, physical compatibility, and chemical interactions. Because they are in liquid form, the content, consistency and pH is very different to normal diet and variable between brands.

Drugs should *never* be added to enteral feeds because this increases the risk of incompatibility, microbial contamination, tube blockage, and underdosing or overdosing if the feed rate is altered.[28] However, complications can still arise from:

- *binding of drugs to the internal surface of the tube reducing absorption*, e.g. **carbamazepine**,[29] **clonazepam**, **diazepam**, **phenytoin**; minimize by diluting with 30–50mL water and flushing as per QCG: Administration of drugs by enteral feeding tube (see p.792)
- *physical interaction with the feed causing coagulation*, particularly if the drug formulation is acidic, i.e. pH<4.[14] This applies to many syrups,[2] and risks tube blockage and reduced drug absorption. Abdominal distension caused by excessive gas production from effervescence has been reported when sodium bicarbonate solutions, used to deliver PPI formulations, have come into contact with the feed[30]
- *chemical interaction between the drug and feed causing a non-absorbable drug–feed complex*, e.g. bezoar (insoluble concretion) formation with **sucralfate**, in the tube or in the stomach.[31,32] Do not prescribe **sucralfate** by EFT
- *chemical interaction between the drug and the feed resulting in reduced drug available for absorption*, e.g. **carbamazepine**, **ciprofloxacin**, **digoxin**, **penicillins**, **phenytoin**, **theophylline**, **warfarin**.[33] A feed break of at least 1h before and after each drug is recommended to minimize the risk of reduced absorption
- *indirect drug or nutrient interactions*, e.g. the **vitamin K** or **eicosapentanoic acid** content of a feed affecting the action of **warfarin**[26](also see p.781).
- *the effects of malnutrition on drug pharmacokinetics.*

Usual considerations for physical and chemical drug–drug interactions must also be taken into consideration, particularly if rationalizing drug administration to once or twice a day.

Flushing the tube effectively, diluting potentially problematic formulations, inserting a feed break as outlined in the QCG: Administration of drugs by enteral feeding tube (see p.792) and choosing an appropriate formulation will reduce the risk of dangerous interactions. Clinically, the most important interactions are those drugs with a narrow therapeutic range, e.g. **digoxin**, **theophylline**, **warfarin**, **phenytoin** and other anti-epileptics; these may warrant monitoring plasma concentrations. Clinical response should also be monitored closely. Appropriate precautionary measures may need to be taken if the feed is discontinued, particularly if dose adjustments were made because of an interaction.

ADMINISTRATION OF E/C (GASTRO-RESISTANT) AND M/R FORMULATIONS BY EFT

Generally, these products should *not* be administered by EFT because of the risk of blocking the tube. However, some capsules/granules/compressed tablets contain e/c or m/r granules for which specific procedures have been developed to allow administration of the coated granules by EFT, e.g. **esomeprazole** gastro-resistant tablets and gastro-resistant granules for oral suspension (Nexium®), **lansoprazole** orodispersible tablets (Zoton FasTab®), certain m/r **morphine** formulations (MST Continus® suspension and Zomorph® capsules) **omeprazole** capsules (Losec®) and **theophylline** m/r capsules (Slo-Phyllin®). See the manufacturer's SPC and/or specialist information for details (Table 2).[1] In order to avoid dangerous dose peaks and troughs or tube blockage, it is essential that:

- the recommended procedure is strictly adhered to and is used only for that *specific* formulation and brand
- the correct tube size and type is used
- extreme care is taken to avoid crushing the coated granules, thereby destroying the coating
- clinical response is monitored closely.

UNBLOCKING EFTS

Tube blockage may be caused by the feed, e.g. stagnant or contaminated feed, or by incorrect drug administration, e.g. particle blockage or interaction between the feed and drug. It can be minimized by effective flushing and choosing an appropriate formulation. It is more likely with narrow lumens; a 35% incidence of blockage in patients with 8 French tubes has been cited.[34] Many tubes can be unblocked using 15–30mL water in a 50mL syringe and a push-pull action, although this may take 20–30min. Excessive force must not be used to unblock a tube because of the danger of perforation. Care must be taken as unblocking a tube may result in bolus drug administration from residual drug in the tube.

Various other agents have anecdotally been used to unblock tubes, e.g. carbonated drinks or cranberry juice. However, these are acidic solutions and can make the situation worse by causing feed coagulation,[14] and are no longer recommended.[1] Pancreatic enzymes, e.g. **pancreatin** (p.58), help only if the blockage is caused by the feed. Sodium bicarbonate needs to be added to activate the enzymes, which may not be practical. Re-insertion of guide-wires is not advisable unless under specialist supervision.[1]

For blockages which do not resolve with water, consult a specialist nutrition nurse if available.

Quick Clinical Guide: Administration of drugs by enteral feeding tube

Before drug administration

1 The administration of drugs by an enteral feeding tube (EFT) is considered a level 3 skill for care workers in care homes. Staff must be adequately trained.

2 Drug charts should state the specific route of administration, e.g. nasogastric (NG), nasojejunal (NJ), and specify the lumen to be used to prevent wrong route errors.

3 Check that there is documented confirmation that the EFT was correctly positioned following insertion. For NG tubes, use CE marked pH paper intended for testing human gastric contents (safe range pH1–5.5 after a 1h break in feeding) or, when there is doubt, by approved radiographic confirmation in accordance with NPSA guidelines.

4 If practical, reconfirm correct NG tube position before each drug administration. For patients on continuous feeding, multiple drug administration times or on acid-suppressants (antacids, H_2 antagonists, PPIs), if correct tube placement confirmed initially and there is no reason to suspect displacement, confirm tube position by observation of the external tube length (in accordance with NPSA guidelines); likewise for NJ tubes.

5 The patient should be in a sitting position to prevent regurgitation and pulmonary aspiration.

6 All EFT lumens should be clearly labelled.

7 To prevent accidental parenteral administration, only use dedicated enteral syringes and connectors.

Drug administration

> Do not add drugs to enteral feeds because this increases the risk of incompatibility, microbial contamination, tube blockage, and underdosing or overdosing if the feed rate is altered.

8 Stop the feed and ensure any other ports are closed and airtight.

9 Flush the EFT using a **push-pause** action with 15–30mL of water (*use sterile water throughout if jejunal tube or immunocompromised patient*). This helps to clear the tube and prevent physical interactions with the feed which could result in coagulation and blockage of the tube.

10 Check if a specific time interval is needed before and after administration to achieve maximal absorption and/or reduce the risk of chemical interactions.

11 Administer the most suitable formulation of each drug separately (see Choosing a suitable formulation, Box A, p.787, and Table 2, p.793):
- a 50mL enteral syringe reduces the risk of rupture of the EFT; a 2mL or smaller enteral syringe can be used for very small quantities to accurately measure the dose
- flush between each drug with 15–30mL of water.

12 After drug administration, flush the EFT using a **push-pause** action with 15–30mL of water.

13 Resume feeding after any necessary feed break (see point 10).

After drug administration

14 Document the total volume of fluid given (including flushes) on a fluid balance chart.

15 Monitor the clinical response, particularly if:
- changing from m/r to immediate-release formulations
- the drug has a narrow therapeutic range
- the bio-availability of the drug differs between solid dose form and liquid.

Table 2 Information on alternative enteral formulations available for administering drugs to patients with swallowing difficulties or by EFT[1,35–39]

Drug	*Authorized soluble tablet or oral liquid available*	*Tablet/capsule contents may disperse sufficiently for 8Fr NG tube*[a,b]	*Oral liquid can be prepared by local pharmacy or special order*	*Injection available and can be diluted and administered PO or by EFT*	*Comments*
Acetylcysteine	No		Yes	Yes	
Amiloride	Yes	Yes	Yes	No	Sugar- and sorbitol-free oral solution
Aminophylline[a]	No	No	Yes	Yes	Consider discontinuing therapy due to dosing complexities Give aminophylline injection orally as a diluted oral solution,[1] take care converting from m/r to immediate-release or convert oral aminophylline total daily dose to oral *unauthorized* theophylline liquid (aminophylline 250mg PO = theophylline 200mg PO) and split into t.d.s regimen (see theophylline below). Monitor blood levels
Amiodarone	No	No	Yes[e,f]	No	Unauthorized 50mg/5mL and 100mg/5mL oral suspension can be obtained via special order A 25mg/5mL suspension[f] or 200mg/5mL suspension can be prepared.[37] Injection contains irritant Tween 80
Amitriptyline	Yes	No	Yes[c]	No	Sugar- and sorbitol-free oral solution
Amlodipine	Yes	Yes	Yes[f]	No	A 1mg/mL suspension can be prepared (90 day shelf-life)[f] or with 1% methylcellulose in syrup (56 day shelf-life).[1] Disperse tablet for intrajejunal administration
Amoxicillin	Yes			Yes	Dilute oral suspensions with an equal volume of water to reduce viscosity for EFT use
Antacids	Yes			No	Not recommended by EFT as can coagulate with feed; not needed with jejunal tube
Ascorbic acid	No	Yes (effervescent)	Yes	No	Add effervescent tablets (only available OTC) to 50mL water

continued

Table 2 Continued

Drug	*Authorized soluble tablet or oral liquid available*	*Tablet/capsule contents may disperse sufficiently for 8Fr NG tube*[a,b]	*Oral liquid can be prepared by local pharmacy or special order*	*Injection available and can be diluted and administered PO or by EFT*	*Comments*
Aspirin	No	Yes (dispersible)	Yes	No	Use dispersible tablet
Baclofen	Yes	Yes	Yes[d]		Authorized oral liquids are viscous and contain sorbitol (2.75g/5mL Lioresal®) dilute with an equal volume of water for EFT use Dispersing tablets is preferable particularly for intrajejunal administration
Bendroflumethiazide	No	Yes (Wockhardt)	Yes[e]	No	Unauthorized 2.5mg/5mL oral suspension can be obtained via special order; viscous liquid, no information of suitability for EFT
Bisacodyl[a]	No	No	Yes[e]	No	Unauthorized 2.5mg/5mL oral suspension can be obtained via special order
Bethanechol	No		Yes	No	A 5mg/mL suspension with cherry syrup can be prepared (60 day shelf-life)[1]
Calcium & vitamin D	No	Yes (effervescent)		No	Use effervescent granules or effervescent tablet and add to 50mL water. The solution can crystallize and calcium can bind to phosphate in enteral feed. Flush EFT well to avoid
Carbamazepine[a]	Yes		Yes	No	Oral liquid contains sorbitol (1.25g/5mL Tegretol®) Dilute with an equal volume of water to reduce adherence to EFT. Monitor for increased undesirable effects particularly with intrajejunal administration
Carbocisteine	Yes			No	
Cefalexin	Yes			No	Dilute oral suspensions with equal volume of water to reduce viscosity for EFT use. Avoid opening capsules/crushing tablets due to risk of cephalosporin sensitization

continued

Table 2 Continued

Drug	*Authorized soluble tablet or oral liquid available*	*Tablet/capsule contents may disperse sufficiently for 8Fr NG tube*[a,b]	*Oral liquid can be prepared by local pharmacy or special order*	*Injection available and can be diluted and administered PO or by EFT*	*Comments*
Cefradine	Yes			No	Avoid opening capsules/crushing tablets due to risk of cephalosporin sensitization
Celecoxib	No	Yes		No	Capsule contents are authorized to be sprinkled onto applesauce, yoghurt or mashed banana
Chlorphenamine	Yes			Yes	
Chlorpromazine	Yes	No	Yes[d]		Some oral liquids contain sorbitol Handle with care to avoid contact sensitization; do not crush tablets
Cimetidine	Yes	Yes (effervescent)		Yes (Tagamet®)	Some oral liquids contain sorbitol (Dyspamet® 2.8g/5mL, Tagamet® negligible). Use effervescent tablet added to 30mL water, or diluted liquid for intrajejunal administration. Tagamet® and Dyspamet® disperse but no information on suitability for EFT
Cinnarizine	No	Yes	Yes	No	
Ciprofloxacin	Yes	Yes (Ranbaxy, Generics)	Yes[c]		Authorized oral suspension not recommended for EFT because too viscous and granular. Disperse tablet with 30–50mL sterile water *not tap water* (to avoid ion chelation). Stop feed for 1h before and 1–2h after dose. Do not administer with iron or zinc
Citalopram	Yes	Yes (Generics)	Yes	No	10mg of tablet equivalent to 8mg of oral liquid (4 drops). Oral liquid should be mixed with water for EFT, or water/orange/apple juice for PO use; contains alcohol (0.01units/mL)
Clarithromycin[a]	Yes			No	Dilute oral liquid with an equal volume of water for EFT. Do not use EFT less than 9Fr gauge

continued

Table 2 Continued

Drug	*Authorized soluble tablet or oral liquid available*	*Tablet/capsule contents may disperse sufficiently for 8Fr NG tube*[a,b]	*Oral liquid can be prepared by local pharmacy or special order*	*Injection available and can be diluted and administered PO or by EFT*	*Comments*
Clindamycin	No	Yes (capsules)	Yes[e]		Unauthorized 75mg/5mL oral suspension can be obtained via special order Avoid inhalation of the capsule contents
Clomipramine[a]	No	Yes	Yes[e]	No	Unauthorized 50mg/5mL oral suspension can be obtained via special order
Clonazepam	Yes	Yes (Rivotril®)	Yes[d, e, f]	Yes	Authorized oral solutions 500microgram/5mL and 2mg/5mL contain alcohol (0.01 units/5mL) and must *not* be diluted. No information on suitability via EFT Dilute all other formulations with 30–50mL water to reduce risk of binding to the tube. Disperse tablets for intrajejunal administration. Injection contains alcohol and other excipients Unauthorized 2.5mg/mL oral drops and 0.5mg orodispersible tablets can be imported
Clonidine	No	Yes (100microgram Catapres®)	Yes[d,e]	Yes (Catapres®)	Unauthorized 50microgram/5mL oral solution and suspension can be obtained via special order. A 100microgram/mL formulation with simple syrup can be prepared (1 month shelf-life)[1]
Co-amoxiclav	Yes	No			Oral liquid not recommended for EFT because too viscous
Co-codamol	No	Yes (effervescent or dispersible)	Yes	No	Add effervescent or dispersible tablet to 50mL water
Co-codaprin	No	Yes (dispersible)		No	Add dispersible tablet to 50mL water
Co-danthramer	Yes			No	Slightly viscous liquid; may require a larger flush volume

continued

Table 2 Continued

Drug	*Authorized soluble tablet or oral liquid available*	*Tablet/capsule contents may disperse sufficiently for 8Fr NG tube*[a,b]	*Oral liquid can be prepared by local pharmacy or special order*	*Injection available and can be diluted and administered PO or by EFT*	*Comments*
Co-danthrusate	Yes			No	No information on suitability via EFT
Co-dydramol	No		Yes[e]	No	Unauthorized 10mg/500mg/5mL oral suspension can be obtained via special order
Codeine phosphate	Yes		Yes[d]		Dilute authorized oral liquid with an equal volume of water to reduce viscosity for EFT use. Tablets disperse but no information on suitability by EFT Some dispersible or effervescent formulations contain 20mmol sodium per tablet
Co-phenotrope	No	Yes (Lomotil®)		No	
Co-trimoxazole	Yes				Oral liquid (Septrin®) contains sorbitol and needs diluting 3 times to reduce viscosity for EFT use
Cyclizine	No	Yes (Valoid®)	Yes[c,e]	Yes	Unauthorized 50mg/5mL oral solution and suspension can be obtained via special order
Cyproheptadine	No	Yes	Yes	No	
Cyproterone	No		Yes[d]	No	Tablets disperse but no information on suitability by EFT
Dantrolene	No		Yes[d,e]	No	Injection formulation may hydrolyze in the stomach Capsule contents disperse but no information on suitability by EFT Unauthorized 10mg/5mL, 25mg/5mL or 100mg/5mL oral suspension can be obtained via special order
Demeclocycline	No	No	Yes	No	Capsule contents are irritant and only sparingly soluble. Absorption is reduced by calcium

continued

Table 2 Continued

Drug	*Authorized soluble tablet or oral liquid available*	*Tablet/capsule contents may disperse sufficiently for 8Fr NG tube*[a,b]	*Oral liquid can be prepared by local pharmacy or special order*	*Injection available and can be diluted and administered PO or by EFT*	*Comments*
Desmopressin	Yes	Yes (Desmotabs, DDAVP®)	Yes		DesmoMelt®, DDAVP Melt®, Noqdirna® and generic desmopressin oral lyophilisates are for SL use only, not for EFT administration
Dexamethasone	Yes	Yes (Organon)	Yes[d]	Yes	Authorized oral liquid contains sorbitol 500microgram/5mL
Dexamfetamine[a]	Yes		Yes	No	
Diamorphine	No		Yes		
Diazepam	Yes	Yes (APS)	Yes[d]	Yes	Dilute authorized oral liquid with an equal volume of water to reduce viscosity and risk of binding to the EFT. Disperse tablets for intrajejunal administration. Anecdotal evidence of using injection enterally; drug loss may occur due to binding to tube
Diclofenac[a]	No	Yes (dispersible)	Yes	No	Use authorized dispersible tablet for EFT. Alternative unauthorized 10mg dispersible tablets or 50mg/5mL oral liquid (1 year shelf-life) available
Dicycloverine	Yes			No	Dilute oral liquid with an equal volume of water for EFT use
Digoxin	Yes		Yes	Yes	In theory 50microgram Lanoxin® oral liquid = 62.5microgram tablet, however in practice unlikely to be clinically important, monitor plasma concentrations if changing formulation or using a high-fibre feed. Oral liquid may cause diarrhoea Lanoxin® tablets disperse but no information on suitability by EFT Bio-availability of the injection PO or EFT is unpredictable and not recommended
Dihydrocodeine[a]	Yes		Yes		Dilute oral liquid with an equal volume of water for EFT use

continued

Table 2 Continued

Drug	*Authorized soluble tablet or oral liquid available*	*Tablet/capsule contents may disperse sufficiently for 8Fr NG tube*[a,b]	*Oral liquid can be prepared by local pharmacy or special order*	*Injection available and can be diluted and administered PO or by EFT*	*Comments*
Docusate sodium	Yes			No	Dilute oral liquid with an equal volume of water for EFT use
Domperidone	Yes	Yes (Co-Pharma, CP)	Yes[d]	No	Dilute oral liquid with an equal volume of water for EFT use. Contains sorbitol 2.3g/5mL. Consider dispersing tablets for intrajejunal administration
Doxepin	No	Yes (Sinepin®)	Yes	No	
Doxycycline	No	Yes (dispersible)	Yes		Use dispersible tablets, do not open capsules as contents are irritant
Erythromycin[a]	Yes	No			Dilute oral liquid with an equal volume of water for EFT use , some brands contain sorbitol. Tablets and capsule contents are e/c therefore not suitable for EFT
Esomeprazole	No	Yes (Nexium®)	Yes		Nexium® tablets and granules for suspension are authorized for administration via a gastric tube. The tablet contains a compressed core of e/c microgranules which can be dispersed and flushed via an 8Fr gauge NG tube. Do not crush. Strictly follow the procedure in the SPC to prevent tube blockage
Etamsylate (not UK)	No		Yes[d]		
Ferrous sulfate	Yes	No	Yes[e]	No	Ironorm® 625mg/5mL oral drops available Unauthorized 60mg/5mL oral solution or suspension can be obtained via special order Convert to an alternative iron salt oral liquid preparation Ferrous sulfate 200mg = 3.3mL Niferex® *or* 7mL Galfer® *or* 12mL Sytron® (contains sorbitol 2g/5mL); dilute with an equal volume of water for EFT use

continued

Table 2 Continued

Drug	*Authorized soluble tablet or oral liquid available*	*Tablet/capsule contents may disperse sufficiently for 8Fr NG tube*[a,b]	*Oral liquid can be prepared by local pharmacy or special order*	*Injection available and can be diluted and administered PO or by EFT*	*Comments*
Flecainide	No	Yes (Generics)	Yes[c, e]	Yes	Use de-ionized/sterile water, *not tap water.* Note crushed tablets have a local anaesthetic effect. *Do not* dilute the injection or mix with alkaline solutions, e.g. chlorides, phosphates, sulfates Unauthorized10mg/5mL oral suspension and 25mg/5mL oral solution and suspension can be obtained via special order
Flucloxacillin	Yes	No		Yes (Berk, CP)	Dilute oral liquid with an equal volume of water for EFT use. Stop feed for 1h before and after dose. Avoid opening capsules due to risk of sensitization
Fluconazole	Yes	Yes (50mg capsule)	Yes[d]	No	Do not use the 150mg capsule contents
Fludrocortisone	No	Yes (Florinef®)	Yes[e]	No	Unauthorized 50microgram/5mL and 100microgram/5mL oral suspension can be obtained via special order
Fluoxetine	Yes		Yes	No	Capsule contents can be dispersed but no information on suitability via EFT
Furosemide	Yes		Yes[d]		Frusol® oral solutions are authorized for NG and PEG administration see SPC for details Oral liquids may be alkaline and may coagulate with other acidic preparations. Flush EFT well to avoid Lasix® tablets disperse but no information on suitability via EFT. SL use may be an option (see p.61)
Gabapentin	Yes	Yes (Neurontin®)	Yes	No	The authorized oral solution contains propylene glycol and other excipients which in high doses, may exceed WHO daily intake limits Gabapentin Rosemont 50mg/mL oral solution is authorized for NG and PEG administration, see SPC for details

continued

Table 2 Continued

Drug	*Authorized soluble tablet or oral liquid available*	*Tablet/capsule contents may disperse sufficiently for 8Fr NG tube*[a,b]	*Oral liquid can be prepared by local pharmacy or special order*	*Injection available and can be diluted and administered PO or by EFT*	*Comments*
Glibenclamide	No	Yes (APS)	Yes[d]	No	Daonil® tablets disperse but no information on suitability via EFT
Gliclazide[a]	No	Yes (Alpharma, CP, Generics)	Yes[d,e]	No	When administering dispersed tablets by EFT, there may be residue left in the oral syringe, which is unlikely to be active drug due to high solubility. Flush EFT well to avoid blockage. Unauthorized 40mg/5mL and 80mg/5mLoral suspension can be obtained via special order
Glycopyrronium	Yes	No	Yes[e]	Yes	Unauthorized tablets disperse coarsely and may leave sediment. Unauthorized oral formulations can be obtained via special order or can be made locally from glycopyrronium powder or injection (see p.13). Cost of bulk powder may be prohibitive
Granisetron	No	Yes (Kytril®)	Yes[f]	Yes	250microgram/5mL suspension can be prepared.[f] TD patch available
Haloperidol	Yes		Yes		Serenace® tablets disperse but no information on suitability by EFT
Hydrocortisone	No	Yes	Yes[e]	Yes (Efcortesol®)	Injection contains significant amounts of phosphate. Unauthorized 5mg/5mL or 10mg/5mL oral suspension can be obtained via special order
Hydromorphone[a]	No		Yes		Do not administer contents of m/r capsules by EFT due to high risk of blockage
Hyoscine *butylbromide*	No	No	Yes[e]	Yes	Injection may be stored for 24h in a refrigerator once opened. Unauthorized 10mg/5mL oral solution and suspension can be obtained via special order

continued

Table 2 Continued

Drug	*Authorized soluble tablet or oral liquid available*	*Tablet/capsule contents may disperse sufficiently for 8Fr NG tube*[a,b]	*Oral liquid can be prepared by local pharmacy or special order*	*Injection available and can be diluted and administered PO or by EFT*	*Comments*
Hyoscine *hydrobromide*	No		Yes[e]	Yes	Unauthorized 300microgram/5mL or 500micorgram/5mL oral solution and suspension can be obtained via special order. TD patch available
Ibandronic acid	No	No	No		Consider alternative route of administration
Ibuprofen[a]	Yes	No	Yes	No	Oral liquid contains sorbitol 500microgram/5mL, dilute with an equal volume of water (more for intrajejunal administration) to reduce viscosity for EFT use
Imipramine	Yes		Yes[c]	No	Dilute commercially available oral solution with an equal volume of water to reduce viscosity for EFT use Tofranil® disperse but particles may be too large for EFT use
Ispaghula husk				No	Do not administer due to high risk of blockage, consider using a high-fibre feed
Itraconazole	Yes		Yes		Stop the feed for 2h before and after dose. Oral liquid contains sorbitol and is acidic. Flush EFT well to avoid coagulation. Absorption via jejunum may be reduced
Ketamine	No	No	Yes[e]	Yes	A 50mg/5mL oral solution using the injection formulation can be prepared by pharmacy, 7 day shelf-life (see p.641). Unauthorized 50mg/5mL oral solution and suspension can be obtained via special order
Ketorolac	No		No		
Lactulose	Yes			No	Dilute oral liquid with 2–3 times volume of water for EFT use
Lamotrigine	No	Yes	Yes[d, f]	No	Use authorized dispersible tablet. A 5mg/5mL suspension can be prepared[f]

continued

Table 2 Continued

Drug	*Authorized soluble tablet or oral liquid available*	*Tablet/capsule contents may disperse sufficiently for 8Fr NG tube*[a,b]	*Oral liquid can be prepared by local pharmacy or special order*	*Injection available and can be diluted and administered PO or by EFT*	*Comments*
Lansoprazole	No	Yes (FasTab®), and capsules	Yes[e]	No	Add orodispersible tablet (FasTab®) to10mL of water and administer by EFT using a push-pull technique to keep the granules suspended. *Do not crush* For tubes smaller than 8Fr, open capsules and mix e/c granules with 10mL of 8.4% sodium bicarbonate, (14 day shelf-life in a refrigerator if locally prepared by pharmacy)[1] Unauthorized 5mg/5mL, 15mg/5mL and 30mg/5mL oral suspension can be obtained via special order
Levetiracetam	Yes	Yes (500mg Keppra®)	Yes		Use the oral liquid for EFT
Levomepromazine	No	Yes (Nozinan®)	Yes[d,e]	Yes	Tablet dispersion is coarse and may block tubes smaller than 8Fr Unauthorized 2.5mg/5mL oral suspension can be obtained via special order
Lofepramine	Yes		Yes	No	Dilute oral liquid with an equal volume of water for EFT use; contains sorbitol 1.4g/5mL
Loperamide	Yes		Yes[e]	No	Oral solution contains alcohol Unauthorized 25mg/5mL oral suspension (alcohol free) can be obtained via special order
Loratadine	Yes			No	Dilute oral liquid with an equal volume of water for jejunal administration to reduce osmolarity
Lorazepam	No	No	Yes[d,e]		Tablets do not disperse easily. Tablets (Genus brand) and injection can be used sublingually. Unauthorized 500microgram/5mL and 1mg/5mL oral solution and suspension can be obtained via special order

continued

Table 2 Continued

Drug	*Authorized soluble tablet or oral liquid available*	*Tablet/capsule contents may disperse sufficiently for 8Fr NG tube*[a,b]	*Oral liquid can be prepared by local pharmacy or special order*	*Injection available and can be diluted and administered PO or by EFT*	*Comments*
Macrogols	Yes			No	May not be suitable for EFT use due to the large volume required to dissolve the powder
Magnesium glycerophosphate	Yes		Yes[e]		Unauthorized 4mmol/5mL and 5mmol/5mL oral solution and suspension can be obtained via special order[e] Various unauthorized tablets available, some will disperse but no information on suitability by EFT
Mebeverine[a]	Yes			No	135mg tablet = 15mL oral liquid 50mg/5mL. Most effective when given 20min before food
Medroxyprogesterone acetate	No	Yes (Provera® 5mg, 100mg)	Yes[d]	Yes (Depo-Provera®)	
Megestrol acetate	No	Yes (Megace®)	Yes[d]		Unauthorized 40mg/mL oral suspension can be imported
Melatonin[a]	No		Yes[e]	No	Unauthorized oral solutions and suspensions can be obtained via special order
Menadiol sodium phosphate	No		Yes[d,e]	No	Tablets disperse but no information on suitability by EFT. Unauthorized 5mg/5mL oral suspension can be obtained via special order
Metformin[a]	Yes	Yes (Glucophage® sachets)	Yes[d]	No	Sachets disperse fully in 20mL of water for EFT, (manufacturer recommends 150mL for PO use)
Methadone	Yes		Yes		No information on suitability via EFT

continued

Table 2 Continued

Drug	*Authorized soluble tablet or oral liquid available*	*Tablet/capsule contents may disperse sufficiently for 8Fr NG tube*[a,b]	*Oral liquid can be prepared by local pharmacy or special order*	*Injection available and can be diluted and administered PO or by EFT*	*Comments*
Methenamine	No			No	Tablets are authorized to be crushed and mixed with milk or fruit juice for swallowing difficulties. No information on suitability by EFT
Methylphenidate[a]	No		Yes[e]	No	Unauthorized 5mg/5mL oral suspension can be obtained via special order
Methylprednisolone	No	Yes (Medrone®)	Yes	Yes (Solu-Medrone®)	
Metoclopramide[a]	Yes		Yes	Yes	Some liquids may contain sorbitol. Maxolon® tablets disperse but no information on suitability by EFT
Metronidazole	Yes	No	Yes		Dilute authorized oral liquid with an equal volume of water for NG use and stop feed for 1h before the dose to allow gastric pH to recover to metabolize the benzoate salt. The benzoate salt is metabolized in the stomach, therefore *not* suitable for jejunal use. A 50mg/mL suspension with cherry syrup can be prepared (60 day shelf-life);[1] it does not require a break in feeding and is more suitable for intrajejunal administration
Midazolam	No		Yes	Yes	Authorized 5mg/mL oromucosal solution for *buccal* use available as unit dose preparation Unauthorized 10mg/mL oromucosal solution for *buccal* use available via special order. Injection can be used via PO, buccal, intranasal and PR routes; injection can be diluted with apple/blackcurrant juice, chocolate sauce or cola for PO administration Unauthorized 2.5mg/mL oral liquid available via special order

continued

Table 2 Continued

Drug	*Authorized soluble tablet or oral liquid available*	*Tablet/capsule contents may disperse sufficiently for 8Fr NG tube*[a,b]	*Oral liquid can be prepared by local pharmacy or special order*	*Injection available and can be diluted and administered PO or by EFT*	*Comments*
Mirtazapine	Yes	No	Yes	No	Use oral liquid; orodispersible tablets (Zispin SolTab®) are *not* recommended for EFT use because too granular
Moclobemide	No	Yes (APS)	Yes	No	
Modafinil	No		Yes[e]	No	Unauthorized 100mg/5mL oral suspension available via special order
Morphine[a]	Yes		Yes		Oral liquid can be used; 10mg/5mL contains alcohol (0.05 units/5mL). Dilute with an equal volume of water, for intrajejunal administration to reduce osmolarity Unauthorized 10mg/5mL oral solution (alcohol free) available via special order M/r granules in Zomorph® capsules are authorized for gastric administration via a 16Fr tube (internal diameter 2.5mm) with an open distal end or lateral pores (see SPC). Certain tubes cause problems[g]. The m/r granules should be mixed (*do not crush*) with 30mL water. Ensure the m/r granules are not crushed by the syringe plunger and that all are administered; add extra water if necessary. There is some anecdotal data on using 8Fr tubes[l]
Morphone (continued)					The m/r granules in MST Continus® suspension sachets have been administered as above in tubes with 8Fr gauge or minimum internal diameter 1.05mm The m/r granules in MXL® capsules are *not* suitable for EFT administration
Nabilone	No			No	The capsule contents disperse but no information on suitability by EFT
Nabumetone	No	No		No	

continued

Table 2 Continued

Drug	*Authorized soluble tablet or oral liquid available*	*Tablet/capsule contents may disperse sufficiently for 8Fr NG tube*[a,b]	*Oral liquid can be prepared by local pharmacy or special order*	*Injection available and can be diluted and administered PO or by EFT*	*Comments*
Naltrexone	No		Yes[e]	No	Unauthorized 5mg/5mL oral solution and suspension can be obtained via special order
Naproxen[a]	No	Yes	Yes[e]	No	Unauthorized 200mg/5mL oral suspension can be obtained via special order
Nefopam	No	Yes (Acupan®)	Yes	No	High risk of sediment when dispersing tablets, may not be suitable for EFT
Nifedipine[a]	No		Yes[e,f]	No	Consider an alternative product, e.g. amlodipine. Drawing up contents of liquid capsules *not* recommended, volumes vary between manufacturers, liquid is light sensitive, and risk of profound hypotension, particularly if converting from m/r preparation. Unauthorized 5mg/5mL and 10mg/5mL oral suspension can be obtained via special order A 20mg/5mL suspension can be prepared using capsule contents[f,37]
Nitrazepam	Yes		Yes	No	Dilute authorized oral liquid to reduce osmolality for intrajejunal use. Unauthorized 5mg/5mL oral suspension can be obtained via special order
Nitrofurantoin[a]	Yes	Yes	Yes[d]	No	Dilute authorized oral liquid with an equal volume of water for EFT use
Olanzapine	No	Yes (Zyprexa Velotab®)	Yes[e]	No	Unauthorized 2.5mg/5mL oral suspension can be obtained via special order

continued

Table 2 Continued

Drug	*Authorized soluble tablet or oral liquid available*	*Tablet/capsule contents may disperse sufficiently for 8Fr NG tube*[a,b]	*Oral liquid can be prepared by local pharmacy or special order*	*Injection available and can be diluted and administered PO or by EFT*	*Comments*
Omeprazole	No	Yes (Alpharma or Dexcel tablets); Losec MUPS®	Yes[e]	Yes	A 2mg/mL formulation with 20mg capsule contents and 10mL 8.4% sodium bicarbonate can be prepared by pharmacy (45 day shelf-life in a refrigerator)[1] Unauthorized oral suspensions can be obtained via special order Orodispersible tablet (Losec MUPS®) can be added to 25mL of water and administered by EFT using a push-pull technique to keep the granules suspended. *Do not crush*. Suitable for 8Fr gauge *Tablets* (Alpharma, Dexcel) disperse; larger doses may be required in gastric administration as this method destroys the e/c coating Contact Astra Zeneca for details of use of injection or infusion via EFT
Ondansetron	Yes		Yes	Yes	Oral liquid contains sorbitol 3g/5mL. Zofran® tablets disperse but no information on suitability by EFT or of the orodispersible tablet (Zofran Melt®). The injection is acidic, flush well to avoid coagulation with feed
Orphenadrine	Yes		Yes[c]	No	Authorized oral liquids contain sorbitol, 0.45g/5mL (Rosemont) and 1.75g/5ml (Biorphen®). Disipal® tablets disperse but no information on suitability by EFT
Oxybutynin[a]	Yes	Yes (Tillomed)	Yes[d]	No	Authorized oral liquid contains sorbitol 1.3g/5mL. Ditropan® may disperse but no information on suitability by EFT. Cystrin® may leave sediment and be unsuitable for EFT use. TD patch available
Oxycodone[a]	Yes		Yes		Anecdotal reports of use of liquid preparation by EFT
Paracetamol	Yes	Yes (dispersible or effervescent)	Yes		Add dispersible tablet to 50mL of water; consider sodium content

continued

Table 2 Continued

Drug	*Authorized soluble tablet or oral liquid available*	*Tablet/capsule contents may disperse sufficiently for 8Fr NG tube*[a,b]	*Oral liquid can be prepared by local pharmacy or special order*	*Injection available and can be diluted and administered PO or by EFT*	*Comments*
Paroxetine	Yes		Yes	No	Dilute oral liquid with an equal volume of water for EFT use, contains sorbitol
Phenobarbital	Yes		Yes[d, f]		Authorized elixir contains alcohol (0.38units/10mL dose). An unauthorized 50mg/5mL alcohol-free suspension can be obtained via special order or locally prepared Dilute oral liquids with an equal volume of water for intrajejunal administration to reduce osmolarity Tablets may disperse but no information on suitability by EFT
Phenoxymethyl-penicillin	Yes				Stop feed for 2h before and 1h after dose
Phenytoin	Yes	Yes (Flynn; capsules)	Yes[e]		Stop feed for 2h before and after dose and flush tube with 50mL water to minimize interaction with feed. Convert to once daily dose. Phenytoin *base* 30mg/5mL oral suspension (Epanutin®); 90mg (15mL) = 100mg phenytoin *sodium* tablet/capsule, shake liquid well, then dilute dose with 30–50mL water, administer and flush An unauthorized concentrated oral liquid 90mg/5mL is available Flynn hard capsule contents will disperse Monitor plasma levels and adhere to a consistent protocol Jejunal absorption is poor
Phytomenadione	No		Yes	Yes (Konakion MM®)	The injection is incompatible with certain types of siliconized syringes. Braun syringes are known to be compatible
Piroxicam	No			No	Add dispersible tablet (Feldene Melt®) to 50mL water, no information on suitability by EFT

continued

Table 2 Continued

Drug	*Authorized soluble tablet or oral liquid available*	*Tablet/capsule contents may disperse sufficiently for 8Fr NG tube[a,b]*	*Oral liquid can be prepared by local pharmacy or special order*	*Injection available and can be diluted and administered PO or by EFT*	*Comments*
Pilocarpine	No		Yes	No	Eyedrops 4% can be used orally (see p.618)
Potassium supplements[a]	Yes	Yes (effervescent)			Flush EFT well to prevent physical interaction with feed. Add effervescent tablets to 50mL water. Oral liquid contains sorbitol 2g/5mL and may cause diarrhoea, dilute with 50–100mL water, not recommended for intrajejunal administration
Prednisolone[a]	Yes	No	Yes[d]		
Pregabalin	Yes	Yes (Lyrica® capsules)	Yes	No	
Prochlorperazine	Yes	Yes (APS, Meridian)			Dilute oral liquid with an equal volume of water for EFT use. Use effervescent granules or disperse tablets for intrajejunal administration. Stemetil® tablets disperse but no information on use by EFT
Promethazine	Yes	Yes (Phenergan®)	Yes		Dilute oral liquid with an equal volume of water for EFT use
Propantheline	No		Yes	No	
Quetiapine[a]	No		Yes[e]	No	Unauthorized oral suspensions (various strengths) can be obtained via special order
Ranitidine	Yes	Yes (effervescent)	Yes[d,e]	Yes	Add effervescent tablets to 30mL water, consider sodium content. Authorized oral liquid contains alcohol (0.04units/5mL) and sorbitol An unauthorized 5mg/5mL oral solution (alcohol free) can be obtained via special order

continued

Table 2 Continued

Drug	*Authorized soluble tablet or oral liquid available*	*Tablet/capsule contents may disperse sufficiently for 8Fr NG tube*[a,b]	*Oral liquid can be prepared by local pharmacy or special order*	*Injection available and can be diluted and administered PO or by EFT*	*Comments*
Rifampicin	Yes		Yes[f]		Stop feed for 2h before and 30min after dose. Dilute authorized oral liquid with equal volume of water. Do not open capsules; risk of contact sensitization. A 125mg/5mL suspension can be prepared (7 day shelf-life)[f]
Risperidone	Yes	Yes (Risperdal®)	Yes	No	No information on suitability of orodispersible tablets (Quicklet®) via EFT
Senna	Yes		Yes[d]	No	Granules not suitable for administration by EFT
Sertraline	No	Yes (Lustral®)	Yes[e]	No	Coarse tablet dispersion may block tube, consider alternative drug Note crushed tablets have a local anaesthetic effect Unauthorized 50mg/5mL and 100mg/5mL oral suspension can be obtained via special order
Sodium clodronate	No	Yes (Bonefos®)		No	Stop feed for 1h before and after dose. Both capsule contents and tablets disperse in water
Sodium fusidate	Yes				Sodium fusidate tablets 500mg = 750mg oral suspension. Oral liquid contains sorbitol
Sodium valproate[a]	Yes	Yes (Epilim® Crushable)	Yes	No	Dilute oral liquid with an equal volume of water for EFT use. Some formulations contain sorbitol. Consider dispersing crushable tablets for intrajejunal administration or dilute oral liquid 3–4 times
Spironolactone	No	Yes (Most generics, Aldactone®)	Yes[d, e, f]	No	Unauthorized oral formulations can be obtained via special order; dilute with an equal volume of water for EFT use. Disperse tablet for intrajejunal administration. A 125mg/5mL suspension can be prepared[f]. Other suspension formulae are also available[37]

continued

Table 2 Continued

Drug	*Authorized soluble tablet or oral liquid available*	*Tablet/capsule contents may disperse sufficiently for 8Fr NG tube*[a,b]	*Oral liquid can be prepared by local pharmacy or special order*	*Injection available and can be diluted and administered PO or by EFT*	*Comments*
Sucralfate	Yes		Yes	No	Do not use sucralfate via EFT. Oral liquid *not* recommended due to high viscosity, bezoar formation and binding with feed; likely to block tube. Need to stop feed for 1h before and after dose; impractical for q4h schedule
Tapentadol[a]	Yes			No	
Temazepam	Yes		Yes	No	Oral liquid contains sorbitol
Tetracycline	No		Yes[f]	No	A 125mg/5mL suspension can be prepared (7day shelf-life).[f] Significant interaction with enteral feed makes four times a day dosing difficult by EFT
Theophylline[a]	No		Yes	No	Convert total daily dose of m/r preparations to oral *unauthorized* liquid and split into t.d.s. regimen. Stop feed for 1h before and 1h after dose. Dilute oral liquid with an equal volume of water. Monitor plasma levels closely The m/r granules of Slo-phyllin® capsules can be administered via EFT, although may block smaller tubes. Take care not to crush There is some information on giving aminophylline injection orally[1]
Tizanidine	No	Yes (Zanaflex®)	Yes[e]	No	Unauthorized 2mg/5mL oral solution and suspension can be obtained via special order
Tolbutamide	No	No	Yes[d]	No	

continued

Table 2 Continued

Drug	*Authorized soluble tablet or oral liquid available*	*Tablet/capsule contents may disperse sufficiently for 8Fr NG tube*[a,b]	*Oral liquid can be prepared by local pharmacy or special order*	*Injection available and can be diluted and administered PO or by EFT*	*Comments*
Topiramate	No	Yes (Topamax® tablets)	Yes[e]	No	Do not use Topamax® Sprinkle capsules by EFT as the beads stick to the tube causing blockage Unauthorized oral suspensions (various strengths) can be obtained via special order
Tramadol[a]	Yes	Yes (Ranbaxy capsules, Zydol® soluble, Zamadol Melt®)	Yes[f]		Use authorized dispersible tablets. Oral drops 100mg/mL available; further dilute with water. Zydol® capsule contents may disperse but no information on suitability by EFT A 25mg/5mL suspension can be prepared
Tranexamic acid	No	Yes (Cyklokapron®, Manx)	Yes[d,e]	Yes	Unauthorized 250mg/5mL and 500mg/5mL oral solution and suspension can be obtained via special order
Trazodone	Yes	Yes (Molipaxin 50mg capsules)	Yes	No	Dilute oral liquid with an equal volume of water
Trimethoprim	Yes		Yes[d]	No	Administer the dose during a break in feeding if practical. Dilute authorized oral liquid with an equal volume of water, some formulations contain sorbitol
Vancomycin	No	No	Yes	Yes	The reconstituted injection is authorized for oral and NG tube use (24h shelf-life time in fridge for enteral use); flavoring syrups may be added immediately prior to use
Venlafaxine[a]	No	Yes (Efexor®)	Yes[e]	No	Unauthorized 37.5mg/5mL or 75mg/5mL oral solution and suspension can be obtained via special order
Warfarin	Yes	Yes	Yes[d]	No	Stop feed for 1h before and 1–2h after dose. INR may be affected by the varying content of vitamin K in feeds

continued

Table 2 Continued

Drug	*Authorized soluble tablet or oral liquid available*	*Tablet/capsule contents may disperse sufficiently for 8Fr NG tube*[a,b]	*Oral liquid can be prepared by local pharmacy or special order*	*Injection available and can be diluted and administered PO or by EFT*	*Comments*
Zinc sulfate	No	Yes (effervescent)			Add effervescent tablet to 10mL water. Jejunal administration may reduce bio-availability
Zopiclone	No	No	Yes[e]	No	Unauthorized 3.75mg/5mL and 7.5mg/5mL oral solution and suspension can be obtained via special order

a. do not use m/r or e/c preparations unless specifically indicated. Take care if converting from m/r to immediate-release preparations because dose, frequency and clinical effect may be different

b. use the brand or manufacturer if specified; different brands may not disperse sufficiently for 8Fr NG tube administration; dispersion time may take up to 5min and require agitation

c. a simple suspension using Diluent C suspending agent can be prepared by some local pharmacies with a 7 day shelf-life

d. a simple suspension using Keltrol (Diluent A) suspending agent can be prepared by some local pharmacies with a 7 day shelf-life

e. unauthorized product listed in part VIIIB of the NHS drug tariff, available from 'specials' manufacturers or imported (see Chapter 24, p.751)

f. a simple suspension using 1:1 mixture of Ora-Plus and Ora-Sweet as a vehicle can be prepared by some local pharmacies, 28 day shelf-life unless otherwise stated[37]

g. tubes which should *not* be used for administration of Zomorph® capsules include; Mallinkrodt enral 205-09-1, Bioser 1147221, Vygon 39110 and Vygon 2395.09. Tubes known to be successful in administering Zomorph® capsules include Pharma Plast LEVIN CH/FG 18, Vygon 391.16, Ventrol 15016IT 85753, Ventrol 82316 16A, Bioser 1147239 and Sherwood 90L100A.

1 White R and Bradnam V (2015) *Handbook of Drug Administration via Enteral Feeding Tubes 3e.* London: Pharmaceutical Press www.medicinescomplete.com
2 Williams NT (2008) Medication administration through enteral feeding tubes. *American Journal of Health-System Pharmacy.* **65**: 2347–2357.
3 BAPEN (British Association of Parenteral and Enteral Nutrition) (2004) Administering drugs via enteral feeding tubes. A practical guide. BAPEN. Available from: www.bapen.org.uk
4 Royal Pharmaceutical Society (2012) Keeping patients safe when they transfer between care providers - getting the medicines right. www.rpharms.com
5 Royal Pharmaceutical Society (2016) Prescribing specials. Guidance for the prescribers of specials. www.rpharms.com
6 NHS England (2015) Never Events List 2015/2016. www.england.nhs.uk
7 NPSA (National Patient Safety Agency) (2007) Promoting safer measurement and administration of liquid medicines via oral and other enteral routes. *Patient Safety Alert.* NPSA/2007/PSA/ www.nrls.npsa.nhs.uk
8 NPSA (National Patient Safety Agency) (2011) Reducing the harm caused by misplaced nasogastric feeding tubes in adults and infants *Patient Safety Alert and Supporting Information.* NPSA/2011/PSA2002. www.nrls.npsa.nhs.uk
9 UK Medicines Information (2013) What are the therapeutic options for patients unable to take solid oral dosage forms. 294.3. *Drugs Q&As.* www.evidence.nhs.uk
10 NPSA (National Patient Safety Agency) (2012) Harm from flushing of nasogastric tubes before confirmation of placement. *Rapid Response Report.* NPSA/2012/RRR www.nrls.npsa.nhs.uk
11 Jackson LD *et al.* (2008) Safe medication swallowing in dysphagia: a collaborative improvement project. *Healthcare Quarterly.* **11**: 110–116.
12 Wright D (2011) How to help if a patient can't swallow. *Pharmaceutical Journal.* **286**: 272–274.
13 Adams D (1994) Administration of drugs through a jejunostomy tube. *British Journal of Intensive Care.* **4**: 10–17.
14 Thomson F *et al.* (2000) Enteral and parenteral nutrition. *Hospital Pharmacist.* **7**: 155–164.
15 Gilbar P (1999) A guide to drug administration in palliative care. *Journal of Pain and Symptom Management.* **17**: 197–207.
16 Royal Pharmaceutical Society of Great Britain (2015) Professional guidance for the procurement and supply of pharmaceutical specials. www.rpharms.com
17 Royal Pharmaceutical Society (2011) Pharmaceutical issues when crushing, opening or splitting oral dosage forms. www.rpharms.com
18 Schier JG *et al.* (2003) Fatality from administration of labetalol and crushed extended-release nifedipine. *Annals of Pharmacotherapy.* **37**: 1420–1423.
19 Cornish P (2005) "Avoid the crush": hazards of medication administration in patients with dysphagia or a feeding tube. *Canadian Medical Association Journal.* **172**: 871–872.
20 Wright DN *et al.* (2006) Consensus guideline on the medication management of adults with swallowing difficulties. *Guidelines London Connect Medical.*
21 Sanofi Aventis (2008) *Medical information. Data on file.*
22 NHS England (2013) Placement devicesd for nasogastric tube insertion DO NOT replace initial position checks. *Patient Safety Alert.* NHS/PSA/W/2013/. www.england.nhs.uk/patientsafety
23 National Patient Safety Agency (2012) Harm from flushing of nasogastric tubes before confirmation of placement. *Rapid Response Report.* NPSA/2012/RRR2001: www.nrls.npsa.nhs.uk
24 McFarland A (2017) A cost utility analysis of the clinical algorithm for nasogastric tube placement confirmation in adult hospital patients. *Journal of Advanced Nursing.* **73**: 201–216.
25 Phillips NM and Nay R (2008) A systematic review of nursing administration of medication via enteral tubes in adults. *Journal of Clinical Nursing.* **17**: 2257–2265.
26 Baxter K and Preston CL Stockley's Drug Interactions London: Pharmaceutical Press, www.medicinescomplete.com (accessed March 2016).
27 Schmidt LE and Dalhoff K (2002) Food-drug interactions. *Drugs.* **62**: 1481–1502.
28 Engle KK and Hannawa TE (1999) Techniques for administering oral medications to critical care patients receiving continuous enteral nutrition. *American Journal of Health System Pharmacy* **56**: 1441–1444.
29 Clark-Schmidt AL *et al.* (1990) Loss of carbamazepine suspension through nasogastric feeding tubes. *American Journal of Hospital Pharmacy.* **47**: 2034–2037.
30 Freeman KL and Trezevant MS (2009) Interaction between liquid protein solution and omeprazole suspension. *American Journal of Health System Pharmacy.* **66**: 1901–1902.
31 Garcia-Luna PP *et al.* (1997) Esophageal obstruction by solidification of the enteral feed: a complication to be prevented. *Intensive Care Medicine.* **23**: 790–792.
32 Chugai Pharma UK (2013) Antepsin 1g/5mL oral suspension. *SPC.* www.medicines.org.uk
33 Wohlt PD *et al.* (2009) Recommendations for the use of medications with continuous enteral nutrition. *American Journal of Health System Pharmacy.* **66**: 1458–1467.
34 Marcuard SP and Stegall KS (1990) Unclogging feeding tubes with pancreatic enzyme. *Journal of Parenteral Enteral Nutrition.* **14**: 198–200.
35 Nottingham City Hospital NHS Trust Pharmacy (1998) Administering drugs to patients by artifical enteral methods. Data on file.
36 Palliativedrugs.com (2003) July Newsletter. Available from: www.palliativedrugs.com
37 Smyth J (2010) *The NEWT guidelines for administration of medication to patients with enteral feeding tubes or swallowing difficulties* (2e). Pharmacy Department, North East Wales NHS Trust.
38 BNF for Children (2010-2011). Available from: www.bnfc.org
39 UK Medicines Information (2016) Which injections can be given enterally? *Medicines Q&A* www.evidence.nhs.uk

Updated April 2017

29: CONTINUOUS SUBCUTANEOUS DRUG INFUSIONS

29

CSCI IN CLINICAL PRACTICE

The administration of drugs by continuous subcutaneous infusion (CSCI) is common in palliative care in the UK, particularly in patients for whom swallowing medication has become increasingly difficult or impossible.[1–3]

Ambulatory battery-powered infusion devices are generally used to administer the CSCI.[2] CSCI is as effective as continuous IV infusion (CIVI),[4] and at least as good as intermittent bolus injections.[5] In settings where it is difficult to be certain that intermittent regular injections will be administered on time, CSCI is likely to provide better round-the-clock comfort.

Indications for CSCI

CSCI is *not* 'Step 4' on the analgesic ladder; it is a useful alternative route of administration in various circumstances,[6] including:

- persistent nausea and vomiting
- dysphagia
- bowel obstruction
- coma
- poor absorption of oral drugs (rare)
- patient preference.

Before setting up a CSCI, it is important to explain to the patient and family:

- the reason(s) for using this route
- how the infusion device works
- the advantages and possible disadvantages of CSCI (Box A).

Drugs used by CSCI

For most drugs, this route of administration is off-label (see p.xix).[7] However, there is extensive documented clinical experience of CSCI with many drugs used in palliative care.[3,8] In addition, there are reports of other drugs given less frequently by this route, e.g. **diclofenac** (p.332), **furosemide** (p.61), **levetiracetam** (p.287), **ranitidine** (p.29), **valproate** (p.282).

For CSCI, the injectable formulation must be of a suitable concentration to deliver the required dose in a relatively small volume and also be relatively non-irritant (see p.825).

Although often administered by CSCI, several drugs with a long duration of action, e.g. **dexamethasone, levomepromazine** can be given as a bolus SC or IV injection once daily or b.d. (Table 1).[1]

Bolus SC injections should be given via a separate SC butterfly needle/cannula and *not* via a side-arm or port of a CSCI cannula or infusion line. This avoids potential problems with drug incompatibility or loss of symptom control caused by the flush replacing the CSCI contents of the infusion tubing.

Box A Advantages and disadvantages of CSCI

Advantages
Saving nurses' time.
Round-the-clock comfort because plasma drug concentrations are maintained without peaks and troughs.
Less need for repeated injections.
Generally needs to be loaded once daily.
Control of multiple symptoms with a combination of drugs.
Independence and mobility maintained because the infusion device is lightweight and can be worn in a holster.
Patient preference.

Disadvantages
Initial cost of infusion devices.
Training of staff, together with need to maintain competency.
Lack of flexibility if more than one drug is being administered.
Lack of reliable compatibility data for some mixtures.
Possible inflammation and pain at the infusion site.
Although uncommon, problems with the infusion device can lead to break-through pain (or other symptom) if the problem is not resolved quickly.

Table 1 Drugs which can be given once daily or b.d. instead of by CSCI

Drug	*Plasma halflife (h)*	*Duration of action (h)*
Clonazepam[a] (not UK)	20–60	≤12–24
Dexamethasone	3–4.5	36–54
Furosemide	0.5–2	6–8
Granisetron	10–11	≤24
Haloperidol	13–35	≤24
Levomepromazine[b]	15–30	≤24
Methadone[b]	8–75	≤12

a. for SC/IV bolus doses, dilute each 1mg/mL amp with 1mL WFI
b. relatively irritant SC.

PRESCRIBING CSCI

CSCI must be prescribed in the relevant section of the patient's drug chart. Some specialist units have separate CSCI drug charts (examples are available in the Document library of www.palliativedrugs.com); these must be linked or referred to in the patient's main drug chart. The prescription should specify:

- the dose of each drug to be administered over the infusion period (generally 24h)
- the diluent
- the final volume of the infusion.

Compatibility of the drug(s) and the diluent should be confirmed before the CSCI is set up (see Mixing drugs); if it is not a routine combination, ideally, this should be documented in the patient's notes (see p.xix).

If symptoms are controlled, start the CSCI 2–4h before the next dose of PO opioid would have been given. If symptoms are uncontrolled, set up the CSCI immediately with stat doses of the same drugs.

Rescue medication

Appropriate doses of p.r.n. medication must also be prescribed. These are given via a separate SC needle/ cannula (left *in situ* for this purpose) and flushed with compatible diluent (see below). The side-arm or port of the CSCI infusion line must *not* be used because of potential problems with drug incompatibility or loss of symptom control caused by the flush replacing the CSCI contents of the infusion tubing.

Converting from PO to CSCI

Drugs are generally *more* bio-available by injection than PO. This means that the dose of a drug given by CSCI will be *less* than the dose previously given PO, generally between 1/3 and 2/3 of the PO dose. The bio-availability data given at the end of the pharmacology section in the individual drug monographs serve as a guide to the appropriate reduction.

Thus, the dose of a drug with oral bio-availability of 75% should be reduced by a quarter when given SC, halved if 50% bio-available, and so on. Particular care should be taken with strong opioids (see Appendix 2, Table 3, p.861).

Converting from CSCI to PO

Some patients are able to revert from CSCI to PO medication, e.g. those being treated for nausea and vomiting. When this seems possible, convert the drugs sequentially rather than all at once. For example, convert the anti-emetic medication first and, if the nausea and vomiting do not recur, change the other medication 1–2 days later.

Remember: just as drug doses were reduced when starting CSCI, doses will generally need to be increased when reverting to PO. This is particularly the case with strong opioid analgesics, e.g. **morphine** 15mg/24h CSCI will need to be increased to **morphine** 30mg/24h PO.

The CSCI is generally discontinued when the first dose of the PO medication is administered. It is important to review p.r.n. medication, and to adjust it appropriately.

Converting from TD patches to CSCI (or vice versa)

The TD and CSCI routes are considered equipotent in terms of total daily dose, see Appendix 2, p.855.

As a general rule, TD **buprenorphine** or **fentanyl** patches should be continued when the need for supplemental opioid via CSCI is short-term, e.g. in the last days of life. It is simpler to supplement the patch with a CSCI of **morphine** or other opioid than to convert completely to a single alternative opioid. See the respective QCGs for **buprenorphine** or **fentanyl** for more information, including the conversion of a CSCI opioid to a TD patch (p.407 and p.417).

DILUENT

PCF recommends that generally WFI is used as the standard diluent of choice. However, 0.9% saline should be considered if there is a potential or actual problem with inflammatory reactions at the skin injection site (see p.825).

The main purpose of diluents is to help reduce site irritation and enable drug delivery over a prescribed time. It is essential that the diluent is compatible with the drug(s) in the syringe. The SPC may indicate compatible diluents, particularly if a drug is authorized for CSCI. However, the information may not be comprehensive, and is unlikely to cover compatibility when drugs are mixed. Generally, either WFI or 0.9% saline can be used. They both have advantages and disadvantages (Table 2).

Table 2 Comparison of diluents

WFI	*0.9% saline*[9]
Advantages	**Advantages**
Less chance of incompatibility	Isotonic. Preferable for diluting irritant drugs (potentially less infusion site-reaction)
Generally more compatibility data available for commonly used drugs	
Disadvantages	**Disadvantages**
Large volumes are hypotonic, which may cause infusion site pain or skin reaction (generally not a problem in practice because infusion rates are so slow)	Incompatible with some drugs, e.g. cyclizine; higher concentrations of diamorphine >40mg/mL or haloperidol >1mg/mL
	Generally less compatibility data available for commonly used drugs

In the UK, WFI is widely used as the first-line diluent because it can be used to dilute all commonly used drugs in palliative care, including **cyclizine *lactate*** (see p.249) and higher concentrations of **diamorphine *hydrochloride*** (>40mg/mL) or **haloperidol** (>1mg/mL). There is also a wealth of supporting compatibility data and clinical experience for WFI (see Appendix 3, p.863).

For some drugs, e.g. **granisetron**, **hydromorphone**, **ketamine**, **ketorolac**, **octreotide** and **ondansetron**, more compatibility data exists with 0.9% saline and some prefer to use this as the diluent. Further, 0.9% saline would be a reasonable first-line diluent in those countries where **cyclizine *lactate*** or **diamorphine** are unavailable or not used.

Some centres in the USA use 5% glucose in water as the first-line diluent. However, this is acidic and unsuitable for very alkaline drugs, e.g. **dexamethasone**, **furosemide**, **ketorolac**, and **phenobarbital**.

To avoid confusion, consistency of practice within individual units is important.[10]

INFUSION VOLUME

Factors influencing the final volume of the CSCI include the total volume of the drugs, the infusion device being used, the maximum rate of delivery, the intended infusion time and local guidelines. Greater dilution reduces:

- the risk of incompatibility
- the impact of priming a line (less drug in the 'dead space')
- injection site skin reactions from the drug.

For these reasons, 20mL syringes are now generally recommended as the minimum standard size to be used.

In deciding how much diluent to use, one approach, applicable to CME McKinley T34 syringe pumps, is to dilute the contents to a standard volume, e.g.:

- for a total drug volume <10mL, dilute to 15mL in a 20mL luerlock syringe
- for a total drug volume >10mL, dilute to 20mL in a 30mL luerlock syringe.

Additional dilution may be necessary when mixing drugs where compatibility depends on the final drug concentrations e.g. **cyclizine**, **dexamethasone**, **haloperidol**, **ketorolac** (see Drug compatibility, p.822, and footnotes of Charts 1–7, p.866–p.879).

In some situations, the total volume of drugs may exceed the maximum volume/24h that an infusion device can deliver, i.e. about 22mL or 34mL in a 30mL or 50mL syringe respectively for a CME McKinley T34 syringe pump. This is most likely with combinations which include higher doses of **fentanyl**, **metoclopramide**, **midazolam**, **morphine** or **oxycodone**. This problem can generally be circumvented by:

- using a more concentrated formulation (see below)

- switching from **morphine** → **diamorphine** or **hydromorphone**; **fentanyl** → **alfentanil**
- changing the contents of the syringe driver more frequently, e.g. every 12h
- using a different infusion device with a larger capacity.[11]

When a cartridge/cassette/bag infusion system is used, a larger final volume is possible. Even so, some centres standardize to 50mL volume with a maximum rate of 2mL/h.

Caution is required when using a more concentrated formulation, e.g. **fentanyl** 5mg/mL, **oxycodone** 50mg/mL, **midazolam** 5mg/mL, because compatibility can differ from the normal strength formulation (Box B). Further, confusion between the normal and the more concentrated formulations has resulted in overdoses. Consequently, some organizations restrict their availability.[12]

INFUSION DURATION

In the UK, CSCI syringes are generally timed to empty over 24h.[3] The main reasons for this are:

- extrapolation of sterility guidelines from CIVI
- availability of stability and compatibility data
- standardization of practice (for safety reasons)
- tradition based on the limitations of older syringe drivers.

Generally, 24h is satisfactory in terms of both sterility, stability and practicality.[13,14]

For certain infusion devices, e.g. CADD pumps, elastomeric devices, stability and compatibility data may exist for a longer duration of infusion, e.g. 48–72h. Generally, these solutions are made up in aseptically controlled environments, e.g. pharmacy aseptic units to ensure sterility.

Infusion stability

Drug stability and compatibility are closely related. Stability describes how much of the drug remains in its original form in a given period of time. Compatibility describes whether the addition of a diluent or a drug causes a physical or chemical interaction. Various factors affect the stability of the drug in the CSCI and potentially could lead to incompatibility and impaired symptom control (Box B).

Box B Factors affecting CSCI drug stability or compatibility[15–18]

Diluent (see p.819).

Final concentration of drug

The *concentration* of the drug in the solution (the *quantity* of the drug divided by the *total final volume*) should be checked against stability and compatibility data (see p.863).

Order of mixing

Particularly when compatibility is concentration dependent, e.g. dexamethasone and ranitidine should always be the last drug added to an already diluted and mixed syringe to reduce the risk of incompatibility.

Brand/formulation/strength of the drug

Injections contain various excipients, e.g. preservatives, diluents, stabilizing compounds, which can differ between brands, countries, and even between different strengths of the same drug, e.g. oxycodone (see p.866).

Duration of infusion

Note. The rate at which drugs degrade can be increased by:

Higher temperature: do not wear the infusion device under clothes

Exposure to light: e.g. levomepromazine turns pink/yellow; cover the infusion.

Adsorption onto delivery system material

E.g. ≤50% of a dose of clonazepam onto PVC tubing

MIXING DRUGS

The combination of two or more authorized (licensed) drugs results in a new unauthorized (unlicensed) product being formed. Doctors and other independent prescribers (nurse, pharmacist) can mix, and direct others to mix, drugs (including controlled drugs) for administration to a particular patient. Supplementary prescribers can mix and direct others to mix when part of a Clinical Management Plan (also see p.xxi).[19]

In the UK, it is common practice to administer 2–3 different drugs in the same infusion device.[1,2,20] Some centres mix four or more drugs. However, the greater the number of drugs mixed, the greater the probability of compatibility problems. Accordingly, *PCF* recommends that generally no more than three drugs should be mixed in one syringe.

Drug compatibility

When mixing drugs it is essential to consider drug compatibility (Box C). Physical and/or chemical changes can occur which could lead to reduced efficacy.[21]

Box C Drug compatibility data

Physical compatibility

If mixing two or more drugs does not result in a physical change, e.g. discolouration, clouding or crystallization, they are said to be physically compatible.

Observational data

Data from many palliative care services about the visual appearance of various drug mixtures over the infusion period (generally 24h) have been collated for use in Appendix 3. However, observational data are subjective and imprecise; generally, only major incompatibilities can be identified in this way.

Laboratory data

These are generally derived from microscopic examination of a drug mixture under polarized light at specified concentrations and several time points when kept under controlled conditions. Although more robust, these are not definitive; a solution may remain physically clear even when there is chemical incompatibility.[22]

Chemical compatibility

If mixing two or more drugs does not result in a chemical change leading to loss or degradation of one or more of the drugs, the mixture is said to be chemically compatible. Chemical compatibility data are generally obtained by analyzing the drug mixture by high-performance liquid chromatography (HPLC) at specified concentrations and several time points when kept under controlled conditions.

Occasionally, a drug combination has been shown to be chemically compatible but physically incompatible.

Ideally both physical and chemical compatibility data should be known. However, because of the infinite number of possible drug combinations, and a dearth of published chemical compatibility studies, generally, decisions are taken on the basis of physical compatibility, based on observational data and clinical experience.

Information sources

Information on CSCI compatibility can be obtained from several sources:

- *for infusions with WFI as a diluent:* charts 1–7 (see Appendix 3, p.863) summarize the compatibility data for the more commonly used 2- and 3-drug combinations. They have been compiled from clinical observations in palliative care services in the UK, New Zealand and Australia, and from published compatibility data

- *for infusions with 0.9% saline as a diluent:* charts 8–14 (see Appendix 3, p.863) summarize the compatibility data for the more commonly used 2- and 3-drug combinations. They have been compiled from clinical observations in palliative care services in the UK, New Zealand and Australia, and from published compatibility data. They are available in the extended appendix section of the on-line *PCF* on www.palliativedrugs.com
- *Syringe Driver Survey Database* (SDSD) on www.palliativedrugs.com. This is a continually updated resource and contains observational compatibility data on mixing combinations of drugs reported by health professionals. For this to be of maximum benefit, members are urged to donate information about both *successful* and *unsuccessful* combinations for which there are no previously published data
- *The Syringe Driver: Continuous Subcutaneous Infusions in Palliative Care*[20]
- www.pallcare.info
- *Handbook on Injectable Drugs.*[15]

Generally, these sources can only indicate if a drug combination is likely to be stable and compatible. Many factors affect drug compatibility and/or stability (see Box B) which helps explain conflicting reports. If there is doubt about the relevance of the compatibility data to the situation in which a given drug combination is to be used, advice should be obtained from a clinical pharmacist. Regular checks of the CSCI together with the patient's condition should always be undertaken (see p.826).

General principles for compatibility

When there is a lack of robust compatibility data for the prescribed drugs, the following general principles should be noted:

- generally, drugs with a similar pH are more likely to be compatible than those with widely differing ones (Table 3)
- most drugs are acidic in solution, however, **dexamethasone, diclofenac, furosemide**, **ketorolac**, **omeprazole** and **phenobarbital** are alkaline in solution and often cause compatibility problems (Table 3); as a result **diclofenac, furosemide**, **omeprazole** and **phenobarbital** should be administered separately and not be mixed with other drugs
- dilute to the maximum volume possible
- compatibility with **cyclizine** or **haloperidol** is often concentration dependent and they are more likely to cause problems at higher concentrations
- the risk of precipitation with **dexamethasone** is reduced if it is added last to an already dilute drug mixture. On the other hand, as already noted, **dexamethasone** has a long duration of action. Thus, except when it is being given to reduce the risk of skin reactions (see p.825), there is no real need to give it by CSCI (Table 1)
- the risk of precipitation of some combinations of **ranitidine** can be reduced by adding it last to an already dilute drug mixture (see p.29)
- occasionally, initial cloudiness or separation (precipitation) may occur which resolves on full mixing; however, ensure it fully resolves and monitor the infusion closely (Note. Delayed cloudiness can be caused by chemicals from the syringe or tubing leaching out)
- protect from direct sunlight (particularly **levomepromazine**) and heat
- the more drugs combined, the greater the risk of incompatibility; generally, *PCF* recommends a maximum of three drugs in one syringe
- checks in use should be undertaken more regularly (see p.826) monitoring both the infusion and expected clinical outcome. Where incompatibilities are found e.g. crystal formation, details should be submitted to the SDSD, to help build a database of evidence for drug combinations.

Table 3 Approximate pH values of parenteral drug formulations[15,23]

Drug[a]	*pH*	*Drug*[a]	*pH*
Alfentanil	4–6	Ketamine	3.5–5.5
Buprenorphine	4–6	Ketorolac	6.9–7.9
Clonazepam	3.6	Levetiracetam	5–7
Clonidine	4–4.5	Levomepromazine	4.5
Cyclizine lactate	3.3–3.7	Lidocaine	5–7
Dexamethasone *sodium phosphate*	7–10.5	Methadone	3–6.5
Diamorphine[b]		Metoclopramide	4.5–6.5
Diclofenac	7.8–9	Midazolam	3
Fentanyl	4–7.5	Morphine *sulfate*	2.5–6.5
Furosemide	8–9.3	Octreotide	3.9–4.5
Glycopyrronium	2–3	Omeprazole	8.8–10.3
Granisetron	4.7–7.3	Ondansetron	3.3–4
Haloperidol	3–3.8	Oxycodone	4.5–5.5
Hydromorphone	4–5.5	Phenobarbital	9.2–10.2
Hyoscine *butylbromide*	3.7–5.5	Ranitidine	6.7–7.3
Hyoscine *hydrobromide*	5–7		

a. pH values may vary between each strength and different brands

b. powder for reconstitution; most stable when reconstituted so that the pH is 3.8–4.5.

SITE OF CSCI

See Box D. Plastic/teflon cannulae are preferred to metal cannulae because they reduce the risk of site reactions and needle stick injury.[24–26] A 20mm 21-gauge cannula is used for a patient of average build, but a smaller 25-gauge is more appropriate for smaller or emaciated patients.[27] Insert at an angle of approximately 45° and ensure placement into SC tissue.

Where possible use fine bore tubing with a small priming volume (preferably less than 0.3mL) and secure the tubing to the skin with a transparent semipermeable adhesive dressing (e.g. Tegaderm®), with a loop to reduce the likelihood of needle/cannula displacement.

An infusion site may be satisfactory for ≥1 week (and occasionally 2–3 weeks).[25,28] However, generally, prophylactic site rotation is advised, e.g. every 3–5 days, with the exact duration varying between centres.

Box D Siting a CSCI[8]

Preferred sites
Anterior chest wall[a]
Anterolateral aspects of upper arms[b]
Supra- or interscapular area[c]

Alternative sites
Anterior abdominal wall
Anterior surface of the thighs

Areas to avoid
Oedematous areas
Skin folds
Breast
Broken, inflamed or infected skin
Recently irradiated skin sites
Cutaneous tumour sites
Bony prominences
Near a joint
Scarring

a. ideally avoid in cachectic patients

b. ideally avoid in ambulatory patients or bedbound patients who need turning

c. useful when risk of inadvertent removal, e.g. patient with terminal agitation.

Infusion site problems

These occur in ≤25% of patients (Box E).[1,25] The risk of local irritation is increased when injectable formulations have an osmolality of >600mOsmol/kg, a pH <4 or >11, or contain excipients which may themselves be irritant, e.g. ethanol, glycerin. propylene glycol.[8,29]

Apart from discomfort, local inflammation may impair drug absorption and thereby symptom control.

Box E Causes of infusion site problems[20,30,31]

Anatomical site
Local bruising (caused by needle/cannula)
Irritant drug(s)
Tonicity/osmolality of the solution
pH of the solution
Incompatible drug–diluent mixture
Allergy to nickel needle
Glass particles from ampoules
Sterile abscess
Infection
Infrequent resiting

Site reactions can be reduced by:

- using a less irritant parenteral drug formulation, e.g. **haloperidol** instead of **prochlorperazine** (Box F)
- considering the use of 0.9% saline as a diluent, when compatibility data exists (see p.819)
- diluting the solution as much as practical, this may include changing the syringe q12h instead of q24h to permit further dilution
- using a plastic cannula instead of a butterfly needle (always use in patients with a known metal allergy)
- changing the site prophylactically every 2–3 days; particularly if using irritant drugs
- applying **hydrocortisone** 1% cream to the skin around the needle entry site, and covering it with an occlusive dressing
- adding **dexamethasone** 1mg to the solution if compatibility data permits.[28]

Although the routine addition of **dexamethasone** has been recommended on the grounds that it extends the life of an infusion site by about 50%, the fact that some sites have lasted 2–3 weeks without **dexamethasone** means that routine use cannot be recommended.[28]

Box F Parenteral drug formulations which are irritant CSCI

Strongly irritant, do *not* give by CSCI
Chlorpromazine
Diazepam
Prochlorperazine (sometimes given by SC bolus)

Relatively irritant by CSCI, precautions may be necessary[a]
Cyclizine
Diclofenac
Ketamine
Ketorolac
Levomepromazine
Methadone
Octreotide[b]
Ondansetron
Phenobarbital[c]
Promethazine[c]

a. see text and respective monographs
b. painful if given as SC bolus; this is reduced if warmed to body temperature before injection
c. strongly irritant with risk of tissue necrosis if given by SC bolus injection.

INFUSION DEVICES

In the UK, ambulatory syringe drivers/pumps are the most commonly used devices for delivering drugs by CSCI. The use of cartridges/cassettes prepared by a pharmacist adds significantly to the cost.

The CME McKinley T34 is the most frequently used syringe driver.[32,33] The older Graseby MS16A and MS26 syringe drivers lacked the recommended safety features and were removed from use in the UK in December 2015.[34,35]

Setting up the infusion device

Full instructions can be found in the manufacturer's instruction manuals. See also the Quick Clinical Guide for setting up the CME McKinley T34 syringe pump. A Quick Clinical Guide for using the Graseby MS16A and MS26 syringe drivers is available on the www.palliativedrugs.com Document library, for use by health professionals in countries where these are still used.

PCF recommends priming the infusion line before attaching it to the syringe pump. This uses approx. 0.3mL volume depending on the type of infusion line. This means that a small proportion of the dose drawn up for the patient will be lost in the 'dead space' when a new infusion is first set up. The final volume in the syringe should be noted and used to check the infusion rate (automatically calculated by some syringe drivers/pumps). Subsequent infusions given by the same line will not need priming, therefore the final volume and thus the infusion rate will be slightly different.

It is recommended that the syringe and infusion device is covered if using in direct sunlight to minimise the risk of stability problems, particularly for levomepromazine (see Box B), and/or pump malfunctions.[36] Note, the syringe and infusion device should also be protected from excessive heat, i.e. avoid covering with excessive layers of clothes/bedclothes.

Checks in use

Specific record charts should be used for checking a CSCI; examples are available in the Document library of www.palliativedrugs.com. These record charts should be used in addition to the prescription chart. Checks should be documented within 1h of setting up the CSCI, and then q4h:

- is the device still working?
- is the correct rate still infusing?
- amount of time and volume of solution left, and whether the infusion is running to time (based on the preceding 4h)
- appearance of the solution in the tubing and syringe/cartridge/bag
- condition of the skin site
- battery status.

Do not remove the syringe/cartridge/bag from the infusion device to perform these checks. If checking indicates a problem, action should be taken and then documented, e.g. if the infusion needs to be resited (and hence reprimed), the time, the new site and the new infusion volume/syringe length should be recorded. Other comments might include details of incompatibility and mention of any mishaps, e.g. the delivery device found disconnected.

Quick Clinical Guide: Setting up a CME McKinley T34 syringe pump for CSCI

For full instructions, see the manufacturer's operation manual.

PCF recommends 'Lock on' mode for general use; this automatically provides an infusion duration of 24h.

PCF does *not* recommend the use of the automatic purge. Although designed to reduce the slack in the pump mechanism and achieve the correct flow rate more quickly (about 20min vs. 2h), it is more complex to set up and the clinical relevance of the time difference is unknown. Further, patients should have access to p.r.n. medication for the relief of any symptoms.

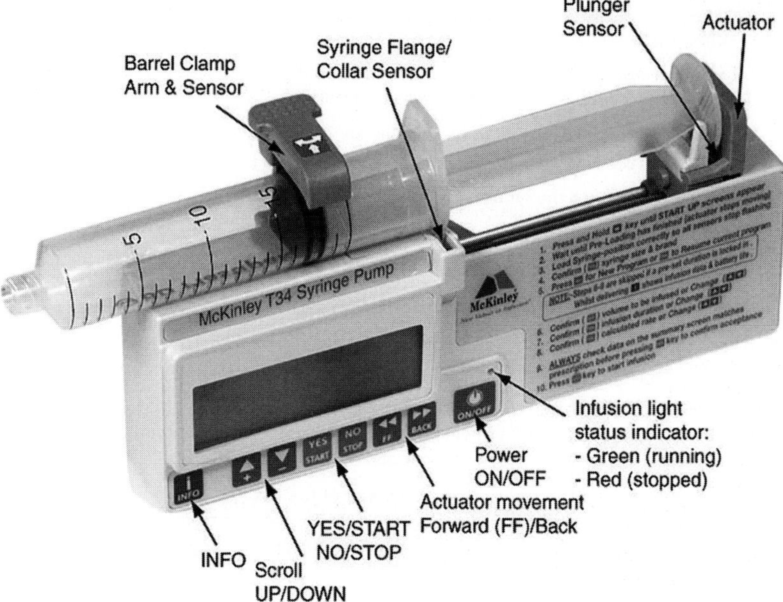

Figure The CME McKinley T34 syringe pump

Additional equipment

- battery, PP3: 9V Alkaline/Lithium + spare battery (each lasts about 3–4 days)
- 20mL or 30mL luerlock syringe
- 100cm McKinley SC infusion line with integrated anti-free flow and anti-siphon valve (0.3mL priming volume)
- lock-box and key
- transparent adhesive dressing.

1 A CSCI may take several hours to provide effective symptom control. SC bolus doses of the appropriate rescue medication should be available to relieve any symptoms.

2 Fill a luerlock syringe with the drugs and dilute the contents to a standard volume, e.g. 15mL in a 20mL syringe with WFI, or when the volume of the undiluted drugs is >10mL, to 20mL in a 30mL syringe. A larger final volume may also be required to ensure compatibility. For maximum fill volumes, see table below.

Syringe size	*Maximum fill volume*[a]
20mL syringe	17mL
30mL syringe	22mL
50mL syringe[b]	34mL

a. for a BD Plastipak luerlock syringe; volumes can vary between manufacturers
b. the lock-box does not accommodate a 50mL syringe.

Note. Dexamethasone should be the last drug added to an already dilute combination of drugs in order to reduce the risk of incompatibility.

3 The syringe should be made up immediately before use, using strict aseptic technique. Ensure adequate mixing has occurred; the solution should be clear and free from discoloration, crystals or precipitate.

4 Label the syringe, taking care not to completely obscure the solution. The label should be flat and unfolded to avoid obstructing the pump mechanism.

5 Attach the syringe to a McKinley infusion line and prime manually (this uses about 0.3mL) and note the remaining volume.

6 Insert the battery into the syringe driver.

7 Ensure the barrel clamp is down and the syringe is *not* connected.

8 Press and hold the **black** ON/OFF key until START UP screens appear.

9 Wait until pre-loading has finished (actuator stops moving).

10 Check the battery capacity by pressing the blue INFO key (use +/- keys to scroll to the battery status option) and the green YES key to view battery status.

At least 40% battery capacity is required for 24 hours. Change the battery if necessary, e.g. for community use. Switch off by holding down the **black** ON/OFF key until the screen goes blank, discard the battery, insert a new one and repeat steps 7–10.

11 The actuator will move automatically to the size of the last syringe used. If a different size syringe is required, use the FF/BACK keys to move the actuator to the correct position for syringe loading. Once the actuator has stopped moving, lift and rotate the barrel clamp arm, load the syringe (ensuring the plunger and syringe barrel are in the correct slots) and rotate and replace the barrel arm clamp.

12 The display screen will show if any of the 3 positioning points are not aligned correctly. If this is the case, remove the syringe and repeat step 11.

13 Ensure the pump has detected the correct syringe type and size, press the **green** YES key to confirm or use +/- keys to scroll and select the correct option.

14 A new programme *must* be set for each new syringe. If the pump gives the option of resuming a previous programme, it has been set up incorrectly. Do *not* take this option (press **red** NO key). Turn off the pump, remove the syringe and start again.

15 Check the correct infusion volume (as documented after priming) and duration (24 hours) is shown on the display. The rate is automatically calculated, but it is good practice to double check this by dividing the volume by the time. Press the **green** YES key if settings are correct.

16 Insert the cannula subcutaneously in the patient in a suitable position; secure and attach the syringe and infusion line to the cannula.

17 Press the **green** YES key to start the infusion.

The screen will continually show the time remaining for the infusion, the rate (mL/h) and the syringe selected.

18 Lock the keypad by pressing and holding the **blue** INFO key until the display shows Keypad LOCK ON.

19 Secure the pump in the lockbox provided.

20 Protect the syringe from excessive sunlight and heat, e.g. electric blankets.

21 Regular checks on the progress, the visual appearance of the infusion and administration site should be performed and documented during the infusion. Do not remove the syringe from the pump to perform these checks. If checking indicates a problem, action should be taken and then documented. An infusion progress summary can be obtained whilst infusing by pressing the **blue** INFO key.

22 If there is a problem, an alert (short audible alarm and a screen message, infusion continues) or an alarm (continuous alarm, infusion stops and a red light appears above the **black** ON/OFF key) will activate. Refer to the trouble-shooting guide and manufacturer's operation manual for implications and actions.

23 Do not add drugs to a syringe or infusion line once the infusion has been commenced. Additional bolus drugs needed should be administered by a separate cannula.

Temporarily stopping and disconnecting the infusion

The infusion may sometimes need to be temporarily stopped (e.g. to change the battery) or disconnected (e.g. when the patient bathes/showers):

- unlock the keypad by pressing and holding the **blue** INFO key until the display shows LOCK OFF
- press the **red** STOP key to stop the infusion
- press and hold the **black** ON/OFF key to switch the pump off; leave the syringe attached to the pump
- *when temporarily disconnecting the infusion*: disconnect the infusion line at the cannula end; cap off both the infusion line and the cannula
- store syringe and infusion line safely; lock in a CD cupboard if it contains a CD.

After interruption:

- check patient details and prescription are correct
- reconnect the infusion line to the cannula
- turn on the pump by pressing and holding the **black** ON/OFF key
- confirm the syringe size and brand
- press the **green** YES key to resume the infusion
- check and confirm the volume, duration and rate
- press the **green** YES key to start the infusion.

24 When the infusion is completed an alarm will sound and the infusion will stop. Unlock the keypad by pressing and holding the **blue** INFO key until the display shows keypad LOCK OFF. Press the **red** STOP key. Press and hold the **black** ON/OFF key to switch the pump off.

25 *If the next prescription is to be repeated exactly*, the same infusion line may be re-used as per local policy. Follow the guidance from step 1; at step 5 priming is not needed, remove the completed syringe from the pump, but leave it connected to the patient; at step 16, remove the old syringe from the infusion line and reconnect the infusion line to the new syringe; complete the remaining steps in the set up as before.

26 *If the next prescription is different (or changed mid-infusion)*, stop the infusion as in step 24, disconnect the infusion line from the patient *before* removing the syringe from the pump. Set up the next prescription from step 1 of the guidelines, using a new syringe and new infusion line.

1 Wilcock A *et al.* (2006) Drugs given by a syringe driver: a prospective multicentre survey of palliative care services in the UK. *Palliative Medicine*. **20**: 661–664.
2 O'Doherty CA *et al.* (2001) Drugs and syringe drivers: a survey of adult specialist palliative care practice in the United Kingdom and Eire. *Palliative Medicine*. **15**: 149–154.
3 Dickman A *et al.* (2017) Identification of drug combinations administered by continuous subcutaneous infusion that require analysis for compatibility and stability. *BMC Palliative Care*. **16**: 22.
4 Nelson KA *et al.* (1997) A prospective within-patient crossover study of continuous intravenous and subcutaneous morphine for chronic cancer pain. *Journal of Pain and Symptom Management*. **13**: 262–267.
5 Watanabe S *et al.* (2008) A randomized double-blind crossover comparison of continuous and intermittent subcutaneous administration of opioid for cancer pain. *Journal of Palliative Medicine*. **11**: 570–574.
6 Anderson SL and Shreve ST (2004) Continuous subcutaneous infusion of opiates at end-of-life. *Annals of Pharmacotherapy*. **38**: 1015–1023.
7 Fonzo-Christe C *et al.* (2005) Subcutaneous administration of drugs in the elderly: survey of practice and systematic literature review. *Palliative Medicine*. **19**: 208–219.
8 Duems-Noriega O and Arino-Blasco (2015) Subcutaneous fluid and drug delivery: safe, efficient and inexpensive. *Reviews in Clinical Gerontology*. **25**: 117–146.
9 Schneider J *et al.* (1997) A study of the osmolality and pH of subcutaneous drug infusion solutions. *Australian Journal of Hospital Pharmacy*. **27**: 29–31.
10 Flowers C and McLeod F (2005) Diluent choice for subcutaneous infusion: a survey of the literature and Australian practice. *International Journal of Palliative Nursing*. **11**: 54–60.
11 Fudin J *et al.* (2000) Use of continuous ambulatory infusions of concentrated subcutaneous (s.q.) hydromorphone versus intravenous (i.v.) morphine: cost implications for palliative care. *American Journal of Hospice and Palliative Care*. **17**: 347–353.
12 Department of Health (2015) Never events list for 2015/2016. www.gov.uk
13 British National Formulary Prescribing in palliative care and guidance on intravenous infusions. London: BMJ Group and Pharmaceutical Press. www.medicinescomplete.com (accessed March 2017).
14 NPSA (National Patient Safety Agency) (2007) Promoting safer use of injectable medicines. Patient safety alert. NPSA/2007/20. www.npsa.nhs.uk
15 Trissel LA. *Handbook on Injectable Drugs*. Maryland, USA: American Society of Health System Pharmacists (accessed March 2017).
16 Kohut J, 3rd *et al.* (1996) Don't ignore details of drug-compatibility reports. *American Journal of Health System Pharmacy*. **53**: 2339.
17 Vermeire A and Remon JP (1999) Stability and compatibility of morphine. *Int J Pharm*. **187**: 17–51.
18 Schneider JJ *et al.* (2006) Effect of tubing on loss of clonazepam administered by continuous subcutaneous infusion. *Journal of Pain and Symptom Management*. **31**: 563–567.
19 UK Government (2012) The Human Medicines Regulations . SI 2012/1916. London. www.legislation.gov.uk
20 Dickman A and Schneider J (2016) *The Syringe Driver: Continuous Subcutaneous Infusions in Palliative Care* (4e). Oxford University Press, Oxford.
21 Foinard A *et al.* (2012) Impact of physical incompatibility on drug mass flow rates: example of furosemide-midazolam incompatibility. *Annals of Intensive Care*. **2**: 28.
22 Good PD et *al.* (2004) The compatibility and stability of midazolam and dexamethasone in infusion solutions. *Journal of Pain and Symptom Management*. **27**: 471–475.
23 Gray A et *al. Injectable Drugs Guide*. London: Pharmaceutical Press. www.medicinescomplete.com (accessed November 2013).
24 Dawkins L et *al.* (2000) A randomized trial of winged Vialon cannulae and metal butterfly needles. *International Journal of Palliative Nursing*. **6**: 110–116.
25 Mitchell K et *al.* (2012) Incidence and causes for syringe driver site reactions in palliative care: A prospective hospice-based study. *Palliative Medicine*. **26**: 979–985.
26 Ross JR *et al.* (2002) A prospective, within-patient comparison between metal butterfly needles and Teflon cannulae in subcutaneous infusion of drugs to terminally ill hospice patients. *Palliative Medicine*. **16**: 13–16.
27 Khan M and Younger G (2007) Promoting safe administration of subcutaneous infusions. *Nursing Standard*. **21**: 50–58.
28 Reymond L *et al.* (2003) The effect of dexamethasone on the longevity of syringe driver subcutaneous sites in palliative care patients. *Medical Journal of Australia*. **178**: 486–489.
29 Wang W (2015) Tolerability of hypertonic injectables. *International Journal of Pharmaceutics*. **490**: 308–315.
30 Oliver D (1991) The tonicity of solutions used in continuous subcutaneous infusions. The cause of skin reactions? *Hospital Pharmacy Practice*. **Sept**: 158–164.
31 Graham F (2006) Syringe drivers and subcutaneous sites: a review. *European Journal of Palliative Care*. **13**: 138–141.
32 Palliativedrugs.com (2014) Which syringe driver do you use? *Latest additions (March)*. www.palliativedrugs.com
33 Freemantle A *et al.* (2011) Safer ambulatory syringe drivers: experiences of one acute hospital trust. *International Journal of Palliative Nursing*. **17**: 86–91.
34 NHS England (2013) Safer use of syringe drivers. Quality Care Commission. www.cgq.org.uk
35 NPSA (National Patient Safety Agency) (2010) Safer ambulatory syringe drivers. In: Rapid Reponse Report RRR019. www.npsa.nhs.uk
36 Field Safety Notice (2016) CME Medical: CME ambulatory syringe pumps - T34, T60 and TPCA. FSN2016-004. www.gov.uk

Updated April 2017

30: TRANSDERMAL PATCHES

Transdermal (TD) patches can be used to administer highly lipid-soluble drugs. Conventional TD patches come in one of two formulations:

- *reservoir:* drug in a reservoir with a rate-limiting membrane to control release
- *matrix:* drug embedded in an adhesive matrix with the release rate determined by the physical properties of the matrix.

The high concentration of drug in the patch relative to the skin provides a concentration gradient which maintains the relatively constant drug-release rate over the application period.

Conventional TD patches are *not* suitable for use when a rapid effect is required, e.g. acute or uncontrolled pain requiring rapid titration, because of the time taken for the drug to reach the systemic circulation (hours) and steady state (days). Conversely, following removal of the patch, because of the reservoir of drug within the skin, significant plasma concentrations may exist for ≤24h.

Cautions

After reports of serious adverse events (overdoses and deaths), regulatory authorities in the UK, USA and Canada have issued safety warnings about the use of TD **fentanyl** which are also applicable to TD **buprenorphine**. For full details see p.409 and p.397 respectively.[1–5] However, contributing factors include:

- inappropriate use for short-term (e.g. postoperative) pain
- lack of patient education about safe use, storage and disposal, leading to accidental exposure and deaths in others, particularly children
- lack of awareness of the impact of increased temperature or direct external heat.

External heat sources and/or increase in body temperature

The rate of absorption of drugs can increase if the skin under the patch becomes vasodilated, e.g. in febrile patients, high ambient temperatures,[6] or by an external heat source, e.g. electric blanket, hot water bottle, heat lamps, saunas, hot tubs. For **buprenorphine** and **fentanyl**, this has resulted in fatal overdoses.

Note. Patients may swim or shower with a patch but should avoid soaking in a hot bath.

TD patches and MRI

National and speciality guidance advises that patches known to contain or possibly contain metal and/or affected by heat should be removed before the patient enters the scan room and replaced afterwards.[7,8] Patients should be advised to bring a replacement patch with them to facilitate this.

The two main risks from wearing patches during MRI are skin burns and drug toxicity (Box A).

Although some patches will be safe, confirmation of this is difficult because:

- the SPC may not contain comprehensive information on excipients
- of limited testing; manufacturers are generally unwilling to comment on patch safety during MRI
- visual inspection of a patch to see if it contains metal can be deceptive; clear patches may contain metal ions.[10]

Because of these difficulties and recent guidance,[7,8] most MRI units have a policy of removing all TD patches before MRI.

Box A Risks from wearing TD patches during MRI

Direct contact burn to the skin underneath the TD patch

Some patches contain metal:

- in the backing, e.g. aluminium (Hapocatsin®) *or*
- as metal salts in other parts of the patch, e.g. aluminium acetylacetonate in the adhesive layer (Butrans®, Transtec®).

The magnetic field from the scanner heats up the metal, and burns have been reported to the MHRA and FDA.[7,9]

Drug toxicity due to increase in body temperature ± direct heating

MRI can heat up the patch and also increase body temperature from the absorption of energy from the magnetic field. Generally, the increase in body temperature is limited to 0.5–1°C depending on the type of scan. However, for certain applications with small or surface coils, local temperature can rise to ≤39°C for the trunk and ≤40°C for limbs. Increased absorption can lead to a serious overdose for **buprenorphine** or **fentanyl** patches.[4,7,8]

Use of TD patches

Prescribing

TD **buprenorphine** and TD **fentanyl** are available for analgesia. Their use is summarized in the respective individual monographs (see p.397 and p.409) and Quick Clinical Guides (see p.407 and p.417).

Further information on dose conversion ratios from PO opioids to TD **buprenorphine** and **fentanyl** can also be found in Appendix 2, p.855.

For **buprenorphine** and **fentanyl** patches, a variety of branded generic formulations is available. Apart from differences in appearance, there are also differences between formulations in the length of time the patch should be applied. Prescribing by brand is recommended to avoid confusion.[1]

Application and disposal

Under *no* circumstances should a *reservoir* patch be cut in an attempt to reduce the dose. Leakage from the cut reservoir could result in either the patient receiving minimal or no drug or, alternatively, an overdose from the rapid absorption of drug through the surrounding skin.

PCF does not generally recommend cutting *matrix* patches, because of similar concerns. The increased range of available strengths has made the need for this less likely. However, in a few situations this may be necessary, e.g. **hyoscine *hydrobromide*** patches in children.[11]

A new site of application should be used each time a patch is changed. Application should be to dry, non-inflamed, non-irradiated, hairless skin on the upper trunk or arm – unless otherwise specified in the SPC, e.g. **hyoscine *hydrobromide*** patches are applied behind the ear.

Body hair may be clipped with scissors (*not* shaved). If the skin is washed beforehand, only water should be used; soap, oils, creams or ointments should *not* be applied as they may interfere with drug absorption. The patch should be pressed firmly in place for at least 30 seconds. Micropore® or Tegaderm® can be used to aid adherence. The date of application and/or date of renewal should be written on the patch, if possible.

Careful removal of the patch helps to minimize local skin irritation. It should be noted that used patches will still contain some drug, and must be disposed of carefully. Patches should be folded in half with the adhesive side inwards and discarded in a sharps container (hospital) or a dustbin (home), and hands washed. In hospital, disposal of controlled drugs should be witnessed and documented.

For patients undergoing MRI, adequate arrangements should be in place for safe disposal of the removed patches, particularly controlled drugs. Rescue medication should be available (where necessary), and a new patch applied as soon as possible after the scan.

Monitoring

Monitoring is essential to ensure patches:

- remain firmly attached to the skin to prevent loss of efficacy *and*
- old patches are removed when new patches are applied.

The date and time the patch was applied, the strength, number of patches, and the site of application, should be recorded and monitored at least twice daily. In addition, the date and time of removal and destruction should also be recorded.

For strong opioids, palliativedrugs.com has developed a specific TD patch monitoring chart which can be downloaded from the Document library (Pain, Strong opioids).

1 Care Quality Commission and NHS England (2013) Safer use of controlled drugs - preventing harms from fentanyl and buprenorphine transdermal patches. *Use of controlled drugs supporting information.* www.cqc.org.uk

2 Health Canada (2008) Fentanyl transdermal patch and fatal adverse reactions. *Canadian Adverse Reaction Newsletter.* **18**: 1–2.

3 FDA (2007) Fentanyl transdermal system (marketed as Duragesic) information. *Post Market Drug Safety Information for Patients and Providers.* www.fda.gov/Drugs/DrugsSafety/default.htm

4 MHRA (2008) Fentanyl patches: serious and fatal overdose from dosing errors, accidental exposure, and inappropriate use. *Drug Safety Update.* 2 www.mhra.gov.uk/safetyinformation

5 Jumbelic MI (2010) Deaths with transdermal fentanyl patches. *American Journal of Forensic Medicine and Pathology.* **31**: 18–21.

6 Sindali K *et al.* (2012) Life-threatening coma and full-thickness sunburn in a patient treated with transdermal fentanyl patches: a case report. *Journal of Medical Case Reports.* **6**: 220

7 MHRA (2015) Safety guidelines for magnetic resonance imaging equipment in clinical use. www.gov.uk

8 Society of Radiographers (2016) Safety in magnetic resonance imaging. www.sor.org

9 Institute for Safe Medication Practices (2004) Medication Safety Alert. Burns in MRI patients wearing transdermal patches. Available from: www.ismp.org/Newsletters/acutecare/articles/20040408.asp?ptr=y

10 Anderton D and Cary P (2009) Medicated patches and MRI imaging - a burning issue. Poster presentation 20. *35th UKMI Practice Development Seminar.*

11 Jassal S and Aindow A (2017) APPM Master Formulary 4th edition. *Association of Paediatric Palliative Medicine.* www.appm.org.uk

Added April 2017

31: NEBULIZED DRUGS

31

Nebulizers are used in asthma and COPD for both acute exacerbations and long-term prophylaxis (see Bronchodilators, p.107).[1–3] Other uses include the pulmonary delivery of antimicrobial drugs for cystic fibrosis, bronchiectasis and AIDS-related pneumonia. For the supplementary role of nebulized bronchodilators in anaphylaxis, see Appendix 1, Box C, p.853.

Nebulizers are also used in palliative care (see below). The aim is to deliver a therapeutic dose of a drug as an aerosol in particles small enough to be inspired within 5–10min. A nebulizer is preferable to a hand-held metered dose inhaler (MDI) when:
- a large drug dose is needed
- co-ordinated breathing is difficult
- MDIs + a spacer are ineffective
- a drug is unavailable in an inhaler.

In these circumstances, by improving drug delivery, a nebulizer can result in better symptom relief.[4] However, nebulizers are noisy, more expensive and less convenient than an MDI; they are also ineffective in patients with shallow breathing, and in those unable to sit up to at least 45°, i.e. semi-upright or more. The higher doses administered can also increase the risk of undesirable effects and their use should be carefully monitored to ensure ongoing efficacy and tolerability.

Commonly used nebulizers are:

Jet: the aerosol is generated by a flow of gas from, for example, an electrical compressor or piped air. At least 50% of the aerosol produced at the recommended driving gas flow should be particles small enough to inhale.

Ultrasonic: the aerosol is generated by ultrasonic vibrations of a piezo-electric crystal.

Aerosol output (the mass of particles in aerosol form produced/min) is not necessarily the same as drug output (the mass of drug produced/min as an aerosol). Ideally, the drug output of a nebulizer should be known for each of the different drugs given. Various factors affect the drug output and deposition:
- gas flow rate; the optimum is 6–8L/min of air or oxygen (see below)
- chamber design
- volume (commonly 2–2.5mL, up to 4mL)
- residual volume (commonly 0.5mL)
- physical properties of the drug in solution
- breathing pattern of the patient.

The choice of gas can be crucial. Air via an electrical compressor or piped air is generally used, and *always* in a patient at risk of hypercapnia; if they are dependent on low concentration oxygen, give this simultaneously via nasal cannulae. Oxygen is *always* used when treating acute asthma, delivered via piped oxygen or a large oxygen cylinder.

The choice of nebulizer can also be crucial, particularly when trying to produce an aerosol small enough to deliver a drug to the alveoli. Services that provide nebulizers will generally offer information, education and support for patients and their families (Box A). Information should include:
- a description of the equipment and its use
- drugs used, doses and frequencies
- equipment maintenance/cleaning
- action to take if treatment becomes less effective
- action to take and emergency telephone number to use if equipment breaks down.

Patients should be instructed to take steady normal breaths (interspersed with occasional deep ones) and nebulization time should be less than 10min or 'to dryness'. Because there is always a residual volume, 'dryness' should be taken as 1min after spluttering starts.

Whereas a mask can be used for bronchodilators, *a mouthpiece should generally be used for other drugs to limit environmental contamination and/or contact with the patient's eyes.* However, a mask may be preferable in patients who are acutely ill, fatigued or very young, regardless of the nature of the drug. Patients' nebulizer technique should be checked periodically.[5]

Nebulizers can also be used in patients with long-term tracheostomies (via a tracheostomy mask or T-piece circuit) or receiving non-invasive ventilation (via the ventilator tubing). However, for patients not completely dependent on non-invasive ventilation, nebulized bronchodilators are more effective when given during breaks from ventilation.[6]

Portable battery-operated nebulizers may be used in aircraft at the discretion of the cabin crew, but the airline must be notified in advance (also see Oxygen, p.130).

In England and Wales nebulizers and electrical compressors are not available on the NHS (but are VAT free). In Scotland, some nebulizers can be prescribed.

Box A Advice about using a nebulizer at home

To help your breathing, your doctor has prescribed a drug to be used with a nebulizer. The nebulizer converts the drug into a fine mist which you inhale.

The apparatus

Your nebulizer system consists of the following parts:

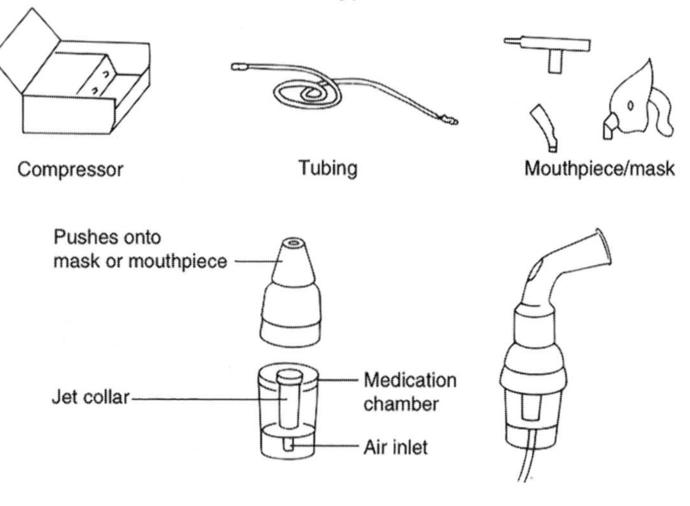

The compressor is the portable pump which pumps air along the tubing into the nebulizer. The nebulizer is a small chamber for the liquid medicine, through which air is blown to make a mist.

The nebulizer has a screw-on top onto which the mask or mouthpiece is attached.

How to use your nebulizer

Place the medication in the nebulizer, replace the screw-on top and turn the compressor on. Inhale by mouthpiece or mask while breathing at a normal rate. Stop 1 minute after the nebulizer contents start spluttering or after a maximum of 10 minutes.

General advice

If you have a cough, the nebulizer may help you to expectorate, so have some tissues nearby.

You may wish to use the nebulizer before attempting an activity which makes you feel out of breath.

If the effects of the nebulizer wear off or you have any questions or concerns about it, please speak to your doctor or nurse.

Cleaning

Wash the mouthpiece/mask and nebulizer in warm water and detergent, then rinse and dry well. Ideally this should be done after every use, but *once a day as a minimum.* Attach the tube and run the nebulizer empty for a few moments after cleaning it to make sure the equipment is dry. Once a week, unplug and wipe the compressor and tubing with a damp cloth.

Nebulizers in palliative care

For the use of nebulized **tranexamic acid** in haemoptysis, see Haemostatics, p.101.

Various drugs have been given by nebulizer to ease cough and breathlessness in advanced cancer (Table 1 and Table 2). However, apart from the use of bronchodilators for reversible airflow obstruction, there is often little evidence to support their use. Thus, some are *not* recommended by *PCF* for routine use (Table 1). The remainder should be considered only when other avenues have failed (Table 2), and reviewed after 2 days to check effectiveness.

In patients with asthma, when using **lidocaine** or **bupivacaine** for a dry cough (not recommended for breathlessness), consider pretreating with **salbutamol** because of the risk of initial bronchospasm.[7] After nebulized local anaesthetic, patients should be advised not to eat or drink for 1h because the reduced gag/cough reflex increases the risk of aspiration (also see Antitussives, p.144).

Because of lack of data about physico-chemical compatibility and aerodynamic properties, manufacturers generally do not recommend mixing nebulizer solutions. Further, when mixing products in this way, the combination is considered an unauthorized product (see Box A p.751). However, some ready-mixed combinations are commercially available, e.g. **salbutamol** + **ipratropium bromide** (generic and Combivent®).

Table 1 Nebulized drugs and cancer-related cough or breathlessness[2,14]

Class of drug[a]	*Indications*	*Scientific evidence*	*Comments*
0.9% saline	Loosening of tenacious secretions	Limited[15]	Probably underused in this setting; may also help breathlessness
Mucolytic agents e.g. hypertonic saline	To thin viscous sputum	Enhances airway clearance in chronic lung diseases characterized by sputum retention	May result in copious liquid sputum which the patient may still not be able to cough up. May cause bronchospasm; begin with a low concentration, i.e. 3% and pretreat at-risk patients with a bronchodilator[16]
Corticosteroids e.g. budesonide	Stridor, lymphangitis, radiation pneumonitis, cough after the insertion of a stent	None	Very limited clinical experience only; may not be more beneficial than use of inhaler or oral routes.
†Local anaesthetics e.g. lidocaine, bupivacaine	Cough, particularly if caused by lymphangitis carcinomatosa	Conflicting evidence for both breathlessness[17,18] and cough[7]	May cause bronchospasm; consider pretreating at risk patients with a bronchodilator.[7] Reduces gag reflex; risk of aspiration immediately after treatment
†Opioids e.g. morphine, fentanyl	Breathlessness associated with diffuse lung disease	Despite anecdotal reports of benefit, the evidence does not support routine use[19]	Not recommended; risk of bronchospasm
Bronchodilators e.g. salbutamol	Treatment of severe reversible airway obstruction	Extrapolated from patients with asthma and COPD	Try MDI + spacer first.[20,21] Use nebulizers only if trial of therapy shows real benefit
†Furosemide	Breathlessness	Despite anecdotal reports of benefit, the evidence does not support routine use (see Furosemide, p.61)	Not recommended

a. mask can be used for bronchodilators; a mouthpiece should be used for all other drugs to limit environmental contamination and/or contact with the patient's eyes. However, a mask may be unavoidable in those incapable of using a mouthpiece, e.g. when acutely ill, fatigued or very young.

Table 2 Recommended uses of nebulized drugs in palliative care

Indication	*Drug*	*Initial regimen*	*Dose titration*	*Comments*
Tenacious secretions	Saline 0.9%	5mL p.r.n.	Up to q2h	
	Hypertonic saline 3%	4mL p.r.n.	Up to q.d.s.	Risk of bronchospasm
	Hypertonic saline 6 or 7%	4mL p.r.n.	Up to b.d.	
Reversible airway obstruction	Salbutamol	2.5mg q6h–q4h	Up to 5mg q4h	Risk of sensitivity to cardiac stimulant effects
Cough	*†Lidocaine 2%	5mL p.r.n.	Up to q.d.s.	Risk of bronchospasm
	*†Bupivacaine 0.25%	5mL p.r.n.	Up to q.d.s.	Loss of gag reflex; nil by mouth for 1h after nebulization

There are limited data indicating that 2-drug mixtures comprising one drug from any two of the classes below will be physically and/or chemically compatible (for all strengths):

- *β_2-adrenergic receptor agonists (β_2 agonists)*, **salbutamol** or **terbutaline** (Bricanyl®)
- *antimuscarinic*, **ipratropium bromide**
- *corticosteroids*, **budesonide** (Pulmicort®) or **fluticasone** (Flixotide®).[8–13]

Solutions should be mixed immediately before use, using aseptic technique. If the colour changes or cloudiness/precipitation occurs, the mixture should be discarded. If dilution is necessary, sterile 0.9% saline is generally best. There is no information on 3-drug mixtures, and these cannot be recommended.

1 The Nebulizer Project Group of the British Thoracic Society Standards of Care Committee (1997) Current best practice for nebuliser treatment. *Thorax*. **52 (Suppl 2)**: S1–3.
2 European Respiratory Society (2001) Guidelines on the use of nebulizers. *European Respiratory Journal*. **18**: 228–242.
3 NICE (2010) Chronic obstructive pulmonary disease in over 16s: diagnosis and management. *Clinical Guideline*. CG101. www.nice.org.uk
4 Tashkin DP *et al.* (2007) Comparing COPD treatment: nebulizer, metered dose inhaler, and concomitant therapy. *American Journal of Medicine*. **120**: 435–441.
5 Ari A and Restrepo RD (2012) Aerosol delivery device selection for spontaneously breathing patients: 2012. *Respiratory Care*. **57**: 613–626.
6 Davidson AC *et al.* (2016) BTS/ICS guideline for the ventilatory management of acute hypercapnic respiratory failure in adults. *Thorax*. **71 (Suppl 2)**: ii1–35.
7 Slaton RM *et al.* (2013) Evidence for therapeutic uses of nebulized lidocaine in the treatment of intractable cough and asthma. *Annals of Pharmacotherapy*. **47**: 578–585.
8 Roberts G and Rossi S (1993) Compatibility of nebuliser solutions. *Australian Journal of Hospital Pharmacy*. **23**: 35–37.
9 McKenzie JE and Cruz-Rivera M (2004) Compatibility of budesonide inhalation suspension with four nebulizing solutions. *Annals of Pharmacotherapy*. **38**: 967–972.
10 Burchett DK *et al.* (2010) Mixing and compatibility guide for commonly used aerosolized medications. *American Journal of Health System Pharmacy*. **67**: 227–230.
11 Joseph JC (1997) Compatibility of nebulizer solution admixtures. *Annals of Pharmacotherapy*. **31**: 487–489.
12 Harriman A-M *et al.* (1996) Can we mix nebuliser solutions? Stability of drug admixtures in solutions for nebulisation. *Pharmacy in Practice*. Oct. 347–348.
13 UK Medicines Information (2016) Which commonly used nebuliser solutions are compatible? *Medicines Q&A* 100.8. www.evidence.nhs.uk
14 Ahmedzai S and Davis C (1997) Nebulised drugs in palliative care. *Thorax*. **52 (Suppl 2)**: s75–77.
15 Tarrant BJ *et al.* (2017) Mucoactive agents for chronic, non-cystic fibrosis lung disease: A systematic review and meta-analysis. *Respirology*. **22**: 1084–1092.
16 Pasteur MC *et al.* (2010) British Thoracic Society guideline for non-CF bronchiectasis. *Thorax*. **65 (Suppl 1)**: i1–58.
17 Winning A *et al.* (1988) Ventilation and breathlessness on maximal exercise in patients with interstitial lung disease after local anaesthetic aerosol inhalation. *Clinical Science*. **74**: 275–281.
18 Wilcock A *et al.* (1994) Safety and efficacy of nebulized lignocaine in patients with cancer and breathlessness. *Palliative Medicine*. **8**: 35–38.
19 Barnes H *et al.* (2016) Opioids for the palliation of refractory breathlessness in adults with advanced disease and terminal illness. *Cochrane Database of Systematic Reviews*. **3**: CD011008. www.thecochranelibrary.com
20 Congleton J and Muers MF (1995) The incidence of airflow obstruction in bronchial carcinoma, its relation to breathlessness, and response to bronchodilator therapy. *Respiratory Medicine*. **89**: 291–296.
21 Colacone A *et al.* (1993) A comparison of albuterol administered by metered dose inhaler (and holding chamber) or wet nebulizer in acute asthma. *Chest*. **104**: 835–841.

Updated (minor update) April 2017

32: SPINAL ANALGESIA

INDICATIONS

Spinal analgesia is used extensively for obstetric or peri-operative pain relief, but is uncommon in palliative care.[1] Only 2–4% of cancer patients receiving specialist palliative care proceed to spinal analgesia because of inadequate relief with systemic analgesia.[2–4] Spinal analgesia is effective in >50% of patients. Good communication between the palliative care, pain, and primary care teams is essential. Typical indications for spinal analgesia include:

- systemic opioid intolerance (an unacceptable balance between efficacy and toxicity)
- refractory neuropathic pain (e.g. lumbosacral plexopathy, visceral neuropathic pain)
- refractory nociceptive pain from progressive tumour or bone metastases.

The aim is to provide optimum pain relief in a patient with a short life expectancy. Rapid disease progression and a changing pain picture is typical, and the combination of drugs used and/or their doses may need to be changed frequently.[5]

CONTRA-INDICATIONS

Uncorrected coagulopathy, systemic or local infection, raised intracranial pressure. Extra caution is necessary when there is:

- spinal deformity
- incipient spinal cord compression
- myelosuppressive chemotherapy
- intracranial metastases.

ROUTE, PLACEMENT AND DELIVERY DEVICE CONSIDERATIONS

Before insertion of a spinal catheter, baseline blood tests help to evaluate renal, hepatic, bone marrow and metabolic function and exclude, for example, coagulopathies and any significant infection. Neurological and cardiopulmonary examination provide a baseline for future reference, and a spinal MRI provides useful anatomical information.

Clinical services caring for patients receiving spinal analgesia need clear procedures to be in place to minimize risk at all stages of treatment. Maintaining staff competence is challenging when such approaches are used infrequently. Guidelines and 'refresher' training are both important.

Analgesics are delivered to the intrathecal (IT) or epidural (ED) space via an indwelling catheter placed by an anaesthetist (or spinal or neurosurgeon in some centres). Options include:

- 'blind' (without radiological screening) sited catheters
- catheters tunnelled subcutaneously away from the spine
- fully implanted systems (IT only).

Tunnelled and fully implanted systems reduce the risk of displacement and infection. Fluoroscopically screened catheter placement ensures drug placement at the optimal dermatome level. Simple placement under local anaesthetic, without tunnelling or radiological screening, can be satisfactory for external pumps.

The preferred route and delivery device are influenced by local custom and the likely duration of use (Table 1). Although ED catheters are sometimes left in place for several months, the preferred route is IT for spinal analgesia expected to be needed for more than a few weeks. Devices vary in relation to fixed vs. variable delivery rates, patient-controlled boluses, and cost.

Table 1 Suggested route and delivery device

Likely duration of use	*Route and device*	*Comments*
≤3 weeks	External ED device (re-usable)	Fewer initial complications than IT (8% vs. 25%); less headache from CSF leakage[6]
3 weeks–3 months	External IT device (re-usable)	Fewer later complications than ED (5% vs. 55%); less catheter occlusion or migration[6]
≥ 3 months	Implantable IT device	More expensive initially, lower running costs; more cost-effective long-term

The use of implanted IT pumps is not widespread in the UK, and there are only a few regional centres. There will be at least one responsible treating physician at each centre, with 24h access to advice and a clear plan for emergency admissions. *Inexperienced staff should never make significant changes to a patient's infusion without advice and support from a senior experienced clinician.*

Opioids administered IT act locally on opioid receptors in the superficial laminae of the dorsal horn of the spinal cord. Thus, compared with the ED route, lower doses are needed, e.g. a woman having a caesarean section might be given ED **diamorphine** 3mg compared with IT 300microgram. Smaller doses permit the use of smaller devices and/or reducing the frequency of refilling (see below). IT administration generally also provides better pain relief than the ED route.

For *implanted IT systems*, because of the slow infusion rate and the tiny volumes used, drugs delivered into the CSF do *not* diffuse rostrally to the brain stem, whether given by infusion or as a bolus. CSF flow is pulsatile with oscillatory displacements, but no net bulk flow.[7–9] Taking samples of **morphine** at points away from the catheter tip demonstrates a steep reducing concentration gradient.[10]

Studies of porcine IT drug delivery (ITDD) using **bupivacaine** at rates reflecting human implanted ITDD (20–1000microL/h and boluses at 1000microL/h) also showed that most of the drug is recovered <1cm of the site of administration.[11] Drug diffusion within the spinal cord parenchyma was higher with boluses and the higher rates of infusion.[12]

Thus, the area of analgesia is completely dependent on the site of the catheter, which must be at or above the dermatomal level of the patient's pain and posterior in the spinal canal. For bilateral pain, it is best in the midline and, for unilateral pain, slightly to the side of the pain.

In contrast, IT drugs from an *external pump* use high volumes and infusion rates, and there is more potential for rostral spread in the CSF. Additional rostral and caudal areas of pain can be covered, and a blindly sited catheter (without fluoroscopy) can be effective.

Drugs administered as a single IT bolus as part of an anaesthetic technique involve relatively big volumes and forces of injection, and often barbotage, to facilitate drug spread either rostrally or caudally. The fluid mechanics here are completely different from those at work in an implanted system. On occasion, opioids have reached the brain stem with consequent adverse effects (see below). However, this does *not* happen with implanted systems even at the maximum rate of infusion. *For a Synchromed II pump, this is 1mL/h compared with an anaesthetic bolus of up to 3.5mL in a few seconds.*

Drugs delivered to the ED space must diffuse through the meninges in order to reach the spinal cord and adjacent nerve roots. The level of the spinal cord at which the catheter is sited determines the area over which maximal analgesia is obtained. Because an ED dose is much higher than an IT one, migration or misplacement of ED catheters into the IT space (a rare event) will deliver an excessive dose resulting in significant toxicity. Unless this is recognized and treated urgently, it can lead to respiratory arrest and death.

Although theoretically the same delivery devices can be used for SC, IV and spinal infusion, for maximum safety it is best to use a device specifically designed for spinal delivery.[2] Distinct pumps and connectors will reduce the potential for confusion in a patient receiving concurrent spinal and SC/IV infusions.[13] However, such recommendations must be weighed against the considerable advantage of staff using a delivery device with which they are familiar from frequent SC/IV use.

BOLUS VS. CONTINUOUS INFUSION

Bolus based regimens are best for break-through pain, and pain not responsive to opioids. Most implanted IT pumps for cancer pain will contain both an opioid and a local anaesthetic. The development of tolerance seen with *continuous* infusions is delayed or prevented by a bolus based regimen.

Patient Therapy Manager

This is a hand-held device for a patient to self-administer boluses from the Medtronic Synchromed II pump (the only implanted pump currently available with this facility). It can be used for opioid, local anaesthetic, and mixed regimens. The device is a 'slave' unit to the pump, i.e. it will work only with the pump to which it was first bonded. The physician programmes the pump, detailing the dose of the primary drug, the duration of the infusion, the lock-out interval and the maximum activations/24h.

CHOICE OF DRUGS FOR IT USE

Parenteral formulations of the same drug vary between manufacturers and it is essential to confirm that a specific brand is suitable for IT use. This requires it to meet a more stringent endotoxin limit and it must *not*:

- be irritant or toxic to the CNS
- contain anti-microbial preservatives
- be at extremes of pH or osmotic strength
- contain other excipients, unless accepted for IT use, e.g. some pH adjusters.

For some drugs, no commercially available formulations are suitable and unauthorized products for IT administration have to be obtained via special order (see Chapter 24, p.751). Seek specialist pharmacist advice.

Opioids (**morphine** or **hydromorphone** for implanted IT pumps and the option of **diamorphine** for external systems), local anaesthetics (**bupivacaine**) and α_2 agonists (**clonidine**) are the most commonly used drugs. A solo opioid infusion may be appropriate for someone with stable pain, e.g. from stable bone metastases, but *most patients with progressive cancer pain need either a combination of drugs or a local anaesthetic alone.*

Health professionals and pharmacists should familiarize themselves with the guidance and supporting material about the legal implication of mixing medicines before administration,[14,15] together with any local policy and practice.

In the UK, specific brands of **baclofen**, **bupivacaine**, **levobupivacaine** and **ziconotide** are authorized for IT use. Other drugs are used 'off label' in accordance with the recommendations of the Polyanalgesic Consensus Conference (PACC).[3,4] These recommendations primarily apply to non-cancer pain, and physicians will need to use their own clinical judgement when making treatment decisions for patients with cancer pain. It is essential that the parenteral formulation of the drug used is suitable for IT administration (see above).

Because each patient's complex pain is different, drug regimens have to be individualized. There is little or no place for predetermined (slow-moving) algorithms. For example, to manage worsening pain, a previously stable continuous opioid infusion may need to be up-titrated (± the addition of **clonidine**), followed by a decision to add in or switch to **bupivacaine**, with a low background infusion and boluses for break-through pain.

For opioid-naïve patients, recommended IT starting doses are shown in Table 2. Recommended maximum opioid concentrations and daily doses are shown in Table 3. The maximum opioid doses aim to minimize the risk of catheter tip granuloma formation (see p.847); these are less relevant with relatively short-term use, although granulomas have been reported after 4 weeks.[16]

Table 2 Opioid-naïve patients: recommended IT starting doses[3]

Drug	*Starting doses/24h*
Bupivacaine	10microgram–4mg
Clonidine	20–100microgram
Hydromorphone	1–150microgram
Morphine	100–500microgram
Ziconotide	0.5–1.2microgram

Table 3 Recommended maximum IT concentrations and doses[3,4]

Drug	*Maximum concentration (mg/mL)*	*Maximum daily dose (mg)*
Bupivacaine	30[a]	15–20[a]
Clonidine	1	600*microgram*
Hydromorphone	15	10
Morphine	20	15
Ziconotide	100*microgram/mL*	19.2*microgram*

a. may be exceeded in end of life care and in complicated cases.

Opioids

In the UK, **morphine**, **hydromorphone** and **diamorphine** are widely used; the latter because of its solubility and lack of preservatives. However, because of a risk of precipitation, **diamorphine** should *not* be used in Medtronic Synchromed® pumps (see p.844), but can be used in Flowonix Prometra® pumps.

The advantages of IT administration are greatest with hydrophilic opioids, e.g. **diamorphine**, **morphine** and **hydromorphone**, because they remain longer in the CSF.[17] In contrast, **fentanyl** is highly lipid-soluble, and has no effect at the spinal cord level because it is rapidly absorbed and redistributed systemically. Thus, spinal administration has no advantages over systemic use, and should be discouraged.[17]

There is much uncertainty about dose equivalents between routes. Most centres have their own conversion tables based on the oral morphine equivalent (OME) dose in mg/24h, which is then converted to an IT dose.

Experience at one centre suggests, for example, that an appropriate starting dose for someone who has been receiving:

- OME 300mg/24h is about IT **morphine** 1mg/24h
- OME 200mg/24h is about IT **hydromorphone** 1mg/24h.[5]

Note. These are recommended *starting doses*, and should *not* be confused with 'equivalent doses' recommended when switching PO to SC/IV or vice versa (Appendix 2, p.855).

Local anaesthetics

Bupivacaine is the most widely used local anaesthetic for spinal analgesia. It has inherent bactericidal properties which theoretically reduces the risk of infection. Alternatives include **levobupivacaine** and **ropivacaine**. Motor weakness can be a limiting undesirable effect; predisposing factors include pre-existing neurological damage.

Self-administered boluses of **bupivacaine** using a Patient Therapy Manager can be particularly effective for progressive cancer pain. Doses of as little as 0.5–2mg may be effective. The maximum bolus dose is 20mg and the shortest duration of administration for this is 30min, using a concentration of 40mg/mL infused at a maximum rate of 1mL/hour (i.e. 20mg in 30min).

32

The motor and sensory changes can be predicted according to the level of the catheter. For example, a bolus through a catheter sited at:

- S2 (the bottom of the dural sac): will cause perineal and buttock numbness, but is unlikely to cause leg weakness
- T12: leg weakness is expected
- T6: there may be some leg weakness, but not as profound as at T12
- T4 (or thereabouts): may affect cardiac nerves with resultant bradycardia and hypotension (opioids can also do this).

Hypotension can occur with both infusions and boluses, and relates to vasodilation caused by the drug's impact on the sympathetic nervous system. It is more likely:

- with higher catheters (above the lumbar sympathetic chain at L2–4)
- with higher bolus doses (e.g. 5–20mg)
- if the patient is septic, hypovolaemic, or generally unwell.

The patient should be sitting or lying and monitored when they first use the bolus facility. Downward dose adjustments may be necessary during episodes of infection, sepsis, bleeding, and hypovolaemia.

Numbness and weakness can last for ≤3h, but there is generally a period of usable pain-free time after that before the local anaesthetic wears off altogether. It is possible to adjust doses and duration of infusion to a certain extent in an attempt to reduce undesirable effects. However, often numbness = pain relief and the patient has to learn to time their boluses to minimize functional limitations.

A starting bolus dose would be **bupivacaine** 1–2mg, which can be given by the single bolus facility on the pump and, depending on the response, can be titrated up or down. This dose is unlikely to cause any cardiovascular effect or profound numbness or weakness, although it can significantly augment pre-existing weakness in the frail.

α-Adrenergic receptor agonists

IT **clonidine** 15–600microgram/24h is generally given concurrently with an opioid and a local anaesthetic. Experience with ED **clonidine** is more limited, and the recommended dose range is narrower, i.e. 150–300microgram/24h. Bigger doses would be more likely cause (dose-dependent) hypotension and bradycardia because of systemic absorption (see p.77).[2]

Benefit is seen particularly in neuropathic pain. Abrupt cessation (e.g. because of pump failure) may cause severe rebound hypertension. Administer oral **clonidine** while seeking specialist advice.[3]

Ziconotide

Ziconotide is an intrathecal calcium channel blocker, acting on presynaptic N-type calcium channels in the dorsal horn of the spinal cord.[18,19] Consequently, it is useful for opioid-tolerant patients. It is recommended as first-line therapy for both nociceptive and neuropathic pain, and there is good evidence to support its use in cancer pain.[20,21] It is a big highly ionized protein molecule and, unlike the other spinally applied drugs, distributes widely throughout central neural tissue independent of the site of the catheter.

However, undesirable effects are common, and can be both dose- and treatment-limiting. The titration schedule is slow, with increases ranging from 0.5–1.2microgram/day *every 1–2 weeks* or longer. Consequently, it may take several months to reach an effective dose. **Ziconotide** is only available in the UK with an authorized 'individual funding request'.

Other drugs

Ketamine is a non-competitive NMDA-receptor-channel blocker (see p.641) but has been shown to be neurotoxic in both animal IT infusion models and in humans.[22,23] Nonetheless, it may have a role if all else has failed in the last days–weeks of life, although sourcing a suitable product may be difficult.

A **baclofen** (see p.608) product is authorized for IT use for spasticity, but not for pain. The spinal use of several other drugs has been reported, but no others are recommended either because of toxicity (e.g. **dexmedetomidine, droperidol, methadone, methylprednisolone, midazolam, ondansetron, pethidine, tramadol, tetracaine**) or inefficacy (e.g. **gabapentin, octreotide, ropivacaine**).

DRUG COMPATIBILITY

Combinations of **morphine** or **diamorphine** with **bupivacaine** ± **clonidine** are widely used, particularly with external devices. Long-term compatibility data for drug combinations in both external devices (at room temperature) and implanted pump reservoirs (at body temperature) are limited.[2] Several factors can affect drug stability and compatibility (see Chapter 29, Box B, p.821). It is important to check with a pharmacist that the compatibility data are relevant to spinal use, and to confirm the appropriate diluent.

When mixing drugs for long periods it is important to consider the material the delivery device is made of because this can affect drug stability, e.g. **diamorphine** should not be used in Synchromed pumps because of reports of precipitation.

Compatibility data at room temperature

There are compatibility data on the following combinations at *room temperature*:

- **diamorphine** with **bupivacaine** 4 weeks[24]
- **morphine sulfate** with **bupivacaine** or **clonidine** 2 months[25,26]
- **hydromorphone** with **bupivacaine** 3 days[27]
- **clonidine** with **bupivacaine** 2 weeks[28]

Compatibility data at body temperature

There are compatibility data on the following combinations at *body temperature*:

- **morphine sulfate** with **clonidine** ± **bupivacaine** ≤3 months in a SynchroMed pump[29,30]
- **hydromorphone** 4 months in a SynchroMed pump[31]
- **clonidine** with **hydromorphone** 1.5 months (only **clonidine** evaluated).[32]

Delivery devices with mixtures for administration over >24h should be prepared in a sterile environment, e.g. a licensed pharmacy. Drugs should be preservative-free.[2]

UNDESIRABLE EFFECTS AND COMPLICATIONS OF SPINAL ANALGESIA

These relate to:

- the drugs (Table 4)
- medical complications, e.g. bleeding, infection (Table 5)
- the delivery system (Table 5).[33]

Respiratory failure is either the result of central depression of respiratory drive (opioids) or impaired motor output to the respiratory muscles at the spinal level (**bupivacaine**). Rate of onset varies: systemic redistribution of the spinally administered opioid causes respiratory depression within minutes or hours, whereas diffusion through the CSF causes a delayed onset, occurring after 6–48h.

When using an implanted IT system, because the drugs do not spread rostrally, respiratory depression is likely to be the result of opioid given by another route, e.g. PO/SL opioid before using an IT bolus for break-through pain.

Table 4 Drug-related undesirable effects

Drug	*Undesirable effect*	*Comment*
Withdrawal of systemic opioids	Diarrhoea and intestinal colic	Partly avoidable if laxatives stopped and then re-titrated after switch to spinal route
Opioids	Nausea and vomiting	Uncommon in patietnts previously on systemic opioids
Opioids	Pruritus	Rare when given to patients who are switching from systemic opioids, and when spinal opioid combined with bupivacaine
Bupivacaine	Motor or sensory disturbance; dose-dependent	Persistent motor impairment 5–10%
Opioids, bupivacaine	Urinary retention	Removal of the urinary catheter after 3–4 days is successful in most patients; if persistent, may relate to underlying pathology
Opioids, bupivacaine	Respiratory depression	Rare
Opioid, bupivacaine, clonidine	Hypotension	Site dependent, see text. Clonidine also causes bradycardia
Opioids[a]	Catheter tip granulomas	Seen in about 3% of long-term IT infusions, mostly asymptomatic;[34] more common with ED infusions
Opioids	Decreased libido, ± disturbed menstruation	Seen in most patients with IT opioids given for >1 year but can occur sooner.[35] Measure testosterone and LH at baseline and annually in men; estradiol, progesterone, LH, FSH in women[2]
Opioids	Hypocorticalism or growth hormone deficiency	Seen in about 15%[35]
Opioids	Oedema	Common; possibly 10–20%
Opioids	Immunomodulation	Frequency and significance uncertain. May be more pronounced with systemic opioids[36]

a. less common with non-opioids.

Table 5 Non-drug complications of spinal analgesia[37]

Undesirable effect	*Comment*
Traumatic catheter placement	
CSF leakage headache	Uncommon
ED haematoma	Rare
Neurological tissue damage	Rare
Infection[38]	
Exit site infection ED abscess Meningitis	Occasional
Delivery system	
Device-related complications	E.g. catheter-related (fracture, kinking, displacement or withdrawal); pump failure (battery failure, mechanical failure, programming or refilling error)

MRI will cause programmable implanted pumps to malfunction. The rotor arm of the Medtronic Synchromed II pump is inactivated by a magnetic field but should restart when removed from it.[39,40] The Flowonix Prometra pump[41] needs to be emptied, filled with saline and turned off, because there is a risk that the pump contents will be dumped into the CSF. Guidance for the radiologist is available from the manufacturers; this includes safe MRI tesla ranges and pump orientation. The Medtronic pump will need to be interrogated after a scan to check that it has restarted; and the Flowonix refilled and restarted.

MANAGEMENT OF LIFE-THREATENING COMPLICATIONS

Clinicians caring for patients with spinal analgesia should be aware of potential life-threatening drug-related complications. Clinical areas should have resuscitation equipment including IV fluids, **naloxone** and **ephedrine** (Box A). However, hypotension and collapse in terminally ill patients with implantable IT pumps is more likely to be caused by other conditions, e.g. sepsis, CVS events.

Box A Emergency management of life-threatening complications

Stop spinal infusion.
Administer oxygen.
Obtain IV access.
If patient arrests, follow local resuscitation procedures.

Respiratory depression (sedation often precedes bradypnoea)
Sit the patient up.
If respiratory rate ≤8 breaths/min, the patient is barely rousable, and/or cyanosed, administer 100microgram boluses of IV naloxone every 2min until respiratory status is satisfactory (see p.457).
Further boluses may be necessary because naloxone is shorter acting than morphine and other spinal opioids.

Hypotension (systolic <80mmHg)
Lay patient flat (not head down).
Check heart rate: if <40 beats/min, treat bradycardia (below) *or*
If no evidence of fluid overload, give an IV fluid challenge, e.g. 500mL of a colloidal plasma expander over 30min.
Examine for alternative causes such as bleeding.
If no response to fluids, give ephedrine 6mg IV.

Bradycardia
ECG monitoring, if available.
Administer atropine (0.6mg boluses IV, up to total 3mg).
If atropine ineffective, give ephedrine 6mg IV.

MANAGEMENT OF UNDESIRABLE OPIOID EFFECTS

The transient undesirable effects seen when starting systemic opioids are also seen when starting spinal opioids *de novo* (see Strong opioids, Box B, p.365).[42] However, some undesirable effects are particularly associated with starting spinal opioid analgesia either *de novo* or after switching from a more traditional route.

Opioid discontinuation (diarrhoea, colic, sweating, restlessness)

Spinal delivery results in a massive reduction in the patient's total opioid dose. Laxatives should be discontinued and re-titrated. If peripheral withdrawal symptoms occur, approximately 25% of the pre-spinal systemic opioid should be given p.r.n.

Opioid-induced pruritus

This is generally a central reaction to opioids, and largely histamine-independent.[43] In surgical (opioid-naïve) patients who receive spinal opioids pre-operatively, the incidence is ≤80% but it is uncommon in patients with cancer pain.

If spinal opioid-induced pruritus occurs in a palliative care patient, consider:

- **ondansetron** 8mg IV stat and p.r.n. (or 8mg b.d. PO for 2 days)
- switching to an alternative opioid
- if all else fails, ultra-low dose **naloxone**:
  - ▷ titrate to effect using repeat IV bolus doses of 40microgram
  - ▷ if pruritus recurs, give 1microgram/kg/h by IVI (also see Chapter 26, p.757).[43]

Note. Ondansetron appears effective for pruritus associated with **morphine**, but not **fentanyl** or **sufentanil**.[44,45]

32

OTHER COMPLICATIONS

Suspected infection

Catheter-related infections can occur, often with coagulase + or – *Staphylococci.*

Exit site infection: transparent dressings allow the early identification of exit site erythema. Systemic and topical antibacterials should be started promptly; this reduces the incidence of deeper infection/meningitis. However, prophylactic antibacterials should *not* be routinely used.

ED abscesses: present with fever, escalating pain (this is invariable; either the original pain or back pain at the ED site, or both), and new neurological impairment. Evaluation includes blood cultures, aspiration of fluid from the spinal catheter for microscopy and culture, neurological examination, identification of other potential sources of fever and MRI (see warning about MRI above). Seek early advice from a microbiologist and spinal or neurosurgeon. The risk increases with time. Distant non-healing wounds may be a risk factor.

Meningitis: presents with fever and/or meningeal irritation (neck stiffness, stretch signs). Evaluation includes blood and line microscopy and cultures, WBC, neurological examination, and identification of other potential sources of fever. Also consider MRI, particularly if new neurological impairment is present (but see warning about MRI above). Spinal catheters need not be automatically removed and allow a means of obtaining CSF for culture. Mild meningeal irritation can be a normal phenomenon post-procedure, and patients can be safely observed while awaiting CSF cultures if they are systemically well and the above reveal no evidence of infection. A prolonged operation time when placing the catheter is a risk factor for serious catheter-related infection.

New neurological impairment

It can be difficult to distinguish between new neurological signs and symptoms caused by complications of spinal analgesia and those caused by disease progresssion (Box B). Disease-related neurological impairment is common: spinal cord compression occurs in ≤6% of patients receiving spinal analgesia. ED metastases are present in ≤70% of patients with refractory cancer pain. They are associated with motor impairment, and higher **morphine** and **bupivacaine** dose requirements (although not higher pain scores). Those with spinal canal stenosis (>50%) also have higher IT insertion complication rates.[46]

Catheter tip granulomas are lumps of inflammatory tissue formed in the lining of the thecal sac as a reaction to opioids. Granulomas may present as catheter occlusion (manifesting as renewed and increasing pain) or local mass effects (spinal cord or cauda equina compression with associated pain). They generally occur several months–years after starting a spinal infusion, with the risk increasing over time.[48] Pain typically precedes neurological impairment, which develops gradually over days–weeks.[49]

Granulomas are more common with ED infusions, and occur particularly with (less lipid soluble) **morphine** or **hydromorphone** at higher concentrations.[3] Animal studies indicate that using the *lowest concentration* of opioid and the *highest infusion rate* reduces the chance of granuloma formation. Granulomas often resolve spontaneously within a few weeks of stopping an infusion.

Box B Differential diagnosis of new neurological impairment in patients receiving spinal analgesia

Neurological damage caused by insertion of the catheter.
Bupivacaine-induced; dose-dependent, generally seen only when IT doses exceed 15mg/day, but unmasking of incipient spinal cord compression can occur with lower doses.[2,47]
Disease progression, e.g. cauda equina or spinal cord compression.
Catheter complication, e.g. ED abscess or haematoma, catheter tip granuloma.

Evaluation

Neurological examination: to confirm the location of the problem: is it related to the catheter or could it be a separate second phenomenon?

Time of onset (after starting infusion):
- immediate: spinal medication, 'unmasking' of subclinical impairment, or neurological damage at insertion
- after days–weeks or longer: ED abscess, haematoma, or disease progression
- after several months–years: catheter tip granuloma.

Investigation: MRI = optimum (but see warning on p.844).

The risk of a granuloma may also be lowered by using:
- a bolus-based regimen
- **clonidine** as an opioid-sparing agent.

In the absence of neurological impairment, treatment options include catheter tip relocation, opioid dose reduction and/or considering a non-opioid. Surgical excision may be necessary if symptoms persist or there is neurological impairment.[16]

Exacerbation of pain

A sudden increase in pain should be initially treated with p.r.n. opioid medication PO/SC while the cause is investigated. Possibilities include:
- worsening of the original pain
- development of a new pain because of:
  - ▷ disease progression or co-morbidity
  - ▷ spinal catheter-related abscess, haematoma or granuloma
- reduced effect of the infusion
  - ▷ catheter dislodgement or disconnection
  - ▷ delivery device malfunction
  - ▷ tolerance developing to the drugs; seen with both opioids and **bupivacaine** when given as continuous infusions.

Plain radiographs may show a kinked, dislodged or disconnected catheter. Catheter position and patency can be confirmed by injection of a radiological contrast agent after first aspirating the catheter dead-space to avoid delivery of the dead-space contents as a bolus. The contrast agent must be appropriate for CSF use; *IT delivery of inappropriate radiological contrast agents can cause arachnoiditis and death.*

Delivery device malfunction may involve:
- a problem with the catheter (kinking, fracture, displacement, occlusion)
- an empty syringe (problem with last refill, altered delivery rate or calendar error about next refill date)
- a problem with the pump itself (battery failure, mechanical failure).

The function of the rotor arm of the Medtronic Synchromed II pump can be checked using fluoroscopy. After a static image is taken, the pump is programmed to deliver at the maximum rate of infusion, and another static image is taken a few minutes later. If the rotor arm is turning then it will be in a different position on the second image. It moves too slowly to be visible on a continuous screening mode. The infusion can then be reprogrammed to the rate intended.

RECORD KEEPING

It is recommended that monitoring charts are used with spinal infusions, comparable with those widely used for checking CSCI (see p.826). The use of a spinal chart should be cross-referenced on the patient's main prescription chart, and should list the drugs being infused.

The National Neuromodulation Registry for record keeping with implanted IT pumps includes patient demographics, drug doses, outcome data (global perceived effect with standardized measures of pain and quality of life), complications and revisions. The Royal College of Anaesthetists also has suggestions for monitoring and auditing spinal analgesia in its compendium of audit recipes.[50]

1 Kurita GP *et al.* (2011) Spinal opioids in adult patients with cancer pain: a systematic review: a European Palliative Care Research Collaborative (EPCRC) opioid guidelines project. *Palliative Medicine.* **25**: 560–577.

2 British Pain Society (2007) Intrathecal drug delivery for the management of pain and spasticity in adults; recommendations for best clinical practice. The British Pain Society. Available from: www.britishpainsociety.org

3 Deer TR *et al.* (2012) Polyanalgesic Consensus Conference 2012: recommendations for the management of pain by intrathecal (intraspinal) drug delivery: report of an interdisciplinary expert panel. *Neuromodulation.* **15**: 436–466.

4 Deer TR *et al.* (2017) The Polyanalgesic Consensus Conference (PACC): Recommendations on intrathecal drug infusion systems best practices and guidelines. *Neuromodulation.* **20**: 96–132.

5 Lynch L (2014) Intrathecal drug delivery for cancer pain. In: *Practical Management of Complex Cancer Pain.* Eds. Manohar Sharma, Karen Simpson, Michael Bennett, and Sanjeeva Gupta. Oxford, Oxford University Press, pp. 197–225.

6 Crul BJP and Delhaas EM (1991) Technical complications during long term subarachnoid or epidural administration of morphine in terminally ill cancer patients: A review of 140 cases. *Regional Anesthesia.* **16**: 209–213.

7 Hsu Y *et al.* (2012) The frequency and magnitude of cerebrospinal fluid pulsations influence intrathecal drug distribution: key factors for interpatient variability. *Anesthesia and Analgesia.* **115**: 386–394.

8 Tagen KM (2015) CNS wide simulation of low resistance and drug transport due to spinal microanatomy. *Journal Biomechanics.* **48**: 2144–2154.

9 Hettiarachchi HD *et al.* (2011) The effect of pulsatile flow on intrathecal drug delivery in the spinal canal. *Annals of Biomedical Engineering.* **39**: 2592–2602.

10 Wallace M and Yaksh TL (2012) Characteristics of distribution of morphine and metabolites in cerebrospinal fluid and plasma with chronic intrathecal morphine infusion in humans. *Anesthesia and Analgesia.* **115**: 797–804.

11 Bernards CM (2006) Cerebrospinal fluid and spinal cord distribution of baclofen and bupivacaine during slow intrathecal infusion in pigs. *Anesthesiology.* **105**: 169–178.

12 Flack SH *et al.* (2011) Morphine distribution in the spinal cord after chronic infusion in pigs. *Anesthesia and Analgesia.* **112**: 460–464.

13 NPSA (National Patient Safety Agency) (2011) Safer spinal (intrathecal), epidural and regional devices. In: Patient Safety Alert Update PSA001. Available from: www.nrls.npsa.nhs.uk

14 Department of Health (2010) Mixing of medicines prior to administration in clinical practice: medical and non-medical prescribing. HMSO, London. Available from: www.gov.uk

15 National Prescribing Centre (2010) Mixing of medicines prior to administration in clinical practice - responding to legislative changes. Liverpool.

16 Deer TR *et al.* (2012) Polyanalgesic Consensus Conference--2012: consensus on diagnosis, detection, and treatment of catheter-tip granulomas (inflammatory masses). *Neuromodulation.* **15**: 483–495.

17 Bujedo BM (2014) Spinal opioid bioavailability in postoperative pain. *Pain Practice.* **14**: 350–364.

18 Zamponi GW *et al.* (2015) The physiology, pathology, and pharmacology of voltage-gated calcium channels and their future therapeutic potential. *Pharmacological Reviews.* **67**: 821–870.

19 Takasusuki T and Yaksh TL (2011) Regulation of spinal substance P release by intrathecal calcium channel blockade. *Anesthesiology.* **115**: 153–164.

20 Smith TJ *et al.* (2002) Randomized clinical trial of an implantable drug delivery system compared with comprehensive medical management for refractory cancer pain: impact on pain, drug-related toxicity, and survival. *Journal of Clinical Oncology.* **20**: 4040–4049.

21 Staats PS *et al.* (2004) Intrathecal ziconotide in the treatment of refractory pain in patients with cancer or AIDS: a randomized controlled trial. *JAMA.* **291**: 63–70.

22 Vranken JH *et al.* (2005) Neuropathological findings after continuous intrathecal administration of S(+)-ketamine for the management of neuropathic cancer pain. *Pain.* **117**: 231–235.

23 Vranken JH *et al.* (2006) Severe toxic damage to the rabbit spinal cord after intrathecal administration of preservative-free S(+)-ketamine. *Anesthesiology.* **105**: 813–818.

24 Mehta A and Kay E (1996) Admixtures' storage is extended. *Pharmacy in Practice.* **6**: 113–118.

25 Trissel LA *et al.* (2002) Physical and chemical stability of low and high concentrations of morphine sulfate with bupivacaine hydrochloride packaged in plastic syringes. *International Journal of Pharmaceutical Compounding.* Jan-Feb: 70–73.

26 Xu Quanyun A *et al.* (2002) Physical and chemical stability of low and high concentrations of morphine sulfate with clonidine hydrochloride packaged in plastic syringes. *International Journal of Pharmaceutical Compounding.* Jan-Feb: 66–69.

27 Christen C *et al.* (1996) Stability of bupivacaine hydrochloride and hydromorphone hydrochloride during simulated epidural coadministration. *American Journal of Health System Pharmacy.* **53**: 170–173.

28 Trissel LA. *Handbook on Injectable Drugs.* Maryland, USA: American Society of Health System Pharmacists (accessed March 2017).

29 Hildebrand KR *et al.* (2003) Stability and compatibility of morphine-clonidine admixtures in an implantable infusion system. *Journal of Pain and Symptom Management.* **25**: 464–471.

30 Classen AM *et al.* (2004) Stability of admixture containing morphine sulfate, bupivacaine hydrochloride, and clonidine hydrochloride in an implantable infusion system. *Journal of Pain and Symptom Management.* **28**: 603–611.

31 Hildebrand KR *et al.* (2001) Stability and compatibility of hydromorphone hydrochloride in animplantable infusion system. *Journal of Pain and Symptom Management.* **22**: 1042–1047.
32 Rudich Z *et al.* (2004) Stability of clonidine in clonidine-hydromorphone mixture from implanted intrathecal infusion pumps in chronic pain patients. *Journal of Pain and Symptom Management.* **28**: 599–602.
33 Naumann C (1999) Drug adverse events and system complications of intrathecal opioid delivery for pain: origins, detection, manifestations and management. *Neuromodulation.* **2**: 92–107.
34 Paice JA *et al.* (1996) Intraspinal morphine for chronic pain: a retrospective, multicenter study. *Journal of Pain and Symptom Management.* **11**: 71–80.
35 Abs R *et al.* (2000) Endocrine consequences of long-term intrathecal administration of opioids. *Journal of Clinical Endocrinology and Metabolism.* **85**: 2215–2222.
36 Budd K and Shipton E (2004) Acute pain and the immune system and opioimmunosuppression. *Acute Pain.* **6**: 123–135.
37 Cook TM *et al.* (2009) Major complications of central neuraxial block: report on the Third National Audit Project of the Royal College of Anaesthetists. *British Journal of Anaesthesia.* **102**: 179–190.
38 Holmfred A *et al.* (2006) Intrathecal catheters with subcutaneous port systems in patients with severe cancer-related pain managed out of hospital: the risk of infection. *Journal of Pain and Symptom Management.* **31**: 568–572.
39 Nitescu P *et al.* (1995) Complications of intrathecal opioids and bupivacaine in the treatment of "refractory" cancer pain. *Clinical Journal of Pain.* **11**: 45–62.
40 MHRA (2008) Implantable drug pumps manufactured by Medtronic - Synchro EL models 8626 and 8627 and SynchroMed II model 8637. *Medical Device Alert.* MDA/2008/2087. www.gov.uk/drug-device-alerts
41 MHRA (2009) Effects of MRI on implantable drug pumps. *Drug Safety Update.* www.gov.uk/drug-safety-update
42 Rawal N *et al.* (1987) Present state of extradural and intrathecal opioid analgesia in Sweden. A nationwide follow-up survey. *British Journal of Anaesthesia.* **59**: 791–799.
43 Reich A and Szepietowski JC (2010) Opioid-induced pruritus: an update. *Clinical Experimental Dermatology.* **35**: 2–6.
44 Borgeat A and Stimemann H-R (1999) Ondansetron is effective to treat spinal or epidural morphine-induced pruritus. *Anesthesiology.* **90**: 432–436.
45 Prin M *et al.* (2016) Prophylactic ondansetron for the prevention of intrathecal fentanyl- or sufentanil-mediated pruritus: a meta-analysis of randomized trials. *Anesthesia and Analgesia.* **122**: 402–409.
46 Appelgren L *et al.* (1997) Spinal epidural metastasis: implications for spinal analgesia to treat "refractory" cancer pain. *Journal of Pain and Symptom Management.* **13**: 25–42.
47 van Dongen RTM *et al.* (1997) Neurological impairment during long-term intrathecal infusion of bupivacaine in cancer patients: a sign of spinal cord compression. *Pain.* **69**: 205–209.
48 Deer TR (2004) A prospective analysis of intrathecal granulomas in chronic pain patients: a review of the literature and report of a surveillance study. *Pain Physician.* **7**: 225–228.
49 Miele VJ *et al.* (2006) A review of intrathecal morphine therapy related granulomas. *European Journal of Pain.* **10**: 251–261.
50 Lynch L and Grady K (2012) Intrathecal drug delivery in the management of cancer-related pain. In: *Raising the Standard: a compendium of audit recipes.* Colvin JR and Peden CJ. London, Royal College of Anaesthetists, pp 336–337.

Updated September 2017

Appendix 1: Anaphylaxis

Anaphylaxis is an acute, life-threatening, systemic allergic or hypersensitivity reaction. It develops rapidly in minutes or, at most, a few hours. It manifests as hypotension (fainting, collapse, loss of consciousness), and/or respiratory difficulty (laryngeal and bronchial constriction).[1]

Pathophysiology

Anaphylaxis is caused by the sudden release of numerous inflammatory mediators from mast cells and basophils into the systemic circulation. This results in:

- vasodilation, hypotension, capillary leakage (leading to cardiovascular collapse)
- mucosal and laryngeal oedema, bronchoconstriction (leading to respiratory difficulty).[1]

Most commonly, the allergic reaction results from the interaction of an allergen with specific IgE antibodies bound to mast cells and basophils, leading to the release of:

- preformed chemical mediators, e.g. chymase, histamine, tryptase
- newly synthesized mediators, e.g. cytokines, leukotrienes, platelet activating factor, prostaglandins.

Anaphylaxis may also be caused by other immunological mechanisms, e.g. IgG-antigen complexes. Some drugs, e.g. NSAIDs, can cause direct activation of mast cells. Other non-immunological triggers of anaphylaxis include exercise and cold.[2] Non-IgE reactions are sometimes called *anaphylactoid reactions*. However, in Europe, the term is no longer used. In terms of management, it is *not* necessary to identify the precise trigger; the difference is relevant only when investigations are being considered.[3]

Anaphylaxis is:

- specific to a given drug or chemically-related class of drugs
- more likely after parenteral drug administration
- more frequent in patients taking β-blockers (see p.853), or who have **aspirin**-induced asthma or systemic lupus erythematosus
- more severe in patients with concomitant illness, particularly upper respiratory tract infections, chronic respiratory diseases.

Anaphylaxis is rare in palliative care. When it occurs, it is generally associated with antibacterials (see p.471) or an NSAID (see p.321). Although refined arachis (peanut) oil is unlikely to cause an allergic reaction, a possible case has been recorded in a woman with known peanut allergy who received an **arachis oil** enema.[4] **Chlorhexidine** has also been implicated, including after the use of a **chlorhexidine** skin wipe.[5]

Clinical features

Anaphylaxis is likely when the following criteria are met after exposure to a possible trigger:

- sudden onset and rapid progression (minutes–few hours)
- life-threatening circulatory or respiratory problems
- skin and/or mucosal changes (Box A).[1,6]

Before progressing to life-threatening respiratory or circulatory problems, patients with a history of anaphylaxis may present with:

- sudden onset and rapidly progressing skin and/or mucosal changes plus GI symptoms (abdominal pain, colic, vomiting) *or*
- hypotension alone.[1,7]

The differential diagnosis of anaphylaxis is extensive but includes:

- life-threatening conditions, e.g. severe asthma, septic shock, seizure
- non life-threatening conditions, e.g. urticaria or angioedema, vasovagal episode, panic attack.[8]

Lack of a complete history or definite diagnosis should not delay initial treatment.

Box A Clinical features of anaphylaxis

Essential

Sudden onset of life-threatening circulatory *and/or* respiratory problems, e.g.

Circulatory problems	**Respiratory problems**
Tachycardia	Airway
Hypotension	pharyngeal/laryngeal oedema
Shock	hoarse voice
Decreased consciousness	stridor
Cardiac arrest	Breathing
	breathlessness
	wheeze/bronchospasm (10%)
	cyanosis
	respiratory arrest

Probable	**Possible**
Skin/mucosal changes (80%):	Agitation
flushing or pallor	Confusion
erythema of skin	Abdominal pain
itching	Vomiting
urticaria	Diarrhoea
angioedema[a], mostly face, hands, feet	Incontinence
	Tingling of the extremities
	Rhinitis
	Conjunctivitis

a. angioedema is swelling in the dermis, subcutaneous and submucosal tissues.

Management

National guidelines vary; the advice here is based on guidance published by the UK Resuscitation Council[6] and NICE.[9,10] Drugs and basic resuscitation equipment for treatment of anaphylaxis must be available in all clinical settings, either as part of a resuscitation kit or in an 'anaphylaxis box'. Urgent treatment with three drugs is required:

1. **Adrenaline** (epinephrine); *of paramount importance because it saves lives*
2. **Chlorphenamine** (or other H_1-antihistamine)
3. **Hydrocortisone** (Box B).

Adrenaline (epinephrine), a direct-acting sympathomimetic, is effective in attenuating anaphylaxis if given promptly and in sufficient dose.[6] Through its α_1-receptor agonist effects, it causes vasoconstriction, increases peripheral vascular resistance and reduces mucosal oedema. As a β_1 agonist, it increases the rate and force of myocardial contraction. As a β_2 agonist, it dilates bronchial airways, increases glycogenolysis and suppresses activity of mast cells, reducing the release of histamine and other inflammatory mediators.

Adrenaline is given by IM injection (Box B). If there is doubt about the adequacy of the circulation, **adrenaline** can be given as a dilute IV solution, i.e. 1 in 10,000 (100microgram/mL), *using 50microgram (0.5mL) boluses, titrated to response.*

If given too rapidly, IV **adrenaline** can cause ventricular arrhythmias, cardiac ischaemia, and hypertension. Thus, IV **adrenaline** should be given only by doctors experienced in its use and where full intensive care facilities are available.[6,11]

Box B Management of anaphylaxis in adults

1 Discontinue administration of any potential causal agent, e.g. IVI antibacterial or blood product.

2 **Adrenaline (epinephrine)** IM *every 5min* until blood pressure, pulse and breathing are satisfactory:
- use 1:1,000 (1mg/1mL), give 500microgram (0.5mL) *or*
- give 300microgram (0.3mL) if an adrenaline (epinephrine) auto-injector is used.

Administer into the anterolateral aspect of the middle third of the thigh.[4] If given promptly, patients rarely need >3 doses of 500microgram.[2]

3 Position patient on back (or semi-reclining if breathless or vomiting) with legs elevated

4 **Chlorphenamine** IM or IV to counter histamine-induced vasodilation and bronchoconstriction:
- give 10mg over 1min
- if necessary, repeat up to a maximum of 40mg/24h.[11]

5 **Hydrocortisone sodium succinate** IM or slowly IV over 1–10min:
- give 200mg for patients with bronchospasm, and for all severe or recurrent reactions to prevent further deterioration
- *takes up to 6h to act.*

6 In severe cases of anaphylaxis, additional treatment (Box C) and transfer to hospital will be necessary.

7 If cardiorespiratory arrest occurs, start cardiopulmonary resuscitation if appropriate to the patient's circumstances (e.g. taking prognosis, stated wishes into consideration). Use doses of *diluted IV* adrenaline as recommended in Advanced Life Support guidelines; *IM* adrenaline is not recommended after a cardiac arrest.

Box C Supplementary measures for anaphylaxis

Patients should be treated using the Airway, Breathing, Circulation, Disability, Exposure (ABCDE approach).

Administer oxygen (>10L/min).

Insert an IV cannula or butterfly needle. If the patient is hypotensive give 0.9% saline 500mL–1L IV fluid over 10min.[12] Repeat if blood pressure remains low.

If bronchospasm does not respond to three-drug management (see Box B), give a nebulized β_2 agonist, e.g. salbutamol 5mg, every 20min or as necessary.

If bronchospasm does not respond to nebulized salbutamol, consider a slow IV injection of salbutamol 250microgram diluted to 5mL with WFI, or a nebulized antimuscarinic bronchodilator, e.g. ipratropium bromide 500microgram, repeated as necessary.[3,11]

Occasionally, emergency tracheotomy and assisted respiration are necessary.

Because 5% patients have biphasic anaphylactic reactions, monitor pulse, blood pressure, pulse oximetry and ECG tracings for 6–12h, ideally in a clinical area with full resuscitation facilities.

Patients taking β-blockers (β-adrenergic receptor blocking drugs), TCAs or MAOIs

Patients taking β-blockers, particularly non-cardioselective ones, are at increased risk of severe anaphylaxis because the β-receptor-mediated effects of **adrenaline** are blunted. Further, unopposed stimulation of α-receptors, with reflex vagotonic effects, may lead to bradycardia, coronary artery constriction, *hypertension* and intracerebral haemorrhage. TCAs and MAOIs potentiate **adrenaline** and increase the risk of cardiac arrhythmias.

Previous UK anaphylaxis guidelines recommended halving the dose of **adrenaline** given to patients on β-blockers, TCAs and MAOIs. However, current guidelines note the large inter-individual variation in response to **adrenaline**, and this recommendation has been withdrawn. Patients on these drugs should be given a full initial dose of **adrenaline**, and further doses titrated according to the initial response.[6]

For patients taking β-blockers and unresponsive to **adrenaline**, give **glucagon** 1–2mg SC, IM or IV every 5min, or as an IV infusion. **Glucagon** has β-receptor independent inotropic, chronotropic and vaso-active effects.[6,10] These patients in particular may not respond to nebulized **salbutamol** and may require IV **salbutamol** or nebulized **ipratropium bromide** (see Box C).[6,11]

Follow-up

After the successful treatment of the acute event, other measures need to be considered (Box D).

Box D Follow-up

If the patient's prognosis is months rather than weeks, take serial blood samples for mast cell tryptase, the first as soon as possible after starting emergency treatment, a second sample 1–2 hours after the onset of symptoms and a third sample after 24 hours or at specialist follow up. Tryptase levels are elevated in only about 60% adults with clinically confirmed anaphylaxis. Refer to an allergy clinic prior to discharge.[6,9]

To reduce the chance of a further anaphylactic reaction, particularly in patients with a history of urticaria, consider prescribing a 3 day course of:

- chlorphenamine 4mg PO q6h (maximum 24mg/24h) *and*
- dexamethasone 8mg once daily for 1 week.[6,13]

If a patient has frequent idiopathic anaphylaxis, e.g. ≥2 in two months or ≥6 episodes in a year, continue both:

- chlorphenamine 4mg PO q6h (maximum 24mg/24h) for 2–3 months *and*
- dexamethasone 8mg once daily for 1 week and, then, if no further episodes of anaphylaxis or urticaria/angioedema occur, tail off over 2 weeks.[13]

Advise patients to avoid the suspected environmental, dietary or drug trigger.

Provide information about recognizing and managing an anaphylactic reaction.

Unless definitely caused by a drug or blood product, supply the patient with an adrenaline auto-injector, e.g. EpiPen, and demonstrate how to use it.[9]

Adrenaline auto-injectors are device-specific in terms of injection technique, thus the patient should continue to use the same brand.

1 Simons FE *et al.* (2015) 2015 update of the evidence base: World Allergy Organization anaphylaxis guidelines. *World Allergy Organization Journal*. **8**: 32–47.
2 Simons FE and Sheikh A (2013) Anaphylaxis: the acute episode and beyond. *British Medical Journal*. **346**: f602.
3 Khan BQ and Kemp SF (2011) Pathophysiology of anaphylaxis. *Current Opinion in Allergy and Clinical Immunology*. **11**: 319–325.
4 Pharmax (1998) *Data on file*.
5 MHRA (2012) All medical devices and medicinal products containing chlorhexidine. *Medical Devices Alert*. MDA/2012/2075 www.mhra.gov.uk/Safetyinformation
6 Resuscitation Council (UK) (2008) Emergency treatment of anaphylactic reactions *Guidelines for healthcare providers*. www.resus.org.uk/pages/mediMain.htm
7 Simons FE *et al.* (2011) World Allergy Organization anaphylaxis guidelines: summary. *Journal of Allergy and Clinical Immunology*. **127**: 587-593 e581–522.
8 Rutkowski K *et al.* (2012) Anaphylaxis: current state of knowledge for the modern physician. *Postgraduate Medical Journal*. **88**: 458–464.
9 NICE (2011) Anaphylaxis. Assessment to confirm an anaphylactic episode and the decision to refer after emergency treatment for a suspected anaphylactic episode. *Clinical Guideline*. CG134 www.nice.org.uk
10 Soar J (2009) Emergency treatment of anaphylaxis in adults: concise guidance. *Clinical Medicine*. **9**: 181–185.
11 British National Formulary Section 3.4.3 Anaphylaxis. London : BMJ Group and Pharmaceutical Press www.medicinescomplete.com (accessed February 2017).
12 Perel P *et al.* (2013) Colloids versus crystalloids for fluid resuscitation in critically ill patients. *Cochrane Database of Systematic Reviews*. **2**: CD000567. www.thechochranelibrary.com
13 Poon M and Reid C (2004) Best evidence topic reports. Oral corticosteroids in acute urticaria. *Emergency Medical Journal*. **21**: 76–77.

Updated March 2017

Appendix 2: Opioid dose conversion ratios

A2

General approach

It is crucial to appreciate that conversion ratios are *never* more than an approximate guide. Thus, careful monitoring during conversion is necessary to avoid both underdosing and excessive dosing. Also see Opioid switching ('rotation'), p.370.

This chapter provides a summary of selected opioid dose conversion ratios. These can be used to calculate equivalent doses of opioids when switching from a weak opioid to **morphine**, or from one strong opioid to another. Caution is always necessary. Conversion ratios are *never* more than an approximate guide because of:

- wide interindividual variation in opioid pharmacokinetics; influencing factors include age, ethnicity, renal or hepatic impairment
- other variables including dose and duration of opioid treatment, direction of switch in opioid, nutritional status and concurrent medications
- their method of derivation, e.g. single dose rather than chronic dose studies using a range of clinical doses.

Careful monitoring is particularly necessary when:

- switching at high doses
- there has been a recent rapid escalation of the first opioid
- switching to **methadone**.

Explicit guidance on switching opioids is difficult because both the reasons for switching and the patient's circumstances differ. One guideline, based on expert consensus, recommends routinely reducing the calculated equivalent dose of the new opioid by 25–50% (see p.370). Various patient factors are then taken into account to modify the rule, e.g. no reduction in a young patient in severe pain switching at low dose, or an even bigger reduction in an older delirious patient in moderate pain switching at high dose.

Certainly, a dose reduction of at least 50% would seem prudent when switching at high doses (e.g. **morphine** or equivalent doses of ≥1g/24h), in elderly or frail patients, because of intolerable undesirable effects (e.g. delirium), or when there has been a recent rapid escalation of the first opioid (possibly due to opioid-induced hyperalgesia). In such circumstances, p.r.n. doses can be relied on to make up any deficit while re-titrating to a satisfactory dose of the new opioid.

A separate strategy is necessary for **methadone** (see p.437).

Determining the dose of the second opioid

Select the appropriate Table based on the routes of administration:

Route	*Table*	*Page*
PO to PO	1	857
PO to TD	2	858
PO to SC/IV	3	861
SC/IV to SC/IV	4	862

The Tables relate mainly to switching to or from **morphine**. If switching from an opioid other than **morphine** to another opioid, it will be necessary to convert the dose of the first opioid to **morphine** equivalents, and then use that quantity to determine the dose of the second opioid.
With any switch:

- round the calculated dose up or down to the nearest convenient dose of the formulation concerned, e.g. tablet, TD patch, ampoule
- decide on an appropriate p.r.n. dose.

The conversion ratios in this chapter are based on referenced sources given in the various individual opioid monographs. Where these differ significantly from the manufacturers' recommended ratios, the latter are included for comparison.

Table 1 *PCF* recommended dose conversion ratios: PO to PO. Before use, see General approach (p.855)

Conversion	*Ratio*	*Calculation*	*Example*	*Monograph*
Codeine to morphine	10:1	Divide 24h codeine dose by 10	Codeine 240mg/24h PO → morphine 24mg/24h PO	Codeine, p.349
Dihydrocodeine to morphine	10:1	Divide 24h dihydrocodeine dose by 10	Dihydrocodeine 240mg/24h PO → morphine 24mg/24h PO	Dihydrocodeine, p.352
Hydrocodone to morphine	1.5:1	Divide 24h hydrocodone dose by 1.5 (i.e. decrease dose by 1/3)	Hydrocodone 60mg/24h PO → morphine 40mg/24h PO	Not UK
Tramadol to morphine	10:1	Divide 24h tramadol dose by 10	Tramadol 400mg/24h PO → morphine 40mg/24h PO	Tramadol, p.354
Morphine to hydromorphone	5:1	Divide 24h morphine dose by 5	Morphine 60mg/24h PO → hydromorphone 12mg/24h PO	Hydromorphone, p.434
	7.5:1[a]	*Divide 24h morphine dose by 7.5*	*Morphine 60mg/24h PO* *→ hydromorphone 8mg/24h PO*	Hydromorphone, p.434
Morphine to methadone	Variable	See methadone, p.437		
Morphine to oxycodone	1.5:1	Divide 24h morphine dose by 1.5 (i.e. decrease dose by 1/3)	Morphine 60mg/24h PO → oxycodone 40mg/24h PO	Oxycodone, p.447
	2:1[a]	*Divide 24h morphine dose by 2*	*Morphine 60mg/24h PO* → oxycodone 30mg/24h PO	Oxycodone, p.447

a. italicized entries = manufacturers' recommendations.

A2

Table 2 *PCF* recommended dose conversion ratios: PO to TD. Before use, see General approach (p.855)

Conversion	*Ratio*	*Calculation*	*Example*	*Monograph*
Morphine to buprenorphine	100:1	Multiply 24h morphine dose in mg by 10 to obtain 24h buprenorphine dose in microgram; divide answer by 24 to obtain microgram/h patch strength	Morphine 300mg/24h PO → buprenorphine 3,000microgram/24h →125microgram/h; *round up* to 70microgram/h x 2 or *round down* to 70 + 35microgram/h patches	Buprenorphine, p.397
	75–115:1[a]	*Use the manufacturer's guidelines in SPC, summarized in Box A, p.859*		Buprenorphine, p.397
Morphine to fentanyl	100:1	Multiply 24h morphine dose in mg by 10 to obtain 24h fentanyl dose in microgram; divide answer by 24 to obtain microgram/h patch strength	Morphine 300mg/24h PO → fentanyl 3,000microgram/24h → 125microgram/h; give as 100+25microgram/h patches	Fentanyl, p.409
	100:1 or 150:1[a,b]	*Use the manufacturer's guidelines in SPC, summarized in Box B, p.860*	*For 150:1, the fentanyl dose will be smaller than that obtained with 100:1*	Fentanyl, p.409

a. italicized entries = manufacturers' recommendations

b. recommended ratio varies according to the duration of use of the previous strong opioid, see Box B, p.860.

For determining the appropriate p.r.n. morphine dose for patients receiving TD buprenorphine or TD fentanyl, see p.397 and 409 respectively.

Box A Summary of manufacturers' recommendations for starting TD buprenorphine (for full details, see specific SPC)[a]

BuTrans® 5, 10, 15 and 20microgram/h TD buprenorphine patch

Patients aged 18 years and over

The lowest BuTrans® dose (BuTrans® 5microgram/h TD patch) should be used as the initial dose. Consideration should be given to the previous opioid history of the patient as well as to the current general condition and medical status of the patient.

Conversion from opioids

BuTrans® can be used as an alternative to treatment with other opioids. Such patients should be started on the lowest available dose (BuTrans® 5microgram/h TD patch) and continue taking short-acting supplemental analgesics during titration, as required.

Transtec® 35, 52.5 and 70microgram/h TD buprenorphine patch

Patients over 18 years of age

The dose should be adapted to the condition of the individual patient (pain intensity, suffering, individual reaction). The lowest possible dose providing adequate pain relief should be given.

Conversion from opioids

Patients on a Step II (weak opioid) analgesic should begin with buprenorphine 35microgram/h TD. The administration of a non-opioid analgesic can be continued, depending on the patient's overall medical condition.

When switching from a Step III (strong opioid) analgesic to buprenorphine TD, the nature of the previous medication, administration and the mean daily dose should be taken into account in order to avoid the recurrence of pain. It is generally advisable to titrate the dose individually, starting with the lowest TD patch strength (35microgram/h). Clinical experience has shown that patients who were previously treated with higher doses of a strong opioid (approximately 120mg oral morphine per day) may start therapy with the next higher TD patch strength (i.e. 52.5microgram/h).

Sufficient supplementary immediate release analgesics should be made available during dose titration.

The necessary strength of buprenorphine TD must be adapted to the requirements of the individual patient and checked at regular intervals.

After application of the first buprenorphine TD patch the buprenorphine serum concentrations rise slowly and there is unlikely to be a rapid onset of effect. Consequently, a first evaluation of the analgesic effect should only be made after 24h.

The previous analgesic medication (with the exception of transdermal opioids) should be given in the same dose during the first 12h after switching to TD and appropriate rescue medication given on demand in the following 12h.

a. several branded generic products are available which follow the same recommendations; see individual SPC.

Box B Summary of manufacturer's recommendations for starting Durogesic DTrans® (for full details see SPC)[a]

Durogesic DTrans® 12/25/50/75/100microgram/h TD fentanyl patch

Adults:

Initial dose selection

The initial Durogesic DTrans® dose should be based on the patient's current opioid use, degree of opioid tolerance and the stability of their clinical status.

In opioid-naïve patients, generally, the TD route is not recommended and patients should be titrated with an immediate-release opioid to a dose equivalent to Durogesic Dtrans® 12–25microgram/h before switching to Durogesic DTrans®. When this is not possible, use an initial dose of 12microgram/h.

In opioid-tolerant patients, the initial dose of Durogesic DTrans® should be based on the previous 24h opioid analgesic requirement, expressed as the oral 24h morphine equivalent. The dose of Durogesic DTrans® is then derived from Tables 1 and 2 according to the patient's clinical status:

Table 1 Adults who have a need for opioid rotation (e.g. because of undesirable effects) or who are less clinically stable (conversion ratio of morphine PO to fentanyl TD of about 150:1)

Oral 24h morphine (mg/24h)	*Durogesic DTrans® (microgram/h)*
<90	12
90–134	25
135–224	50
225–314	75
315–404	100
405–494	125
495–584	150
585–674	175
675–764	200
765–854	225
855–944	250
945–1034	275
1035–1124	300

Table 2 Adults on a stable and well-tolerated opioid regimen (conversion ratio of morphine PO to fentanyl TD of about 100:1)

Oral 24h morphine (mg/24h)	*Durogesic DTrans® (microgram/h)*
≤44	12
45–89	25
90–149	50
150–209	75
210–269	100
270–329	125
330–389	150
390–449	175
450–509	200
510–569	225
570–629	250
630–689	275
690–749	300

Previous analgesic therapy should be phased out gradually from the time of the first patch application until analgesic efficacy with Durogesic DTrans® is attained. The initial evaluation of the analgesic effect of Durogesic DTrans® should not be made until the patch has been worn for 24h due to the gradual increase in serum fentanyl concentrations up to this time.

a. guidance varies between brands of TD fentanyl; see individual SPC.

Table 3 *PCF* recommended dose conversion ratios; PO to SC/IV. Before use, see General approach (p.855)

Conversion	*Ratio*	*Calculation*	*Example*	**Monograph**
Hydromorphone to hydromorphone	2:1[a]	Divide 24h hydromorphone dose by 2	Hydromorphone 32mg/24h PO → hydromorphone 16mg/24h SC/IV	Hydromorphone, p.434
	3:1[b]	*Divide 24h hydromorphone dose by 3*	*Hydromorphone 32mg/24h PO → hydromorphone 10mg/24h SC/IV*	Hydromorphone, p.434
Methadone to methadone	2:1[c]	Divide 24h methadone dose by 2	Methadone 30mg/24h PO → methadone 15mg/24h SC/IV	Methadone, p.437
Morphine to alfentanil	30:1	Divide 24h morphine dose by 30	Morphine 60mg/24h PO → alfentanil 2mg/24h SC/IV	Alfentanil, p.390
Morphine to diamorphine	3:1	Divide 24h morphine dose by 3	Morphine 60mg/24h PO → diamorphine 20mg/24h SC/IV	Diamorphine, p.387
Morphine to fentanyl	Variable[d,e]	Divide 24h morphine dose in mg by 100–150	Morphine 60mg/24h PO → fentanyl 400microgram/24h SC/IV	Fentanyl, p.409
Morphine to hydromorphone	10:1	Divide 24h morphine dose by 10	Morphine 60mg/24h PO → hydromorphone 6mg/24h SC/IV	Hydromorphone, p.434
Morphine to methadone	Variable	See methadone, p.437		
Morphine to morphine	2:1	Divide 24h morphine dose by 2	Morphine 60mg/24h PO → morphine 30mg/24h SC/IV	Morphine, p.375
Morphine to oxycodone	2:1	Divide 24h morphine dose by 2	Morphine 60mg/24h PO → oxycodone 30mg/24h SC/IV	Oxycodone, p.447
Oxycodone to oxycodone	1.5:1[f]	Divide 24h oxycodone dose by 1.5 (i.e. decrease dose by 1/3)	Oxycodone 30mg/24h PO → oxycodone 20mg/24h SC/IV	Oxycodone, p.447
	2:1[b]	*Divide 24h oxycodone dose by 2*	*Oxycodone 30mg/24h PO → oxycodone 15mg/24h SC/IV*	Oxycodone, p.447

a. because mean oral bio-availability is 50% (range 35–60%), some centres use a conversion ratio of 2:1 rather than 3:1
b. italicized entry = manufacturer's recommendation
c. because mean oral bio-availability is 80% (range 40–100%), some centres use 1:1, e.g. methadone 30mg/24h PO g methadone 30mg/24h SC/IV, see p.437
d. the same conversion ratios as for morphine PO to fentanyl TD can be used for morphine PO to fentanyl SC/IV, see Table 2, p.858
e. volume constraints for a syringe driver may prevent doses >500microgram/24h being used; alfentanil is an alternative
f. because mean oral bio-availability is 75% (range 60–87%), some centres use a conversion ratio of 1.5:1 rather than 2:1.

A2

Table 4 *PCF* recommended dose conversion ratios; SC/IV to SC/IV. Before use, see General approach (p.855)

Conversion	*Ratio*	*Calculation*	*Example*	*Monograph*
Morphine to alfentanil	15:1	Divide 24h morphine dose by 15	Morphine 30mg/24h SC/IV → alfentanil 2mg/24h SC/IV	Alfentanil, p.390
Morphine to buprenorphine	30–40:1	Divide 24h morphine dose in mg by 30–40	Morphine 40mg/24h SC/IV → buprenorphine 1mg/24h SC/IV	Buprenorphine, p.397
Morphine to diamorphine	1.5:1	Divide 24h morphine dose by 1.5 (i.e. decrease dose by 1/3)	Morphine 30mg/24h SC/IV → diamorphine 20mg/24h SC/IV	Diamorphine, p.387
Morphine to fentanyl	50–75:1[a,b]	Divide 24h morphine dose in mg by 50–75	Morphine 30mg/24h SC/IV → fentanyl 400microgram/24h SC/IV	Fentanyl, p.409
Morphine to hydromorphone	5:1	Divide 24h morphine dose by 5	Morphine 30mg/24h SC/IV → hydromorphone 6mg/24h SC/IV	Hydromorphone, p.434
Morphine to methadone	Variable	See methadone, p.437		
Morphine to oxycodone	1:1	Use same dose as 24h morphine dose	Morphine 30mg/24h SC/IV → oxycodone 30mg/24h SC/IV	Oxycodone, p.447

a. extrapolated from the manufacturer's recommended ratios for morphine PO to fentanyl TD, which varies according to the duration of use of the previous strong opioid, see Table 2 (p.858) and Box B (p.860)

b. volume constraints for a syringe driver may prevent doses >500microgram/24h being used; alfentanil is an alternative.

Updated (minor change) August 2017

Appendix 3: Compatibility charts

PCF recommends that generally water for injection (WFI) is used as the standard diluent of choice because there is less likelihood of incompatibility. However, 0.9% saline should be considered when there is actual or potential for inflammation at the injection site (see Chapter 29, p.817).

Charts 1–7 and Table 1 summarize the compatibility data available for the more commonly used 2-drug and 3-drug combinations given by CSCI in WFI. Charts summarizing the compatibility data available for the more commonly used 2-drug and 3-drug combinations given by CSCI in 0.9% saline can be found in the extended appendix section of the on-line *PCF* on *www.palliativedrugs.com*. For compatibility information for drugs given less frequently by this route, e.g. **fentanyl** (p.409), **levetiracetam** (p.287), **ranitidine** (p.29), see individual drug monographs.

The charts have been compiled from clinical observations in palliative care services submitted to the www.palliativedrugs.com Syringe Driver Survey Database (SDSD) from the UK, New Zealand and Australia, and from published compatibility data (see reference list). The SDSD is a continually updated resource and contains more detailed observational compatibility data on mixing up to four drugs in either WFI or 0.9% saline.

A traffic light system has been devised for use in the clinical setting as a practical summary of the data available:

- *red* = do not use (available information indicates a compatibility problem)
- *amber* = proceed with caution (possible compatibility problem, depending on the order of mixing or drug concentrations)
- *green* = reported compatible (data may be observational, physical or chemical, i.e. may be practice- or evidence-based).

Multiple factors affect drug stability and compatibility, including drug concentration, brand/formulation of the drug (e.g. compatibility for oxycodone 10mg/mL and 50mg/mL formulations differ), diluent, infusion time, exposure to light, ambient temperature, order of mixing and delivery system material (see Chapter 29, Box B p.821). These factors probably explain why conflicting reports occur. *Regular monitoring of all CSCI drug combinations is essential*, even for those coded green. If there is doubt about the relevance of the compatibility data in any particular situation, e.g. at the extremes of dose and concentration, advice should be obtained from a clinical pharmacist.

Dexamethasone often causes compatibility problems. It should always be the last drug to be added to an already dilute combination of drugs, thus reducing the risk of precipitation. However, because **dexamethasone** has a long duration of action, it can generally be given as a bolus SC injection once daily.

Health professionals are urged to contact hq@palliativedrugs.com if their experience indicates that the code for a combination should be changed. Submissions to the SDSD of details of successful combinations for which there are no published data are also welcome.

Most of the information in these charts relates to the use of drugs outside the scope of their Marketing Authorization and health professionals using this information must satisfy themselves as to its appropriateness in any given clinical situation (see also p.xix). Further, health professionals should familiarize themselves with the guidance and supporting material relating to the legal implications of mixing medicines before administration (Department of Health, 2010) together with any local policy and practice (see also p.xix).

Allwood M (1984) Diamorphine mixed with antiemetic drugs in plastic syringes. *British Journal of Pharmaceutical Practice*. **6**: 88–90.

Allwood M (1991) The stability of diamorphine alone and in combination with anti-emetics in plastic syringes. *Palliative Medicine*. **5**: 330–333.

Allwood M *et al.* (1994) Stability of injections containing diamorphine and midazolam in plastic syringes. *International Journal of Pharmacy Practice*. **3**: 57–59.

Al-Tannak NF *et al.* (2012) A stability indicating assay for a combination of morphine sulphate with levomepromazine hydrochloride used in palliative care. *Journal Clinical Pharmacy and Therapeutics*. **37**: 71-73.

Ambados F (1995) Compatibility of morphine and ketamine for subcutaneous infusion. *Australian Journal of Hospital Pharmacy*. **25**: 352.

Back I *Syringe driver database.* www.pallcare.info (accessed May 2013).

Barcia E *et al.* (2003) Compatibility of haloperidol and Hyoscine-N-butylbromide in mixtures for subcutaneous infusion to cancer patients in palliative care. *Supportive Care in Cancer.* **11**: 107-113.

Chin A *et al.* (1996) Stability of Granisetron hydrochloride with dexamethasone sodium phosphate for 14 days. *American Journal of Health-System Pharmacy.* **53**: 1174-1176.

Department of Health (2010) Mixing of medicines prior to administration in clinical practice: medical and non-medical prescribing. Department of Health Gateway reference 14330. www.gov.uk

Dickman A and Schneider J (2016) *The Syringe Driver: Continuous Subcutaneous Infusions in Palliative Care* (4e). Oxford University Press, Oxford.

Fawcett J *et al.* (1994) Compatibility of cyclizine lactate and haloperidol lactate. *American Journal of Hospital Pharmacy.* **51**: 2292–2294.

Fielding H *et al.* (2000) The compatibility and stability of octreotide acetate in the presence of diamorphine hydrochloride in polypropylene syringes. *Palliative Medicine.* **14**: 205–207.

Frimley Park Hospital NHS Trust (1998) *Personal communication.*

Gardiner P (2003) Compatibility of an injectable oxycodone formulation with typical diluents, syringes, tubings, infusion bags and drugs for potential co-administration. *Hospital Pharmacist.* **10**: 354–361.

Good PD *et al.* (2004) The compatibility and stability of midazolam and dexamethasone in infusion solutions. *Journal of Pain and Symptom Management.* **27**: 471–475.

Grassby P and Hutchings L (1997) Drug combinations in syringe drivers: the compatibility and stability of diamorphine with cyclizine and haloperidol. *Palliative Medicine.* **11**: 217–224.

Grassby PF (1995) *UK stability database (Apr 1995 and Jul 1997).* Welsh Pharmaceutical Services, St. Mary's Pharmaceutical Unit, Corbett Road, Penarth, South Glamorgan.

Hagan R *et al.* (1996) Stability of ondansetron hydrochloride and dexamethasone sodium phosphate in infusion bags and syringes for 32 days. American *Journal of Health-System Pharmacy.* **53**: 1431-1435.

Hines S and Pleasance S (2009) Compatibility of an injectable high strength oxycodone formulation with typical diluents, syringes, tubings, infusion bags and drugs for potential co-administration. *European Journal of Hospital Pharmacy Practice* **15**: 32–38.

Hines S and Pleasance S (2011) Compatibility of injectable hydromorphone formulations with typical diluents, components of giving sets and drugs for potential co-administration. *European Journal of Hospital Pharmacy Practice.* **17**: 47-53.

Huang E and Anderson RP (1994) Compatibility of hydromorphone hydrochloride with haloperidol lactate and ketorolac tromethamine. *American Journal of Hospital Pharmacy.* **51**: 2963.

Hughes A *et al.* (1997) Ketorolac: continuous subcutaneous infusion for cancer pain. *Journal of Pain and Symptom Management.* **13**: 315–317.

Ingallinera TS *et al.* (1979) Compatibility of glycopyrrolate injection with commonly used infusion solutions and additives. *American Journal of Hospital Pharmacy.* **36**: 508–510.

Lau M-H *et al.* (1998) Compatibility of ketamine and morphine injections. *Pain.* **75**: 389–390.

Lawson WA *et al.* (1991) Stability of hyoscine in mixtures with morphine for continuous subcutaneous administration. *Australian Journal of Hospital Pharmacy.* **21**: 395–396.

LeBelle MJ *et al.* (1995) Compatibility of morphine and midazolam or haloperidol in parenteral admixtures. *Canadian Journal of Hospital Pharmacy.* **48**: 155–160.

Mehta AC and Kay EA (1997) Storage time can be extended: A stability study of alfentanil and midazolam admixture stored in plastic syringes. *Pharmacy in Practice.* **7**: 305-308.

Mendenhall A and Hoyt DB (1994) Incompatibility of ketorolac tromethamine with haloperidol lactate and thiethylperazine maleate. *American Journal of Hospital Pharmacy.* **51**: 2964.

Middleton M and Reilly CS (1994) Do morphine and ketamine keep? The stability of morphine and ketamine separately and combined for use as an infusion. *Hospital Pharmacy Practice.* **4**: 57-58.

Napp (2010) *Personal communication.*

Napp (2014) OxyNorm 10mg/mL solution for injection or infusion. *SPC.* www.medicines.org.uk.

Negro S *et al.* (2002) Physical compatibility and in vivo evaluation of drug mixtures for subcutaneous infusion to cancer patients in palliative care. *Supportive Care in Cancer.* **10**: 65-70.

NHS Argyll and Clyde (2005) Syringe driver guidelines for Graseby MS26 (mm/24h). *Document library: Syringe drivers and infusion pumps (Syringe driver guidelines).* www.palliativedrugs.com

NUH (Nottingham University Hospitals) NHS Trust (2002) *Data on file.* Hayward House, Nottingham.

Palliativedrugs.com (2006) Syringe Driver Survey Results. *Newsletter archive (June/July).* www.palliativedrugs.com

Palliativedrugs.com *Syringe Driver Survey Database.* www.palliativedrugs.com (accessed January 2014).

Pesko LJ *et al.* (1988) Physical compatibility and stability of metoclopramide injection. *Parenterals.* **5**: 1–3, 6–8.

Peterson G *et al.* (1991) A preliminary study of the stability of midazolam in polypropylene syringes, *Australian Journal of Hospital Pharmacy.* **21**: 115-118.

Pinguet F *et al.* (1995) Compatibility and stability of granisetron, dexamethasone, and methylprednisolone in injectable solutions. *Journal of Pharmaceutical Sciences.* **84**: 267–268.

Regnard C *et al.* (1986) Antiemetics/diamorphine mixture compatibility in infusion pumps. *British Journal of Pharmaceutical Practice.* **8**: 218–220.

Riley and Fallon (1994) Octreotide in terminal malignant obstruction of the gastrointestinal tract. *European Journal of Palliative Care.* **1**: 23-25.

Sample E (2001) *Personal communication.* Burnaby Hospital, British Columbia, Canada.

Sanofi (2014) Nozinan injection. *SPC.* www.medicines.org.uk.

Schneider JJ (2001) *Personal communication.* Pharmacy Department, University of Newcastle, Callaghan, Australia.

Smith JC *et al.* (2000) The stability of diamorphine and glycopyrrolate in PCA syringes. *Pharmaceutical Journal.* **265 (Suppl. R69)**.

Stewart JT *et al.* (1998) Stability of ondansetron hydrochloride and 12 medications in plastic syringes. *American Journal of the Health-System Pharmacy.* **55**: 2630-2634.

Storey P *et al.* (1990) Subcutaneous infusions for control of cancer symptoms. *Journal of Pain and Symptom Management.* **5**: 33–41.

Thomas B (2011) *Personal communication.* Pharmacist, LOROS (Leicestershire and Rutland Organisation for the Relief of Suffering) Hospice, UK.

Trissel LA *Handbook on Injectable Drugs.* Maryland, USA: American Society of Health-System Pharmacists www.medicinescomplete.com (accessed May 2013).

Trissel LA *et al.* (1994) Compatibility and stability of ondansetron hydrochloride with morphine sulphate and with hydromorphone hydrochloride in 0.9% sodium chloride injection at 4,22 and 32 degrees C. *American Journal of Hospital Pharmacy.* **51**: 2138-2142.

Virdee H *et al.* (1997) The chemical stability of diamorphine and ketorolac in 0.9% sodium chloride stored in plastic syringes. *Pharmacy in Practice*. February: 82-83.

Walker SE *et al.* (1991) Compatibility of dexamethasone sodium phosphate with hydromorphone hydrochloride or diphenhydramine hydrochloride. *American Journal of Hospital Pharmacy*. **48**: 2161-2166.

Watson DG et al. (2005) Compatibility and stability of dexamethasone sodium phosphate and ketamine hydrochloride subcutaneous infusions in polypropylene syringes. *Journal of Pain and Symptom Management*. **31**: 80-86.

General key for charts

[dark grey box]	Do *not* use, *incompatible* at usual concentrations
[light grey box]	Use with caution, compatibility may depend on order of mixing or drug concentrations
a,b,c, etc.	Some reports of *incompatibility*, but may be compatible at other concentrations (see footnotes)
[mid grey box]	Reported compatible (data may be observational, physical or chemical, i.e. practice- or evidence-based)
?	No data. Please provide information on this combination to the Syringe Driver Survey Database (SDSD), www.palliativedrugs.com
[black box]	Not applicable or not generally recommended, e.g. seek specialist advice when combining multiple anti-emetics
#	Use non-PVC tubing; up to 50% of a dose of clonazepam is adsorbed by PVC tubing
##	Dexamethasone sodium phosphate can generally be given once daily by SC bolus injection. If given by CSCI, to minimize the risk of incompatibility, always add it last to a maximally diluted syringe
####	Compatibility data for oxycodone 10mg/mL formulation only; for 50mg/mL formulation, see Table 1, p.880.

Alf	Alfentanil
Clzm	Clonazepam (not UK)
Cyc	Cyclizine
Dex/Dexamethasone	Dexamethasone sodium phosphate
Dia	Diamorphine
Gly	Glycopyrronium
Gra	Granisetron
Hal	Haloperidol
HBBr	Hyoscine butylbromide
HHBr	Hyoscine hydrobromide
Hyd	Hydromorphone
Keta	Ketamine
Ketor	Ketorolac
Levo	Levomepromazine
Meto	Metoclopramide
Mid	Midazolam
MS	Morphine sulfate
MT	Morphine tartrate (not UK)
Oct	Octreotide
Ond	Ondansetron
Oxy	Oxycodone 10mg/mL

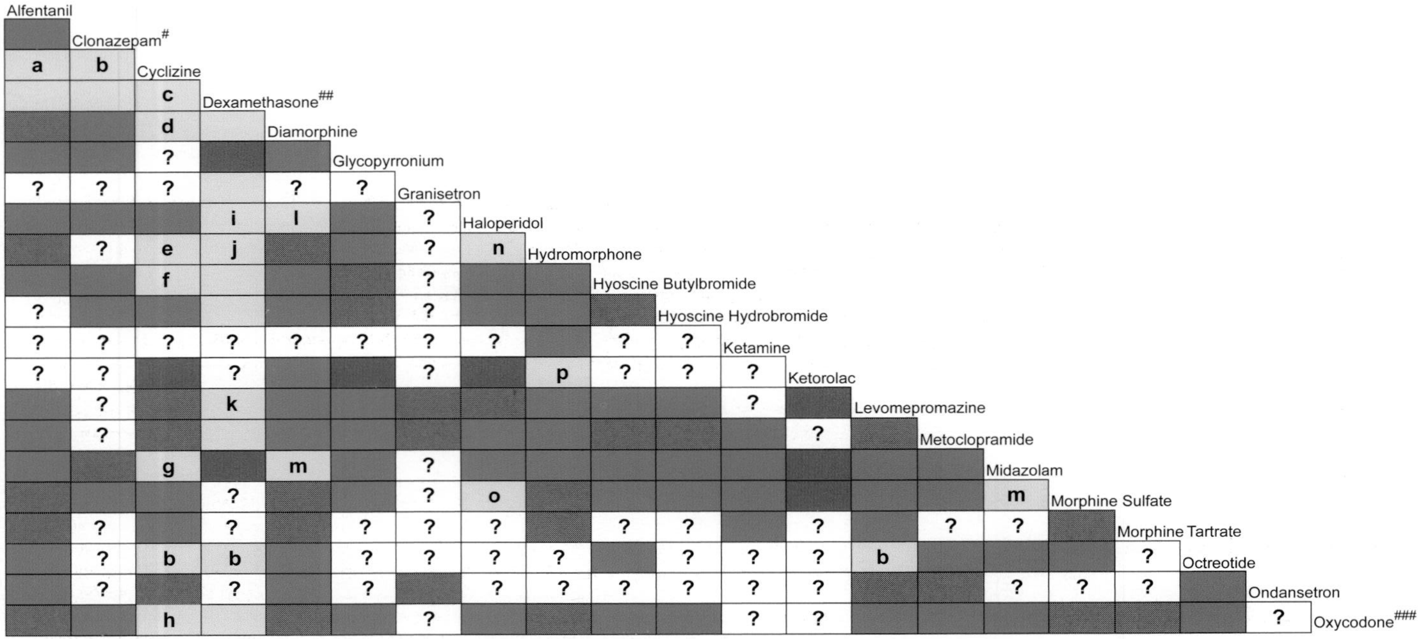

	Alfentanil	Clonazepam#	Cyclizine	Dexamethasone##	Diamorphine	Glycopyrronium	Granisetron	Haloperidol	Hydromorphone	Hyoscine Butylbromide	Hyoscine Hydrobromide	Ketamine	Ketorolac	Levomepromazine	Metoclopramide	Midazolam	Morphine Sulfate	Morphine Tartrate	Octreotide	Ondansetron
Clonazepam#																				
Cyclizine	a	b																		
Dexamethasone##			c																	
Diamorphine			d																	
Glycopyrronium			?																	
Granisetron	?	?	?		?	?														
Haloperidol				i	l		?													
Hydromorphone		?	e	j			?	n												
Hyoscine Butylbromide			f				?													
Hyoscine Hydrobromide	?						?													
Ketamine	?	?	?	?	?	?	?	?		?	?									
Ketorolac	?	?		?			?		p	?	?	?								
Levomepromazine		?		k								?								
Metoclopramide		?											?							
Midazolam			g		m		?													
Morphine Sulfate				?			?	o								m				
Morphine Tartrate		?		?		?	?	?		?	?		?		?	?				
Octreotide		?	b	b		?	?	?	?		?	?	?	b				?		
Ondansetron		?		?		?		?	?	?	?	?	?			?	?	?		
Oxycodone###			h				?					?	?							?

Note. This chart summarizes the compatibility information available for drug combinations in **WFI** used for CSCI over 24h in palliative care units and the literature (see p.863). It includes compatibility data for oxycodone 10mg/mL formulation only; for 50mg/mL, see Table 1, p.880. It should be used in conjunction with the key and the footnotes. Further information about each combination may be found on the www.palliativedrugs.com Syringe Driver Survey Database (SDSD). Charts with drug combinations diluted in 0.9% saline can be found in the extended appendix section of the on-line *PCF*.

Chart 1 Compatibility chart for *two* drugs in ***WFI.***

Chart 1 footnotes

All drug concentration values (mg/mL) specified below are the maximum *final* concentrations of each drug in the syringe after mixing and dilution reported compatible; at higher concentrations *incompatibility* has either been reported or may occur. For full reference details, see p.863.

a. alfentanil 0.24mg/mL + cyclizine 8.8mg/mL (Dickman *et al.* 2011, palliativedrugs.com 2014)
b. some observational reports of *incompatibility* from miscellaneous sources
c. cyclizine 8.33mg/mL + dexamethasone sodium phosphate 0.33mg/mL (Dickman *et al.* 2011, palliativedrugs.com 2014)
d. cyclizine up to 20mg/mL + diamorphine up to 20mg/mL, or cyclizine maximum 10mg/mL + diamorphine **>**20mg/mL, or cyclizine >20mg/mL + diamorphine maximum 15mg/mL (Grassby and Hutchings 1997)
e. cyclizine 8.82mg/mL + hydromorphone 5.8mg/mL(Hines and Pleasance 2011); one report of *incompatibility* at *lower* concentrations (Back 2013)
f. generally regarded as *incompatible*; one report of compatibility of low concentrations for a *12h* infusion of cyclizine 3.7mg/mL + hyoscine *butylbromide* 1.5mg/mL (palliativedrugs.com 2014)
g. cyclizine 8.82mg/mL + midazolam 0.88mg/mL (Back 2013, palliativedrugs.com 2014)
h. cyclizine 3mg/mL + oxycodone 9mg/mL; cyclizine concentrations between 3mg/mL and 8mg/mL may be used as long as the oxycodone concentration is reduced to below 3mg/mL by diluting with WFI (Napp 2010, Napp 2014)
i. dexamethasone sodium phosphate 0.15mg/mL + haloperidol 0.38mg/mL (Dickman *et al.* 2011, palliativedrugs.com 2014)
j. dexamethasone sodium phosphate 2mg/mL + hydromorphone 20mg/mL, or dexamethasone sodium phosphate >2mg/mL + hydromorphone 10mg/mL (Walker *et al.* 1991, Hines and Pleasance 2011)
k. dexamethasone sodium phosphate 0.11mg/mL + levomepromazine 2.78mg/mL (Dickman *et al.* 2011, palliativedrugs.com 2014)
l. diamorphine up to 50mg/mL + haloperidol 4mg/mL, or diamorphine 50–100mg/mL + haloperidol 3mg/mL (Grassby and Hutchings 1997)
m. diamorphine or morphine sulfate + midazolam generally regarded as compatible (palliativedrugs.com 2014, Dickman *et al.* 2011); one report *of incompatibility* for diamorphine (palliativedrugs.com 2014); microscopic precipitation may occur with morphine (LeBelle *et al.* 1995)
n. variable reports at higher concentrations, e.g. haloperidol 2.5mg/mL + hydromorphone 5mg/mL compatible (Huang and Anderson 1994), haloperidol 3mg/mL + hydromorphone 20mg/mL compatible (Hines and Pleasance 2011) but haloperidol 2mg/mL + hydromorphone 10mg/mL *incompatible* (Storey *et al.* 1990)
o. haloperidol <1mg/mL + morphine sulfate <10mg/mL (palliativedrugs.com 2014, Storey *et al.* 1990, Trissel 2006, LeBelle *et al.* 1995)
p. hydromorphone 0.5mg/mL + ketorolac 15mg/mL (Huang and Anderson 1994).

	Alf + Clzm#	Alf + Cyc	Alf + Dex##	Alf + Gly	Alf + Gra	Alf + Hal	Alf + HBBr	Alf + HHBr	Alf + Keta	Alf + Ketor	Alf + Levo	Alf + Meto	Alf + Mid	Alf + Oct
Cyclizine	a													
Dexamethasone##	?	?												
Glycopyrronium		?	?											
Granisetron	?	?	?	?										
Haloperidol		b	?		?									
Hyoscine Butylbromide	?	?	?		?									
Hyoscine Hydrobromide		?	?		?	?								
Ketamine	?	?	?	?	?	?	?	?						
Ketorolac	?	?	?	?	?	?	?	?	?					
Levomepromazine	?		?					?	?	?				
Metoclopramide	?		?			?			?	?				
Midazolam		c	?		?				?	?				
Octreotide	?	?	?	?	?	?	?	?	?	?			?	
Ondansetron	?	?	?	?		?	?	?	?	?			?	?

Note. This chart summarizes the compatibility information available for drug combinations in **WFI** used for CSCI over 24h in palliative care units and the literature (see p.863). It should be used in conjunction with the key and the footnotes. Further information about each combination may be found on the www.palliativedrugs.com Syringe Driver Survey Database (SDSD). Charts with drug combinations diluted in 0.9% saline can be found in the extended appendix section of the on-line *PCF*.

Chart 2 Compatibility chart for alfentanil: *three* drugs in ***WFI.***

Chart 2 footnotes

All drug concentration values (mg/mL) specified below are the maximum *final* concentrations of each drug in the syringe after mixing and dilution reported compatible; at higher concentrations *incompatibility* has either been reported or may occur. For full reference details, see p.863.

Concentration dependent *incompatibility* reported with 2-drug combinations of **alfentanil** + **cyclizine** (see 2-drug chart, p.866).

a. alfentanil 0.53mg/mL + clonazepam 0.24mg/mL + cyclizine 8.82mg/mL (Dickman *et al.* 2011)
b. one report of *incompatibility* (Back 2013) but several other reports of compatibility (Dickman *et al.* 2011, palliativedrugs.com 2014)
c. alfentanil 3mg/mL + cyclizine 6mg/mL + midazolam 1.2mg/mL (Dickman et al. 2011).

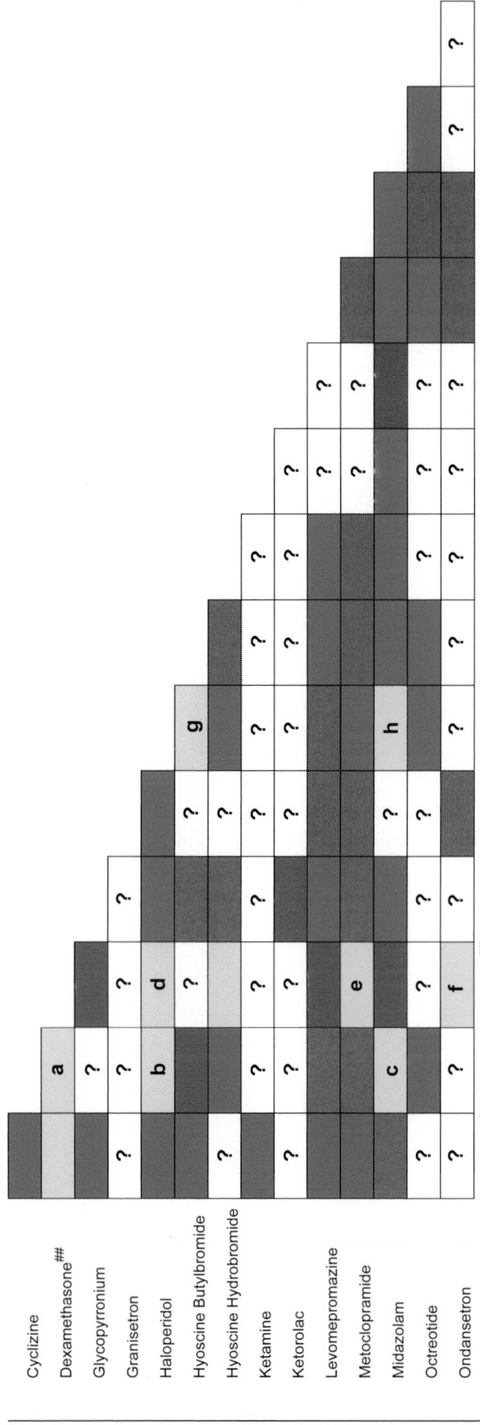

	Dia + Clzm#	Dia + Cyc	Dia + Dex##	Dia + Gly	Dia + Gra	Dia + Hal	Dia + HBBr	Dia + HHBr	Dia + Keta	Dia + Ketor	Dia + Levo	Dia + Meto	Dia + Mid	Dia + Oct
Cyclizine														
Dexamethasone##		a												
Glycopyrronium		?												
Granisetron	?	?	?	?										
Haloperidol		b	d											
Hyoscine Butylbromide			?		?	g								
Hyoscine Hydrobromide	?				?									
Ketamine		?	?	?	?	?	?	?						
Ketorolac	?	?	?		?	?	?	?	?					
Levomepromazine									?	?				
Metoclopramide			e						?	?				
Midazolam		c			?	h								
Octreotide	?		?	?	?			?	?	?				
Ondansetron	?	?	f	?		?	?	?	?	?			?	?

Note. This chart summarizes the compatibility information available for drug combinations in **WFI** used for CSCI over 24h in palliative care units and the literature (see p.863). It should be used in conjunction with the key and the footnotes. Further information about each combination may be found on the www.palliativedrugs.com Syringe Driver Survey Database (SDSD). Charts with drug combinations diluted in 0.9% saline can be found in the extended appendix section of the on-line *PCF*.

Chart 3 Compatibility chart for diamorphine: *three* drugs in ***WFI***.

Chart 3 footnotes

All drug concentration values (mg/mL) specified below are the maximum *final* concentrations of each drug in the syringe after mixing and dilution reported compatible; at higher concentrations *incompatibility* has either been reported or may occur. For full reference details, see p.863.

Concentration dependent *incompatibility* reported with 2-drug combinations of **diamorphine** + **cyclizine** or **haloperidol** (see 2-drug chart, p.866).

a. diamorphine 5.88mg/mL + cyclizine 8.82mg/mL + dexamethasone sodium phosphate 0.71mg/mL (Dickman *et al.* 2011, palliativedrugs.com 2014)
b. diamorphine 56mg/mL + cyclizine 13mg/mL + haloperidol 2.1mg/mL (Grassby 1995, palliativedrugs.com 2014)
c. diamorphine 37mg/mL + cyclizine 8.82mg/mL + midazolam 2.35mg/mL (palliativedrugs.com 2014)
d. diamorphine 25mg/mL + dexamethasone sodium phosphate 0.35mg/mL + haloperidol 0.59mg/mL (Dickman *et al.* 2011)
e. diamorphine 3.53mg/mL + dexamethasone sodium phosphate 0.59mg/mL + metoclopramide 2.35mg/mL (Dickman *et al.* 2011)
f. diamorphine 35mg/mL + dexamethasone sodium phosphate 0.06mg/mL + ondansetron 1.41mg/mL (Dickman *et al.* 2011)
g. diamorphine 117.7mg/mL + haloperidol 0.59mg/mL + hyoscine *butylbromide* 3.53mg/mL (palliativedrugs.com 2014)
h. diamorphine 28mg/mL+ haloperidol 2mg/mL + midazolam 1mg/mL (palliativedrugs.com 2014).

	Hyd + Clzm[#]	Hyd + Cyc	Hyd + Dex[##]	Hyd + Gly	Hyd + Gra	Hyd + Hal	Hyd + HBBr	Hyd + HHBr	Hyd + Keta	Hyd + Ketor	Hyd + Levo	Hyd + Meto	Hyd + Mid	Hyd + Oct
Cyclizine	?													
Dexamethasone[##]	?	?												
Glycopyrronium	?	?	?											
Granisetron	?	?	?	?										
Haloperidol	?	?	?	?	?									
Hyoscine Butylbromide	?	?	?		?	?								
Hyoscine Hydrobromide	?	?	?		?	?								
Ketamine	?	?	?	?	?	c	?	?						
Ketorolac	?	?	?	?	?		?	?	?					
Levomepromazine	?		?	?			?	?	?	?				
Metoclopramide	?		?			?			?	?				
Midazolam		?	b	?	?	d	?	?	?	?				
Octreotide	?	a	?	?	?	?	?	?	?	?	?		?	
Ondansetron	?	?	?	?		?	?	?	?	?			?	?

Note. This chart summarizes the compatibility information available for drug combinations in **WFI** used for CSCI over 24h in palliative care units and the literature (see p.863). It should be used in conjunction with the key and the footnotes. Further information about each combination may be found on the www.palliativedrugs.com Syringe Driver Survey Database (SDSD). Charts with drug combinations diluted in 0.9% saline can be found in the extended appendix section of the on-line *PCF*.

Chart 4 Compatibility chart for hydromorphone: *three* drugs in ***WFI***.

Chart 4 footnotes

All drug concentration values (mg/mL) specified below are the maximum *final* concentrations of each drug in the syringe after mixing and dilution reported compatible; at higher concentrations *incompatibility* has either been reported or may occur. For full reference details, see p.863.

Concentration dependent *incompatibility* reported with 2-drug combinations of **hydromorphone** + **cyclizine**, **dexamethasone**, **haloperidol** or **ketorolac** (see 2-drug chart, p.866).

a. hydromorphone 1.67mg/mL + cyclizine 16.67mg/mL + octreotide 0.02mg/mL; *incompatibility* has been reported with cyclizine and octreotide see 2-drug chart (Dickman 2011)
b. generally regarded as *incompatible,* despite observational reports of compatibility, as dexamethasone + midazolam 2-drug combination are *incompatible* although may be visually clear, see Chapter 29, Box C, p.822 (Good P 2004)
c. hydromorphone 3.75mg/mL + haloperidol 0.16mg/mL + ketamine 31.25mg/mL (palliativedrugs.com 2014)
d. hydromorphone 0.35mg/mL + haloperidol 0.06mg/mL + midazolam 0.23mg/mL (palliativedrugs.com 2014).

	MS + Clzm[#]	MS + Cyc	MS + Dex[##]	MS + Gly	MS + Gra	MS + Hal	MS + HBBr	MS + HHBr	MS + Keta	MS + Ketor	MS + Levo	MS + Meto	MS + Mid	MS + Oct
Cyclizine														
Dexamethasone[##]	?													
Glycopyrronium	?	?	?											
Granisetron	?	?	?	?										
Haloperidol	?		?	?	?									
Hyoscine Butylbromide	?		?		?									
Hyoscine Hydrobromide	?	?	?		?	?								
Ketamine	?	?	?	?	?	?	?	?						
Ketorolac	?	?	?	?	?	?	?	?	?					
Levomepromazine	?		?	?				?	?	?				
Metoclopramide	?								?	?				
Midazolam			?		?				?	?				
Octreotide	?	?	?	?	?		?	?	?	?	?		?	
Ondansetron	?	?	?	?		?	?	?	?	?			?	?

Note. This chart summarizes the compatibility information available for drug combinations in **WFI** used for CSCI over 24h in palliative care units and the literature (see p.863). It should be used in conjunction with the key and the footnotes. Further information about each combination may be found on the www.palliativedrugs.com Syringe Driver Survey Database (SDSD). Charts with drug combinations diluted in 0.9% saline can be found in the extended appendix section of the on-line *PCF*.

Chart 5 Compatibility chart for morphine sulfate: *three* drugs in ***WFI***.

Chart 5 footnote

Concentration dependent *incompatibility* reported with 2-drug combinations of **morphine sulfate** + **haloperidol** (see 2-drug chart, p.866).

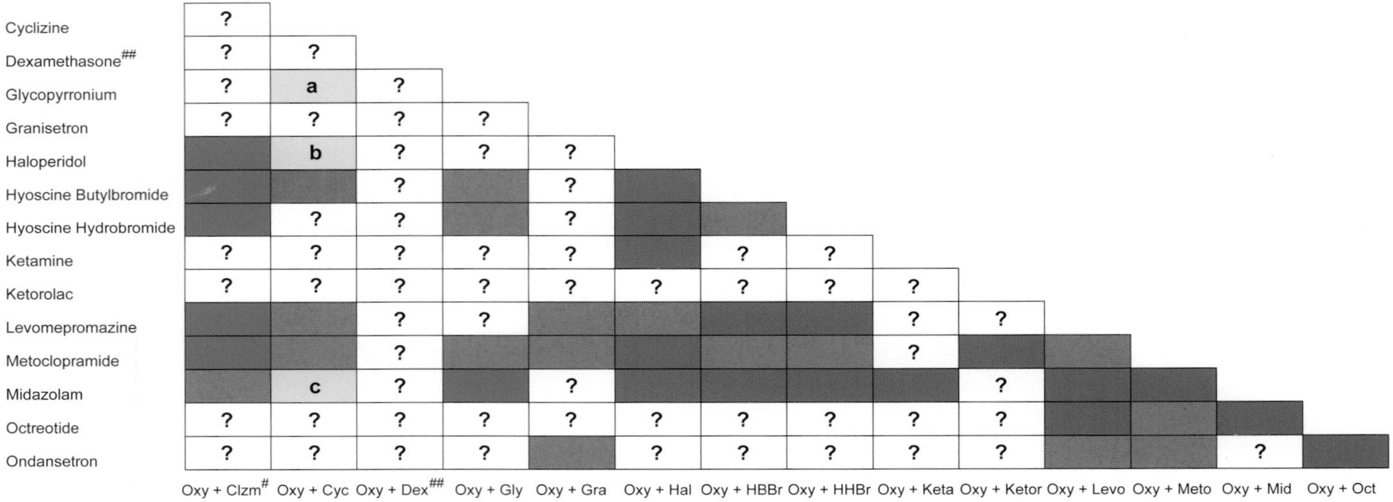

	Oxy + Clzm[#]	Oxy + Cyc	Oxy + Dex[##]	Oxy + Gly	Oxy + Gra	Oxy + Hal	Oxy + HBBr	Oxy + HHBr	Oxy + Keta	Oxy + Ketor	Oxy + Levo	Oxy + Meto	Oxy + Mid	Oxy + Oct
Cyclizine	?													
Dexamethasone[##]	?	?												
Glycopyrronium	?	a	?											
Granisetron	?	?	?	?										
Haloperidol		b	?	?	?									
Hyoscine Butylbromide			?		?									
Hyoscine Hydrobromide		?	?		?									
Ketamine	?	?	?	?	?		?	?						
Ketorolac	?	?	?	?	?	?	?	?	?					
Levomepromazine			?	?					?	?				
Metoclopramide			?						?					
Midazolam		c	?		?					?				
Octreotide	?	?	?	?	?	?	?	?	?	?				
Ondansetron	?	?	?	?		?	?	?	?	?			?	

Note. Compatibility data for oxycodone 10mg/mL formulation only; for 50mg/mL formulation, see Table 1, p.880. This chart summarizes the compatibility information available for drug combinations in **WFI** used for CSCI over 24h in palliative care units and the literature (see p.863). It should be used in conjunction with the key and the footnotes. Further information about each combination may be found on the www.palliativedrugs.com Syringe Driver Survey Database (SDSD). Charts with drug combinations diluted in 0.9% saline can be found in the extended appendix section of the on-line *PCF*.

Chart 6 Compatibility chart for oxycodone 10mg/mL formulation: *three* drugs in ***WFI***.

Chart 6 footnotes

All drug concentration values (mg/mL) specified below are the maximum *final* concentrations of each drug in the syringe after mixing and dilution reported compatible; at higher concentrations *incompatibility* has either been reported or may occur. For full reference details, see p.863.

Concentration dependent *incompatibility* reported with 2-drug combinations of **oxycodone** + **cyclizine** (see 2-drug chart, p.866).

a. oxycodone 3.5mg/mL + cyclizine 7.5mg/mL + glycopyrronium 0.06mg/mL (Dickman *et al* 2011, Napp 2010)
b. oxycodone 1.9mg/mL + cyclizine 7.14mg/mL + haloperidol 0.95mg/mL; higher concentrations have been reported compatible, but it is unclear whether the higher strength oxycodone formulation has been used (50mg/mL) which has a different compatibility profile (palliativedrugs.com 2014, Dickman *et al.* 2011, Napp 2010)
c. oxycodone 2.22mg/mL + cyclizine 8.33mg/mL + midazolam 0.28mg/mL; *incompatibility* with some 2-drug combinations of cyclizine + midazolam (Back 2013, palliativedrugs.com 2014, Napp 2010).

	Clzm[#] + Meto	Cyc + Dex[##]	Cyc + Hal	Cyc + HBBr	Dex[##] + Mid	Gly + Keta	Gly + Levo	Hal + Mid	HBBr + Ketor	Levo + Mid
Haloperidol		?		b	d	?				
Hyoscine Butylbromide		a	b							
Hyoscine Hydrobromide		?	?		?					
Ketamine	?	?	?	?	?		?		?	?
Ketorolac	?	?	?	?	?	?	?			?
Metoclopramide					?	?			?	
Midazolam		?		c			?			
Octreotide	?	?	?	?	?	?		?	?	?

Note. This chart summarizes the compatibility information available for drug combinations in **WFI** used for CSCI over 24h in palliative care units and the literature (see p.863). It should be used in conjunction with the key and the footnotes. Further information about each combination may be found on the www.palliativedrugs.com Syringe Driver Survey Database (SDSD). Charts with drug combinations diluted in 0.9% saline can be found in the extended appendix section of the on-line *PCF*.

Chart 7 Compatibility chart for non-opioids: *three* drugs in ***WFI***.

Chart 7 footnotes

All drug concentration values (mg/mL) specified below are the maximum *final* concentrations of each drug in the syringe after mixing and dilution reported compatible; at higher concentrations *incompatibility* has either been reported or may occur. For full reference details, see p.863.

a. cyclizine 8.82mg/mL + dexamethasone sodium phosphate 0.71mg/mL + hyoscine *butylbromide* 2.35mg/mL (Dickman *et al.* 2011)
b. generally regarded as *incompatible* (NUH 2002); one report of compatibility (Back 2013)
c. generally regarded as *incompatible*; *incompatibility* reported with 2-drug combinations of cyclizine + hyoscine *butylbromide* and some 2-drug combinations of cyclizine + midazolam (NUH 2002, palliativedrugs.com 2014)
d. generally regarded as *incompatible*, despite observational reports of compatibility, as dexamethasone + midazolam 2-drug combination are *incompatible* although may be visually clear, see Chapter 29, Box C, p.822 (Good P 2004).

Compatibility information for oxycodone 50mg/mL formulation

When mixed with other drugs some differences in compatibility have been demonstrated for the 10mg/mL and 50mg/mL formulations of oxycodone solution for injection, e.g. with cyclizine (Gardiner 2003, Hines and Pleasance 2009). This may be due to the different ratios of excipients in each formulation. The manufacturer recommends that the compatibility information for each formulation is considered separately and not extrapolated from one formulation to another.

Chemical compatibility data between oxycodone 50mg/mL solution for injection and other drugs over 24h at room temperature are summarized in Table 1. Full details are available on the SDSD on www.palliativedrugs.com. Please submit details to the SDSD of successful combinations containing oxycodone 50mg/mL and, more important, details of combinations which were incompatible.

Table 1 Oxycodone 50mg/mL formulation compatibility with other drugs (Hines and Pleasance 2009)

	Oxycodone 250mg diluted[a]		*Oxycodone 500mg undiluted*	
	Dose (mg)	*Concentration (mg/mL)*	*Dose (mg)*	*Concentration (mg/mL)*
Cyclizine[b,c,d]	150	8.8	50	4.5
Dexamethasone sodium phosphate	20	1.2	40	2
Glycopyrronium	1.2	0.07	2.4	0.1
Haloperidol	7.5	0.4	15	1.2
Hyoscine butylbromide	30	1.8	60	4.6
Hyoscine hydrobromide	1.2	0.07	2.4	0.15
Ketamine	400	23.5	800	44.4
Levomepromazine	100	5.9	200	11.1
Metoclopramide	50	2.9	100	3.3
Midazolam	50	2.9	100	3.3

a. oxycodone 50mg/mL formulation, 5mL (250mg) mixed with the drug and diluted to 17mL with WFI or 0.9% saline; oxycodone final concentration 14mg/mL

b. use WFI only, *incompatible* with 0.9% saline

c. maximum concentrations found compatible for cyclizine and oxycodone 50mg/mL formulation; concentration dependent *incompatibility* found above this

d. for practical purposes, a cyclizine concentration of >4mg/mL to a maximum of 8mg/mL may be used if the oxycodone concentration is kept ≤14mg/mL by diluting with WFI (Napp, 2010).

Updated May 2017

Drug Index

Note. Main references are in **bold**.

Supplementary Topic Index

A textbook on pain and symptom management should be consulted for a full discussion on these topics.

Note:
1. **Words** in **bold type** indicate a chapter or an appendix.
2. **Numbers** in **bold type** indicate the main entry for that topic.